Biological Psychology

13th Edition

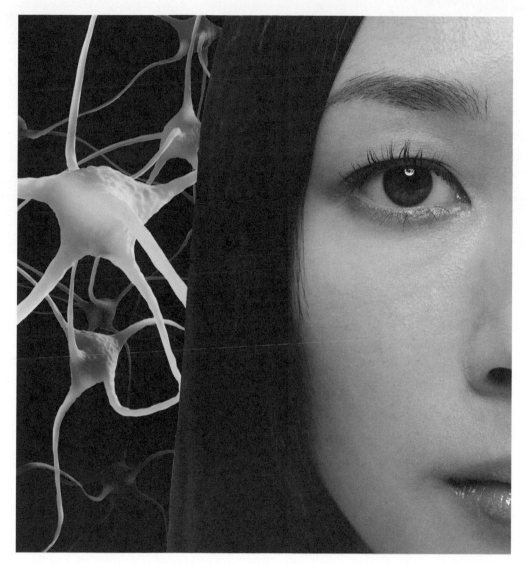

James W. Kalat
North Carolina State University

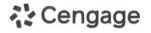 Cengage

Australia • Brazil • Canada • Mexico • Singapore • United Kingdom • United States

Cengage

Biological Psychology, **Thirteenth Edition**
James W. Kalat

Product Director: Marta Lee-Perriard

Product Team Manager: Star Burruto

Product Manager: Erin Schnair

Content Developer: Linda Man

Product Assistant: Leah Jenson

Marketing Manager: Heather Thompson

Content Project Manager: Rita Jaramillo

Production Service: Lori Hazzard, MPS Limited

Photo Researcher: Nisha Bhanu Beegum,
Lumina Datamatics, Ltd.

Text Researcher: Ramya Selvaraj,
Lumina Datamatics, Ltd.

Art Director: Vernon Boes

Cover/Text Designer: Cheryl Carrington

Cover Image: Image Source/Getty Images;
BeholdingEye/Getty Images

Compositor: MPS Limited

For product information and technology assistance, contact us at
**Cengage Customer & Sales Support, 1-800-354-9706
or support.cengage.com.**

For permission to use material from this text or product, submit all requests online at **www.copyright.com.**

Library of Congress Control Number: 2017945649

Student Edition:
ISBN: 978-1-337-40820-2

Loose-leaf Edition:
ISBN: 978-1-337-61861-8

Cengage
200 Pier 4 Boulevard
Boston, MA 02210
USA

Cengage is a leading provider of customized learning solutions with employees residing in nearly 40 different countries and sales in more than 125 countries around the world. Find your local representative at:
www.cengage.com.

To learn more about Cengage platforms and services, register or access your online learning solution, or purchase materials for your course, visit **www.cengage.com.**

Printed in the United States of America
Print Number: 10   Print Year: 2022

About the Author

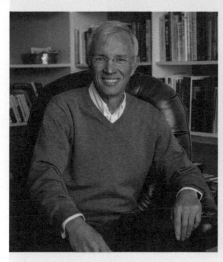

James W. Kalat (rhymes with ballot) is professor emeritus of psychology at North Carolina State University, where he taught courses in introduction to psychology and biological psychology from 1977 through 2012. Born in 1946, he received a BA summa cum laude from Duke University in 1968, and a PhD in psychology from the University of Pennsylvania in 1971. He is also the author of *Introduction to Psychology* (11th edition) and co-author with Michelle Shiota of *Emotion* (3rd edition). In addition to textbooks, he has written journal articles on taste-aversion learning, the teaching of psychology, and other topics. He was twice the program chair for the annual convention of the American Psychological Society, now named the Association for Psychological Science. A remarried widower, he has three children, two stepsons, and four grandchildren.

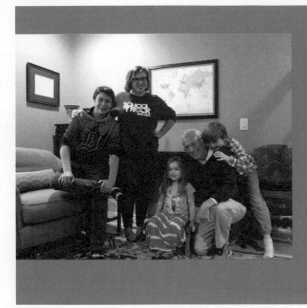

To my grandchildren.

Brief Contents

Contents

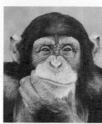
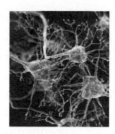
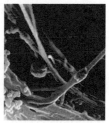

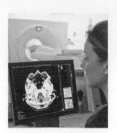
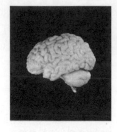

Chapter 5

Vision   147

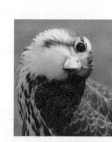

Chapter 6

Other Sensory Systems   187

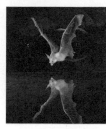

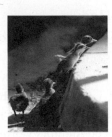
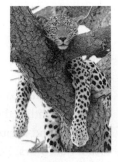

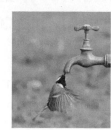

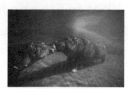

Chapter 11

Emotional Behaviors   351

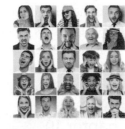

Chapter 12

Learning, Memory, and Intelligence   383

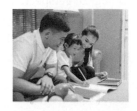

Chapter 13
Cognitive Functions   423

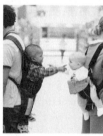

Chapter 14
Psychological Disorders   459

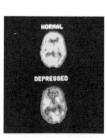

Preface

In the first edition of this text, published in 1981, I remarked, "I almost wish I could get parts of this text . . . printed in disappearing ink, programmed to fade within 10 years of publication, so that I will not be embarrassed by statements that will look primitive from some future perspective." I would say the same thing today, except that I would like for the ink to fade faster. Biological psychology progresses rapidly, and much that we thought we knew becomes obsolete.

Biological psychology is the most interesting topic in the world. No doubt many people in other fields think their topic is the most interesting, but they are wrong. This really is the most interesting. Unfortunately, it is easy to get so bogged down in memorizing facts that one loses the big picture. The big picture here is fascinating and profound: Your brain activity *is* your mind. I hope that readers of this book will remember that message even after they forget many of the details.

Each chapter is divided into modules that begin with an introduction and end with a summary, a list of key terms, and some review questions. This organization makes it easy for instructors to assign part of a chapter per day instead of a whole chapter per week. Modules can also be covered in a different order, or of course omitted.

I assume that readers have a basic background in psychology and biology, and understand such terms as *classical conditioning, reinforcement, vertebrate, mammal, gene, chromosome, cell,* and *mitochondrion.* I also assume at least a high school chemistry course. Those with a weak background in chemistry or a fading memory of it may consult Appendix A.

MindTap for Biological Psychology, 13e

MindTap for Biological Psychology, 13th edition, engages students to produce their best work. By integrating course material with videos, activities, and much more, MindTap provides an opportunity for increased comprehension and retention.

For students, MindTap provides:

- activities and assignments that build critical thinking and analytic skills that can transfer to other domains.
- guidance to focus on what the instructor emphasizes, with tools for mastering the content.
- feedback on progress, compared to the student's own past performance and the performance of other students in the class.

For faculty, MindTap provides:

- the ability to specify what the students read and when, matched to the course syllabus.
- an opportunity to assign relevant activities.
- the ability to supplement the MindTap Reader with your own documents or sources such as RSS feeds, YouTube videos, websites, or Google Docs.
- reports on students' progress and completion of assignments.

Changes in This Edition

Reflecting the rapid changes in biological psychology, this edition includes revised content throughout, with almost 700 new references, including more than 550 from 2014 or later. Some of the figures are new or revised, and most of the review questions at the end of modules are new. The most extensive changes are in the later chapters. These organizational changes are worth notice: Chapter 9 ("Internal Regulation") includes a new section about anorexia nervosa. Chapter 12 ("Learning, Memory, and Intelligence") now has four modules instead of two. What used to be the first module has been split into two, and a new module has been added about intelligence. That module includes some material previously in the anatomy chapter, plus more, and all of it reorganized. In Chapter 13 ("Cognitive Functions"), the previous modules on lateralization and language have been shortened and combined into one module. The previous module on social neuroscience has been expanded with the addition of a section on the neurobiology of making decisions. In Chapter 14 ("Psychological Disorders"), the first module ("Substance Abuse") has been reorganized and reordered.

With regard to new or revised content, here are some of the highlights:

- This edition continues the tradition of including photographs and quotes of some prominent researchers, now adding Karl Deisseroth, Margaret McCarthy, May-Britt Moser and Edvard Moser, and Stanislas Dehaene. Students can name hundreds of singers, actors, and athletes. I think they should be able to identify some important researchers too, especially in the field in which they chose to major.
- Neuroscientists no longer believe that glia outnumber neurons in the human brain.
- Although many psychologists and others have explained risky adolescent behavior in terms of an

immature prefrontal cortex, that explanation looks less plausible. Between early adolescence and age 20, most risky behaviors *increase,* even while the prefrontal cortex is approaching maturity. Risky behavior more likely reflects increased drive for excitement.

- Current research indicates that astrocytes and scar tissue are more helpful than harmful for regrowth of axons.
- A new study found that people who lose a sensation as a result of brain damage also have trouble thinking about concepts related to that sensation. For example, someone with damage to the auditory cortex might regard "thunder" as a nonword.
- Previous data showed that acetaminophen decreases emotional pain. New data say that it also decreases pleasant experiences.
- The text includes updated information about the genetic basis of Parkinson's disease, substance abuse, depression, schizophrenia, and autism.
- Certain bird species sleep while they are flying over great distances. Frigate birds, which are large enough for researchers to monitor in the air, sometimes sleep in one hemisphere at a time, sometimes sleep briefly in both hemispheres at once, but overall get very little sleep on days when they are at sea.
- Thirst anticipates needs, and so does satiation of thirst. We stop drinking long before the water we have drunk reaches the cells that need it.
- New research sheds important light on male–female differences in brain anatomy. Because the mechanisms controlling male–female differences vary from one brain area to another, it is common for someone to have a patchwork of male-typical, female-typical, and approximately neutral anatomy in different brain areas.
- A new hypothesis holds that the rapid formation of new neurons in an infant hippocampus is responsible for both the ease of new learning and the phenomenon of infant amnesia. That is, infants learn rapidly, but also tend to forget episodic memories.
- Chapter 12 includes a new section about the role of the hippocampus and surrounding areas in control of navigation.
- Accumulating data cast doubt on the central role of dopamine in addictive behaviors.
- The previous belief that later episodes of depression get shorter and shorter was based on a methodological artifact. Many people have only one episode, possibly a very long one. Only people with short episodes get as far as, say, a 10th episode. Therefore, the mean duration of all first episodes is not comparable to the mean delay of later episodes.

I would also like to mention certain points about my writing style. You would not have noticed these points, and I know that you don't care either, but I shall mention them anyway: I avoid the term *incredible,* which has been so overused that it has lost its original meaning of "not believable." I also avoid the terms *intriguing, involved,* and *outrageous,* which are also overused and misused. Finally, I avoid the term *different* after a quantifier. For example, I would not say, "They offered four different explanations." If they offered four explanations, we can take it for granted that the explanations were different!

Instructor Ancillaries

Biological Psychology, **13th edition,** is accompanied by an array of supplements developed to facilitate both instructors' and students' best experience inside as well as outside the classroom. All of the supplements continuing from the 12th edition have been revised and updated. Cengage invites you to take full advantage of the teaching and learning tools available to you and has prepared the following descriptions of each.

Online Instructor's Manual

The manual includes learning objectives, key terms, a detailed chapter outline, a chapter summary, lesson plans, discussion topics, student activities, media tools, a sample syllabus, and an expanded test bank. The learning objectives are correlated with the discussion topics, student activities, and media tools.

Online PowerPoints

Helping you make your lectures more engaging while effectively reaching your visually oriented students, these handy Microsoft PowerPoint® slides outline the chapters of the main text in a classroom-ready presentation. The PowerPoint® slides are updated to reflect the content and organization of the new edition of the text.

Cengage Learning Testing, Powered by Cognero®

Cengage Learning Testing, Powered by Cognero®, is a flexible online system that allows you to author, edit, and manage test bank content. You can create multiple test versions in an instant and deliver tests from your LMS in your classroom.

Acknowledgments

Let me tell you something about researchers in this field: As a rule, they are amazingly cooperative with textbook authors. Many colleagues and students sent me comments and helpful suggestions. I thank all of these instructors who have reviewed one or more editions of the text:

Text Reviewers and Contributors:

- John Agnew, *University of Colorado at Boulder*
- John Dale Alden III, *Lipscomb University*
- Joanne Altman, *Washburn University*
- Kevin Antshel, *SUNY–Upstate Medical University*
- Bryan Auday, *Gordon College*
- Susan Baillet, *University of Portland*
- Teresa Barber, *Dickinson College*
- Christie Bartholomew, *Kent State University*
- Howard Bashinski, *University of Colorado*
- Bakhtawar Bhadha, *Pasadena City College*
- Chris Brill, *Old Dominion University*
- J. Timothy Cannon, *The University of Scranton*
- Lorelei Carvajal, *Triton College*
- Sarah Cavanagh, *Assumption College*
- Linda Bryant Caviness, *La Sierra University*
- Cathy Cleveland, *East Los Angeles College*
- Elie Cohen, *Lander College for Men (Touro College)*
- Howard Cromwell, *Bowling Green State University*
- David Crowley, *Washington University*
- Carol DeVolder, *St. Ambrose University*
- Jaime L. Diaz-Granados, *Baylor University*
- Carl DiPerna, *Onondaga Community College*
- Francine Dolins, *University of Michigan–Dearborn*
- Timothy Donahue, *Virginia Commonwealth University*
- Michael Dowdle, *Mt. San Antonio College*
- Jeff Dyche, *James Madison University*
- Gary Felsten, *Indiana University–Purdue University Columbus*
- Erin Marie Fleming, *Kent State University*
- Lauren Fowler, *Weber State University*
- Deborah Gagnon, *Wells College*
- Jonathan Gewirtz, *University of Minnesota*
- Jackie Goldstein, *Samford University*
- Peter Green, *Maryville University*
- Jeff Grimm, *Western Washington University*
- Amy Clegg Haerich, *Riverside Community College*
- Christopher Hayashi, *Southwestern College*
- Suzanne Helfer, *Adrian College*
- Alicia Helion, *Lakeland College*
- Jackie Hembrook, *University of New Hampshire*
- Phu Hoang, *Texas A&M International University*
- Richard Howe, *College of the Canyon*
- Barry Hurwitz, *University of Miami*
- Karen Jennings, *Keene State College*
- Craig Johnson, *Towson University*
- Robert Tex Johnson, *Delaware County Community College*
- Kathryn Kelly, *Northwestern State University*
- Shannon Kundey, *Hood College*
- Craig Kinsley, *University of Richmond*
- Philip Langlais, *Old Dominion University*
- Jerry Lee, *Albright College*
- Robert Lennartz, *Sierra College*
- Hui-Yun Li, *Oregon Institute of Technology*
- Cyrille Magne, *Middle Tennessee State University*
- Michael Matthews, *U.S. Military Academy (West Point)*
- Estelle Mayhew, *Rutgers University–New Brunswick*
- Daniel McConnell, *University of Central Florida*
- Maria McLean, *Thomas More College*
- Elaine McLeskey, *Belmont Technical College*
- Corinne McNamara, *Kennesaw State University*
- Brian Metcalf, *Hawaii Pacific University*
- Richard Mills, *College of DuPage*
- Daniel Montoya, *Fayetteville State University*
- Paulina Multhaupt, *Macomb Community College*
- Walter Murphy, *Texas A&M University–Central Texas*
- Joseph Nedelec, *Florida State University*
- Ian Norris, *Murray State University*
- Marcia Pasqualini, *Avila University*
- Susana Pecina, *University of Michigan–Dearborn*
- Linda Perrotti, *University of Texas–Arlington*
- Terry Pettijohn, *The Ohio State University*
- Jennifer Phillips, *Mount St. Mary's University*
- Edward Pollak, *West Chester University*
- Brian Pope, *Tusculum College*
- Mark Prendergast, *University of Kentucky*
- Jean Pretz, *Elizabethtown College*
- Mark Prokosch, *Elon University*
- Adam Prus, *Northern Michigan University*
- Khaleel Razak, *University of California–Riverside*
- John Rowe, *Florida Gateway College*
- David Rudek, *Aurora University*
- Jeffrey Rudski, *Muhlenberg College*
- Karen Sabbah, *California State University–Northridge*
- Sharleen Sakai, *Michigan State University*
- Ron Salazar, *San Juan College*

XVIII ACKNOWLEDGMENTS

- Shannon Saszik, *Northeastern Illinois University*
- Steven Schandler, *Chapman University*
- Sue Schumacher, *North Carolina A&T State University*
- Vicki Sheafer, *LeTourneau University*
- Timothy Shearon, *College of Idaho*
- Stephanie Simon-Dack, *Ball State University*
- Steve Smith, *University of California–Santa Barbara*
- Suzanne Sollars, *University of Nebraska–Omaha*
- Gretchen Sprow, *University of North Carolina–Chapel Hill*
- Jeff Stowell, *Eastern Illinois University*
- Gary Thorne, *Gonzaga University*
- Chris Tromborg, *Sacramento City College and University of California–Davis*
- Lucy Troup, *Colorado State University*
- Joseph Trunzo, *Bryant University*
- Sandy Venneman, *University of Houston–Victoria*
- Beth Venzke, *Concordia University*
- Ruvanee Vilhauer, *Felician College*
- Jacquie Wall, *University of Indianapolis*
- Zoe Warwick, *University of Maryland–Baltimore County*
- Jon Weimer, *Columbia College*
- Rosalyn Weller, *The University of Alabama–Birmingham*
- Adam Wenzel, *Saint Anselm College*
- David Widman, *Juniata College*
- Steffen Wilson, *Eastern Kentucky University*
- Joseph Wister, *Chatham University*
- Jessica Yokley, *University of Pittsburgh*

I thank my product manager, Erin Schnair, for her support, encouragement, and supervision. Linda Man, my content developer for this edition, carefully oversaw this complex project, and has my highest respect and appreciation. Lori Hazzard supervised the production, a major task for a book like this one. As art director, Vernon Boes's considerable artistic abilities helped to compensate for my complete lack. The production phases of the 13th edition were skillfully overseen by Rita Jaramillo, content project manager. Betsy Hathaway had charge of permissions, a major task for a book like this. I thank the rest of the entire team at Cengage for their contributions, including Heather Thompson, marketing manager; and Leah Jenson, product assistant. All of these people have been splendid colleagues, and I thank them immensely.

And, emphatically, I thank my wife and family for their constant support.

I welcome correspondence from both students and faculty. Write James W. Kalat, Department of Psychology, Box 7650, North Carolina State University, Raleigh, NC 27695–7801, USA. E-mail: james_kalat@ncsu.edu

James W. Kalat

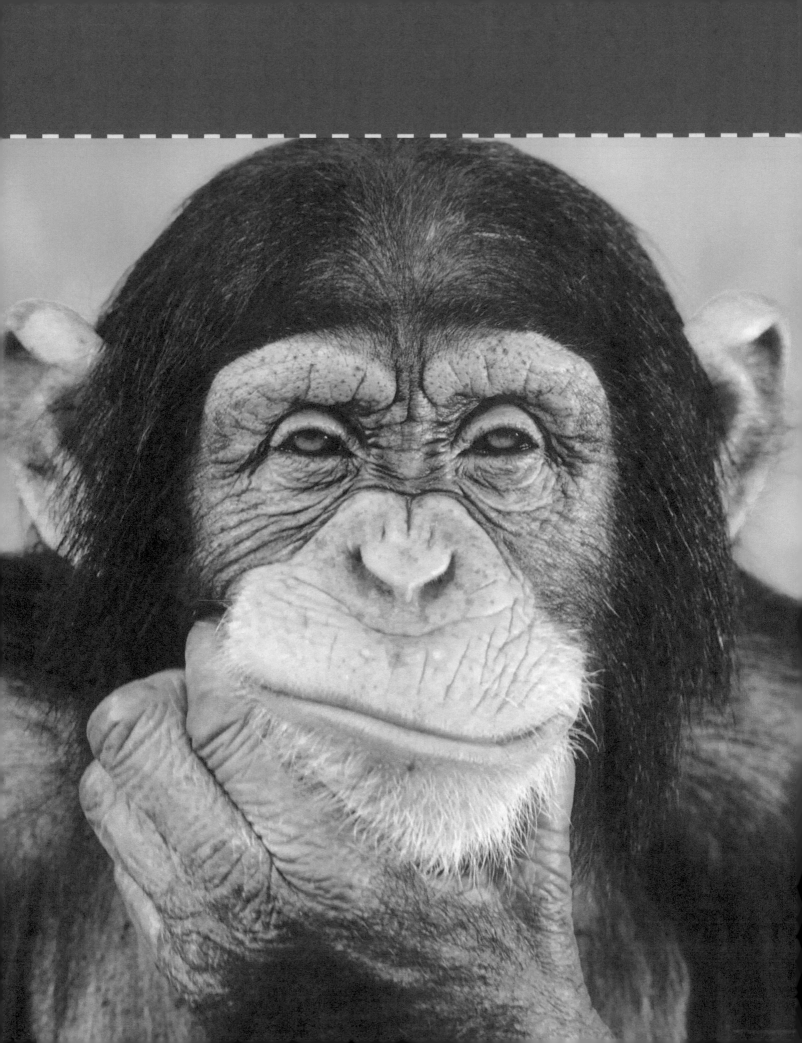

Overview and Major Issues

It is often said that Man is unique among animals. It is worth looking at this term *unique* before we discuss our subject proper. The word may in this context have two slightly different meanings. It may mean: Man is strikingly different—he is not identical with any animal. This is of course true. It is true also of all other animals: Each species, even each individual, is unique in this sense. But the term is also often used in a more absolute sense: Man is so different, so "essentially different" (whatever that means) that the gap between him and animals cannot possibly be bridged—he is something altogether new. Used in this absolute sense, the term is scientifically meaningless. Its use also reveals and may reinforce conceit, and it leads to complacency and defeatism because it assumes that it will be futile even to search for animal roots. It is prejudging the issue.

Niko Tinbergen (1973, p. 161)

What is meant by the term *biological psychology*? In a sense, all psychology is biological. You are a biological organism, and everything you do or think is part of your biology. However, it is helpful to distinguish among levels of explanation. All of biology is chemical, and all of chemistry is physics, but we do not try to explain every biological observation in terms of protons and electrons. Similarly, much of psychology is best described in terms of cultural, social, and cognitive influences. Nevertheless, much of psychology is also best understood in terms of genetics, evolution, hormones, body physiology, and brain mechanisms. This textbook concentrates mostly on brain mechanisms, but also discusses the other biological influences. In this chapter, we consider three major issues: the relationship between mind and brain, the roles of nature and nurture, and the ethics of research. We also briefly consider career opportunities in this and related fields.

Learning Objectives

After studying this introduction, you should be able to:

1. State the mind–brain problem and contrast monism with dualism.
2. List three general points that are important to remember from this text.
3. Give examples of physiological, ontogenetic, evolutionary, and functional explanations of behavior.
4. Discuss the ethical issues of research with laboratory animals.

Opposite:

It is tempting to try to "get inside the mind" of people and other animals, to imagine what they are thinking or feeling. In contrast, biological psychologists try to explain behavior in terms of its physiology, development, evolution, and function. (© Renee Lynn/Corbis/VCG/Getty Images)

The Biological Approach to Behavior

Of all the questions that people ask, two stand out as the most profound and the most difficult. One of those questions deals with physics. The other pertains to the relationship between physics and psychology.

Gottfried Leibniz (1714/1989) posed the first of these questions: "Why is there something rather than nothing?" It would seem that nothingness would be the default state. Evidently, the universe—or whoever or whatever created the universe—had to be self-created.

So . . . how did that happen?

That question is supremely baffling, but a subordinate question is more amenable to discussion: Given the existence of a universe, why this particular kind of universe? Could the universe have been fundamentally different? Our universe has protons, neutrons, and electrons with particular dimensions of mass and charge. It has four fundamental forces—gravity, electromagnetism, the strong nuclear force, and the weak nuclear force. What would happen to the universe if any of these properties had been different?

Beginning in the 1980s, specialists in a branch of physics known as *string theory* set out to prove mathematically that this is the only possible way the universe could be. Succeeding in that effort would have been theoretically satisfying, but alas, as string theorists worked through their equations, they concluded that this is not the only possible universe. The universe could have taken a vast number of forms with different laws of physics. How vast a number? Imagine the number 1 followed by about 500 zeros. And that's the *low* estimate.

Of all those possible universes, how many could have supported life? Very few. Consider the following (Davies, 2006):

- If gravity were weaker, matter would not condense into stars and planets. If it were stronger, stars would burn brighter and use up their fuel too quickly for life to evolve.
- If the electromagnetic force were stronger, the protons within an atom would repel one another so strongly that atoms would burst apart.
- In the beginning was hydrogen. The other elements formed by fusion within stars. The only way to get those elements out of stars and into planets is for a star to explode as a supernova and send its contents out into the galaxy. If the weak nuclear force were *either* a bit stronger *or* a bit weaker, a star could not explode.
- Because of the exact ratio of the electromagnetic force to the strong nuclear force, helium (element 2 on the periodic table) and beryllium (element 4) go into resonance within a star, enabling them to fuse easily into carbon (element 6), which is essential to life as we know it. (It's hard to talk about life as we don't know it.) If either the electromagnetic force or the strong nuclear force changed slightly (less than one percent), the universe would have almost no carbon.
- The electromagnetic force is 10^{40} times stronger than gravity. If gravity were a bit stronger relative to the electromagnetic force, planets would not form. If it were a bit weaker, planets would consist of only gases.

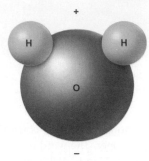

Figure Intro.1 A water molecule Because of the hydrogen-oxygen-hydrogen angle, one end of a water molecule is more positive and the other negative. The exact difference in charge causes water molecules to attract one another just enough to be a liquid.

- The mass of a neutron is 0.14 percent greater than that of a proton. If the difference had been a little larger, all the hydrogen would have fused into helium, but the helium would not have fused into any of the heavier elements (Wilczek, 2015).
- Why is water (H_2O) a liquid? Similar molecules such as carbon dioxide, nitric oxide, ozone, and methane are gases except at extremely low temperatures. In a water molecule, the two hydrogen ions form a 104.5° angle (see Figure Intro.1). As a result, one end of the water molecule has a slight positive charge and the other has a slight negative charge. The difference is enough for water molecules to attract one another electrically. If they attracted one another a bit less, all water would be a gas (steam). But if water molecules attracted one another a bit more strongly, water would always be a solid (ice).

In short, the universe could have been different in many ways, nearly all of which would have made life impossible. Why is the universe the way it is? Maybe it's just a coincidence. (Lucky for us, huh?) Or maybe intelligence of some sort guided the formation of the universe. That hypothesis clearly goes beyond the reach of empirical science. A third possibility that many physicists favor is that a huge number of other universes (perhaps an infinite number) really *do* exist, and we of course know about only the kind of universe in which we could evolve. That hypothesis, too, goes beyond the reach of empirical science, as we cannot know about other universes. Will we ever know why the universe is the way it is? Maybe or maybe not, but the question is fascinating.

At the start I mentioned two profound and difficult questions. The second one is called the **mind–brain problem** or the **mind–body problem**, the question of how mind relates to brain activity. Put another way: Given a universe composed of matter and energy, why is there such a thing as consciousness? We can imagine how matter came together to form molecules, and how certain kinds of carbon compounds came together to form a primitive type of life, which then evolved into animals with brains and complex behaviors. But why are certain types of brain activity conscious?

So far, no one has offered a convincing explanation of consciousness. A few scholars have suggested that we abandon the concept of consciousness altogether (Churchland, 1986; Dennett, 1991). That proposal avoids the question, rather than answering it. Consciousness is something we experience, and it calls for an explanation, even if we do not yet see how to explain it. Chalmers (2007) and Rensch (1977) proposed,

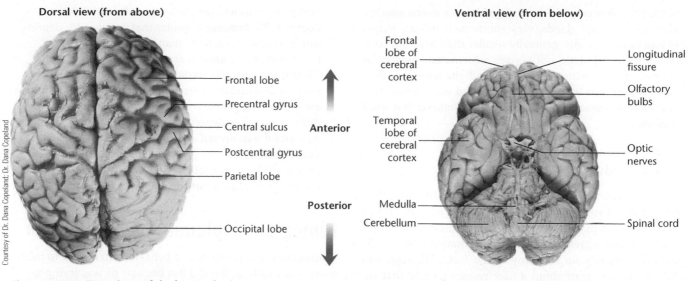

Dorsal view (from above)

- Frontal lobe
- Precentral gyrus
- Central sulcus
- Postcentral gyrus
- Parietal lobe
- Occipital lobe

Anterior

Posterior

Courtesy of Dr. Dana Copeland; Dr. Dana Copeland

Ventral view (from below)

- Frontal lobe of cerebral cortex
- Longitudinal fissure
- Olfactory bulbs
- Temporal lobe of cerebral cortex
- Optic nerves
- Medulla
- Cerebellum
- Spinal cord

Figure Intro.2 Two views of the human brain
The brain has an enormous number of divisions and subareas; the labels point to a few of the main ones on the surface of the brain.

instead, that we regard consciousness as a fundamental property of matter. A fundamental property is one that cannot be reduced to something else. For example, mass and electrical charge are fundamental properties. Maybe consciousness is like that.

However, that is an unsatisfying answer. First, consciousness isn't like other fundamental properties. Matter has mass all the time, and protons and electrons have charge all the time. So far as we can tell, consciousness occurs only in certain parts of a nervous system, just some of the time—not when you are in a dreamless sleep, and not when you are in a coma. Besides, it's unsatisfying to call *anything* a fundamental property, even mass or charge. To say that mass is a fundamental property doesn't mean that there is no reason. It means that we have given up on finding a reason. And, in fact, contemporary physicists have not given up. They are trying to explain mass and charge in terms of the Higgs boson and other principles of the universe. To say that consciousness is a fundamental property would mean that we have given up on explaining it. Certainly it is too soon to give up. After we learn as much as possible about the nervous system, perhaps we shall understand what consciousness is all about. Even if not, the research will teach us much that is important and interesting.

The Field of Biological Psychology

Biological psychology is the study of the physiological, evolutionary, and developmental mechanisms of behavior and experience. It is approximately synonymous with the terms *biopsychology, psychobiology, physiological psychology,* and *behavioral neuroscience.* The term *biological psychology* emphasizes that the goal is to relate biology to issues of psychology. *Neuroscience* includes much that is relevant to behavior but also includes more detail about anatomy and chemistry.

Biological psychology is not only a field of study, but also a point of view. It holds that we think and act as we do because of brain mechanisms, and that we evolved those brain mechanisms because ancient animals built this way survived and reproduced.

Biological psychology deals mostly with brain activity. Figure Intro.2 offers a view of the human brain from the top (what anatomists call a *dorsal* view) and from the bottom (a *ventral* view). The labels point to a few important areas that will become more familiar as you proceed through this text. An inspection of a brain reveals distinct subareas. At the microscopic level, we find two kinds of cells: the *neurons* (Figure Intro.3)

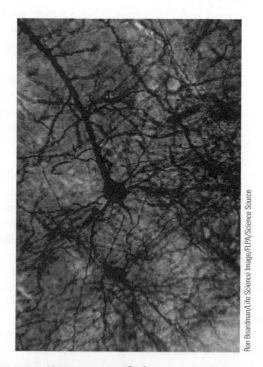

Ron Boardman/Life Science Image/FLPA/Science Source

Figure Intro.3 Neurons, magnified
The brain is composed of cells called neurons and glia.

and the *glia.* Neurons, which convey messages to one another and to muscles and glands, vary enormously in size, shape, and functions. The glia, generally smaller than neurons, have many functions but do not convey information over great distances. The activities of neurons and glia somehow produce an enormous wealth of behavior and experience. This book is about researchers' attempts to elaborate on that word *somehow.*

Three Main Points to Remember from This Book

This book presents a great deal of factual information. How much of it will you remember a few years from now? If you enter a career in psychology, biology, or medicine, you might continue using a great deal of the information. Otherwise, you will inevitably forget many of the facts, although you will occasionally read about a new research study that refreshes your memory. Regardless of how many details you remember, at least three general points should stick with you forever:

1. Perception occurs in your brain. When something contacts your hand, the hand sends a message to your brain. You feel it in your brain, not your hand. (Electrical stimulation of your brain could produce a hand experience even if you had no hand. A hand disconnected from your brain has no experience.) Similarly, you see when light comes into your eyes. The experience is in your head, not "out there." You do NOT send "sight rays" out of your eyes, and even if you did, they wouldn't do you any good. The chapter on vision elaborates on this point.

2. Mental activity and certain types of brain activity are, so far as we can tell, inseparable. This position is known as **monism,** the idea that the universe consists of only one type of being. (The opposite is **dualism,** the idea that minds are one type of substance and matter is another.) Nearly all neuroscientists and philosophers support the position of monism. You should understand monism and the evidence behind it. The chapter on consciousness considers this issue directly, but nearly everything in the book pertains to the mind–brain relationship in one way or another.

   It is not easy to get used to the concept of monism. According to monism, your thoughts or experiences are the same thing as your brain activity. People sometimes ask whether brain activity causes thoughts, or whether thoughts direct the brain activity (e.g., Miller, 2010). According to monism, that question is like asking whether temperature causes the movement of molecules, or whether the movement of molecules causes temperature. Neither causes the other; they are just different ways of describing the same thing.

3. We should be cautious about what is an explanation and what is not. For example, people with depression have less than usual activity in certain brain areas. Does that evidence tell us *why* people became depressed? No, it does not. To illustrate, consider that people with depression also have less activity than normal in their legs. (They don't move around as much as other people do.) Clearly, the inactive legs did not cause depression. Suppose we also find that certain genes are less common than average among people with depression. Does that genetic difference explain depression? Again, it does not. It might be a useful step toward explaining depression, after we understand what those genes do, but the genetic difference itself does not explain anything. In short, we should avoid overstating the conclusions from any research study.

Biological Explanations of Behavior

Commonsense explanations of behavior often refer to intentional goals such as, "He did this because he was trying to . . ." or "She did that because she wanted to. . . ." But often, we have

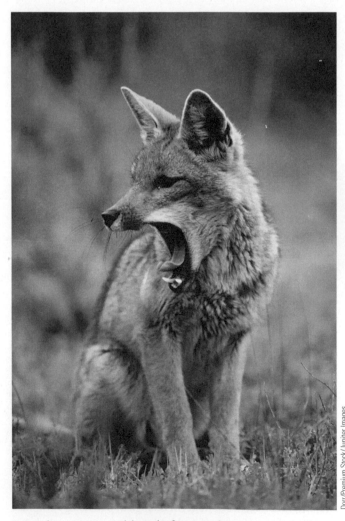

Researchers continue to debate the function of yawning. Brain mechanisms produce many behaviors that we engage in without necessarily knowing why.

no reason to assume intentions. A 4-month-old bird migrating south for the first time presumably does not know why. The next spring, when she lays an egg, sits on it, and defends it from predators, again she doesn't know why. Even humans don't always know the reasons for their own behaviors. Yawning and laughter are two examples. You do them, but can you explain what they accomplish? Intentions are, at best, a weak form of explanation.

In contrast to commonsense explanations, biological explanations of behavior fall into four categories: physiological, ontogenetic, evolutionary, and functional (Tinbergen, 1951). A **physiological explanation** relates a behavior to the activity of the brain and other organs. It deals with the machinery of the body—for example, the chemical reactions that enable hormones to influence brain activity and the routes by which brain activity controls muscle contractions.

The term *ontogenetic* comes from Greek roots meaning the origin (or genesis) of being. An **ontogenetic explanation** describes how a structure or behavior develops, including the influences of genes, nutrition, experiences, and their interactions. For example, males and females differ on average in several ways. Some of those differences can be traced to the effects of genes or prenatal hormones, some relate to cultural influences, many relate partly to both, and some await further research.

An **evolutionary explanation** reconstructs the evolutionary history of a structure or behavior. The characteristic features of an animal are almost always modifications of something found in ancestral species. For example, bat wings are modified arms, and porcupine quills are modified hairs.

In behavior, monkeys use tools occasionally, and humans evolved elaborations on those abilities that enable us to use tools even better (Peeters et al., 2009). Evolutionary explanations call attention to behavioral similarities among related species.

A **functional explanation** describes *why* a structure or behavior evolved as it did. Within a small, isolated population, a gene can spread by accident through a process called *genetic drift*. For example, a dominant male with many offspring spreads all his genes, including some that may have been irrelevant to his success or even disadvantageous. However, a gene that is prevalent in a large population probably provided some advantage—at least in the past, though not necessarily today. A functional explanation identifies that advantage. For example, many species have an appearance that matches their background (see Figure Intro.4). A functional explanation is that camouflaged appearance makes the animal inconspicuous to predators. Some species use their behavior as part of the camouflage. For example, zone-tailed hawks, native to Mexico and the southwestern United States, fly among vultures and hold their wings in the same posture as vultures. Small mammals and birds run for cover when they see a hawk, but they learn to ignore vultures, which pose no threat to healthy animals. Because the zone-tailed hawks resemble vultures in both appearance and flight behavior, their prey disregard them, enabling the hawks to pick up easy meals (Clark, 2004).

To contrast the four types of biological explanation, consider how they all apply to one example, birdsong (Catchpole & Slater, 1995):

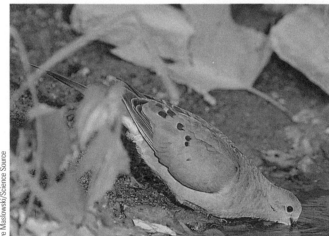

Unlike other birds, doves and pigeons can drink with their heads down. Others fill their mouths and then raise their heads. A physiological explanation would describe these birds' nerves and throat muscles. An evolutionary explanation states that all doves and pigeons share this behavioral capacity because they inherited their genes from a common ancestor.

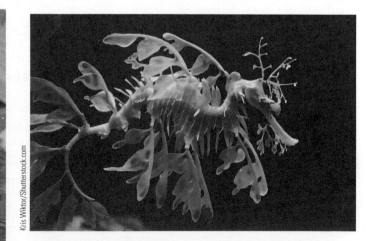

Figure Intro.4 A seadragon, an Australian fish related to the seahorse, lives among kelp plants, looks like kelp, and usually drifts slowly, *acting* like kelp.
A functional explanation is that potential predators overlook a fish that resembles inedible plants. An evolutionary explanation is that genetic modifications expanded smaller appendages that were present in these fish's ancestors.

Type of Explanation	Example from Birdsong
Physiological	A particular area of a songbird brain grows under the influence of testosterone; hence, it is larger in breeding males than in females or immature birds. That brain area enables a mature male to sing.
Ontogenetic	In certain species, a young male bird learns its song by listening to adult males. Development of the song requires certain genes and the opportunity to hear the appropriate song during a sensitive period early in life.
Evolutionary	Certain pairs of species have similar songs. For example, dunlins and Baird's sandpipers, two shorebird species, give their calls in distinct pulses, unlike other shorebirds. The similarity suggests that the two evolved from a single ancestor.
Functional	In most bird species, only the male sings. He sings only during the reproductive season and only in his territory. The functions of the song are to attract females and warn away other males.

STOP & CHECK

1. How does an evolutionary explanation differ from a functional explanation?

ANSWER

1. An evolutionary explanation states what evolved from what. For example, humans evolved from earlier primates and therefore have certain features that we inherited from those ancestors, even if the features are not useful to us today. A functional explanation states why something was advantageous and therefore favored by natural selection.

Career Opportunities

If you want to consider a career related to biological psychology, you have a range of options relating to research and therapy. Table Intro.1 describes some of the major fields.

A research position ordinarily requires a PhD in psychology, biology, neuroscience, or other related field. People with a master's or bachelor's degree might work in a research laboratory but would not direct it. Many people with a PhD hold college or university positions, where they perform some combination of teaching and

Table Intro.1 | Fields of Specialization

Specialization	Description
Research Fields	**Research positions ordinarily require a PhD. Researchers are employed by universities, hospitals, pharmaceutical firms, and research institutes.**
Neuroscientist	Studies the anatomy, biochemistry, or physiology of the nervous system. (This broad term includes any of the next five, as well as other specialties not listed.)
Behavioral neuroscientist (almost synonyms: psychobiologist, biopsychologist, or physiological psychologist)	Investigates how functioning of the brain and other organs influences behavior.
Cognitive neuroscientist	Uses brain research, such as scans of brain anatomy or activity, to analyze and explore people's knowledge, thinking, and problem solving.
Neuropsychologist	Conducts behavioral tests to determine the abilities and disabilities of people with various kinds of brain damage, and changes in their condition over time. Most neuropsychologists have a mixture of psychological and medical training; they work in hospitals and clinics.
Psychophysiologist	Measures heart rate, breathing rate, brain waves, and other body processes and how they vary from one person to another or one situation to another.
Neurochemist	Investigates the chemical reactions in the brain.
Comparative psychologist (almost synonyms: ethologist, animal behaviorist)	Compares the behaviors of different species and tries to relate them to their ways of life.
Evolutionary psychologist (almost synonym: sociobiologist)	Relates behaviors, especially social behaviors, including those of humans, to the functions they have served and, therefore, the presumed selective pressures that caused them to evolve.
Practitioner Fields of Psychology	**Require a PhD, PsyD, or master's degree. In most cases, their work is not directly related to neuroscience. However, practitioners often need to understand it enough to communicate with a client's physician.**
Clinical psychologist	Employed by hospital, clinic, private practice, or college; helps people with emotional problems.
Counseling psychologist	Employed by hospital, clinic, private practice, or college. Helps people make educational, vocational, and other decisions.

Table Intro.1 | **Fields of Specialization** (*Continued*)

Specialization	Description
School psychologist	Most are employed by a school system. Identifies educational needs of schoolchildren, devises a plan to meet the needs, and then helps teachers implement it.
Medical Fields	**Require an MD plus about four years of additional specialized study and practice. Physicians are employed by hospitals, clinics, medical schools, and in private practice. Some conduct research in addition to seeing patients.**
Neurologist	Treats people with brain damage or diseases of the brain.
Neurosurgeon	Performs brain surgery.
Psychiatrist	Helps people with emotional distress or troublesome behaviors, sometimes using drugs or other medical procedures.
Allied Medical Field	**Ordinarily require a master's degree or more. Practitioners are employed by hospitals, clinics, private practice, and medical schools.**
Physical therapist	Provides exercise and other treatments to help people with muscle or nerve problems, pain, or anything else that impairs movement.
Occupational therapist	Helps people improve their ability to perform functions of daily life, for example, after a stroke.
Social worker	Helps people deal with personal and family problems. The activities of a social worker overlap those of a clinical psychologist.

research. Others have pure research positions in laboratories sponsored by the government, drug companies, or other industries.

Fields of therapy include clinical psychology, counseling psychology, school psychology, medicine, and allied medical practice such as physical therapy. These fields range from neurologists (who deal exclusively with brain disorders) to social workers and clinical psychologists, who need to recognize possible signs of brain disorder so they can refer a client to a proper specialist.

Anyone who pursues a career in research needs to stay up to date on new developments by attending conventions, consulting with colleagues, and reading research journals, such as *The Journal of Neuroscience, Neurology, Behavioral Neuroscience, Brain Research*, and *Nature Neuroscience*. But what if you are entering a field on the outskirts of neuroscience, such as clinical psychology, school psychology, social work, or physical therapy? In that case, you probably don't want to wade through technical journal articles, but you do want to stay current on major developments, at least enough to converse intelligently with medical colleagues. You can find much information in the magazine *Scientific American Mind* or at websites such as the Dana Foundation at www.dana.org.

The Use of Animals in Research

Certain ethical disputes resist agreement. One is abortion. Another is the use of animals in research. In both cases, well-meaning people on each side of the issue insist that their position is proper and ethical. The dispute is not a matter of the good guys against the bad guys. It is between two views of what is good.

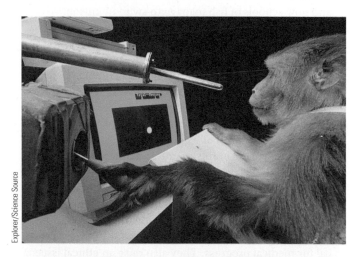

Explorer/Science Source

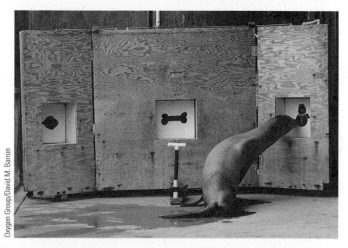

Oxygen Group/David M. Barron

Animals are used in many kinds of research studies, some dealing with behavior and others with the functions of the nervous system.

Given that most biological psychologists and neuroscientists are primarily interested in the human brain and human behavior, why do they study nonhumans? Here are four reasons:

1. *The underlying mechanisms of behavior are similar across species and sometimes easier to study in a nonhuman species.* If you want to understand a complex machine, you might begin by examining a simpler machine. We also learn about brain–behavior relationships by starting with simpler cases. For example, much research has been conducted on squid nerves, which are thicker than human nerves and therefore easier to study. The roundworm *Caenorhabditis elegans* has only 302 neurons, the same for all individuals, enabling researchers to map all the cells and all their interconnections. The brains and behavior of nonhuman vertebrates resemble those of humans in their chemistry and anatomy, but are smaller and easier to study (see Figure Intro.5).

2. *We are interested in animals for their own sake.* Humans are naturally curious. We would love to know about life, if any, elsewhere in the universe, regardless of whether that knowledge might be useful. Similarly, we would like to understand how bats chase insects in the dark, how migratory birds find their way over unfamiliar territory, and how schools of fish manage to swim in unison.

3. *What we learn about animals sheds light on human evolution.* How did we come to be the way we are? How do we resemble chimpanzees and other primates, and how do we differ from them? Why and how did primates evolve larger brains than other species? Researchers approach such questions by comparing species.

4. *Legal or ethical restrictions prevent certain kinds of research on humans.* For example, investigators insert electrodes into the brains of rats and other animals to determine the relationship between brain activity and behavior. They also inject chemicals, extract brain chemicals, and study the effects of brain damage. Such experiments answer questions that investigators cannot address in any other way, including some questions that are critical for medical progress. They also raise an ethical issue: If the research is unacceptable with humans, is it acceptable with other species? If so, under what circumstances?

✓ STOP & CHECK

2. Describe reasons biological psychologists conduct much of their research on nonhuman animals.

ANSWER

2. Sometimes the mechanisms of behavior are easier to study in a nonhuman species. We are curious about animals for their own sake. We study animals to understand human evolution. Certain procedures that might lead to important knowledge are illegal or unethical with humans.

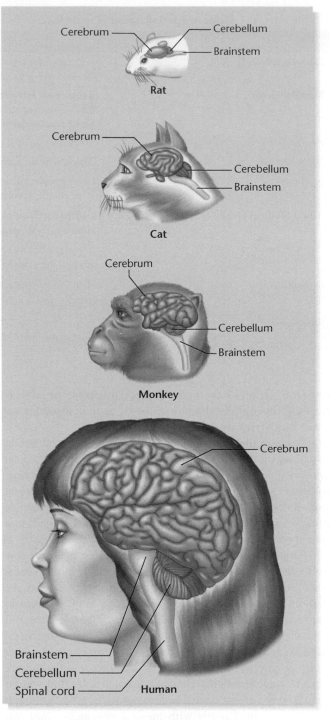

Figure Intro.5 Brains of several species
The general plan and organization of the brain are similar for all mammals, even though the size varies from species to species.

In some cases, researchers simply observe how animal behavior in nature varies as a function of times of day, seasons of the year, changes in diet, and so forth. These procedures raise no ethical problems. In other studies, however, including many discussed in this book, animals have been subjected to brain damage, electrode implantation, injections of drugs or hormones, and other procedures that are clearly not for their own benefit. Anyone with a conscience, including scientists, is distressed by this fact. Nevertheless, experimentation with animals has been critical to the medical research that led to methods for the prevention or treatment of polio, diabetes, measles, smallpox, massive burns, heart disease, and other serious conditions. Progress toward treating or preventing AIDS, Alzheimer's disease, stroke, and other disorders depends largely on animal research. In much of medicine and biological psychology, research would progress slowly or not at all without animals.

Degrees of Opposition

Opposition to animal research ranges considerably in degree. "Minimalists" tolerate certain types of animal research but wish to limit or prohibit others depending on the probable value of the research, the amount of distress to the animal, and the type of animal. (Few people have serious qualms about hurting an insect, for example.) They favor firm regulations on research. Researchers agree in principle, although they often differ in where they draw the line between acceptable and unacceptable research.

The legal standard emphasizes "the three R's": *reduction* of animal numbers (using fewer animals), *replacement* (using computer models or other substitutes for animals, when possible), and *refinement* (modifying the procedures to reduce pain and discomfort). In the United States, every college or other institution that receives government research funds is required to have an Institutional Animal Care and Use Committee, composed of veterinarians, community representatives, and scientists that evaluate proposed experiments, decide whether they are acceptable, and specify procedures to minimize pain and discomfort. Similar regulations and committees govern research on human subjects. In addition, research laboratories must abide by national laws requiring standards of cleanliness and animal care. Scientific journals accept publications only after researchers state that they followed all the laws and regulations. Professional organizations such as the Society for Neuroscience publish guidelines for the use of animals in research (see Appendix B). Rules do differ, however, from one country to another. For example, research on treatments for Ebola, Zika, and other viruses requires studies on monkeys, but political pressures in the United States and Europe block nearly all such research, leaving the world to rely on researchers in China, where the government is more permissive ("Monkeying around," 2016).

In contrast to "minimalists," the "abolitionists" see no room for compromise. Abolitionists maintain that all animals have the same rights as humans. They regard killing an animal as murder, regardless of whether the intention is to eat it, use its fur, or gain scientific knowledge. Keeping an animal in a cage (presumably even a pet) is, in their view, slavery. Because animals cannot give informed consent to research, abolitionists insist it is wrong to use them in any way, regardless of the circumstances. According to one opponent of animal research, "We have no moral option but to bring this research to a halt. Completely. . . . We will not be satisfied until every cage is empty" (Regan, 1986, pp. 39–40). Advocates of this position sometimes claim that most animal research is painful and that it never leads to important results. However, for a true abolitionist, neither of those points really matters. Their moral imperative is that people have no right to use animals at all, even if the research is highly useful and totally painless.

The disagreement between abolitionists and animal researchers is a dispute between two ethical positions: "Never knowingly harm an innocent" and "Sometimes a little harm leads to a greater good." On the one hand, permitting research has the undeniable consequence of inflicting pain or distress. On the other hand, banning all use of animals would mean a great setback in medical research as well as the end of animal-to-human transplants (e.g., transplanting pig heart valves to prolong lives of people with heart diseases).

It would be nice to say that this ethical debate has always proceeded in an intelligent and mutually respectful way. Unfortunately, it has not. Over the years, abolitionists have sometimes advanced their cause through intimidation. Examples include vandalizing laboratories, placing a bomb under a professor's car, placing a bomb on a porch (intended for a researcher but accidentally placed on the neighbor's porch), banging on a researcher's children's windows at night, and inserting a garden hose through a researcher's window to flood the house (Miller, 2007a). Michael Conn and James Parker (2008, p. 186) quote a spokesperson for the Animal Defense League as follows: "I don't think you'd have to kill—assassinate—too many [doctors involved with animal testing]. . . . I think for 5 lives, 10 lives, 15 human lives, we could save a million, 2 million, 10 million nonhuman lives." One researcher, Dario Ringach, finally agreed to stop his research on monkeys, if animal-rights extremists would stop harassing and threatening his children. He emailed them, "You win." In addition to researchers who quit in the face of attacks, many colleges and other institutions have declined to open animal research laboratories because of their fear of violence. Researchers have replied to attacks with campaigns such as the one illustrated in Figure Intro.6.

The often fervent and extreme nature of the opposition makes it difficult for researchers to express intermediate or nuanced views. Many of them remark that they really do care about animals, despite using them for research. Some neuroscientists are even vegetarians

Figure Intro.6 In defense of animal research
For many years, opponents of animal research have been protesting against experimentation with animals. This ad defends such research. (*Source: Courtesy of the Foundation for Biomedical Research*)

(Marris, 2006). But admitting to doubts seems almost like giving in to intimidation. The result is extreme polarization that interferes with open-minded contemplation of the difficult issues.

We began this chapter with a quote from the Nobel Prize–winning biologist Niko Tinbergen, who argued that no fundamental gulf separates humans from other animal species. Because we are similar in many ways to other species, we learn much about ourselves from animal studies. Also because of that similarity, we wish not to hurt them. Neuroscience researchers who decide to conduct animal research do not, as a rule, take this decision lightly. They believe it is better to inflict distress under controlled conditions than to permit ignorance and disease to inflict greater distress. In some cases, however, it is a difficult decision.

STOP & CHECK

3. What are the "three R's" in the legal standards for animal research?
4. How does the "minimalist" position differ from the "abolitionist" position?

ANSWERS

3. Reduction, replacement, and refinement.
4. A "minimalist" wishes to limit animal research to studies with little discomfort and much potential value. An "abolitionist" wishes to eliminate all animal research regardless of how the animals are treated or how much value the research might produce.

Introduction | In Closing

Your Brain and Your Experience

The goal in this introduction has been to preview the kinds of questions biological psychologists hope to answer. In the next several chapters, we shall go through a great deal of technical information of the type you need to know before we can start applying it to questions about why people do what they do and experience what they experience.

Biological psychologists are ambitious, hoping to explain as much as possible of psychology in terms of brain processes, genes, and the like. The guiding assumption is that the pattern of activity that occurs in your brain when you see something *is* your perception. The pattern that occurs when you feel fear *is* your fear. This is not to say "your brain physiology controls you" any more than "you control your brain." Rather, your brain *is* you! The rest of this book explores how far we can go with this guiding assumption.

Summary

1. Two profound, difficult questions are why the universe exists, and why consciousness exists. Regardless of whether these questions are answerable, they motivate research on related topics. **4**

2. Three key points are important to remember: First, perception occurs in your brain, not in your skin or in the object you see. Second, as far as we can tell, brain activity is inseparable from mental activity. Third, it is important

to be cautious about what is or is not an explanation of behavior. **6**

3. Biological psychologists address four types of questions about any behavior. Physiological: How does the behavior relate to the physiology of the brain and other organs? Ontogenetic: How does it develop within the individual? Evolutionary: How did the capacity for the behavior evolve? Functional: Why did the capacity for this behavior evolve? That is, what function does it serve or did it serve? **7**

4. Many careers relate to biological psychology, including various research fields, certain medical specialties, and counseling and psychotherapy. **8**

5. Researchers study animals because the mechanisms are sometimes easier to study in nonhumans, because they are interested in animal behavior for its own sake, because they want to understand the evolution of behavior, and because certain kinds of experiments are difficult or impossible with humans. **9**

6. Using animals in research is ethically controversial. Some research does inflict stress or pain on animals. However, many research questions can be investigated only through animal research. **10**

7. Animal research today is conducted under legal and ethical controls that attempt to minimize animal distress. **11**

Key Terms

Terms are defined in the module on the page number indicated. They're also presented in alphabetical order with definitions in the book's Subject Index/Glossary, which begins on page 589. Interactive flash cards, audio reviews, and crossword puzzles are among the online resources available to help you learn these terms and the concepts they represent.

biological psychology **(p. 5)**
dualism **(p. 6)**
evolutionary explanation **(p. 7)**

functional explanation **(p. 7)**
mind–body or mind–brain
    problem **(p. 4)**

monism **(p. 6)**
ontogenetic explanation **(p. 7)**
physiological explanation **(p. 7)**

Thought Question

Thought questions are intended to spark thought and discussion. In most cases, there is no clearly right answer.

1. Is consciousness useful? What, if anything, can we do because of consciousness that we couldn't do otherwise?

2. What are the special difficulties of studying the evolution of behavior, given that behavior doesn't leave fossils (with a few exceptions such as footprints showing an animal's gait)?

End of Introduction Quiz

1. What is meant by "monism"?

    A. The idea that all forms of life evolved from a single ancestor
    B. The idea that conscious and unconscious motivations combine to produce behavior
    C. The idea that the mind is made of the same substance as the rest of the universe
    D. The idea that the mind is one type of substance as matter is another

2. An ontogenetic explanation focuses on which of the following?

    A. How a behavior develops
    B. The brain mechanisms that produce a behavior
    C. The conscious experience that accompanies a behavior
    D. The procedures that measure a behavior

3. Of the following, which one is an example of an evolutionary explanation (as opposed to a functional explanation)?

    A. People evolved a fear of snakes because many snakes are dangerous.
    B. Humans have a (tiny) tailbone because our ancient monkey-like ancestors had a tail.
    C. People evolved an ability to recognize faces because that ability is essential for cooperative social behaviors.
    D. People evolved a tendency to form long-term male–female bonds because human infants benefit from the help of two parents during their long period of dependence.

4. Of the following, which is a reason favoring the use of animals in biological psychology research aimed at solving human problems?

   A. Nonhuman animals engage in all the same behaviors as humans.

   B. One human differs from another, but nonhumans are nearly the same as one another.

   C. The nervous system of nonhuman animals resembles that of humans in many ways.

   D. Researchers can study nonhuman animals without any legal restraints.

5. What does a "minimalist" favor with regard to animal research?

   A. All research should have a minimum of at least 10 animals per group.

   B. A minimum of three people should review each research proposal.

   C. Interference with animal research should be held to a minimum.

   D. Animal research is permissible but should be held to a minimum.

Answers: 1C, 2A, 3B, 4C, 5D.

Suggestions for Further Reading

Books

de Waal, F. B. M. (2016). *Are we smart enough to know how smart animals are?* New York: W. W. Norton. An exploration of the intelligence of animals and the difficulties in estimating it accurately.

Morrison, A. R. (2009). *An odyssey with animals: A veterinarian's reflections on the animal rights & welfare debate.* New York: Oxford University Press. A defense of animal research that acknowledges the difficulties of the issue and the competing values at stake.

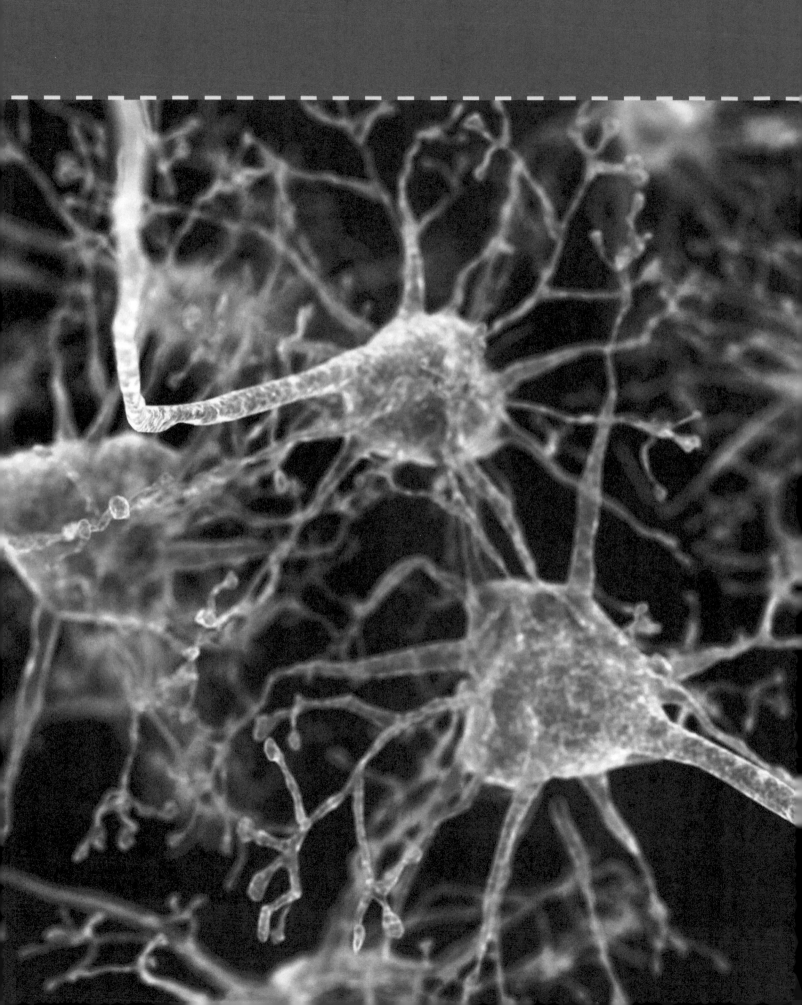

Nerve Cells and Nerve Impulses

Chapter 1

People talk about growing into adulthood and becoming independent, but in fact almost no human life is truly independent. How often do you hunt your own meat and cook it on a fire you made from scratch? Do you grow your own vegetables? Could you build your own house (with tools you made yourself)? Have you ever made your own clothing (with materials you gathered in the wild)? Of all the activities necessary for your survival, which ones—if any—could you do completely on your own, other than breathe? People can do an enormous amount together, but very little by themselves.

The cells of your nervous system are like that, too. Together they accomplish amazing things, but one cell by itself is helpless. We begin our study of the nervous system by examining single cells. Later, we examine how they act together.

Advice: Parts of this chapter and the next assume that you understand the basics of chemistry. If you have never studied chemistry or if you have forgotten what you did study, read Appendix A.

Learning Objectives

After studying this chapter, you should be able to:

1. Describe neurons and glia, the cells that constitute the nervous system.
2. Summarize how the blood–brain barrier relates to protection and nutrition of neurons.
3. Explain how the sodium–potassium pump and the properties of the membrane lead to the resting potential of a neuron.
4. Discuss how the movement of sodium and potassium ions produces the action potential and recovery after it.
5. State the all-or-none law of the action potential.

Opposite:

An electron micrograph of neurons, magnified tens of thousands of times. The color is added artificially. For objects this small, it is impossible to focus light to obtain an image. It is possible to focus an electron beam, but electrons do not show color. (© Juan Gaertner/Shutterstock.com)

The Cells of the Nervous System

No doubt you think of yourself as an individual. You don't think of your mental experience as being composed of pieces . . . but it is. Your experiences depend on the activity of a huge number of separate but interconnected cells. To understand the nervous system, the place to begin is to examine the cells that compose it.

Neurons and Glia

The nervous system consists of two kinds of cells, neurons and glia. **Neurons** receive information and transmit it to other cells. Glia serve many functions that are difficult to summarize, and we shall defer that discussion until later in this module. The adult human brain contains approximately 86 billion neurons, on average (Herculano-Houzel, Catania, Manger, & Kaas, 2015; see Figure 1.1). The exact number varies from person to person.

We now take it for granted that the brain is composed of individual cells, but the idea was in doubt as recently as the early 1900s. Until then, the best microscopic views revealed little detail about the brain. Observers noted long, thin fibers between one cell body and another, but they could not see whether a fiber merged into the next cell or stopped before it. In the late 1800s, Santiago Ramón y Cajal used newly developed staining techniques to show that a small gap separates the tip of a neuron's fiber from the surface of the next neuron. The brain, like the rest of the body, consists of individual cells.

Santiago Ramón y Cajal, a Pioneer of Neuroscience

Two scientists of the late 1800s and early 1900s are widely recognized as the main founders of neuroscience—Charles Sherrington, whom we shall discuss in Chapter 2, and the Spanish investigator Santiago Ramón y Cajal (1852–1934). Cajal's early education did not progress smoothly. At one point, he was imprisoned in a solitary cell, limited to one meal a day, and taken out daily for public floggings—at the age of 10—for the crime of not paying attention during his Latin class (Cajal, 1901–1917/1937). (And *you* complained about *your* teachers!)

Cerebral cortex:
16 billion neurons

Rest of the brain:
Less than 1 billion

Cerebellum:
69 billion neurons

Spinal cord:
1 billion neurons

Figure 1.1 Estimated numbers of neurons in humans
The numbers differ from one person to another.
(Source: Herculano-Houzel et al., 2015)

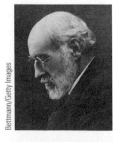

Bettmann/Getty Images

Santiago Ramón y Cajal (1852–1934)

How many interesting facts fail to be converted into fertile discoveries because their first observers regard them as natural and ordinary things! . . . It is strange to see how the populace, which nourishes its imagination with tales of witches or saints, mysterious events and extraordinary occurrences, disdains the world around it as commonplace, monotonous and prosaic, without suspecting that at bottom it is all secret, mystery, and marvel. (Cajal, 1937, pp. 46–47)

Cajal wanted to become an artist, but his father insisted that he study medicine as a safer way to make a living. He managed to combine the two fields, becoming an outstanding anatomical researcher and illustrator. His detailed drawings of the nervous system are still considered definitive today.

Before the late 1800s, microscopy revealed few details about the nervous system. Then the Italian investigator Camillo Golgi found a way to stain nerve cells with silver salts. This method, which completely stains some cells without affecting others at all, enabled researchers to examine the structure of a single cell. Cajal used Golgi's methods but applied them to infant brains, in which the cells are smaller and therefore easier to examine on a single slide. Cajal's research demonstrated that nerve cells remain separate instead of merging into one another. (Oddly, when Cajal and Golgi shared the 1906 Nobel Prize for Physiology or Medicine, they used their acceptance lectures to defend contradictory positions. In spite of Cajal's evidence, which had persuaded almost everyone else, Golgi clung to the theory that all nerve cells merge directly into one another.)

Philosophically, we see the appeal of the old idea that neurons merge. We describe our experience as undivided, not the sum of separate parts, so it seemed right that all the cells in the brain might be joined together as one unit. How the separate cells combine their influences is a complex and still mysterious process.

The Structures of an Animal Cell

Figure 1.2 illustrates a neuron from the cerebellum of a mouse (magnified enormously, of course). Neurons have much in common with the rest of the body's cells. The surface of a cell is its **membrane** (or *plasma membrane*), a structure that separates the inside of the cell from the outside environment. Most chemicals cannot cross the membrane, but protein channels in the membrane permit a controlled flow of water, oxygen, sodium, potassium, calcium, chloride, and other important chemicals.

Except for mammalian red blood cells, all animal cells have a **nucleus**, the structure that contains the chromosomes. A **mitochondrion** (plural: mitochondria) is the structure that performs metabolic activities, providing the energy that the cell uses for all activities. Mitochondria have genes separate from those in the nucleus of a cell, and mitochondria differ from one another genetically. People with overactive mitochondria tend to burn their fuel rapidly and overheat, even in a cool environment. People whose mitochondria are less active than normal are predisposed to depression and pains. Mutated mitochondrial genes are a possible cause of autism (Aoki & Cortese, 2016).

Ribosomes are the sites within a cell that synthesize new protein molecules. Proteins provide building materials for the cell and facilitate chemical reactions. Some ribosomes float freely within the cell, but others are attached to the **endoplasmic reticulum**, a network of thin tubes that transport newly synthesized proteins to other locations.

The Structure of a Neuron

The most distinctive feature of neurons is their shape, which varies enormously from one neuron to another (see Figure 1.3). Unlike most other body cells, neurons have long branching extensions. All neurons include a soma (cell body), and most also have dendrites, an axon, and presynaptic terminals. The tiniest neurons lack axons, and some lack well-defined dendrites. Contrast the motor neuron in Figure 1.4 and the sensory neuron in Figure 1.5. A **motor neuron**, with its soma in the spinal cord, receives excitation through its dendrites and conducts impulses along its axon to a muscle. A **sensory neuron** is specialized at one end to be highly sensitive to a particular type of stimulation, such as light, sound, or touch. The sensory

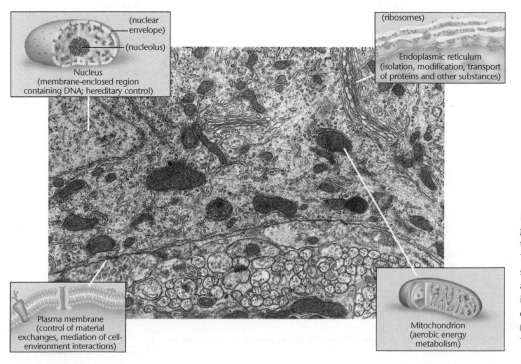

(nuclear envelope)

(nucleolus)

Nucleus
(membrane-enclosed region containing DNA; hereditary control)

(ribosomes)

Endoplasmic reticulum
(isolation, modification, transport of proteins and other substances)

Plasma membrane
(control of material exchanges, mediation of cell-environment interactions)

Mitochondrion
(aerobic energy metabolism)

Figure 1.2 An electron micrograph of parts of a neuron from the cerebellum of a mouse
The nucleus, membrane, and other structures are characteristic of most animal cells. The plasma membrane is the border of the neuron. Magnification approximately x 20,000.
(*Source: Courtesy of Dr. Dennis M. D. Landis*)

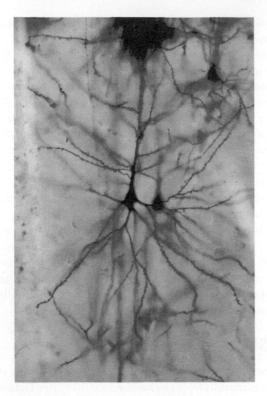

Figure 1.3 Neurons, stained to appear dark
Note the small fuzzy-looking spines on the dendrites.
(Source: Photo courtesy of Bob Jacobs, Colorado College)

neuron shown in Figure 1.5 conducts touch information from the skin to the spinal cord. Tiny branches lead directly from the receptors into the axon, and the cell's soma is located on a little stalk off the main trunk.

Dendrites are branching fibers that get narrower near their ends. (The term *dendrite* comes from a Greek root word meaning "tree." A dendrite branches like a tree.) The dendrite's surface is lined with specialized *synaptic receptors*, at which the dendrite receives information from other neurons. (Chapter 2 concerns synapses.) The greater the surface area of a dendrite, the more information it can receive. Many dendrites contain **dendritic spines**, short outgrowths that increase the surface area available for synapses (see Figure 1.6).

The **cell body**, or **soma** (Greek for "body"; plural: somata), contains the nucleus, ribosomes, and mitochondria. Most of a neuron's metabolic work occurs here. Cell bodies of neurons range in diameter from 0.005 millimeter (mm) to 0.1 mm in mammals and up to a millimeter in certain invertebrates. In many neurons, the cell body is like the dendrites—covered with synapses on its surface.

The **axon** is a thin fiber of constant diameter. (The term *axon* comes from a Greek word meaning "axis.") The axon conveys an impulse toward other neurons, an organ, or a muscle. Axons can be more than a meter in length, as in the case of axons from your spinal cord to your feet. The length of an axon is enormous in comparison to its width, and in comparison

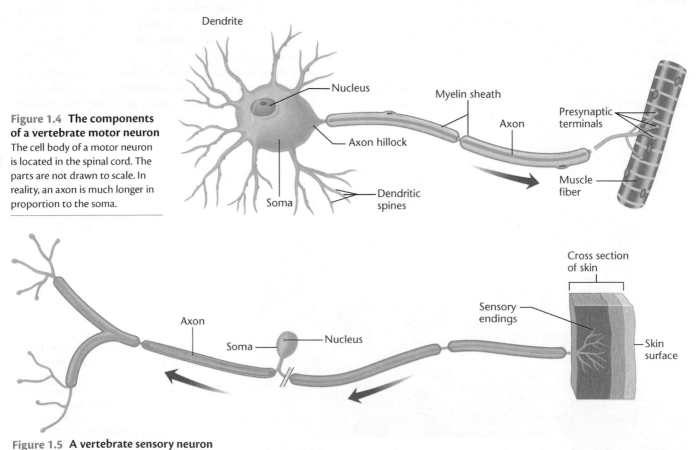

Figure 1.4 The components of a vertebrate motor neuron
The cell body of a motor neuron is located in the spinal cord. The parts are not drawn to scale. In reality, an axon is much longer in proportion to the soma.

Dendrite

Nucleus

Myelin sheath

Presynaptic terminals

Axon

Axon hillock

Muscle fiber

Soma

Dendritic spines

Figure 1.5 A vertebrate sensory neuron
Note that the soma is located on a stalk off the main trunk of the axon. As in Figure 1.4, the structures are not drawn to scale.

Axon

Soma

Nucleus

Cross section of skin

Sensory endings

Skin surface

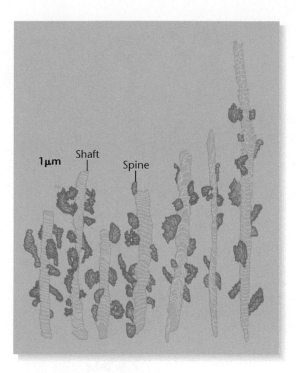

Figure 1.6 Dendritic spines
Many dendrites are lined with spines, short outgrowths that receive incoming information.
(Source: From K. M. Harris and J. K. Stevens, Society for Neuroscience, "Dendritic Spines of CA1 Pyramidal Cells in the Rat Hippocampus: Serial Electron Microscopy with Reference to Their Biophysical Characteristics." Journal of Neuroscience, 9 (1989), 2982–2997. Copyright © 1989 Society for Neuroscience. Reprinted by permission.)

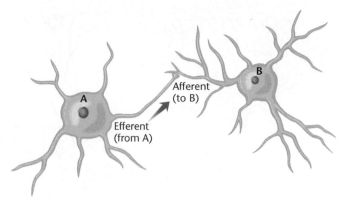

Figure 1.7 Cell structures and axons
It all depends on the point of view. An axon from A to B is an efferent axon from A and an afferent axon to B, just as a train from Washington to New York is exiting Washington and approaching New York.

to the length of dendrites. Giorgio Ascoli (2015) offers the analogy that if you could expand the dendrite of a reasonably typical neuron to the height of a tree, the cell's axon and its branches would extend for more than 25 city blocks.

Many vertebrate axons are covered with an insulating material called a **myelin sheath** with interruptions known as **nodes of Ranvier** (RAHN-vee-ay). Invertebrate axons do not have myelin sheaths. Although a neuron can have many dendrites, it can have only one axon, but the axon may have branches. The end of each branch has a swelling, called a **presynaptic terminal**, also known as an *end bulb* or *bouton* (French for "button"). At that point the axon releases chemicals that cross through the junction between that neuron and another cell.

Other terms associated with neurons are *afferent, efferent,* and *intrinsic.* An **afferent axon** brings information into a structure; an **efferent axon** carries information away from a structure. Every sensory neuron is an afferent to the rest of the nervous system, and every motor neuron is an efferent from the nervous system. Within the nervous system, a given neuron is an efferent from one structure and an afferent to another (see Figure 1.7). You can remember that *efferent* starts with *e* as in *exit*; *afferent* starts with *a* as in *admit*. If a cell's dendrites and axon are entirely contained within a single structure, the cell is an **interneuron** or **intrinsic neuron** of that structure. For example, an intrinsic neuron of the thalamus has its axon and all its dendrites within the thalamus.

STOP & CHECK

1. What are the widely branching structures of a neuron called? And what is the long, thin structure that carries information to another cell called?
2. Which animal species would have the longest axons?
3. Compared to other neurons, would an interneuron's axon be relatively long, short, or about the same?

ANSWERS

1. The widely branching structures of a neuron are called *dendrites,* and the long thin structure that carries information to another cell is called an *axon.* 2. The longest axons occur in the largest animals. For example, giraffes and elephants have axons that extend from the spinal cord to the feet, nearly 2 meters away. 3. Because an interneuron is contained entirely within one part of the brain, its axon is short.

Variations among Neurons

Neurons vary enormously in size, shape, and function. The shape of a neuron determines its connections with other cells and thereby determines its function (see Figure 1.8). For example, the widely branching dendrites of the Purkinje cell in the cerebellum (see Figure 1.8a) enable it to receive input from up to 200,000 other neurons. By contrast, bipolar neurons in the retina (see Figure 1.8d) have only short branches, and some receive input from as few as two other cells.

Glia

Glia (or neuroglia), the other components of the nervous system, perform many functions (see Figure 1.9). The term *glia,* derived from a Greek word meaning "glue," reflects early investigators' idea that glia were like glue that held the neurons together. Although that concept is obsolete, the term remains. Glia outnumber neurons in the cerebral cortex, but neurons outnumber glia in several other brain areas,

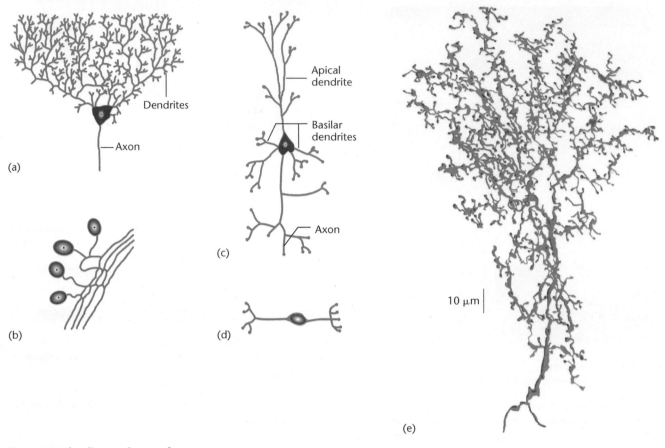

Figure 1.8 The diverse shapes of neurons
(a) Purkinje cell, a cell type found only in the cerebellum; **(b)** sensory neurons from skin to spinal cord; **(c)** pyramidal cell of the motor area of the cerebral cortex; **(d)** bipolar cell of retina of the eye; **(e)** Kenyon cell, from a honeybee.
(Source: Part e courtesy of R. G. Goss)

especially the cerebellum (Herculano-Houzel et al., 2015; Khakh & Sofroniew, 2015). Overall, the numbers are almost equal.

The brain has several types of glia. The star-shaped **astrocytes** wrap around the synapses of functionally related axons, as shown in Figure 1.10. By surrounding a connection between neurons, an astrocyte shields it from chemicals circulating in the surround (Nedergaard & Verkhatsky, 2012). Also, by taking up the ions and transmitters released by axons and then releasing them back, an astrocyte helps synchronize closely related neurons, enabling their axons to send messages in waves (Martín, Bajo-Grañeras, Moratalla, Perea, & Araque, 2015). Astrocytes are therefore important for generating rhythms, such as your rhythm of breathing (Morquette et al., 2015).

Astrocytes dilate the blood vessels to bring more nutrients into brain areas that have heightened activity (Filosa et al., 2006; Takano et al., 2006). A possible role in information processing is also likely but less certain. According to a popular hypothesis known as the *tripartite synapse*, the tip of an axon releases chemicals that cause the neighboring astrocyte to release chemicals of its own, thus magnifying or modifying

the message to the next neuron (Ben Achour & Pascual, 2012). This process is a possible contributor to learning and memory (De Pitta, Brunel, & Volterra, 2016). In some brain areas, astrocytes also respond to hormones and thereby influence neurons (Kim et al., 2014). In short, astrocytes are active partners of neurons in many ways.

Tiny cells called **microglia** act as part of the immune system, removing viruses and fungi from the brain. They proliferate after brain damage, removing dead or damaged neurons (Brown & Neher, 2014). They also contribute to learning by removing the weakest synapses (Zhan et al., 2014). **Oligodendrocytes** (OL-i-go-DEN-druh-sites) in the brain and spinal cord and **Schwann cells** in the periphery of the body build the myelin sheaths that surround and insulate certain vertebrate axons. They also supply an axon with nutrients necessary for proper functioning (Y. Lee et al., 2012). **Radial glia** guide the migration of neurons and their axons and dendrites during embryonic development. When embryological development finishes, most radial glia differentiate into neurons, and a smaller number differentiate into astrocytes and oligodendrocytes (Pinto & Götz, 2007).

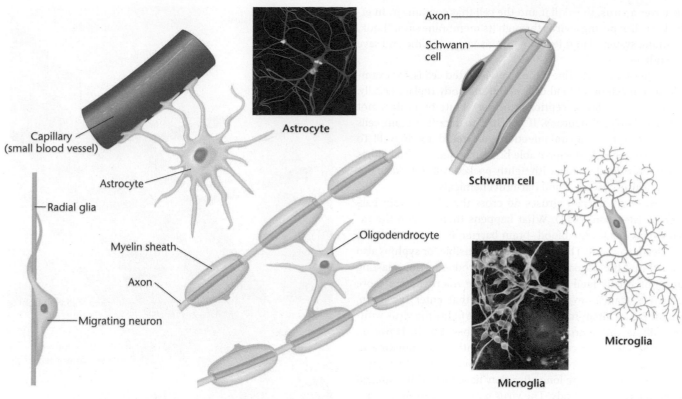

Figure 1.9 Shapes of some glia cells
Oligodendrocytes produce myelin sheaths that insulate certain vertebrate axons in the central nervous system; Schwann cells have a similar function in the periphery. The oligodendrocyte is shown here forming a segment of myelin sheath for two axons; in fact, each oligodendrocyte forms such segments for 30 to 50 axons. Astrocytes pass chemicals back and forth between neurons and blood and among neighboring neurons. Microglia proliferate in areas of brain damage and remove toxic materials. Radial glia guide the migration of neurons during embryological development. Glia have other functions as well.

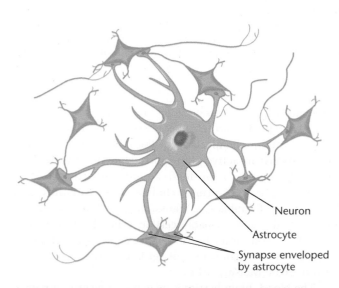

Figure 1.10 How an astrocyte synchronizes associated axons
Branches of the astrocyte (in the center) surround the presynaptic terminals of related axons. If a few of them are active at once, the astrocyte absorbs some of the chemicals they release. It then temporarily inhibits all the axons to which it is connected. When the inhibition ceases, all of the axons are primed to respond again in synchrony.
(Source: Based on Antanitus, 1998)

STOP & CHECK

4. What are the four major structures that compose a neuron?
5. Which kind of glia cell wraps around the synaptic terminals of axons?

ANSWERS

4. Dendrites, soma (cell body), axon, and presynaptic terminal. **5.** Astrocytes.

The Blood–Brain Barrier

Although the brain, like any other organ, needs to receive nutrients from the blood, many chemicals cannot cross from the blood to the brain (Hagenbuch, Gao, & Meier, 2002). The mechanism that excludes most chemicals from the vertebrate brain is known as the **blood–brain barrier.** Before we examine how it works, let's consider why we need it.

Why We Need a Blood–Brain Barrier

When a virus invades a cell, mechanisms within the cell extrude virus particles through the membrane so that the immune system can find them. When the immune system cells discover a virus, they kill it and the cell that contains it. In effect, a cell exposing a virus through its membrane says, "Look, immune system, I'm infected with this virus. Kill me and save the others."

This plan works fine if the virus-infected cell is, for example, a skin cell or a blood cell, which the body replaces easily. However, with few exceptions, the vertebrate brain does not replace damaged neurons. If you had to sacrifice brain cells whenever you had a viral infection, you would not do well! To minimize the risk of irreparable brain damage, the body lines the brain's blood vessels with tightly packed cells that keep out most viruses, bacteria, and harmful chemicals.

However, certain viruses do cross the blood–brain barrier (Kristensson, 2011). What happens then? When the rabies virus evades the blood–brain barrier, it infects the brain and leads to death. The spirochete responsible for syphilis also penetrates the blood–brain barrier, producing long-lasting and potentially fatal consequences. The microglia are more effective against several other viruses that enter the brain, mounting an inflammatory response that fights the virus without killing the neuron (Ousman & Kubes, 2012). However, this response may control the virus without eliminating it. When the chicken pox virus enters spinal cord cells, virus particles remain there long after they have been exterminated from the rest of the body. The virus may emerge from the spinal cord decades later, causing a painful condition called shingles. Similarly, the virus responsible for genital herpes hides in the nervous system, producing little harm there but periodically emerging to cause new genital infections.

How the Blood–Brain Barrier Works

The blood–brain barrier (see Figure 1.11) depends on the endothelial cells that form the walls of the capillaries (Bundgaard, 1986; Rapoport & Robinson, 1986). Outside the brain, such cells are separated by small gaps, but in the brain, they are joined so tightly that they block viruses, bacteria, and other harmful chemicals from passage.

"If the blood–brain barrier is such a good defense," you might ask, "why don't we have similar walls around all our other organs?" The answer is that the barrier keeps out useful chemicals as well as harmful ones. Those useful chemicals include all fuels and amino acids, the building blocks for proteins. For these chemicals to cross the blood–brain barrier, the brain needs special mechanisms not found in the rest of the body.

No special mechanism is required for *small, uncharged molecules* such as oxygen and carbon dioxide that cross through cell walls freely. Also, *molecules that dissolve in the fats of the membrane* cross easily. Examples include vitamins A and D and all the drugs that affect the brain—from antidepressants and other psychiatric drugs to illegal drugs such as heroin. How fast a drug takes effect depends largely on how readily it dissolves in fats and therefore crosses the blood–brain barrier.

Water crosses through special protein channels in the wall of the endothelial cells (Amiry-Moghaddam &

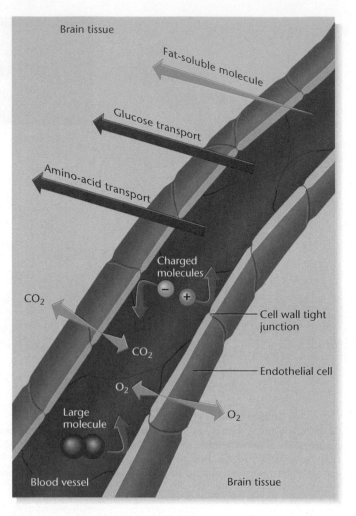

Figure 1.11 The blood–brain barrier
Most large molecules and electrically charged molecules cannot cross from the blood to the brain. A few small, uncharged molecules such as O_2 and CO_2 cross easily, as can certain fat-soluble molecules. Active transport systems pump glucose and amino acids across the membrane.

Ottersen, 2003). For certain other chemicals, the brain uses **active transport**, a protein-mediated process that expends energy to pump chemicals from the blood into the brain. Chemicals that are actively transported into the brain include glucose (the brain's main fuel), amino acids (the building blocks of proteins), purines, choline, a few vitamins, and iron (Abbott, Rönnback, & Hansson, 2006; Jones & Shusta, 2007). Insulin and probably certain other hormones also cross the blood–brain barrier, at least in small amounts, although the mechanism is not yet known (Gray, Meijer, & Barrett, 2014; McNay, 2014).

The blood–brain barrier is essential to health. In people with Alzheimer's disease or similar conditions, the endothelial cells lining the brain's blood vessels shrink, and harmful chemicals enter the brain (Zipser et al., 2007). However, the barrier poses a difficulty for treating brain cancers, because nearly all the drugs used for chemotherapy fail to cross the blood–brain barrier.

STOP & CHECK

6. Identify one major advantage and one disadvantage of having a blood–brain barrier.
7. Which chemicals cross the blood–brain barrier passively?
8. Which chemicals cross the blood–brain barrier by active transport?

ANSWERS

6. The blood-brain barrier keeps out viruses (an advantage) and also keeps out most nutrients (a disadvantage). 7. Small, uncharged molecules such as oxygen, carbon dioxide, and water cross the blood-brain barrier passively. So do chemicals that dissolve in the fats of the membrane. 8. Glucose, amino acids, purines, choline, certain vitamins, and iron.

Nourishment of Vertebrate Neurons

Most cells use a variety of carbohydrates and fats for nutrition, but vertebrate neurons depend almost entirely on **glucose**, a sugar. (Cancer cells and the testis cells that make sperm also rely overwhelmingly on glucose.) Because metabolizing glucose requires oxygen, neurons need a steady supply of oxygen. Although the human brain constitutes only about 2 percent of the body's weight, it uses about 20 percent of its oxygen and 25 percent of its glucose (Bélanger, Allaman, & Magistretti, 2011).

Why do neurons depend so heavily on glucose? They can and sometimes do use ketones (a kind of fat) and lactate for fuel. However, glucose is the only nutrient that crosses the blood–brain barrier in large quantities.

Although neurons require glucose, glucose shortage is rarely a problem, except during starvation. The liver makes glucose from many kinds of carbohydrates and amino acids, as well as from glycerol, a breakdown product from fats. A more likely problem is an inability to *use* glucose. To use glucose, the body needs vitamin B_1, **thiamine.** Prolonged thiamine deficiency, common in chronic alcoholism, leads to death of neurons and a condition called *Korsakoff's syndrome,* marked by severe memory impairments.

Module 1.1 | In Closing
Neurons

What does the study of individual neurons tell us about behavior? Everything the brain does depends on the detailed anatomy of its neurons and glia. In a later chapter we consider the physiology of learning, where one slogan is that "cells that fire together, wire together." That is, neurons active at the same time become connected. However, that is true only if the neurons active at the same time are also in approximately the same place (Ascoli, 2015). The brain cannot connect dendrites or axons that cannot find each other. In short, the locations, structures, and activities of your neurons are the basis for everything you experience, learn, or do.

However, nothing in your experience or behavior follows from the properties of any one neuron. The nervous system is more than the sum of its individual cells, just as water is more than the sum of oxygen and hydrogen. Our behavior emerges from the communication among neurons.

Summary

1. Neurons receive information and convey it to other cells. The nervous system also contains *glia,* cells that enhance and modify the activity of neurons in many ways. **18**
2. In the late 1800s, Santiago Ramón y Cajal used newly discovered staining techniques to establish that the nervous system is composed of separate cells, now known as neurons. **18**
3. Neurons contain the same internal structures as other animal cells. **19**
4. Neurons have these major parts: a cell body (or soma), dendrites, an axon with branches, and presynaptic terminals. Neurons' shapes vary greatly depending on their functions and their connections with other cells. **19**
5. Because of the blood–brain barrier, many molecules cannot enter the brain. The barrier protects the nervous system from viruses and many dangerous chemicals. **23**
6. The blood–brain barrier consists of an unbroken wall of cells that surround the blood vessels of the brain and spinal cord. A few small, uncharged molecules such as water, oxygen, and carbon dioxide cross the barrier freely. So do molecules that dissolve in fats. Active transport proteins pump glucose, amino acids, and a few other chemicals into the brain and spinal cord. Certain hormones, including insulin, also cross the blood–brain barrier. **24**
7. Neurons rely heavily on glucose, the only nutrient that crosses the blood–brain barrier in large quantities. They need thiamine (vitamin B_1) to use glucose. **25**

Key Terms

Terms are defined in the module on the page number indicated. They are also presented in alphabetical order with definitions in the book's Subject Index/Glossary, which begins on page 589. Interactive flash cards, audio reviews, and crossword puzzles are among the online resources available to help you learn these terms and the concepts they represent.

active transport **24**

afferent axon **21**

astrocytes **22**

axon **20**

blood–brain barrier **23**

cell body (soma) **20**

dendrites **20**

dendritic spines **20**

efferent axon **21**

endoplasmic reticulum **19**

glia **21**

glucose **25**

interneuron **21**

intrinsic neuron **21**

membrane **19**

microglia **22**

mitochondrion **19**

motor neuron **19**

myelin sheath **21**

neurons **18**

nodes of Ranvier **21**

nucleus **19**

oligodendrocytes **22**

presynaptic terminal **21**

radial glia **22**

ribosomes **19**

Schwann cells **22**

sensory neuron **19**

thiamine **25**

Thought Question

Although heroin and morphine are similar in many ways, heroin exerts faster effects on the brain. What can we infer about those drugs with regard to the blood–brain barrier?

Module 1.1 | End of Module Quiz

1. Santiago Ramón y Cajal was responsible for which of these discoveries?

   A. The human cerebral cortex has many specializations to produce language.

   B. The brain's left and right hemispheres control different functions.

   C. The nervous system is composed of separate cells.

   D. Neurons communicate at specialized junctions called synapses.

2. Which part of a neuron has its own genes, separate from those of the nucleus?

   A. The ribosomes

   B. The mitochondria

   C. The axon

   D. The dendrites

3. What is most distinctive about neurons, compared to other cells?

   A. Their temperature

   B. Their shape

   C. Their internal components, such as ribosomes and mitochondria

   D. Their color

4. Which of these do dendritic spines do?

   A. They synthesize proteins.

   B. They increase the surface area available for synapses.

   C. They hold the neuron in position.

   D. They metabolize fuels to provide energy for the rest of the neuron.

5. What does an efferent axon do?

   A. It controls involuntary behavior.

   B. It controls voluntary behavior.

   C. It carries output from a structure.

   D. It brings information into a structure.

6. Which of the following is a function of astrocytes?

   A. Astrocytes conduct impulses over long distances.

   B. Astrocytes build myelin sheaths that surround and insulate axons.

   C. Astrocytes create the blood–brain barrier.

   D. Astrocytes synchronize activity for a group of neurons.

7. Which of the following is a function of microglia?
    A. Microglia remove dead cells and weak synapses.
    B. Microglia build myelin sheaths that surround and insulate axons.
    C. Microglia dilate blood vessels to increase blood supply to active brain areas.
    D. Microglia synchronize activity for a group of neurons.

8. Which of these can easily cross the blood–brain barrier?
    A. Fat-soluble molecules
    B. Chemotherapy drugs
    C. Proteins
    D. Viruses

9. Which of these chemicals cross the blood–brain barrier by active transport?
    A. Oxygen, water, and fat-soluble molecules
    B. Glucose and amino acids
    C. Proteins
    D. Viruses

10. What is the brain's main source of fuel?
    A. Glucose
    B. Glutamate
    C. Chocolate
    D. Proteins

11. For the brain to use its main source of fuel, what does it also need?
    A. Steroid hormones
    B. Vitamin C
    C. Thiamine
    D. Acetylsalicylic acid

Answers: 1C, 2B, 3B, 4B, 5C, 6D, 7A, 8A, 9B, 10A, 11C.

The Nerve Impulse

Think about the axons that convey information from the touch receptors in your hands or feet toward your spinal cord and brain. If the axons used electrical conduction, they could transfer information at a velocity approaching the speed of light. However, given that your body is made of water and carbon compounds instead of copper wire, the strength of an impulse would decay rapidly as it traveled. A touch on your shoulder would feel stronger than a touch on your abdomen. Short people would feel their toes more strongly than tall people could—if either could feel their toes at all.

The way your axons actually function avoids these problems. Instead of conducting an electrical impulse, the axon regenerates an impulse at each point. Imagine a long line of people holding hands. The first person squeezes the second person's hand, who then squeezes the third person's hand, and so forth. The impulse travels along the line without weakening because each person generates it anew.

Although the axon's method of transmitting an impulse prevents a touch on your shoulder from feeling stronger than one on your toes, it introduces a different problem: Because axons transmit information at only moderate speeds (varying from less than 1 meter/second to about 100 m/s), a touch on your shoulder reaches your brain sooner than will a touch on your toes, although you will not ordinarily notice the difference. Your brain is not set up to register small differences in the time of arrival of touch messages. After all, why should it be? You almost never need to know whether a touch on one part of your body occurred slightly before or after a touch somewhere else.

In vision, however, your brain *does* need to know whether one stimulus began slightly before or after another one. If two adjacent spots on your retina—let's call them A and B—send impulses at almost the same time, an extremely small difference between them in timing tells your brain whether light moved from A to B or from B to A. To detect movement as accurately as possible, your visual system compensates for the fact that some parts of the retina are slightly closer to your brain than other parts are. Without some sort of compensation, simultaneous flashes arriving at two spots on your retina would reach your brain at different times, and you might perceive movement inaccurately. What prevents this illusion is the fact that axons from more distant parts of your retina transmit impulses slightly faster than those closer to the brain (Stanford, 1987)!

In short, the properties of impulse conduction in an axon are amazingly well adapted to your needs for information transfer. Let's examine the mechanics of impulse transmission.

The Resting Potential of the Neuron

Messages in a neuron develop from disturbances of the resting potential. Let's begin by understanding the resting potential.

All parts of a neuron are covered by a membrane about 8 nanometers (nm) thick. That is about one ten-thousandth the width of an average human hair. The membrane is composed of two layers (free to float relative to each other) of phospholipid molecules (containing chains of fatty acids and a phosphate group). Embedded among the phospholipids are cylindrical protein molecules through which certain chemicals can pass (see Figure 1.12).

When at rest, the membrane maintains an **electrical gradient**, also known as **polarization**—a difference in

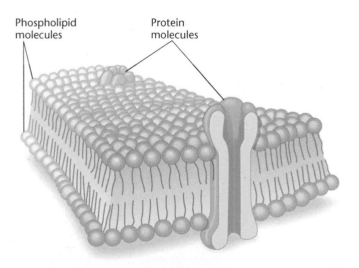

Phospholipid molecules

Protein molecules

Figure 1.12 The membrane of a neuron
Embedded in the membrane are protein channels that permit certain ions to cross through the membrane at a controlled rate.

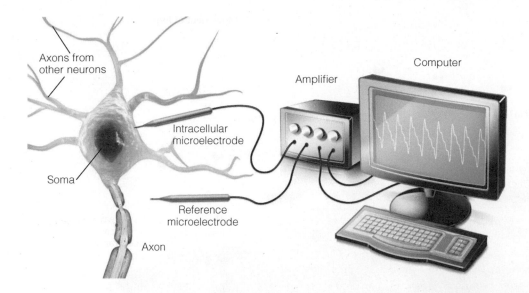

Figure 1.13 **Methods for recording activity of a neuron** Diagram of the apparatus and a sample recording. (*Source: Fritz Goro*)

electrical charge between the inside and outside of the cell. The electrical potential inside the membrane is slightly negative with respect to the outside, mainly because of negatively charged proteins inside the cell. This difference in voltage is called the **resting potential**.

Researchers measure the resting potential by inserting a very thin *microelectrode* into the cell body, as in Figure 1.13. The diameter of the electrode must be small enough to enter without damaging the cell. The most common electrode is a fine glass tube filled with a salt solution, tapering to a tip diameter of 0.0005 mm or less. A reference electrode outside the cell completes the circuit. Connecting the electrodes to a voltmeter, we find that the neuron's interior has a negative potential relative to its exterior. The magnitude varies, but a typical level is −70 millivolts (mV).

Forces Acting on Sodium and Potassium Ions

If charged ions could flow freely across the membrane, the membrane would depolarize, eliminating the negative potential inside. However, the membrane has **selective permeability**. That is, some chemicals pass through it more freely than others do. Oxygen, carbon dioxide, urea, and water cross freely through channels that are always open. Several biologically important ions, including sodium, potassium, calcium, and chloride, cross through membrane channels (or gates) that are sometimes open and sometimes closed, as shown in Figure 1.14. When the membrane is at rest, the sodium and potassium channels are closed, permitting almost no flow of sodium and only a small flow of potassium. Certain types of stimulation can open these channels, permitting freer flow of either or both ions.

The **sodium–potassium pump**, a protein complex, repeatedly transports three sodium ions out of the cell while drawing two potassium ions into it. The sodium–potassium pump is an active transport that requires energy. As a result

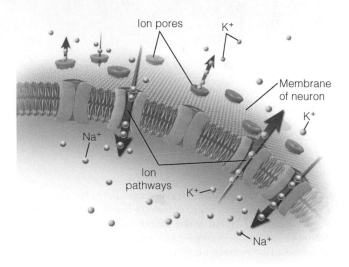

Figure 1.14 **Ion channels in the membrane of a neuron** When a channel opens, it permits some type of ion to cross the membrane. When it closes, it prevents passage of that ion.

of the sodium–potassium pump, sodium ions are more than 10 times more concentrated outside the membrane than inside, and potassium ions are more concentrated inside than outside.

The sodium–potassium pump is effective only because of the selective permeability of the membrane, which prevents the sodium ions that were pumped out of the neuron from leaking right back in again. When sodium ions are pumped out, they stay out. However, some of the potassium ions in the neuron slowly leak out, carrying a positive charge with them. That leakage increases the electrical gradient across the membrane, as shown in Figure 1.15.

When the neuron is at rest, two forces act on sodium, both tending to push it *into* the cell. First, consider the electrical gradient. Sodium is positively charged and the inside of the

Distribution of Ions   Movement of Ions

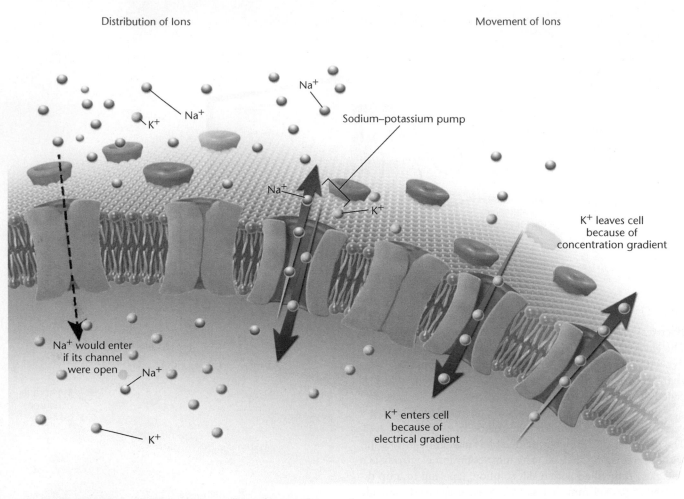

Figure 1.15 The sodium and potassium gradients for a resting membrane
Sodium ions are more concentrated outside the neuron, and potassium ions more concentrated inside. Protein and chloride ions (not shown) bear negative charges inside the cell. At rest, almost no sodium ions cross the membrane except by the sodium–potassium pump. Potassium tends to flow into the cell because of an electrical gradient but tends to flow out because of the concentration gradient. However, potassium gates retard the flow of potassium when the membrane is at rest.

cell is negatively charged. Opposite electrical charges attract, so the electrical gradient tends to pull sodium into the cell. Second, consider the **concentration gradient**, the difference in distribution of ions across the membrane. Sodium is more concentrated outside than inside, so just by the laws of probability, sodium is more likely to enter the cell than to leave it. Given that both the electrical gradient and the concentration gradient tend to move sodium ions into the cell, sodium would enter rapidly if it could. However, because the sodium channels are closed when the membrane is at rest, almost no sodium flows except for what the sodium–potassium pump forces *out of* the cell.

Potassium is subject to competing forces. Potassium is positively charged and the inside of the cell is negatively charged, so the electrical gradient tends to pull potassium in. However, potassium is more concentrated inside the cell than outside, so the concentration gradient tends to drive it out. (For an analogy, imagine a number of women inside

a room. Men can enter the room or leave through a narrow door. They are attracted to the women, but when the men get too crowded, some of them leave. The concentration gradient counteracts the attraction.)

If the potassium channels were wide open, potassium would have a small net flow out of the cell. That is, the electrical gradient and concentration gradient for potassium are almost in balance, but not quite. The sodium–potassium pump continues pulling potassium into the cell, counteracting the ions that leak out.

The cell has negative ions, too. Negatively charged proteins inside the cell sustain the membrane's polarization. Chloride ions, being negatively charged, are mainly outside the cell. When the membrane is at rest, the concentration gradient and electrical gradient balance, so opening the chloride channels would produce little effect. However, chloride does have a net flow when the membrane's polarization changes.

9. When the membrane is at rest, are the sodium ions more concentrated inside the cell or outside? Where are the potassium ions more concentrated?

10. When the membrane is at rest, what tends to drive the potassium ions out of the cell? What tends to draw them into the cell?

ANSWERS
9. Sodium ions are more concentrated outside the cell, and potassium is more concentrated inside. 10. When the membrane is at rest, the concentration gradient tends to drive potassium ions out of the cell, and the electrical gradient draws them into the cell. The sodium–potassium pump also draws them into the cell.

Why a Resting Potential?

The body invests much energy to operate the sodium–potassium pump, which maintains the resting potential. Why is it worth so much energy? The resting potential prepares the neuron to respond rapidly. As we shall see in the next section, excitation of the neuron opens channels that allow sodium to enter the cell rapidly. Because the membrane did its work in advance by maintaining the concentration gradient for sodium, the cell is prepared to respond vigorously to a stimulus.

Compare the resting potential of a neuron to a poised bow and arrow: An archer who pulls the bow in advance is ready to fire at the appropriate moment. The neuron uses the same strategy. The resting potential remains stable until the neuron is stimulated. Ordinarily, stimulation of the neuron takes place at synapses, which we consider in Chapter 2. In the laboratory, it is also possible to stimulate a neuron by inserting an electrode into it and applying current.

The Action Potential

Messages sent by axons are called **action potentials**. To understand action potentials, let's begin by considering what happens when the resting potential is disturbed. We can measure a neuron's potential with a microelectrode, as shown in Figure 1.13. When an axon's membrane is at rest, the recordings show a negative potential inside the axon. If we now use a different electrode to apply a negative charge, we can further increase the negative charge inside the neuron. The change is called **hyperpolarization**, which means increased polarization. When the stimulation ends, the charge returns to its original resting level. The recording looks like this:

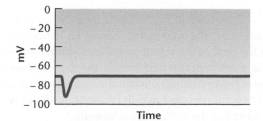

Now let's apply a current to **depolarize** the neuron—that is, reduce its polarization toward zero. If we apply a small depolarizing current, we get a result like this:

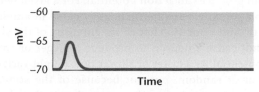

With a slightly stronger depolarizing current, the potential rises slightly higher but again returns to the resting level as soon as the stimulation ceases:

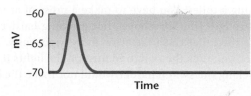

Now let's apply a still stronger current: Stimulation beyond the **threshold** of excitation produces a massive depolarization of the membrane. When the potential reaches the threshold, the membrane opens its sodium channels and lets sodium ions flow into the cell. The potential shoots up far beyond the strength that the stimulus provided:

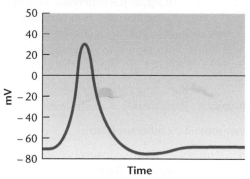

Any *subthreshold* stimulation produces a small response that quickly decays. Any stimulation beyond the threshold, regardless of how far beyond, produces a big response like the one shown, known as the action potential. The peak of the action potential, shown as +30 mV in this illustration, varies from one axon to another.

11. What is the difference between a hyperpolarization and a depolarization?

12. What happens if the depolarization does or does not reach the threshold?

ANSWERS
11. A hyperpolarization is an exaggeration of the usual negative charge within a cell, to a more negative level than usual. A depolarization is a decrease in the amount of negative charge within the cell. 12. If the depolarization reaches or passes the threshold, the cell produces an action potential. If it is less than threshold, no action potential arises.

The All-or-None Law

Note that any depolarization that reaches or passes the threshold produces an action potential. For a given neuron, all action potentials are approximately equal in amplitude (intensity) and velocity. That is, the intensity of the stimulus cannot cause a neuron to produce a bigger or smaller action potential, or a faster or slower one. (Slight variations can occur at random, but not because of the stimulus.) More properly stated, the **all-or-none law** is that the amplitude and velocity of an action potential are independent of the intensity of the stimulus that initiated it, provided that the stimulus reaches the threshold. By analogy, imagine flushing a toilet: You have to make a press of at least a certain strength (the threshold), but pressing harder does not make the toilet flush faster or more vigorously. Similarly, when you flick the switch to turn on the lights in your room, flicking the switch harder would not make the lights brighter.

Although the amplitude, velocity, and shape of action potentials are consistent over time for a given axon, they vary from one neuron to another. Thicker axons convey action potentials at greater velocities. Thicker axons can also convey more action potentials per second.

The all-or-none law puts constraints on how an axon can send a message. To signal the difference between a weak stimulus and a strong stimulus, the axon cannot send bigger or faster action potentials. All it can change is the timing. By analogy, you might send signals to someone by flashing the lights in your room on and off, varying the speed or rhythm of flashing.

Flash-flash . . . [long pause] . . . flash-flash

might mean something different from

Flash . . . [pause] . . . flash . . . [pause] . . . flash . . . [pause] . . . flash.

The nervous system uses both kinds of coding. For example, a taste axon shows one rhythm of responses for sweet tastes and a different rhythm for bitter tastes (Di Lorenzo, Leshchinskiy, Moroney, & Ozdoba, 2009).

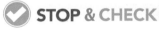 **STOP & CHECK**

13. State the all-or-none law.
14. Does the all-or-none law apply to dendrites? Why or why not?

ANSWERS 13. According to the all-or-none law, the size and shape of the action potential are independent of the intensity of the stimulus that initiated it. That is, every depolarization beyond the threshold of excitation produces an action potential of about the same amplitude and velocity for a given axon. 14. The all-or-none law does not apply to dendrites, because they do not have action potentials.

The Molecular Basis of the Action Potential

The chemical events behind the action potential may seem complex, but they make sense if you remember three principles:

1. At the start, sodium ions are mostly outside the neuron, and potassium ions are mostly inside.
2. When the membrane is depolarized, sodium and potassium channels in the membrane open.
3. At the peak of the action potential, the sodium channels close.

A neuron's membrane contains cylindrical proteins, like the ones in Figure 1.12. Opening one of these proteins allows a particular type of ion to cross the membrane. (Which ion crosses depends on the size and shape of the opening.) A protein that allows sodium to cross is called a sodium channel (or gate), and one that allows potassium to cross is a potassium channel. The axon channels regulating sodium and potassium are **voltage-gated channels**. That is, their permeability depends on the voltage difference across the membrane. At the resting potential, the sodium channels are fully closed and the potassium channels are almost closed, allowing only a little flow of potassium. As the membrane becomes depolarized, both the sodium and the potassium channels begin to open, allowing freer flow. At first, opening the potassium channels makes little difference, because the concentration gradient and electrical gradient are almost in balance anyway. However, opening the sodium channels makes a big difference, because both the electrical gradient and the concentration gradient tend to drive sodium ions into the neuron. When the depolarization reaches the threshold of the membrane, the sodium channels open wide enough for sodium to flow freely. Driven by both the concentration gradient and the electrical gradient, the sodium ions enter the cell rapidly, until the electrical potential across the membrane passes beyond zero to a reversed polarity, as shown in the following diagram:

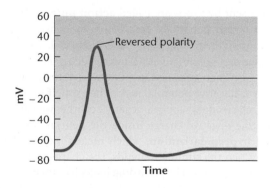

Of the total number of sodium ions near the axon, less than 1 percent cross the membrane during an action potential. Even at the peak of the action potential, sodium ions continue to be far more concentrated outside the neuron than inside. Because of the persisting concentration gradient, sodium ions still tend to diffuse into the cell. However, at the peak of the action potential, the sodium gates snap shut.

Then what happens? Remember that depolarizing the membrane also opens potassium channels. At first, opening those channels made little difference. However, after so many sodium ions have crossed the membrane, the inside of the cell has a slight positive charge instead of its usual negative charge. At this point both the concentration gradient and the electrical gradient drive potassium ions out of the cell. As they flow out of the axon, they carry with them a positive charge. Because the potassium channels remain open after the sodium channels close, enough potassium ions leave to drive the membrane beyond its usual resting level to a temporary hyperpolarization. Figure 1.16 summarizes the key movements of ions during an action potential.

At the end of this process, the membrane has returned to its resting potential, but the inside of the neuron has slightly more sodium ions and slightly fewer potassium ions than before. Eventually, the sodium–potassium pump restores the original distribution of ions, but that process takes time. After an unusually rapid series of action potentials, the pump cannot keep up with the action, and sodium accumulates within the axon. Excessive buildup of sodium can be toxic to a cell. (Excessive stimulation occurs only under abnormal conditions, however, such as during a stroke or after the use of certain drugs. Don't worry that thinking too hard will explode your brain cells!)

Action potentials require the flow of sodium and potassium. **Local anesthetic** drugs, such as Novocain and Xylocaine, attach to the sodium channels of the membrane, preventing sodium ions from entering. When a dentist administers Novocain before drilling into one of your teeth, your receptors are screaming, "pain, pain, pain!" but the axons cannot transmit the message to your brain, and so you don't feel it.

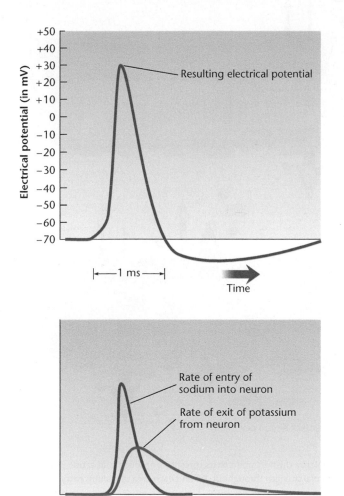

Figure 1.16 The movement of sodium and potassium ions during an action potential
Sodium ions cross during the peak of the action potential, and potassium ions cross later in the opposite direction, returning the membrane to its original polarization.

STOP & CHECK

15. During the rise of the action potential, do sodium ions move into the cell or out of it? Why?
16. As the membrane reaches the peak of the action potential, what brings the membrane down to the original resting potential?

ANSWERS 15. During the action potential, sodium ions move into the cell. The voltage-dependent sodium gates have opened, so sodium can move freely. Sodium is attracted to the inside of the cell by both an electrical and a concentration gradient. 16. After the peak of the action potential, potassium ions exit the cell, driving the membrane back to the resting potential. Important note: The sodium–potassium pump is NOT responsible for returning the membrane to its resting potential. The sodium–potassium pump is too slow for this purpose.

Propagation of the Action Potential

Up to this point, we have considered how the action potential occurs at one point on the axon. Now let us consider how it moves down the axon. Remember, it is important for axons to convey impulses without any loss of strength over distance.

During an action potential, sodium ions enter a point on the axon. Temporarily, that spot is positively charged in comparison with neighboring areas along the axon. The positive ions flow within the axon to neighboring regions. The positive charges slightly depolarize the next area of the membrane, causing it to reach its threshold and open its voltage-gated sodium channels. Then the membrane regenerates the action potential at that point. In this manner, the action potential travels along the axon, as in Figure 1.17.

The term **propagation of the action potential** describes the transmission of an action potential down an axon. The propagation of an animal species is the production of offspring. In a sense, the action potential gives birth to a new action potential at each point along the axon.

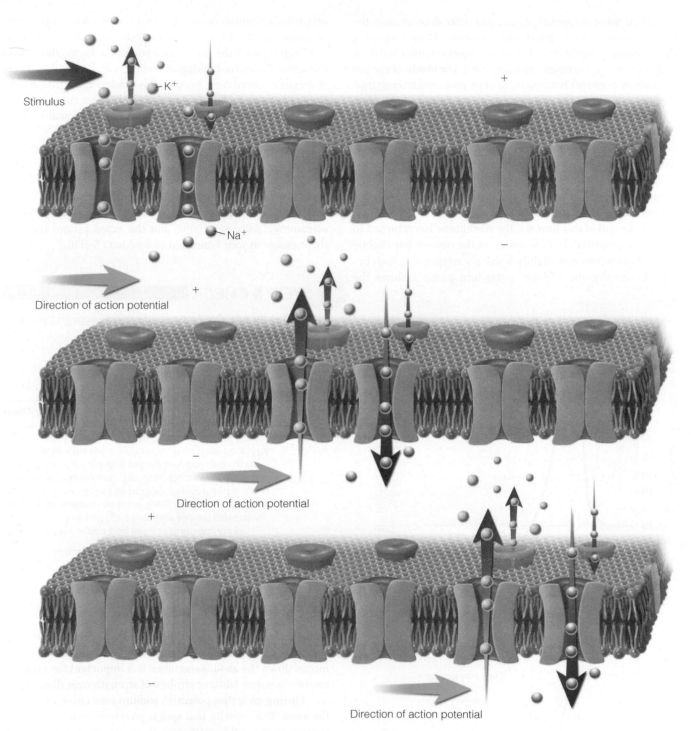

Figure 1.17 Propagation of an action potential
As an action potential occurs at one point on the axon, enough sodium enters to depolarize the next point to its threshold, producing an action potential at that point. In this manner the action potential flows along the axon, remaining at equal strength throughout. Behind each area of sodium entry, potassium ions exit, restoring the resting potential.

An action potential always starts in an axon and propagates without loss from start to finish. However, at its start, it "back-propagates" into the cell body and dendrites (Lorincz & Nusser, 2010). The cell body and dendrites do not conduct action potentials in the same way that axons do, but they passively register the electrical event that started in the nearby axon. This back-propagation is important: When an action potential back-propagates into a dendrite, the dendrite becomes more susceptible to the structural changes responsible for learning.

Let's review the action potential:

- When an area of the axon membrane reaches its threshold of excitation, sodium channels and potassium channels open.

- At first, the opening of potassium channels produces little effect.
- Opening sodium channels lets sodium ions rush into the axon.
- Positive charge flows down the axon and opens voltage-gated sodium channels at the next point.
- At the peak of the action potential, the sodium gates snap shut. They remain closed for the next millisecond or so, despite the depolarization of the membrane.
- Because voltage-gated potassium channels remain open, potassium ions flow out of the axon, returning the membrane toward its original depolarization.
- A few milliseconds later, the voltage-dependent potassium channels close.

All of this may seem like a lot to memorize, but it is not. Everything follows logically from the facts that voltage-gated sodium and potassium channels open when the membrane is depolarized and that sodium channels snap shut at the peak of the action potential.

The Myelin Sheath and Saltatory Conduction

In the thinnest axons, action potentials travel at a velocity of less than 1 meter/second. Increasing the diameter brings conduction velocity up to about 10 m/s. At that speed, an impulse along an axon between a giraffe's spinal cord and its foot takes about half a second. To increase the speed still more, vertebrate axons evolved a special mechanism: sheaths of **myelin**, an insulating material composed of fats and proteins.

Consider the following analogy. Suppose your job is to take written messages over a long distance without using any mechanical device. Taking each message and running with it would be reliable but slow, like the propagation of an action potential along an unmyelinated axon. If you tied each message to a ball and threw it, you could increase the speed, but your throws would not travel far enough. The best solution would be to station people at moderate distances along the route and throw the message-bearing ball from person to person until it reaches its destination.

The same principle applies to **myelinated axons**, those covered with a myelin sheath. Myelinated axons, found only in vertebrates, are covered with layers of fats and proteins. The myelin sheath is interrupted periodically by short sections of axon called nodes of Ranvier, each one about 1 micrometer wide, as shown in Figure 1.18. In myelinated axons, the action potential starts at the first node of Ranvier (Kuba, Ishii, & Ohmari, 2006).

Suppose an action potential occurs at the first myelin segment. The action potential cannot regenerate along the membrane between nodes because sodium channels are virtually absent between nodes (Catterall, 1984). After an action potential occurs at a node, sodium ions enter the axon and diffuse, pushing a chain of positive charge along the axon to the next node, where they regenerate the action potential (see Figure 1.19).

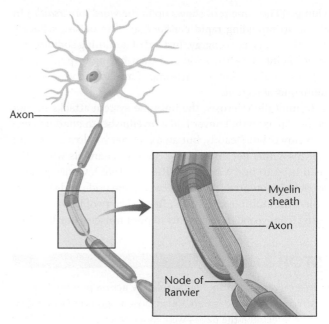

Cutaway view of axon wrapped in myelin

Figure 1.18 An axon surrounded by a myelin sheath and interrupted by nodes of Ranvier
The inset shows a cross section through both the axon and the myelin sheath. The anatomy is distorted here to show several nodes; in fact, the distance between nodes is generally at least 100 times as long as a node.

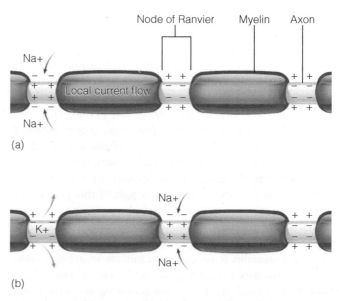

Figure 1.19 Saltatory conduction in a myelinated axon
An action potential at the node triggers flow of current to the next node, where the membrane regenerates the action potential. In reality, a myelin sheath is much longer than shown here, relative to the size of the nodes of Ranvier and to the diameter of the axon.

This flow of charge moves considerably faster than the regeneration of an action potential at each point along the axon. The jumping of action potentials from node to node is referred to as **saltatory conduction**, from the Latin word *saltare*, meaning "to jump." (The same root shows up in the word *somersault*.) In addition to providing rapid conduction of impulses, saltatory conduction conserves energy: Instead of admitting sodium ions at every point along the axon and then having to pump them out via the sodium–potassium pump, a myelinated axon admits sodium only at its nodes.

In multiple sclerosis, the immune system attacks myelin sheaths. An axon that never had a myelin sheath conducts impulses slowly but steadily, but an axon that has lost its myelin is not the same, because it lacks sodium channels where the myelin used to be (Waxman & Ritchie, 1985). Consequently, most action potentials die out between one node and the next. People with multiple sclerosis suffer a variety of impairments, ranging from visual impairments to poor muscle coordination.

STOP & CHECK

17. In a myelinated axon, how would the action potential be affected if the nodes were much closer together? How might it be affected if the nodes were much farther apart?

ANSWER

17. If the nodes were closer, the action potential would travel more slowly. If they were much farther apart, the action potential would travel faster *if it could success-fully jump from one node to the next*. When the distance becomes too great, the current cannot diffuse from one node to the next and still remain above threshold, so the action potentials would stop.

The Refractory Period

Consider the action potential while it is returning from its peak. At that point, the electrical potential across the membrane is still above the threshold. Why doesn't the cell produce another action potential during this period? (If it did, of course, it would endlessly repeat one action potential after another.) Remember, at the peak of the action potential, the sodium gates snap shut. As a result, the cell is in a **refractory period** during which it resists the production of further action potentials. In the first part of this period, the **absolute refractory period**, the membrane cannot produce another action potential, regardless of the stimulation. During the second part, the **relative refractory period**, a stronger-than-usual stimulus is necessary to initiate an action potential. The refractory period depends on two facts: The sodium channels are closed, and potassium is flowing out of the cell at a faster-than-usual rate.

In most of the neurons that researchers have tested, the absolute refractory period is about 1 millisecond (ms), and the relative refractory period is another 2 to 4 ms. (A toilet is similar. During a short time right after you flush a toilet, you cannot make it flush again—an absolute refractory period. Then follows a period when it is possible but difficult to flush it again—a relative refractory period—before it returns to normal.)

Let's reexamine Figure 1.17 for a moment. As the action potential travels down the axon, what prevents the electrical

charge from flowing in the direction opposite that in which the action potential is traveling? Nothing. In fact, the electrical charge does flow in both directions. Then what prevents an action potential near the center of an axon from reinvading the areas that it has just passed? The answer is that the areas it just passed are still in their refractory period.

STOP & CHECK

18. Suppose researchers find that axon A can produce up to 1,000 action potentials per second (at least briefly, with maximum stimulation), but axon B can never produce more than 100 per second (regardless of the strength of the stimulus). What could we conclude about the refractory periods of the two axons?

ANSWER

18. Axon A must have a shorter absolute refractory period, about 1 ms, whereas B has a longer absolute refractory period, about 10 ms.

Local Neurons

Axons produce action potentials. However, many small neurons have no axon. Neurons without an axon exchange information with only their closest neighbors. We therefore call them **local neurons**. Because they do not have an axon, they do not follow the all-or-none law. When a local neuron receives information from other neurons, it has a **graded potential**, a membrane potential that varies in magnitude in proportion to the intensity of the stimulus. The change in membrane potential is conducted to adjacent areas of the cell, in all directions, gradually decaying as it travels. Those various areas of the cell contact other neurons, which they excite or inhibit.

Local neurons are difficult to study because it is almost impossible to insert an electrode into a tiny cell without damaging it. Most of our knowledge, therefore, has come from large neurons, and that bias in our research methods may have led to a misconception. Many years ago, all that neuroscientists knew about local neurons was that they were small. Given their focus on larger neurons, many scientists assumed that the small neurons were immature. As one textbook author put it, "Many of these [neurons] are small and apparently undeveloped, as if they constituted a reserve stock not yet utilized in the individual's cerebral activity" (Woodworth, 1934, p. 194). In other words, the small cells would contribute to behavior only if they grew.

Perhaps this misunderstanding was the origin of that widespread, nonsensical belief that "they say we use only 10 percent of our brain." (Who are "they," incidentally?) Other origins have also been suggested for this belief. No one is sure where it originated, but people have been quoting it to one another since the early 1900s. This belief has been remarkably persistent, given its total lack of justification. What does it mean? Does it mean that you could lose 90 percent of your brain and still behave normally? Good luck with that one.

Perhaps it means that only 10 percent of your neurons are active at any given moment. Depending on how we define a "given moment," 10 percent could be either an overestimate or an underestimate, but in any case irrelevant. If you could contract all your muscles at one time, you would not be a great athlete; you would just have spasms. If you could activate all your neurons at one time, you would not have brilliant thoughts; you would have an epileptic seizure. Any meaningful thought or activity requires activating some neurons and inhibiting others, and the inhibition is just as important as the excitation. You use all of your brain, regardless of whether you are using it well.

Module 1.2 | In Closing
Neurons and Messages

As you have been reading about action potentials and sodium gates and so forth, it probably seems that all this is remote from most issues in psychology. Well, you are right, but all these physiological mechanisms are the building blocks that we need to understand before delving into synapses, the connections between neurons. Synapses are the decision makers of your brain, but the input into these decision makers is the on/off messages transmitting down axons. All of the glories of human experience originate in the simple chemical processes we have seen in this chapter.

Summary

1. The action potential transmits information without loss of intensity over distance. The cost is a delay between the stimulus and its arrival in the brain. **28**

2. The inside of a resting neuron has a negative charge with respect to the outside, mainly because of negatively charged proteins inside the neuron. The sodium–potassium pump moves sodium ions out of the neuron, and potassium ions in. **28**

3. When the membrane is at rest, both the electrical gradient and the concentration gradient would act to move sodium ions into the cell, except that its gates are closed. The electrical gradient tends to move potassium ions into the cell, but the concentration gradient tends to move it out. The two forces almost balance out, but not quite, leaving a net tendency for potassium to exit the cell. **29**

4. The all-or-none law: For any stimulus greater than the threshold, the amplitude and velocity of the action potential are independent of the size of the stimulus that initiated it. **32**

5. When the membrane is sufficiently depolarized to reach the cell's threshold, sodium and potassium channels open. Sodium ions enter rapidly, reducing and reversing the charge across the membrane. This event is known as the action potential. **32**

6. After the peak of the action potential, the membrane returns toward its original level of polarization because of the outflow of potassium ions. **33**

7. The action potential is regenerated at successive points along the axon as sodium ions flow through the core of the axon and stimulate the next point along the axon to its threshold. The action potential maintains a constant magnitude as it passes along the axon. **33**

8. In axons that are covered with myelin, action potentials form only in the nodes that separate myelinated segments. Transmission in myelinated axons is faster than in unmyelinated axons. **35**

9. Immediately after an action potential, the membrane enters a refractory period during which it is resistant to starting another action potential. **36**

10. Local neurons are small, with no axon. They convey information over short distances. **36**

11. Contrary to a popular belief, people use all of their brain, not some smaller percentage. **36**

Key Terms

Terms are defined in the module on the page number indicated. They're also presented in alphabetical order with definitions in the book's Subject Index/Glossary, which begins on page 589. Interactive flash cards, audio reviews, and crossword puzzles are among the online resources available to help you learn these terms and the concepts they represent.

absolute refractory period **36**
action potential **31**
all-or-none law **32**
concentration gradient **30**
depolarize **31**
electrical gradient **28**
graded potential **36**
hyperpolarization **31**
local anesthetic **33**
local neurons **36**
myelin **35**
myelinated axons **35**

Thought Questions

1. Suppose the threshold of a neuron were the same as the neuron's resting potential. What would happen? At what frequency would the cell produce action potentials?

2. In the laboratory, researchers can apply an electrical stimulus at any point along the axon, making action potentials travel in both directions from the point of stimulation. An action potential moving in the usual direction, away from the axon hillock, is said to be traveling in the *orthodromic* direction. An action potential traveling toward the axon hillock is traveling in the *antidromic* direction. If we started an orthodromic action potential at the start of the axon and an antidromic action potential at the opposite end of the axon, what would happen when they met at the center? Why?

3. If a drug partly blocks a membrane's potassium channels, how does it affect the action potential?

Module 1.2 | End of Module Quiz

1. When the neuron's membrane is at rest, where are the sodium ions and potassium ions most concentrated?
   - **A.** Sodium is mostly outside and potassium is mostly inside.
   - **B.** Sodium is mostly inside and potassium is mostly outside.
   - **C.** Both ions are mostly inside the cell.
   - **D.** Both ions are mostly outside the cell.

2. When the membrane is at rest, what are the forces acting on sodium ions?
   - **A.** Both the concentration gradient and the electrical gradient tend to move sodium ions into the cell.
   - **B.** Both the concentration gradient and the electrical gradient tend to move sodium ions out of the cell.
   - **C.** The concentration gradient tends to move sodium ions into the cell, and the electrical gradient tends to move them out of the cell.
   - **D.** The concentration gradient tends to move sodium ions out of the cell, and the electrical gradient tends to move them into the cell.

3. When the membrane is at rest, what are the forces acting on potassium ions?
   - **A.** Both the concentration gradient and the electrical gradient tend to move potassium ions into the cell.
   - **B.** Both the concentration gradient and the electrical gradient tend to move potassium ions out of the cell.
   - **C.** The concentration gradient tends to move potassium ions into the cell, and the electrical gradient tends to move them out of the cell.
   - **D.** The concentration gradient tends to move potassium ions out of the cell, and the electrical gradient tends to move them into the cell.

4. Which direction does the sodium–potassium pump move ions?
   - **A.** It moves both sodium and potassium ions into the cell.
   - **B.** It moves both sodium and potassium ions out of the cell.
   - **C.** It moves sodium ions into the cell and potassium ions out of the cell.
   - **D.** It moves sodium ions out of the cell and potassium ions into the cell.

5. Under what conditions does an axon produce an action potential?
   - **A.** Whenever the membrane is hyperpolarized
   - **B.** Whenever the membrane's potential reaches the threshold
   - **C.** Whenever the membrane is depolarized
   - **D.** Whenever the membrane's potential reaches zero

6. If a membrane is depolarized to twice its threshold, what happens?

   A. The neuron produces an action potential at twice as much strength as usual.

   B. The neuron produces an action potential that travels twice as fast as usual.

   C. The neuron produces an action potential slightly stronger and slightly faster than usual.

   D. The neuron produces the same action potential it would at the threshold.

7. To which part or parts of a neuron does the all-or-none law apply?

   A. Axons

   B. Dendrites

   C. Both axons and dendrites

   D. Neither axons nor dendrites

8. During the rising portion of the action potential, which ions are moving across the membrane and in which direction?

   A. Sodium ions move out.

   B. Sodium ions move in.

   C. Both sodium and potassium ions move in.

   D. Potassium ions move in.

9. After the action potential reaches its peak, the potential across the membrane falls toward its resting level. What accounts for this recovery?

   A. The sodium–potassium pump removes the extra sodium.

   B. Sodium ions move out because their channels are open and the concentration gradient pushes them out.

   C. Potassium ions move out because their channels are open and the concentration gradient pushes them out.

   D. Potassium ions move in.

10. What does the myelin sheath of an axon accomplish?

    A. It enables an axon to communicate with other axons.

    B. It enables action potentials to travel both directions along an axon.

    C. It enables nutrients to enter the axon.

    D. It enables action potentials to travel more rapidly.

11. What causes the refractory period of an axon?

    A. The sodium–potassium pump becomes inactive.

    B. The sodium–potassium pump increases its activity.

    C. The potassium channels are closed.

    D. The sodium channels are closed.

12. About what percentage of the brain does an average person use?

    A. 10 percent

    B. 30 percent

    C. 50 percent

    D. 100 percent

Answers: 1A, 2A, 3D, 4D, 5B, 6D, 7A, 8B, 9C, 10D, 11D, 12D.

Suggestion for Further Reading

Ascoli, G. A. (2015). *Trees of the brain, roots of the mind.* Cambridge, MA: MIT Press. A richly illustrated description of axons, dendrites, and what they have to do with psychology.

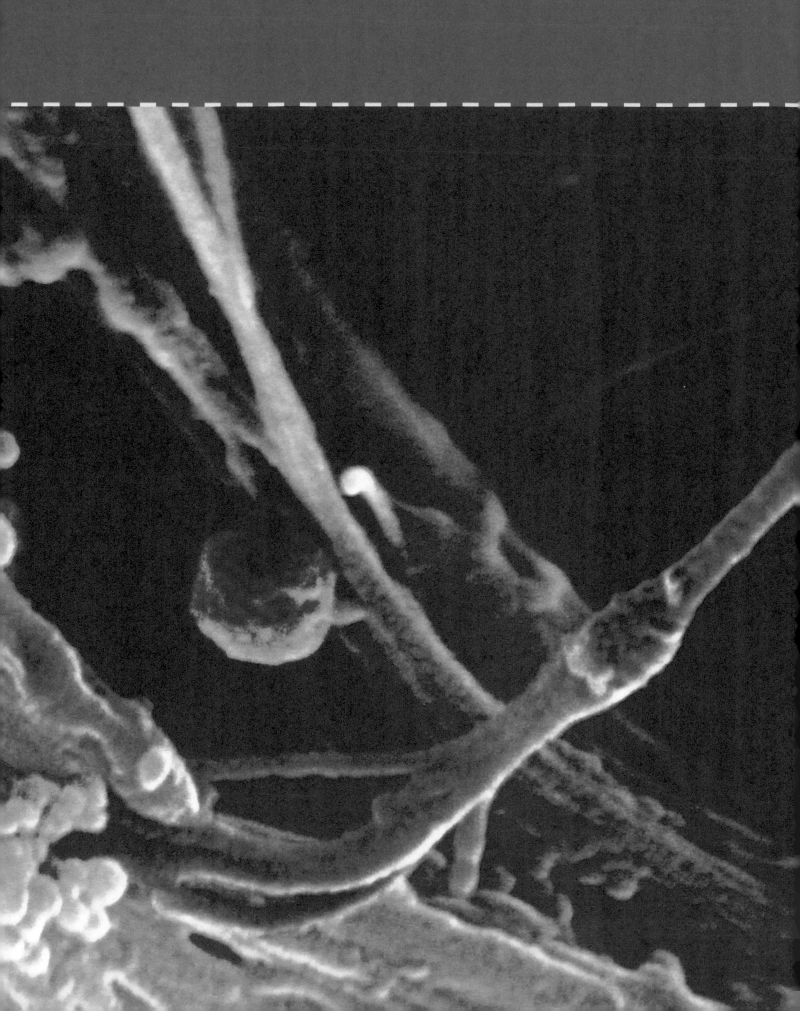

Synapses

I f you had to communicate with someone without sight or sound, what would you do? Chances are, your first choice would be a touch code or a system of electrical impulses. You might not even think of passing chemicals back and forth. Chemicals are, however, the main way your neurons communicate. They communicate by transmitting chemicals at specialized junctions called *synapses.*

Learning Objectives

After studying this chapter, you should be able to:

1. Describe how Charles Sherrington used behavioral observations to infer the major properties of synapses.
2. Relate the activities at a synapse to the probability of an action potential.
3. List and explain the sequence of events at a synapse, from synthesis of neurotransmitters, through stimulation of receptors, to the disposition of the transmitter molecules.
4. Discuss how certain drugs affect behavior by altering events at synapses.
5. Contrast neurotransmitters, neuropeptides, and hormones.

Opposite:
This electron micrograph, with color added artificially, shows branches of an axon making contact with other cells. (Eye of Science/Science Source)

The Concept of the Synapse

In the late 1800s, Ramón y Cajal anatomically demonstrated a narrow gap separating one neuron from another. In 1906, Charles Scott Sherrington physiologically demonstrated that communication between one neuron and the next differs from communication along a single axon. He inferred a specialized gap between neurons and introduced the term **synapse** to describe it. Cajal and Sherrington are regarded as the great pioneers of modern neuroscience, and their nearly simultaneous discoveries supported each other: If communication between neurons is special in some way, then there can be no doubt that neurons are anatomically separate from one another. Sherrington's discovery was an amazing feat of scientific reasoning, as he used behavioral observations to infer the major properties of synapses half a century before researchers had the technology to measure those properties directly.

Properties of Synapses

Sherrington studied **reflexes**, automatic muscular responses to stimuli. In a leg flexion reflex, a sensory neuron excites a second neuron, which in turn excites a motor neuron, which excites a muscle, as in Figure 2.1. The circuit from sensory neuron to muscle response is called a **reflex arc**. If one neuron is separate from another, as Cajal had demonstrated, a reflex must require communication between neurons, and therefore, measurements of reflexes might reveal some of the special properties of that communication.

Sherrington strapped a dog into a harness above the ground and pinched one of the dog's feet. After a fraction of a second, the dog *flexed* (raised) the pinched leg and *extended* the other legs. Sherrington found the same reflexive movements

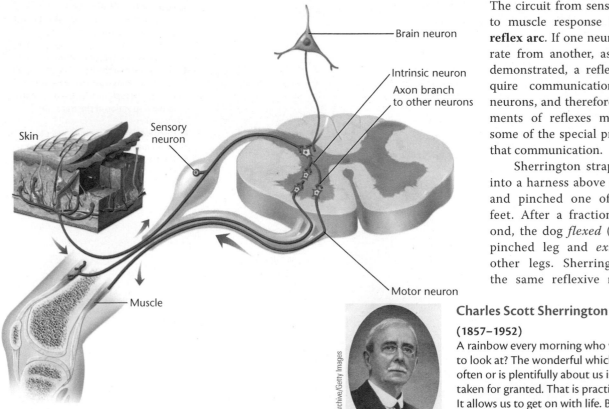

Figure 2.1 A reflex arc for leg flexion
The anatomy has been simplified to show the relationship among sensory neuron, intrinsic neuron, and motor neuron.

Labels: Brain neuron; Intrinsic neuron; Axon branch to other neurons; Skin; Sensory neuron; Muscle; Motor neuron

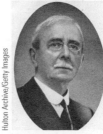

Charles Scott Sherrington
(1857–1952)
A rainbow every morning who would pause to look at? The wonderful which comes often or is plentifully about us is soon taken for granted. That is practical enough. It allows us to get on with life. But it may stultify if it cannot on occasion be thrown off. To recapture now and then childhood's wonder is to secure a driving force for occasional grown-up thoughts. (Sherrington, 1941, p. 104)

after he made a cut that disconnected the spinal cord from the brain. Evidently, the spinal cord controlled the flexion and extension reflexes. In fact, the movements were more consistent after he separated the spinal cord from the brain. In an intact animal, messages descending from the brain modify the reflexes, making them stronger at some times and weaker at others.

Sherrington observed several properties of reflexes that suggest special processes at the junctions between neurons: (1) Reflexes are slower than conduction along an axon. (2) Several weak stimuli presented at nearby places or times produce a stronger reflex than one stimulus alone does. (3) When one set of muscles becomes excited, a different set becomes relaxed. Let's consider each of these points and their implications.

Speed of a Reflex and Delayed Transmission at the Synapse

When Sherrington pinched a dog's foot, the dog flexed that leg after a short delay. During that delay, an impulse had to travel up an axon from the skin receptor to the spinal cord, and then an impulse had to travel from the spinal cord back down the leg to a muscle. Sherrington measured the total distance that the impulse traveled from skin receptor to spinal cord to muscle and calculated the speed at which the impulse traveled to produce the response. He found that the speed of conduction through the reflex arc varied but was never more than about 15 meters per second (m/s). In contrast, previous research had measured action potential velocities along sensory or motor nerves at about 40 m/s. Sherrington concluded that some process must be slowing conduction through the reflex, and he inferred that the delay occurs where one neuron communicates with another (see Figure 2.2). This idea is critical, as it established the existence of synapses. Sherrington, in fact, introduced the term *synapse.*

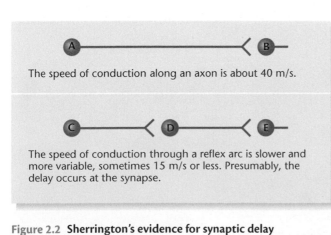

Figure 2.2 **Sherrington's evidence for synaptic delay**
An impulse traveling through a synapse in the spinal cord is slower than one traveling a similar distance along an uninterrupted axon.

1. What evidence led Sherrington to conclude that transmission at a synapse is not the same as transmission along an axon?

ANSWER

1. Sherrington found that the velocity of conduction through a reflex arc was slower than the velocity of an action potential along an axon. Therefore, some delay must occur at the junction between one neuron and the next.

Temporal Summation

Sherrington found that repeated stimuli within a brief time have a cumulative effect. He referred to this phenomenon as **temporal summation**, meaning summation over time. A light pinch of the dog's foot did not evoke a reflex, but a few rapidly repeated pinches did. Sherrington surmised that a single pinch did not reach the threshold of excitation for the next neuron. The neuron that delivers transmission is the **presynaptic neuron**, and the one that receives it is the **postsynaptic neuron**. Sherrington proposed that although the subthreshold excitation in the postsynaptic neuron decays over time, it can combine with a second excitation that follows it quickly. With a rapid succession of pinches, each adds its effect to what remained from the previous ones, until the combination exceeds the threshold of the postsynaptic neuron, producing an action potential.

Decades later, Sherrington's former student, John Eccles (1964), attached microelectrodes to stimulate axons of presynaptic neurons while he recorded from the postsynaptic neuron. For example, after he had briefly stimulated an axon, Eccles recorded a slight depolarization of the membrane of the postsynaptic cell (point 1 in Figure 2.3).

Note that this partial depolarization is a graded potential. Unlike action potentials, which are always depolarizations, graded potentials may be either depolarizations (excitatory) or hyperpolarizations (inhibitory). A graded depolarization is known as an **excitatory postsynaptic potential (EPSP)**. It results from a flow of sodium ions into the neuron. If an EPSP does not cause the cell to reach its threshold, the depolarization decays quickly.

When Eccles stimulated an axon twice, he recorded two EPSPs. If the delay between EPSPs was short enough, the second EPSP added to what was left of the first one (point 2 in Figure 2.3), producing temporal summation. At point 3 in Figure 3.3, a quick sequence of EPSPs combines to exceed the threshold and produce an action potential.

Spatial Summation

Sherrington also found that synapses have the property of **spatial summation**—that is, summation over space. Synaptic inputs from separate locations combine their effects on a neuron. Sherrington again began with a pinch too weak to elicit a reflex. This time, instead of pinching one point twice, he pinched two points at once. Although neither pinch alone

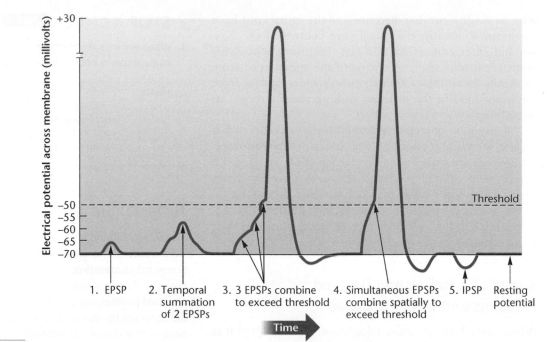

Figure 2.3 **Recordings from a postsynaptic neuron during synaptic activation**

1. EPSP
2. Temporal summation of 2 EPSPs
3. 3 EPSPs combine to exceed threshold
4. Simultaneous EPSPs combine spatially to exceed threshold
5. IPSP
Resting potential

Time

produced a reflex, together they did. Sherrington concluded that pinching two points activated separate sensory neurons, whose axons converged onto one neuron in the spinal cord. Excitation from either sensory axon excited that spinal neuron, but not enough to reach the threshold. A combination of excitations exceeded the threshold and produced an action potential (point 4 in Figure 2.3). Again, Eccles confirmed Sherrington's inference, demonstrating that EPSPs from several axons summate their effects on a postsynaptic cell (see Figure 2.4).

Spatial summation is critical to brain functioning. In most cases, sensory input at a single synapse produces only a weak effect. However, if a neuron receives many incoming axons with synchronized input, spatial summation excites the neuron enough to activate it.

Temporal summation and spatial summation ordinarily occur together. That is, a neuron might receive input from several axons in close succession. Integrating these inputs provides complexity. As Figure 2.5 shows, a series of axons active in one order can have a different result from the same axons

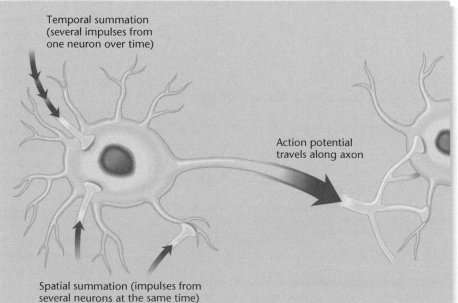

Figure 2.4 **Temporal and spatial summation**

Temporal summation (several impulses from one neuron over time)

Action potential travels along axon

Spatial summation (impulses from several neurons at the same time)

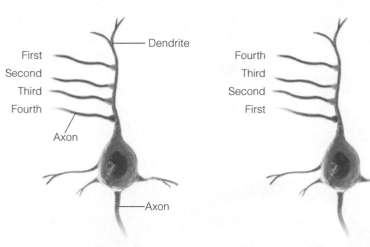

Summation in this direction produces greater depolarization.

Summation in this direction produces less depolarization.

Figure 2.5 Summation effects can depend on the order of stimuli.

in a different order. For example, a neuron in the visual system could respond to light moving in one direction and not another (Branco, Clark, & Häusser, 2010).

STOP & CHECK

2. What is the difference between temporal summation and spatial summation?

ANSWER

2. Temporal summation is the combined effect of quickly repeated stimulation at a single synapse. Spatial summation is the combined effect of several nearly simultaneous stimulations at several synapses onto one neuron.

Inhibitory Synapses

When Sherrington vigorously pinched a dog's foot, the flexor muscles of that leg contracted, and so did the extensor muscles of the other three legs (see Figure 2.6). You can see how this arrangement would be useful. A dog raising one leg needs to extend the other legs to maintain balance. At the same time, the dog relaxed the extensor muscles of the stimulated leg and the flexor muscles of the other legs. Sherrington's explanation assumed certain connections in the spinal cord: A pinch on the foot sends a message along a sensory neuron to an *interneuron* (an intermediate neuron) that excites the motor neurons connected to the flexor muscles of that leg and the extensor muscles of the other legs (see Figure 2.7). Also, the interneuron sends messages to inhibit the extensor muscles in that leg and the flexor muscles of the three other legs.

Later researchers physiologically demonstrated the inhibitory synapses that Sherrington had inferred. At these synapses, input from an axon hyperpolarizes the postsynaptic

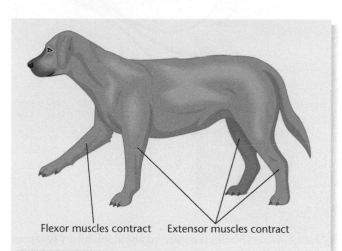

Flexor muscles contract   Extensor muscles contract

Figure 2.6 Antagonistic muscles
Flexor muscles draw an extremity toward the trunk of the body, whereas extensor muscles move an extremity away from the body.

cell. That is, it increases the negative charge within the cell, moving it farther from the threshold and decreasing the probability of an action potential (point 5 in Figure 2.3). This temporary hyperpolarization of a membrane—called an **inhibitory postsynaptic potential** (**IPSP**)—resembles an EPSP. An IPSP occurs when synaptic input selectively opens the gates for potassium ions to leave the cell (carrying a positive charge with them) or for chloride ions to enter the cell (carrying a negative charge).

Today, we take for granted the concept of inhibition, but at Sherrington's time, the idea was controversial, as no one could imagine a mechanism to accomplish it. Establishing the idea of inhibition was critical not just for neuroscience but for psychology as well. Whenever we talk about inhibiting an impulse, we use a concept first demonstrated by Sherrington.

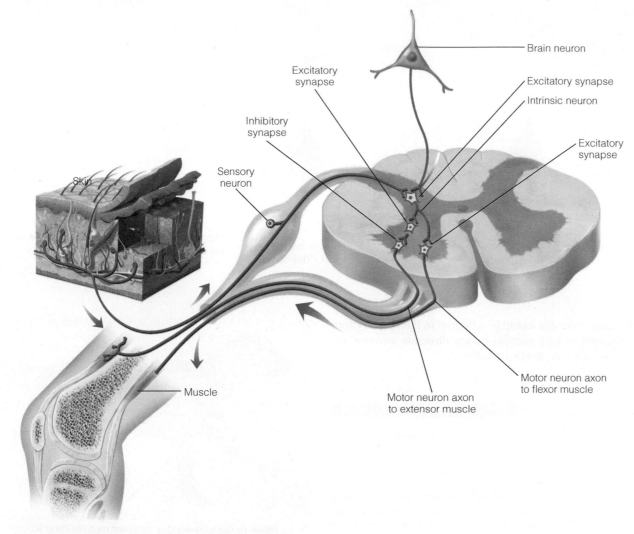

Figure 2.7 What Sherrington inferred about inhibitory synapses
When a flexor muscle is excited, input to the extensor muscle is inhibited. Sherrington inferred that the interneuron that excited a motor neuron to the flexor muscle also inhibited a motor neuron connected to the extensor muscle. Not shown here are the connections to motor neurons controlling the other three legs.

STOP & CHECK

3. What was Sherrington's evidence for inhibition in the nervous system?
4. What ion gates in the membrane open during an EPSP? What gates open during an IPSP?
5. Can an inhibitory message flow along an axon?

ANSWERS

3. Sherrington found that a reflex that stimulates a flexor muscle prevents contraction of the extensor muscles of the same limb. He therefore inferred that an interneuron that excited motor neurons connected to the flexor muscle also inhibited the input to the extensor muscle. 4. During an EPSP, sodium gates open. During an IPSP, potassium or chloride gates open. 5. No. Only action potentials propagate along an axon. Inhibitory messages—IPSPs—decay over time and distance.

Relationship among EPSP, IPSP, and Action Potentials

Sherrington's work opened the way to exploring the wiring diagram of the nervous system. Consider the neurons shown in Figure 2.8. When neuron 1 excites neuron 3, it also excites neuron 2, which inhibits neuron 3. The excitatory message reaches neuron 3 faster because it goes through just one synapse instead of two. The result is a burst of excitation (EPSP) in neuron 3, which quickly slows or stops. You see how inhibitory messages can regulate the timing of activity.

To see how the wiring diagram in the nervous system controls the outcome, consider Figure 2.9. The axon from either cell A or cell B stimulates cell X with +1 unit. If the threshold of cell X is +1, then cell X responds to "A or B." If the threshold

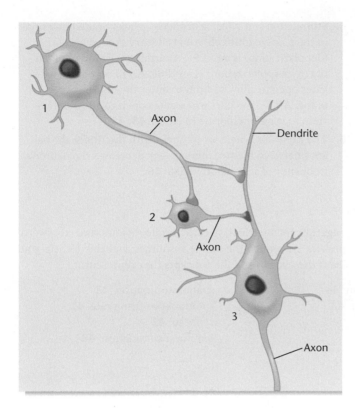

Figure 2.8 A possible wiring diagram for synapses
Excitatory synapses are in green, and inhibitory synapses in red. In the circuit shown here, excitation reaches the dendrite before inhibition. (Remember, any transmission through a synapse produces a delay.) The result is brief excitation of the dendrite.
(Source: Based on Kullmann & Lamsa, 2007)

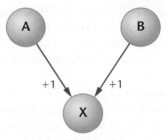

Figure 2.9 A simple wiring diagram for three neurons
Depending on whether the threshold for cell X is 1 or 2, it responds to "A or B" or it responds to "A and B."

is +2, then cell X responds to "A and B." With a little effort you can imagine other constructions.

Many mathematical models of the nervous system are based on connections like these. However, researchers have discovered complexities that Sherrington did not anticipate. Some synapses produce fast, brief effects, and others produce slow, long-lasting effects. In many cases, the effect of two synapses at the same time can be more than double the effect of either one, or less than double (Silver, 2010). Certain combinations of synapses summate with one another more strongly than others do (Lavzin, Rapoport, Polsky, Garion, & Schiller, 2012). Also, the strength of a synapse can vary from one time to another. The nervous system is indeed complex.

Most neurons have a **spontaneous firing rate**, a periodic production of action potentials even without synaptic input. In such cases, the EPSPs increase the frequency of action potentials above the spontaneous rate, whereas IPSPs decrease it. For example, if the neuron's spontaneous firing rate is 10 action potentials per second, a stream of EPSPs might increase the rate to 15 or more, whereas a preponderance of IPSPs might decrease it to 5 or fewer.

Module 2.1 | In Closing
The Neuron as Decision Maker

Transmission along an axon merely sends information from one place to another. Synapses determine whether to send the message. The EPSPs and IPSPs reaching a neuron at a given moment compete with one another, and the net result is a complicated, not exactly algebraic summation of their effects. We could regard the summation of EPSPs and IPSPs as a decision because it determines whether or not the postsynaptic cell fires an action potential. However, do not imagine that any single neuron decides what you will eat for breakfast. Complex behaviors depend on the contributions from a huge network of neurons.

Summary

1. The synapse is the point of communication between two neurons. Charles S. Sherrington's observations of reflexes enabled him to infer the existence of synapses and many of their properties. **42**

2. Because transmission through a reflex arc is slower than transmission through an equivalent length of axon, Sherrington concluded that some process at the synapses delays transmission. **43**

3. Graded potentials (EPSPs and IPSPs) summate their effects. The summation of graded potentials from stimuli at different times is temporal summation. The summation of potentials from different locations is spatial summation. **43**

4. Inhibition is more than just the absence of excitation. It is an active brake that suppresses excitation. For effective functioning of the nervous system, inhibition is just as important as excitation. **45**

5. Stimulation at a synapse produces a brief graded potential in the postsynaptic cell. An excitatory graded potential (depolarization) is an EPSP. An inhibitory graded potential (hyperpolarization) is an IPSP. An EPSP occurs when gates open to allow sodium to enter the neuron's membrane. An IPSP occurs when gates open to allow potassium to leave or chloride to enter. **43, 45**

6. The EPSPs on a neuron compete with the IPSPs; the balance between the two increases or decreases the neuron's frequency of action potentials. **46**

Key Terms

Terms are defined in the module on the page number indicated. They're also presented in alphabetical order with definitions in the book's Subject Index/Glossary, which begins on page 589. Interactive flash cards, audio reviews, and crossword puzzles are among the online resources available to help you learn these terms and the concepts they represent.

excitatory postsynaptic potential (EPSP) **43**

inhibitory postsynaptic potential (IPSP) **45**

postsynaptic neuron **43**

presynaptic neuron **43**

reflex arc **42**

reflexes **42**

spatial summation **43**

spontaneous firing rate **47**

synapse **42**

temporal summation **43**

Thought Questions

1. When Sherrington measured the reaction time of a reflex (i.e., the delay between stimulus and response), he found that the response occurred faster after a strong stimulus than after a weak one. Can you explain this finding? Remember that all action potentials—whether produced by strong or weak stimuli—travel at the same speed along a given axon.

2. Suppose neuron X has a synapse onto neuron Y, which has a synapse onto Z. Presume that no other neurons or synapses are present. An experimenter finds that stimulating neuron X causes an action potential in neuron Z after a short delay. However, she determines that the synapse of X onto Y is inhibitory. Explain how the stimulation of X might produce excitation of Z.

3. Figure 2.9 shows synaptic connections to produce a cell that responds to "A or B" or "A and B." Construct a diagram for a cell that responds to "A and B if not C."

4. Construct a wiring diagram for a cell that responds to "A *or* B if not C." This is trickier than it sounds. If you simply shift the threshold of cell X to 1, it will respond to "A if not C, or B if not C, or A and B even if C." Can you get X to respond to either A or B, but only if C is inactive? (Hint: You might need to introduce more than just cells A, B, and C.)

Module 2.1 | End of Module Quiz

1. How well did Sherrington's inferences about synapses harmonize with Cajal's conclusions about the anatomy of neurons?

   A. The two conclusions supported each other.
   B. Sherrington's conclusions were incompatible with Cajal's conclusions.
   C. The two conclusions were irrelevant to each other.

2. Sherrington based his conclusions on what type of evidence?

   A. Microscopic examination of synapses
   B. Results of injecting drugs into the spinal cord
   C. Electrical recordings from inside neurons
   D. Observations of reflexive responses

3. Although one pinch did not cause a dog to flex its leg, a rapid sequence of pinches did. Sherrington cited this observation as evidence for what?

   A. Temporal summation
   B. Spatial summation
   C. Inhibitory synapses
   D. Refractory period

4. Although one pinch did not cause a dog to flex its leg, several simultaneous pinches at nearby locations did. Sherrington cited this observation as evidence for what?

A. Temporal summation

B. Spatial summation

C. Inhibitory synapses

D. Refractory period

5. According to Sherrington, why do the extensor muscles of a leg relax when the flexor muscles contract?

A. Voluntary control by the cerebral cortex

B. Inhibitory connections in the spinal cord

C. Direct connections between the muscles themselves

D. Control by different chemical neurotransmitters

6. In the membrane of a neuron, what happens during an IPSP?

A. All the ion gates in the membrane close.

B. The sodium gates open.

C. The potassium or chloride gates open.

D. All the ion gates in the membrane open.

7. In what way were Sherrington's conclusions important for psychology as well as neuroscience?

A. He demonstrated the importance of unconscious motivations.

B. He demonstrated the importance of inhibition.

C. He demonstrated the phenomenon of classical conditioning.

D. He demonstrated the evolution of intelligence.

Answers: 1A, 2D, 3A, 4B, 5B, 6C, 7B.

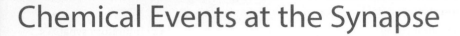

Module 2.2

Chemical Events at the Synapse

Although Charles Sherrington accurately inferred many properties of the synapse, he was wrong about one important point: Although he knew that synaptic transmission was slower than transmission along an axon, he thought it was still too fast to depend on a chemical process, and he therefore concluded that it must be electrical. We now know that the great majority of synapses rely on chemical processes, which are much faster and more versatile than Sherrington or anyone else of his era would have guessed. Over the years, our concept of activity at synapses has grown in many ways.

The Discovery of Chemical Transmission at Synapses

A set of nerves called the sympathetic nervous system accelerates the heartbeat, relaxes the stomach muscles, dilates the pupils of the eyes, and regulates other organs. T. R. Elliott, a young British scientist, reported in 1905 that applying the hormone *adrenaline* directly to the surface of the heart, the stomach, or the pupils produces the same effects as those of the sympathetic nervous system. Elliott therefore suggested that the sympathetic nerves stimulate muscles by releasing adrenaline or a similar chemical.

However, this evidence was not decisive. Possibly adrenaline just mimicked effects that are ordinarily electrical in nature. At the time, Sherrington's prestige was so great that most scientists ignored Elliott's results and continued to assume that synapses transmitted electrical impulses. Otto Loewi, a German physiologist, liked the idea of chemical synapses but did not see how to demonstrate it more conclusively. In 1920, he awakened one night with an idea about what research to do. He wrote himself a note and went back to sleep. Unfortunately, the next morning he could not read his note! The following night he awoke at 3 A.M. with the same idea, rushed to the laboratory, and performed the experiment.

Loewi repeatedly stimulated the vagus nerve, thereby decreasing a frog's heart rate. He then collected fluid from around that heart, transferred it to a second frog's heart, and found that the second heart also decreased its rate of beating, as shown in Figure 2.10. Then Loewi stimulated the accelerator nerve to the first frog's heart, increasing the heart rate.

When he collected fluid from that heart and transferred it to the second frog's heart, its heart rate increased. That is, stimulating one nerve released something that inhibited heart rate, and stimulating a different nerve released something that increased heart rate. He knew he was collecting and transferring chemicals, not loose electricity. Therefore, Loewi concluded, nerves send messages by releasing chemicals.

Loewi later remarked that if he had thought of this experiment in the light of day, he probably would have dismissed it as unrealistic (Loewi, 1960). Even if synapses did release chemicals, his daytime reasoning went, they probably did not release much. Fortunately, by the time he realized that the experiment should not work, he had already completed it, and it did work. It earned him a Nobel Prize.

Despite Loewi's work, most researchers over the next three decades continued to believe that most synapses were electrical and that chemical synapses were the exception. Finally, in the 1950s, researchers established that chemical transmission predominates throughout the nervous system. That discovery revolutionized our understanding and encouraged

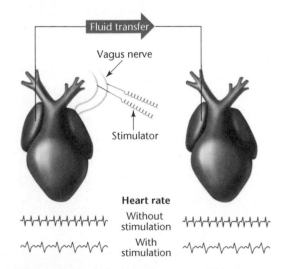

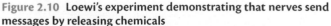

Figure 2.10 Loewi's experiment demonstrating that nerves send messages by releasing chemicals
Loewi stimulated the vagus nerve to one frog's heart, decreasing the heartbeat. When he transferred fluid from that heart to another frog's heart, he observed a decrease in its heartbeat.

50

research that developed drugs for psychiatric uses (Carlsson, 2001). A small number of electrical synapses do exist, however, as discussed later in this module.

✅ **STOP** & CHECK ▮▮▮▮▮▮▮▮▮▮

6. What was Loewi's evidence that neurotransmission depends on the release of chemicals?

ANSWER

6. When Loewi stimulated a nerve that increased or decreased a frog's heart rate, he could withdraw fluid from the area around the heart, transfer it to another frog's heart, and thereby increase or decrease its rate also.

The Sequence of Chemical Events at a Synapse

Understanding the chemical events at a synapse is fundamental to understanding the nervous system. Every year, researchers discover more and more details about synapses, their structure, and how those structures relate to function. Here are the major events:

1. The neuron synthesizes chemicals that serve as neurotransmitters. It synthesizes the smaller neurotransmitters in the axon terminals and synthesizes neuropeptides in the cell body.
2. Action potentials travel down the axon. At the presynaptic terminal, an action potential enables calcium to enter the cell. Calcium releases neurotransmitters from the terminals and into the *synaptic cleft*, the space between the presynaptic and postsynaptic neurons.
3. The released molecules diffuse across the narrow cleft, attach to receptors, and alter the activity of the postsynaptic neuron. Mechanisms vary for altering that activity.
4. The neurotransmitter molecules separate from their receptors.
5. The neurotransmitter molecules may be taken back into the presynaptic neuron for recycling or they may diffuse away.
6. Some postsynaptic cells send reverse messages to control the further release of neurotransmitter by presynaptic cells.

Figure 2.11 summarizes these steps. Let's now consider each step in more detail. As we do, we shall also consider drugs that affect certain steps in this process. Nearly all drugs that affect behavior or experience do so by altering synaptic transmission.

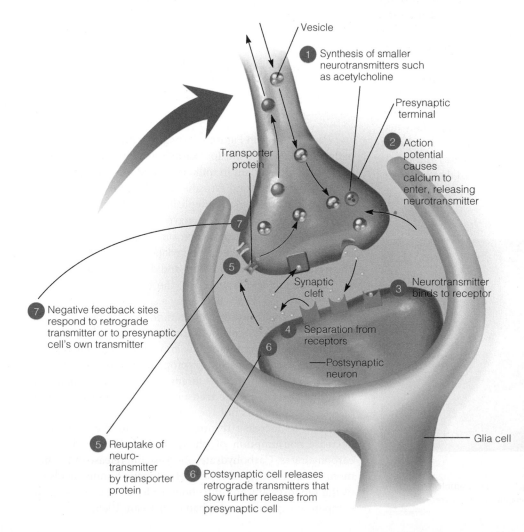

Vesicle

1 Synthesis of smaller neurotransmitters such as acetylcholine

Presynaptic terminal

2 Action potential causes calcium to enter, releasing neurotransmitter

Transporter protein

Neurotransmitter binds to receptor

7 Negative feedback sites respond to retrograde transmitter or to presynaptic cell's own transmitter

Synaptic cleft

4 Separation from receptors

Postsynaptic neuron

5 Reuptake of neuro-transmitter by transporter protein

6 Postsynaptic cell releases retrograde transmitters that slow further release from presynaptic cell

Glia cell

Figure 2.11 Some major events in transmission at a synapse
The structure shown in green is an astrocyte that shields the synapse from outside chemicals. The astrocyte also exchanges chemicals with the two neurons.

Table 2.1 | **Neurotransmitters**

Amino Acids	glutamate, GABA, glycine, aspartate, maybe others
A Modified Amino Acid	acetylcholine
Monoamines (also modified from amino acids)	indoleamines: serotonin
	catecholamines: dopamine, norepinephrine, epinephrine
Neuropeptides (chains of amino acids)	endorphins, substance P, neuropeptide Y, many others
Purines	ATP, adenosine, maybe others
Gases	NO (nitric oxide), maybe others

Types of Neurotransmitters

At a synapse, a neuron releases chemicals that affect another neuron. Those chemicals are known as **neurotransmitters**. A hundred or so chemicals are known or suspected to be neurotransmitters, as shown in Table 2.1 (Borodinsky et al., 2004). Ctenophores (see Figure 2.12), possibly representative of the earliest, most primitive animals, apparently have only one neurotransmitter, glutamate (Moroz et al., 2014). Most of the rest of the animal kingdom has all or nearly all of the same transmitters that humans have.

The oddest transmitter is **nitric oxide** (chemical formula NO), a gas released by many small local neurons. (Do not confuse nitric oxide, NO, with nitrous oxide, N_2O, sometimes known as "laughing gas.") Nitric oxide is poisonous in large quantities and difficult to make in a laboratory. Yet, many neurons contain an enzyme that enables them to make it efficiently. Many neurons release nitric oxide when they are stimulated. In addition to influencing other neurons, nitric oxide dilates the nearby blood vessels, thereby increasing blood flow to that brain area (Dawson, Gonzalez-Zulueta, Kusel, & Dawson, 1998).

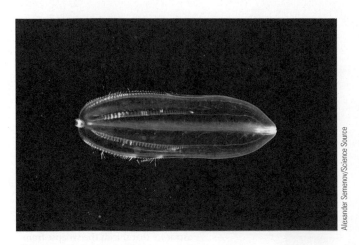

Figure 2.12 A ctenophore
Ctenophores, otherwise known as comb jellies, have a simple nervous system with reportedly only one neurotransmitter, glutamate.

7. Blood flow increases to the most active brain areas. How does the blood "know" which areas are most active?

ANSWER

7. In a highly active brain area, many stimulated neurons release nitric oxide, which dilates the blood vessels in the area and thereby makes it easier for blood to flow to the area.

Synthesis of Transmitters

Neurons synthesize nearly all neurotransmitters from amino acids, which the body obtains from proteins in the diet. Figure 2.13 illustrates the chemical steps in the synthesis of acetylcholine, serotonin, dopamine, epinephrine, and norepinephrine. Note the relationship among epinephrine, norepinephrine, and dopamine—compounds known as **catecholamines**, because they contain a catechol group and an amine group, as shown here:

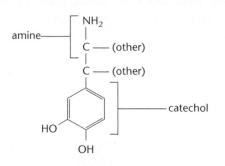

Each pathway in Figure 2.13 begins with substances found in the diet. Acetylcholine, for example, is synthesized from choline, which is abundant in milk, eggs, and peanuts. The amino acids phenylalanine and tyrosine, present in proteins, are precursors of dopamine, norepinephrine, and epinephrine. People with phenylketonuria lack the enzyme that converts phenylalanine to tyrosine. They can get tyrosine from their diet, but they need to minimize intake of phenylalanine, because excessive phenylalanine would accumulate and damage the brain.

The amino acid *tryptophan*, the precursor to serotonin, crosses the blood–brain barrier by a special transport system that it shares with other large amino acids. Your serotonin levels rise after you eat foods richer in tryptophan, such as soy, and fall after something low in tryptophan, such as maize (American corn). However, tryptophan has to compete with other, more abundant large amino acids, such as phenylalanine, that share the same transport system, so increasing intake of tryptophan is not the best way to increase serotonin. One way to increase tryptophan entry to the brain is to decrease consumption of phenylalanine. Another is to eat carbohydrates. Carbohydrates increase the release of the hormone *insulin*, which takes several competing amino acids out of the bloodstream and into body cells, thus decreasing the competition against tryptophan (Wurtman, 1985).

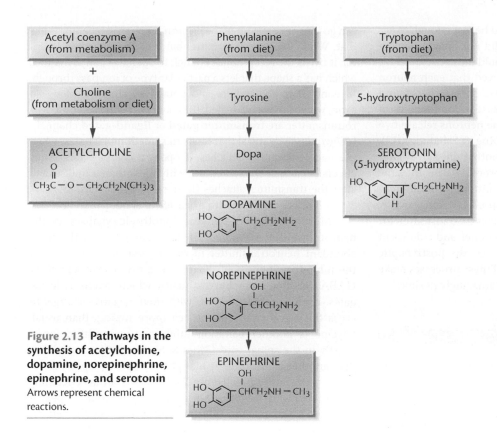

Figure 2.13 **Pathways in the synthesis of acetylcholine, dopamine, norepinephrine, epinephrine, and serotonin** Arrows represent chemical reactions.

Several drugs act by altering the synthesis of transmitters. L-dopa, a precursor to dopamine, helps increase the supply of dopamine. It is a helpful treatment for people with Parkinson's disease. AMPT (alpha-methyl-para-tyrosine) temporarily blocks the production of dopamine. It has no therapeutic use, but researchers sometimes use it to study the functions of dopamine.

✓ STOP & CHECK

8. Name the three catecholamine neurotransmitters.

ANSWER   confuse the term catecholamine with acetylcholine.
8. Epinephrine, norepinephrine, and dopamine. Do not

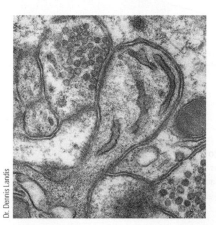
Dr. Dennis Landis

(a)

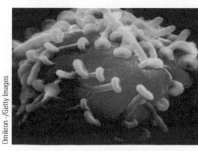
Omikron-/Getty Images

(b)

Storage of Transmitters

Most neurotransmitters are synthesized in the presynaptic terminal, near the point of release. The presynaptic terminal stores high concentrations of neurotransmitter molecules in **vesicles**, tiny nearly spherical packets (see Figure 2.14). (Nitric oxide is an exception to this rule. Neurons release nitric oxide as soon as they form it instead of storing it.) The presynaptic terminal also maintains much neurotransmitter outside the vesicles.

Neurons that release serotonin, dopamine, or norepinephrine contain an enzyme, **MAO** (monoamine oxidase), that breaks down these transmitters into inactive chemicals, thereby preventing the transmitters to accumulate to harmful levels. The first antidepressant drugs that psychiatrists discovered were MAO inhibitors. By blocking MAO, they increase the brain's supply of serotonin, dopamine, and norepinephrine. However, MAO inhibitors also have other effects, and exactly how they help relieve depression is still not certain.

Release and Diffusion of Transmitters

At the end of an axon, an action potential itself does not release the neurotransmitter. Rather, depolarization opens voltage-dependent calcium gates in the presynaptic terminal. Within 1 or 2 milliseconds (ms) after calcium enters the terminal, it causes **exocytosis**—bursts of release of neurotransmitter from the presynaptic neuron. An action potential often fails to release any transmitter, and even when it does, the amount varies (Craig & Boudin, 2001).

After its release from the presynaptic cell, the neurotransmitter diffuses across the synaptic cleft to the postsynaptic membrane, where it attaches to a receptor. The neurotransmitter takes no more than 0.01 ms to diffuse across the cleft, which is only 20 to 30 nanometers (nm) wide. Remember, Sherrington

Figure 2.14 **Anatomy of a synapse**
(a) An electron micrograph showing a synapse from the cerebellum of a mouse. The small round structures are vesicles. (b) Electron micrograph showing axon terminals onto the soma of a neuron.

did not believe chemical processes could be fast enough to account for the activity at synapses. He did not imagine such a narrow gap through which chemicals could diffuse so quickly.

For many years, investigators believed that each neuron released just one neurotransmitter, but later researchers found that many, perhaps most, neurons release a combination of two or more transmitters at a time. Some neurons release two transmitters at the same time (Tritsch, Ding, & Sabatini, 2012), whereas some release one at first and another one slowly later (Borisovska, Bensen, Chong, & Westbrook, 2013). In some cases a neuron releases different transmitters from different branches of its axon (Nishimaru, Restrepo, Ryge, Yanagawa, & Kiehn, 2005). Sometimes a neuron changes its transmitter, for example releasing one transmitter in summer and a different one in winter (Spitzer, 2015). Presumably, the postsynaptic neuron changes its receptors as well. All these processes make it possible for the nervous system to be amazingly flexible.

✓ STOP & CHECK

9. When the action potential reaches the presynaptic terminal, which ion must enter the presynaptic terminal to evoke release of the neurotransmitter?

ANSWER   9. Calcium

Activating Receptors of the Postsynaptic Cell

Sherrington's concept of the synapse was simple: Input produced excitation or inhibition—in other words, an on/off system. When Eccles recorded from individual cells, he happened to choose cells that produced only brief EPSPs and IPSPs—again, just on/off. The discovery of chemical transmission at synapses didn't change that, at first. Researchers discovered more and more neurotransmitters and wondered, "Why does the nervous system use so many chemicals, if they all produce the same type of message?" Eventually they found that the messages are more complicated and more varied.

The effect of a neurotransmitter depends on its receptor on the postsynaptic cell. When the neurotransmitter attaches to its receptor, the receptor may open a channel—exerting an *ionotropic* effect—or it may produce a slower but longer effect—a *metabotropic* effect.

Ionotropic Effects

At one type of receptor, neurotransmitters exert **ionotropic effects**, corresponding to the brief on/off effects that Sherrington and Eccles studied. Imagine a paper bag that is twisted shut at the top. If you untwist it, the opening grows larger so that something

can go into or come out of the bag. An ionotropic receptor is like that. When the neurotransmitter binds to an ionotropic receptor, it twists the receptor just enough to open its central channel, which has a shape that lets a particular type of ion pass through. In contrast to the sodium and potassium channels along an axon, which are voltage-gated, the channels controlled by a neurotransmitter are **transmitter-gated** or **ligand-gated** channels. (A *ligand* is a chemical that binds to something.) That is, when the neurotransmitter attaches, it opens a channel. Ionotropic effects begin quickly, sometimes within less than a millisecond after the transmitter attaches (Lisman, Raghavachari, & Tsien, 2007). The effects decay with a half-life of about 5 ms.

Most of the brain's excitatory ionotropic synapses use the neurotransmitter *glutamate.* In fact, glutamate is the most abundant neurotransmitter in the nervous system. Most of the inhibitory ionotropic synapses use the neurotransmitter GABA (gamma-aminobutyric acid), which opens chloride gates, enabling chloride ions, with their negative charge, to cross the membrane into the cell more rapidly than usual. Glycine is another common inhibitory transmitter, found mostly in the spinal cord (Moss & Smart, 2001). Acetylcholine, another transmitter at many ionotropic synapses, is excitatory in most cases. Figure 2.15a shows an acetylcholine receptor (hugely magnified, of course), as it would appear if you were looking down at it from within the synaptic cleft. Its

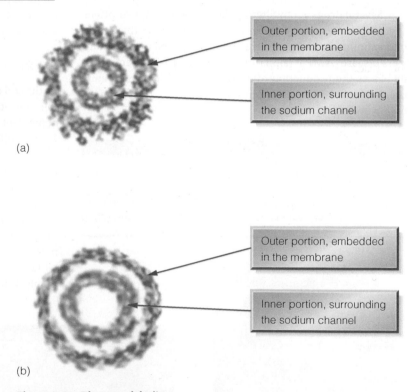

(a)

Outer portion, embedded in the membrane

Inner portion, surrounding the sodium channel

(b)

Outer portion, embedded in the membrane

Inner portion, surrounding the sodium channel

Figure 2.15 The acetylcholine receptor
(a) A cross section of the receptor at rest, as viewed from the synaptic cleft. The membrane surrounds it. **(b)** A similar view after acetylcholine has attached to the side of the receptor, opening the central channel wide enough for sodium to pass through.
(Source: From "Structure and gating mechanism of the acetylcholine receptor pore," by A. Miyazawa, Y. Fujiyoshi, and N. Unwin, 2003, Nature, 423, pp. 949–955.)

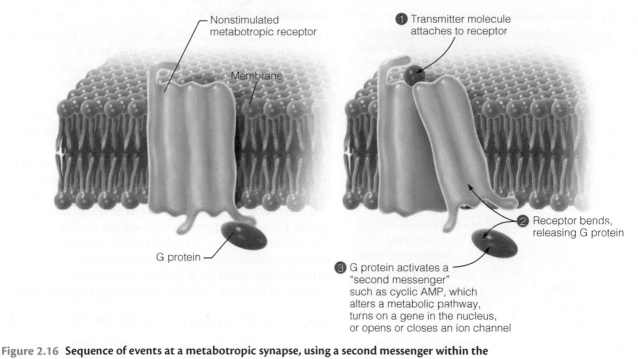

Figure 2.16 **Sequence of events at a metabotropic synapse, using a second messenger within the postsynaptic neuron**

outer portion (in red) is embedded in the neuron's membrane; its inner portion (in purple) surrounds the sodium channel. When the receptor is at rest, the inner portion coils together tightly enough to block sodium passage. When acetylcholine attaches as in Figure 2.15b, the receptor folds outward, widening the sodium channel (Miyazawa, Fujiyoshi, & Unwin, 2003).

Metabotropic Effects and Second Messenger Systems

At other receptors, neurotransmitters exert **metabotropic effects** by initiating a sequence of metabolic reactions that start slowly but last longer than ionotropic effects. Metabotropic effects emerge 30 ms or more after the release of the transmitter (North, 1989). Typically, they last up to a few seconds, sometimes longer. Whereas most ionotropic effects depend on either glutamate or GABA, metabotropic synapses use many neurotransmitters, including dopamine, norepinephrine, and serotonin . . . and sometimes glutamate and GABA too.

Apologies if you find this analogy silly, but it might help clarify metabotropic synapses: Imagine a large room. You are outside the room holding a stick that goes through a hole in the wall and attaches to the hinge of a cage. If you shake the stick, you open that cage and release an angry dog. The dog runs around waking up all the rabbits in the room, which then scurry around causing all kinds of further action. A metabotropic receptor acts a little like that. When a neurotransmitter attaches to a metabotropic receptor, it bends the receptor protein that goes through the membrane of the cell. The other side of that receptor is attached to a **G protein**—that is, a protein coupled to guanosine triphosphate (GTP), an energy-storing molecule. Bending the receptor protein detaches that

G protein, which is then free to take its energy elsewhere in the cell, as shown in Figure 2.16. The result of that G protein is increased concentration of a **second messenger**, such as cyclic adenosine monophosphate (cyclic AMP), inside the cell. Just as the "first messenger" (the neurotransmitter) carries information to the postsynaptic cell, the second messenger communicates to areas within the cell. It may open or close ion channels in the membrane or activate a portion of a chromosome. Note the contrast: An ionotropic synapse has effects localized to one point on the membrane, whereas a metabotropic synapse, by way of its second messenger, influences activity in much or all of the cell and over a longer time.

Ionotropic and metabotropic synapses contribute to different aspects of behavior. For vision and hearing, the brain needs rapid, up-to-date information, the kind that ionotropic synapses bring. In contrast, metabotropic synapses are better suited for more enduring effects such as taste (Huang et al., 2005), smell, and pain (Levine, Fields, & Basbaum, 1993), where the exact timing isn't important anyway. Metabotropic synapses are also important for many aspects of arousal, attention, pleasure, and emotion—again, functions that arise more slowly and last longer than a visual or auditory stimulus.

Neuropeptides

Researchers often refer to the neuropeptides as **neuromodulators**, because they have properties that set them apart from other transmitters (Ludwig & Leng, 2006). Whereas the neuron synthesizes most other neurotransmitters in the presynaptic terminal, it synthesizes neuropeptides in the cell body and then slowly transports them to other parts of the cell. Whereas other neurotransmitters are released at the axon terminal, the

Table 2.2 | Distinctive Features of Neuropeptides

	Neuropeptides	Neurotransmitters
Place synthesized	Cell body	Presynaptic terminal
Place released	Mostly from dendrites, also cell body and sides of axon	Axon terminal
Released by	Repeated depolarization	Single action potential
Effect on neighboring cells	They release the neuropeptide too	No effect on neighbors
Spread of effects	Diffuse to wide area	Effect mostly on receptors of the adjacent postsynaptic cell
Duration of effects	Minutes	Milliseconds to seconds

neuropeptides are released mainly by dendrites, and also by the cell body and by the sides of the axon. A single action potential can release a neurotransmitter, but neuropeptide release requires repeated stimulation. However, after a few dendrites release a neuropeptide, the released chemical primes other nearby dendrites, including those on other cells, to release the same neuropeptide also. Thus, neurons containing neuropeptides do not release them often, but when they do, they release substantial amounts. Furthermore, unlike other transmitters that are released immediately adjacent to their receptors, neuropeptides diffuse widely, slowly affecting many neurons in their region of the brain. In that way they resemble hormones. Because many of them exert their effects by altering gene activity, their effects often last 20 minutes or more. Neuropeptides are important for hunger, thirst, and other long-term changes in behavior and experience. Table 2.2 summarizes differences between neurotransmitters and neuropeptides.

✓ STOP & CHECK

10. How do ionotropic and metabotropic synapses differ in speed and duration of effects?

11. What are second messengers, and which type of synapse relies on them?

12. How do neuropeptides compare to other transmitters?

ANSWERS

10. Ionotropic synapses act more quickly and more briefly. 11. Second messengers are chemicals that alter metabolism or gene expression within a postsynaptic neuron. At metabotropic synapses, the neurotransmitter attaches to a receptor and thereby releases a second messenger. 12. Neuropeptides are released only after prolonged stimulation, but when they are released, they are released in large amounts by all parts of the neuron, not just the axon terminal. Neuropeptides diffuse widely, producing long-lasting effects on many neurons.

Variation in Receptors

The brain has a variety of receptor types for each neurotransmitter. Receptors for a given transmitter differ in their chemical structure, responses to drugs, and roles in behavior. Because of this variation in properties, it is possible to devise drugs with specialized effects on behavior. For example, the serotonin receptor type 3 mediates nausea, and the drug *ondansetron* that blocks this receptor helps cancer patients undergo treatment without nausea.

A given receptor can have different effects for different people, or even in different parts of one person's brain, because of differences in the hundreds of proteins associated with the synapse (O'Rourke, Weiler, Micheva, & Smith, 2012). The synapse is a complicated place, where dozens of proteins tether the presynaptic neuron to the postsynaptic neuron and guide neurotransmitter molecules to their receptors (Wilhelm et al., 2014). Genetic variations in synaptic proteins have been linked to variation in anxiety, sleep, and other aspects of behavior.

Drugs That Act by Binding to Receptors

A drug that chemically resembles a neurotransmitter can bind to its receptor. Many **hallucinogenic drugs**—that is, drugs that distort perception, such as lysergic acid diethylamide (LSD)—chemically resemble serotonin (see Figure 2.17). They attach to serotonin type 2A ($5\text{-}HT_{2A}$) receptors and provide stimulation at inappropriate times or for longer-than-usual durations. LSD increases the connections among brain areas that ordinarily do not communicate much with one another. A possible explanation for the hallucinogenic effect is that the increased spontaneous communication within the brain dominates over the input coming from the sense organs (Carhart-Harris et al., 2016; Tagliazucchi et al., 2016).

Nicotine, a compound present in tobacco, stimulates a family of acetylcholine receptors, conveniently known as *nicotinic receptors*. Because nicotinic receptors are abundant on neurons that release dopamine, nicotine increases dopamine release (Levin & Rose, 1995; Pontieri, Tanda, Orzi, & DiChiara, 1996). Because dopamine release is associated with reward, nicotine stimulation is rewarding also.

Opiate drugs are derived from, or chemically similar to those derived from, the opium poppy. Familiar opiates include

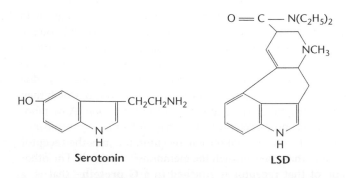

Figure 2.17 Resemblance of the neurotransmitter serotonin to LSD, a hallucinogenic drug

morphine, heroin, and methadone. People used morphine and other opiates for centuries without knowing how the drugs affected the brain. Then researchers found that opiates attach to specific receptors in the brain (Pert & Snyder, 1973). It was a safe guess that vertebrates had not evolved such receptors just to enable us to become drug addicts. Soon investigators found that the brain produces its own neuropeptides, now known as *endorphins* (a contraction of *endo*genous m*orphines*), that bind to the same receptors as endorphins. This discovery was important because it indicated that opiates relieve pain by acting on receptors in the brain as well as in the skin. This finding also paved the way for the discovery of other neuropeptides that regulate emotions and motivations.

STOP & CHECK

13. How do LSD, nicotine, and opiate drugs influence behavior?

ANSWER

13. LSD binds to one type of serotonin receptor. Nicotine binds to one type of acetylcholine receptor. Opiates bind to endorphin receptors.

Inactivation and Reuptake of Neurotransmitters

A neurotransmitter does not linger at the postsynaptic membrane, where it might continue exciting or inhibiting the receptor. Various neurotransmitters are inactivated in different ways. The neuropeptides, however, are not inactivated. They simply diffuse away. Because resynthesizing these large molecules takes time, a neuron can temporarily exhaust its supply.

After acetylcholine activates a receptor, the enzyme **acetylcholinesterase** (a-SEE-til-ko-lih-NES-teh-raze) breaks it into two fragments: acetate and choline. The choline diffuses back to the presynaptic neuron, which takes it up and reconnects it with acetate already in the cell to form acetylcholine again. Although this recycling process is highly efficient, it takes time, and the presynaptic neuron does not reabsorb every molecule it releases. A sufficiently rapid series of action potentials at any synapse depletes the neurotransmitter faster than the presynaptic cell replenishes it, thus slowing or interrupting transmission (Liu & Tsien, 1995).

Serotonin and the catecholamines (dopamine, norepinephrine, and epinephrine) do not break down into inactive fragments at the postsynaptic membrane. They simply detach from the receptor. At that point, the next step varies. The presynaptic neuron takes up much or most of the released neurotransmitter molecules intact and reuses them. This process, called **reuptake**, occurs through special membrane proteins called **transporters**. The activity of transporters varies among individuals and from one brain area to another. Any transmitter molecules that the transporters do not take will instead break down by an enzyme called **COMT**

(catechol-o-methyltransferase). The breakdown products wash away and eventually show up in the blood and urine.

Stimulant drugs, including **amphetamine** and **cocaine**, inhibit the transporters for dopamine, serotonin, and norepinephrine, thus decreasing reuptake and prolonging the effects of the neurotransmitters (Beuming et al., 2008; Schmitt & Reith, 2010; Zhao et al., 2010). Most antidepressant drugs also block reuptake of one or more neurotransmitters, but more weakly than amphetamine and cocaine do.

When stimulant drugs increase the accumulation of dopamine in the synaptic cleft, COMT breaks down the excess dopamine faster than the presynaptic cell can replace it. A few hours after taking a stimulant drug, a user has a deficit of dopamine and enters a withdrawal state, marked by reduced energy, reduced motivation, and mild depression.

Methylphenidate (Ritalin), another stimulant drug, is often prescribed for people with attention deficit/hyperactivity disorder. Methylphenidate and cocaine block the reuptake of dopamine in the same way at the same brain receptors. The differences between the drugs relate to dose and time course. Cocaine users typically sniff it or inject it to produce a rapid rush of effect on the brain. People taking methylphenidate pills experience a gradual increase in the drug's concentration over an hour or two, followed by a slow decline. Therefore, methylphenidate does not produce the sudden rush of excitement that cocaine does. However, anyone who injects methylphenidate experiences effects similar to cocaine's, including a risk of addiction.

STOP & CHECK

14. What happens to acetylcholine molecules after they stimulate a postsynaptic receptor?
15. What happens to serotonin and catecholamine molecules after they stimulate a postsynaptic receptor?
16. How do amphetamine and cocaine influence synapses?
17. Why is methylphenidate generally less disruptive to behavior than cocaine is despite the drugs' similar mechanisms?

ANSWERS

14. The enzyme acetylcholinesterase breaks acetylcholine molecules into two smaller molecules, acetate and choline, which are then reabsorbed by the presynaptic terminal. 15. Most serotonin and catecholamine molecules are reabsorbed by the presynaptic terminal. Some of their molecules are broken down into inactive chemicals, which then diffuse away. 16. They block reuptake of released dopamine, serotonin, and norepinephrine. 17. The effects of a methylphenidate pill develop and decline in the brain much more slowly than do those of cocaine.

Negative Feedback from the Postsynaptic Cell

Suppose someone sends you an email message and then, worried that you might not have received it, sends it again and again. To prevent cluttering your inbox, you might add a system that provides an automatic answer, "Yes, I got your message. Don't send it again."

A couple of mechanisms in the nervous system serve that function. First, many presynaptic terminals have receptors sensitive to the same transmitter they release. These receptors are known as **autoreceptors**—receptors that respond to the released transmitter by inhibiting further synthesis and release. That is, they provide negative feedback (Kubista & Boehm, 2006).

Second, some postsynaptic neurons respond to stimulation by releasing chemicals that travel back to the presynaptic terminal to inhibit further release of transmitter. Nitric oxide is one such transmitter. Certain cells in the retina emit hydrogen ions (that is, protons) to inhibit further transmission (Wang, Holzhausen, & Kramer, 2014). Two other reverse transmitters are **anandamide** (from

the Sanskrit word *anana*, meaning "bliss") and **2-AG** (*sn*-2 arachidonylglycerol).

Cannabinoids, the active chemicals in marijuana, bind to anandamide or 2-AG receptors on presynaptic neurons, indicating, "The cell got your message. Stop sending it." The presynaptic cell, unaware that it hadn't sent any message at all, stops sending. In this way, the chemicals in marijuana decrease both excitatory and inhibitory messages from neurons that release glutamate, GABA, and other transmitters. In various cases the result can be either brief or more long-lasting suppression of release (Lutz, Marsicano, Maldonado, & Hillard, 2015). The behavioral results vary, but usually include decreased anxiety.

Figure 2.18 summarizes some of the ways in which drugs affect dopamine synapses, including effects on synthesis,

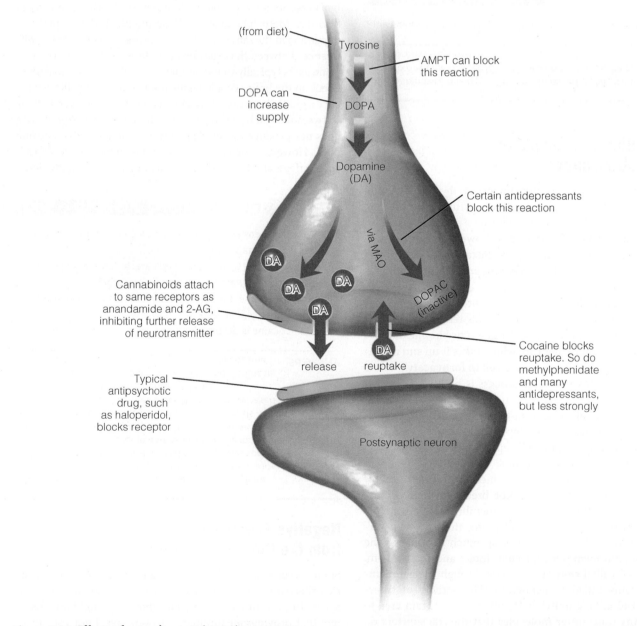

Figure 2.18 Effects of some drugs at dopamine synapses

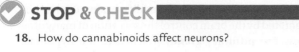
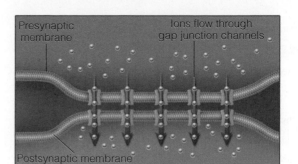

Figure 2.19 **A gap junction for an electrical synapse**

release, action on postsynaptic receptors, reuptake, and breakdown. Table 2.3 also summarizes effects of some common drugs.

Electrical Synapses

At the start of this module, you learned that Sherrington was wrong to assume that synapses convey messages electrically. Well, he wasn't completely wrong. A few special-purpose synapses do operate electrically. Because electrical transmission is faster than even the fastest chemical transmission, electrical synapses have evolved in cases where exact synchrony between two cells is important. For example, some of the cells that control your rhythmic breathing are synchronized by electrical synapses. (It's important to inhale on the left side at the same time as on the right side.) Also, many animal species have electrical synapses in their system responsible for coordinating rapid escape movements (Pereda, 2014).

At an electrical synapse, the membrane of one neuron comes into direct contact with the membrane of another, as shown in Figure 2.19. This contact is called a **gap junction**. Fairly large pores of the membrane of one neuron line up precisely with similar pores in the membrane of the other cell. These pores are large enough for sodium and other ions to pass readily, and unlike the other membrane channels we have considered, these pores remain open constantly. Therefore, whenever one of the neurons is depolarized, sodium ions from that cell can pass immediately into the other neuron and depolarize it, too. As a result, the two neurons act as if they were a single neuron. Again we see the great variety of synapses in the nervous system.

Hormones

Hormonal influences resemble synaptic transmission in many ways, including the fact that many chemicals serve both as hormones and as neurotransmitters. A **hormone** is a chemical secreted by cells in one part of the body and conveyed by the blood to influence other cells. A neurotransmitter is like a telephone signal: It conveys a message from the sender to the intended receiver. Hormones function more like a radio station: They convey a message to any receiver tuned to the right station. Neuropeptides are intermediate. They diffuse within part of the brain, but not to other parts of the body. Figure 2.20 shows the major **endocrine** (hormone-producing) **glands**. Table 2.4 lists those hormones that become relevant in other chapters of this book. (A complete list of hormones would be lengthy.)

Hormones are particularly useful for coordinating long-lasting changes in multiple parts of the body. For example, birds that are preparing for migration secrete hormones that change their eating and digestion to store extra energy for a long journey. Two types of hormones are **protein hormones** and **peptide hormones**, composed of chains of amino acids. (Proteins are longer chains and peptides are shorter.) Protein and peptide hormones attach to membrane receptors, where they activate a second messenger within the cell—exactly like a metabotropic synapse.

Table 2.3 | **Summary of Some Drugs and Their Effects**

Drugs	Main Synaptic Effects
Amphetamine	Blocks reuptake of dopamine and several other transmitters
Cocaine	Blocks reuptake of dopamine and several other transmitters
Methylphenidate (Ritalin)	Blocks reuptake of dopamine and others, but gradually
MDMA ("Ecstasy")	Releases dopamine / Releases serotonin
Nicotine	Stimulates nicotinic-type acetylcholine receptor, which (among other effects) increases dopamine release in nucleus accumbens
Opiates (e.g., heroin, morphine)	Stimulates endorphin receptors
Cannabinoids (marijuana)	Excites negative-feedback receptors on presynaptic cells; those receptors ordinarily respond to anandamide and 2AG
Hallucinogens (e.g., LSD)	Stimulates serotonin type 2A receptors (5-HT_{2A})

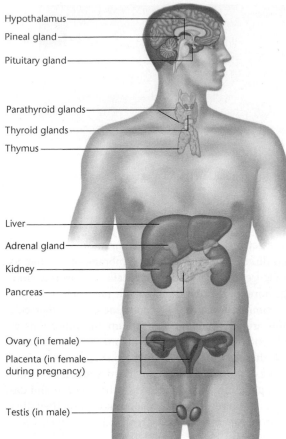

Hypothalamus

Pineal gland

Pituitary gland

Parathyroid glands

Thyroid glands

Thymus

Liver

Adrenal gland

Kidney

Pancreas

Ovary (in female)

Placenta (in female during pregnancy)

Testis (in male)

Figure 2.20 Location of some major endocrine glands
(*Source: Starr & Taggart, 1989*)

Just as circulating hormones modify brain activity, hormones secreted by the brain control the secretion of many other hormones. The **pituitary gland**, attached to the hypothalamus (see Figure 2.21), has two parts, the **anterior pituitary** and the **posterior pituitary**, which release different sets of hormones. The posterior pituitary, composed of neural tissue, can be considered an extension of the hypothalamus. Neurons in the hypothalamus synthesize the hormones **oxytocin** and **vasopressin** (also known as antidiuretic hormone), which migrate down axons to the posterior pituitary, as shown in Figure 2.22. Later, the posterior pituitary releases these hormones into the blood.

The anterior pituitary, composed of glandular tissue, synthesizes six hormones, although the hypothalamus controls their release (see Figure 2.22). The hypothalamus secretes **releasing hormones**, which flow through the blood to the anterior pituitary. There they stimulate or inhibit the release of other hormones.

The hypothalamus maintains fairly constant circulating levels of certain hormones through a negative feedback system. For example, when the level of thyroid hormone is low, the hypothalamus releases *TSH-releasing hormone*, which stimulates the anterior pituitary to release TSH, which in turn causes the thyroid gland to secrete more thyroid hormones (see Figure 2.23).

Table 2.4 | **Selective List of Hormones**

Organ	Hormone	Hormone Functions (partial)
Hypothalamus	Various releasing hormones	Promote/inhibit release of hormones from pituitary
Anterior pituitary	Thyroid-stimulating hormone	Stimulates thyroid gland
	Luteinizing hormone	Stimulates ovulation
	Follicle-stimulating hormone	Promotes ovum maturation (female), sperm production (male)
	ACTH	Increases steroid hormone production by adrenal gland
	Prolactin	Increases milk production
	Growth hormone	Increases body growth
Posterior pituitary	Oxytocin	Uterine contractions, milk release, sexual pleasure
	Vasopressin	Raises blood pressure, decreases urine volume
Pineal	Melatonin	Sleepiness; also role in puberty
Adrenal cortex	Aldosterone	Reduces release of salt in the urine
	Cortisol	Elevated blood sugar and metabolism
Adrenal medulla	Epinephrine, norepinephrine	Similar to actions of sympathetic nervous system
Pancreas	Insulin	Helps glucose enter cells
	Glucagon	Helps convert stored glycogen into blood glucose
Ovary	Estrogens and progesterone	Female sexual characteristics and pregnancy
Testis	Testosterone	Male sexual characteristics and pubic hair
Kidney	Renin	Regulates blood pressure, contributes to hypovolemic thirst
Fat cells	Leptin	Decreases appetite, increases activity

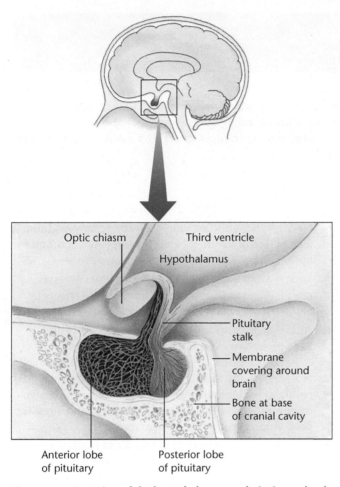

Figure 2.21 **Location of the hypothalamus and pituitary gland in the human brain**
(Source: Starr & Taggart, 1989)

Hypothalamus secretes releasing hormones and inhibiting hormones that control anterior pituitary. Also synthesizes vasopressin and oxytocin, which travel to posterior pituitary.

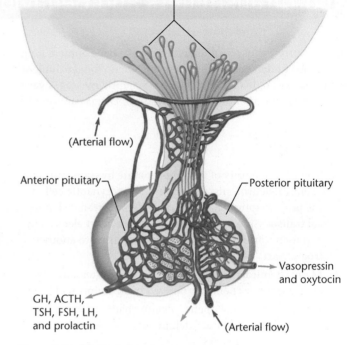

Figure 2.22 **Pituitary hormones**
The hypothalamus produces vasopressin and oxytocin, which travel to the posterior pituitary (really an extension of the hypothalamus). The posterior pituitary releases those hormones in response to neural signals. The hypothalamus also produces releasing hormones and inhibiting hormones, which travel to the anterior pituitary, where they control the release of six hormones synthesized there.

✅ **STOP & CHECK**

19. Which part of the pituitary—anterior or posterior—is neural tissue, similar to the hypothalamus? Which part is glandular tissue and produces hormones that control the secretions by other endocrine organs?
20. In what way is a neuropeptide intermediate between neurotransmitters and hormones?

ANSWERS

19. The posterior pituitary is neural tissue, like the hypothalamus. The anterior pituitary is glandular tissue and produces hormones that control several other endocrine organs. **20.** Ordinary neurotransmitters are released in small amounts close to their receptors. Neuropeptides are released into a brain area in larger amounts or not at all. When released, they diffuse more widely. Hormones are released into the blood for diffuse delivery throughout the body.

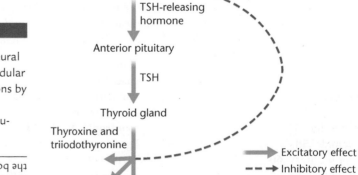

Figure 2.23 **Negative feedback in the control of thyroid hormones**
The hypothalamus secretes a releasing hormone that stimulates the anterior pituitary to release TSH, which stimulates the thyroid gland to release its hormones. Those hormones, in turn, act on the hypothalamus to decrease its secretion of the releasing hormone.

Module 2.2 | In Closing

Neurotransmitters and Behavior

In the century-plus since Sherrington, we have come a long way in our understanding of synapses. We no longer think of synapses as simple on/off messages. Synaptic messages vary in intensity, speed of onset, and duration. Drugs can modify them in many ways, for good or bad, but so can experiences. Understanding how the nervous system produces our behavior and experiences is largely a matter of understanding synapses.

Summary

1. The great majority of synapses operate by transmitting a chemical neurotransmitter from the presynaptic cell to the postsynaptic cell. Otto Loewi demonstrated chemical transmission by stimulating a frog's heart electrically and then transferring fluids from that heart to another frog's heart. **50**

2. Many chemicals are used as neurotransmitters. Most are amino acids or chemicals derived from amino acids. **52**

3. An action potential opens calcium channels in the axon terminal, and the calcium enables release of neurotransmitters. **53**

4. At ionotropic synapses, a neurotransmitter attaches to a receptor that opens the gates to allow a particular ion, such as sodium, to cross the membrane. Ionotropic effects are fast and brief. Most excitatory ionotropic synapses use glutamate, and most inhibitory ionotropic synapses use GABA. **54**

5. At metabotropic synapses, a neurotransmitter activates a second messenger inside the postsynaptic cell, leading to slower but longer-lasting changes. **55**

6. Neuropeptides diffuse widely, affecting many neurons for a period of minutes. Neuropeptides are important for hunger, thirst, and other slow, long-term processes. **55**

7. Several drugs including LSD, antipsychotic drugs, nicotine, and opiate drugs exert their behavioral effects by binding to receptors on the postsynaptic neuron. **56**

8. After a neurotransmitter (other than a neuropeptide) has activated its receptor, many of the transmitter molecules reenter the presynaptic cell through transporter molecules in the membrane. This process, known as reuptake, enables the presynaptic cell to recycle its neurotransmitter. Stimulant drugs and many antidepressant drugs inhibit reuptake of certain transmitters. **57**

9. Postsynaptic neurons send chemicals to receptors on the presynaptic neuron to inhibit further release of neurotransmitter. Cannabinoids, found in marijuana, mimic these chemicals. **58**

10. Hormones travel through the blood, affecting receptors in many organs. Their mechanism of effect resembles that of a metabotropic synapse. **59**

Key Terms

Terms are defined in the module on the page number indicated. They are also presented in alphabetical order with definitions in the book's Subject Index/Glossary, which begins on page 589. Interactive flash cards, audio reviews, and crossword puzzles are among the online resources available to help you learn these terms and the concepts they represent.

2-AG **58**
acetylcholine **52**
acetylcholinesterase **57**
amino acids **52**
amphetamine **57**
anandamide **58**
anterior pituitary **60**
autoreceptors **58**
cannabinoids **58**
catecholamines **52**
cocaine **57**
COMT **57**
endocrine glands **59**
exocytosis **53**
gap junction **59**

G protein **55**
gases **52**
hallucinogenic drugs **56**
hormone **59**
ionotropic effects **54**
ligand-gated channels **54**
MAO **53**
metabotropic effects **55**
methylphenidate **57**
monoamines **52**
neuromodulators **55**
neuropeptides **52**
neurotransmitters **52**
nicotine **56**
nitric oxide **52**

opiate drugs **56**
oxytocin **60**
peptide hormones **59**
pituitary gland **60**
posterior pituitary **60**
protein hormones **59**
purines **52**
releasing hormones **60**
reuptake **57**
second messenger **55**
transmitter-gated channels **54**
transporters **57**
vasopressin **60**
vesicles **53**

Thought Questions

1. Suppose axon A enters a ganglion (cluster of neurons) and axon B leaves on the other side. Shortly after an experimenter stimulates A, an impulse travels down B. We want to know whether B is just an extension of axon A or whether A formed an excitatory synapse on some neuron in the ganglion, whose axon is axon B. How could an experimenter determine the answer? Try to think of more than one good method. Presume that the anatomy within the ganglion is so complex that you cannot simply observe the course of an axon through it.

2. If incoming serotonin axons were destroyed, LSD would still have its full effects. However, if incoming dopamine axons were destroyed, amphetamine and cocaine would lose their effects. Explain the difference.

Module 2.2 | End of Module Quiz

1. Loewi's evidence for chemical transmission at a synapse used observations of what?

   A. Electrical potentials across a membrane
   B. Heart rate in frogs
   C. Chemical analysis of fluids in the brain
   D. Reflexes in dogs

2. Which of the following is NOT one of the brain's neurotransmitters?

   A. Glutamate
   B. GABA
   C. Glucose
   D. Serotonin

3. Which of these is a catecholamine?

   A. GABA
   B. Glutamate
   C. Acetylcholine
   D. Dopamine

4. What does MAO (monoamine oxidase) do in the brain?

   A. It stimulates certain types of serotonin receptors.
   B. It sends a message to the presynaptic neuron to decrease its firing rate.
   C. It converts catecholamine transmitters into inactive chemicals.
   D. It blocks the reuptake of certain neurotransmitters.

5. Suppose you want to cause the presynaptic terminal of an axon to release its transmitter. How could you do so *without* an action potential?

   A. Decrease the temperature at the synapse.
   B. Use an electrode to produce IPSPs in the postsynaptic neuron.
   C. Inject water into the presynaptic terminal.
   D. Inject calcium into the presynaptic terminal.

6. Which type of synapse is better suited for vision and hearing, and why?

   A. Metabotropic synapses because they produce quick, brief effects
   B. Metabotropic synapses because they produce longer-lasting effects
   C. Ionotropic synapses because they produce quick, brief effects
   D. Ionotropic synapses because they produce longer-lasting effects

7. What is the most abundant excitatory ionotropic neurotransmitter?

   A. Dopamine
   B. Serotonin
   C. Glutamate
   D. GABA

8. What is a second messenger?

   A. A chemical released by the presynaptic neuron a few milliseconds after release of the first neurotransmitter
   B. A chemical released inside a cell after stimulation at a metabotropic synapse
   C. A chemical that travels from the postsynaptic neuron back to the presynaptic neuron
   D. A neuropeptide that affects all neurons in a given area

9. Which of the following is true of neuropeptides?

   A. They produce effects that last for minutes.
   B. They are chemically similar to the genes on a chromosome.
   C. They are released close to their receptors.
   D. They are released from the tip of an axon.

10. How does LSD exert its effects on the nervous system?

A. It attaches to serotonin receptors.

B. It blocks reuptake of serotonin.

C. Neurons convert it to dopamine.

D. It tells the presynaptic neuron to stop releasing its transmitter.

11. The serotonin transporter is responsible for which of these processes?

A. Exocytosis

B. Reuptake

C. Inhibition

D. Synthesis

12. Except for the magnitude and speed of effects, methylphenidate (Ritalin) affects synapses the same way as which other drug?

A. Heroin

B. Cocaine

C. Nicotine

D. Marijuana

13. In what way do cannabinoids differ from other drugs that affect the nervous system?

A. Cannabinoids produce their effects in only one brain area.

B. Cannabinoids act without attaching to any receptor.

C. Cannabinoids act on the presynaptic neuron.

D. Cannabinoids travel through the blood from one brain area to another.

14. Electrical synapses are important when the nervous system needs to accomplish which of the following?

A. Inhibition of competing behaviors

B. Synchrony between neurons

C. Complex reasoning

D. Long-lasting activation

15. Which of these is composed of neural tissue, as opposed to glandular tissue?

A. The anterior pituitary

B. The posterior pituitary

C. The pancreas

D. The adrenal gland

16. In what way is a neuropeptide intermediate between neurotransmitters and hormones?

A. A neuropeptide diffuses more widely than other neurotransmitters but less than a hormone.

B. A neuropeptide is larger than other neurotransmitters but smaller than a hormone.

C. A neurotransmitter produces excitatory effects, a neuropeptide produces neutral effects, and a hormone produces negative effects.

D. A neurotransmitter produces slow effects, a neuropeptide produces faster effects, and a hormone produces still faster effects.

Answers: 1B, 2C, 3D, 4C, 5D, 6C, 7C, 8B, 9A, 10A, 11B, 12B, 13C, 14B, 15B, 16A.

Suggestion for Further Reading

Berkowitz, A. (2016). *Governing behavior: How nerve cell dictatorships and democracies control everything we do.* Cambridge, MA: Harvard University Press. Discusses many examples illustrating how synaptic connections decide between one course of action and another.

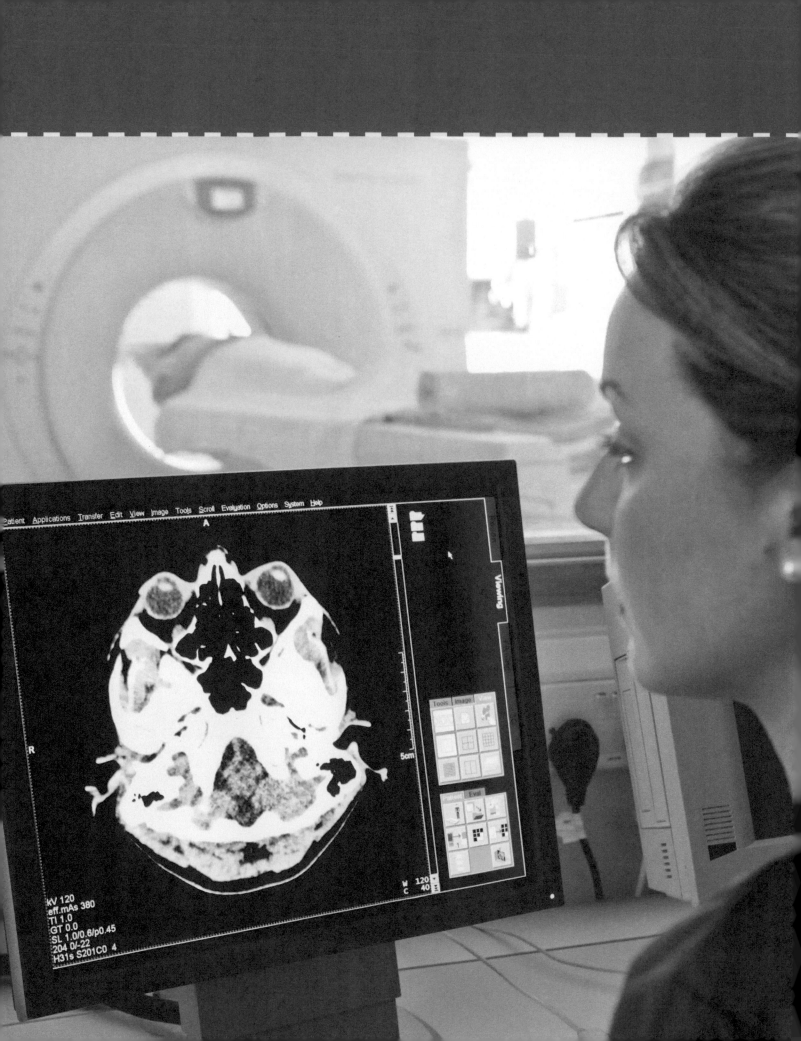

Anatomy and Research Methods

Chapter 3

Trying to learn **neuroanatomy** (the anatomy of the nervous system) from a book is like trying to learn geography from a road map. A map can tell you that Mystic, Georgia, is about 40 km north of Enigma, Georgia. Similarly, a book can tell you that the habenula is about 4.6 mm from the interpeduncular nucleus in a rat's brain (proportionately farther in a human brain). But these little gems of information will seem both mysterious and enigmatic unless you are interested in that part of Georgia or that area of the brain.

This chapter does not provide a detailed road map of the nervous system. It is more like a world globe, describing the large, basic structures, analogous to the continents, and some distinctive features of each.

The first module introduces key neuroanatomical terms and outlines overall structures of the nervous system. In the second module, we concentrate on the cerebral cortex, the largest part of the mammalian central nervous system. The third module deals with the main methods that researchers use to discover the functions of brain areas.

Be prepared: This chapter contains a huge number of new terms. You should not expect to memorize all of them at once, and you should review this chapter repeatedly.

Learning Objectives

After studying this chapter, you should be able to:

1. Define the terms used to describe brain anatomy.
2. Describe the principal functions of certain brain areas.
3. List the four lobes of the cerebral cortex and name their principal functions.
4. Describe the binding problem and explain its theoretical importance.
5. Cite examples of several methods for studying the relationship between brain activity and behavior.

Opposite:
New methods allow researchers to examine living brains. (Dorsal view of brain)
(Source: Jupiter Images/Getty Images)

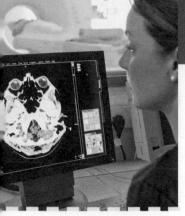

Module 3.1

Structure of the Vertebrate Nervous System

Your nervous system includes a huge number of neurons, and an even huger number of synapses. How do all the parts work together to make one behaving unit? Does each neuron have a unique function? Or does the brain operate as an undifferentiated whole?

The answer is something between those extremes. Consider an analogy to human society: Each individual has a specialty, such as teacher, farmer, or nurse, but no one performs any function without the cooperation of many other people. Similarly, brain areas and neurons have specialized functions, but they perform those roles by means of connections with other areas.

Terminology to Describe the Nervous System

For vertebrates, we distinguish the central nervous system from the peripheral nervous system (see Figure 3.1). The **central nervous system (CNS)** is the brain and the spinal cord. The **peripheral nervous system (PNS)** connects the brain and spinal

Figure 3.1 The human nervous system
The central nervous system consists of the brain and spinal cord. The peripheral nervous system is the nerves outside the brain and spinal cord.

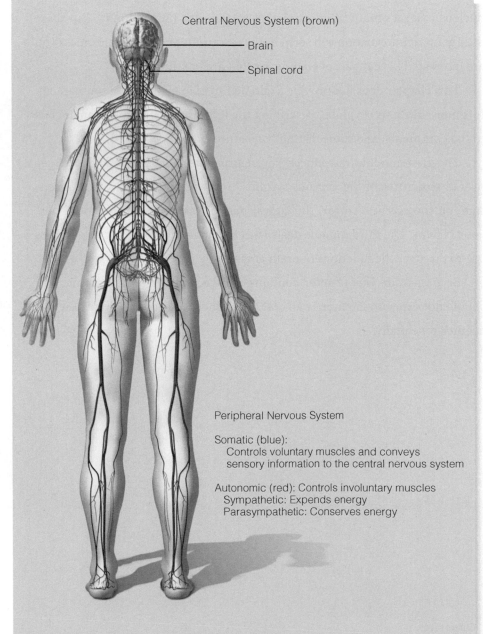

Central Nervous System (brown)
— Brain
— Spinal cord

Peripheral Nervous System

Somatic (blue):
   Controls voluntary muscles and conveys sensory information to the central nervous system

Autonomic (red): Controls involuntary muscles
   Sympathetic: Expends energy
   Parasympathetic: Conserves energy

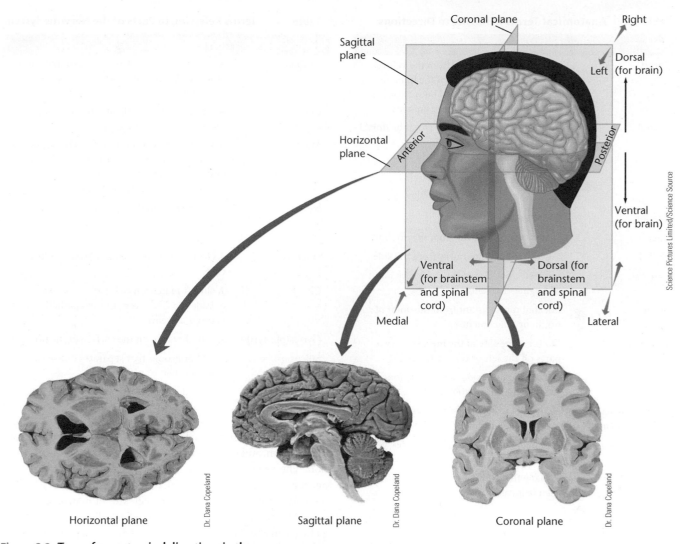

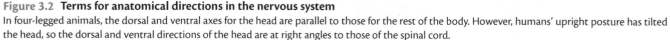

Figure 3.2 Terms for anatomical directions in the nervous system
In four-legged animals, the dorsal and ventral axes for the head are parallel to those for the rest of the body. However, humans' upright posture has tilted the head, so the dorsal and ventral directions of the head are at right angles to those of the spinal cord.

cord to the rest of the body. Part of the PNS is the **somatic nervous system,** which consists of the axons conveying messages from the sense organs to the CNS and from the CNS to the muscles. Another part of the PNS, the **autonomic nervous system,** controls the heart, intestines, and other organs. The autonomic nervous system has some of its cell bodies within the brain or spinal cord and some in clusters along the sides of the spinal cord.

To follow a map, you must understand *north, south, east,* and *west.* Because the nervous system is three-dimensional, we need more terms to describe it. As Figure 3.2 and Table 3.1 indicate, **dorsal** means toward the back and **ventral** means toward the stomach. (A *ventri*loquist is literally a "stomach talker.") In a four-legged animal, the top of the brain is dorsal (on the same side as the animal's back),

and the bottom of the brain is ventral (on the stomach side). The same would be true for you if you crawled on your hands and knees. However, when humans evolved upright posture, the position of the head changed relative to the spinal cord. For convenience, we still apply the terms *dorsal* and *ventral* to the same parts of the human brain as other vertebrate brains. Consequently, the dorsal–ventral axis of the human brain is at a right angle to the dorsal–ventral axis of the spinal cord. Figure 3.2 also illustrates the three ways of taking a plane through the brain, known as horizontal, sagittal, and coronal (or frontal).

Table 3.2 introduces additional terms that are worth learning. Tables 3.1 and 3.2 require careful study and review. After you think you have mastered the terms, check yourself with the following "Stop & Check" questions.

Table 3.1 | Anatomical Terms Referring to Directions

Term	Definition
Dorsal	Toward the back, away from the ventral (stomach) side. The top of the human brain is considered dorsal because it has that position in four-legged animals.
Ventral	Toward the stomach, away from the dorsal (back) side
Anterior	Toward the front end
Posterior	Toward the rear end
Superior	Above another part
Inferior	Below another part
Lateral	Toward the side, away from the midline
Medial	Toward the midline, away from the side
Proximal	Located close (approximate) to the point of origin or attachment
Distal	Located more distant from the point of origin or attachment
Ipsilateral	On the same side of the body (e.g., two parts on the left or two on the right)
Contralateral	On the opposite side of the body (one on the left and one on the right)
Coronal plane (or frontal plane)	A plane that shows brain structures as seen from the front
Sagittal plane	A plane that shows brain structures as seen from the side
Horizontal plane (or transverse plane)	A plane that shows brain structures as seen from above

Table 3.2 | Terms Referring to Parts of the Nervous System

Term	Definition
Lamina	A row or layer of cell bodies separated from other cell bodies by a layer of axons and dendrites
Column	A set of cells perpendicular to the surface of the cortex, with similar properties
Tract	A set of axons within the CNS, also known as a *projection*. If axons extend from cell bodies in structure A to synapses onto B, we say that the fibers "project" from A onto B.
Nerve	A set of axons in the periphery, either from the CNS to a muscle or gland or from a sensory organ to the CNS
Nucleus	A cluster of neuron cell bodies within the CNS
Ganglion	A cluster of neuron cell bodies, usually outside the CNS (as in the sympathetic nervous system)
Gyrus (pl.: gyri)	A protuberance on the surface of the brain
Sulcus (pl.: sulci)	A fold or groove that separates one gyrus from another
Fissure	A long, deep sulcus

was that the entering dorsal roots (axon bundles) carry sensory information, and the exiting ventral roots carry motor information. The cell bodies of the sensory neurons are in clusters of neurons outside the spinal cord, called the **dorsal root ganglia.** (*Ganglia* is the plural of *ganglion,* a cluster of neurons. In most cases, a neuron cluster outside the CNS is called a ganglion, and a cluster inside the CNS is called a nucleus.) Cell bodies of the motor neurons are inside the spinal cord.

In the cross section through the spinal cord shown in Figures 3.4 and 3.5, the H-shaped **gray matter** in the center

STOP & CHECK

1. What does *ventral* mean, and what is its opposite?
2. What term means *toward the midline*, and what is its opposite?
3. If two structures are both on the left side of the body, they are _____ to each other. If one is on the left and the other is on the right, they are _____ to each other.
4. The bulges in the cerebral cortex are called _____. The grooves between them are called ____.

ANSWERS 1. Ventral means toward the stomach side. Its opposite is dorsal. 2. medial; lateral 3. ipsilateral; contralateral 4. gyri; sulci. To remember sulcus, think of the word sulk, meaning "to pout" (and therefore lie low).

The Spinal Cord

The **spinal cord** is the part of the CNS within the spinal column. The spinal cord communicates with all the sense organs and muscles except those of the head. It is a segmented structure, and each segment has on both the left and right sides a sensory nerve and a motor nerve, as Figure 3.3 shows. One of the earliest discoveries about the functions of the nervous system

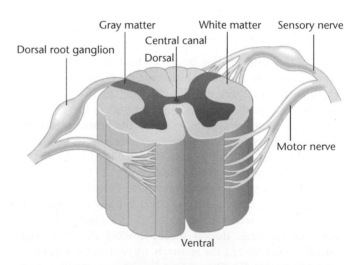

Gray matter　　White matter　　Sensory nerve

Dorsal root ganglion　　Central canal

Dorsal

Motor nerve

Ventral

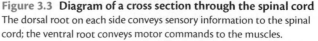

Figure 3.3　Diagram of a cross section through the spinal cord
The dorsal root on each side conveys sensory information to the spinal cord; the ventral root conveys motor commands to the muscles.

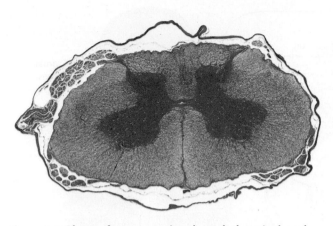

Figure 3.4 **Photo of a cross section through the spinal cord**
The H-shaped structure in the center is gray matter, composed largely of cell bodies. The surrounding white matter consists of axons.
(Source: Dr. Keith Wheeler/Science Source)

of the cord is densely packed with cell bodies and dendrites. Many neurons from the gray matter of the spinal cord send axons to the brain or to other parts of the spinal cord through the **white matter,** containing myelinated axons.

Each segment of the spinal cord sends sensory information to the brain and receives motor commands from the brain. All that information passes through tracts of axons in the spinal cord. If the spinal cord is cut at a given segment, the brain loses sensation from that segment and below. The brain also loses motor control over all parts of the body served by that segment and the lower ones.

The Autonomic Nervous System

The autonomic nervous system consists of neurons that receive information from and send commands to the heart, intestines, and other organs. Its two parts are the sympathetic

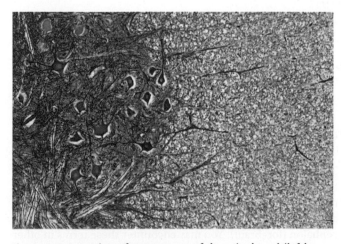

Figure 3.5 **A section of gray matter of the spinal cord (left) and white matter surrounding it**
Cell bodies and dendrites reside entirely in the gray matter. Axons travel from one area of gray matter to another in the white matter.
(Source: Ed Reschke/Photolibrary/Getty Images)

and parasympathetic nervous systems (see Figure 3.6). The **sympathetic nervous system,** a network of nerves that prepare the organs for a burst of vigorous activity, consists of chains of ganglia just to the left and right of the spinal cord's central regions (the thoracic and lumbar areas). These ganglia have connections back and forth with the spinal cord. Sympathetic axons prepare the organs for "fight or flight," such as by increasing breathing and heart rate and decreasing digestive activity. Because the sympathetic ganglia are closely linked, they often act as a single system "in sympathy" with one another, although certain events activate some parts more than others. The sweat glands, the adrenal glands, the muscles that constrict blood vessels, and the muscles that erect the hairs of the skin have sympathetic input but no parasympathetic input.

The **parasympathetic nervous system**, sometimes called the "rest and digest" system, facilitates vegetative, nonemergency responses. The term *para* means "beside" or "related to," and parasympathetic activities are related to, and generally the opposite of, sympathetic activities. For example, the sympathetic nervous system increases heart rate, and the parasympathetic nervous system decreases it. The parasympathetic nervous system increases digestive activity, whereas the sympathetic nervous system decreases it. The parasympathetic system also promotes sexual arousal, including erection in males. Although the sympathetic and parasympathetic systems produce contrary effects, both are constantly active to varying degrees, and many stimuli arouse parts of both systems.

The parasympathetic nervous system is also known as the craniosacral system because it consists of the cranial nerves and nerves from the sacral spinal cord (see Figure 3.6). Unlike the ganglia in the sympathetic system, the parasympathetic ganglia are not arranged in a chain near the spinal cord. Rather, long *preganglionic* axons extend from the spinal cord to parasympathetic ganglia close to each internal organ. Shorter *postganglionic* fibers then extend from the parasympathetic ganglia into the organs themselves. Because the parasympathetic ganglia are not linked to one another, they act more independently than the sympathetic ganglia do. Parasympathetic activity decreases heart rate, increases digestive rate, and in general, conserves energy.

The parasympathetic nervous system's axons release the neurotransmitter acetylcholine onto the organs. Most sympathetic nervous system axons release norepinephrine, although a few, such as those onto the sweat glands, use acetylcholine. Because the two systems use different transmitters, certain drugs excite or inhibit one system or the other. For example, over-the-counter cold remedies exert most of their effects by blocking parasympathetic activity or increasing sympathetic activity. Because the flow of sinus fluids is a parasympathetic response, drugs that block the parasympathetic system inhibit sinus flow. The side effects of cold remedies stem from their pro-sympathetic, anti-parasympathetic activities: They increase heart rate, blood pressure, and arousal. They inhibit salivation and digestion. Certain decongestant pills containing pseudoephedrine have been withdrawn or restricted because of their potential for abuse.

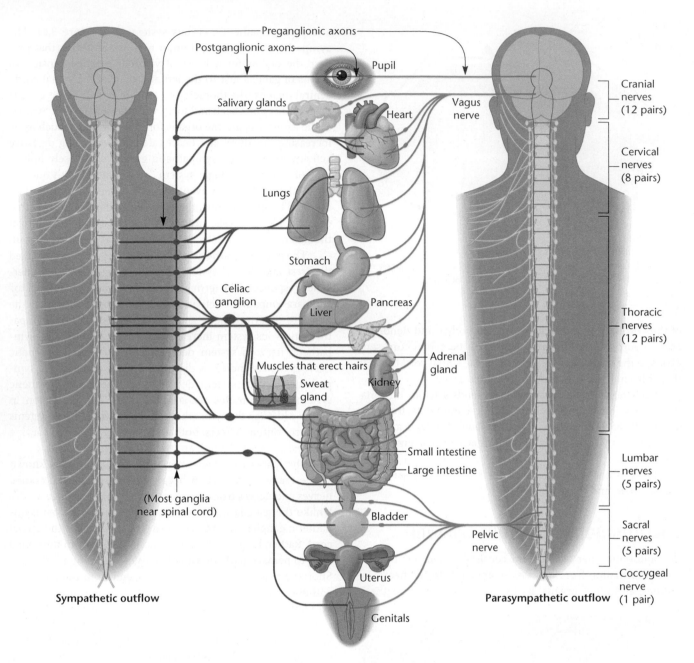

Figure 3.6 **The sympathetic nervous system (red lines) and parasympathetic nervous system (blue lines)**
Note that the adrenal glands, sweat glands, and hair erector muscles receive sympathetic input only.
(*Source: Starr & Taggart, 1989*)

✓ STOP & CHECK

5. Motor nerves leave from which side of the spinal cord, dorsal or ventral?
6. Which functions are controlled by the sympathetic nervous system? Which are controlled by the parasympathetic nervous system?

ANSWERS

5. Ventral. 6. The sympathetic nervous system prepares the organs for vigorous fight-or-flight activity. The parasympathetic system increases vegetative responses such as digestion.

The Hindbrain

The brain has three major divisions—the hindbrain, the midbrain, and the forebrain (see Figure 3.7 and Table 3.3). Some neuroscientists prefer terms with Greek roots: rhombencephalon (hindbrain), mesencephalon (midbrain), and prosencephalon (forebrain). You may encounter these terms in other reading.

The **hindbrain,** the posterior part of the brain, consists of the medulla, the pons, and the cerebellum. The medulla and pons, the midbrain, and certain central structures of the forebrain constitute the **brainstem** (see Figure 3.8).

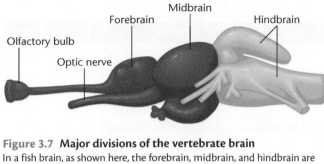

Figure 3.7 Major divisions of the vertebrate brain
In a fish brain, as shown here, the forebrain, midbrain, and hindbrain are clearly visible as separate bulges. In adult mammals, the forebrain grows and surrounds the entire midbrain and part of the hindbrain.

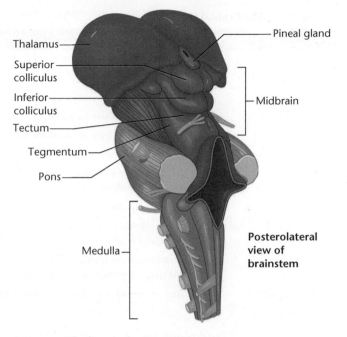

Figure 3.8 The human brainstem
This composite structure extends from the top of the spinal cord into the center of the forebrain. The cerebral cortex surrounds the thalamus, pineal gland, and midbrain.

The **medulla,** or medulla oblongata, can be regarded as an enlarged extension of the spinal cord. Just as the lower parts of the body connect to the spinal cord via sensory and motor nerves, the head and the organs connect to the medulla and adjacent areas by 12 pairs of **cranial nerves** (one of each pair on the right side and one on the left), as shown in Table 3.4 and Figure 3.9. The cranial nerves originating in the medulla control vital reflexes such as breathing, heart rate, vomiting, salivation, coughing, and sneezing. Because opiate receptors, which suppress activity, are abundant in the medulla, opiates can produce a dangerous decrease in breathing and heart rate.

The **pons** lies anterior and ventral to the medulla. Like the medulla, it contains nuclei for several cranial nerves. The term *pons* is Latin for "bridge," reflecting the fact that in the pons, axons from each half of the brain cross to the opposite side of the spinal cord so that the left hemisphere controls the muscles of the right side of the body and the right hemisphere controls the left side.

The **cerebellum** is a large hindbrain structure with many deep folds. It has long been known for its contributions to the control of movement, and many older textbooks describe the cerebellum as important for "balance and coordination." True, people with cerebellar damage are clumsy and lose their balance, but the functions of the cerebellum extend far beyond balance and coordination. People with damage to the cerebellum have trouble shifting their attention back and forth between auditory and visual stimuli (Courchesne et al., 1994). They have difficulty with timing, such as judging whether one rhythm is faster than another. The cerebellum is also critical for certain types of learning and conditioning.

The Midbrain

As the name implies, early in development the **midbrain** is in the middle of the brain, although in adult mammals it is dwarfed and surrounded by the forebrain. The midbrain is more prominent in reptiles, amphibians, and fish. The roof of the midbrain is called the **tectum.** (*Tectum* is the Latin word for "roof." The same root occurs in the geological term *plate tectonics.*) The swellings on each side of the tectum are the **superior colliculus** and the **inferior colliculus** (see Figures 3.8 and 3.10). Both are important for sensory processing—the inferior colliculus for hearing and the superior colliculus for vision.

Under the tectum lies the **tegmentum,** the intermediate level of the midbrain. (In Latin, *tegmentum* means a "covering," such as a rug on the floor. The tectum covers the tegmentum, but the tegmentum covers several other midbrain structures.) Another midbrain structure, the **substantia nigra,** gives rise to a dopamine-containing

Table 3.3 | Major Divisions of the Vertebrate Brain

Area	Also Known as	Major Structures
Forebrain	Prosencephalon ("forward-brain")	
	Diencephalon ("between-brain")	Thalamus, hypothalamus
	Telencephalon ("end-brain")	Cerebral cortex, hippocampus, basal ganglia
Midbrain	Mesencephalon ("middle-brain")	Tectum, tegmentum, superior colliculus, inferior colliculus, substantia nigra
Hindbrain	Rhombencephalon (literally, "parallelogram-brain")	Medulla, pons, cerebellum

Table 3.4 | The Cranial Nerves

Number and Name	Major Functions
I. Olfactory	Smell
II. Optic	Vision
III. Oculomotor	Control of eye movements; pupil constriction
IV. Trochlear	Control of eye movements
V. Trigeminal	Skin sensations from most of the face; control of jaw muscles for chewing and swallowing
VI. Abducens	Control of eye movements
VII. Facial	Taste from the anterior two thirds of the tongue; control of facial expressions, crying, salivation, and dilation of the head's blood vessels
VIII. Statoacoustic	Hearing; equilibrium
IX. Glossopharyngeal	Taste and other sensations from throat and posterior third of the tongue; control of swallowing, salivation, throat movements during speech
X. Vagus	Sensations from neck and thorax; control of throat, esophagus, and larynx; parasympathetic nerves to stomach, intestines, and other organs
XI. Accessory	Control of neck and shoulder movements
XII. Hypoglossal	Control of muscles of the tongue

Cranial nerves III, IV, and VI are coded in red to highlight their similarity: control of eye movements. Cranial nerves VII, IX, and XII are coded in green to highlight their similarity: taste and control of tongue and throat movements. Cranial nerve VII has other important functions as well. Nerve X (not highlighted) also contributes to throat movements, although it is primarily known for other functions.

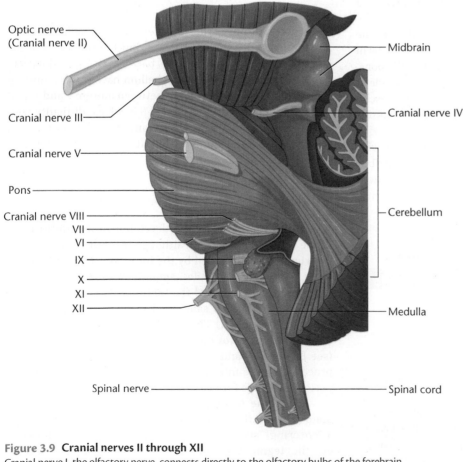

Figure 3.9 Cranial nerves II through XII
Cranial nerve I, the olfactory nerve, connects directly to the olfactory bulbs of the forebrain.
(Source: Based on Braus, 1960)

pathway that facilitates readiness for movement.

The Forebrain

The **forebrain**, the most prominent part of the mammalian brain, consists of two cerebral hemispheres, one on the left and one on the right (see Figure 3.11). Each hemisphere is organized to receive sensory information, mostly from the contralateral (opposite) side of the body. It controls muscles, mostly on the contralateral side, by way of axons to the spinal cord and the cranial nerve nuclei.

The outer portion is the cerebral cortex. (*Cerebrum* is a Latin word for "brain." *Cortex* is a Latin word for "bark" or "shell.") Under the cerebral cortex are other structures, including the thalamus and the basal ganglia. Several interlinked structures, known as the **limbic system**, form a border (or *limbus*, the Latin word for "border") around the brainstem. The limbic system includes the olfactory bulb, hypothalamus, hippocampus, amygdala, and cingulate

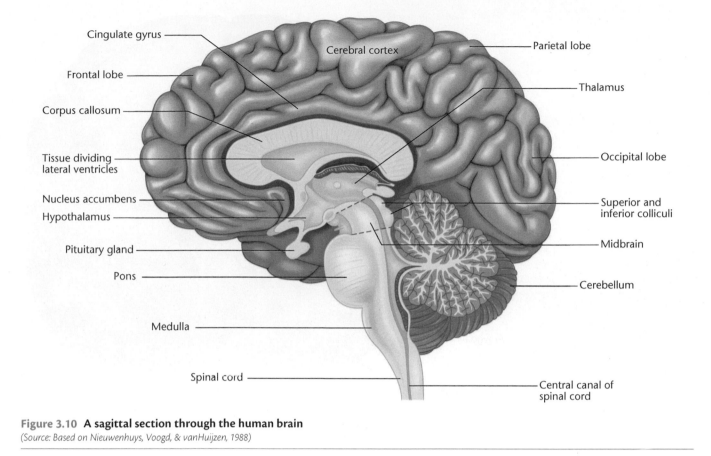

Figure 3.10 A sagittal section through the human brain
(*Source: Based on Nieuwenhuys, Voogd, & vanHuijzen, 1988*)

gyrus of the cerebral cortex. The hypothalamus is essential for control of eating, drinking, temperature control, and reproductive behaviors. The **amygdala** is part of the circuit that is most central for evaluating emotional information, especially with regard to fear. Figure 3.12 shows the positions of these structures in three-dimensional perspective. Figures 3.13 and 3.10 show coronal (from the front) and sagittal (from the side) sections through the human brain.

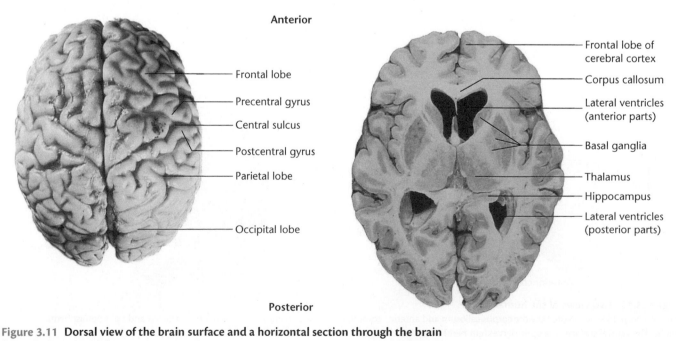

Figure 3.11 Dorsal view of the brain surface and a horizontal section through the brain
(*Source: Dr. Dana Copeland*)

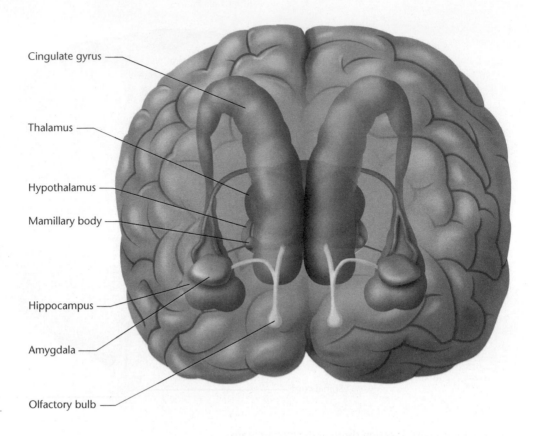

Figure 3.12 The limbic system is a set of subcortical structures that form a border (or limbus) around the brainstem.

Figure 3.13 also includes a view of the ventral surface of the brain.

In describing the forebrain, let's begin with the subcortical areas. The next module focuses on the cerebral cortex. Later chapters discuss certain areas in more detail as they become relevant.

Thalamus

The thalamus and hypothalamus form the *diencephalon,* a section distinct from the *telencephalon,* which is the rest of the forebrain. The **thalamus** is a pair of structures (left and right) in the center of the forebrain. The term derives from a

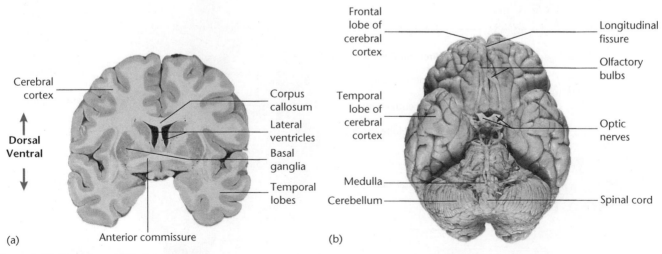

Figure 3.13 Two views of the human brain
Left: A coronal section. Note how the corpus callosum and anterior commissure provide communication between the left and right hemispheres.
Right: The ventral surface. The optic nerves (cut here) extend to the eyes.
(Source: Dr. Dana Copeland)

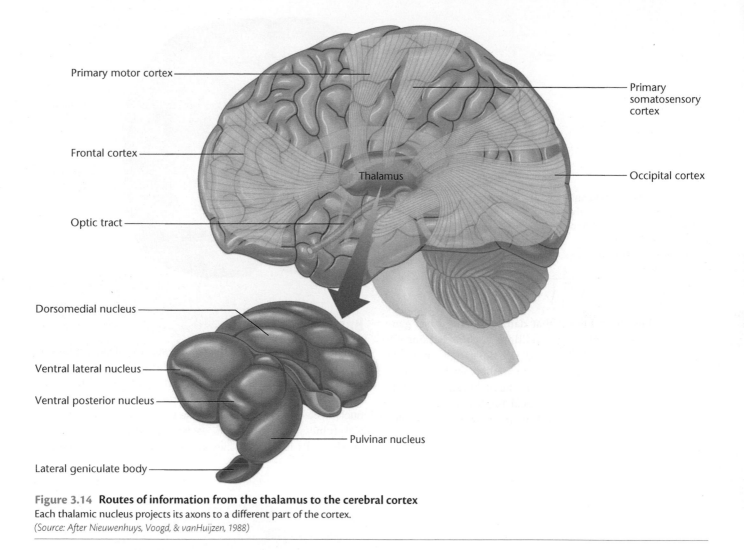

Primary motor cortex

Frontal cortex

Optic tract

Thalamus

Primary somatosensory cortex

Occipital cortex

Dorsomedial nucleus

Ventral lateral nucleus

Ventral posterior nucleus

Pulvinar nucleus

Lateral geniculate body

Figure 3.14 **Routes of information from the thalamus to the cerebral cortex**
Each thalamic nucleus projects its axons to a different part of the cortex.
(*Source: After Nieuwenhuys, Voogd, & vanHuijzen, 1988*)

Greek word meaning "anteroom," "inner chamber," or "bridal bed." It resembles two small avocados joined side by side, one in the left hemisphere and one in the right. Most sensory information goes first to the thalamus, which processes it and sends output to the cerebral cortex. An exception to this rule is olfactory information, which goes from the olfactory receptors to the olfactory bulbs and then directly to the cerebral cortex.

Many nuclei of the thalamus receive their input from a sensory system, such as vision, and transmit information to a single area of the cerebral cortex, as in Figure 3.14. The cerebral cortex sends information back to the thalamus, prolonging and magnifying certain kinds of input and focusing attention on particular stimuli (Komura et al., 2001).

Hypothalamus and Pituitary Gland

The **hypothalamus**, a small area near the base of the brain just ventral to the thalamus (see Figures 3.10 and 3.12), has widespread connections with the rest of the brain. The hypothalamus contains distinct nuclei, which we examine in the chapters on motivation and emotion. Partly through nerves and partly by releasing hormones, the hypothalamus conveys messages to the pituitary gland, altering its release of hormones. Damage to any hypothalamic nucleus leads to abnormalities in motivated behaviors, such as feeding, drinking, temperature regulation, sexual behavior, fighting, or activity level. Because of these important behavioral effects, the small hypothalamus attracts much research attention.

The **pituitary gland** is an endocrine (hormone-producing) gland attached to the base of the hypothalamus (see Figure 3.10). In response to messages from the hypothalamus, the pituitary synthesizes hormones that the blood carries to organs throughout the body.

Basal Ganglia

The **basal ganglia,** a group of subcortical structures lateral to the thalamus, include three major structures: the caudate nucleus, the putamen, and the globus pallidus (see Figure 3.15). Some authorities include other structures as well.

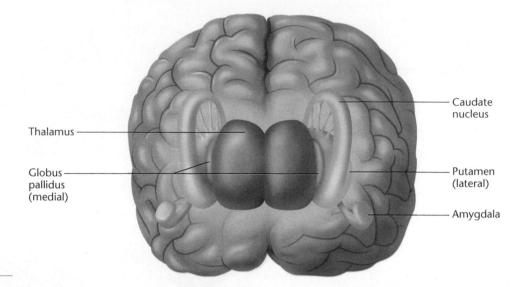

Thalamus

Globus pallidus (medial)

Caudate nucleus

Putamen (lateral)

Amygdala

Figure 3.15 The basal ganglia
The thalamus is in the center, the basal ganglia are lateral to it, and the cerebral cortex is on the outside.
(*Source: Based on Nieuwenhuys, Voogd, & vanHuijzen, 1988*)

It has long been known that damage to the basal ganglia impairs movement, as in conditions such as Parkinson's disease and Huntington's disease. The basal ganglia integrate motivational and emotional behavior to increase the vigor of selected actions. However, the role of the basal ganglia extends beyond movement. They are critical for learned skills and habits, as well as other types of learning that develop gradually with extended experience. We return to the basal ganglia in more detail in the chapters on movement and memory.

Basal Forebrain

One of the structures on the ventral surface of the forebrain, the **nucleus basalis,** receives input from the hypothalamus and basal ganglia and sends axons that release acetylcholine to widespread areas in the cerebral cortex (see Figure 3.16). The nucleus basalis is a key part of the brain's system for arousal, wakefulness, and attention, as we consider in the chapter on sleep. Patients with Parkinson's disease and Alzheimer's

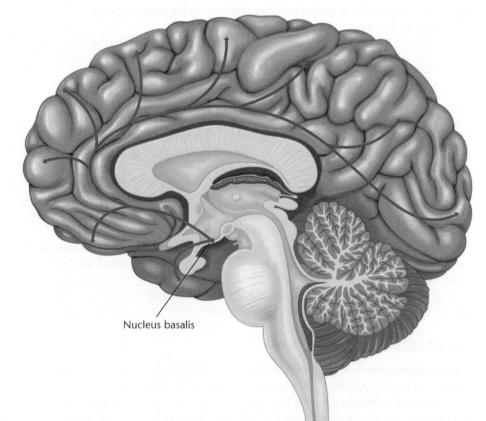

Nucleus basalis

Figure 3.16 The basal forebrain
The nucleus basalis and other structures in this area send axons throughout the cortex, increasing its arousal and wakefulness through release of the neurotransmitter acetylcholine.
(*Source: Based on Woolf, 1991*)

disease have impairments of attention and intellect because of inactivity or deterioration of their nucleus basalis.

Hippocampus

The **hippocampus** (from the Latin word meaning "sea horse," a shape suggested by the hippocampus) is a large structure between the thalamus and the cerebral cortex, mostly toward the posterior of the forebrain, as shown in Figure 3.12. We consider the hippocampus in more detail in the chapter on memory. The gist of that discussion is that the hippocampus is critical for certain types of memories, especially memories for individual events. It is also essential for monitoring where you are and where you are going.

✓ STOP & CHECK ▬▬▬▬

7. Of the following, which are in the hindbrain, which in the midbrain, and which in the forebrain: basal ganglia, cerebellum, hippocampus, hypothalamus, medulla, pituitary gland, pons, substantia nigra, superior and inferior colliculi, tectum, tegmentum, thalamus?
8. Which area is the main source of input to the cerebral cortex?

ANSWERS   **8.** Thalamus. hypothalamus, pituitary, and thalamus. and tegmentum. Forebrain: basal ganglia, hippocampus, substantia nigra, superior and inferior colliculi, tectum, **7.** Hindbrain: cerebellum, medulla, and pons. Midbrain:

The Ventricles

The nervous system begins its development as a tube surrounding a fluid canal. The canal persists into adulthood as the central canal in the center of the spinal cord, and as the **ventricles,** four fluid-filled cavities within the brain. Each hemisphere contains one of the two large lateral ventricles (see Figure 3.17). Toward their posterior, they connect to the third ventricle, positioned at the midline, separating the left thalamus from the right thalamus. The third ventricle connects to the fourth ventricle in the center of the medulla.

Cells called the *choroid plexus* along the walls of the four ventricles produce **cerebrospinal fluid (CSF)**, a clear fluid similar to blood plasma. CSF fills the ventricles, flowing from the lateral ventricles to the third and fourth ventricles. From the fourth ventricle, some of it flows into the central canal of the spinal cord, but more goes into the narrow spaces between the brain and the thin **meninges,** membranes that surround the brain and spinal cord. In one of those narrow spaces, the subarachnoid space, the blood gradually reabsorbs the CSF. Although the brain has no pain receptors, the meninges do, and meningitis—inflammation of the meninges—is painful. Swollen blood vessels in the meninges are responsible for the pain of a migraine headache (Hargreaves, 2007).

Cerebrospinal fluid cushions the brain against mechanical shock when the head moves. It also provides buoyancy. Just as a person weighs less in water than on land, cerebrospinal fluid

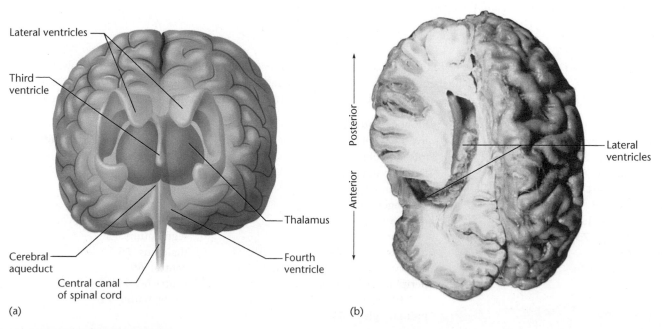

Figure 3.17 The cerebral ventricles
(a) Diagram showing positions of the four ventricles. **(b)** Photo of a human brain, viewed from above, with a horizontal cut through one hemisphere to show the position of the lateral ventricles.
(Source: Photo courtesy of Dr. Dana Copeland)

helps support the weight of the brain. It also provides a reservoir of hormones and nutrition for the brain and spinal cord.

If the flow of CSF is obstructed, it accumulates within the ventricles or in the subarachnoid space, increasing pressure on the brain. When this occurs in infants, the skull bones spread, causing an overgrown head. This condition, known as *hydrocephalus* (HI-dro-SEFF-ah-luss), can lead to mental retardation, although the results vary from one person to another.

Module 3.1 | In Closing

Learning Neuroanatomy

The brain is a complex structure. This module has introduced a great many terms and facts. Do not be discouraged if you have trouble remembering them. It will help to return to this module to review anatomy as you encounter structures again in later chapters. Gradually, the material will become more familiar.

Summary

1. The vertebrate nervous system has two main divisions, the central nervous system and the peripheral nervous system. **68**

2. Each segment of the spinal cord has a sensory nerve and a motor nerve on both the left and right sides. Spinal pathways convey information to the brain. **70**

3. The sympathetic nervous system (one of the two divisions of the autonomic nervous system) activates the body's internal organs for vigorous activities. The parasympathetic system (the other division) promotes digestion and other nonemergency processes. **71**

4. The central nervous system consists of the spinal cord, the hindbrain, the midbrain, and the forebrain. **72**

5. The hindbrain consists of the medulla, pons, and cerebellum. The medulla and pons control breathing, heart rate, and other vital functions through the cranial nerves. The cerebellum contributes to movement, timing short intervals, and certain types of learning and conditioning. **72**

6. The cerebral cortex receives its sensory information, except for olfaction, from the thalamus. **76**

7. The subcortical areas of the forebrain include the thalamus, hypothalamus, pituitary gland, basal ganglia, and hippocampus. **76**

8. The cerebral ventricles contain fluid that provides buoyancy and cushioning for the brain. **79**

Key Terms

Terms are defined in the module on the page number indicated. They're also presented in alphabetical order with definitions in the book's Subject Index/Glossary, which begins on page 589. Interactive flash cards, audio reviews, and crossword puzzles are among the online resources available to help you learn these terms and the concepts they represent.

amygdala **75**

autonomic nervous system **69**

basal ganglia **77**

brainstem **72**

central nervous system **68**

cerebellum **73**

cerebrospinal fluid (CSF) **79**

cranial nerves **73**

dorsal **69**

dorsal root ganglia **70**

forebrain **74**

gray matter **70**

hindbrain **72**

hippocampus **79**

hypothalamus **77**

inferior colliculus **73**

limbic system **74**

medulla **73**

meninges **79**

midbrain **73**

neuroanatomy **67**

nucleus basalis **78**

parasympathetic nervous system **71**

peripheral nervous system (PNS) **68**

pituitary gland **77**

pons **73**

somatic nervous system **69**

spinal cord **70**

substantia nigra **73**

superior colliculus **73**

sympathetic nervous system **71**

tectum **73**

tegmentum **73**

thalamus **76**

ventral **69**

ventricles **79**

white matter **71**

Thought Question

Being nervous interferes with sexual arousal. Explain why, with reference to the sympathetic and parasympathetic nervous systems.

Module 3.1 | End of Module Quiz

1. What does *ventral* mean?

    A. Toward the side
    B. Toward the front

    C. Toward the stomach
    D. Toward the head

2. If two structures are both on the left side, or both on the right, what is their relationship?

    A. Medial
    B. Ventral

    C. Ipsilateral
    D. Contralateral

3. What is a *sulcus* in the brain?

    A. A groove that separates one gyrus from another
    B. A fluid-filled cavity

    C. A set of axons from one brain structure to another
    D. A temporary decrease in activity

4. What is the function of the dorsal roots of the spinal cord?

    A. They receive sensory input.
    B. They control motor output.

    C. They convey information from the brain to the spinal cord.
    D. They convey information from the spinal cord to the brain.

5. What does the parasympathetic nervous system control?

    A. Fight-or-flight activities
    B. Vegetative activities

    C. Social behavior
    D. Learned habits

6. Which of these controls breathing, heart rate, and salivation?

    A. The hippocampus
    B. The cranial nerves

    C. The basal ganglia
    D. The pituitary gland

7. Which of these is part of the forebrain?

    A. Hippocampus
    B. Medulla

    C. Pons
    D. Cerebellum

8. Which structure provides most of the direct input to the cerebral cortex?

    A. Cranial nerves
    B. Medulla

    C. Thalamus
    D. Pineal gland

9. What do the ventricles contain?

    A. Densely packed neuron cell bodies
    B. Glia

    C. Cerebrospinal fluid
    D. Long axons

Answers: 1C, 2C, 3A, 4A, 5B, 6B, 7A, 8C, 9C.

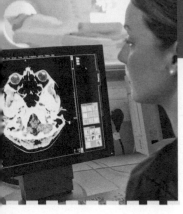

The Cerebral Cortex

The most prominent part of the mammalian brain is the **cerebral cortex**. The cells on the outer surface of the cerebral cortex are gray matter, and their axons extending inward are white matter (see Figure 3.13a). Neurons in each hemisphere communicate with neurons in the corresponding part of the other hemisphere through two bundles of axons, the **corpus callosum** (see Figures 3.10, 3.11, and 3.13) and the smaller **anterior commissure** (see Figure 3.13). Several other commissures (pathways across the midline) link subcortical structures.

The basic organization of the cerebral cortex is remarkably similar across vertebrate species (Harris & Shepherd, 2015). The visual cortex is in the same place, the auditory cortex is in the same place, and so forth. However, brains vary enormously in size. The largest mammalian brains are 100,000 times larger than the smallest ones (Herculano-Houzel, 2011).

If we compare mammalian species, we see differences in the size of the cerebral cortex and the degree of folding (see Figure 3.18). Compared to other mammals of comparable size, the **primates**—monkeys, apes, and humans—have a larger cerebral cortex, more folding, and more neurons per unit of volume (Herculano-Houzel, 2011). Larger animals, such as elephants, have larger brain size but also larger neurons and fewer neurons per unit of volume. Humans have almost three times as many neurons in the cerebral cortex as elephants

have, although the elephant brain is more than twice as large (Herculano-Houzel et al., 2015). In Figure 3.19, the investigators arranged the insectivores and primates from left to right in terms of what percentage of their brain was devoted to the forebrain, including the cerebral cortex (Clark, Mitra, & Wang, 2001). They also inserted tree shrews, a species often considered intermediate between insectivores and primates. Note that as the proportion devoted to the forebrain increases, the relative sizes of the midbrain and medulla decrease. That is, humans and other primates have a larger cerebral cortex than other species do, in proportion to the rest of the brain.

Curiously, the cerebellum occupies a nearly constant percentage—about 10 to 14 percent of the brain in most species (Herculano-Houzel et al., 2015). Most species have about four (mostly tiny) neurons in the cerebellum for every one in the cerebral cortex (Herculano-Houzel, 2011). Why? Good question. Elephants, however, have a much larger number of neurons in the cerebellum, proportional to the rest of the brain (Herculano-Houzel et al., 2015). Why? Another good question.

Organization of the Cerebral Cortex

The microscopic structure of the cells of the cerebral cortex varies from one cortical area to another, as does the density of neurons per volume (Collins, 2011). Much research has

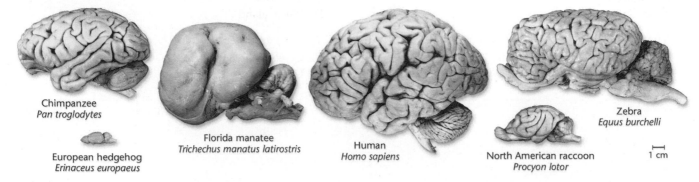

Chimpanzee
Pan troglodytes

European hedgehog
Erinaceus europaeus

Florida manatee
Trichechus manatus latirostris

Human
Homo sapiens

North American raccoon
Procyon lotor

Zebra
Equus burchelli

1 cm

Figure 3.18 Comparison of mammalian brains
All mammals have the same brain subareas in the same locations.
(*Source: From the University of Wisconsin-Madison Comparative Mammalian Brain Collection, Wally Welker, Curator. Project supported by the National Science Foundation*)

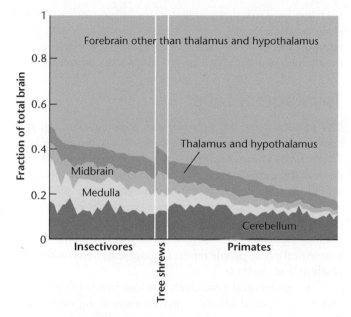

Figure 3.19 Relative sizes of five brain components in insectivores and primates
The forebrain composes a larger percentage of primate than insectivore brains. Note also the nearly constant fraction devoted to the cerebellum.
(*Source: Figure 1, p. 189, from "Scalable architecture in mammalian brains," by D. A. Clark, P. P. Mitra, & S. S-H. Wang, 2001, Nature, 411, pp. 189–193. Reprinted with permission from Nature. Copyright © 2001 Macmillan Magazine Limited.*)

laminae vary in thickness and prominence from one part of the cortex to another, and a given lamina may be absent from certain areas. Lamina V, which sends long axons to the spinal cord and other distant areas, is thickest in the motor cortex, which has the greatest control of the muscles. Lamina IV, which receives axons from the sensory nuclei of the thalamus, is prominent in the sensory areas of the cortex (visual, auditory, and somatosensory) but absent from the motor cortex.

The cells of the cortex are also organized into **columns** of cells perpendicular to the laminae. Figure 3.21 illustrates the idea of columns, although in nature they are not so straight. The cells within a given column have similar properties to one another. For example, if one cell in a column responds to touch on the palm of the left hand, then the other cells in that column do, too. If one cell responds to a horizontal pattern of light at a particular location, then other cells in the column respond to the same pattern in nearby locations.

We now turn to specific parts of the cortex. Researchers make fine distinctions among areas of the cerebral cortex based on the structure and function of cells. For convenience, we group these areas into four *lobes* named for the skull bones that lie over them: occipital, parietal, temporal, and frontal.

been directed toward understanding the relationship between structure and function.

In humans and most other mammals, the cerebral cortex contains up to six distinct **laminae,** layers of cell bodies that are parallel to the surface of the cortex and separated from each other by layers of fibers (see Figure 3.20). The

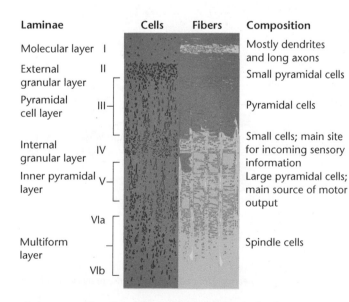

Figure 3.20 The six laminae of the human cerebral cortex
(*Source: Adapted from Ranson & Clark, 1959*)

Figure 3.21 Columns in the cerebral cortex
Each column extends through several laminae. Neurons within a given column have similar properties. For example, in the somatosensory cortex, all the neurons within a given column respond to stimulation of the same area of skin.

9. If several neurons of the visual cortex all respond best when the retina is exposed to horizontal lines of light, then those neurons are probably in the same _____.

ANSWER   ˙column ·6

The Occipital Lobe

The **occipital lobe**, at the posterior (caudal) end of the cortex (see Figure 3.22), is the main target for visual information. The posterior pole of the occipital lobe is known as the *primary visual cortex,* or *striate cortex,* because of its striped appearance in cross section. Destruction of any part of the striate cortex causes *cortical blindness* in the related part of the visual field. For example, extensive damage to the striate cortex of the right hemisphere causes blindness in the left visual field (that is, the left side of the world from the viewer's perspective). A person with cortical blindness has normal eyes and pupillary reflexes, but no conscious visual perception and no visual imagery (not even in dreams). People who suffer eye damage become blind, but if they have an intact occipital cortex and previous visual experience, they can still imagine visual scenes and can still have visual dreams (Sabo & Kirtley, 1982). In short, the eyes provide the stimulus, and the visual cortex provides the experience.

The Parietal Lobe

The **parietal lobe** lies between the occipital lobe and the **central sulcus**, a deep groove in the surface of the cortex (see Figure 3.23). The area just posterior to the central sulcus, the **postcentral gyrus**, or *primary somatosensory cortex,* receives sensations from touch receptors, muscle-stretch receptors, and joint receptors. Brain surgeons sometimes use only local anesthesia—that is, anesthetizing the scalp but leaving the brain awake. If during this process they lightly stimulate the postcentral gyrus, people report tingling sensations on the opposite side of the body.

The postcentral gyrus includes four bands of cells parallel to the central sulcus. Separate areas along each band receive simultaneous information from different parts of the body, as shown in Figure 3.23a (Nicolelis et al., 1998). Two of the bands receive mostly light-touch information, one receives deep-pressure information, and one receives a combination of both (Kaas, Nelson, Sur, Lin, & Merzenich,

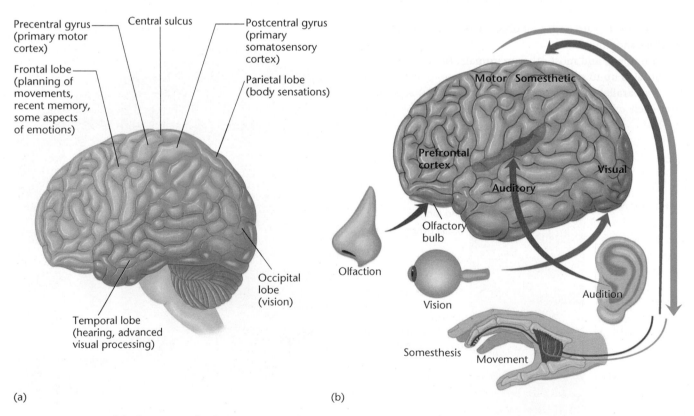

(a)   (b)

Figure 3.22 Areas of the human cerebral cortex
(a) The four lobes: occipital, parietal, temporal, and frontal. **(b)** The primary sensory cortex for vision, hearing, and body sensations; the primary motor cortex; and the olfactory bulb, responsible for the sense of smell.
(Source for part b: Deacon, 1990)

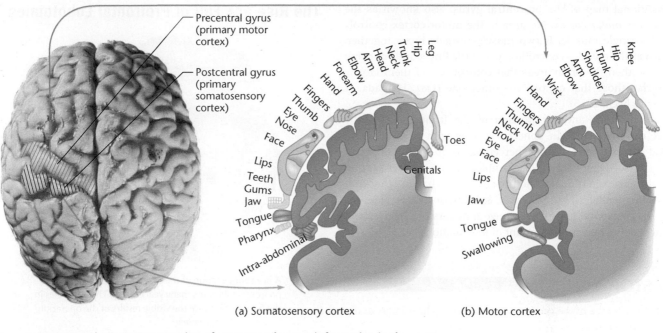

Figure 3.23 Approximate representation of sensory and motor information in the cortex
(a) Each location in the somatosensory cortex represents sensation from a different body part. **(b)** Each location in the motor cortex regulates movement of a different body part.
(*Source: Based on Penfield & Rasmussen, 1950*)

1979). In effect, the postcentral gyrus represents the body four times.

Information about touch and body location is important not only for its own sake but also for interpreting visual and auditory information. For example, if you see something in the upper-left portion of the visual field, your brain needs to know which direction your eyes are turned, the position of your head, and the tilt of your body before it can determine the location of whatever you see. The parietal lobe monitors all the information about eye, head, and body positions and passes it on to brain areas that control movement. The parietal lobe is essential not only for spatial information but also numerical information (Hubbard, Piazza, Pinel, & Dehaene, 2005). That overlap makes sense when you consider all the ways in which numbers relate to space—including the fact that we initially use our fingers to count.

The Temporal Lobe

The **temporal lobe** is the lateral portion of each hemisphere, near the temples (see Figure 3.22). It is the primary cortical target for auditory information. The human temporal lobe—in most cases, the left temporal lobe—is essential for understanding spoken language. The temporal lobe also contributes to complex aspects of vision, including perception of movement and recognition of faces. A tumor in the temporal lobe may give rise to elaborate auditory or visual hallucinations, whereas a tumor in the occipital lobe

ordinarily evokes only simple sensations, such as flashes of light. When psychiatric patients report hallucinations, brain scans detect much activity in the temporal lobes (Dierks et al., 1999).

The temporal lobes are also important for emotional and motivational behaviors. Temporal lobe damage can lead to a set of behaviors known as the **Klüver-Bucy syndrome** (named for the investigators who first described it). Previously wild and aggressive monkeys fail to display normal fears and anxieties after temporal lobe damage (Klüver & Bucy, 1939). They put almost anything they find into their mouths and attempt to pick up snakes and lighted matches (which intact monkeys consistently avoid). Interpreting this behavior is difficult. For example, a monkey might handle a snake because it is no longer afraid (an emotional change) or because it no longer recognizes what a snake is (a cognitive change). We explore these issues in the chapter on emotion.

The Frontal Lobe

The **frontal lobe**, containing the primary motor cortex and the prefrontal cortex, extends from the central sulcus to the anterior limit of the brain (see Figure 3.22). The posterior portion of the frontal lobe, the **precentral gyrus**, is specialized for the control of fine movements, such as moving a finger. Separate areas are responsible for different parts of the body, mostly on the contralateral (opposite) side but also with slight control of the ipsilateral (same) side. Figure 3.23b shows the traditional map of the precentral gyrus, also known as the *primary motor cortex*. No area in the motor cortex controls just a single muscle. If two muscles usually move together, such as the muscles controlling your little finger and your ring finger, then the brain areas that control one of them largely overlap those that control the other one (Ejaz, Hamada, & Diedrichsen, 2015).

The most anterior portion of the frontal lobe is the **prefrontal cortex**. In general, species with a larger cerebral cortex devote a larger percentage of it to the prefrontal cortex (see Figure 3.24). For example, it forms a larger portion of the cortex in humans and the great apes than in other species (Semendeferi, Lu, Schenker, & Damasio, 2002). Neurons in the prefrontal cortex have huge numbers of synapses and integrate an enormous amount of information.

✓ STOP & CHECK

10. Which lobe of the cerebral cortex includes the primary auditory cortex?
11. Which lobe of the cerebral cortex includes the primary somatosensory cortex?
12. Which lobe of the cerebral cortex includes the primary visual cortex?
13. Which lobe of the cerebral cortex includes the primary motor cortex?

ANSWERS

10. Temporal lobe 11. Parietal lobe 12. Occipital lobe 13. Frontal lobe

The Rise and Fall of Prefrontal Lobotomies

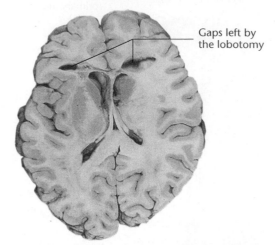

A horizontal section of the brain of a person who had a prefrontal lobotomy many years earlier. The two holes in the frontal cortex are the visible results of the operation. *(Source: Dr. Dana Copeland)*

You probably have heard of the infamous procedure known as **prefrontal lobotomy**—surgical disconnection of the prefrontal cortex from the rest of the brain. The surgery consisted of damaging the prefrontal cortex or cutting its connections to the rest of the cortex. Lobotomy began with a report that damaging the prefrontal cortex of laboratory primates made them tamer without noticeably impairing their sensations or coordination. A few physicians reasoned loosely (!) that the

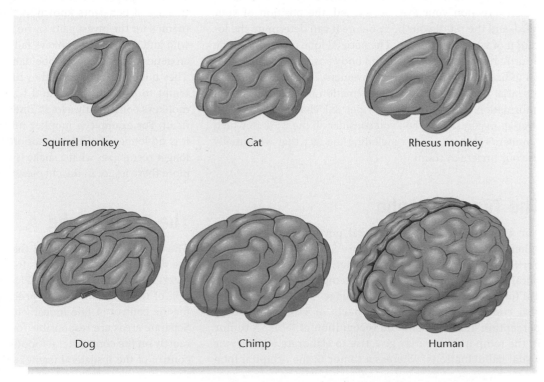

Figure 3.24 Species differences in prefrontal cortex Note that the prefrontal cortex (blue area) constitutes a larger proportion of the human brain than of these other species. *(Source: Based on Fuster, 1989)*

same operation might help people who suffered from severe, untreatable psychiatric disorders.

In the late 1940s and early 1950s, at a time when legal and ethical restraints in medicine were lax, about 40,000 prefrontal lobotomies were performed in the United States (Shutts, 1982), many of them by Walter Freeman, a medical doctor untrained in surgery. His techniques were crude, even by the standards of the time, using such instruments as an electric drill and a metal pick. He performed many operations in his office or other nonhospital sites. (Freeman carried his equipment in his car, which he called his "lobotomobile.")

At first, Freeman and others limited the technique to people with severe schizophrenia, for which no effective treatment was available at the time. Later, Freeman lobotomized people with less serious disorders, including some people whom we would consider normal by today's standards. After drug therapies became available in the mid-1950s, lobotomies quickly dropped out of favor.

Among the common consequences of prefrontal lobotomy were apathy, a loss of the ability to plan and take initiative, memory disorders, distractibility, and a loss of emotional expressions (Stuss & Benson, 1984). People with prefrontal damage lost their social inhibitions, ignoring the rules of polite, civilized conduct. They often acted impulsively because they failed to calculate adequately the probable outcomes of their behaviors.

Functions of the Prefrontal Cortex

An analysis of thousands of studies concluded that the prefrontal cortex has three major regions (de la Vega, Chang, Banich, Wager, & Yarkoni, 2016). The posterior portion is associated mostly with movement. The middle zone pertains to working memory, cognitive control, and emotional reactions. Working memory is the ability to remember recent events, such as where you parked your car or what you were talking about before an interruption. People with damage to the prefrontal cortex have trouble on the **delayed-response task,** in which they see or hear something, and then have to respond to it after a delay.

The anterior zone of the prefrontal cortex is important for making decisions, evaluating which of several courses of action is likely to achieve the best outcome. When you decide whether to do something, you consider the difficulty of the action, the probabilities of success and failure, and how valuable the possible reward would be to you, all things considered. For example, the chance to win a pizza becomes less valuable if you have just finished a meal. An opportunity to win a few extra-credit points is valuable if you think you are on the borderline between two grades, but less valuable otherwise. If you have a choice between spending money now and saving it for later, you try to compare the possibility of current pleasure and the possible need for money later. Cells in the prefrontal cortex respond to all these complex factors (Hunt et al., 2012; Wallis, 2012). People with prefrontal cortical damage often make decisions that seem impulsive, because they failed to weigh all the likely pros and cons.

14. What are the functions of the prefrontal cortex?

ANSWER

14. The posterior portion contributes to control of movement. The middle portion pertains to working memory, cognitive control, and emotion. The anterior portion compares various types of information for making a decision.

How Do the Parts Work Together?

Here is a theoretical issue that researchers hardly even considered before about 1990: How do various brain areas combine to produce a unified experience? When you eat something, you experience the smell in the nose, and the taste and touch on the tongue as a single experience (Stevenson, 2014). If you shake something that makes a noise, you perceive that what you see is also what you feel and what you hear. But how do you do that? Each of the senses activates a different area of the cortex, and those areas have only weak connections with one another.

The question of how various brain areas produce a perception of a single object is known as the **binding problem,** or *large-scale integration* problem. In an earlier era, researchers thought that various kinds of sensory information converged onto what they called the association areas of the cortex. Their guess was that those areas associate one sensation with another, or current sensations with memories of previous experiences. Later research found that relatively few cells combine one sense with another (Blanke, 2012). Even when they do, they don't fully answer the question of how we bind sensory information together. For example, certain neurons in the posterior temporal cortex both when you see a chain saw and when you hear the sound it makes, or both when you see a jackhammer and when you hear a jackhammer sound (Man, Kaplan, Damasio, & Meyer, 2012). But surely you weren't born knowing what sound a chain saw or a jackhammer makes. Somehow those cells had to develop those properties through experience. Similarly, many neurons in the superior colliculus respond to more than one sensory system, but they constantly change their properties based on experience (Stein, Stanford, & Rowland, 2014).

Although researchers cannot fully explain binding, they know what is necessary for it to occur: It occurs if you perceive two sensations as happening at the same time and in approximately the same place. For example, when a skilled ventriloquist says something and makes the dummy's mouth move at the same time, you perceive the sound as coming from the dummy. As part of this illusion, the visual stimulus alters the response of the auditory cortex, so that the sound really does seem to come from the same location as the dummy's mouth (Bonath et al., 2007; Bruns, Liebnau, & Röder, 2011). In contrast, if you watch a poorly dubbed foreign-language film, the lips do not move at the same time as the speech, and you perceive that the words did *not* come from those lips.

Applying these principles, researchers arranged a camera to video someone's back, and simultaneously sent the pictures to a three-dimensional display mounted to the person's head,

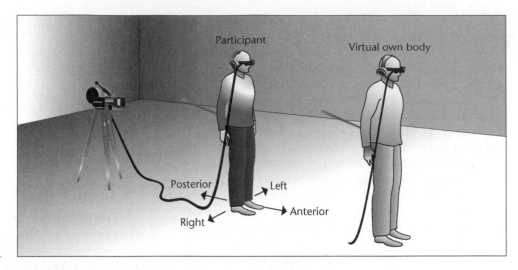

Figure 3.25 Where Am I?
As someone stroked the person's back, a video camera relayed the information so the person could view it, appearing to be a few feet ahead. After a few minutes, the person felt as if the body were in fact a few feet ahead of where it was. *(Source: From "Video ergo sum: Manipulating bodily self-consciousness," by B. Lenggenhager, T. Tadi, T. Metzinger, & O. Blanke, 2007, Science, 317, pp. 1096–1099.)*

as in Figure 3.25. Imagine that you are the participant. As you view the video of your back, it appears to be 2 meters in front of you. Then someone strokes your back. You simultaneously feel the touch and see the action that appears to be 2 meters in front. After a while, you start perceiving your body as being 2 meters in front of you! When asked, "please return to your seat," you walk to a spot displaced from the actual seat, as if you were actually 2 meters forward from your current position (Lenggenhager, Tadi, Metzinger, & Blanke, 2007).

Suppose you see a light flash once while you hear two beeps. You will sometimes think you saw the light flash twice. If the tone is soft, you may experience the opposite: The tone beeps twice during one flash of light, and you think you heard only one beep. If you saw three flashes of light, you might think you heard three beeps (Andersen, Tiippana, & Sams, 2004). The near simultaneity of lights and sounds causes you to bind them and perceive an illusion that alters your perception of one or the other. Binding often fails if the displays are flashed very briefly or while the viewer is distracted (Holcombe & Cavanagh, 2001; Lehky, 2000).

Here is another great demonstration (Robertson, 2005). Position yourself parallel to a large mirror, as in Figure 3.26, so that you see your right hand and its reflection in the mirror. Keep your left hand out of sight. Now repeatedly clench and unclench both hands in unison. Wiggle your fingers, touch your thumb to each finger, and so forth, in each case doing the same thing with both hands at the same time. You will continually feel your left hand doing the same thing you see the hand in the mirror doing, which (being the mirror image of your right hand) looks like your left hand. After 2 or 3 minutes, you may start to feel that the hand in the mirror is your own left hand.

TRY IT YOURSELF

In a variant of this procedure, researchers arranged to touch someone's real right hand and a rubber hand next to it, both at the same time and in the same way, allowing the person to see both hands. Within minutes, people reported feeling that they had two right hands, in addition to the unseen left hand (Guterstam, Petkova, & Ehrsson, 2011). So, the evidence indicates that we bind two experiences that occur at the same time. Still, the theoretical question remains of exactly how we do so.

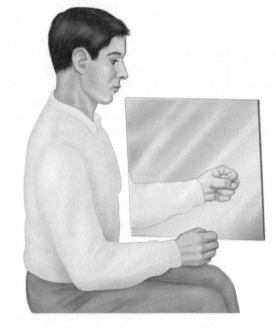

Figure 3.26 An illusion to demonstrate binding
Clench and unclench both hands while looking at your right hand and its reflection in the mirror. Keep your left hand out of sight. After a couple of minutes, you may start to experience the hand in the mirror as being your own left hand.

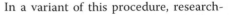

✔ STOP & CHECK

15. What is meant by the binding problem, and what is necessary for binding to occur?

ANSWER

15. The binding problem is the question of how the brain combines activity in different brain areas to produce unified perception and coordinated behavior. Binding requires identifying the location of an object and perceiving sight, sound, and other aspects of a stimulus as being simultaneous. When the sight and sound appear to come from the same location at the same time, we bind them as a single experience.

Functions of the Cerebral Cortex

The cerebral cortex is the largest portion of the human brain, but it is not the entire brain. What is its function? The primary function seems to be one of elaborating sensory information and organizing sequences of behaviors. Even fish, which have no cerebral cortex, can see, hear, and so forth, but the cerebral cortex enables us to add great complexity to our behavior.

Summary

1. Although brain size varies among mammalian species, the overall organization is similar. **82**

2. The cerebral cortex has six laminae (layers) of neurons. A given lamina may be absent from certain parts of the cortex. For example, the lamina responsible for sensory input is absent from the motor cortex. The cortex is organized into columns of cells arranged perpendicular to the laminae. **83**

3. The occipital lobe of the cortex is primarily responsible for vision. Damage to part of the occipital lobe leads to blindness in part of the visual field. **84**

4. The parietal lobe processes body sensations. The postcentral gyrus contains four representations of the body. **84**

5. The temporal lobe contributes to hearing, complex aspects of vision, and processing of emotional information. **85**

6. The frontal lobe includes the precentral gyrus, which controls fine movements. It also includes the prefrontal cortex. **85**

7. The prefrontal cortex is important for planning actions, working memory, certain aspects of emotion, and decision making. **87**

8. The binding problem is the question of how we connect activities in different brain areas, such as sights and sounds. Binding requires perceiving that two aspects of a stimulus (such as sight and sound) occurred at the same place at the same time. **87**

Key Terms

Terms are defined in the module on the page number indicated. They're also presented in alphabetical order with definitions in the book's Subject Index/Glossary, which begins on page 589.

Interactive flash cards, audio reviews, and crossword puzzles are among the online resources available to help you learn these terms and the concepts they represent.

anterior commissure **82**
binding problem **87**
central sulcus **84**
cerebral cortex **82**
columns **83**
corpus callosum **82**

delayed-response task **87**
frontal lobe **85**
Klüver-Bucy syndrome **85**
laminae **83**
occipital lobe **84**
parietal lobe **84**

postcentral gyrus **84**
precentral gyrus **85**
prefrontal cortex **86**
prefrontal lobotomy **86**
primates **82**
temporal lobe **85**

Thought Question

When monkeys with Klüver-Bucy syndrome pick up lighted matches and snakes, we do not know whether they are displaying an emotional deficit or an inability to identify the object. What kind of research method might help answer this question?

Module 3.2 | End of Module Quiz

1. What is the main way in which mammalian species vary in their cerebral cortex?

   A. The locations of visual and auditory cortex vary among species.

   B. Some mammals have a cerebral cortex and some do not.

   C. Brains differ in their size and degree of folding.

   D. The number of laminae varies from 2 to 12.

2. In which of these ways do primates differ from elephants in their cerebral cortex?
    A. Primates have more neurons per unit volume.
    B. Primates have a larger volume of cerebral cortex.
    C. The average size of neurons is greater in primates.
    D. The average length of axons is greater in primates.

3. What is the relationship between columns and laminae in the cerebral cortex?
    A. Each column contains one and only one lamina.
    B. Each column crosses through one lamina after another.
    C. Some parts of the cortex have columns and others have laminae.
    D. A column is just another word for a lamina.

4. Where is the primary visual cortex?
    A. Temporal lobe
    B. Frontal lobe
    C. Parietal lobe
    D. Occipital lobe

5. Where is the primary somatosensory cortex?
    A. Temporal lobe
    B. Frontal lobe
    C. Parietal lobe
    D. Occipital lobe

6. Where is the primary auditory cortex?
    A. Temporal lobe
    B. Frontal lobe
    C. Parietal lobe
    D. Occipital lobe

7. Where is the primary motor cortex?
    A. Temporal lobe
    B. Frontal lobe
    C. Parietal lobe
    D. Occipital lobe

8. The main functions of the prefrontal cortex include which of the following?
    A. Perceiving the location of body parts in space
    B. Providing a pool of immature neurons to replace those damaged in other brain areas
    C. Controlling reflexes
    D. Working memory and weighing the pros and cons of a possible action

9. What is the binding problem?
    A. The difficulty of coordinating the left side of the body with the right side
    B. The difficulty of synchronizing output from a population of axons
    C. The question of how we perceive separate sensations as part of a single object
    D. The question of how a bilingual person shifts from one language to another

Answers: 1C, 2A, 3B, 4D, 5C, 6A, 7B, 8D, 9C.

Research Methods

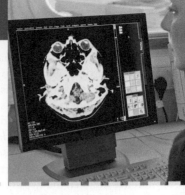

Describing the structure of the brain does not advance our knowledge of biological psychology until we discover how it works. Throughout this text, we shall consider many methods of relating the brain's structure to its function. However, most methods fall into a few categories. This module provides an overview of those categories and the logic behind them:

1. *Examine the effects of brain damage.* After damage or temporary inactivation, what aspects of behavior are impaired?
2. *Examine the effects of stimulating a brain area.* Ideally, if damaging some area impairs a behavior, stimulating that area should enhance the behavior.
3. *Record brain activity during behavior.* We might record changes in brain activity during fighting, sleeping, finding food, solving a problem, or any other behavior.
4. *Correlate brain anatomy with behavior.* Do people with some unusual behavior also have unusual brains? If so, in what way?

Effects of Brain Damage

In 1861, the French neurologist Paul Broca found that a patient who had lost the ability to speak had damage in part of his left frontal cortex. Additional patients with loss of speech also showed damage in and around that area, now known as *Broca's area*. Although much more research was necessary to explore the functions of that area, its discovery revolutionized neurology, as many other physicians at the time had doubted that different brain areas had different functions at all.

Since then, researchers have made countless reports of behavioral impairments after brain damage. Brain damage can produce an inability to recognize faces, an inability to perceive motion, a shift of attention to the right side of the world, changes in motivation and emotion, memory impairments, and a host of other specialized effects. The implications are deep: If you lose part of your brain, you lose part of your mind.

Many of the most interesting results come from humans with brain damage, but human studies have their limitations. Few people have damage confined to just one brain area, and each person's pattern of brain damage is unique. Therefore,

researchers often turn to producing carefully localized damage in laboratory animals. An **ablation** is the removal of a brain area, generally with a surgical knife. Because surgical removal is difficult for tiny structures below the surface of the brain, researchers sometimes make a **lesion**, meaning damage, by means of a **stereotaxic instrument,** a device for the precise placement of electrodes in the brain (see Figure 3.27). By consulting a stereotaxic atlas (map) of a species' brain, a researcher aims an electrode at the desired position relative to landmarks on the skull. The researcher anesthetizes an animal, drills a small hole in the skull, inserts the electrode (insulated except at the tip), lowers it to the target, and passes an electrical current just sufficient to damage that area. For example, researchers have made lesions in parts of the hypothalamus to explore their contributions to eating and drinking. After the death of the animal, someone takes slices of its brain, applies stains, and verifies the actual location of the damage.

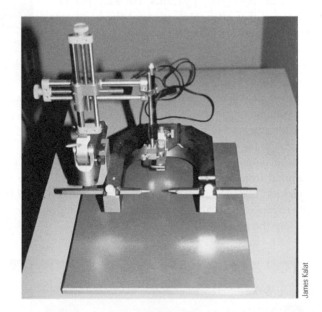

Figure 3.27 A stereotaxic instrument for locating brain areas in small animals
Using this device, researchers can insert an electrode to stimulate, record from, or damage any point in the brain.

Suppose a researcher makes a lesion and reports some behavioral deficit. You might ask, "How do we know the deficit wasn't caused by anesthetizing the animal, drilling a hole in its skull, and lowering an electrode to this target?" To test this possibility, an experimenter produces a *sham lesion* in a control group, performing all the same procedures except for passing the electrical current. Any behavioral difference between the two groups must result from the lesion and not the other procedures.

An electric lesion is a crude technique that damages the axons passing through as well as the neurons in the area itself. Researchers use this method less often today than in the past. Instead, they might inject a chemical that kills neurons, or disables them temporarily, without harming the passing axons. They can also inject a chemical that disables a particular type of synapse. Another option is the *gene-knockout approach* that directs a mutation to a gene that regulates one type of cell, transmitter, or receptor.

Transcranial magnetic stimulation (TMS), the application of magnetic stimulation to a portion of the scalp, can stimulate neurons in the area below the magnet, if the stimulation is sufficiently brief and mild. With stronger stimulation it inactivates the neurons, producing a "virtual lesion" that outlasts the magnetic stimulation itself (Dayan, Censor, Buch, Sandrini, & Cohen, 2013). This procedure enables researchers to study behavior with some brain area active, then inactive, and then active again. Figure 3.28 shows the apparatus. For example, one study found that after TMS silenced the hand area of the motor cortex, people had trouble with a task of mentally rotating the hand in a picture to imagine how it would look from a different angle (Ganis, Keenan, Kosslyn, & Pascual-Leone, 2000). That is, when you imagine seeing your hand from a different angle, you imagine *moving* it, not just seeing it move.

After any kind of brain damage or inactivation, the problem for psychologists is to specify the exact behavioral deficit. For example, if you damage a brain area and the animal stops eating, you don't know why. Did it lose its hunger? Its ability to taste food? Its ability to find the food? Its ability to move at all? You would need further behavioral tests to explore the possibilities.

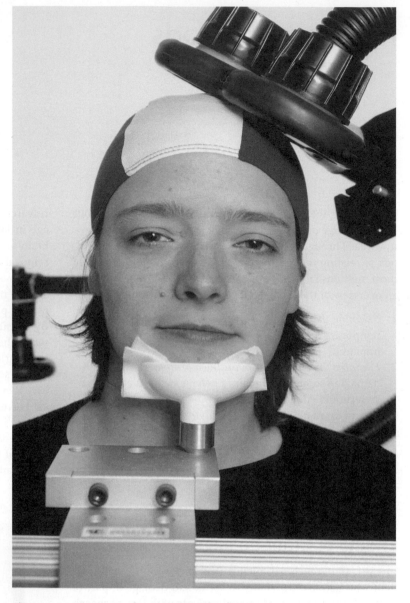

Figure 3.28 Apparatus for magnetic stimulation of a human brain
The procedure is known as transcranial magnetic stimulation, or TMS.
(*BSIP SA/Alamy Stock Photo*)

Effects of Brain Stimulation

If brain damage impairs some behavior, stimulation should increase it. The old-fashioned way is to insert an electrode into an animal's brain and deliver brief, mild currents to stimulate one area or another. That method has limited value, because a given area has many types of neurons with varying functions. The electrical current stimulates all of them, as well as passing axons.

A popular approach today is **optogenetics**, using light to control a limited population of neurons. Development of this method required three steps, each of which would be useless without the others, and each of which seemed almost impossible. Despite the enormous reasons for pessimism, Karl Deisseroth and his colleagues persisted in efforts for years, until the method was ready for wide use in 2009 (Deisseroth, 2015).

✓ STOP & CHECK

16. What is the difference between a lesion and an ablation?

ANSWER

16. A lesion is damage to a structure. An ablation is removal of the structure. For example, a blood clot might produce a lesion, whereas surgery could produce an ablation.

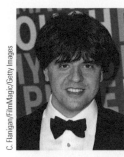

Karl Deisseroth

[A] final point [is] the essential value of exploratory basic science research.... It seems unlikely that the initial experiments described here would have been fundable, as such, by typical grant programs focusing on a disease state.... [T]he advances brought by microbial opsin-based optogenetics may inform the pathophysiology of neurological and psychiatric disease states ... in addition to the broad basic science discoveries. (Deisseroth, 2015, p. 1224)

The first step was to discover or invent a protein that responds to light by producing an electrical current. Certain microbes do produce such proteins, which researchers have found ways to modify. One protein reacts to light by opening a sodium channel, exciting the neuron, and another reacts by opening a chloride channel, producing inhibition. The second step was to develop viruses that insert one of these proteins into a certain type of neuron, or even to just one part of the neuron, such as the axon or the dendrites (Packer, Roska, & Häusser, 2013). The third step was to develop very thin optical fibers that can shine just the right amount of light onto neurons in a narrowly targeted brain area.

Using these methods, an investigator can control the excitation or inhibition of one type of neuron in a small brain area with millisecond accuracy. Thus, researchers can study the function of given cells in greater detail than ever before. A few physicians have begun applying optogenetics to human patients to try to control narcolepsy (a sleep disorder) and other medical or psychiatric conditions.

The success of optogenetics has inspired related methods that can stimulate particular types of neurons by magnetic fields or by chemical injections (Smith, Bucci, Luikart, & Mahler, 2016; Wheeler et al., 2016). These methods activate larger numbers of neurons at one time than optogenetic methods do.

✓ STOP & CHECK

17. What determines whether optogenetic stimulation excites a neuron or inhibits it?

ANSWER

17. Optogenetic stimulation activates a light-sensitive protein. If that protein opens a sodium channel in the membrane, the result is excitation of the neuron. If it opens a chloride channel, the result is inhibition.

Recording Brain Activity

Suppose damage to some brain area impairs a behavior (eating, for example) and stimulation of that area increases the behavior. We can strengthen the conclusion by showing that the area increases its activity during spontaneous occurrences

of the behavior. We might also use brain recordings for exploratory purposes: During a given behavior or cognitive activity, which brain areas increase their activity?

With laboratory animals, one method is to insert an electrode to record activity from a single neuron. We shall consider examples of this method in the chapter on vision. New technologies enable researchers to record from tens to hundreds of neurons simultaneously (Luczak, McNaughton, & Harris, 2015).

On rare occasions, researchers insert an electrode into a human neuron to record its activity, when the brain is exposed preliminary to brain surgery. Much more frequently, human research relies on noninvasive methods—that is, recordings from outside the skull. An **electroencephalograph (EEG)** records electrical activity of the brain through electrodes—ranging from just a few to more than a hundred—attached to the scalp (see Figure 3.29). Electrodes glued to the scalp measure the average activity at any moment for the population of cells under the electrode. The output is then amplified and recorded. An EEG is useful for distinguishing between wakefulness and various stages of sleep. It can also help with the diagnosis of epilepsy, although a physician may need to conduct the test repeatedly or test the person under special conditions before seeing the abnormal EEG pattern that is characteristic of epilepsy (Renzel, Baumann, & Poryazova, 2016; Salinsky, Kanter, & Dasheiff, 1987).

The same device used for an EEG can also record brain activity in response to a stimulus, in which case we call the results **evoked potentials** or **evoked responses**. Evoked responses are useful for many purposes, including studies of infants too young to give verbal answers (Parise & Csibra, 2012).

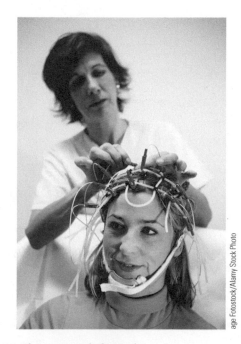

Figure 3.29 Electroencephalography
An electroencephalograph records the overall activity of neurons under various electrodes attached to the scalp.

A **magnetoencephalograph (MEG)** is similar, but instead of measuring electrical activity, it measures the faint magnetic fields generated by brain activity (Hari, 1994). Like EEG, an MEG recording identifies the approximate location of activity to within about a centimeter. An MEG has excellent temporal resolution, showing changes from one millisecond to the next.

Figure 3.30 shows an MEG record of brain responses to a brief tone heard in the right ear. The diagram represents a human head as viewed from above, with the nose at the top (Hari, 1994). Researchers using an MEG can identify the times at which various brain areas respond and thereby trace a wave of brain activity from its point of origin to the other areas that process it (Salmelin, Hari, Lounasmaa, & Sams, 1994).

Positron-emission tomography (PET) provides a high-resolution image of activity in a living brain by recording the emission of radioactivity from injected chemicals. First, the person receives an injection of glucose or some other chemical containing radioactive atoms. Because the most active brain areas increase their use of glucose, tracking the levels of glucose tells us something about brain activity. When a radioactive atom decays, it releases a positron that immediately

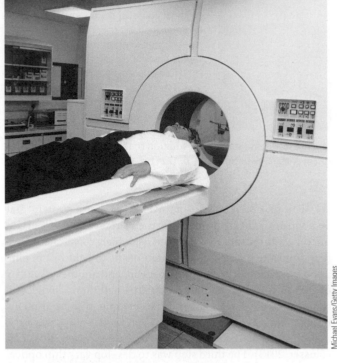

Michael Evans/Getty Images

Figure 3.31 A PET scanner
A person engages in a cognitive task while attached to this apparatus that records which areas of the brain become more active and by how much.

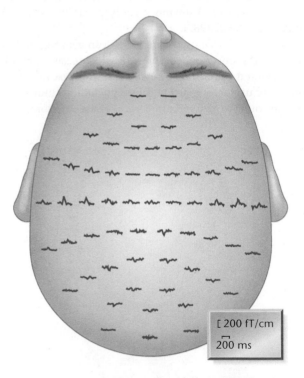

[200 fT/cm
⌐ ⌐
200 ms

Figure 3.30 A result of magnetoencephalography, showing responses to a tone in the right ear
The nose is shown at the top. For each spot on the diagram, the display shows the changing response over a few hundred milliseconds following the tone. (Note calibration at lower right.) The tone evoked responses in many areas, with the largest responses in the temporal cortex, especially on the left side.
(*Source: Reprinted from* Neuroscience: From the Molecular to the Cognitive, *by R. Hari, 1994, p. 165, with kind permission from Elsevier Science—NL, Sara Burgerhartstraat 25, 1055 KV Amsterdam, The Netherlands.*)

collides with a nearby electron, emitting two gamma rays in opposite directions. The person's head is surrounded by a set of gamma ray detectors (see Figure 3.31). When two detectors record gamma rays at the same time, they identify a spot halfway between those detectors as the point of origin of the gamma rays. A computer uses this information to determine how many gamma rays came from each spot in the brain and therefore how much of the radioactive chemical is located in each area (Phelps & Mazziotta, 1985). The areas with the most radioactivity are presumably the ones with the most active neurons.

PET scans use radioactive chemicals with a short half-life, made in a device called a cyclotron. Because cyclotrons are expensive, PET is available only at research hospitals. Furthermore, PET requires exposing the brain to radioactivity, a potential hazard. For most purposes, researchers have replaced PET scans with **functional magnetic resonance imaging (fMRI)**, which is less expensive and less risky. Standard MRI scans record the energy released by water molecules after removal of a magnetic field. (We consider more details about this method later.) An fMRI is a modified version of MRI based on hemoglobin (the blood protein that binds oxygen) instead of water (Detre & Floyd, 2001). Hemoglobin with oxygen reacts to a magnetic field differently from hemoglobin without oxygen. Researchers set the fMRI scanner to detect the amount of hemoglobin with oxygen (Viswanathan & Freeman, 2007). When a brain area becomes more active, two relevant changes occur: First, blood vessels dilate to allow more blood flow to

reading and during a comparison task and then subtract the brain activity during the comparison task to determine which areas are more active during reading. As a comparison task, for example, researchers might ask you to look at a page written in a language you do not understand. That task would activate visual areas just as the reading task did, but it presumably would not activate the language areas of your brain. Figure 3.33 illustrates the idea.

The fMRI method produces spectacular pictures, but difficulties arise when we interpret the results (Rugg & Thompson-Schill, 2013). Researchers often examine the mean results for a group of participants, ignoring important differences among individuals (Finn et al., 2015). More importantly, researchers sometimes make the mistake of assuming that if an area is active during some psychological process, then its activity always indicates that process. For example, certain types of reward activate a brain area called the dorsal striatum (part of the basal ganglia). If the dorsal striatum becomes active while people are doing something, does that activity mean that people find the activity rewarding? Not necessarily, unless we know that the dorsal striatum is active *only* as a function of reward (Poldrack, 2006). Most brain areas participate in several functions.

The best way to test our understanding of fMRI results is to see whether the inference we make from a recording matches what someone is actually doing or thinking. That is, we should be able to use it to read someone's mind, to a limited degree. A few examples of success have been reported. For example, researchers used fMRI to record brain activity from people as they were falling asleep. People typically have

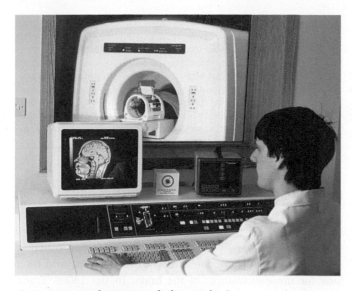

Figure 3.32 An fMRI scan of a human brain
An fMRI produces an image with a spatial resolution of 1 to 2 mm and temporal resolution of about a second.
(*Source: Simon Fraser, Dept. of Neuroradiology, Newcastle General Hosptial/Science Photo Library/Science Source*)

the area. Second, as the brain area uses oxygen, the percentage of hemoglobin with oxygen decreases. An fMRI scan responds to both of these processes (Sirotin, Hillman, Bordier, & Das, 2009). Figure 3.32 shows an example.

An fMRI while you were, for example, reading would mean nothing without a comparison to something else. Researchers would record your brain activity while you were

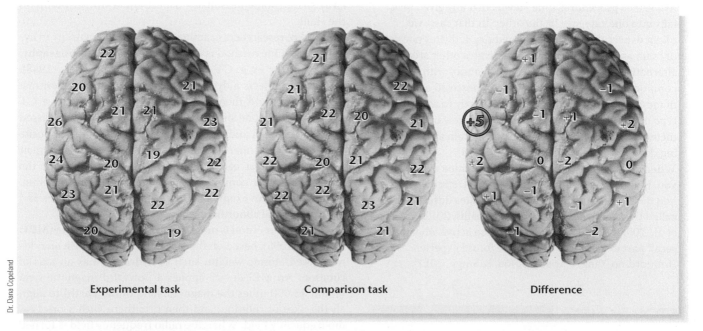

Figure 3.33 Subtraction for a brain scan procedure
Numbers on the brain at the left show hypothetical levels of arousal during some task, measured in arbitrary units. The brain at the center shows activity during the same brain areas during a comparison task. The brain at the right shows the differences. The highlighted area shows the largest difference. In actual data, the largest increases in activity would be one-tenth or two-tenths of a percent.

some visual imagery at that time, but not quite a dream. The researchers repeatedly awakened these people, asked them to report their visual images, and compared the reports to the fMRI data. After enough repetitions, they were able to use the fMRI data to predict approximately what imagery the people were about to report (Horikawa, Tamaki, Miyawaki, & Kamitani, 2013). In another study, people learned to use a mental code to spell out words. For example, if you waited 10 seconds and then performed mental math calculations for 20 seconds, that combination meant the letter M. Using an fMRI, researchers could identify the word the person wanted to express (Sorger, Reithler, Dahmen, & Goebel, 2012). Don't worry. No one could use this method to read your mind without your enthusiastic cooperation. Researchers need to calibrate the equipment over many trials to know what your particular fMRI results mean. The main point is that under limited circumstances, we can indeed use an fMRI to infer someone's psychological processes.

Most fMRI studies have concentrated on identifying the functions of brain areas, rather than contributing to our understanding of psychology (Coltheart, 2013). Nevertheless, fMRI does sometimes provide valuable psychological information. Here are a few examples:

1. Many people in pain report decreased pain after they receive a placebo (a drug with no pharmacological activity). Do they really feel less pain, or are they just saying so? Studies with fMRI show that brain areas responsible for pain really do decrease their response (Wager & Atlas, 2013).
2. Psychologists find it useful to distinguish several types of memory, such as implicit versus explicit and declarative versus procedural. One view is that any given task falls into one category or the other. In that case, we might expect that one type of memory activates one set of brain areas and another type activates other areas. An alternative view is that we process memory with several components, some of which pertain mostly to one type of memory and others that pertain mostly to a different type of memory. The fMRI data fit that view better: Most memory tasks activate a wide array of brain areas to varying degrees (Cabeza & Moscovitch, 2013).
3. When you are just sitting there with nothing expected of you, is your brain really doing nothing? Definitely not. You do "mind wandering," which activates diffuse areas called the brain's *default system* (Corballis, 2012b; Mason et al., 2007). These same areas are also active when people recall past experiences or imagine future experiences (Immordino-Yang, Christodoulou, & Singh, 2012).

STOP & CHECK

18. What does fMRI measure?
19. Suppose someone demonstrates that a particular brain area becomes active when people are listening to music. When that area becomes active later, what if anything can we conclude?

Correlating Brain Anatomy with Behavior

One of the first ways ever used for studying brain function sounds easy: Find someone with unusual behavior and then look for unusual features of the brain. In the 1800s, Franz Gall observed some people with excellent verbal memories who had protruding eyes. He inferred that verbal memory depended on brain areas behind the eyes that had pushed the eyes forward. Gall then examined the skulls of people with other talents or personalities. He assumed that bulges and depressions on their skull corresponded to the brain areas below them. His process of relating skull anatomy to behavior is known as **phrenology**. One of his followers made the phrenological map in Figure 3.34.

Phrenology was invalid for many reasons. One problem was that skull shape does not match brain anatomy. The skull is thicker in some places than others and thicker in some people than others. Another problem was that they based many conclusions on small numbers of people who apparently shared some personality aspect and a similar bump on the skull.

Today, researchers examine detailed brain anatomy in living people. One method is **computerized axial tomography**, better known as a **CT** or **CAT scan** (Andreasen, 1988). A physician injects a dye into the blood to increase contrast in the image, and then places the person's head into a CT scanner like the one shown in Figure 3.35a. X-rays are passed through the head and recorded by detectors on the opposite side. The CT scanner is rotated slowly until a measurement has been taken at each angle over 180 degrees. From the measurements, a computer constructs images of the brain. Figure 3.35b is an example. CT scans help detect tumors and other structural abnormalities.

Another method is **magnetic resonance imaging (MRI)** (Warach, 1995), based on the fact that any atom with an odd-numbered atomic weight, such as hydrogen, has an axis of rotation. An MRI device applies a powerful magnetic field (about 25,000 times the magnetic field of the Earth) to align all the axes of rotation, and then tilts them with a brief radio frequency field. When the radio frequency field is turned off, the atomic nuclei release electromagnetic energy as they relax and return to their original axis. By measuring that energy, MRI devices form an image of the brain, such as the one in Figure 3.36. MRI shows anatomical details smaller

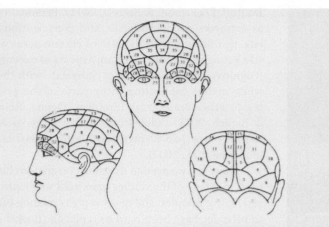

Affective Faculties

Propensities	Sentiments
? Desire to live	10 Cautiousness
• Alimentiveness	11 Approbativeness
1 Destructiveness	12 Self-esteem
2 Amativeness	13 Benevolence
3 Philoprogenitiveness	14 Reverence
4 Adhesiveness	15 Firmness
5 Inhabitiveness	16 Conscientiousness
6 Combativeness	17 Hope
7 Secretiveness	18 Marvelousness
8 Acquisitiveness	19 Ideality
9 Constructiveness	20 Mirthfulness
	21 Imitation

Intellectual Faculties

Perceptive	Reflective
22 Individuality	34 Comparison
23 Configuration	35 Causality
24 Size	
25 Weight and resistance	
26 Coloring	
27 Locality	
28 Order	
29 Calculation	
30 Eventuality	
31 Time	
32 Tune	
33 Language	

Figure 3.34 A phrenologist's map of the brain
Neuroscientists today also try to localize functions in the brain, but they use more careful methods and they study such functions as vision and hearing, not "secretiveness" and "marvelousness."
(*Source: From Spurzheim, 1908*)

than a millimeter in diameter. One drawback is that the person must lie motionless in a confining, noisy apparatus. The procedure is usually not suitable for children or anyone who fears enclosed places.

Researchers using these methods sometimes find that a particular brain area is enlarged in certain types of people. For example, it has been reported that people with a larger amygdala tend to have more social contacts (Bickart, Wright,

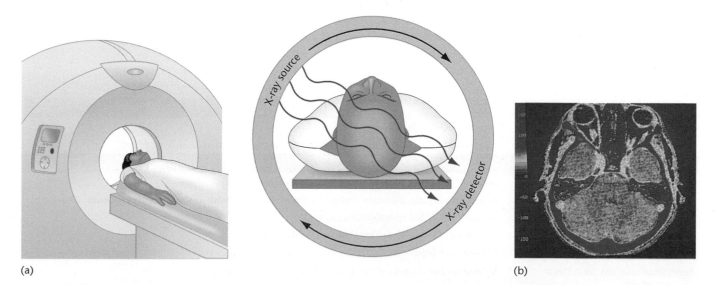

(a)   (b)

Figure 3.35 CT scanner
(a) A person's head is placed into the device and then a rapidly rotating source sends X-rays through the head while detectors on the opposite side make photographs. A computer then constructs an image of the brain. **(b)** A view of a normal human brain generated by computerized axial tomography (CT scanning).
(*Source: Dan McCoy/Rainbow*)

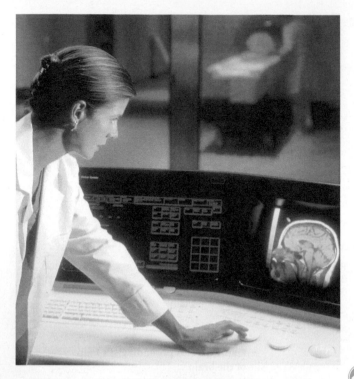

Figure 3.36 A view of a living brain generated by magnetic resonance imaging
Any atom with an odd-numbered atomic weight, such as hydrogen, has an inherent rotation. An outside magnetic field can align the axes of rotation. A radio frequency field can then make all these atoms move like tiny gyros. When the radio frequency field is turned off, the atomic nuclei release electromagnetic energy as they relax. By measuring that energy, we can obtain an image of a structure such as the brain without damaging it.
(Source: Will & Deni McIntyre/Science Source)

Dautoff, Dickerson, & Barrett, 2011). Personality traits such as extraversion, neuroticism, and conscientiousness correlate significantly with the size of certain areas of the cortex (De Young et al., 2010). Certain aspects of executive function (cognitive control of behavior) correlate with the amount of white matter connecting three parts of the prefrontal cortex to other brain areas (Smolker, Depue, Reineberg, Orr, & Banich, 2015). Adolescents with a large vocabulary tend to have more than average gray matter in part of the parietal lobe (Lee et al., 2007).

However, we need to examine correlations like these with caution. Many of the studies have used small, possibly unrepresentative samples, and many reports relating brain anatomy to behavior have been hard to replicate (Boekel et al., 2015). Because of the tendency to publish what appear to be positive results and ignore negative results, conclusions based on small samples are sometimes wrong, or at least overstatements of small effects. Table 3.5 summarizes various methods of studying brain-behavior relationships.

STOP & CHECK

20. What are the similarities and differences between MRI and fMRI?

ANSWER
20. Both methods measure the responses of brain chemicals to a magnetic field. MRI shows the anatomy of the brain. The fMRI method shows which brain areas are most active at the moment.

Table 3.5 | Methods of Studying Brain-Behavior Relationships

Examine Effects of Brain Damage	
Study victims of stroke, etc.	Used with humans; each person has different damage
Lesion	Controlled damage in laboratory animals
Ablation	Removal of a brain area
Gene knockout	Affects wherever that gene is active (e.g., a receptor)
Transcranial magnetic stimulation	Intense application temporarily inactivates a brain area
Examine Effects of Stimulating a Brain Area	
Stimulating electrodes	Invasive; used with laboratory animals, rarely with humans
Optogenetic stimulation	Mostly with laboratory animals; can indicate function of a particular type of cell
Record Brain Activity during Behavior	
Record from electrodes in brain	Invasive; used with laboratory animals, rarely with humans
Electroencephalograph (EEG)	Records from scalp; measures changes by milliseconds, but with low resolution of location of the signal
Evoked potentials	Similar to EEG but in response to stimuli
Magnetoencephalograph (MEG)	Similar to EEG but measures magnetic fields
Positron emission tomography (PET)	Measures changes over both time and location but requires exposing brain to radiation
Functional magnetic resonance imaging (fMRI)	Measures changes over about 1 second, identifies location within 1 to 2 mm
Correlate Brain Anatomy with Behavior	
Computerized axial tomography (CAT)	Maps brain areas, but requires exposure to X-rays
Magnetic resonance imaging (MRI)	Maps brain areas in detail, using magnetic fields

Research Methods and Progress

In any scientific field—indeed, any field of knowledge—progress almost always depends on improvements in measurement. In astronomy, for example, improvements in both ground-based and satellite-based astronomy have established conclusions that even science-fiction writers couldn't have imagined a few decades ago. Weather prediction is vastly more accurate than it used to be. Similarly, our understanding of the brain has advanced greatly because of the introduction of PET scans, fMRI, optogenetics, and other modern technologies. Future progress will continue to depend on improvements in our methods of measurement.

Summary

1. One way to study brain-behavior relationships is to examine the effects of brain damage. If someone suffers a loss after some kind of brain damage, then that area contributes in some way to that behavior. 91

2. If stimulation of a brain area increases some behavior, presumably that area contributes to the behavior. Optogenetics is a relatively new method that enables researchers to stimulate a particular type of cell at a particular moment. 92

3. Researchers try to understand brain-behavior relationships by recording activity in various brain areas during a given behavior. Many methods are available, including EEG, MEG, PET, and fMRI. 93

4. People who differ with regard to some behavior sometimes also differ with regard to their brain anatomy. MRI is one modern method of imaging a living brain. However, correlations between behavior and anatomy should be evaluated cautiously until they have been replicated. 96

Key Terms

Terms are defined in the module on the page number indicated. They're also presented in alphabetical order with definitions in the book's Subject Index/Glossary, which begins on page 589. Interactive flash cards, audio reviews, and crossword puzzles are among the online resources available to help you learn these terms and the concepts they represent.

ablation **91**
computerized axial tomography
     (CT or CAT scan) **96**
electroencephalograph (EEG)
     93 lesion
evoked potentials or evoked
     responses **93**

functional magnetic resonance
     imaging (fMRI) **94**
lesion **91**
magnetic resonance imaging (MRI)
     96
magnetoencephalograph (MEG) **94**
optogenetics **92**

phrenology **96**
positron-emission tomography
     (PET) **94**
stereotaxic instrument **91**
transcranial magnetic stimulation
     (TMS) **92**

Thought Question

Certain unusual aspects of brain structure were observed in the brain of Albert Einstein (Falk, Lepore, & Noe, 2013). One interpretation is that he was born with certain specialized brain features that encouraged his scientific and intellectual abilities. What is an alternative interpretation?

Module 3.3 | End of Module Quiz

1. The first demonstration that a brain area controlled a particular aspect of behavior pertained to which type of behavior?

    A. Criminal activity
    B. Language

    C. Hunger
    D. Sexual arousal

2. Which of the following is a method to inactivate a brain area temporarily?

    A. Stereotaxic instrument
    B. Transcranial magnetic stimulation

    C. Lesion
    D. Ablation

3. What does the optogenetic technique enable researchers to test?

   A. The evolution of brain anatomy
   B. The functions of a particular type of neuron

   C. The relationship between brain anatomy and intelligence
   D. How people bind one type of sensation with another

4. EEG and MEG are advantageous for measuring which of the following?

   A. The functions of different neurotransmitters
   B. The brain areas receiving the greatest amount of blood flow during some activity

   C. Effects of hormones on behavior
   D. Changes in brain activity over very short periods of time

5. Which of these is the first step for positron-emission tomography (PET)?

   A. Inject a radioactive chemical into the blood.
   B. Insert an electrode into the brain.

   C. Subject the brain to a strong magnetic field.
   D. Attach light-sensitive proteins to a virus.

6. What is one advantage of fMRI over PET scans?

   A. The fMRI technique measures activity on a millisecond-by-millisecond basis.
   B. The fMRI technique does not require inserting an electrode into the head.

   C. The fMRI technique does not expose the brain to radioactivity.
   D. The fMRI technique identifies which brain areas are most active at a given moment.

7. Comparing MRI and fMRI, which one(s) measure the responses of brain chemicals to a magnetic field? Which one(s) show which brain areas are most active at the moment?

   A. Only MRI measures responses of brain chemicals to a magnetic field. Both show which brain areas are most active at the moment.
   B. Only fMRI measures responses of brain chemicals to a magnetic field. Only MRI shows which brain areas are most active at the moment.

   C. Both measure responses of brain chemicals to a magnetic field. Only fMRI shows which brain areas are most active at the moment.
   D. Both measure responses of brain chemicals to a magnetic field. Both show which brain areas are most active at the moment.

8. Why should we be cautious when interpreting many of the reports linking certain aspects of brain anatomy to behavior?

   A. Many published studies used inaccurate measures of brain anatomy.
   B. Many published studies studied people varying widely in their ages.

   C. Many published studies were based on small samples.
   D. Many published studies used unethical methods.

Answers: 1B, 2B, 3B, 4D, 5A, 6C, 7C, 8C.

Suggestions for Further Reading

Burrell, B. (2004). *Postcards from the brain museum.* New York: Broadway Books. Fascinating history of the attempts to collect brains of successful people and try to relate their brain anatomy to their success.

Klawans, H. L. (1988). *Toscanini's fumble and other tales of clinical neurology.* Chicago: Contemporary Books. Description of illustrative cases of brain damage and their behavioral consequences.

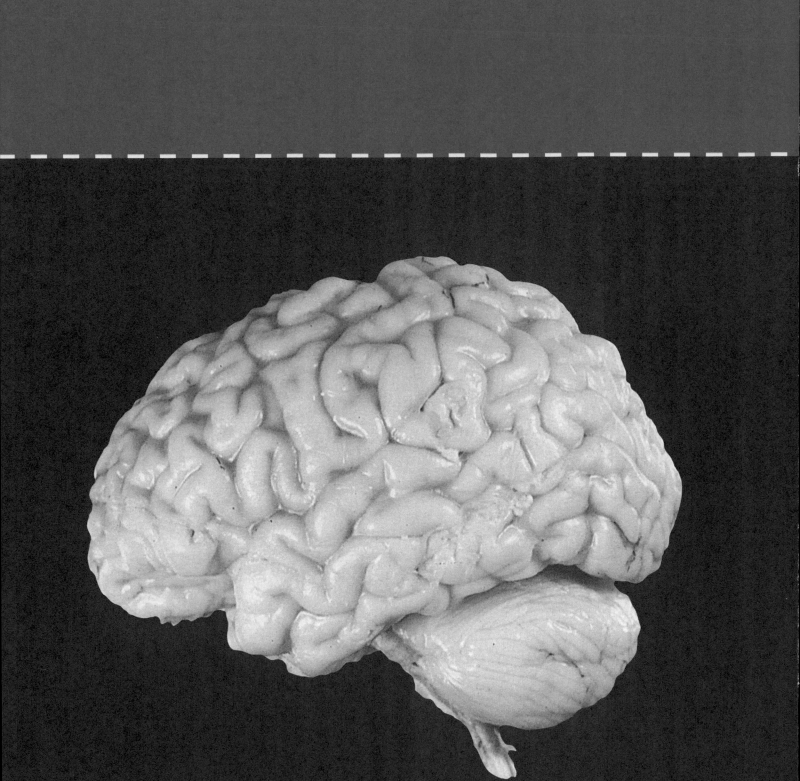

Genetics, Evolution, Development, and Plasticity

"**S**ome assembly required." Have you ever bought a package with those ominous words? Sometimes, all you have to do is attach a few parts, but other times, you face page after page of barely comprehensible instructions.

The human nervous system requires an enormous amount of assembly, and the instructions are different from those for the objects we assemble from a kit. Instead of "Put this piece here and that piece there," the instructions are, "Put these axons here and those dendrites there, and then wait to see what happens. Keep the connections that work the best and discard the others. Continue making new connections and keeping only the successful ones."

Therefore, we say that the brain's anatomy is *plastic*. It changes rapidly in early development and continues changing throughout life.

Module 4.1

Genetics and Evolution of Behavior
Mendelian Genetics
Heredity and Environment
The Evolution of Behavior
In Closing: Genes and Behavior

Module 4.2

Development of the Brain
Maturation of the Vertebrate Brain
Pathfinding by Axons
Determinants of Neuronal Survival
The Vulnerable Developing Brain
Differentiation of the Cortex
Fine-Tuning by Experience
Brain Development and Behavioral
  Development
In Closing: Brain Development

Module 4.3

Plasticity after Brain Damage
Brain Damage and Short-Term Recovery
Later Mechanisms of Recovery
In Closing: Brain Damage and Recovery

Learning Objectives

After studying this chapter, you should be able to:

1. Distinguish between genetic and epigenetic influences on development.
2. Describe the types of evidence researchers use to infer heritability.
3. Give examples of evolutionary explanations in psychology.
4. Discuss the formation of new neurons in a mature brain.
5. Describe the evidence showing that axons seek specific targets.
6. Define apoptosis, and explain how neurotrophins prevent it.
7. Cite examples of how experiences alter brain anatomy and function.
8. Evaluate possible explanations of risky behavior in adolescents.
9. List several possible mechanisms of recovery after brain damage.
10. Explain how remodeling in the cerebral cortex produces the phantom limb experience.

Opposite:
An enormous amount of brain development occurs by the time a person is 1 year old.
(Source: Dr. Dana Copeland)

Genetics and Evolution of Behavior

Everything you do depends on both your genes and your environment. Consider facial expressions. A contribution of the environment is obvious: You smile more when the world is treating you well and frown when things are going badly. Does heredity influence your facial expressions? Researchers examined facial expressions of people who were born blind and therefore could not have learned to imitate facial expressions. The facial expressions of the people born blind were remarkably similar to those of their sighted relatives, as shown in Figure 4.1 (Peleg et al., 2006). These results suggest a role for genetics in controlling facial expressions.

Controversies arise when we move beyond the generalization that both heredity and environment are important. For example, do differences in human intelligence depend mostly on genetic differences, mostly on environmental influences, or both equally? Similar questions arise for sexual orientation, alcoholism, weight gain, mental illness, and much else that interests psychologists and the general public. This module should help you understand these issues, even when the answer remains uncertain. We begin with a review of genetics, a field that has become more and more complicated as research has progressed.

Mendelian Genetics

Prior to the work of Gregor Mendel, a late 19th-century monk, scientists thought that inheritance was a blending process in which the properties of the sperm and the egg simply mixed, like two colors of paint.

Mendel demonstrated that inheritance occurs through **genes**, units of heredity that maintain their structural identity from one generation to another. As a rule, genes come in pairs because they are aligned along **chromosomes** (strands of genes) that also come in pairs. The exception to this rule is that a male mammal has unpaired X and Y chromosomes with different genes. Classically, a gene has been defined as part of a chromosome composed of the double-stranded molecule **deoxyribonucleic acid (DNA)**. However, many genes do not have the discrete locations we once imagined (Bird, 2007). Sometimes several genes overlap on a stretch of chromosome. Sometimes a genetic outcome depends on parts of two or more chromosomes. In many cases, part of a chromosome

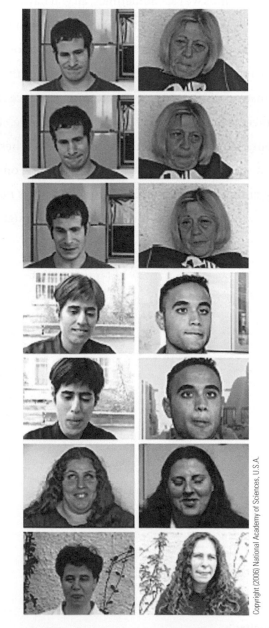

Copyright (2006) National Academy of Sciences, U.S.A.

Figure 4.1 Facial expressions by people born blind (left) and their sighted relatives (right)
The similarities imply a genetic contribution to facial expressions.

alters the expression of another part without coding for any protein of its own.

A strand of DNA serves as a template (model) for the synthesis of **ribonucleic acid (RNA)** molecules, a single-strand chemical. One type of RNA molecule—messenger RNA—serves as a template for the synthesis of protein molecules. DNA contains four "bases"—adenine, guanine, cytosine, and thymine. The order of those bases determines the order of corresponding bases along an RNA molecule—adenine, guanine, cytosine, and uracil. The order of bases along an RNA molecule in turn determines the order of amino acids that compose a protein. For example, if three RNA bases are in the order cytosine, adenine, and guanine, then the protein adds the amino acid *glutamine.* If the next three RNA bases are uracil, guanine, and guanine, the next amino acid on the protein is *tryptophan.* Any protein consists of some combination of 20 amino acids, in an order that depends on the order of DNA and RNA bases. It's an amazingly simple code, considering the complexity of body structures and functions that result from it.

Figure 4.2 summarizes the main steps in translating information from DNA through RNA into proteins. Some proteins form part of the structure of the body. Others serve as *enzymes,* biological catalysts that regulate chemical reactions in the body. Not all RNA molecules code for proteins. Many RNA molecules perform regulatory functions.

If you have the same genes on your two copies of some chromosome, you are **homozygous** for that gene. If you have an unmatched pair of genes, you are **heterozygous** for that gene. For example, you might have a gene for blue eyes on one chromosome and a gene for brown eyes on the other.

Genes are dominant, recessive, or intermediate. A **dominant gene** shows a strong effect in either the homozygous or heterozygous condition. A **recessive gene** shows its effects only in the homozygous condition. For example, a gene for brown eyes is dominant and a gene for blue eyes is recessive. If you have one gene for brown eyes and one for blue, the result is brown eyes. The gene for high sensitivity to the taste of phenylthiocarbamide (PTC) is dominant, and the gene for low sensitivity is recessive. Only someone with two recessive genes has trouble tasting it (Wooding et al., 2004). Figure 4.3 illustrates the possible results of a mating between people who are both heterozygous for the PTC-tasting gene. Because each has one high taste sensitivity gene—let's abbreviate it "T"—both parents readily taste PTC. However, each parent transmits either a high taste sensitivity gene (T) or a low taste sensitivity gene (t) to any child. Therefore, a child in this family has a 25 percent chance of two T genes, a 50 percent chance of the heterozygous condition, and a 25 percent chance of being homozygous for the t gene.

However, an example like this can be misleading, because it implies that a single gene produces a single outcome. Even in the case of eye color, that is not true. Researchers have identified at least 10 genes that contribute to variations in eye color (Liu et al., 2010). At least 180 genes contribute to differences in people's height (Allen et al., 2010). Each gene that contributes to eye color or height affects other characteristics as well. Furthermore, you express most of your genes in certain cells and not others, and changes in the environment can increase or decrease the expression of a gene. Genetic influences are more complex than we once imagined.

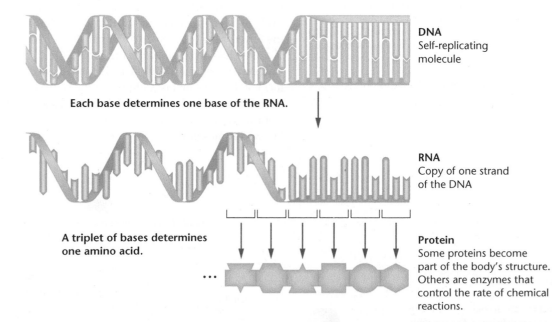

DNA
Self-replicating molecule

Each base determines one base of the RNA.

RNA
Copy of one strand of the DNA

A triplet of bases determines one amino acid.

Protein
Some proteins become part of the body's structure. Others are enzymes that control the rate of chemical reactions.

Figure 4.2 How DNA controls development of the organism
The sequence of bases along a strand of DNA determines the order of bases along a strand of RNA; RNA in turn controls the sequence of amino acids in a protein molecule.

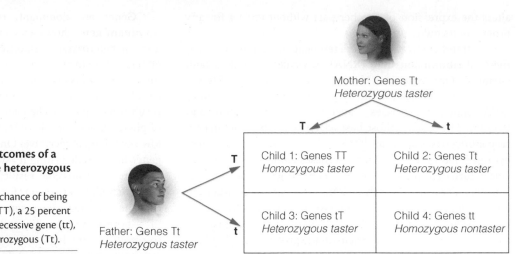

Figure 4.3 Four equally likely outcomes of a mating between parents who are heterozygous for a given gene (Tt)
A child in this family has a 25 percent chance of being homozygous for the dominant gene (TT), a 25 percent chance of being homozygous for the recessive gene (tt), and a 50 percent chance of being heterozygous (Tt).

Mother: Genes Tt
Heterozygous taster

Father: Genes Tt
Heterozygous taster

	T	t
T	Child 1: Genes TT *Homozygous taster*	Child 2: Genes Tt *Heterozygous taster*
t	Child 3: Genes tT *Heterozygous taster*	Child 4: Genes tt *Homozygous nontaster*

✅ STOP & CHECK

1. Suppose you have high sensitivity to tasting PTC. If your mother can also taste it easily, what (if anything) can you predict about your father's ability to taste it?

2. Suppose you have high sensitivity to the taste of PTC. If your mother has low sensitivity, what (if anything) can you predict about your father's taste sensitivity?

3. Suppose someone identifies a "gene for" certain aspects of development. How might that statement be misleading?

ANSWERS

1. If your mother has high sensitivity to the taste of PTC, we can make no predictions about your father. You may have inherited a high-sensitivity gene from your mother, and because the gene is dominant, you need only one copy of the gene to taste PTC. 2. If your mother has low sensitivity, you must have inherited your high-sensitivity gene from your father, so he must have high sensitivity. 3. Almost any characteristic depends on more than one gene, as well as influences from the environment.

Sex-Linked and Sex-Limited Genes

The genes on the sex chromosomes (designated X and Y in mammals) are known as **sex-linked genes.** All other chromosomes are autosomal chromosomes, and their genes are known as **autosomal genes**.

A female mammal has two X chromosomes, whereas a male has an X and a Y. During reproduction, the female necessarily contributes an X chromosome, and the male contributes either an X or a Y. If he contributes an X, the offspring is female; if he contributes a Y, the offspring is male. (Exceptions to this rule are possible, but uncommon.)

When biologists speak of sex-linked genes, they usually mean X-linked genes. The Y chromosome is small, with relatively few genes of its own, but it also has sites that influence the functioning of genes on other chromosomes.

One human sex-linked gene controls red-green color vision deficiency (see Figure 4.4). Any man with the recessive form of this gene on his X chromosome is red-green color deficient because he has no other X chromosome. A woman is color deficient only if she has that recessive gene on both of her X chromosomes. So, for example, if 8 percent of human

Figure 4.4 Red-green color deficiency, a sex-linked gene
RG represents normal red-green color vision, and rg represents red-green color deficiency. Any son who receives an rg gene from his mother is red-green color deficient, because the Y gene has no gene for color vision. A daughter could be color deficient only if her father has color deficiency and her mother is a carrier for the condition.

Mother: X chromosome with RG gene; X chromosome with rg gene
Normal color vision, but carrier for color deficiency

Father: X chromosome with RG gene; Y chromosome with no relevant gene
Normal color vision

	X with RG	X with rg
X with RG	Daughter (XX) RG, RG *Normal color vision*	Daughter (XX) RG, rg *Normal color vision, but carrier for color deficiency*
Y	Son (XY) RG *Normal color vision*	Son (XY) rg *Red-green color deficient*

X chromosomes contain the gene for color vision deficiency, then 8 percent of men will be color deficient, but less than one percent of women will be (0.08 × 0.08).

Distinct from sex-linked genes are the **sex-limited genes**, present in both sexes but active mainly in one sex. Examples include the genes that control the amount of chest hair in men, breast size in women, amount of crowing in roosters, and rate of egg production in hens. Both sexes have the genes, but sex hormones activate them in one sex and not the other, or one sex much more than the other. Many sex-limited genes show their effects at puberty.

⊘ STOP & CHECK

4. How does a sex-linked gene differ from a sex-limited gene?

ANSWER

4. A sex-linked gene is on the X or Y chromosome. A sex-limited gene is on an autosomal chromosome, but activated in one sex more than the other.

Genetic Changes

Genes change in several ways. One way is by **mutation**, a heritable change in a DNA molecule. Changing just one base in DNA to any of the other three types means that the mutant gene will code for a protein with a different amino acid at one location in the molecule. Given that evolution has already had eons to select the best makeup of each gene, a mutation is rarely advantageous. Still, those rare exceptions are important. The human *FOXP2* gene differs from the chimpanzee version of that gene in just two bases, but those two mutations modified the human brain and vocal apparatus in several ways that facilitate language development (Konopka et al., 2009).

Another kind of mutation is a duplication or deletion. During the process of reproduction, part of a chromosome that ordinarily appears once might instead appear twice or not at all. When this process happens to just a tiny portion of a chromosome, we call it a microduplication or microdeletion. Although it is possible for a microduplication to be helpful, most are not. Microduplications and microdeletions of brain-relevant genes are responsible for several psychological or neurological disorders, probably including some cases of schizophrenia.

Epigenetics

In addition to mutations that cause permanent changes in genes, the field of **epigenetics** deals with changes in gene expression. Every cell in your body has the same DNA as every other cell (except your red blood cells, that have no DNA). However, the activity of a gene can vary. The genes that are most active in your brain are not the same as those active in your lungs or kidneys, and those most active in one part of your brain are not the most active in another part. Many genes that are essential to a developing fetus become less active after birth, and others that did little for the fetus become important after birth (Hannon et al., 2016; Jaffe et al., 2016). At puberty, certain genes that had been almost silent become much more active (Lomniczi et al., 2013). A gene may be active in one person and not another. After all, monozygotic ("identical") twins sometimes differ in handedness, mental health, or other aspects.

Various experiences can turn a gene on or off. Even forming a new memory or habit increases the activity of certain genes in particular neurons (Feng, Fouse, & Fan, 2007). If a mother rat is malnourished during pregnancy, her offspring alter the expression of certain genes to conserve energy and adjust to a world in which food will presumably be hard to find. If in fact rich food becomes abundant later in life, those offspring are predisposed, because of their gene expression, to a high probability of obesity and heart disease (Godfrey, Lillycrop, Burdge, Gluckman, & Hanson, 2007). Epigenetic changes can be inherited, at least for a generation or two. When mice were conditioned to fear a particular odor, the first and second generations of offspring showed increased sensitivity to that odor (Dias & Ressler, 2014). When male mice were exposed to chronic stressful experiences, their offspring showed a weakened hormonal response to stresses and altered gene expression in part of the brain. The effect was traced to RNA molecules in the father's sperm (Rodgers, Morgan, Leu, & Bale, 2015).

Epigenetic changes in humans are also critical. Drug addiction produces epigenetic changes in the brain (Sadri-Vakili et al., 2010; Tsankova, Renthal, Kumar, & Nestler, 2007). The experience of feeling socially isolated or rejected alters the activity of hundreds of genes (Slavich & Cole, 2013). How well one of your grandparents was nourished or malnourished in childhood correlates with your chances for a long, healthy life, apparently because of changes in your father's sperm cells (Pembrey et al., 2006).

How could an experience modify gene expression? First, let's look at how gene expression is regulated, and then see how environmental factors can influence that regulation. Standard illustrations of the DNA molecule, as in Figure 4.2, show it as a straight line, which is an oversimplification. In fact, proteins called **histones** bind DNA into a shape that is more like string wound around a ball (see Figure 4.5). The histone molecules in the ball have loose ends to which certain chemical groups can attach. To activate a gene, the DNA must partially unwind from the histones.

The result of an experience—maternal deprivation, cocaine exposure, new learning, or whatever—in some way alters the chemical environment within a cell. In some cases the outcome adds acetyl groups ($COCH_3$) to the histone tails near a gene, causing the histones to loosen their grip on the DNA, and facilitating the expression of that gene. Removal of the acetyl group causes the histones to tighten their grip on the DNA, and turns the gene off. Another possibility is to add or remove methyl groups from DNA, usually at the promoter regions at the beginning of a gene. Adding methyl groups (CH_3) to a promoter turns off a gene, and removing them turns on

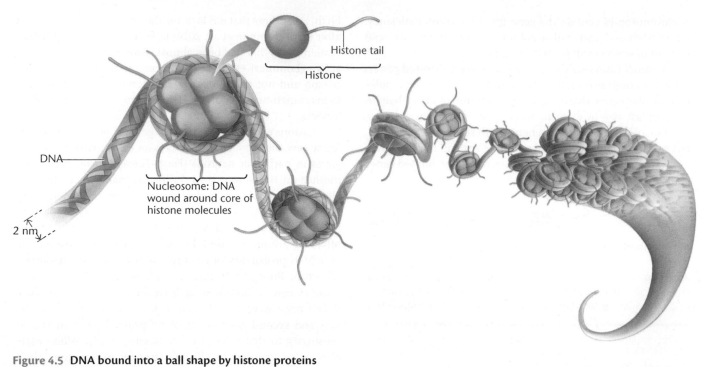

Figure 4.5 DNA bound into a ball shape by histone proteins
Acetyl groups that attach to a loose end of a histone molecule loosen the histone's grip on DNA, exposing more genes to the possibility of being active.

a gene (Tsankova et al., 2007). For example, severe traumatic experiences in early childhood decrease methylation of many brain genes, increasing the later risk of depression, posttraumatic stress disorder, and so forth (Klengel et al., 2013).

The general point is that what you do at any moment not only affects you now, but also produces epigenetic effects that alter gene expression for longer periods of time. Furthermore, the distinction between "genetic" effects and "experiential" effects has become blurrier than ever. Experiences act by altering the activity of genes.

✓ STOP & CHECK ▮▮▮▮▮▮▮▮▮

5. How does an epigenetic change differ from a mutation?
6. How does adding a methyl or acetyl group to a histone protein alter gene activity?

ANSWERS
5. A mutation is a permanent change in part of a chromosome. An epigenetic change is an increase or decrease in the activity of a gene or group of genes. 6. Adding a methyl group turns genes off. An acetyl group loosens histone's grip and increases gene activation.

Heredity and Environment

Does singing ability depend on heredity or environment? That question as stated is meaningless. Unless you had both heredity and environment, you couldn't sing at all. However, we can rephrase the question meaningfully: Do the observed *differences* among individuals depend more on *differences* in heredity or *differences* in environment? For example, if you

sing better than someone else, the reason could be different genes, better training, or both. If the variations in some characteristic depend largely on genetic differences, the characteristic has high **heritability**. Heritability ranges from zero, indicating no genetic contribution to the variation, to one, indicating complete control.

But how could we determine the heritability of a characteristic? Researchers rely mainly on three kinds of evidence. First, they compare **monozygotic** ("from one egg") **twins** and **dizygotic** ("from two eggs") **twins**. People usually call **monozygotic twins** "identical" twins, but that term is misleading, because they sometimes differ in important ways. For example, some are mirror images of each other, one of them right-handed and the other one left-handed. Still, they have the same genes, whereas dizygotic twins do not. A stronger resemblance between monozygotic than dizygotic twins suggests a genetic contribution. However, that evidence by itself is not totally decisive, because the way you look influences the way people treat you, and therefore the way you act. Researchers sometimes also examine "virtual twins"—children of the same age, adopted at the same time into a single family. They grow up in the same environment from infancy, but without any genetic similarity. Any similarities in behavior imply environmental influences. However, the behavioral differences—which are in many cases substantial—suggest genetic influences (Segal, 2000).

A second kind of evidence is studies of adopted children. Any tendency for adopted children to resemble their biological parents suggests a hereditary influence. However, again the evidence is not always decisive. The biological mother contributes not only her genes, but also the prenatal environment.

A mother's health, diet, and smoking and drinking habits during pregnancy can greatly influence her child's development, especially the brain development. A similarity between an adopted child and the genetic mother could reflect either genetic influences or prenatal environment.

Using twin studies and adoption studies, researchers have found evidence for significant heritability of almost every behavior they have tested, including loneliness (McGuire & Clifford, 2000), neuroticism (Lake, Eaves, Maes, Heath, & Martin, 2000), television watching (Plomin, Corley, DeFries, & Fulker, 1990), childhood misbehavior (Burt, 2009), social attitudes (Posner, Baker, Heath, & Martin, 1996), cognitive performance (Plomin et al., 2013), educational attainment (Rietveld et al., 2013), and speed of learning a second language (Dale, Harlaar, Haworth, & Plomin, 2010). About the only behavior that has *not* shown a significant heritability is religious affiliation—such as Protestant or Catholic (Eaves, Martin, & Heath, 1990).

Any estimate of the heritability of a trait is specific to a given population. Consider alcohol abuse, which has moderate heritability in the United States. Imagine a population somewhere in which some families teach very strict prohibitions on alcohol use, perhaps for religious reasons, and other families are more permissive. With such strong environmental differences, the genetic influences exert less effect, and heritability will be relatively low. Then imagine another population where all families have the same rules, but people happen to differ substantially in genes that affect their reactions to alcohol. In that population, heritability will be higher. In short, any estimate of heritability applies only to a particular population at a particular time.

In addition to twin and adoption studies, a third and potentially most decisive approach is to identify specific genes linked to some behavior. Using the *candidate gene* approach, researchers test a hypothesis, such as "a gene that increases the activity of the serotonin transporter may be linked to an increased risk of depression." The candidate gene approach has identified one gene with a significant influence on the risk of alcohol abuse, and a few other genes with moderate effects, but many studies have yielded small or uncertain effects (Dick et al., 2015). Another approach, a *genome wide association study*, examines all the genes while comparing two groups, such as people with and without schizophrenia. The problem with that approach is that it tests thousands of hypotheses at once (one for each gene) and therefore has a risk of seeing an apparent effect by accident, especially in studies with a small sample. The approach can also have misleading results when applied to an ethnically diverse sample. Suppose some disorder, psychological or otherwise, is more common in one ethnic group than another. Then any other gene that is common in that ethnic group will appear to be a "risk factor," even if in fact the gene has nothing to do with the disorder (Dick et al., 2015).

A review titled "Top 10 replicated findings from behavioral genetics" (Plomin, DeFries, Knopik, & Neiderhiser, 2016) listed statements that are well supported, although not very specific. For example, almost everything in psychology shows an important genetic influence, nothing in psychology has 100 percent heritability, heritability almost always depends on many genes with small effects, and stability of behavior over age is due to genetics. However, as one critic pointed out, we still have few cases of identified genes with major effects, and we rarely know much about how any gene exerts its effects on behavior (Turkheimer, 2016).

If nearly everything in psychology has significant heritability, but nevertheless researchers cannot locate a gene with a strong link to a behavior, what might they be overlooking? In addition to the possibility of a huge number of genes each exerting small effects, another possibility is microduplications or microdeletions, which we know contribute in some cases. Another possibility is mutations that have a large effect but occur too rarely for typical research methods to find them. Still another possibility is that what appear to be genetic effects might actually be epigenetic effects.

STOP & CHECK

7. What are the main types of evidence to estimate the heritability of some behavior?
8. Suppose someone determines the heritability of IQ scores for a given population. Then society changes in a way that provides the best possible opportunity for everyone within that population. Will heritability of IQ increase, decrease, or stay the same?

ANSWERS 7. One type of evidence is greater similarity between monozygotic twins than dizygotic twins. Another is resemblance between adopted children and their biological parents. A third is a demonstration that a particular gene is more common than average among people who show a particular behavior. 8. Heritability will *increase*. Heritability estimates how much of the variation is due to differences in genes. If everyone has the same environment, then differences in environment cannot account for much of the remaining differences in IQ scores. Therefore, the relative role of genetic differences will be greater.

Environmental Modification

Even a trait with high heritability can be modified by environmental interventions. A prime example is **phenylketonuria** (FEE-nil-KEET-uhn-YOOR-ee-uh), or **PKU**, a genetic inability to metabolize the amino acid phenylalanine. If PKU is not treated, phenylalanine accumulates to toxic levels, impairing brain development and leaving a child mentally retarded, restless, and irritable. Approximately one percent of Europeans carry a recessive gene for PKU. Fewer Asians and almost no Africans have the gene (T. Wang et al., 1989).

Although PKU is a hereditary condition, environmental interventions can modify it. Physicians in many countries routinely test the level of phenylalanine or its metabolites in each baby's blood or urine. If a baby has high levels, indicating PKU, physicians advise the parents to put the baby on a strict low-phenylalanine diet to protect the brain (Waisbren, Brown, de Sonneville, & Levy, 1994). The success of this diet shows that *heritable* does not mean *unmodifiable.*

A couple of notes about PKU: The required diet is difficult. People have to avoid meats, eggs, dairy products, grains, and especially aspartame (NutraSweet), which is 50 percent phenylalanine. Instead, they eat an expensive formula containing the other amino acids. Physicians long believed that children with PKU could quit the diet after a few years. Later experience has shown that high phenylalanine levels damage mature brains, too. A woman with PKU should be especially careful during pregnancy and when nursing. Even a genetically normal baby cannot handle the enormous amounts of phenylalanine that an affected mother might pass through the placenta.

✓ STOP & CHECK ▆▆▆▆▆▆▆

9. What example illustrates the point that even if some characteristic is highly heritable, a change in the environment can alter it?

ANSWER

9. Keeping a child with the PKU gene on a strict low-phenylalanine diet prevents the mental retardation that the gene ordinarily causes. The general point is that sometimes a highly heritable condition can be modified environmentally.

How Genes Influence Behavior

No gene produces its effects by itself. A gene produces a protein that interacts with the rest of body chemistry and with the environment. Exactly how a gene might influence behavior is a complex issue, with many answers in different cases. A gene could influence your behavior even without being expressed in your brain. Suppose your genes make you unusually attractive. As a result, strangers smile at you and many people want to get to know you. If their reactions to your appearance influence your personality, then the genes altered your behavior by altering your environment!

For another example, imagine a child born with genes promoting greater than average height and running speed. Because of these factors, the child shows early success at basketball, and soon spends more and more time playing basketball. As a result, the child spends less time than average on other pursuits—watching television, playing chess, or anything else. This is a hypothetical example, but it illustrates the point: Genes can influence behavior in roundabout ways. We should not be amazed by reports that nearly every human behavior has some heritability.

The Evolution of Behavior

Charles Darwin, known as the founder of evolutionary theory, didn't like the term *evolution.* He preferred *descent with modification,* emphasizing the idea of changes without necessarily implying improvement. **Evolution** is a change over generations in the frequencies of various genes in a population.

We distinguish two questions about evolution: How *did* some species evolve, and how *do* species evolve? To ask how a species did evolve is to ask what evolved from what. For example, because humans are more similar to chimpanzees than to other species, biologists infer a common ancestor. Fossils also help to illuminate changes over time. As new evidence becomes available, biologists sometimes change their opinions about the evolutionary relationship between one species and another.

In contrast, the question of how species *do* evolve is a question of how the process works, and that process is a necessary outcome from what we know about reproduction. The reasoning goes as follows:

* Because of genetic influences, offspring generally resemble their parents. That is, "like begets like."
* Mutations, recombinations, and microduplications of genes introduce new heritable variations that help or harm an individual's chance of surviving and reproducing.
* Certain individuals reproduce more than others do, thus passing on their genes to the next generation. Any gene that is associated with greater reproductive success will become more prevalent in later generations. Therefore, the current generation of any species resembles the individuals who reproduced in the past. If a change in the environment causes a different gene to increase the probability of survival and reproduction, then that gene will spread in the population.

Because plant and animal breeders have long understood this idea, they choose individuals with a desired trait and make them the parents of the next generation through a process called **artificial selection**. Over many generations, breeders have produced exceptional racehorses, chickens that lay huge numbers of eggs, hundreds of kinds of dogs, and so forth. Darwin's (1859) insight was that nature also selects. If certain individuals are more successful than others in finding food, escaping enemies, resisting illness, attracting mates, or protecting their offspring, then their genes will become more prevalent in later generations. Given a huge amount of time, this process can produce the wide variety of life that we in fact observe.

Common Misunderstandings about Evolution

Let's clarify the principles of evolution by addressing a few misconceptions:

* *Does the use or disuse of some structure or behavior cause an evolutionary increase or decrease in that feature?* You may have heard people say something like, "Because we hardly ever use our little toes, they get smaller and smaller in each succeeding generation." This idea is a carryover of biologist Jean-Baptiste Lamarck's theory of evolution through the inheritance of acquired characteristics, known as **Lamarckian evolution.** According to this idea, if you exercise your arm muscles, your children will be born with bigger arm muscles, and if you fail to use your

little toes, your children's little toes will be smaller than yours. However, biologists have found no mechanism for Lamarckian evolution to occur and no evidence that it does. Using or failing to use some body structure does not change the genes. People's little toes will shrink in future generations only if people with genes for smaller little toes manage to reproduce more than other people do.

- *Have humans stopped evolving?* Because modern medicine can keep almost anyone alive, and because welfare programs in prosperous countries provide the necessities of life for almost everyone, some people assert that humans are no longer subject to the principle of "survival of the fittest." Therefore, the argument goes, human evolution has slowed or stopped.

The flaw in this argument is that evolution depends on reproduction, not just survival. If people with certain genes have more than the average number of children, their genes will spread in the population.

- *Does "evolution" mean "improvement"?* It depends on what you mean by "improvement." By definition, evolution improves **fitness**, which is operationally defined as *the number of copies of one's genes that endure in later generations.* If you have more children than average, and they survive long enough to reproduce, you are evolutionarily fit, regardless of whether you are successful in any other way. You also increase your fitness by supporting your relatives, who share many of your genes and spread them by their own reproduction. Any gene that spreads is, by definition, fit. However, genes that increase fitness at one time and place might be disadvantageous after a change in the environment. For example, the colorful tail feathers of the male peacock enable it to attract females

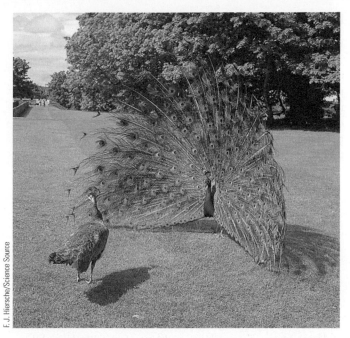

Sometimes, a sexual display, such as a peacock's spread of its tail feathers, improves reproductive success and spreads the associated genes. In a changed environment, this gene could become maladaptive.

but might become disadvantageous in the presence of a new predator that responds to bright colors. In other words, the genes of the current generation evolved because they were fit for *previous* generations. They may or may not be adaptive in the future.

- *Does evolution benefit the individual or the species?* Neither: It benefits the genes! In a sense, you don't use your genes to reproduce yourself. Rather, your genes use *you* to reproduce *themselves* (Dawkins, 1989). Imagine a gene that causes you to risk your life to protect your children. If that gene enables you to leave behind more surviving children than you would have otherwise, then that gene will increase in prevalence within your population.

Natural selection cannot favor a gene that benefits the species while disadvantaging the individuals with the gene. Some people have claimed—incorrectly—that when lemming populations become too high, some of the lemmings jump off cliffs to decrease the overpopulation problem. If that were true (and it is not!), the next generation would all descend from those lemmings that failed to jump. The "self-sacrificing" gene would die out with those who had it.

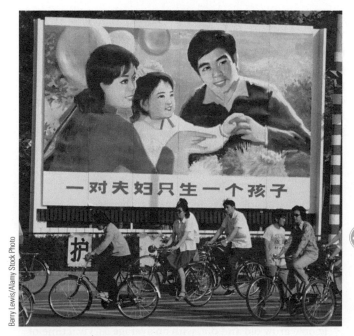

China's policy to limit each family to one child decreases the possibility of genetic changes between generations.

✓ STOP & CHECK

10. Many people believe the human appendix is useless. Will it become smaller and smaller with each generation?

ANSWER

10. No. Failure to need a structure does not make it smaller in the next generation. The appendix will shrink only if people with a gene for a smaller appendix reproduce more successfully than other people do.

Evolutionary Psychology

Evolutionary psychology concerns how behaviors evolved. The emphasis is on *evolutionary* and *functional* explanations—that is, how our genes reflect those of our ancestors and why natural selection might have favored the genes that promote certain behaviors. The assumption is that any behavior characteristic of a species arose through natural selection and presumably provided some advantage, at least in ancestral times. Consider these examples:

- Some animal species have better color vision than others, and some have better peripheral vision. Species evolve the kind of vision they need for their way of life (Chapter 5).
- Animals that are in danger of being attacked while they sleep get by with little sleep per night, as compared to seldom-attacked species like lions, bats, and armadillos, that sleep many hours (Chapter 8).
- Bears eat all the food they can find, storing fat to help them survive during times when food is scarce. Small birds eat only enough to satisfy their immediate needs, because any extra weight would interfere with their ability to fly away from predators. Eating habits relate to the needs of each species (Chapter 9).

Several human behaviors make no sense except in terms of evolution. For example, people get "goose bumps"—erections of the hairs, especially on their arms and shoulders—when they are cold or frightened. Goose bumps produce little if any benefit to humans because our shoulder and arm hairs are short and usually covered by clothing. In most other mammals, however, erected hairs make a frightened animal look larger and more intimidating (see Figure 4.6). They also provide extra insulation when the air is cold. We explain human goose bumps by saying that the behavior evolved in our remote ancestors and we inherited the mechanism.

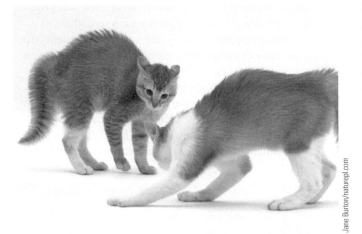

Figure 4.6 A frightened cat with erect hairs
For animals with long hairs, erecting those hairs increases insulation from cold and makes the animal look larger and more dangerous. We humans continue to erect our hairs in those same situations as a remnant from our evolutionary past.

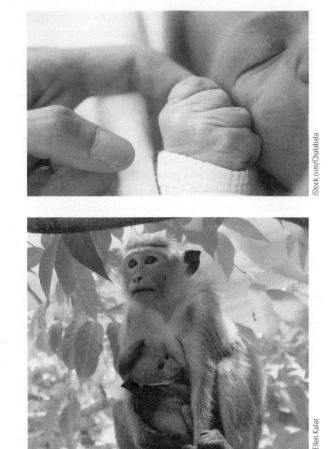

Figure 4.7 Grasp reflex in human and monkey infants
The grasp reflex, which accomplishes little or nothing for human infants, makes sense as an evolutionary remnant of a behavior necessary for the survival of our monkey-like ancestors.

Also consider the infant grasp reflex (see Figure 4.7). An infant will grasp tightly onto a finger, pencil, or similar object placed in the palm of the hand. What good does that accomplish? Little or none for humans, but for our monkey-like ancestors, it was critical. A mother monkey often needs all four limbs to climb a tree for food or to run away from a predator. An infant monkey that couldn't hold on would jeopardize its life.

Certain other proposed evolutionary explanations are more controversial. Consider two examples:

- More men than women enjoy the prospect of casual sex with multiple partners. Theorists have related this tendency to the fact that a man can spread his genes by impregnating many women, whereas a woman cannot multiply her children by having more sexual partners (Buss, 1994). Are men and women prewired to have different sexual behaviors? To what extent is this behavior biologically driven and to what extent culturally driven? We shall explore this topic in a later chapter.
- People grow old and die, with an average survival time of 70 to 80 years under favorable circumstances. However, people vary in how rapidly they deteriorate in old age, and

part of that variation is under genetic control. Researchers have identified several genes that are significantly more common among people who remain healthy and alert at ages 85 and beyond (Halaschek-Wiener et al., 2009; Poduslo, Huang, & Spiro, 2009; Puca et al., 2001). Why don't we all have those genes? Perhaps living many years after the end of your reproductive years is evolutionarily disadvantageous. Did we evolve a tendency to grow old and die in order to get out of the way and stop competing with our children and grandchildren? Curiously, a few species of turtles and fish continue reproducing throughout their long lives, and they do not seem to deteriorate with age. Greenland sharks can live for 400 years, maybe more (Nielsen et al., 2016). On the opposite extreme, some insects die of old age within weeks. Again, the idea is that human life span may be an evolved adaptation, rather than a physical necessity.

To further illustrate evolutionary psychology, consider the theoretically interesting example of **altruistic behavior**, an action that benefits someone other than the actor. A gene that encourages altruistic behavior would help *other* individuals survive and spread *their* genes, at a possible cost to the altruistic individual. Could a gene for altruism spread, and if so, how?

How common is altruism? It certainly occurs in humans: We contribute to charities. We try to help people in distress. A student may explain something to a classmate who is competing for a good grade in a course. Some people donate a kidney to save the life of someone they didn't even know (MacFarquhar, 2009).

Among nonhumans, altruism is less common. Cooperation occurs, certainly. A pack of animals may hunt together or forage together. A flock of small birds may "mob" an owl or hawk to drive it away. Chimpanzees sometimes share food (Hamann, Warneken, Greenberg, & Tomasello, 2011). But real altruism, in the sense of helping a nonrelative without quickly getting something in return, is unusual for nonhumans (Cheney, 2011). In one study, a chimpanzee could pull one rope to bring food into its own cage or a second rope that would bring food to itself and additional food to a familiar but unrelated chimpanzee in a neighboring cage. Most often, chimps pulled whichever rope happened to be on the right at the time—suggesting right-handedness—apparently indifferent to the welfare of the other chimpanzee, even when the other made begging gestures (Silk et al., 2005).

Even when animals do appear altruistic, they often have a selfish motive. When a crow finds food on the ground, it caws loudly, attracting other crows that will share the food. Altruism? Not really. A bird on the ground is vulnerable to attack by cats and other enemies. Having other crows around means more eyes to watch for dangers.

Also consider meerkats (a kind of mongoose). Periodically, one or another member of a meerkat colony stands and, if it sees danger, emits an alarm call that warns the others (see Figure 4.8). Its alarm call helps the others (including its relatives), but the one who sees the danger first and emits the alarm call is the one most likely to escape (Clutton-Brock et al., 1999).

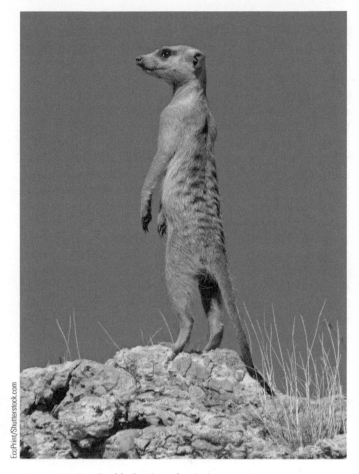

EcoPrint/Shutterstock.com

Figure 4.8 Sentinel behavior: altruistic or not?
As in many other prey species, meerkats sometimes show sentinel behavior in watching for danger and warning the others. However, the meerkat that emits the alarm is the one most likely to escape the danger.

For the sake of illustration, let's suppose—without evidence—that some gene increases altruistic behavior—a behavior that helps others and not yourself. Could it spread within a population? One common reply is that most altruistic behaviors cost very little. True, but costing little is not good enough. A gene spreads only if the individuals with it reproduce more than those without it. Another common reply is that the altruistic behavior benefits the species. True again, but the rebuttal is the same. A gene that benefits the species but fails to help the individual dies out with that individual.

A better explanation is **kin selection**—selection for a gene that benefits the individual's relatives. A gene spreads if it causes you to take great efforts, even risking your life, to protect your children, because they share many of your genes, including perhaps a gene for protecting their own children. Natural selection can also favor altruism toward other relatives—such as brothers and sisters, cousins, nephews, and nieces (Dawkins, 1989; Hamilton, 1964; Trivers, 1985). In both humans and nonhumans, helpful behavior is more common toward relatives than toward unrelated individuals (Bowles & Posel, 2005; Krakauer, 2005).

Another explanation is **reciprocal altruism**, the idea that individuals help those who will return the favor. Researchers find that people are prone to help not only those who helped them but also people whom they observed helping someone else. Even young children show this tendency (Martin & Olson, 2015). The idea is not just "you scratched my back, so I'll scratch yours," but also "you scratched someone else's back, so I'll scratch yours." By helping others, you build a reputation for helpfulness, and others are willing to cooperate with you. This system works only if individuals recognize one another. Otherwise, an uncooperative individual can accept favors, prosper, and never repay the favors. In other words, reciprocal altruism requires an ability to identify individuals and remember them later. Humans, of course, are excellent at recognizing one another even over long delays.

A third hypothesis is **group selection**. According to this idea, altruistic groups thrive better than less cooperative ones (Bowles, 2006; Kohn, 2008). Although this idea is certainly true, it faces a problem: Even if cooperative groups do well, wouldn't an uncooperative individual within the cooperative group gain an advantage? Nevertheless, theorists have concluded that group selection does work under certain circumstances, such

as when cooperative individuals do most of their interactions with one another (Simon, Fletcher, & Doebeli, 2013). Group selection works especially well for humans, because of our ability to punish or expel uncooperative people.

At its best, evolutionary psychology leads to research that helps us understand a behavior. The search for a functional explanation directs researchers to explore species' different habitats and ways of life until we understand why they behave differently. The approach is criticized when its practitioners propose explanations without testing them (Schlinger, 1996).

STOP & CHECK

11. What are plausible ways for possible altruistic genes to spread in a population?

ANSWER

11. Altruistic genes could spread because they facilitate care for one's kin or because they facilitate exchanges of favors with others (reciprocal altruism). Group selection may also work under some circumstances, especially if the cooperative group has a way to punish or expel an uncooperative individual.

Module 4.1 | In Closing

Genes and Behavior

In the control of behavior, genes are important but not all-important. Certain behaviors have a high heritability, such as the ability to taste PTC. Many other behaviors are influenced by genes but also subject to strong influence by experience. Our genes and our evolution make it possible for humans to be what we are today, but they also give us the flexibility to change our behavior as circumstances warrant.

Understanding the genetics of human behavior is important but also especially difficult, because researchers have such

limited control over environmental influences and no control over who mates with whom. Inferring how human behavior evolved is also difficult, partly because we do not know enough about the lives of our ancient ancestors.

Finally, we should remember that the way things *are* is not necessarily the same as the way they *should be*. Even if our genes predispose us to behave in a particular way, we can still decide to try to overcome those predispositions if they do not suit the needs of modern life.

Summary

1. Genes are chemicals that maintain their integrity from one generation to the next and influence the development of the individual. A dominant gene affects development regardless of whether a person has pairs of that gene or only a single copy per cell. A recessive gene affects development only in the absence of the dominant gene. **104**

2. Genes can change by mutations, microduplications, and microdeletions. **107**

3. Gene expression can also change in a process called epigenetics, as chemicals activate or deactivate parts of chromosomes. Experiences can cause epigenetic changes, and in some cases an epigenetic change can influence the next generation. **107**

4. Most behavioral variations reflect the combined influences of genes and environmental factors. Heritability is an estimate of the amount of variation that is due to genetic variation as opposed to environmental variation. **108**

5. Researchers estimate heritability of a human condition by comparing monozygotic and dizygotic twins and by comparing adopted children to their biological and adoptive parents. They also search for genes that are more common in people with one type of behavior than another. **108**

6. Even if some behavior shows high heritability for a given population, a change in the environment might significantly alter the behavioral outcome. **109**

7. Genes influence behavior directly by altering brain chemicals and indirectly by affecting other aspects of the body and therefore the way other people react to us. **110**

8. The process of evolution through natural selection is a necessary outcome, given what we know about reproduction: Mutations sometimes occur in genes, and individuals with certain sets of genes reproduce more successfully than others do. **110**

9. Evolution spreads the genes of the individuals who have reproduced the most. Therefore, if some characteristic is widespread within a population, it is reasonable to look for ways in which that characteristic is or has been adaptive. However, we need to evaluate the relative contributions of genetics and cultural influences. **112**

Key Terms

Terms are defined in the module on the page number indicated. They're also presented in alphabetical order with definitions in the book's Subject Index/Glossary, which begins on page 589. Interactive flash cards, audio reviews, and crossword puzzles are among the online resources available to help you learn these terms and the concepts they represent.

Thought Questions

1. For what human behaviors, if any, are you sure that heritability would be extremely low?
2. Certain genes influence the probability of developing Alzheimer's disease or other conditions that occur mostly in old age. Given that the genes controlling old age have their onset long after people have stopped having children, how could evolution have any effect on such genes?

Module 4.1 | End of Module Quiz

1. What is a sex-linked gene?
   A. A gene that influences sexual behavior
   B. A gene that has greater effects on one sex than the other
   C. A gene on either the X or Y chromosome –
   D. A gene that becomes activated during sexual behavior

2. What is a sex-limited gene?
   A. A gene that influences sexual behavior
   B. A gene that has greater effects on one sex than the other —
   C. A gene on either the X or Y chromosome
   D. A gene that becomes activated during sexual behavior

3. What does a microdeletion remove?
   A. Part of a protein
   B. Part of a brain wave
   C. Part of a chromosome
   D. Part of a neuron

4. How does an epigenetic change differ from a mutation?
   A. An epigenetic change is a duplication or deletion of part of a gene.
   B. An epigenetic change alters gene activity without replacing any gene.
   C. An epigenetic change alters more than one gene at a time.
   D. An epigenetic change is beneficial, whereas a mutation is harmful.

5. How does adding a methyl or acetyl group to a histone protein alter gene activity?
   - **A.** A methyl group turns genes off. An acetyl group loosens histone's grip and increases gene activation.
   - **B.** A methyl group turns genes on. An acetyl group tightens histone's grip and decreases gene activation.
   - **C.** A methyl group increases the probability of a mutation, whereas an acetyl group decreases the probability.
   - **D.** A methyl group decreases the probability of a mutation, whereas an acetyl group increases the probability.

6. Most estimates of heritability of human behavior use what type(s) of evidence?
   - **A.** Studies of changes in behavior as people grow older
   - **B.** Studies of similarities between parents and children
   - **C.** Comparisons of twins and studies of adopted children
   - **D.** Comparisons of people living in different cultures

7. What is the difference between monozygotic (MZ) and dizygotic (DZ) twins?
   - **A.** MZ twins develop from two eggs, whereas DZ twins develop from a single egg.
   - **B.** MZ twins develop from a single egg, whereas DZ twins develop from two eggs.
   - **C.** MZ twins are one male and one female, whereas DZ twins are of the same gender.
   - **D.** MZ twins are of the same gender, whereas DZ twins are one male and one female.

8. Which of the following offers strong evidence that environmental changes can largely counteract the effect of a gene?
   - **A.** The effects of temperature on children with autism spectrum disorder
   - **B.** The effects of diet on children with phenylketonuria (PKU)
   - **C.** The effects of muscle training on children who have suffered a concussion
   - **D.** The effects of sleep on children with malaria

9. Which of these is responsible for evolutionary changes in a species?
   - **A.** Using or failing to use part of the body increases or decreases its size for the next generation.
   - **B.** A gene that has long-term benefits to the species will become more common.
   - **C.** Individuals with certain genes reproduce more than average.
   - **D.** Evolutionary changes anticipate the adaptations that will be advantageous in the future.

10. What, if anything, can we predict about the future of human evolution?
    - **A.** People will get smarter, wiser, and more cooperative.
    - **B.** People will not change, because evolution no longer affects humans.
    - **C.** People will become more like whichever people tend to have the most children.
    - **D.** We cannot make any of these predictions.

11. Why do human infants show a grasp reflex?
    - **A.** The reflex is an accidental by-product of brain development.
    - **B.** The reflex is an imitation of actions the infant sees adults doing.
    - **C.** The reflex helps the infant develop motor skills that will be helpful later.
    - **D.** The reflex was advantageous to infants of our remote ancestors.

Answers: 1C, 2B, 3C, 4B, 5A, 6C, 7B, 8B, 9C, 10C, 11D.

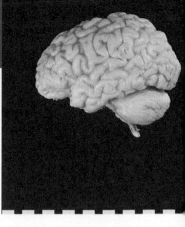

Development of the Brain

Think of all the things you can do that you couldn't have done a few years ago—analyze statistics, read a foreign language, write brilliant critiques of complex issues, and so on. Have you developed these new skills because of brain growth? Many of your dendrites have grown new branches, but your brain as a whole hasn't grown.

Now think of all the things that 1-year-old children can do that they could not do at birth. Have *they* developed their new skills because of brain growth? To a large extent, yes, although the results depend on experiences as well. In this module, we consider how neurons develop, how their axons connect, and how experience modifies development.

Maturation of the Vertebrate Brain

The earliest stages of development are remarkably similar across species. A series of genes known as *homeobox genes*—found in vertebrates, insects, plants, even fungi and yeast—regulate the expression of other genes and control the start of anatomical development, including such matters as which end is the front and which is the rear. All these genes share a large sequence of DNA bases. A mutation in one homeobox gene causes insects to form legs where their antennas should be, or to form an extra set of wings. In humans, mutations in homeobox genes have been linked to many brain disorders including mental retardation, as well as physical deformities (Conti et al., 2011).

The human central nervous system begins to form when the embryo is about 2 weeks old. The dorsal surface thickens and then long thin lips rise, curl, and merge, forming a neural tube that surrounds a fluid-filled cavity (see Figure 4.9). As the tube sinks under the surface of the skin, the forward end enlarges and differentiates into the hindbrain, midbrain, and forebrain (see Figure 4.10). The rest becomes the spinal cord. The fluid-filled cavity within the neural tube becomes the central canal of the spinal cord and the four ventricles of the brain, containing the cerebrospinal fluid (CSF). The first muscle movements start at age 7½ weeks, and their only accomplishment is to stretch the muscles. At that age, spontaneous activity in the spinal cord drives all the muscle movements, as the sensory organs are not yet functional (Provine, 1972). That is, contrary to what we might guess, we start making movements before we start receiving sensations.

At birth, the average human brain weighs about 350 grams. By the end of the first year, it weighs 1,000 g, close to the adult weight of 1,200 to 1,400 g. In early infancy, the primary sensory areas of the cortex—responsible for registering vision, hearing,

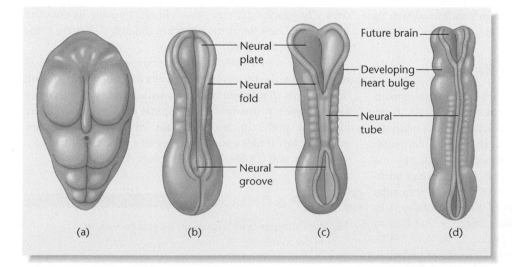

Figure 4.9 Early development of the human central nervous system The brain and spinal cord begin as folding lips surrounding a fluid-filled canal. The stages shown occur at approximately 2 to 3 weeks after conception.

117

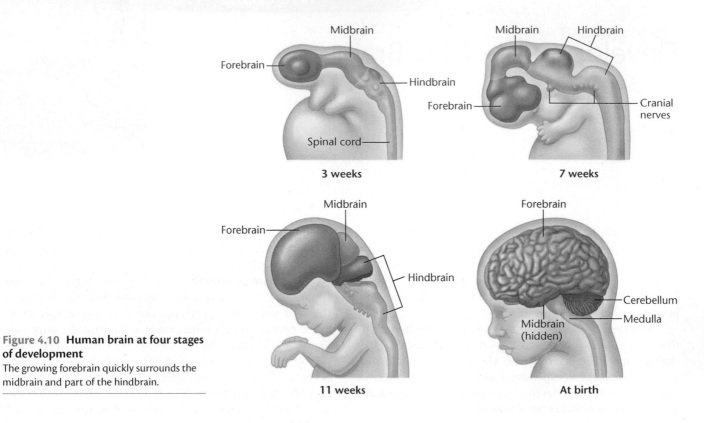

Figure 4.10 Human brain at four stages of development
The growing forebrain quickly surrounds the midbrain and part of the hindbrain.

and other senses—are more mature than the rest of the cortex. Their gyri and sulci are mostly formed, and their connections with the thalamus are fairly well established. They continue to develop, of course, but the greatest changes over the first couple of years happen in the prefrontal cortex and other cortical areas responsible for attention, working memory, and decision making (Alcuter et al., 2014; G. Li et al., 2014). In short, the infant brain is set up to see, hear, and so forth, but limited in its ability to interpret that information or to decide what to do about it. The human prefrontal cortex continues slowly maturing through the teenage years and beyond. In general, the brain areas that are slowest to develop, such as the prefrontal cortex, are the ones most likely to deteriorate in conditions such as Alzheimer's disease (Douaud et al., 2014).

Growth and Development of Neurons

Neuroscientists distinguish several stages in the development of neurons. **Proliferation** is the production of new cells. Early in development, the cells lining the ventricles of the brain divide. Some cells remain where they are as **stem cells**, continuing to divide, whereas others migrate to other parts of the nervous system. In humans, most of the migration occurs before birth, but a small number continue to migrate for the first few months after birth (Paredes et al., 2016). One of the major differences between human brains and chimpanzee brains is that human neurons continue proliferating longer (Rakic, 1998; Vrba, 1998). Nearly all neurons form within the first 28 weeks of gestation, and premature birth before that time inhibits neuron formation (Malik et al., 2013).

Early in development, the primitive cells, not yet identifiable as neurons or glia, begin to **migrate** (move). Chemicals known as *immunoglobulins* and *chemokines* guide neuron migration. A deficit in these chemicals leads to impaired migration, decreased brain size, and mental retardation (Berger-Sweeney & Hohmann, 1997; Crossin & Krushel, 2000; Tran & Miller, 2003). The brain has many kinds of immunoglobulins and chemokines, reflecting the complexity of brain development.

As a cell **differentiates** into a neuron, it begins to form its dendrites, axon, and synapses. **Synaptogenesis**, the formation of synapses, begins long before birth, but it continues throughout life, as neurons form new synapses and discard old ones. The process generally slows in older people, as does the formation of new dendritic branches (Buell & Coleman, 1981; Jacobs & Scheibel, 1993).

A later and slower stage of neuronal development is **myelination**, the process by which glia produce the insulating fatty sheaths that accelerate transmission in many vertebrate axons. Myelin forms first in the spinal cord and then in the hindbrain, midbrain, and forebrain. Myelination continues gradually for decades and increases as a result of learning a new motor skill (Fields, 2015; McKenzie et al., 2014).

✓ **STOP & CHECK** ▬▬▬▬▬▬

12. Which comes first: migration, synaptogenesis, or myelination?

ANSWER   12. Migration occurs first.

New Neurons Later in Life

Can the adult vertebrate brain generate new neurons? The traditional belief, dating back to Cajal's work in the late 1800s, as discussed in Chapter 1, was that vertebrate brains formed all their neurons in embryological development or early infancy at the latest. Beyond that point, neurons could modify their shape, but the brain could not develop new neurons. Later researchers found exceptions.

The first exceptions were the olfactory receptors, which are exposed to the outside world and its toxic chemicals. The nose contains stem cells that remain immature throughout life. Periodically, they divide, with one cell remaining immature while the other differentiates to replace a dying olfactory receptor. It grows its axon back to the appropriate site in the brain (Gogos, Osborne, Nemes, Mendelsohn, & Axel, 2000; Graziadei & deHan, 1973).

The olfactory receptors send axons to the olfactory bulb, and later researchers also demonstrated the formation of new neurons in the olfactory bulb for many species (Gage, 2000). However, new neurons do not form in this area for humans, at least after the first year or so of life (Bergmann et al., 2012; Sanai et al., 2011).

In songbirds, one brain area that is necessary for singing loses neurons in fall and winter and regains them the next spring (mating season) (Nottebohm, 2002; Wissman & Brenowitz, 2009). Also, new neurons form in the adult hippocampus of birds (Smulders, Shiflett, Sperling, & DeVoogd, 2000) and mammals (Song, Stevens, & Gage, 2002; van Praag et al., 2002). The hippocampus is an important area for memory formation. A supply of new neurons keeps the hippocampus "young" for learning new tasks (Ge, Yang, Hsu, Ming, & Song, 2007; Schmidt-Hieber, Jonas, & Bischofberger, 2004). Blocking the formation of new neurons (such as by exposing the hippocampus to X-rays) impairs the formation of new memories (Clelland et al., 2009; Meshi et al., 2006).

How could researchers determine whether new neurons form in the adult brain in humans? A clever method relies on a radioactive isotope of carbon, ^{14}C. The concentration of ^{14}C in the atmosphere, compared with other isotopes of carbon, was nearly constant over time until the era of nuclear bomb testing released much radioactivity. That era ended with the Test Ban Treaty of 1963. The concentration of ^{14}C peaked in 1963 and has been declining since then. If you examine tree rings, you find that a ring that formed in 1963 has the ^{14}C content typical of 1963, a ring that formed in 1990 has the ^{14}C content typical of 1990, and so forth. Researchers examined carbon in the DNA of various human cells. Every cell acquires DNA molecules when it forms and keeps them until it dies. When researchers examined people's skin cells, they found a concentration of ^{14}C corresponding to the year in which they did the test. That is, skin cells turn over rapidly, and your skin cells are less than a year old. When they examined skeletal muscle cells, they found a ^{14}C concentration corresponding to 15 years ago, indicating that skeletal muscles are replaced slowly, making the average cell 15 years old. Cells of the heart are, on average, almost as old as the person, indicating that the body replaces no more than one percent of heart cells per year (Bergmann et al., 2009). When researchers examined neurons in the cerebral cortex (of dead people at autopsy), they found a ^{14}C concentration corresponding to the year of the person's birth. These results indicate that the mammalian cerebral cortex forms few or no new neurons after birth (Spalding, Bhardwaj, Buchholz, Druid, & Frisén, 2005). Further research confirmed that suffering a stroke does not prompt the human cortex to form new neurons (Huttner et al., 2014). However, the ^{14}C concentration of the human hippocampus indicates that we replace almost 2 percent of neurons in that area per year (Spalding et al., 2013). We also replace some of the neurons in parts of the basal ganglia known as the *striatum*, including the caudate nucleus, putamen, and nucleus accumbens (see Figures 3.11 and 3.15) (Ernst et al., 2014). The hippocampus and basal ganglia, the two areas where we make new neurons throughout life, are both important for new learning. The new neurons are invariably small interneurons, not neurons with long axons extending to other brain areas.

STOP & CHECK

13. New receptor neurons form in which sensory system?
14. What evidence indicates that new neurons form in the human hippocampus and basal ganglia?

ANSWERS   13. Olfaction 14. The mean ^{14}C concentration of the DNA of human neurons in the hippocampus and basal ganglia corresponds to a level slightly more recent than the year the person was born, indicating that some of those neurons formed after birth.

Pathfinding by Axons

If you asked someone to run a cable from one place to another in your room, your directions could be simple. But imagine asking someone to run a cable to somewhere on the other side of the country. You would have to give detailed instructions about how to find the right city, building, and location within the building. The developing nervous system faces a similar challenge because it sends axons over great distances. How do they find their way?

Chemical Pathfinding by Axons

A famous biologist, Paul Weiss (1924), conducted an experiment in which he grafted an extra leg to a salamander and then waited for axons to grow into it. Unlike mammals, salamanders and other amphibians accept transplants of extra limbs and generate new axon branches to the extra limbs. Much research requires finding the right species to study. After the axons reached the muscles, the extra leg moved in synchrony with the normal leg next to it.

Weiss dismissed the idea that each axon found its way to the correct muscle in the extra limb. He suggested instead that the nerves attached to muscles at random and then sent a variety of messages, each one tuned to a different muscle.

He supposed that muscles were like radios tuned to different stations: Each muscle received many signals but responded to only one. (The 1920s were the early days of radio, and it was an appealing analogy to think the nervous system might work like a radio. In the 1600s, Descartes thought the nervous system worked like a hydraulic pump, the most advanced technology of the time. Today, many people think the nervous system works like a computer, our own most advanced technology.)

Specificity of Axon Connections

Later evidence supported the interpretation that Weiss had rejected: The salamander's extra leg moved in synchrony with its neighbor because each axon found the correct muscle.

Roger Sperry, a former student of Weiss, performed a classic experiment that showed how sensory axons find their way to their correct targets. The principle is the same as for axons finding their way to muscles. First, Sperry cut the optic nerves of some newts. (Note the importance of choosing the right species: A cut optic nerve grows back in amphibians, but not in mammals or birds.) The damaged optic nerve grew back and connected with the *tectum*, which is amphibians' main visual area (see Figure 4.11), thereby reestablishing normal vision. So then Sperry's question was: Did they grow at random, or did they grow to a specific target?

For the next set of newts, Sperry (1943) cut the optic nerve and rotated the eye by 180 degrees. When the axons grew back to the tectum, the axons from what had originally been the dorsal portion of the retina (which was now ventral) grew back to the area responsible for vision in the dorsal retina. Axons from other parts of the retina also grew back to their original targets. The newt now saw the world upside down and backward, responding to stimuli in the sky as if they were on the ground and to stimuli on the left as if they were on the right (see Figure 4.12). Each axon regenerated to the same

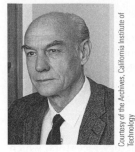

Roger W. Sperry (1913–1994)

When subjective values have objective consequences . . . they become part of the content of science. . . . Science would become the final determinant of what is right and true, the best source and authority available to the human brain for finding ultimate axioms and guideline beliefs to live by, and for reaching an intimate understanding and rapport with the forces that control the universe and created man. (Sperry, 1975)

Courtesy of the Archives, California Institute of Technology

place where it had originally been, presumably by following a chemical trail.

Chemical Gradients

The next question was: How does an axon find its target? The current estimate is that humans have fewer than 30,000 genes total, probably fewer than 20,000—far too few to specify individual targets for each of the brain's billions of neurons.

A growing axon follows a path of cell surface molecules, attracted by certain chemicals and repelled by others, in a process that steers the axon in the correct direction (Yu & Bargmann, 2001). Eventually, axons sort themselves over the surface of their target area by following a gradient of chemicals. One protein in the amphibian tectum is 30 times more concentrated in the axons of the dorsal retina than of the ventral retina and 10 times more concentrated in the ventral tectum than in the dorsal tectum. As axons from the retina grow toward the tectum, the retinal axons with the greatest concentration of this chemical connect to the tectal cells with the highest concentration. The axons with the lowest concentration connect to the tectal cells with the lowest concentration. A similar gradient of another protein aligns the axons along the anterior–posterior

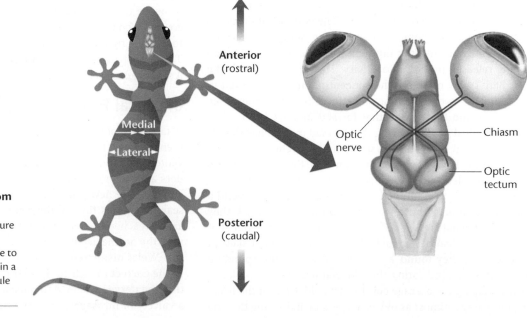

Figure 4.11 Connections from eye to brain in a newt
The optic tectum is a large structure in fish, amphibians, reptiles, and birds. Note: Connections from eye to brain in a newt differ from those in a human, as described in the module on lateralization.

Anterior (rostral)

Medial

Lateral

Posterior (caudal)

Optic nerve

Chiasm

Optic tectum

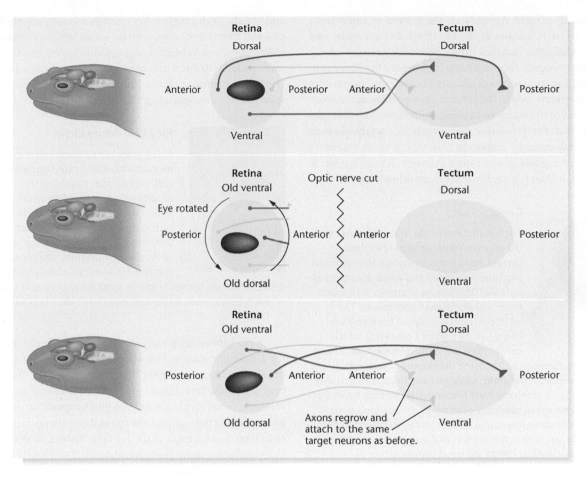

Figure 4.12 Sperry's experiment on nerve connections in newts
After he cut the optic nerve and inverted the eye, the axons grew back to their original targets, not to the targets corresponding to the eye's current position.

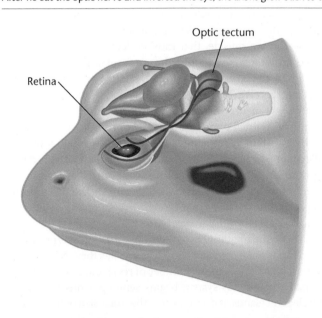

Figure 4.13 Retinal axons find targets in the tectum by following chemical gradients
One protein is concentrated mostly in the dorsal retina and the ventral tectum. Axons rich in that protein attach to tectal neurons that are also rich in that chemical. A second protein directs axons from the posterior retina to the anterior portion of the tectum.

axis (Sanes, 1993) (see Figure 4.13). By analogy, you could think of men lining up from tallest to shortest, pairing up with women who lined up from tallest to shortest.

✅ **STOP & CHECK**

15. What was Sperry's evidence that axons grow to a specific target instead of attaching at random?

ANSWER **15.** If he cut a newt's eye and inverted it, axons grew back to their original targets, even though the connections were inappropriate to their new positions on the eye.

Competition among Axons as a General Principle

When axons initially reach their targets, chemical gradients steer them to approximately their correct location, but it would be hard to imagine that they achieve perfect accuracy. Instead, each axon forms synapses onto many cells in approximately the correct location, and each target cell receives synapses from many axons. Over time, each postsynaptic cell strengthens the most appropriate synapses and eliminates others (Hua & Smith,

2004). This adjustment depends on the pattern of input from incoming axons (Catalano & Shatz, 1998). For example, one part of the thalamus receives input from many retinal axons. During embryological development, long before the first exposure to light, repeated waves of spontaneous activity sweep over the retina from one side to the other. Consequently, axons from adjacent areas of the retina send almost simultaneous messages to the thalamus. Each thalamic neuron selects a group of axons that are simultaneously active. In this way, it finds receptors from adjacent regions of the retina (Meister, Wong, Baylor, & Shatz, 1991). It then rejects synapses from other locations.

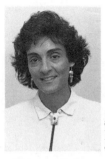

Carla J. Shatz

The functioning of the brain depends upon the precision and patterns of its neural circuits. How is this amazing computational machine assembled and wired during development? The biological answer is so much more wonderful than anticipated! The adult precision is sculpted from an early imprecise pattern by a process in which connections are verified by the functioning of the neurons themselves. Thus, the developing brain is not simply a miniature version of the adult. Moreover, the brain works to wire itself, rather than assembling itself first and then flipping a switch, as might happen in the assembly of a computer. This kind of surprise in scientific discovery opens up new vistas of understanding and possibility and makes the process of doing science infinitely exciting and fascinating. (Shatz, personal communication)

These results suggest a general principle, called **neural Darwinism** (Edelman, 1987). In the development of the nervous system, we start with more neurons and synapses than we can keep, and then a selection process keeps some of the synapses and rejects others. The most successful combinations survive, and the others fail. The principle of competition is an important one, although we should use the analogy with Darwinian evolution cautiously. Mutations in the genes are random events, but neurotrophins steer new axonal branches and synapses in approximately the right direction.

✓ STOP & CHECK

16. If axons from the retina were prevented from showing spontaneous activity during early development, what would be the probable effect on development of the thalamus?

ANSWER 16. The axons would attach based on a chemical gradient but could not fine-tune their adjustment based on experience. Therefore, the connections would be less precise.

Determinants of Neuronal Survival

Getting the right number of neurons for each area of the nervous system is more complicated than it might seem. Consider an example. The sympathetic nervous system sends axons to muscles

and glands. Each ganglion has enough axons to supply the muscles and glands in its area, with no axons left over. How does the match come out so exact? Long ago, one hypothesis was that the muscles sent chemical messages to tell the sympathetic ganglion how many neurons to form. Rita Levi-Montalcini was largely responsible for disconfirming this hypothesis.

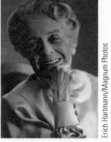

Rita Levi-Montalcini

Many years later, I often asked myself how we could have dedicated ourselves with such enthusiasm to solving this small neuroembryological problem while German armies were advancing throughout Europe, spreading destruction and death wherever they went and threatening the very survival of Western civilization. The answer lies in the desperate and partially unconscious desire of human beings to ignore what is happening in situations where full awareness might lead one to self-destruction.

Levi-Montalcini's early life would seem most unfavorable for a scientific career. She was a young Italian Jewish woman during the Nazi era. World War II destroyed the Italian economy, and at the time almost everyone discouraged women from scientific or medical careers. She had to spend several years in hiding during the war, but she spent those years conducting research on development of the nervous system, as she described in her autobiography (Levi-Montalcini, 1988) and a later interview with Moses Chao (2010). She developed a love for research and eventually discovered that the muscles do not determine how many axons *form;* they determine how many *survive.*

Initially, the sympathetic nervous system forms far more neurons than it needs. When one of its neurons forms a synapse onto a muscle, that muscle delivers a protein called **nerve growth factor (NGF)** that promotes the survival and growth of the axon (Levi-Montalcini, 1987). An axon that does not receive NGF degenerates, and its cell body dies. That is, each neuron starts life with a "suicide program": If its axon does not make contact with an appropriate postsynaptic cell by a certain age, the neuron kills itself through a process called **apoptosis,**[1] a programmed mechanism of cell death. (Apoptosis is distinct from *necrosis,* which is death caused by an injury or a toxic substance.) NGF cancels the program for apoptosis; it is the postsynaptic cell's way of telling the incoming axon, "I'll be your partner. Don't kill yourself."

The sympathetic nervous system's way of overproducing neurons and then applying apoptosis enables the CNS to match the number of axons to the number of receiving cells. When the sympathetic nervous system begins sending axons toward the muscles and glands, it doesn't know the exact size of the muscles

[1]Apoptosis is based on the Greek root *ptosis* (meaning "dropping"), which is pronounced TOE-sis. Therefore, many scholars insist that the second *p* in *apoptosis* should be silent, a-po-TOE-sis. Others argue that *helicopter* is also derived from a root with a silent *p (pteron)*, but we pronounce the *p* in *helicopter*, so we should also pronounce the second *p* in *apoptosis*. Most people today do pronounce the second p, but be prepared for either pronunciation.

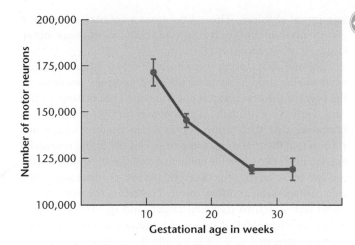

Figure 4.14 Cell loss during development of the nervous system
The number of motor neurons in the spinal cord of human fetuses is
highest at 11 weeks and drops steadily until about 25 weeks. Axons that
fail to make synapses die.
*(Source: From "Motoneuronal death in the human fetus," by N. G. Forger and
S. M. Breedlove, 1987,* Journal of Comparative Neurology, 264, pp. 118–122.
Copyright © 1987 Alan R. Liss, Inc. Reprinted by permission of N. G. Forger..)

or glands. It makes more neurons than necessary and discards the excess. In fact, all areas of the developing nervous system make more neurons than will survive into adulthood. Each brain area has a period of massive cell death, becoming littered with dead and dying cells (see Figure 4.14) (Forger & Breedlove, 1987). This loss of cells is a natural part of development. In fact, loss of cells in a particular brain area often indicates maturation. Maturation of successful cells is linked to simultaneous loss of less successful ones.

Nerve growth factor is a **neurotrophin**, meaning a chemical that promotes the survival and activity of neurons. (The word *trophin* derives from a Greek word for "nourishment.") In addition to NGF, the nervous system responds to *brain-derived neurotrophic factor* (BDNF) and several other neurotrophins (Airaksinen & Saarma, 2002). Neurotrophins are essential for growth of axons and dendrites, formation of new synapses, and learning (Alleva & Francia, 2009; Pascual et al., 2008; Rauskolb et al., 2010). Remember the term *BDNF*, because it becomes important again in the discussion of depression.

Although neurotrophins are essential to the survival of motor neurons in the periphery, they do not control survival of neurons within the brain. When cortical neurons reach a certain age in early development, a certain percentage of them die. How many neurons are present doesn't seem to matter. Experimenters transplanted extra neurons into mouse cortex with no apparent effect on the survival of the neurons already present (Southwell et al., 2012). What controls neuron death in the brain is not yet understood, but one factor is that neurons need input from incoming neurons. In one study, researchers examined mice with a genetic defect that prevented release of neurotransmitters. The brains initially assembled normal anatomies, but then the neurons started dying rapidly (Verhage et al., 2000).

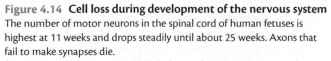

STOP & CHECK

17. What process assures that the spinal cord has the right number of axons to innervate all the muscle cells?
18. What class of chemicals prevents apoptosis in the sympathetic nervous system?
19. At what age does a person have the greatest number of neurons—early in life, during adolescence, or during adulthood?

ANSWERS

17. The nervous system builds more neurons than it needs and discards through apoptosis those that do not make lasting synapses. **18.** Neurotrophins, such as nerve growth factor. **19.** The neuron number is greatest early in life.

The Vulnerable Developing Brain

According to Lewis Wolpert (1991), "It is not birth, marriage, or death, but gastrulation, which is truly the most important time of your life." (Gastrulation is one of the early stages of embryological development.) Wolpert's point was that if you mess up in early development, you have problems from then on. Actually, if you mess up during gastrulation, your life is over.

During early development, the brain is highly vulnerable to malnutrition, toxic chemicals, and infections that would produce milder problems at later ages. For example, impaired thyroid function produces lethargy in adults but mental retardation in infants. (Thyroid deficiency was common in the past because of iodine deficiency. It is rare today because table salt is fortified with iodine.) A fever is a mere annoyance to an adult, but it impairs neuron proliferation in a fetus (Laburn, 1996). Low blood glucose decreases an adult's pep, but before birth, it impairs brain development (Nelson et al., 2000).

The infant brain is highly vulnerable to damage by alcohol. Children of mothers who drink heavily during pregnancy are born with **fetal alcohol syndrome**, a condition marked by hyperactivity, impulsiveness, difficulty maintaining attention, varying degrees of mental retardation, motor problems, heart defects, and facial abnormalities. Drinking during pregnancy leads to thinning of the cerebral cortex that persists to adulthood (Zhou et al., 2011) (see Figure 4.15). More drinking causes greater deficits, but even moderate drinking produces a measurable effect (Eckstrand et al., 2012).

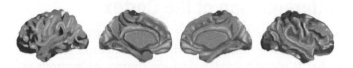

Figure 4.15 Cortical thinning as a result of prenatal alcohol exposure
The cortical areas marked in red are thinner, on average, in adults whose mothers drank alcohol during pregnancy.
(Source: From "Developmental cortical thinning in fetal alcohol spectrum disorders," by D. Zhou et al., 2011, NeuroImage, 58, pp. 16–25.)

Exposure to alcohol damages the brain in several ways. At the earliest stage of pregnancy, it interferes with neuron proliferation. A little later, it impairs neuron migration and differentiation. Still later, it impairs synaptic transmission (Kleiber, Mantha, Stringer, & Singh, 2013). Alcohol kills neurons partly by apoptosis. To prevent apoptosis, a brain neuron must receive input from incoming axons. Alcohol inhibits receptors for glutamate, the brain's main excitatory transmitter, and enhances receptors for GABA, the main inhibitory transmitter. Because of the decrease in net excitation, many neurons undergo apoptosis (Ikonomidou et al., 2000). Further harm occurs *after* a bout of drinking, while the alcohol is washing out of the system. While alcohol was inhibiting the glutamate receptors, many neurons compensated by quickly building more glutamate receptors. Then, when alcohol leaves, glutamate overexcites its receptors, bringing excess sodium and calcium into the cell and poisoning the mitochondria. The result is increased cell death in several brain areas (Clements et al., 2012).

The developing brain is highly responsive to many influences from the mother. If a mother rat is exposed to stressful experiences, she becomes more fearful, she spends less than the usual amount of time licking and grooming her offspring, and her offspring become permanently more fearful in a variety of situations (Cameron et al., 2005). Analogously, the children of impoverished and abused women have, on average, increased problems in both their academic and social lives. The mechanisms in humans are not the same as those in rats, but the overall principles are similar: Stress to the mother changes her behavior in ways that change her offspring's behavior.

STOP & CHECK

20. Anesthetic drugs and anxiety-reducing drugs increase activity of GABA, decreasing brain excitation. Why would we predict that exposure to these drugs might be dangerous to the brain of a fetus?

ANSWER

20. Prolonged exposure to anesthetics or anxiety-reducing drugs might increase apoptosis of developing neurons. Increased GABA activity decreases excitation, and developing neurons undergo apoptosis if they do not receive enough excitation.

Differentiation of the Cortex

Neurons differ in shape and chemistry. When and how does a neuron "decide" which kind of neuron it is going to be? It is not a sudden decision. Immature neurons experimentally transplanted from one part of the developing cortex to another develop the properties characteristic of their new location (McConnell, 1992). However, neurons transplanted at a slightly later stage develop some new properties while retaining some old ones (Cohen-Tannoudji, Babinet, & Wassef, 1994). It is like the speech of

immigrant children: Those who enter a country when very young master the correct pronunciation, whereas older children retain an accent.

In one fascinating experiment, researchers explored what would happen to the immature auditory portions of the brain if they received input from the eyes instead of the ears. Ferrets—mammals in the weasel family—are born so immature that their optic nerves (from the eyes) have not yet reached the thalamus. On one side of the brain, researchers damaged the superior colliculus and the occipital cortex, the two main targets for the optic nerves. On that side, they also damaged the auditory input. Therefore, the optic nerve could not attach to its usual target, and the auditory area of the thalamus lacked its usual input. As a result, the optic nerve attached to what is usually the auditory area of the thalamus. What would you guess happened? Did the visual input cause auditory sensations, or did the auditory areas of the brain turn into visual areas?

The result, surprising to many, was this: What would have been the auditory thalamus and cortex reorganized, developing some (but not all) of the characteristic appearance of visual areas (Sharma, Angelucci, & Sur, 2000). But how do we know whether the animals treated that activity as vision? Remember that the researchers performed these procedures on one side of the brain. They left the other side intact. The researchers presented stimuli to the normal side of the brain and trained the ferrets to turn one direction when they heard something and the other direction when they saw a light, as shown in Figure 4.16. After the ferrets learned this task well, the researchers presented a light that the rewired side could see. The result: The ferrets turned the way they had been taught to turn when they saw something. In short, the rewired temporal cortex, receiving input from the optic nerve, produced visual responses (von Melchner, Pallas, & Sur, 2000).

In a related study with newborn mice, researchers damaged the thalamic nucleus responsible for touch. As a result, axons from the nucleus responsible for pain sent their axons both to their usual target and to the cortical area usually receptive to touch. The cortex then reorganized to be responsive to pain in both areas (Pouchelon et al., 2014). The overall conclusion is that to some extent, the sensory input instructs the cortex about how to develop.

STOP & CHECK

21. In the ferret study, how did the experimenters determine that visual input to the auditory portions of the brain actually produced a visual sensation?

ANSWER

21. They trained the ferrets to respond to stimuli on the normal side, turning one direction in response to sounds and the other direction to lights. Then they presented light to the rewired side and saw that the ferret turned in the direction it had associated with lights.

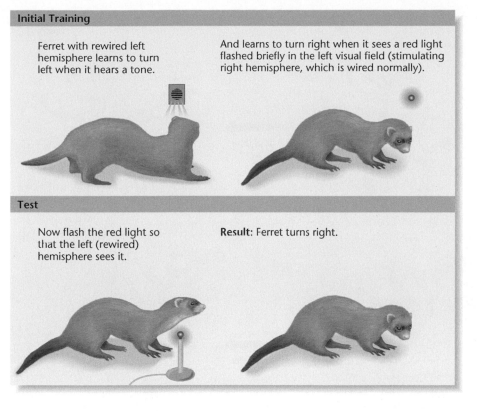

Initial Training

Ferret with rewired left hemisphere learns to turn left when it hears a tone.

And learns to turn right when it sees a red light flashed briefly in the left visual field (stimulating right hemisphere, which is wired normally).

Test

Now flash the red light so that the left (rewired) hemisphere sees it.

Result: Ferret turns right.

Figure 4.16 A ferret with rewired temporal cortex
First, the normal (right) hemisphere is trained to respond to a red light by turning to the right. Then, the rewired (left) hemisphere is tested with a red light. The fact that the ferret turns to the right indicates that it regards the stimulus as light, not sound.

Fine-Tuning by Experience

The blueprints for a house determine its overall plan, but because architects cannot anticipate every detail, construction workers often have to improvise. The same is true for your nervous system. Because of the unpredictability of life, our brains have evolved the ability to remodel themselves in response to experience (Shatz, 1992).

Experience and Dendritic Branching

Decades ago, researchers doubted that adult neurons substantially changed their shape. Although the central structure of a dendrite becomes stable by adolescence, the peripheral branches of a dendrite remain flexible throughout life (Koleske, 2013). Dale Purves and R. D. Hadley (1985) injected a dye that let them watch the structure of a living mouse neuron over days or weeks. They found that some dendritic branches extended between one viewing and another, whereas others retracted or disappeared (see Figure 4.17). About 6 percent of dendritic spines appear or disappear within a month (Xu, Pan, Yang, & Gan, 2007). The gain or loss of spines means a turnover of synapses, which relates to learning (Yang, Pan, & Gan, 2009).

Experiences guide the neuronal changes. Let's start with a simple example. Decades ago, it was typical for a laboratory rat to live alone in a small gray cage. Imagine by contrast several rats in a larger cage with a few objects to explore. Researchers called this an enriched environment, but it was enriched only by comparison to the deprived experience of a typical rat

cage. A rat in the more stimulating environment developed a thicker cortex, more dendritic branching, and improved learning (Greenough, 1975; Rosenzweig & Bennett, 1996). As a result of this research, most rats today are kept in a more enriched environment than was typical in the past. Further research found differences between the brains of laboratory-reared rats and wild rats that someone captured. Here, the difference is not just a matter of less enriched versus more enriched, but different types of stimulation and activities. The wild-caught rats had more neurons in the visual areas of the brain and fewer in the auditory areas (Campi, Collins, Todd, Kaas, & Krubitzer, 2011). A stimulating environment enhances sprouting of axons and dendrites in many other species also (Coss, Brandon, & Globus, 1980) (see Figure 4.18).

We might suppose that the neuronal changes in an enriched environment depend on interesting experiences and social interactions. No doubt some of them do, but much of the enhancement produced by the enriched environment is due to physical activity. Using a running wheel enhances growth of axons and dendrites, as well as learning, even for rodents in isolation (Marlatt, Potter, Lucassen, & van Praag, 2012; Pietropaolo, Feldon, Alleva, Cirulli, & Yee, 2006; Rhodes et al., 2003; Robinson, Buttolph, Green, & Bucci, 2015; van Praag, Kempermann, & Gage, 1999).

Can we extend these results to humans? Physical activity appears to be as beneficial for brain functioning in humans as in laboratory animals. The results on enriched environments are more debatable. Remember, the studies with laboratory rats merely showed that having a bigger cage with something to do was better than a small gray cage with nothing but food

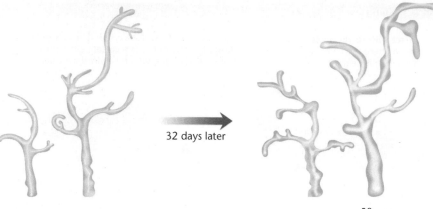

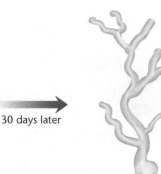

32 days later

50 μm

30 days later

Figure 4.17 Changes in dendritic trees of two mouse neurons
During a month, some branches elongated and others retracted.
Source: Based on the results of "Changes in dendritic branching of adult mammalian neurons revealed by repeated imaging in situ," by D. Purves and R. D. Hadley, 1985, Nature, 315, pp. 404–406.

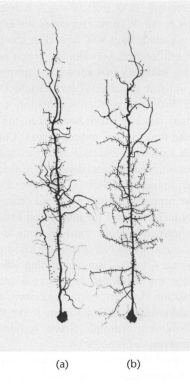

(a)   (b)

Figure 4.18 Effect of a stimulating environment
(a) A jewelfish reared in isolation develops neurons with fewer branches.
(b) A fish reared with others has more dendritic branches.
(Source: Richard Coss)

and water. So far as that goes, yes, humans in a normal environment do better intellectually than children in orphanages where the staff provides little more than minimum care (Helder, Mulder, & Gunnoe, 2016; Loman et al., 2013). But the more important question is how much we could increase intelligence beyond normal by providing special training or enhanced experiences.

Educators have long operated on the assumption that training children to do something difficult will enhance their intellect in general. Long ago, British schools taught children Greek and Latin. Today it might be calculus, but in either case, the idea is to teach something challenging and hope students get smarter in other ways, too. The psychological term is **far transfer**. (*Near transfer* occurs if training on one task produces improvement on a similar task.) In general, far transfer is a weak effect. Many studies have attempted to improve memory or intelligence by computerized tasks that practice verbal and spatial skills. Despite high claims by the publishers of these programs, most studies show little or no improvement in real-world performance (Melby-Lervåg, Redick, & Hulme, 2016; Simons et al., 2016). Typically, people showed clear benefits on the skills they had practiced, especially right after the training, but little improvement of any skills unlike the practiced ones, and declining benefits as time passes. Similarly, many people advise old people to do crossword puzzles or Sudoku puzzles to "exercise their brains." Experimental studies suggest that practicing such puzzles improves their skills at the puzzles, but not much else (Salthouse, 2006).

Computerized training may yet prove to be valuable, but if so it will probably need to include more varied or more difficult skills. Some promising results emerged from a study in which people spent weeks playing a complex three-dimensional video game (Clemenson & Stark, 2015).

⊘ **STOP & CHECK** ▬▬▬▬▬▬

22. An enriched environment promotes growth of axons and dendrites in laboratory rodents. What is known to be one important reason for this effect?

ANSWER 22. Animals in an enriched environment are more active, and their exercise enhances growth of axons and dendrites.

Effects of Special Experiences

So far, generalized training programs to enhance overall intelligence have produced only temporary or modest benefits. However, prolonged practice of a particular activity does produce definite brain changes that enhance the ability to perform the task.

Brain Adaptations in People Blind since Infancy

What happens to the brain if one sensory system is impaired? Recall the experiment on ferrets, in which axons of the visual system, unable to contact their normal targets, attached instead to the brain areas usually devoted to hearing, and managed to convert them into more or less satisfactory visual areas. Might anything similar happen in the brains of people born deaf or blind?

People often say that blind people become better than usual at touch and hearing. That statement is true in a way, but we need to be more specific. Blind people improve their attention to touch and sound, based on practice. Researchers found that blind people have greater than average touch sensitivity in their fingers, especially blind people who read Braille and therefore practice their finger sensitivity extensively. Touch sensitivity does not increase at all for the lips, where blind people pay no more attention to touch than anyone else does (Wong, Gnanakumaran, & Goldreich, 2011).

In several studies, investigators asked sighted people and people blind since infancy to feel Braille letters or other objects and say whether two items were the same or different. On average, blind people performed more accurately than sighted people, as you would guess. More surprisingly, while blind people performed these tasks, brain scans showed substantial activity in the occipital cortex, which is usually limited to visual information (Burton et al., 2002; Sadato et al., 1996, 1998). Evidently, touch information had invaded this cortical area.

To double-check this conclusion, researchers asked people to perform the same kind of task during temporary inactivation of the occipital cortex. Intense magnetic stimulation on the scalp temporarily inactivates neurons beneath the magnet.

Applying this procedure to the occipital cortex of people who are blind interferes with their ability to identify Braille symbols, whereas it does not affect touch perception in sighted people. In short, blind people, unlike sighted people, use the occipital cortex to help identify what they feel (Cohen et al., 1997). In people blind since birth, the occipital cortex also responds to auditory information (Watkins et al., 2013), especially language (Bedny, Richardson, & Saxe, 2015).

Just as people who are blind from an early age become more sensitive to touch and sound, people who are deaf from an early age become more responsive to touch and vision. Just as touch and sound come to activate what would be the visual cortex in blind people, touch and vision come to activate what would be the auditory cortex in deaf people (Karns, Dow, & Neville, 2012). The auditory cortex not only responds to vision, but responds specifically to certain aspects of vision. For example, different cells respond to different locations of visual stimuli (Almeida et al., 2015).

⊘ **STOP & CHECK** ▬▬▬▬▬▬

23. Name two kinds of evidence indicating that touch information from the fingers activates the occipital cortex of people blind since birth.

ANSWER 23. First, brain scans indicate increased activity in the occipital cortex while blind people perform tasks such as feeling two objects and saying whether they are the same or different. Second, temporary inactivation of the occipital cortex blocks blind people's ability to perform that task, without affecting the ability of sighted people.

Music Training

People who develop expertise in any area spend enormous amounts of time practicing, generally beginning in childhood, and it seems reasonable to look for corresponding changes in their brains. Of the various kinds of expertise, which would you want to examine? Researchers' favorite choice has been musicians, for two reasons. First, we have a good idea of where in the brain to look for changes—the brain areas responsible for hearing and finger control. Second, serious musicians are numerous and easy to find. Almost any big city has an orchestra, and so do most colleges.

One study used magnetoencephalography to record responses of the auditory cortex to pure tones. The responses in musicians were about twice as strong as those in nonmusicians. An examination of their brains, using MRI, found that one area of the temporal cortex in the right hemisphere was about 30 percent larger in the musicians (Schneider et al., 2002). Other studies found enhanced responses of subcortical brain structures to musical sounds and speech sounds, compared to nonmusicians (Herdener et al., 2010; Lee, Skoe, Kraus, & Ashley, 2009; Musacchia, Sams, Skoe, & Kraus, 2007). Even as little as three years of musical training in childhood produces a measurable increase in brainstem responses to sounds (Skoe & Kraus, 2012).

These brain changes help musicians attend to slight changes in sounds that other people might not distinguish. For example, older adults who practice music tend to have better speech perception than others of their age (Bidelman & Alain, 2015). Also, on average, musicians are quicker than others to learn to distinguish the sounds of a tonal language, such as Chinese, in which *nián* (with a rising tone) means year, and *niàn* (with a falling tone) means study (Wong, Skoe, Russo, Dees, & Kraus, 2007).

According to a study using MRI, gray matter of several cortical areas was thicker in professional musicians than in amateurs and thicker in amateurs than in nonmusicians, as shown in Figure 4.19 (Gaser & Schlaug, 2003). The most strongly affected areas related to hand control and vision (which is important for reading music). A related study on stringed instrument players found that a larger than normal section of the somatosensory cortex in the right hemisphere was devoted to representing the fingers of the left hand, which they use to control the strings (Elbert, Pantev, Wienbruch, Rockstroh, & Taub, 1995). The area devoted to the left fingers was largest in those who began their music practice early and therefore also continued for more years.

These results suggest that practicing a skill reorganizes the brain to maximize performance of that skill. However, an alternative hypothesis is that brain characteristics that were present from birth attract people to one occupation or another. The structure of the auditory cortex predicts who can learn most quickly to distinguish very similar or unfamiliar speech sounds (Golestani, Molko, Dehaene, LeBihan, & Palier, 2007; Golestani, Price, & Scott, 2011). Might it also be the case that inborn brain features attract certain people to music?

One way to address that question is with a longitudinal study. Researchers examined 15 6-year-olds who were beginning piano lessons and 16 other children not taking music lessons. At the start of training, neither brain scans nor cognitive tests showed any significant difference between the two groups. After 15 months, the trained group performed better on measures of rhythm and melody discrimination, and they showed enlargements of brain areas responsible for hearing and hand movements, similar to those seen in adult musicians (Hyde et al., 2009a, 2009b). These results imply that the brain differences are the result of musical training, not the cause.

Another issue is whether music training produces bigger effects if it begins early in life, while the brain is more easily modified. Several studies found major differences between young adults who started music training in childhood and those who began as teenagers. However, because the adults who started in childhood had practiced for more years, those studies did not separate the effects of age at starting from the effects of total years of practice. Two later studies compared people who started music training before age 7 with people who started later but continued for just as many years. In both studies, those who started younger showed greater changes in sensory discriminations and brain anatomy (Steele, Bailey, Zatorre, & Penhune, 2013; Watanabe, Savion-Lemieux, & Penhune, 2007).

✔ **STOP & CHECK**

24. Which brain area shows expanded representation of the left hand in people who began practicing stringed instruments in childhood and continued for many years?

ANSWER 24. Somatosensory cortex (postcentral gyrus) of the right hemisphere.

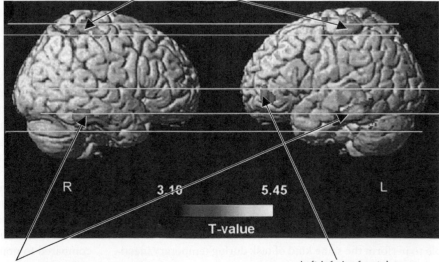

Precentral and postcentral gyri
(Body sensations and motor control, including fingers)

R 3.10 5.45 L

T-value

Inferior visual cortex
(Vision, such as reading music)

Left inferior frontal gyrus

Figure 4.19 Brain correlates of music practice
Areas marked in red showed thicker gray matter among professional keyboard players than in amateurs and thicker among amateurs than in nonmusicians. Areas marked in yellow showed even stronger differences in that same direction. (*Source: Gaser & Schlaug, 2003*)

Brain Changes after Briefer Practice

Being blind or deaf from birth leads to altered brain anatomy, and so does long-term musical training. Might briefer experiences also modify brain anatomy? In a sense, the answer is, "Yes, of course." Anything you learn must have some effect on the brain. Just reading this sentence has rearranged a few molecules in your brain. The issue is whether a relatively brief experience produces a big enough effect that we might observe it with MRI or similar technology.

Many studies have in fact reported changes in adult brain anatomy from tasks such as learning to juggle three balls (Draganski et al., 2004; Zatorre, Fields, & Johansen-Berg, 2012), 16 hours of playing a complex video game (Colom et al., 2012), or 40 hours of playing golf for the first time (Bezzola, Mérillat, Gaser, & Jäncke, 2011). However, skeptics have raised objections (Thomas & Baker, 2013): Many of the studies compared mean MRIs of the entire brains of the trained group to the entire brains of a control group. In effect, they tested a huge number of hypotheses at once—one hypothesis for each brain area. That procedure has a high risk of finding an apparent result by accident, and we should withhold judgment until someone replicates a result. Nevertheless, one study found that two brain areas enlarged after learning to juggle three balls and were also expanded (only more so) in expert jugglers (Gerber et al., 2014). That finding strengthens our confidence that the briefer experience did in fact induce a measurable change in the brain.

When Brain Reorganization Goes Too Far

If playing music or practicing anything else expands a relevant brain area, the change is good, right? Usually it is, but not always. As mentioned, when people play musical instruments many hours a day for years, the representation of the hand increases in the somatosensory cortex. Imagine the normal representation of the fingers in the cortex:

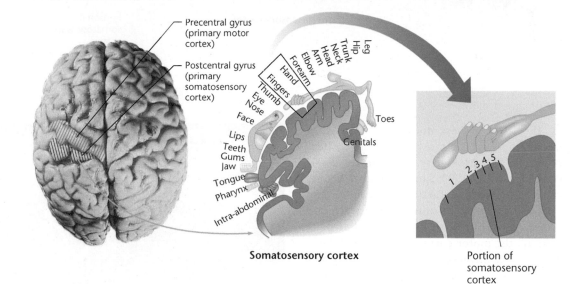

Somatosensory cortex

Portion of somatosensory cortex

With extensive musical practice, the expanding representations of the fingers might spread out like this:

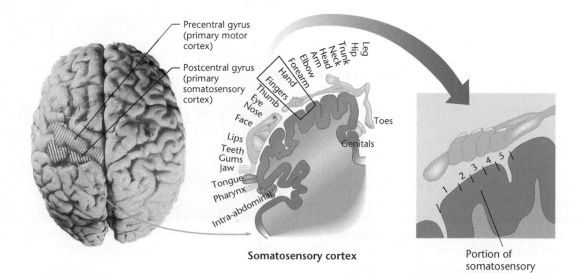

Somatosensory cortex

Portion of somatosensory cortex

Or the representations of all fingers could grow from side to side without spreading out so that representation of each finger overlaps that of its neighbor:

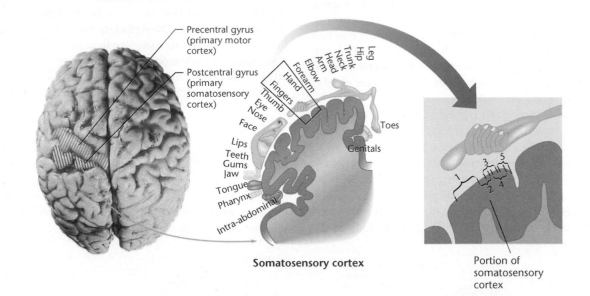

Somatosensory cortex

Portion of somatosensory cortex

In some cases, the latter process does occur, such that stimulation on one finger excites mostly the same cortical areas as another finger (Byl, McKenzie, & Nagarajan, 2000; Elbert et al., 1998; Lenz & Byl, 1999; Sanger, Pascual-Leone, Tarsy, & Schlaug, 2001; Sanger, Tarsy, & Pascual-Leone, 2001). If you cannot clearly feel the difference between one finger and another, it is difficult to move them independently. Furthermore, the motor cortex changes also. Representation of the middle fingers expands, overlapping and displacing representation of the index finger and little finger. One or more fingers may go into constant contraction (Beck et al., 2008; Burman, Lie-Nemeth, Brandfonbrener, Parisi, & Meyer, 2009). Moving one finger without moving another becomes more difficult. This condition, known as "musician's cramp" or more formally as **focal hand dystonia**, can threaten a musician's career. Similar problems sometimes happen to writers, surgeons, golfers, or anyone else who repetitively practices precise hand movements (Furuya & Hanakawa, 2016).

Previously, physicians assumed that musician's cramp was in the hands themselves, in which case the treatment would be hand surgery or injection of some drug into the hand. Now that we have identified brain reorganization as the problem, the approach is to find an appropriate type of retraining. Proprioceptive training provides bursts of vibration to affected muscles or trains the person to reach toward targets. This procedure improves sensation and muscle control for people with musician's cramp and related disabilities (Aman, Elangovan, Yeh, & Konczak, 2015; Rosenkranz, Butler, Williamson, & Rothwell, 2009).

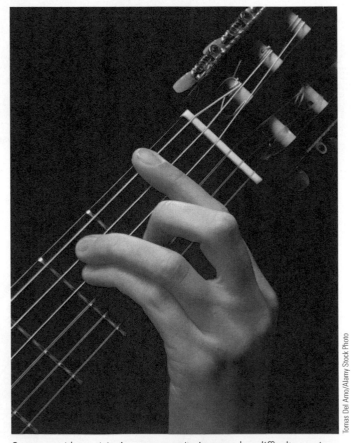

Someone with musician's cramp or writer's cramp has difficulty moving one finger independently of others. One or more fingers may twitch or go into a constant contraction.

25. What change in the brain is responsible for musician's cramp?

ANSWER

25. Extensive practice of violin, piano, or other instruments causes expanded representation of the fingers in the somatosensory cortex, as well as displacement of representation of one or more fingers in the motor cortex. If the sensory representation of two fingers overlaps too much, the person cannot feel them separately or move them separately.

Brain Development and Behavioral Development

As people grow older, their behavior changes. How much of that change has to do with the brain? Let's consider adolescence and old age.

Adolescence

Adolescents are widely regarded as impulsive and prone to seek immediate pleasure, as compared to adults. Impulsiveness is a problem if it leads to risky driving, drinking, sex, spending sprees, and so forth.

In addition to being more impulsive than older adults, children and adolescents tend to "discount the future" more than adults do. Which would you prefer, $100 now or $125 a year from now? What about $100 now versus $150 a year from now? How much bigger would next year's payoff have to be to make you willing to wait? Adolescents are more likely to choose the immediate reward than adults are, in a variety of situations (Steinberg et al., 2009). To be fair, the situation is not the same for people of different ages, especially with regard to money. Adults are more likely to be financially secure and better able to wait for a higher reward. Still, adolescents tend to prefer immediate rewards even with rewards other than money, and adolescent rats and mice show a similar tendency to prefer immediate food instead of a larger portion later (Doremus-Fitzwater, Barretto, & Spear, 2012; Pinkston & Lamb, 2011).

Many studies have found that adolescent humans show weaker responses than adults do in the areas of the prefrontal cortex responsible for inhibiting behaviors (e.g., Geier, Terwilliger, Teslovich, Velanova, & Luna, 2010). Furthermore, the degree of maturity of the prefrontal cortex and its connections correlates positively with restraint of impulses (Gilaie-Dotan et al., 2014; van den Bos, Rodriguez, Schweitzer, & McClure, 2014). That type of evidence influenced the U.S. Supreme Court to rule that the death penalty is unconstitutional for adolescents, because adolescents are less able to restrain their impulses (Steinberg, 2013). However, although the prefrontal cortex is indeed not quite mature in adolescents, its immaturity is only a small part of the explanation for impulsivity. In laboratory tests most adolescents inhibit impulses just as well as adults. Most of the riskiest behaviors, especially antisocial risky behaviors, come from individuals with a lifelong history of troublesome behaviors, beginning in childhood and extending into adulthood (Bjork & Pardini, 2015). Furthermore, if risky, impulsive behavior were the product of an immature prefrontal cortex, we should expect it to decline over the teenage years as the cortex gradually matures. In fact, most types of risky behavior become *more* common toward the later teenage years (see Figure 4.20) (Shulman, 2014). A more likely explanation for risky adolescent behaviors is that the brain's response to rewards, especially anticipation of rewards, increases strongly during the teenage years (Braams, van Duijvenvoorde, Peper, & Crone, 2015; Larsen & Luna, 2015). Adolescents seek excitement, especially when they are trying to impress their peers (Casey & Caudle, 2013; Crone & Dahl, 2012; Luna et al., 2010).

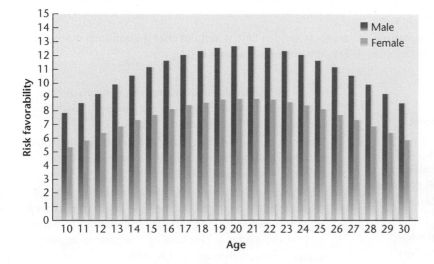

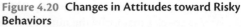

Figure 4.20 Changes in Attitudes toward Risky Behaviors
People of various ages were asked how favorable they felt toward risky actions such as bicycling down a staircase or surfing in very high waves.
(Source: Shulman, 2014)

✓ **STOP & CHECK** ▬▬▬▬▬▬▬▬

26. Why is immaturity of the prefrontal cortex not a satisfactory explanation for risky behaviors in adolescents?

ANSWER

26. As the teenage years progress, risky behavior tends to increase, even though the prefrontal cortex is becoming more mature.

Old Age

Many studies confirm that, on average, old people's memory and reasoning begin to fade. Many neurons lose some of their synapses, and the remaining synapses change more slowly than before in response to experiences (Morrison & Baxter, 2012). The thickness of the temporal cortex shrinks by about half a percent per year, on average (Fjell et al., 2009). The frontal cortex begins thinning at age *30* (Brans et al., 2010)!

The volume of the hippocampus also gradually declines in old age, and certain aspects of memory decline in proportion to the loss of hippocampus (Erickson et al., 2010). Old people are apt to decline rapidly after an injury or illness because of brain inflammation (Barrientos et al., 2011).

Nevertheless, most chief executives of major corporations, world political leaders, and college presidents are over 60 years old. Is this a problem? Should we fire them and replace them with 25-year-olds? Much of the research underestimates older people, for several reasons. The average implies that everyone is decaying a little each year, but averages can be misleading. Some people deteriorate markedly, whereas others show little sign of loss (Barzilai, Alzmon, Derby, Bauman, & Lipton, 2006; Pudas et al., 2013). In general, those who remain physically fit also retain their cognitive abilities (Fletcher et al., 2016). Also, even those who may be slower in certain intellectual activities have developed a great base of knowledge and experience. On certain kinds of questions, older people do significantly better than younger people (Queen & Hess, 2010). Third, many older people find ways to compensate for losses, such as by activating more widespread brain areas to compensate for decreased arousal in one or two areas (Park & McDonough, 2013).

What procedures might help protect against cognitive decline in old age? Experimental studies in which people were randomly assigned to daily exercise or sedentary activities have generally found improvements in cortical activity, attention, and sometimes memory (Hayes, Hayes, Cadden, & Verfaellie, 2013; Hötting & Röder, 2013). Chemical interventions are also worth investigating. After researchers transfused blood from old mice into young mice, the young mice showed a temporary impairment of synaptic plasticity and learning (Villeda et al., 2011). Transferring blood from young mice to old ones increased their number of dendritic spines and improved their learning and memory (Villeda et al., 2014). However, many procedures that work well with rats or mice yield disappointing results with humans, so we need to await further research before getting too excited. (In the meantime, if you need a blood transfusion, hope that you get it from a young person!)

✓ **STOP & CHECK** ▬▬▬▬▬▬▬▬

27. What is one way in which older adults compensate for less efficient brain functioning?

ANSWER

27. Many of them compensate by activating additional brain areas.

Module 4.2 | **In Closing**

Brain Development

Once a machine is built, it might need repair, but the construction is finished. Your brain isn't like that. Although the changes are most rapid at first, structural changes continue throughout life. You are forever a work in progress.

Summary

1. In vertebrate embryos, the central nervous system begins as a tube surrounding a fluid-filled cavity. Developing neurons proliferate, migrate, differentiate, and develop synapses and myelin. Neuron proliferation varies among species mainly by the number of cell divisions. Migration depends on chemicals that guide immature neurons to their destinations. **117**

2. In adult vertebrates, new neurons form only in a few parts of the brain. Adult humans form new olfactory receptors, but the brain develops new neurons only in the hippocampus and the basal ganglia, both of which are important for new learning. **119**

3. Growing axons find their way close to the right locations and then arrange themselves over a target area by following chemical gradients. **119**

4. After axons reach their targets based on chemical gradients, the postsynaptic cell adjusts the connections based on experience, accepting certain combinations of axons and rejecting others. This kind of competition among axons continues throughout life. **120**

5. Initially, the nervous system develops more neurons than will actually survive. Axons of the sympathetic nervous system survive only if they reach a target cell that releases to them nerve growth factor. Otherwise, they die in a process called apoptosis. Apoptosis also occurs in the brain, but the factors controlling it are less well understood. Prenatal exposure to alcohol increases apoptosis. **122**

6. The developing brain is vulnerable to chemical insult. Many chemicals that produce only mild, temporary problems for adults can impair early brain development. **123**

7. At an early stage of development, the cortex is sufficiently plastic that visual input can cause what would have been the auditory cortex to develop different properties and now respond visually. **124**

8. Enriched experience leads to greater branching of axons and dendrites, partly because animals in enriched environments are more active than those in deprived environments. **125**

9. Specialized experiences can alter brain development, especially early in life. For example, in people who are born blind, representation of touch and hearing expands in the brain areas usually reserved for vision. **127**

10. Extensive practice of a skill expands the brain's representation of sensory and motor information relevant to that skill. For example, the representation of fingers expands in people who regularly practice musical instruments. **127**

11. Although controversy remains, several studies report that even brief practice of a skill, such as juggling, can produce measurable changes in brain anatomy. **129**

12. Although expanded representation in the brain is ordinarily a good thing, it can be harmful if carried too far. Some musicians and others who use their hands many hours each day develop brain changes that interfere with their ability to feel or use one finger independently of the others. **129**

13. Compared to adults, adolescents tend to be impulsive and centered more on present pleasures than future prospects. In most cases, risky behaviors in adolescents probably reflect increased drive for excitement, more than lack of ability to inhibit impulses. **131**

14. On average, people in old age show declining memory and reasoning, and shrinkage of certain brain areas. However, these averages do not apply to all individuals or all situations. On average, physically fit people tend to maintain their cognitive abilities. Many older people compensate for inefficiency of certain brain functions by recruiting activity in additional brain areas. **132**

Key Terms

Terms are defined in the module on the page number indicated. They're also presented in alphabetical order with definitions in the book's Subject Index/Glossary, which begins on page 589. Interactive flash cards, audio reviews, and crossword puzzles are among the online resources available to help you learn these terms and the concepts they represent.

apoptosis **122**
differentiates **118**
far transfer **126**
fetal alcohol syndrome **123**
focal hand dystonia **130**

migrate **118**
myelination **118**
nerve growth factor (NGF) **122**
neural Darwinism **122**
neurotrophin **123**

proliferation **118**
stem cells **118**
synaptogenesis **118**

Thought Question

Biologists can develop antibodies against nerve growth factor (i.e., molecules that inactivate nerve growth factor). What would happen if someone injected such antibodies into a developing nervous system?

Module 4.2 | End of Module Quiz

1. In early brain development, what is the relationship between the sensory systems and muscle movements?

   A. The sensory systems develop before the first muscle movements.
   B. The first muscle movements occur at the same time as when the sensory systems develop.
   C. The first muscle movements occur before the sensory systems develop.
   D. First vision develops, then movements, and then the other sensory systems.

2. Which parts of the cerebral cortex are most likely to deteriorate in Alzheimer's disease and other conditions?

   A. The areas that mature at the earliest ages, such as the primary visual cortex.

   B. The areas most distant from the heart, such as the parietal cortex.

   C. The areas responsible for emotional processing, such as the amygdala.

   D. The areas that mature at the latest age, such as the prefrontal cortex.

3. In which areas of the human brain do some new neurons develop during adulthood?

   A. The primary visual cortex and the primary auditory cortex

   B. The hippocampus and the basal ganglia

   C. The olfactory bulbs and the areas responsible for speech

   D. The corpus callosum and the cerebellum

4. When Sperry cut a newt's optic nerve and turned the eye upside down, what happened?

   A. Axons of the optic nerve grew randomly and attached diffusely to target cells.

   B. Axons of the optic nerve grew back to their original targets.

   C. Axons of the optic nerve grew back to targets appropriate to their new location in the eye.

   D. At first the axons grew back randomly, but then they established appropriate connections by learning.

5. In the sympathetic nervous system, which of the following prevents apoptosis?

   A. Steroid hormones

   B. Nerve growth factor

   C. Physical exercise

   D. Myelination

6. Why does the spinal cord have the right number of axons to innervate all the muscle cells?

   A. Each muscle cell sends a chemical message telling the spinal cord to make a neuron.

   B. The genes cause a certain number of neurons to form and the same number of muscles to form.

   C. Immature cells divide, with one daughter cell becoming a neuron and the other becoming a muscle.

   D. The spinal cord makes an excess of neurons, but those that fail to innervate a muscle die.

7. At what age does a person have the largest number of neurons?

   A. Before or shortly after birth

   B. Equally at all times of life

   C. Adolescence

   D. Adulthood

8. If a pregnant woman drinks alcohol, alcohol harms the brain of the fetus not only while it is in the system, but also while it is washing away after drinking. What is the danger while alcohol is washing away?

   A. Temperature in the brain may decrease.

   B. Blood pressure in the brain may decrease.

   C. Excess inhibition at GABA synapses can lead to apoptosis.

   D. Overstimulation at glutamate synapses can poison the mitochondria.

9. In the ferret study, what evidence indicated that visual input to the auditory portions of the brain actually produced a visual sensation?

   A. Bright flashes of light to the rewired eye caused the ferrets to blink both eyes.

   B. Recordings from individual cells of the rewired temporal cortex showed the same patterns usually seen in cells of the occipital cortex.

   C. Ferrets could find their way around an unfamiliar room even with the normal eye closed.

   D. Ferrets that learned to turn one way in response to light in the normal eye turned the same way to light in the rewired eye.

10. An enriched environment including social interactions promotes growth of axons and dendrites in laboratory rodents. What else can produce the same effect?

    A. Improved diet

    B. Physical activity

    C. Exposure to music

    D. Extra sleep

11. According to most research, what are the effects of computerized programs to practice memory skills?

    A. Temporary improvement of the skills that were practiced

    B. Temporary improvement of both the practiced skills and general intelligence ("far transfer")

    C. Long-term improvement of both the practiced skills and general intelligence ("far transfer")

    D. No benefits, not even temporarily

12. If a person is born blind, what happens to the occipital ("visual") cortex?

   A. Its cells shrink and gradually die.
   B. Its cells remain intact but forever inactive.
   C. Its cells become responsive to touch or hearing.
   D. Its cells become spontaneously active, producing hallucinations.

13. In people who practice violin or other stringed instruments for many years, what changes in the cerebral cortex?

   A. Both hemispheres begin controlling speech equally.
   B. Parts of the occipital cortex stop responding to vision and switch to hearing.
   C. A larger than average portion of the cortex responds to the passage of time.
   D. A larger than average portion of the cortex responds to fingers of the left hand.

14. What causes musician's cramp?

   A. Changes in the muscles and tendons of the hand
   B. Rewiring of the cerebral cortex
   C. Loss of myelin on the motor nerves to the hand
   D. Changes in the touch receptors of the hand

15. What is the most likely biological explanation for increased risky behavior among adolescents?

   A. Immaturity of the prefrontal cortex
   B. Increased activity in brain areas that anticipate reward
   C. Increased activity in brain areas responsible for depressed mood
   D. Immaturity of the corpus callosum

16. Why do many older people continue to hold important jobs in spite of the declines in memory and brain function that are known to occur in old age?

   A. Laws prevent them from being fired.
   B. Most of their jobs don't require much brain activity.
   C. Old people take the credit for work that younger people actually do.
   D. The declines on average do not apply to all people.

Answers: 1C, 2D, 3B, 4B, 5B, 6D, 7A, 8D, 9D, 10B, 11A, 12C, 13D, 14B, 15B, 16D.

Plasticity after Brain Damage

An American soldier who suffered a wound to the left hemisphere of his brain during the Korean War was at first unable to speak at all. Three months later, he could speak in short fragments. When he was asked to read the letterhead, "New York University College of Medicine," he replied, "Doctors—little doctors." Eight years later, when someone asked him again to read the letterhead, he replied, "Is there a catch? It says, 'New York University College of Medicine'" (Eidelberg & Stein, 1974).

Almost all survivors of brain damage show behavioral recovery to some degree. Some of the mechanisms rely on the growth of new branches of axons and dendrites, similar to the mechanisms of brain development. Understanding the process leads to better therapies for people with brain damage and contributes to our understanding of brain functioning.

Brain Damage and Short-Term Recovery

Possible causes of brain damage include tumors, infections, exposure to radiation or toxic substances, and degenerative conditions such as Parkinson's disease and Alzheimer's disease. In young people, the most common cause is **closed head injury**, a sharp blow to the head that does not puncture the brain. The effects of closed head injury depend on severity and frequency. Many children and young adults sustain at least one mild blow to the head from a fall, a bicycle or automobile accident, or a sports injury. Most recover without treatment, possibly suffering an occasional headache afterward (Babikian, Merkeley, Savage, Giza, & Levin, 2015). However, about 7 or 8 young people per thousand require hospital treatment, and of those, about 20 percent suffer a persisting disability (Thurman, 2016). If a blow to the head causes a period of confusion and loss of recent memory, then the duration of this period is a strong predictor of long-term problems (Briggs, Brookes, Tate, & Lah, 2015).

One cause of damage after closed head injury is the rotational forces that drive brain tissue against the inside of the skull. Another cause is blood clots that interrupt blood flow to the brain (Kirkpatrick, Smielewski, Czosnyka, Menon, & Pickard, 1995). Given the dangers from a blow to the head,

how do woodpeckers manage to avoid giving themselves concussions? If you banged your head into a tree 20 times per second at a speed strong enough to tear a hole in the bark, you would not be in good shape.

Using slow-motion photography, researchers found that woodpeckers usually start with a couple of quick preliminary taps against the wood, much like a carpenter lining up a nail with a hammer. Then the birds make a hard strike in a straight line, keeping a rigid neck. They almost completely avoid rotational forces and whiplash (May, Fuster, Haber, & Hirschman, 1979). Furthermore, the spongy bone of the woodpecker's head makes an excellent shock absorber (Yoon & Park, 2011).

The implication is that football helmets, race car helmets, and so forth would give more protection if they extended down to the shoulders to prevent rotation and whiplash. Also, if you see a crash about to happen, you should tuck your chin to your chest and tighten your neck muscles.

Reducing the Harm from a Stroke

A common cause of brain damage, especially in older people, is temporary interruption of normal blood flow to a brain area during a **stroke**, also known as a **cerebrovascular accident.** The more common type of stroke is **ischemia** (iss-KEE-me-uh), the result of a blood clot or other obstruction in an artery. The less common type is **hemorrhage** (HEM-oh-rage), the result of a ruptured artery. Effects of strokes vary from barely noticeable to immediately fatal. Figure 4.21 shows the brains of three people: one who died immediately after a stroke, one who survived long after a stroke, and a bullet wound victim.

In ischemia, the neurons deprived of blood lose much of their oxygen and glucose supplies. In hemorrhage, they are flooded with blood and excess oxygen, calcium, and other chemicals. Both ischemia and hemorrhage lead to many of the same problems, including **edema** (the accumulation of fluid), which increases pressure on the brain and the probability of additional strokes (Unterberg, Stover, Kress, & Kiening, 2004). Both ischemia and hemorrhage also impair the sodium–potassium pump, leading to an accumulation of sodium inside neurons. The combination of edema and excess sodium provokes excess release of the transmitter glutamate (Rossi, Oshima, & Attwell, 2000), which overstimulates neurons,

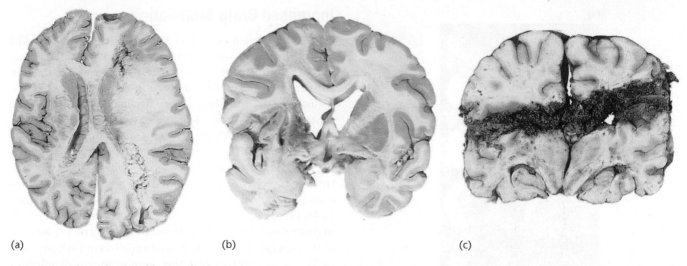

Figure 4.21 Three damaged human brains
(a) Brain of a person who died immediately after a stroke. Note the swelling on the right side. (b) Brain of someone who survived for a long time after a stroke. Note the cavities on the left side, where many cells were lost. (c) Brain of a person who suffered a gunshot wound and died immediately. *(Source: Dr. Dana Copeland)*

damaging both neurons and synapses (Castro-Alvarez, Gutierrez-Vargas, Darnaudéry, & Cardona-Gómez, 2011).

Immediate Treatments

As recently as the 1980s, hospitals had little to offer to stroke patients. Today, prospects are good for ischemia if physicians act quickly. A drug called **tissue plasminogen activator (tPA)** breaks up blood clots. To get a benefit, a patient should receive tPA quickly, at least within 4.5 hours after a stroke. Emergency wards have improved their response times, but the limiting factor is that most stroke victims don't get to the hospital quickly enough, sometimes because they did not realize they had suffered a stroke.

It is difficult to determine whether a stroke was ischemic or hemorrhagic. Given that tPA is useful for ischemia but could only make matters worse in a hemorrhage, what is a physician to do? An MRI scan distinguishes between the two kinds of stroke, but MRIs take time, and time is limited. The usual decision is to give the tPA. Hemorrhage is less common and usually fatal anyway, so the risk of making a hemorrhage worse is small compared to the hope of alleviating ischemia.

What other treatments might be effective shortly after a stroke? Given that strokes kill neurons by overstimulation, one approach has been to decrease stimulation by blocking glutamate synapses or blocking calcium entry. Other approaches include cooling the brain, antioxidants, antibiotics, albumin, and treatments affecting the immune system. Each of these and more have shown promise in studies with laboratory animals, but all of them have produced disappointing results with humans (Moretti, Ferrari, & Villa, 2015). A possible explanation is that the lab animals were young and healthy before

the induced stroke, whereas most human stroke patients are old and have other health problems. Also, the lab animals received the drugs immediately, whereas humans receive them hours later. Furthermore, physicians are reluctant to give humans large doses of experimental drugs, for fear of dangerous side effects. In spite of the discouraging results, research is continuing on many possible remedies.

Another procedure might surprise you: Exposure to cannabinoids (the chemicals found in marijuana) minimizes the damage caused by strokes in laboratory animals. You might wonder how anyone thought of trying such a thing. One theoretical rationale was that cannabinoids decrease the release of glutamate. If excessive glutamate is one of the reasons for cell loss, then cannabinoids might be helpful. They do, in fact, minimize the damage after a stroke in rats, as shown in Figure 4.22, although the explanation for the benefit is not yet clear (Schomacher, Müller, Sommer, Schwab, & Schäbitz, 2008). In addition to putting the brakes on glutamate, cannabinoids exert anti-inflammatory effects and alter brain chemistry in several ways that might protect against damage (Fernández-Ruiz, Moro, & Martínez-Orgado, 2015).

So far, very little research has examined possible effects for human stroke patients. Again the problem is that cannabinoids are helpful only if administered within the first hours after a stroke. In fact, the research on laboratory animals indicates that cannabinoids are most effective if taken shortly *before* the stroke. One study did find that stroke patients with cannabinoids in their blood stream, indicating marijuana use before the stroke, had on average less severe damage from the stroke (Di Napoli et al., 2016). However, the mean age of the marijuana users was 47, and the mean for nonusers was 69.

(a)   (b)

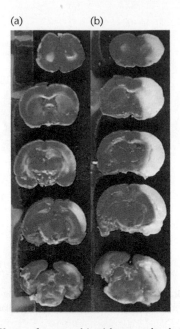

Figure 4.22 Effects of a cannabinoid on stroke damage
Row (a) shows slices through the brains of five rats treated with a high dose of a cannabinoid shortly after a stroke. Row (b) shows slices for rats not treated with cannabinoids. The white areas on the right of each brain show the extent of the damage.
(Source: From "Endocannabinoids mediate neuroprotection after transient focal cerebral ischemia," by M. Schomacher, H. D. Müller, C. Sommer, S. Schwab, & W.-R. Schäbitz, 2008, Brain Research, 1240, pp. 213–220.)

It is difficult to know how much of the difference in outcome was due to a possibly beneficial effect of marijuana, and how much was due to the difference in age. A similar problem relates to reports (Wolff et al., 2013) that marijuana users are more likely than average to have certain physical and mental illnesses: Does marijuana increase the risk of disorders? Or are people with certain disorders more likely than average to use marijuana? In the absence of any random-assignment experiments, we should be wary about drawing conclusions.

✓ STOP & CHECK

28. What are the two kinds of stroke, and what causes each kind?
29. Why is tPA not helpful in cases of hemorrhage?

ANSWERS
28. The more common form, ischemia, is the result of an occlusion of an artery. The other form, hemorrhage, is the result of a ruptured artery. 29. The drug tPA breaks up blood clots, and hemorrhage results from a ruptured blood vessel, not a blood clot.

Later Mechanisms of Recovery

After the first days following brain damage, many of the surviving brain areas increase or reorganize their activity (Nishimura et al., 2007). In most cases the recovery depends mostly on increased activity by the spared cells surrounding the area of damage (Murata et al., 2015).

Increased Brain Stimulation

A behavioral deficit after brain damage reflects more than just the cells that died. After damage to any brain area, other areas that have lost part of their normal input become less active. For example, shortly after damage in one brain hemisphere, its input to the other hemisphere declines, and therefore the other hemisphere shows deficits also (van Meer et al., 2010).

Diaschisis (di-AS-ki-sis, from a Greek term meaning "to shock throughout") refers to the decreased activity of surviving neurons after damage to other neurons. If diaschisis contributes to behavioral deficits following brain damage, then increased stimulation should help. In a series of experiments, D. M. Feeney and colleagues measured the behavioral effects of cortical damage in rats and cats. Depending on the location of the damage, the animals showed impairments in movement or depth perception. Injecting amphetamine significantly enhanced both behaviors, and animals that practiced the behaviors under the influence of amphetamine showed long-lasting benefits. Injecting a drug to block dopamine synapses impaired behavioral recovery (Feeney & Sutton, 1988; Feeney, Sutton, Boyeson, Hovda, & Dail, 1985; Hovda & Feeney, 1989; Sutton, Hovda, & Feeney, 1989). Although amphetamine is too risky for use with human patients, other drugs that increase dopamine release have shown promise in a few studies (Sami & Faruqui, 2015).

✓ STOP & CHECK

30. After someone has had a stroke, would it be best (if possible) to direct stimulant drugs to the cells that were damaged or somewhere else?

ANSWER
30. It is best to direct a stimulant drug to the cells that had been receiving input from the damaged cells. Presumably, the loss of input has produced diaschisis.

Regrowth of Axons

Damage to the brain or spinal cord damages many axons of neurons that survived the damage. Getting those axons to grow back and connect to the correct targets could offer a great benefit. In principle, axon regrowth would seem to be possible. Damaged axons in the peripheral nervous system do grow back at a rate of about 1 mm per day, following its myelin sheath to the original target. Damaged axons also grow back in the spinal cord of a fish, under the control of a gene that is active in glia cells (Mokalled et al., 2016; Zhang, Pizarro, Swain, Kang, & Selzer, 2014). However, axons do not grow back in the mammalian brain or spinal cord, at least not enough to produce any benefit. Many efforts have been made to find ways to promote axon regrowth in mammals.

A cut in the nervous system causes astrocytes to form scar tissue, thicker in mammals than in fish. One hypothesis has been that scar tissue is the main impediment, and that reducing the scar tissue might enable axon regrowth. However, more recent studies indicate that the scar tissue is more help-ful than harmful. The astrocytes release chemicals that keep nearby neurons alive, and procedures that remove the scar lead to tissue degeneration (Anderson et al., 2016; Sabelström et al., 2013).

A damaged axon does not automatically start growing back. Several chemicals can stimulate regrowth, and research with laboratory rats has shown that such chemicals sometimes enable axons to return to their normal targets (Anderson et al., 2016; Ruschel et al., 2015; Wong, Gibson, Arnold, Pepinsky, & Frank, 2015). Even then, behavioral recovery is not automatic. To get proper function, the animal needs much practice of the relevant movements (Hollis et al., 2016; Wahl et al., 2014). If the damaged axons were sensory rather than motor, then extensive sensory experience is necessary for the axons to restore function (Lim et al., 2016).

In short, researchers have made much progress in facilitating regrowth of damaged axons in laboratory animals. However, we do not yet know how well these procedures might work with humans.

Axon Sprouting

Ordinarily, the surface of dendrites and cell bodies is cov-ered with synapses, and a vacant spot doesn't stay vacant for long. After a cell loses input from an axon, it secretes neu-rotrophins that induce other axons to form new branches, or **collateral sprouts**, that take over the vacant synapses (Ramirez, 2001) (see Figure 4.23). In the area near the dam-age, new synapses form at a high rate, especially for the first two weeks (C. E. Brown, Li, Boyd, Delaney, & Murphy, 2007).

Collateral sprouting in the cortex contributes to behav-ioral recovery in some cases (e.g., Li et al., 2015; Siegel, Fink, Strittmatter, & Cafferty, 2015). However, the result depends on whether the sprouting axons convey information similar to those that they replace. For example, the hippocampus re-ceives much input from an area called the entorhinal cortex. If the entorhinal cortex is damaged in one hemisphere, then ax-ons from the entorhinal cortex of the other hemisphere sprout, take over the vacant synapses, and largely restore behavior

(Ramirez, Bulsara, Moore, Ruch, & Abrams, 1999; Ramirez, McQuilkin, Carrigan, MacDonald, & Kelley, 1996). However, if the entorhinal cortex is damaged in both hemispheres, then axons from other locations sprout into the vacant synapses, conveying different information. Under those conditions, the sprouting interferes with behavior and prevents recovery (Ramirez, 2001; Ramirez et al., 2007).

Denervation Supersensitivity

Neurons make adjustments to maintain a nearly constant level of arousal. After learning strengthens one set of syn-apses, other synapses weaken. (If this didn't happen, then ev-ery time you learned something, your brain would get more and more aroused.) Conversely, if a certain set of synapses becomes inactive—perhaps because of damage elsewhere in the brain—the remaining synapses become more responsive, more easily stimulated. This process of enhanced response, known as **denervation supersensitivity** or *receptor supersen-sitivity*, has been demonstrated mostly with dopamine syn-apses (Kostrzewa, Kostrzewa, Brown, Nowak, & Brus, 2008).

Denervation supersensitivity helps compensate for de-creased input. However, when either collateral sprouting or denervation supersensitivity occurs, it can strengthen not only the desirable connections, but also undesirable ones, such as those responsible for pain. Unfortunately, many treatments that facilitate the regrowth of axons in a damaged spinal cord also lead to chronic pain (Brown & Weaver, 2012).

✓ **STOP & CHECK** ▰▰▰▰▰▰

31. Is collateral sprouting a change in axons or dendritic receptors?

32. Is denervation supersensitivity a change in axons or dendritic receptors?

ANSWERS   31. Axons 32. Dendritic receptors

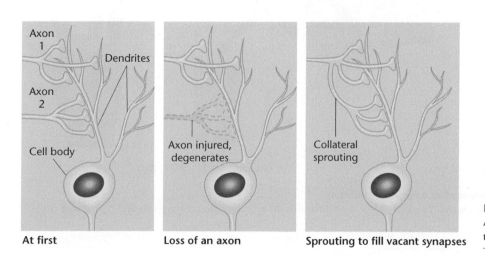

At first   **Loss of an axon**   **Sprouting to fill vacant synapses**

Axon 1, Axon 2, Dendrites, Cell body / Axon injured, degenerates / Collateral sprouting

Figure 4.23 Collateral sprouting
A surviving axon grows a new branch to replace the synapses left vacant by a damaged axon.

Reorganized Sensory Representations and the Phantom Limb

If a brain area loses some of its incoming axons, we can expect denervation supersensitivity, collateral sprouting, or both. The result is either increased response to a synapse that previously produced little effect, or response to an axon that previously did not attach at all. Let's imagine how these processes might apply in the case of an amputation.

Reexamine Figure 3.23. Each section along the somatosensory cortex receives input from part of the body. Within the area marked "fingers" in that figure, a closer examination reveals that each subarea responds more to one finger than to others. Figure 4.24 shows the arrangement for a monkey brain. In one study, experimenters amputated finger 3 of an owl monkey. The cortical cells that previously responded to information from finger 3 lost their input. Soon those cells became more responsive to finger 2, finger 4, or part of the palm, until the cortex developed the pattern of responsiveness shown in Figure 4.24b (Kaas, Merzenich, & Killackey, 1983; Merzenich et al., 1984).

What happens if an entire arm is amputated? For many years, neuroscientists assumed that the cortical area corresponding to that arm would remain permanently silent, because axons from other cortical areas could not sprout far enough to reach the area representing the arm. Then came a surprise. Investigators recorded from the cerebral cortices of monkeys whose sensory nerves from one forelimb had been cut 12 years previously. They found that the stretch of cortex previously responsive to that limb was now responsive to the face (Pons et al., 1991). After loss of sensory input from the forelimb, the axons representing the forelimb degenerated, leaving vacant synaptic sites at several levels

of the CNS. Evidently, axons representing the face sprouted into those sites in the spinal cord, brainstem, and thalamus (Florence & Kaas, 1995; Jones & Pons, 1998). Or perhaps axons from the face were already present but became stronger through denervation supersensitivity. Brain scan studies confirm that the same processes occur with humans. Later studies showed that this process can occur much quicker than 12 years.

Now consider that reorganized cortex. The cells that previously responded to arm stimulation now receive information from the face. Does it feel like stimulation on the face or on the arm? The answer: It feels like the arm (Davis et al., 1998). Evidently the brain areas that start off as arm areas, hand areas, or whatever retain those properties even after decades without normal input. One patient had a hand amputated at age 19; 35 years later, a new hand was grafted in its place. Within months, he started to feel normal sensations in that hand (Frey, Bogdanov, Smith, Watrous, & Breidenbach, 2008).

Physicians have long noted that many people with amputations experience a **phantom limb,** a continuing sensation of an amputated body part. That experience can range from tingling to intense pain, either occasionally or constantly (Giummarra et al., 2010). People can have a phantom hand, foot, or any other body part. The phantom sensation might last days, weeks, or a lifetime (Ramachandran & Hirstein, 1998).

Until the 1990s, no one knew what caused phantom pains, and most physicians believed that the sensations came from the stump of the amputated limb. However, removing more of the limb in an attempt to eliminate the phantom sensations accomplished nothing. Modern methods show that phantom limbs develop when the relevant

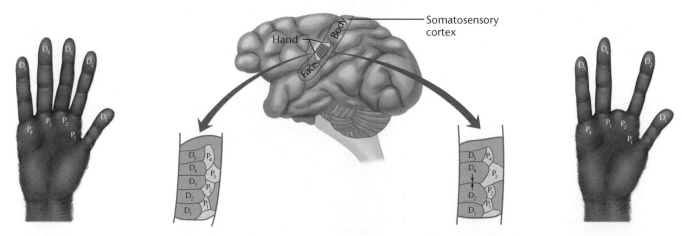

(a) Normal (before amputation)   (b) After amputation of 3rd digit

Figure 4.24 Somatosensory cortex of a monkey after a finger amputation
Note that the cortical area previously responsive to the third finger (D$_3$) becomes responsive to the second and fourth fingers (D$_2$ and D$_4$) and part of the palm (P$_3$).
(Source: Redrawn from the Annual Review of Neuroscience, *Vol. 6, © 1983, by Annual Reviews, Inc. Reprinted by permission of Annual Reviews, Inc. and Jon H. Kaas.)*

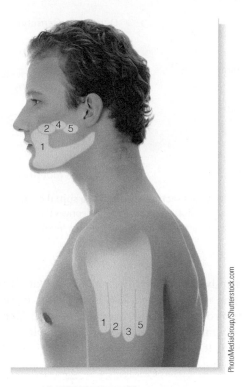

Figure 4.25 Sources of phantom sensation for one person
Stimulation in the areas marked on the cheek produced phantom sensations of digits 1 (thumb), 2, 4, and 5. Stimulation on the shoulder also evoked phantom sensations of digits 1, 2, 3, and 5.
(*Source: Based on* Phantoms in the Brain *by V. S. Ramachandran, M.D., Ph.D. and Sandra Blakeslee. Copyright © 1998 by V. S. Ramachandran and Sandra Blakeslee.*)

portion of the somatosensory cortex reorganizes and becomes responsive to alternative inputs (Flor et al., 1995). For example, suppose axons representing the face come to activate the cortical area previously devoted to an amputated hand. A touch on the face now produces a facial sensation but it also produces a sensation in the phantom hand. Figure 4.25 shows a map of which face area stimulates sensation in which part of the phantom hand, for one person (Aglioti, Smania, Atzei, & Berlucchi, 1997). For some people, seeing someone else being touched can also elicit a sensation in the phantom limb (Goller, Richards, Novak, & Ward, 2013).

Note in Figure 3.23 that the part of the cortex responsive to the feet is adjacent to the part responsive to the genitals. Two patients with foot amputations felt a phantom foot during sexual arousal! One reported feeling orgasm in the phantom foot as well as the genitals—and enjoyed it intensely (Ramachandran & Blakeslee, 1998). Evidently, the representation of the genitals had spread into the cortical area responsible for foot sensation.

Is there any way to relieve a painful phantom sensation? In some cases, yes. Many amputees who learn to use an artificial arm report that their phantom sensations gradually disappear (Lotze et al., 1999). As they start attributing sensations to the artificial arm, they displace the abnormal connections that caused phantom sensations.

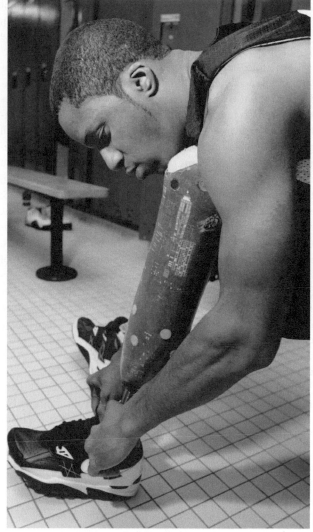

Amputees who feel a phantom limb are likely to lose those phantom sensations if they learn to use an artificial arm or leg.

STOP & CHECK

33. What is responsible for the phantom limb experience?

ANSWER

33. Synapses that used to receive input from the now amputated part become vacant. Axons representing another part of the body take over those synapses. Now stimulation of this other part activates the synapses associated with the amputated area, but that stimulation feels like the amputated area.

Learned Adjustments in Behavior

If you cannot find your keys, perhaps you accidentally dropped them into the trash (so they are gone forever), or perhaps you absentmindedly put them in an unusual place (where you will find them if you keep looking). Similarly, someone with brain damage may have lost some ability totally or may be able to find it with enough effort. Much recovery from brain damage depends on learning to make better use of the abilities that were spared. For example, if you lose your peripheral vision, you learn to move your head from side to side to compensate (Marshall, 1985).

Sometimes, a person or animal with brain damage appears unable to do something but is in fact not trying. Consider an animal that incurred damage to the sensory nerves from a forelimb to the spinal cord, as in Figure 4.26. The animal no longer feels the limb, although the motor nerves still connect to the muscles. We say the limb is **deafferented** because it has lost its afferent (sensory) input. A monkey with a deafferented limb does not spontaneously use it for walking, picking up objects, or any other voluntary behaviors (Taub & Berman, 1968). At first investigators assumed that the monkey was unable to use the deafferented limb. In a later experiment, however, they cut the afferent nerves of both forelimbs. Despite this more extensive damage, the monkey used both of its deafferented limbs to walk, climb, and pick up food. Apparently, a monkey fails to use a deafferented forelimb only because walking on three limbs is easier than using an impaired limb. When it has no choice but to use its deafferented limbs, it does. Similarly, one treatment for people recovering from a stroke is to force them to use the weaker limb by preventing them from using the normal limb (Sens et al., 2012).

Therapy for a person with brain damage begins with careful evaluation of a patient's abilities and disabilities. For example, someone who has trouble carrying out spoken instructions might be impaired in hearing, memory, language, muscle control, or alertness. After identifying the problem, a physical therapist or occupational therapist helps the patient practice the impaired skills.

Behavior recovered after brain damage is effortful, and its recovery is precarious. A person with brain damage who

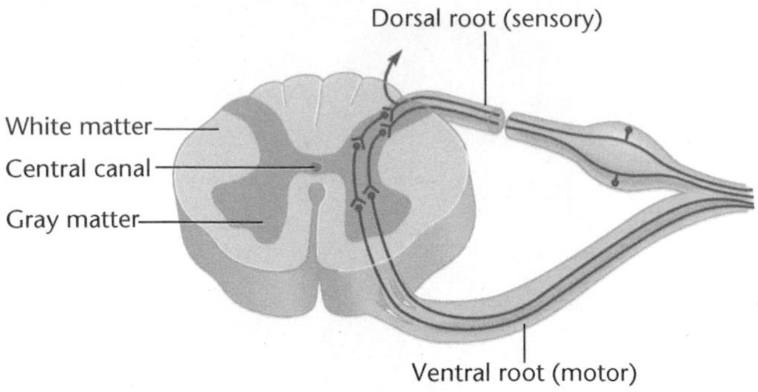

Figure 4.26 Cross section through the spinal cord
A cut through the dorsal root (as shown) deprives the animal of touch sensations from part of the body but leaves the motor nerves intact.

appears to be functioning normally is working harder than usual. The recovered behavior deteriorates markedly after drinking alcohol, physical exhaustion, or other kinds of stress that would minimally affect most other people (Fleet & Heilman, 1986). It also deteriorates in old age (Corkin, Rosen, Sullivan, & Clegg, 1989).

✓ STOP & CHECK

34. A monkey that loses sensation from one arm stops using it, but a monkey that loses sensation from both arms does use them. Why?

ANSWER

34. A monkey that lost sensation in one arm is capable of moving it, but finds it easier to walk with the three intact limbs. When both arms lose their sensations, the monkey is forced to rely on them.

Module 4.3 │ In Closing

Brain Damage and Recovery

The mammalian body is well equipped to replace lost blood cells or skin cells but poorly prepared to deal with lost brain cells. Even the processes that do occur after brain damage, such as collateral sprouting of axons or reorganization of sensory representations, are not always helpful. It is tempting to speculate that we failed to evolve mechanisms to recover from brain damage because, through most of our evolutionary history, an individual with brain damage was not likely to survive long enough to recover. Today, many people with brain and spinal cord damage survive for years, and we need continuing research on how to improve their lives.

Summary

1. Brain damage has many causes, including blows to the head, obstruction of blood flow to the brain, or a ruptured blood vessel in the brain. Strokes kill neurons largely by overexcitation. **136**

2. During the first hours after an ischemic stroke, tissue plasminogen activator (tPA) can reduce cell loss by breaking up the blood clot. However, not many patients get treatment in time for tPA to be helpful. **137**

3. Many procedures for reducing the effects of nervous system injury have shown promise with laboratory animals, but so far none of them have been reliably helpful with humans. One reason is that many of the treatments are

effective only if administered promptly after nervous system damage. Also, many patients have additional health problems, not just the stroke or other damage. **137**

4. When one brain area is damaged, other areas become less active than usual because of their loss of input. Stimulant drugs can help restore normal function of these undamaged areas. **138**

5. After an area of the CNS loses its usual input, other axons begin to excite it as a result of either sprouting or denervation supersensitivity. The anatomical reorganization is helpful in some cases but not always. **138**

6. The phantom limb experience occurs because axons from another body part invade the cortical area ordinarily devoted to sensation from the now lost body part. Stimulation of the other body part now produces sensation as if it had come from the amputated part. **140**

7. Many individuals with brain damage are capable of more than they show because they avoid using skills that have become impaired or difficult. **141**

Key Terms

Terms are defined in the module on the page number indicated. They're also presented in alphabetical order with definitions in the book's Subject Index/Glossary, which begins on page 589. Interactive flash cards, audio reviews, and crossword puzzles are among the online resources available to help you learn these terms and the concepts they represent.

cerebrovascular accident **136**
closed head injury **136**
collateral sprouts **139**
deafferent **142**
denervation supersensitivity **139**

diaschisis **138**
edema **136**
hemorrhage **136**
ischemia **136**
phantom limb **140**

stroke **136**
tissue plasminogen activator (tPA) **137**

Thought Questions

1. Ordinarily, patients with advanced Parkinson's disease (who have damage to dopamine-releasing axons) move very slowly if at all. However, during an emergency (e.g., a fire in the building), they may move rapidly and vigorously. Suggest a possible explanation.

2. Drugs that block dopamine synapses tend to impair or slow limb movements. However, after people have taken such drugs for a long time, some experience involuntary twitches or tremors in their muscles. Based on material in this chapter, propose a possible explanation.

Module 4.3 | End of Module Quiz

1. Tissue plasminogen activator (tPA) is helpful in reducing the effect of a stroke only under which of these conditions?

   A. It is helpful only if the stroke was due to a hemorrhage.

   B. It is helpful only if administered within the first hours after a stroke.

   C. It is helpful only if the patient practices relevant movements while taking the drug.

   D. It is effective only for laboratory animals, not for humans.

2. What would be the purpose of giving a drug that stimulates dopamine receptors to a stroke patient?

   A. To break up blood clots in the nervous system

   B. To increase collateral sprouting

   C. To combat diaschisis

   D. To stimulate regrowth of axons

3. Name two procedures that decrease the damage caused by strokes in laboratory animals, although physicians so far have seldom tried them with people.

   A. Dehydration and lithium

   B. Increased blood flow and antidepressants

   C. Decreased body temperature and cannabinoids

   D. Increased body temperature and tranquilizers

4. In which species, if any, can axons regrow in the spinal cord?

   A. In humans only

   B. In fish

   C. In birds

   D. In no species

5. Where does collateral sprouting take place?

    A. In the cell body

    B. In the axon

    C. In the dendrites

    D. In both the axons and the dendrites

6. Where does denervation supersensitivity take place?

    A. In the blood flow to the brain

    B. In glia cells

    C. At synapses

    D. In axon membranes

7. What causes the phantom limb experience?

    A. Irritation of receptors at the stump where the amputation occurred

    B. Spontaneous activity of receptors at the stump where the amputation occurred

    C. Reorganization of the sensory cortex

    D. A psychiatric reaction based on denial of the amputation

8. Suppose a patient uses only the right arm following injury that blocked all sensation from the left arm. Of the following, which is the most promising therapy?

    A. Electrically stimulate the skin of the left arm.

    B. Tie the right arm behind the person's back.

    C. Blindfold the person.

    D. Increase visual stimulation on the right side of the body.

Answers: 1B, 2C, 3C, 4B, 5B, 6C, 7C, 8B.

Suggestions for Further Reading

Levi-Montalcini, R. (1988). *In praise of imperfection.* New York: Basic Books. Autobiography by the discoverer of nerve growth factor.

Ramachandran, V. S., & Blakeslee, S. (1998). *Phantoms in the brain.* New York: Morrow. One of the most thought-provoking books ever written about human brain damage, including the phantom limb phenomenon.

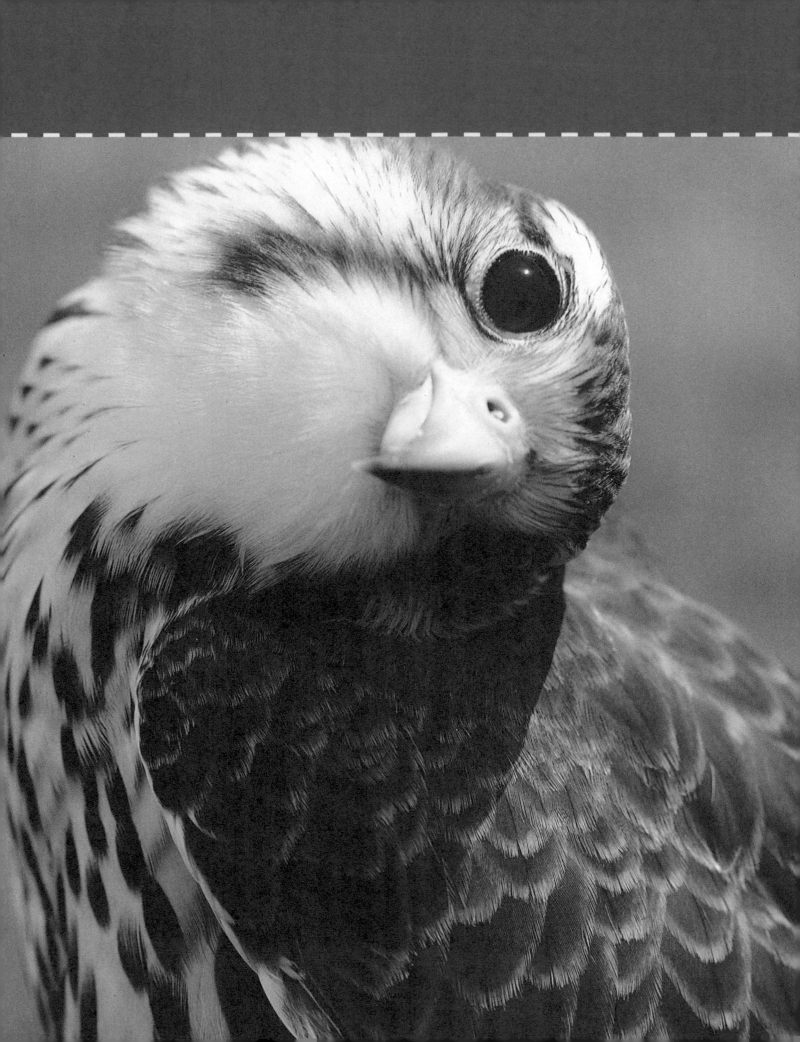

Vision

Chapter 5

Imagine that you are a piece of iron. So there you are, sitting around doing nothing, as usual, when along comes a drop of water. What will be your perception of the water? Yes, of course, a bar of iron doesn't have a brain, and it wouldn't have any perception at all. But let's ignore that inconvenient fact and imagine what it would be like if a bar of iron could perceive the water. From the standpoint of a piece of iron, water is above all *rustish*.

Now return to your perspective as a human. You know that rustishness is not really a property of water itself but of how it reacts with iron. The same is true of human perception. When you see grass as *green*, the green is no more a property of grass than rustish is a property of water. Green is the experience that results when the light bouncing off grass reacts with the neurons in your brain. Greenness is in us—just as rust is in the piece of iron.

Learning Objectives

After studying this chapter, you should be able to:

1. Remember that we see because light strikes the retina, sending a message to the brain.
2. List the properties of cones and rods.
3. Explain the main features of color vision.
4. Trace the route of visual information from the retina to the cerebral cortex.
5. Explain lateral inhibition in terms of the connections among neurons in the retina.
6. Define and give examples of receptive fields.
7. Describe research on how experiences alter development of the visual cortex.
8. Discuss specific deficits that can occur after damage to parts of the visual cortex, such as impaired facial recognition or impaired motion perception.

Opposite:
Later in this chapter, you will understand why this prairie falcon has tilted its head.
(Tom McHugh/Science Source)

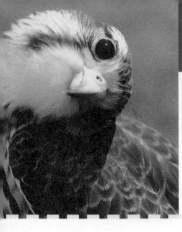

Module 5.1

Visual Coding

Several decades ago, a graduate student taking his final oral exam for a PhD in psychology was asked, "How far can an ant see?" He turned pale. He did not know the answer, and evidently he was supposed to. He tried to remember everything he knew about insect vision. Finally, he gave up and admitted he did not know.

With an impish grin, the professor told him, "Presumably, an ant can see 93 million miles—the distance to the sun." Yes, this was a trick question. However, it illustrates an important point: How far an ant sees, or how far you see, depends on how far the light travels before it strikes the eyes. You do not send out "sight rays." That principle was probably the first scientific discovery in psychology (Steffens, 2007). About a thousand years ago, the Arab philosopher Ibn al-Haytham (965–1040) observed that when you open your eyes at night, you immediately see the distant stars. He reasoned that if you saw by sending out sight rays, they couldn't get to the stars that fast. Then he demonstrated that light rays bounce off an object in all directions, but you see only those rays that reflect off the object and strike your retina (Gross, 1999).

The point is worth emphasizing, because a distressingly large number of college students believe they send out sight rays from their eyes when they see (Winer, Cottrell, Gregg, Fournier, & Bica, 2002). Even some students who have taken courses in physics or visual perception hold that profound misunderstanding. Here is one of the most important principles to remember from this text: When you see a tree, for example, your perception is not in the tree. It is in your brain. You see something only when light from the object alters your brain activity. Even if you did send out rays from your eyes— and you don't—when they struck some object, you wouldn't know about it, unless they bounced back and returned to your eyes. Similarly, you feel something only when touch information reaches your brain. When you feel something *with* your fingers, you don't feel it *in* your fingers. You feel it in your brain.

STOP & CHECK

1. What was Ibn al-Haytham's evidence that we see only because light enters the eyes, not by sending out sight rays?

ANSWER

1. First, you can see distant objects such as stars far faster than we could imagine any sight rays reaching them. Second, when light strikes an object, we see only the light rays that reflect off the object and into the eyes.

General Principles of Perception

You see an object when it emits or reflects light that stimulates receptors that transmit information to your brain. How does your brain make sense of that information? The 17th-century philosopher René Descartes believed that the nerves from the eye would send the brain a pattern of impulses arranged like a picture of the perceived object, right side up. In fact, your brain encodes the information in a way that doesn't resemble what you see. A computer's representation of a triangle is a series of 0s and 1s that are in no way arranged like a triangle. Similarly, your brain stores a representation of a triangle in terms of altered activity in many neurons, and if you examine those neurons, you see nothing that looks like a triangle.

The brain codes information largely in terms of *which* neurons are active, and how active they are at any moment. Impulses in certain neurons indicate light, whereas impulses in others indicate sound, touch, or other sensations. In 1838, Johannes Müller described this insight as the **law of specific nerve energies**. Müller held that whatever excites a particular nerve establishes a special kind of energy unique to that nerve. In modern terms, the brain somehow interprets the action potentials from the auditory nerve as sounds, those from the olfactory nerve as odors, and so forth. Admittedly, that word *somehow* glosses over a deep mystery.

Here is a demonstration: If you rub your eyes, you may see spots or flashes of light even in a totally dark room. You applied mechanical pressure, which excited visual receptors in your eyes. Anything that excites those receptors is perceived as light. (If you try this demonstration, first remove any contact lenses. Shut your eyelids and rub gently.)

TRY IT YOURSELF

✅ STOP & CHECK

2. If someone electrically stimulated the auditory receptors in your ear, what would you perceive?

3. If it were possible to flip your entire brain upside down, without breaking any of the connections to sense organs or muscles, what would happen to your perceptions of what you see, hear, and so forth?

ANSWER

2. Because of the law of specific nerve energies, you would perceive it as sound, not as shock. (Of course, a strong enough shock might spread far enough to excite pain receptors also.) 3. Your perceptions would not change. The way visual or auditory information is coded in the brain does not depend on the physical location within the brain. Seeing something as "on top," or "to the left" depends on which neurons are active but does not depend on the physical location of those neurons.

The Eye and Its Connections to the Brain

Light enters the eye through an opening in the center of the iris called the **pupil** (see Figure 5.1). It is focused by the lens (adjustable) and cornea (not adjustable) and projected onto the **retina**, the rear surface of the eye, which is lined with visual receptors. Light from the left side of the world strikes the right half of the retina, and vice versa. Light from above strikes the bottom half of the retina, and light from below strikes the top half. The inversion of the image poses no problem for the nervous system. Remember, the visual system does not duplicate the image. It codes it by various kinds of neuronal activity. If you find this idea puzzling, think about a computer. Some chip in the computer indicates what to display at the upper left of your screen, but there is no reason why that chip needs to be in the upper left part of the computer.

Route within the Retina

If you were designing an eye, you would probably send the receptors' messages directly back to the brain. In the vertebrate retina, however, messages go from the receptors at the back of the eye to **bipolar cells**, located closer to the center of the eye (see Figure 5.2). The bipolar cells send their messages to **ganglion cells**, located still closer to the center of the eye. The ganglion cells' axons join together and travel back to the brain

(see Figure 5.3). Additional cells called *amacrine cells* get information from bipolar cells and send it to other bipolar, amacrine, and ganglion cells. Amacrine cells refine the input to ganglion cells, enabling certain ones to respond mainly to particular shapes, directions of movement, changes in lighting, color, and other visual features (Masland, 2012). Researchers have identified dozens of types of ganglion and amacrine cells, varying in their chemistry and connections (Kántor et al., 2016).

One consequence of this anatomy is that light passes through the ganglion, amacrine, and bipolar cells en route to the receptors. However, these cells are transparent, and light passes through them without distortion. A more important consequence is the *blind spot*. The ganglion cell axons join to form the **optic nerve** that exits through the back of the eye. The point at which it leaves (also where the blood vessels enter and leave) is a **blind spot** because it has no receptors. You can demonstrate your own blind spot with Figure 5.4. Close your left eye and focus your right eye on the top o. Then move the page forward and back. When the page is about 10 inches (25 cm) away, the x disappears because its image strikes the blind spot.

Now repeat with the lower part of the figure. When the page is again about 10 inches away from your eyes, what do you see? The *gap* disappears! When the blind spot interrupts a straight line or other regular pattern, your brain fills in the gap.

TRY IT YOURSELF

In everyday life, you never notice your blind spot, for two reasons. First, your brain fills in the gap, as you just experienced. Second, anything in the blind spot of one eye is visible to the other eye. Use Figure 5.4 again to locate the

TRY IT YOURSELF

blind spot in your right eye. Then close your right eye and open the left one. You will see the spot that the right eye couldn't see.

✅ STOP & CHECK

4. What makes the blind spot of the retina blind?

ANSWER

4. The blind spot has no receptors because it is occupied by exiting axons and blood vessels.

Fovea and Periphery of the Retina

When you look at details such as letters on this page, you fixate them on the central portion of your retina, especially the **fovea** (meaning "pit"), a tiny area specialized for acute, detailed vision (see Figure 5.1). Because blood vessels and ganglion cell axons are almost absent near the fovea, it has nearly unimpeded vision. The tight packing of receptors aids perception of detail.

More importantly for perceiving detail, each receptor in the fovea connects to a single *bipolar cell*, which in turn connects to a single *ganglion cell* that has an axon to the brain. The ganglion cells in the fovea of humans and other primates are called

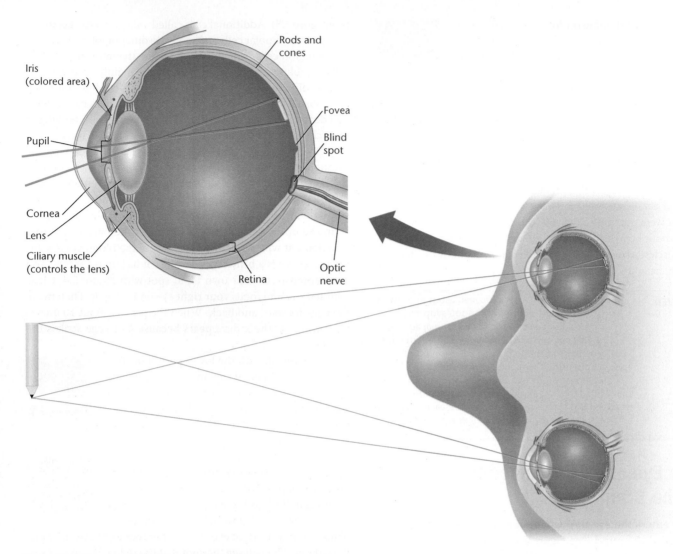

Figure 5.1 Cross section of the vertebrate eye
An object in the visual field produces an inverted image on the retina. The optic nerve exits the eyeball on the nasal side (the side closer to the nose).

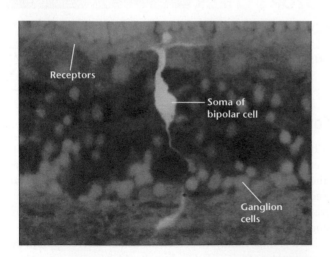

Figure 5.2 A bipolar cell from the retina of a carp, stained yellow
Bipolar cells get their name from the fact that a fibrous process is attached to each end (or pole) of the neuron.
(Source: Dowling, 1987)

midget ganglion cells because each is small and responds to just a single cone. That is, each cone in the fovea has a direct route to the brain. Because the midget ganglion cells provide 70 percent of the input to the brain, your vision is dominated by what you see in and near the fovea (Nassi & Callaway, 2009).

You have heard the expression "eyes like a hawk." Many birds' eyes occupy most of the head, compared to only 5 percent of the head in humans. Furthermore, many bird species have two foveas per eye, one pointing ahead and one pointing to the side (Wallman & Pettigrew, 1985). The extra foveas enable perception of detail in the periphery.

Hawks and other predatory birds have a greater density of visual receptors on the top half of their retinas (looking down) than on the bottom half (looking up). That arrangement is adaptive because predatory birds spend most of their day looking down, either while flying or while perched high in a tree. However, to look up, the bird must turn its head, as in Figure 5.5 (Waldvogel, 1990). Conversely, many prey species such as rats have most of their receptors on the bottom half of the retina, enabling them

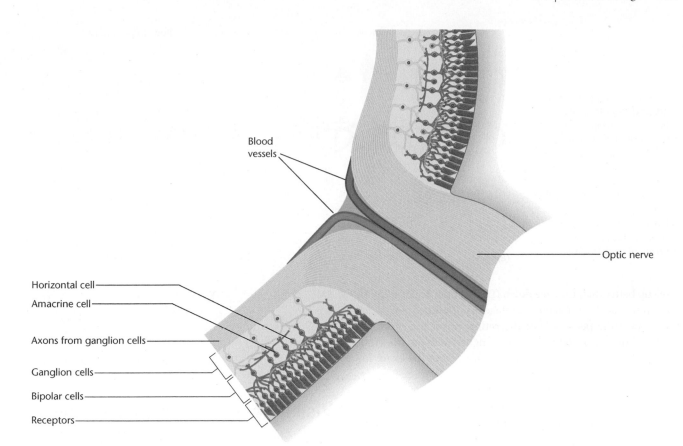

Figure 5.3 Visual path within the eye
Receptors send their messages to bipolar and horizontal cells, which in turn send messages to amacrine and ganglion cells. The axons of the ganglion cells form the optic nerve, which exits the eye at the blind spot and continues to the brain.

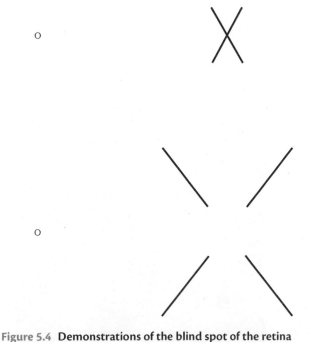

Figure 5.4 Demonstrations of the blind spot of the retina
Close your left eye and focus your right eye on the o in the top part. Move the page toward you and away, noticing what happens to the x. At a distance of about 10 inches (25 cm), the x disappears. Now repeat this procedure with the bottom part. At that same distance, what do you see?

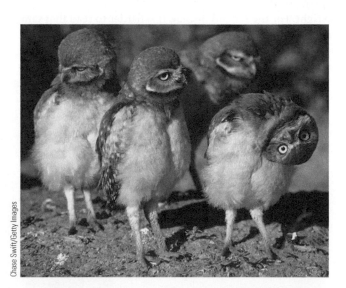

Figure 5.5 A consequence of how receptors are arranged on the retina
One owlet has turned its head almost upside down to look up. Birds of prey have many receptors on the upper half of the retina, enabling them to see down in great detail during flight. But they see objects above themselves poorly, unless they turn their heads. Take another look at the prairie falcon at the start of this chapter. It is not a one-eyed bird; it is a bird that has tilted its head. Do you now understand why?

Cones in fovea

Rods in periphery

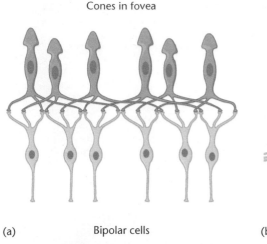

Figure 5.6 Convergence of input onto bipolar cells
In the fovea, each bipolar cell receives excitation from just one cone (and inhibition from a few surrounding cones), and relays its information to a single midget ganglion cell. In the periphery, input from many rods converges onto each bipolar cell, resulting in higher sensitivity to faint light and low sensitivity to spatial location.

(a)   Bipolar cells

(b)   Bipolar cells

to see up better than they see down (Lund, Lund, & Wise, 1974). You can see the evolutionary advantages for these species.

Toward the periphery of the retina, more and more receptors converge onto bipolar and ganglion cells, as shown in Figure 5.6. As a result, the brain cannot detect the exact location or shape of a peripheral light source (Rossi & Roorda, 2010). However, the summation enables perception of fainter lights in the periphery. In short, foveal vision has better *acuity* (sensitivity to detail), and peripheral vision has better sensitivity to dim light.

In the periphery, your ability to detect detail is limited by interference from other nearby objects (Pelli & Tillman, 2008). In the following displays, focus on the x. For the first display, you can probably identify the letter to the right. For the second display, it is harder to read that same letter in the same location, because of interference from the neighboring letters.

TRY IT YOURSELF

X   T

X   ATE

Visual Receptors: Rods and Cones

The vertebrate retina contains two types of receptors: rods and cones (see Figure 5.7). The **rods**, abundant in the periphery of the human retina, respond to faint light but are not useful in daylight because bright light bleaches them. **Cones**, abundant in and near the fovea, are less active in dim light, more useful in bright light, and essential for color vision. Because of the distribution of rods and cones, you have good color vision in the fovea but not in the periphery. Table 5.1 summarizes the differences between foveal and peripheral vision.

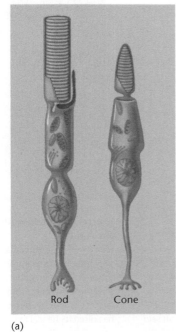

Figure 5.7 Structure of rod and cone
(a) Diagram of a rod and a cone. (b) Photo of rods and a cone, produced with a scanning electron microscope. Magnification x 7000.
(Source: Reprinted from Brain Research, *15(2), E.R. Lewis, Y.Y. Zeevi and F.S. Werblin, Scanning electron microscopy of vertebrate visual receptors, 1969, with permission from Elsevier.)*

Rod   Cone

(a)

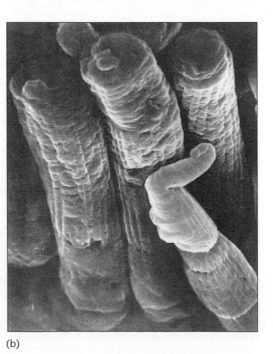

(b)

Table 5.1 | **Human Foveal and Peripheral Vision**

Characteristic	Foveal Vision	Peripheral Vision
Receptors	Cones only	Proportion of rods increases toward periphery
Convergence of input	Each ganglion cell excited by a single cone	Each ganglion cell excited by many receptors
Brightness sensitivity	Distinguishes among bright lights; responds poorly to dim light	Responds to dim light; poor for distinguishing among bright lights
Sensitivity to detail	Good detail vision because each cone's own ganglion cell sends a message to the brain	Poor detail vision because many receptors converge their input onto a given ganglion cell
Color vision	Good (many cones)	Poor (few cones)

Although rods outnumber cones by about 20 to 1 in the human retina, cones provide about 90 percent of the brain's input (Masland, 2001). Remember the midget ganglion cells: In the fovea, each cone has its own line to the brain. In the periphery (mostly rods), each receptor shares a line with tens or hundreds of others. Overall, 120 million rods and 6 million cones converge onto 1 million axons in the optic nerve, on average.

A 20:1 ratio of rods to cones may sound high, but the ratio is much higher in species that are active at night. South American oilbirds, which live in caves and emerge only at night, have about 15,000 rods per cone. As a further adaptation to detect faint lights, their rods are packed three deep throughout the retina (Martin, Rojas, Ramírez, & McNeil, 2004).

People vary substantially in the number of axons in their optic nerve and the size of the visual cortex, largely for genetic reasons (Bakken et al., 2012). Some people have two or three times as many axons from the eyes to the brain as others do. They also have more cells in their visual cortex (Andrews, Halpern, & Purves, 1997; Stevens, 2001; Sur & Leamey, 2001) and greater ability to detect brief, faint, or rapidly changing

visual stimuli (Halpern, Andrews, & Purves, 1999). Heightened visual responses are valuable in many activities, especially in sports that require aim. Researchers find that top performers in tennis, squash, fencing, baseball, and badminton show enhanced processing of visual stimuli, compared to other people (Muraskin, Sherwin, & Sajda, 2015; Nakata, Yoshie, Miura, & Kudo, 2010; C.-H. Wang et al., 2015). Of course, excellent vision is hardly the only ingredient for athletic success, but it helps.

Both rods and cones contain **photopigments**, chemicals that release energy when struck by light. Photopigments consist of 11-*cis*-retinal (a derivative of vitamin A) bound to proteins called *opsins*, which modify the photopigments' sensitivity to different wavelengths of light. Light converts 11-*cis*-retinal to all-*trans*-retinal, thus releasing energy that activates second messengers within the cell (Q. Wang, Schoenlein, Peteanu, Mathies, & Shank, 1994). (The light is absorbed in this process. It does not continue to bounce around the eye.)

STOP & CHECK

5. You sometimes find that you can see a faint star on a dark night better if you look slightly to the side of the star instead of straight at it. Why?

6. If you found a species with a high ratio of cones to rods in its retina, what would you predict about its way of life?

ANSWERS

5. If you look slightly to the side, the light falls on an area of the retina with more rods and more convergence of input. **6.** We should expect this species to be highly active during the day and seldom active at night.

Color Vision

Visible light consists of electromagnetic radiation within the range from less than 400 nm (nanometer, or 10^{-9} m) to more than 700 nm. We perceive the shortest visible wavelengths as violet. Progressively longer wavelengths are perceived as blue, green, yellow, orange, and red (see Figure 5.8). We call these wavelengths "light" only because the receptors in our eyes are tuned to detecting them. If we had different receptors, we would define light differently. Indeed, many species of birds,

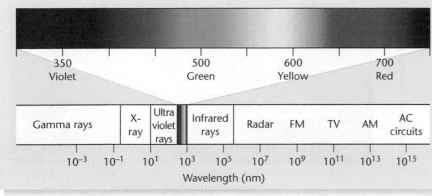

Colin Blakemore/Oxford University

Figure 5.8 A beam of light separated into its wavelengths
Although the wavelengths vary as a continuum, we perceive distinct colors.

fish, and insects have visual receptors sensitive to what we call ultraviolet radiation (Stevens & Cuthill, 2007). Of course, we cannot know what it looks like to them, but so far as they are concerned, ultraviolet radiation is a type of light. In some species of birds, the male and female look alike to us, but different to birds, because the male reflects more ultraviolet light.

The Trichromatic (Young-Helmholtz) Theory

People distinguish red, green, yellow, blue, orange, pink, purple, greenish blue, and so forth. Presuming that we don't have a separate receptor for every possible color, how many receptor types do we have?

The first person to advance our understanding on this question was an amazingly productive man named Thomas Young (1773–1829). Young was the first to start deciphering the Rosetta stone. He also founded the modern wave theory of light, defined energy in its modern form, founded the calculation of annuities, introduced the coefficient of elasticity, discovered much about the anatomy of the eye, and made major contributions to other fields (Martindale, 2001). Previous scientists thought they could explain color by understanding the physics of light. Young recognized that color required a biological explanation. He proposed that we perceive color by comparing the responses across a few types of receptors, each of which was sensitive to a different range of wavelengths.

This theory, later modified by Hermann von Helmholtz, is now known as the **trichromatic theory** of color vision, or the **Young-Helmholtz theory**. According to this theory, we perceive color through the relative rates of response by three kinds of cones, each one maximally sensitive to a different set of wavelengths. (*Trichromatic* means "three colors.") How did Helmholtz decide on the number three? He found that people could match any color by mixing appropriate amounts of just three wavelengths. Therefore, he concluded that three kinds of receptors—we now call them cones—are sufficient to account for human color vision.

Figure 5.9 shows wavelength-sensitivity functions for the *short-wavelength*, *medium-wavelength*, and *long-wavelength*

cone types. Each cone responds to a broad range of wavelengths but to some more than others.

According to the trichromatic theory, we discriminate among wavelengths by the ratio of activity across the three types of cones. For example, light at 550 nm excites the medium-wavelength and long-wavelength receptors about equally and the short-wavelength receptor almost not at all. This ratio of responses among the three cones determines a perception of yellow-green. More intense light increases the activity of all three cones without much change in their ratio of responses. As a result, the light appears brighter but still the same color. When all three types of cones are equally active, we see white or gray.

Think about this example of coding: Your perception of color depends on the frequency of response in each cell *relative to* the frequency of other cells. The response of any one cone is ambiguous. For example, a low response rate by a middle-wavelength cone might indicate low-intensity 540 nm light or brighter 500 nm light or still brighter 460 nm light. The nervous system determines the color of the light by comparing the responses of different types of cones.

Given the desirability of seeing all colors in all locations, we might suppose that the three kinds of cones would be equally abundant and evenly distributed. In fact, they are not. Long- and medium-wavelength cones are far more abundant than short-wavelength (blue) cones. Consequently, it is easier to see tiny red, yellow, or green dots than blue dots (Roorda & Williams, 1999). Try this: Look at the dots in the following display, first from close and then from greater distances. You probably will notice that the blue dots look blue when close but appear black from a greater distance. The other colors remain distinct when the blue is not.

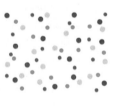

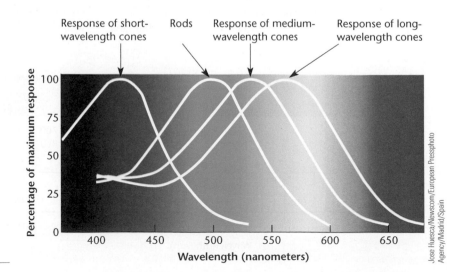

Figure 5.9 Responses of rods and three kinds of cones
Note that each kind responds somewhat to a wide range of wavelengths but best to wavelengths in a particular range.
(*Source: Adapted from Bowmaker & Dartnall, 1980*)

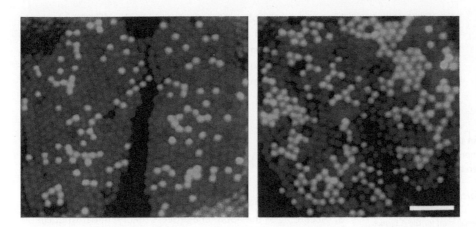

Figure 5.10　Distribution of cones in two human retinas
Investigators artificially colored these images of cones from two people's retinas, indicating short-wavelength cones with blue, medium-wavelength cones with green, and long-wavelength cones with red. Note the difference between the two people, the scarcity of short-wavelength cones, and the patchiness of the distributions.
(*Source: Reprinted by permission from Macmillan Publishers Ltd: Nature, The arrangement of the three cone classes in the living human eye, Roorda & Williams, 1999*)

Although the short-wavelength (blue) cones are about evenly distributed across the retina, the other two kinds are distributed haphazardly, with big differences among individuals (Solomon & Lennie, 2007). Figure 5.10 shows the distribution of short-, medium-, and long-wavelength cones in two people's retinas, with colors artificially added to distinguish them. Note the patches of all medium- or all long-wavelength cones. Some people have more than 10 times as many of one kind as the other. Surprisingly, these variations produce only small differences in people's color perceptions (Solomon & Lennie, 2007).

In the retina's periphery, cones are so scarce that you have no useful color vision (Diller et al., 2004; P. R. Martin, Lee, White, Solomon, & Rütiger, 2001). Try this: Get someone to put a colored dot on the tip of your finger without telling you the color. A spot of colored ink will do. While keeping your eyes straight ahead, slowly move your finger from behind your head into your field of vision and gradually toward your fovea. At what point do you first see your finger? At what point do you see the color? Certainly you see your finger before you see the color. The smaller the dot, the farther you have to move it into your **visual field**—that is, the part of the world that you see—before you can identify the color.

The Opponent-Process Theory

The trichromatic theory is incomplete as a theory of color vision. For example, try the following demonstration: Pick a point near the center of Figure 5.11 and stare at it under a bright light, without moving your eyes, for a minute. (The brighter the light and the longer you stare, the stronger the effect.) Then look at a plain white surface, such as a wall or a blank sheet of paper. Keep your eyes steady. You will see a **negative color afterimage**, a replacement of the red you had been staring at with green, green with red, yellow and blue with each other, and black and white with each other.

To explain this and related phenomena, Ewald Hering, a 19th-century physiologist, proposed the **opponent-process theory**: We perceive color in terms of opposites (Hurvich & Jameson, 1957). That is, the brain has a mechanism that perceives color on a continuum from red to green, another from yellow to blue, and another from white to black. After you stare at one color in one location long enough, you fatigue that response and swing to the opposite.

Part of the explanation for this process pertains to the connections within the retina. For example, imagine a bipolar cell that receives excitation from a short-wavelength cone and inhibition from long- and medium-wavelength cones. It increases its activity in response to short-wavelength (blue) light and decreases it in response to yellowish light. After prolonged exposure to blue light, the fatigued cell decreases its response. Because a low level of response by that cell usually means yellow, you perceive yellow. When researchers around 1950 first demonstrated that certain neurons in the visual system increased their activity in response to one wavelength of light and decreased it to another, they revolutionized our understanding of vision, and of the nervous system in general (Jacobs, 2014).

However, that explanation cannot be the whole story. Try this: Stare at the x in the following diagram for about a minute under a bright light and then look at a white page.

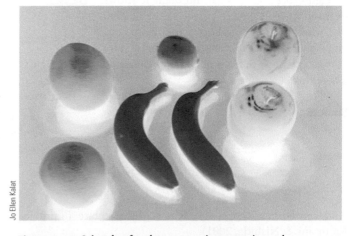

Jo Ellen Kalat

Figure 5.11　Stimulus for demonstrating negative color afterimages
Stare at one point under bright light for about a minute, without moving your eyes, and then look at a white field. You should see two oranges, a lime, two bananas, and two apples, all in their normal color.

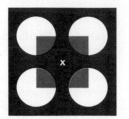

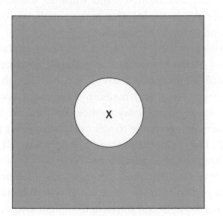

Figure 5.12 An afterimage hard to explain in terms of the retina
Stare at the x under bright light for a minute and then look at a white surface. Many people report an alternation between two afterimages, one of them based on the illusion of a red square.
(Source: Reprinted with permission from "Afterimage of perceptually filled-in surface," by S. Shimojo, Y. Kamitani, and S. Nishida, 2001, Science, 293, 1677–1680, specifically Figure 1A, p. 1678 (left hand). Copyright 2001 American Association for the Advancement of Science.)

For the afterimage of the surrounding area, you saw red, as the theory predicts. But what about the circle inside? Theoretically, you should see a gray or black afterimage (the opposite of white), but in fact, if you used a bright enough light, you saw a green afterimage. What you saw in the surround influenced what you saw in the center.

Here is another demonstration: First, look at Figure 5.12. Note that although it shows four red quarter circles, you have the illusion of a whole red square. (Look carefully to convince yourself that it is an illusion.) Now stare at the x in Figure 5.12 for at least a minute under bright lights. Then look at a white surface.

People usually report that the afterimage fluctuates. Sometimes, they see four green quarter circles:

And sometimes, they see a whole green square (Shimojo, Kamitani, & Nishida, 2001):

If you see a whole green square, it is the afterimage of an illusion! The red square you "saw" wasn't really there. This demonstration suggests that afterimages depend on the whole context, not just the light on individual receptors. The cerebral cortex must be responsible, not the bipolar or ganglion cells.

STOP & CHECK

7. Examine Figure 5.9. According to the trichromatic theory, what causes you to perceive red?
8. According to the opponent-process theory, under what circumstance would you perceive a white object as blue?

ANSWERS

7. Activity of the long-wavelength cone is not sufficient. In fact, notice that the long-wavelength cone responds to what we call yellow more than to what we call red. A perception of red occurs only if the long-wavelength cone has a high ratio of response relative to the other two types of cone. 8. If you stared at a bright yellow object for a minute or so and then looked at a white object, it would appear blue.

The Retinex Theory

The trichromatic theory and the opponent-process theory cannot easily explain **color constancy**, the ability to recognize colors despite changes in lighting (Kennard, Lawden, Morland, & Ruddock, 1995; Zeki, 1980, 1983). If you wear green-tinted glasses or replace your white light bulb with a green one, you still identify bananas as yellow, paper as white, and so forth. Your brain compares the color of one object with the color of another, in effect subtracting a certain amount of green from each.

To illustrate, examine Figure 5.13 (Purves & Lotto, 2003). Although different colors of light illuminate the two objects at the top, you easily identify the squares as red, yellow, blue, and so forth. Note the result of removing context. The bottom part shows the squares that looked blue in the top left part and yellow in the top right part. Without the context that indicated yellow light or blue light, all these squares look gray. For this reason, we should avoid talking about the color of a wavelength of light. A certain wavelength of light can appear as different colors depending on the background.

Similarly, we perceive the brightness of an object by comparing it to other objects. Examine Figure 5.14 (Purves, Shimpi, & Lotto, 1999). The object in the center appears to have a dark gray top and a white bottom. Now cover the border between the top and the bottom with a finger. You see that the top of the object has exactly the same brightness as the bottom! For additional examples like this, visit the

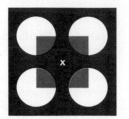
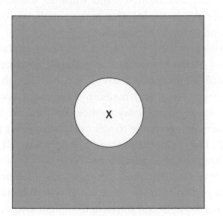

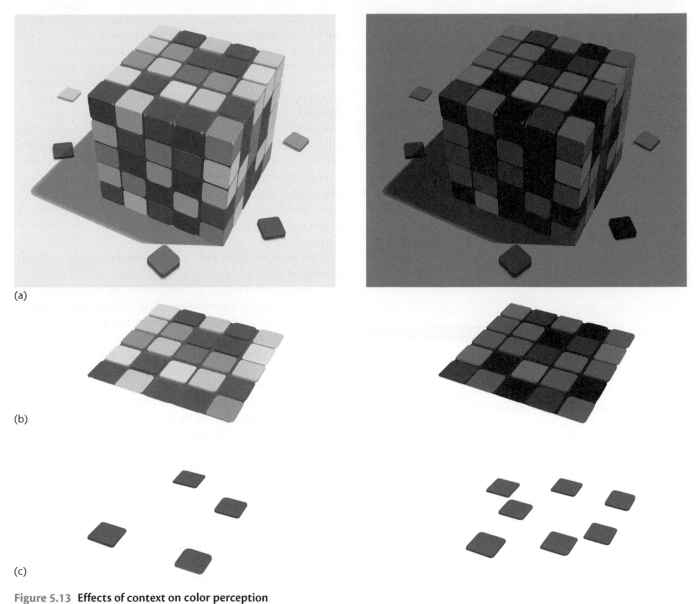

(a)

(b)

(c)

Figure 5.13 Effects of context on color perception
After removal of the context, squares that appeared blue on the left or yellow on the right now appear gray.
(Source: From Why we see what we do, *by D. Purves and R. B. Lotto, Figure 5.10, p. 134. Copyright 2003 Oxford Publishing Limited. Reprinted by permission.)*

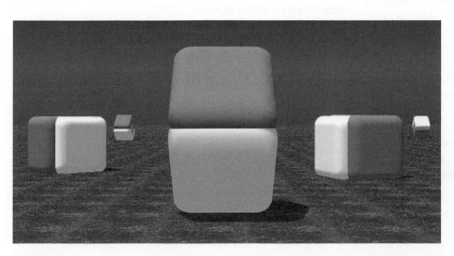

Figure 5.14 Brightness constancy
In the center of this figure, do you see a gray object above and a white object below? Place a finger over the border between them and then compare the objects.
(Source: From "An empirical explanation of cornsweet effect," by D. Purves, A. Shimpi, and R. B. Lotto, Journal of Neuroscience, *19, p. 8542–8551. Copyright 1999 by the Society for Neuroscience.)*

website of Dale Purves, Center for Cognitive Neuroscience, Duke University.

To account for color and brightness constancy, Edwin Land proposed the **retinex theory** (a combination of the words *retin*a and cort*ex*): The cortex compares information from various parts of the retina to determine the brightness and color for each area (Land, Hubel, Livingstone, Perry, & Burns, 1983).

Dale Purves and colleagues have expressed a similar idea in more general terms: Whenever we see anything, we make an inference. For example, when you look at the objects in Figures 5.13 and 5.14, you ask yourself, "On occasions when I have seen something that looked like this, what was it really?" You go through the same process for perceiving shapes, motion, or anything else (Lotto & Purves, 2002; Purves & Lotto, 2003). That is, visual perception requires reasoning and inference, not just retinal stimulation.

STOP & CHECK

9. When a television set is off, its screen appears gray. When you watch a program, parts of the screen appear black, even though more light is actually showing on the screen than when the set was off. What accounts for the black perception?

10. Figure 5.9 shows light at about 510 nm as green. Why should we nevertheless not call it "green light"?

ANSWERS

9. The black experience arises by contrast with the brighter areas around it. 10. Color perception depends not just on the wavelength of light from a given spot but also the light from surrounding areas. As in Figure 5.13, the context can change the color perception.

Color Vision Deficiency

One of the first discoveries in psychology was colorblindness, better described as **color vision deficiency**. (Complete colorblindness, perception of only black and white, is rare.) Today we are familiar with the idea that some people see color better than others do, but before the 1600s, people assumed that everyone sees the same way, and that what we perceive is what the object actually *is* (Fletcher & Voke, 1985). Then investigators demonstrated that some people have otherwise satisfactory vision without seeing all the color that other people do. That is, color is in the brain, not in the light or the object itself. In contrast to our three types of cones, many birds, reptiles, and fish have four types (Bowmaker, 2008). So far as they are concerned, all humans are color deficient.

Color deficiency results because people with certain genes fail to develop one type of cone, or develop an abnormal type of cone (Nathans et al., 1989). In red-green color deficiency, the most common form of color deficiency, people have trouble distinguishing red from green because their long- and medium-wavelength cones have the same photopigment instead of different ones. The gene causing this deficiency is on the X chromosome. About 8 percent of northern European men (and a smaller percentage of men from other backgrounds) are red-green colorblind, compared with less than 1 percent of women (Bowmaker, 1998). Women with one normal gene and one color-deficient gene—and that includes all women with a red-green color-deficient father—are slightly less sensitive to red and green than the average for other people (Bimler & Kirkland, 2009).

Suppose an adult with a red-green deficiency suddenly developed all three types of normal cones. Would the brain start seeing in full color? No one has tested this question for people, but we do know what would happen for monkeys. Researchers took adult monkeys with red-green color deficiency from birth, and used gene therapy to add a third kind of cone to their retinas. They quickly learned to discriminate red from green (Mancuso et al., 2009). Evidently, the brain adapts to use the information it receives.

What would happen if people had a fourth type of cone? Actually, some women do, in a way. The long-wavelength cone shows genetic variation. At one point in the protein, most genes code for the amino acid *serine* but 16 to 38 percent of the genes (depending on people's ethnic background) produce instead the amino acid *alanine*. Because the gene is on the X chromosome, a man has only one or the other. However, because women have two X chromosomes, some women have one long-wavelength receptor with serine and one with alanine. Those two versions of the long-wavelength receptor differ slightly in their responsiveness to light (Deeb, 2005). Women with different versions of that receptor make somewhat finer distinctions between one color and another, compared to other people (Jameson, Highnote, & Wasserman, 2001). Because some women have two types of long-wavelength receptors and others have just one, women's performance on color vision tests is more variable than men's is (Dees & Baraas, 2014).

STOP & CHECK

11. Why is color vision deficiency a better term than color blindness?

ANSWER

11. Very few people see the world entirely in black and white. The more common condition is difficulty discriminating red from green.

Module 5.1 | In Closing

Visual Receptors

I remember once explaining to my then teenage son a newly discovered detail about the visual system, only to have him reply, "I didn't realize it would be so complicated. I thought the light strikes your eyes and then you see it." As you should now be starting to realize—and if not, the rest of the chapter should convince you—vision requires complicated processing. If you tried to equip a robot with vision, you would quickly discover that shining light into its eyes accomplishes nothing, unless its visual detectors are connected to devices that identify the useful information and use it to select the proper action. We have such devices in our brains, and they produce the amazing results that we call vision.

Summary

1. You see because light strikes your retina, causing it to send a message to your brain. You send no sight rays out to the object. **148**

2. According to the law of specific nerve energies, the brain interprets any activity of a given sensory neuron as representing a particular type of sensory information. **148**

3. Sensory information is coded so that the brain can process it. The coded information bears no physical similarity to the stimuli it describes. **148**

4. Light passes through the pupil of a vertebrate eye and stimulates the receptors lining the retina at the back of the eye. **149**

5. The axons from the retina loop around to form the optic nerve, which exits from the eye at a point called the blind spot. **149**

6. Visual acuity is greatest in the fovea, the central area of the retina. Because so many receptors in the periphery converge their messages to their bipolar cells, our peripheral vision is highly sensitive to faint light but poorly sensitive to detail. **149**

7. The retina has two kinds of receptors: rods and cones. Rods, more numerous in the periphery of the retina, are more sensitive to faint light. Cones, more numerous in the fovea, are more useful in bright light. **152**

8. People vary in their number of axons from the retina to the brain. Those with more axons show a greater ability to detect brief, faint, or rapidly changing stimuli. **153**

9. According to the trichromatic (or Young-Helmholtz) theory of color vision, color perception begins with a given wavelength of light stimulating a distinctive ratio of responses by the three types of cones. **154**

10. According to the opponent-process theory of color vision, visual system neurons beyond the receptors respond with an increase in activity to indicate one color of light and a decrease to indicate the opposite color. The three pairs of opposites are red-green, yellow-blue, and white-black. **155**

11. According to the retinex theory, the cortex compares the responses across the retina to determine brightness and color of each object. **156**

12. For genetic reasons, certain people are unable to distinguish one color from another. Red-green color deficiency is the most common type. **158**

Key Terms

Terms are defined in the module on the page number indicated. They're also presented in alphabetical order with definitions in the book's Subject Index/Glossary, which begins on page 589. Interactive flash cards, audio reviews, and crossword puzzles are among the online resources available to help you learn these terms and the concepts they represent.

bipolar cells **149**
blind spot **149**
color constancy **156**
color vision deficiency **158**
cones **152**
fovea **149**
ganglion cells **149**

law of specific nerve energies **148**
midget ganglion cells **150**
negative color afterimage **155**
opponent-process theory **155**
optic nerve **149**
photopigments **153**
pupil **149**

retina **149**
retinex theory **158**
rods **152**
trichromatic theory (or Young-Helmholtz theory) **154**
visual field **155**

Thought Question

How could you test for the presence of color vision in a bee? Examining the retina does not help because invertebrate receptors resemble neither rods nor cones. It is possible to train bees to approach one visual stimulus and not another. However, if you train bees to approach, say, a yellow card and not a green card, you do not know whether they solved the problem by color or by brightness. Because brightness is different from physical intensity, you cannot assume that two colors equally bright to humans are also equally bright to bees. How might you get around the problem of brightness to test color vision in bees?

Module 5.1 | End of Module Quiz

1. What happens when you see something?
   A. You send out sight rays that strike the object.
   B. Light rays reflect off the object and strike your retina.
   C. You send out sight rays, *and* light reflecting off the object strikes your retina.
   D. You neither send out sight rays nor receive light rays onto your retina.

2. What is the route from retinal receptors to the brain?
   A. Receptors send axons directly to the brain.
   B. Receptors connect to bipolars, which connect to ganglion cells, which send axons to the brain.
   C. Receptors connect to ganglion cells, which connect to bipolars, which send axons to the brain.
   D. Receptors connect to amacrine cells, which send axons to the brain.

3. Where does the optic nerve exit from the retina?
   A. At the blind spot
   B. At the fovea
   C. From the edge of the fovea
   D. Diffusely from all parts of the retina

4. Why is vision most acute at the fovea?
   A. The fovea is closest to the pupil.
   B. The fovea has an equal ratio of cones to rods.
   C. The cornea produces the least distortion of light at the fovea.
   D. Each receptor in the fovea has a direct line to the brain.

5. Vision in the periphery of the retina has poor sensitivity to detail but great sensitivity to faint light. Why?
   A. Toward the periphery, the retina has more midget ganglion cells.
   B. Toward the periphery, the retina has more cones and fewer rods.
   C. Toward the periphery, the retina has more convergence of input.
   D. Toward the periphery, the light falls farther from the blind spot.

6. Why do some people have greater than average sensitivity to brief, faint, or rapidly changing visual stimuli?
   A. They do not have a blind spot in their retina.
   B. The blind spot in their retina is smaller than average.
   C. They have more axons from the retina to the brain.
   D. They have four types of cones instead of three.

7. Suppose you perceive something as red. According to the trichromatic theory, what is the explanation?
   A. Light from the object has excited your long-wavelength cones more strongly than your other cones.
   B. Light from the object has excited your short-wavelength cones more strongly than your other cones.
   C. Ganglion cells that increase response to red and decrease their response to green are firing strongly.
   D. The cortex compares activity over all parts of the retina and computes that one area is red.

8. If you stare at a white circle surrounded by a green background, and then look at a white surface, you perceive a green circle surrounded by a red background. What does this observation imply about the opponent-process theory?
   A. We perceive colors based on the pattern of input to the bipolar and ganglion cells of the retina.
   B. The mechanisms of color vision vary from one species to another.
   C. Opponent-process color perception depends on the visual cortex, not just the cells in the retina.
   D. The opponent-process theory is wrong.

9. An object that reflects all wavelengths equally ordinarily appears gray, but it may appear yellow, blue, or any other color, depending on what?

   A. Brightness of the light

   B. Contrast with surrounding objects

   C. The culture in which you grew up

   D. The ratio of cones to rods in your retina

10. Color vision deficiency demonstrates which fundamental point about perception?

    A. Color is in the brain and not in the light itself.

    B. Each sensory system depends on a different part of the cerebral cortex.

    C. Color perception varies because of cultural influences.

    D. Fatiguing a receptor can lead to a negative afterimage.

Answers: 1B, 2B, 3A, 4D, 5C, 6C, 7A, 8C, 9B, 10A.

How the Brain Processes Visual Information

Vision is complicated. We shall go through it in some detail, for two reasons. First, without vision and other senses, you would have no more mental experience than a tree does. Everything in psychology starts with sensations. Second, neuroscientists have investigated vision in more detail than anything else that the brain does. Examining the mechanisms of vision illustrates what it means to explain something in biological terms. It provides a model of what we would like to accomplish eventually for other psychological processes.

An Overview of the Mammalian Visual System

Let's begin with a general outline of the anatomy of the mammalian visual system. The rods and cones of the retina make synapses with **horizontal cells** and bipolar cells (see Figures 5.3 and 5.15). The horizontal cells make inhibitory contact onto bipolar cells, which in turn make synapses onto *amacrine cells* and ganglion cells. All these cells are within the eyeball.

The axons of the ganglion cells form the optic nerve, which leaves the retina and travels along the lower surface of the brain. The optic nerves from the two eyes meet at the optic chiasm (see Figure 5.16a), where, in humans, half of the axons from each eye cross to the opposite side of the brain. As shown in Figure 5.16b, information from the nasal half of each eye (the side closer to the nose) crosses to the contralateral hemisphere. Information from the temporal half (the side toward the temporal cortex) goes to the ipsilateral hemisphere. The percentage of crossover varies from one species to another depending on the location of the eyes. In species with eyes far to the sides of the head, such as rabbits and guinea pigs, nearly all axons cross to the opposite side.

Most ganglion cell axons go to the **lateral geniculate nucleus**, part of the thalamus. (The term *geniculate* comes from the Latin root *genu*, meaning "knee." To *genuflect* is to bend the knee. The lateral geniculate looks somewhat like a knee, if you use some imagination.) A smaller number of axons go to the superior colliculus and other areas, including part of the hypothalamus that controls the waking–sleeping

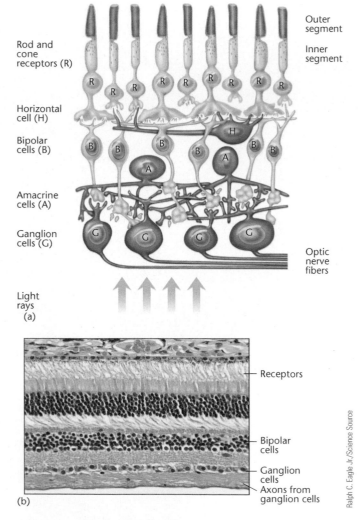

Labels: Rod and cone receptors (R); Outer segment; Inner segment; Horizontal cell (H); Bipolar cells (B); Amacrine cells (A); Ganglion cells (G); Optic nerve fibers; Light rays; (a)

Receptors; Bipolar cells; Ganglion cells; Axons from ganglion cells; (b)

Ralph C. Eagle Jr./Science Source

Figure 5.15 The vertebrate retina
The top of the figure is the back of the retina. The optic nerve fibers group together and exit through the back of the retina, in the "blind spot" of the eye.
(Source: Based on "Organization of the primate retina," by J. E. Dowling and B. B. Boycott, Proceedings of the Royal Society of London, B, 1966, 166, pp. 80–111. *Used by permission of the Royal Society of London and John Dowling.)*

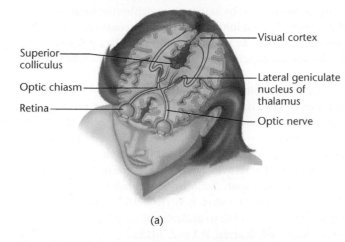

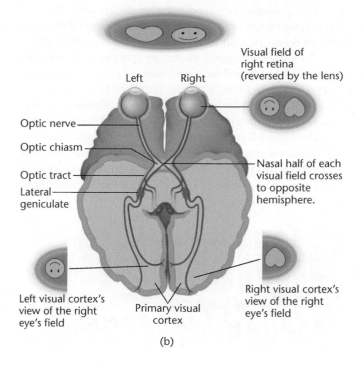

Figure 5.16 Major connections in the visual system
(a) Part of the visual input goes to the thalamus and from there to the visual cortex. Another part goes to the superior colliculus. (b) Axons from the retina maintain their relationship to one another—what we call their *retinotopic organization*—throughout their journey from the retina to the lateral geniculate and then from the lateral geniculate to the cortex.

schedule. The lateral geniculate, in turn, sends axons to other parts of the thalamus and the visual cortex. Axons returning from the cortex to the thalamus modify thalamic activity (Ling, Pratte, & Tong, 2015).

✓ STOP & CHECK

12. Where does the optic nerve start and where does it end?

ANSWER

12. It starts with the ganglion cells in the retina. Most of its axons go to the lateral geniculate nucleus of the thalamus, but some go to the hypothalamus and superior colliculus.

Processing in the Retina

Combined, your two eyes include about a quarter of a billion receptors. Your brain would not be able to handle a quarter of a billion separate messages, nor would that much information be useful. You need to extract the meaningful patterns. To understand how the wiring diagram of your retina highlights those patterns, let's start by exploring one example in detail: lateral inhibition.

Lateral inhibition is the retina's way of sharpening contrasts to emphasize the borders of objects. For analogy, suppose 15 people stand in a line. At first, each holds one cookie. Now someone hands 5 extra cookies to the 5 people in the middle of the line, but then each of those 5 people has to throw away one of his or her own cookies, and throw away one cookie that the person on each side is holding. Presuming that you want as many cookies as possible, where is the best

place to be? You don't want to be in the middle of the group who receive cookies, because after gaining 5 you would have to throw away one of your own and lose one to each of your neighbors (a total loss of 3). But if you're either the first or last person to receive a cookie, you'll throw one away and lose one to just one neighbor (a total loss of 2). The worst place to be is right before or after the group receiving cookies. You would receive none, and lose the one you already had. The result is a sharp contrast at the border between those receiving cookies and those not.

The analogy may sound silly—okay, it *is* silly—but it illustrates something that happens in the retina. The receptors send messages to excite nearby bipolar cells (like giving them cookies) and also send messages to horizontal cells that slightly inhibit those bipolar cells and the neighbors to their sides (like subtracting cookies). The net result is to heighten the contrast between an illuminated area and its darker surround.

Actually, light striking the rods and cones *decreases* their spontaneous output, and the receptors make *inhibitory* synapses onto the bipolar cells. Therefore, light on the rods or cones decreases their inhibitory output. A decrease in inhibition means net excitation, so to avoid double negatives, let's think of the receptors' output as excitation of the bipolar cells.

In the fovea, each cone attaches to just one bipolar cell. We'll consider that simple case. In the following diagram, green arrows represent excitation, and the width of an arrow indicates the amount of excitation. Receptor 8, which is highlighted, excites bipolar cell 8. It also excites a horizontal cell, which *inhibits* a group of bipolar cells, as shown by red arrows. Because the horizontal cell spreads widely, excitation of any receptor inhibits the surrounding bipolar cells. However, because the horizontal cell is a *local cell*, with no axon and no action potentials, its depolarization decays with distance. The horizontal cell inhibits bipolar cells 7 through 9 strongly, bipolars 6 and 10 a bit less, and so on. Bipolar cell 8 shows net excitation, because the excitatory synapse outweighs the effect of the horizontal cell's inhibition. (It's like gaining some cookies and then losing a smaller number.) However, the bipolar cells to the sides (laterally) get no excitation but some inhibition by the horizontal cell. (They gained none and then they lost some.) Bipolar cells 7 and 9 are strongly inhibited, and bipolars 6 and 10 are inhibited less. In this diagram, the thickness of the arrow indicates the amount of excitation or inhibition. The lightness of blue indicates the net amount of excitation in each bipolar cell.

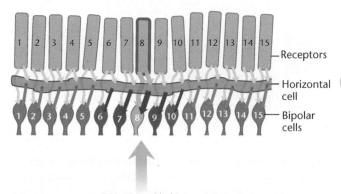

Direction of light

Now imagine that light excites receptors 6 through 10. These receptors excite bipolar cells 6 through 10 and the horizontal cell. Bipolar cells 6 through 10 all receive the same amount of excitation. Bipolar cells 7, 8, and 9 are inhibited by input on both sides, but bipolar cells 6 and 10 are inhibited from one side and not the other. That is, the bipolar cells in the middle of the excited area are inhibited the most, and those on the edges are inhibited the least. Therefore, bipolar cells 6 and 10, the ones on the edges of the field of excitation, respond *more* than bipolars 7 through 9.

Next, consider bipolar cells 5 and 11. What excitation do they receive? None. However, the horizontal cell inhibits them. Therefore, receiving inhibition but no excitation, they respond less than bipolar cells that are farther from the area of excitation.

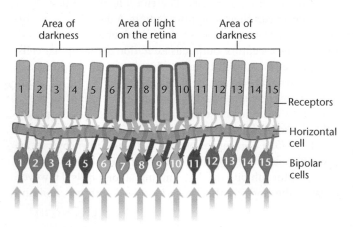

These results illustrate **lateral inhibition**, the reduction of activity in one neuron by activity in neighboring neurons (Hartline, 1949). Lateral inhibition heightens contrast. When light falls on a surface, as shown here, the bipolars just inside the border are most excited, and those outside the border respond the least.

Lateral inhibition is important for many functions in the nervous system. In olfaction, a strong stimulus can suppress the response to another one that follows slightly after it, because of inhibition in the olfactory bulb (Whitesell, Sorensen, Jarvie, Hentges, & Schoppa, 2013). In touch, stimulation of one spot on the skin weakens the response to stimulation of a neighboring spot, again by lateral inhibition (Severens, Farquhar, Desain, Duysens, & Gielen, 2010). In hearing, inhibition makes it possible to understand speech amid irrelevant noise (Bashford, Warren, & Lenz, 2013).

STOP & CHECK

13. When light strikes a receptor, does the receptor excite or inhibit the bipolar cells? What effect does it have on horizontal cells? What effect does the horizontal cell have on bipolar cells?

14. If light strikes only one receptor, what is the net effect (excitatory or inhibitory) on the nearest bipolar cell that is directly connected to that receptor? What is the effect on bipolar cells to the sides? What causes that effect?

15. Examine Figure 5.17. You should see grayish diamonds at the crossroads among the black squares. Explain why.

ANSWERS

13. The receptor excites both the bipolar cells and the horizontal cell. The horizontal cell inhibits the same bipolar cell that was excited plus additional bipolar cells in the surround. **14.** It produces more excitation than inhibition for the nearest bipolar cell. The reason is that the receptor excites a horizontal cell, which inhibits all bipolar cells in the area. **15.** In the parts of your retina that look at the long white arms, each neuron is inhibited by white input on two of its sides (either above and below or left and right). In the crossroads, each neuron is inhibited by input on all four sides. Therefore, the response in the crossroads is decreased compared to that in the arms.

Further Processing

Each cell in the visual system of the brain has a **receptive field**, an area in visual space that excites or inhibits it. The receptive field of a rod or cone is simply the point in space from which light strikes the cell. Other visual cells derive their receptive fields from the connections they receive. This concept is important, so let's spend some time with it. Suppose you keep track of the events on one city block. We'll call that your receptive field. Someone else keeps track of events on the next block, another person on the block after that, and so on. Now suppose that everyone responsible for a block on your street

Figure 5.17 An illustration of lateral inhibition
Do you see dark diamonds at the "crossroads"?

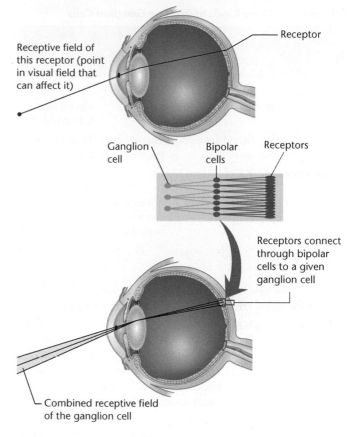

Figure 5.18 Receptive fields
The receptive field of any neuron in the visual system is the area of the visual field that excites or inhibits it. Receptors have tiny receptive fields and later cells have progressively larger receptive fields.

reports to a supervisor. That supervisor's receptive field is the whole street, because it includes reports from each block on the street. The supervisors for several streets report to the neighborhood manager, whose receptive field is the whole neighborhood. The neighborhood manager reports to a district chief, and so on.

The same idea applies to vision and other sensations. A rod or cone has a tiny receptive field in space to which it is sensitive. One or more receptors connect to a bipolar cell, with a receptive field that is the sum of the receptive fields of all those rods or cones connected to it (including both excitatory and inhibitory connections). Several bipolar cells report to a ganglion cell, which therefore has a still larger receptive field, as shown in Figure 5.18. The receptive fields of several ganglion cells converge to form the receptive field at the next level, and so on.

To find a cell's receptive field, an investigator records from the cell while shining light in various locations. If light from a particular spot excites the neuron, then that location is part of the neuron's excitatory receptive field. If it inhibits activity, the location is in the inhibitory receptive field.

A ganglion cell has a receptive field consisting of a circular center and an antagonistic doughnut-shaped surround. That is, the receptive field might be excited by light in the center and inhibited by light in the surround, or the opposite.

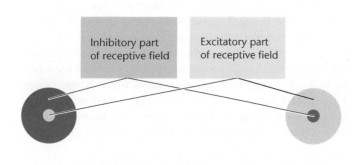

Inhibitory part of receptive field

Excitatory part of receptive field

Primate ganglion cells fall into three categories: parvocellular, magnocellular, and koniocellular (Nassi & Callaway, 2009). The **parvocellular neurons**, with small cell bodies and small receptive fields, are mostly in or near the fovea. (Parvocellular means "small celled," from the Latin root *parv*, meaning "small.") The **magnocellular neurons**, with larger cell bodies and receptive fields, are distributed evenly throughout the retina. (Magnocellular means "large celled," from the Latin root *magn*, meaning "large." The same root appears in *magnify*.) The **koniocellular neurons** have small cell bodies, similar to the parvocellular neurons, but they occur throughout the retina. (Koniocellular means "dust celled," from the Greek root meaning "dust." They got this name because of their granular appearance.)

The parvocellular neurons, with their small receptive fields, are well suited to detect visual details. They also respond to color, each neuron being excited by some wavelengths and inhibited by others. The high sensitivity to detail and color relates to the fact that parvocellular cells are located mostly in and near the fovea, which has many cones. The magnocellular neurons, with larger receptive fields, respond strongly to movement and large overall patterns, but they do not respond to color or fine details. Magnocellular neurons are found throughout the retina, including the periphery. Koniocellular

Table 5.2 | **Three Kinds of Primate Ganglion Cells**

	Parvocellular neurons	Magno-cellular neurons	Koniocellular neurons
Cell bodies	Small	Large	Small
Receptive fields	Small	Large	Mostly small, but variable
Retinal location	In and near fovea	Throughout the retina	Throughout the retina
Color sensitive?	Yes	No	Some are
Respond to	Detailed shape	Movement and broad outlines of shape	Varied

neurons have several functions, and their axons terminate in several locations (Hendry & Reid, 2000). The existence of so many kinds of ganglion cells implies that the visual system analyzes information in many ways from the start. Table 5.2 summarizes the three kinds of primate ganglion cells.

Axons from the ganglion cells form the optic nerve, which proceeds to the optic chiasm, where half of the axons (in humans) cross to the opposite hemisphere. Most of the axons go to the lateral geniculate nucleus of the thalamus. Cells of the lateral geniculate have receptive fields that resemble those of the ganglion cells—an excitatory or inhibitory central portion and a surrounding ring with the opposite effect. After the information reaches the cerebral cortex, the receptive fields become more complicated.

✓ STOP & CHECK

16. As we progress from bipolar cells to ganglion cells to later cells in the visual system, are receptive fields ordinarily larger, smaller, or the same size? Why?

17. What are the differences between the parvocellular and magnocellular systems?

ANSWERS

16. They become larger because each cell's receptive field is made by inputs converging at an earlier level. 17. Neurons of the parvocellular system have small cell bodies with small receptive fields, are located mostly in and near the fovea, and are specialized for detailed color vision. Neurons of the magnocellular system have large cell bodies with large receptive fields, are located in all parts of the retina, and are specialized for perception of large patterns and movement.

The Primary Visual Cortex

Information from the lateral geniculate nucleus of the thalamus goes to the **primary visual cortex** in the occipital cortex, also known as **area V1** or the *striate cortex* because of its striped appearance. If you close your eyes and imagine seeing

something, activity increases in area V1 in a pattern similar to what happens when you actually see that object (Kosslyn & Thompson, 2003; Stokes, Thompson, Cusack, & Duncan, 2009). If you see an optical illusion, the activity in area V1 corresponds to what you think you see, not what the object really is (Sperandie, Chouinard, & Goodale, 2012). Although we do not know the exact role of area V1 in consciousness, V1 is apparently necessary for it. People with damage to area V1 report no conscious vision, no visual imagery, and no visual images in their dreams (Hurovitz, Dunn, Domhoff, & Fiss, 1999). In contrast, adults who lose vision because of eye damage continue to have visual imagery and visual dreams.

Some people with damage to area V1 show a surprising phenomenon called **blindsight**, the ability to respond in limited ways to visual information without perceiving it consciously. Within the damaged part of their visual field, they are unaware of visual input, unable even to distinguish between bright sunshine and utter darkness. Nevertheless, they might be able to point accurately to something in the area where they cannot see, or move their eyes toward it, while insisting that they are "just guessing" (Bridgeman & Staggs, 1982; Weiskrantz, Warrington, Sanders, & Marshall, 1974). Some blindsight patients can reach for an object they cannot consciously see, avoiding obstacles in the way (Striemer, Chapman, & Goodale, 2009). Some can identify an object's color, direction of movement, or approximate shape, also insisting that they are just guessing (Radoeva, Prasad, Brainard, & Aguirre, 2008). Some can identify or copy the emotional expression of a face that they insist they do not see (Gonzalez Andino, de Peralta Menendez, Khateb, Landis, & Pegna, 2009; Tamietto et al., 2009). With practice, blindsight can improve (Das, Tadin, & Huxlin, 2014).

The research supports two explanations for blindsight: First, in some cases, small islands of healthy tissue remain within an otherwise damaged visual cortex, not large enough to provide conscious perception but enough to support limited visual functions (Fendrich, Wessinger, & Gazzaniga, 1992; Radoeva et al., 2008). Second, the thalamus sends visual input to several other brain areas, including parts of the temporal cortex (Schmid et al., 2013). In one study, every patient with blindsight had intact connections from the thalamus to the temporal cortex, whereas blindsight was absent for people without those connections (Ajina, Pestilli, Rokem, Kennard, & Bridge, 2015). In any case, the conclusion remains that conscious visual perception requires activity in area V1.

Even if your brain is intact, you can experience something like blindsight under certain circumstances. Researchers set up an apparatus so that people saw a face or a tool for three-tenths of a second in just one eye, while the other eye was viewing a display that changed 10 times a second. In this procedure, known as *continuous flash suppression*, a viewer is conscious of the rapidly changing stimuli and not the steady picture. However, even though people insisted they did not see a face or tool, when they were asked to guess where it was (upper left, upper right, lower left, or lower right), they were correct almost half the time, as opposed to the one-fourth we could expect by chance (Hesselmann, Hebart, & Malach, 2011).

✅ **STOP & CHECK** ▬▬▬▬▬▬▬

18. If you were in a darkened room and researchers wanted to "read your mind" just enough to know whether you were having visual fantasies, what could they do?

19. What is an example of an unconscious response to visual information?

ANSWERS

18. Researchers could use fMRI, EEG, or other recording methods to see whether activity increased in your primary visual cortex. 19. In blindsight, someone can point toward an object or move the eyes toward the object, despite insisting that he or she sees nothing.

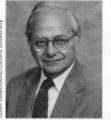
David Hubel (1926–2013)

Brain science is difficult and tricky, for some reason; consequently one should not believe a result (one's own or anyone else's) until it is proven backwards and forwards or fits into a framework so highly evolved and systematic that it couldn't be wrong. *(Hubel, personal communication)*

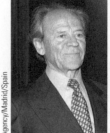
Torsten Wiesel (b. 1924)

Neural connections can be modulated by environmental influences during a critical period of postnatal development.... Such sensitivity of the nervous system to the effects of experience may represent the fundamental mechanism by which the organism adapts to its environment during the period of growth and development. *(Wiesel, 1982, p. 591)*

Simple and Complex Receptive Fields

In the 1950s, David Hubel and Torsten Wiesel (1959) inserted thin electrodes to record activity from cells in cats' and monkeys' occipital cortex while they shined light patterns on the retina. At first, they presented dots of light, using a slide projector and a screen, but they found little response by cortical cells. They wondered why cells were so unresponsive, when they knew the occipital cortex was essential for vision. Then they noticed a big response while they were moving a slide into place. They quickly realized that the cell was responding to the edge of the slide. It had a bar-shaped receptive field, rather than a circular receptive field like cells in the retina and lateral geniculate (Hubel & Wiesel, 1998). Their research, for which they received a Nobel Prize, has often been called "the research that launched a thousand microelectrodes" because it inspired so much further research. By now, it has probably launched a million microelectrodes.

Hubel and Wiesel distinguished several types of cells in the visual cortex. Figure 5.19 illustrates the receptive field of a **simple cell**. A simple cell has a receptive field with fixed excitatory and inhibitory zones. The more light shines in the excitatory zone, the more the cell responds. The more light shines in the inhibitory zone, the less the cell responds. In Figure 5.19, the receptive field is a vertical bar. Tilting the bar slightly decreases the cell's response because light then strikes inhibitory regions as well. Moving the bar left, right, up, or down also reduces the response. Most simple cells have bar-shaped or edge-shaped receptive fields. More of them respond to horizontal or vertical orientations than to diagonals. That disparity makes sense, considering the importance of horizontal

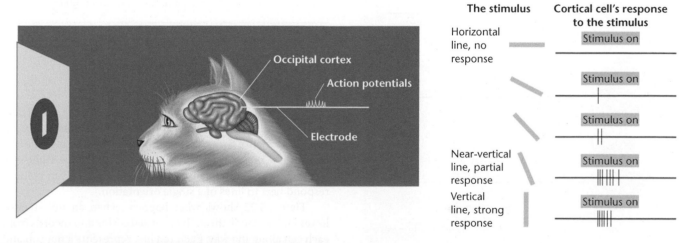

Figure 5.19 Responses of a cat's simple cell to a bar of light
This cell responds best to a vertical line in a particular location. Other simple cells respond to lines at other orientations.
(Source: Right, from D. H. Hubel and T. N. Wiesel, "Receptive fields of single neurons in the cat's striate cortex," Journal of Physiology, 148, 1959, 574–591. Copyright © 1959 Cambridge University Press. Reprinted by permission.)

and vertical objects in our world (Coppola, Purves, McCoy, & Purves, 1998).

Unlike simple cells, **complex cells**, located in areas V1 and V2, do not respond to the exact location of a stimulus. A complex cell responds to a pattern of light in a particular orientation (e.g., a vertical bar) anywhere within its large receptive field (see Figure 5.20). Most complex cells respond most strongly to a stimulus moving in a particular direction—for example, a vertical bar moving horizontally. The best way to classify a cell as simple or complex is to present the stimulus in several locations. A cell that responds to a stimulus in only one location is a simple cell. One that responds equally throughout a large area is a complex cell.

End-stopped, or **hypercomplex**, **cells** resemble complex cells with one exception: An end-stopped cell has a strong inhibitory area at one end of its bar-shaped receptive field. The cell responds to a bar-shaped pattern of light anywhere in its broad receptive field, provided the bar does not extend beyond a certain point (see Figure 5.21). Table 5.3 summarizes the properties of simple, complex, and end-stopped cells.

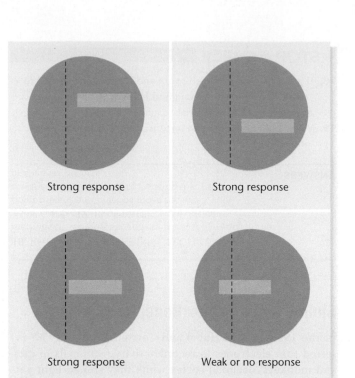

Strong response   Strong response

Strong response   Weak or no response

Figure 5.21 The receptive field of an end-stopped cell
The cell responds to a bar in a particular orientation (in this case horizontal) anywhere in its receptive field, provided the bar does not extend into a strongly inhibitory area.

✓ **STOP & CHECK**

20. How could a researcher determine whether a given neuron in the visual cortex is simple or complex?

ANSWER

20. First identify a stimulus, such as a horizontal line, that stimulates the cell. Then present the stimulus in several locations. If the cell responds strongly in only one location, it is a simple cell. If it responds in several locations, it is a complex cell.

The Columnar Organization of the Visual Cortex

Cells with similar properties group together in the visual cortex in columns perpendicular to the surface (Hubel & Wiesel, 1977) (see Figure 5.22). For example, cells within a given column might respond to only the left eye, only the right eye, or both eyes about equally. Also, cells within a given column respond best to lines of a single orientation.

Figure 5.22 shows what happens when an investigator lowers an electrode through the visual cortex and records from each cell along the way. Each red line represents a neuron and shows the angle of orientation of its receptive field. In electrode path A, the first series of cells are all in one column and show the same orientation preferences. However, after passing through the white matter, the end of path A invades columns

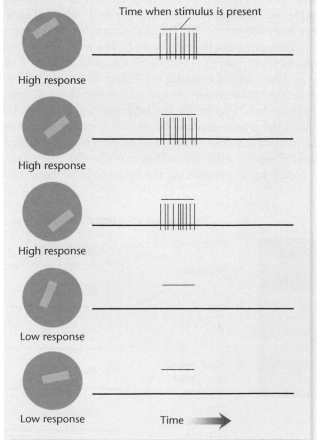

Time when stimulus is present

High response

High response

High response

Low response

Low response

Time →

Figure 5.20 The receptive field of a complex cell
Like a simple cell, its response depends on a bar of light's angle of orientation. However, a complex cell responds the same for a bar in any location within a large receptive field.

Table 5.3 | Cells in the Primary Visual Cortex

	Simple cells	Complex cells	End-stopped cells
Location	V1	V1 and V2	V1 and V2
Binocular input?	Yes	Yes	Yes
Size of receptive field	Smallest	Medium	Largest
Shape of receptive field	Bar- or edge-shaped, with fixed excitatory and inhibitory zones	Bar- or edge-shaped, but responding equally throughout a large receptive field	Same as complex cell, but with a strong inhibitory zone at one end

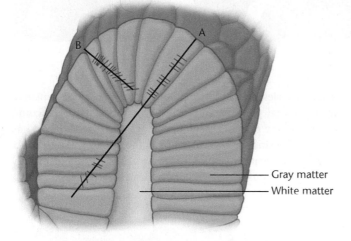

Figure 5.22 Columns of neurons in the visual cortex
When an electrode passes perpendicular to the surface of the cortex (first part of line A), it encounters a sequence of neurons responsive to the same orientation of a stimulus. (The colored lines show the preferred stimulus orientation for each cell.) When an electrode passes across columns (B, or second part of A), it encounters neurons responsive to different orientations. Column borders are drawn here to illustrate the point; no such borders are visible in the real cortex.
(Source: Hubel, 1963)

with different preferred orientations. Electrode path B, which is not perpendicular to the surface of the cortex, crosses through columns and encounters cells with different properties. In short, the cells within a given column process similar information. The existence of columns indicates that the various layers of the cerebral cortex communicate richly with one another, instead of being independent, as researchers at one time thought.

✓ **STOP & CHECK**

21. What do cells within a column of the visual cortex have in common?

ANSWER

21. They respond best to lines in the same orientation. Also, they are similar in their preference for one eye or the other, or both equally.

Are Visual Cortex Cells Feature Detectors?

Given that neurons in area V1 respond strongly to bar- or edge-shaped patterns, we might suppose that the activity of such a cell represents the perception of a bar, line, or edge. That is, such cells might be **feature detectors**—neurons whose responses indicate the presence of a particular feature.

Supporting the idea of feature detectors is the fact that prolonged exposure to a given visual feature decreases sensitivity to that feature, as if it fatigued the relevant detectors. For example, if you stare at a waterfall for a minute or more and then look to the side, the rocks and trees next to the waterfall appear to flow upward. This *waterfall illusion* suggests that you have fatigued the neurons that detect downward motion, leaving unopposed the detectors for the opposite motion.

Long ago, Gestalt psychologists cast doubt on the idea that our vision depends entirely on feature detectors. For example, if you examine Figure 5.23, you might at first see nothing. Then suddenly you exclaim, "Oh, that's a face! [pause] And another face!" Simply looking at these displays (known as Mooney faces) should excite whatever feature detectors your brain has, but seeing them as faces requires interpretation and reorganization of the material. When you start seeing them as faces, the pattern of responses in your visual cortex suddenly changes (Hsieh, Vul, & Kanwisher, 2010). That result implies "top-down" processes in which other brain areas interpret the visual stimulus and send messages back to reorganize the activity in the primary visual cortex. Similarly, when you see an optical illusion, it is due to feedback from other cortical areas to change responses in the primary visual cortex (Wokke, Vandenbroucke, Scholte, & Lamme, 2013). Your brain's response to any visual stimulus depends on your expectations as well as on the stimulus itself (Roth et al., 2016). In other words, excitation of feature detectors is not sufficient to explain all of vision.

Furthermore, later researchers found that a cortical cell that responds well to a single bar or line

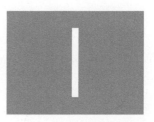

Figure 5.23 Mooney faces
At first glance, you may see only meaningless blobs. With some time and effort you may get an "Aha" experience when you suddenly see them as faces.

responds even more strongly to a sine wave grating of bars or lines:

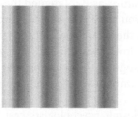

Many cortical neurons respond best to a particular spatial frequency and hardly at all to other frequencies (DeValois, Albrecht, & Thorell, 1982). Most visual researchers therefore believe that neurons in area V1 detect spatial frequencies rather than bars or edges. If so, it is a feature detector for a feature that we don't perceive consciously. How do we translate a series of spatial frequencies into perception? From a mathematical standpoint, sine wave frequencies are easy to work with. A branch of mathematics called Fourier analysis demonstrates that a combination of sine waves can produce an unlimited variety of other patterns. For example, the graph at the top of the following display is the sum of the five sine waves below it:

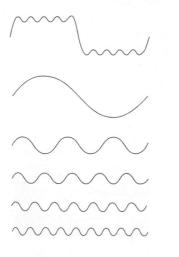

Thus, a series of spatial frequency detectors, some sensitive to horizontal patterns and others to vertical patterns, could represent any possible display. Still, we perceive the world as objects, not sine waves. Output from the primary visual cortex leads to further processing in other brain areas, but exactly how a conscious visual perception emerges remains a fascinating mystery.

✓ STOP & CHECK

22. What is a feature detector?

ANSWER

22. It is a neuron that detects the presence of a particular aspect of an object, such as a shape or a direction of movement.

Development of the Visual Cortex

How do cells in the visual cortex develop their properties? Suppose you had lived all your life in the dark. Then today, for the first time, you came out into the light and looked around. Would you understand anything?

Unless you were born blind, you did have this experience—on the day you were born! At first, presumably you had no idea what you were seeing. Within months, however, you began to recognize faces and crawl toward your favorite toys. How did you learn to make sense of what you saw?

In a newborn mammal, many of the normal properties of the visual system develop normally at first, before birth (Lein & Shatz, 2001; Shatz, 1996). Waves of spontaneous activity sweep over the developing retina, synchronizing the activity of neighboring receptors and enabling appropriate combinations of receptors to establish connections with cells in the brain (Ackman, Burbridge, & Crair, 2012; Zhang, Ackman, Xu, & Crair, 2012). Still, when an animal first opens its eyes, cells of the visual system show patterns of activity that are little more than random noise. Watching a visual stimulus quickly reduces the noise (Smith et al., 2015).

What about connections beyond the primary visual cortex? A study of people who were born without eyes found that the connections from the primary visual cortex to its main targets were more or less normal (Bock et al., 2015). Evidently, certain axon paths develop automatically, without any need for guidance by experience. Nevertheless, visual experience after birth modifies and fine-tunes many of the connections.

Deprived Experience in One Eye

What would happen if a young animal could see with one eye but not the other? When a kitten opens its eyes at about age 9 days, each neuron responds to areas in the two retinas that focus on approximately the same point in space—a process necessary for binocular vision. However, innate mechanisms cannot make the connections exactly right because the exact distance between the eyes varies from one kitten to another, and the distance changes over age. Therefore, experience is necessary for fine-tuning.

If an experimenter sutures one eyelid shut for a kitten's first 4 to 6 weeks of life, synapses in the visual cortex gradually become unresponsive to input from the deprived eye (Rittenhouse, Shouval, Paradiso, & Bear, 1999). After the deprived eye is opened, the kitten does not respond to it. A similar period of deprivation in older animals weakens the response to the deprived eye, but not as strongly as it does in young ones (Wiesel, 1982; Wiesel & Hubel, 1963). After an eye deprived of vision in adults is reopened, cells gradually return to their previous levels of responsiveness (Rose, Jaepel, Hübener, & Bonhoeffer, 2016).

Deprived Experience in Both Eyes

If *both* eyes stayed shut for the first few weeks, what would you expect? You might guess that the kitten would become insensitive to both eyes, but it does not. When just one eye is open, the synapses from the open eye inhibit the synapses from the closed eye (Maffei, Nataraj, Nelson, & Turrigiano, 2006). If neither eye is active, no axon outcompetes any other. For at least 3 weeks, the kitten's cortex remains responsive to visual input, although most cells become responsive to just one eye or the other and not both (Wiesel, 1982). If the eyes remain shut still longer, the cortical responses start to become sluggish and lose their well-defined receptive fields (Crair, Gillespie, & Stryker, 1998). Eventually, the visual cortex starts responding to auditory and touch stimuli instead.

For each aspect of visual experience, researchers identify a **sensitive period**, when experiences have a particularly strong and enduring influence (Lewis & Maurer, 2005; Tagawa, Kanold, Majdan, & Shatz, 2005). The sensitive period depends on inhibitory neurons. In fact, a study with mice found that transplanting inhibitory neurons from an infant into an older mouse could induce a new period of heightened susceptibility to experience (Southwell, Froemke, Alvarez-Buylla, Stryker, & Gandhi, 2010). However, even

long after the sensitive period, a prolonged experience—such as a full week without visual stimulation to one eye—produces a smaller but measurable effect on the visual cortex (Sato & Stryker, 2008). Cortical plasticity is greatest in early life, but it never ends.

STOP & CHECK

23. What is the effect of closing one eye early in life? What is the effect of closing both eyes?

ANSWER

23. If one eye is closed during early development, the cortex becomes unresponsive to it. If both eyes are closed, cortical cells remain somewhat responsive for several weeks and then gradually become sluggish and unselective in their responses.

Uncorrelated Stimulation in the Two Eyes

Most neurons in the human visual cortex respond to both eyes—specifically, to approximately corresponding areas of both eyes. By comparing the inputs from the two eyes, you achieve stereoscopic depth perception.

Stereoscopic depth perception requires the brain to detect **retinal disparity**, the discrepancy between what the left and right eyes see. Experience fine-tunes binocular vision, and abnormal experience disrupts it. Imagine a kitten with weak or damaged eye muscles so that its eyes do not point in the same direction. Both eyes are active, but no cortical neuron consistently receives messages from one eye that match messages from the other eye. Each neuron in the visual cortex becomes responsive to one eye or the other, and few neurons respond to both (Blake & Hirsch, 1975; Hubel & Wiesel, 1965). The behavioral result is poor depth perception.

A similar phenomenon occurs in humans. Certain children are born with **strabismus** (or strabismic amblyopia), also known as "lazy eye," a condition in which the eyes do not point in the same direction. Generally, these children attend to one eye and not the other. The usual treatment is to put a patch over the active eye, forcing attention to the other one. That procedure works to some extent, especially if it begins early (Lewis & Maurer, 2005), but many children refuse to wear an eye patch for as long as they need to. In any case, the child is not learning to use both eyes at the same time.

A promising therapy for lazy eye is to ask a child to play three-dimensional action video games that require attention to both eyes. Good performance requires increasing attention to exactly the kind of input we want to enhance. This procedure appears to improve the use of both eyes better than patching does, although neither procedure has much effect on stereoscopic depth perception (S. Li et al., 2014).

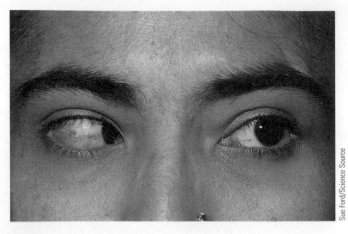

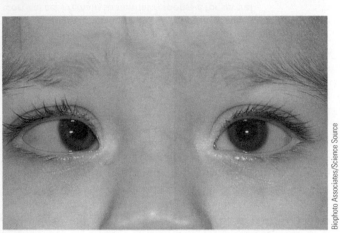

Two examples of lazy eye.

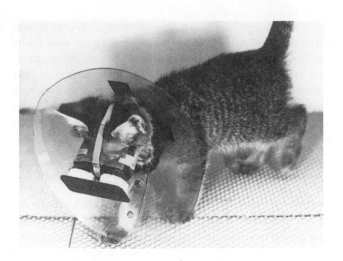

Figure 5.24 **Procedure for restricting a kitten's visual experience**
For a few hours a day, the kitten wears goggles that show just one stimulus, such as horizontal stripes or diagonal stripes. For the rest of the day, the kitten stays with its mother in a dark room without the mask.
(*Source: Photo courtesy of Helmut V. B. Hirsch*)

✔ **STOP & CHECK**

24. What early experience would cause a kitten or human child to lose stereoscopic depth perception?

ANSWER

24. If the eye muscles cannot keep both eyes focused in the same direction, the developing brain loses the ability for any neuron in the visual cortex to respond to input from both eyes. Instead, each neuron responds to one eye or the other. Stereoscopic depth perception requires cells that compare the input from the two eyes.

Early Exposure to a Limited Array of Patterns

If a kitten spends its entire early sensitive period wearing goggles with horizontal lines painted on them (see Figure 5.24), nearly all its visual cortex cells become responsive only to horizontal lines (Stryker & Sherk, 1975; Stryker, Sherk, Leventhal, & Hirsch, 1978). Even after months of later normal experience, the cat does not respond to vertical lines (Mitchell, 1980).

What happens if human infants are exposed mainly to vertical or horizontal lines instead of both equally? They become more sensitive to the kind of line they have seen. You might wonder how such a bizarre thing could happen. No parents would let an experimenter subject their child to such a procedure, and it never happens in nature. Right?

Wrong. In fact, it probably happened to you! About 70 percent of all infants have **astigmatism**, a blurring of vision for lines in one direction (e.g., horizontal, vertical, or one of the diagonals), caused by an asymmetric curvature of the eyes. Normal growth reduces the prevalence of astigmatism to about 10 percent in 4-year-old children.

You can informally test yourself for astigmatism with Figure 5.25. Do the lines in one direction look darker than

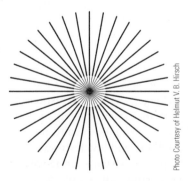

Figure 5.25 **An informal test for astigmatism**
Do the lines in one direction look darker or sharper than the other lines do? If so, notice what happens when you rotate the page. If you wear corrective lenses, try this demonstration both with and without your lenses.

another? If so, rotate the page to demonstrate that the darkness is in you, not in the lines themselves. The appearance of the lines depends on their position. If you wear corrective lenses, try this demonstration with and without them. If you see a difference in the lines only without your lenses, then the lenses have corrected your astigmatism.

Impaired Infant Vision and Long-Term Consequences

At the start of this section, we raised the question of what you would see if you lived all your life in the dark and then suddenly could see. Newborn infants have that experience, and we assume they have no idea what they are seeing. We have to assume, because we cannot ask newborns what they see. However, in some countries, a newborn with dense cataracts (cloudy spots on the lenses that prevent perception of anything other than bright versus dark) may have to wait years for surgery to enable vision. When the cataracts are finally removed, researchers can ask the children about their experience.

At first, these children have only a limited idea of what they are seeing. In one study, children looked at a picture of a toy building block, and another picture with two blocks. The task was to point to the block in the second picture that matched the first. Children did well on this task, indicating that they could see. However, when the task was to feel a building block and point to which of two choices was the picture of that block, performance was only a little better than chance. They could see the pictures, but they didn't understand them. A week later, without any special training, they did much better on this task (Held et al., 2011). Within weeks they could start recognizing faces. With much practice, they began to develop hand–eye coordination. Seeing well enough to ride a bicycle took a year and a half (Chatterjee, 2015; Gandhi, Ganesh, & Sinha, 2014). However, some aspects of vision never fully recovered. Their acuity (ability to see detail) remained poor, and their motion perception and depth perception never reached normal levels (Dormal, Lepore, & Collignon, 2012; Ellemberg, Lewis, Maurer, Brar, & Brent, 2002).

One man had normal vision in early childhood until age 3½, when a chemical explosion destroyed one eye and damaged the cornea of his other eye so badly that he could see nothing more than light versus dark. By adulthood, he had no visual memories and no visual imagery. At age 43, a corneal transplant enabled him to recover vision. Immediately he could see colors and he could soon identify simple shapes. Eventually he learned to recognize common household objects, but unlike most people who identify objects immediately, he had to think about it more carefully (Fine et al., 2003). Even 10 years later, he could not identify whether a face was male or female, happy or sad (Huber et al., 2015).

Various other aspects of vision remained impaired. For example, when viewing something like Figure 5.26, he reported seeing three objects, instead of a partly transparent object overlapping a second one (Fine et al., 2013). As a blind man, he had learned to ski by following directions and memorizing hills. When he tried skiing with his eyes open, the result was frightening. By two years later he was willing to open his eyes while skiing, and he could use vision to estimate the steepness of a hill. However, on the most difficult hills, he insisted on closing his eyes! Evidently, the visual understanding that most of us take for granted depends on practice early in life.

STOP & CHECK

25. What causes astigmatism?
26. If an infant is born with dense cataracts on both eyes and they are surgically removed years later, how well does the child see at first?

ANSWERS

25. Astigmatism results when the eyeball is not quite spherical. As a result, the person sees one direction of lines more clearly than the other. 26. The child sees well enough to identify whether two objects are the same or different, but the child doesn't understand what the visual information means. In particular, the child cannot answer which visual display matches something the child touches. However, understanding of vision improves with practice.

Figure 5.26 How many squares?
Most people immediately see two squares, one overlapping the other. A man who lost vision from age 3½ until 43 sees this display as three objects.

Module 5.2 | In Closing

Understanding Vision by Understanding the Wiring Diagram

Your eyes are bombarded with a complex pattern of light emanating from every source in front of you. Out of all this, your brain needs to extract the most useful information. The nervous system from the start identifies the borders between one object and another through lateral inhibition. It identifies lines and their locations by simple and complex cells in the primary visual cortex. Researchers have gone a long way toward mapping out the excitatory and inhibitory connections that make these cells possible. The visual experiences you have at any moment are the result of an awe-inspiring complexity of connections and interactions among a huge number of neurons. Understanding what you see is also the product of years of experience.

Summary

1. The optic nerves of the two eyes join at the optic chiasm, where half of the axons from each eye cross to the opposite side of the brain. Most of the axons then travel to the lateral geniculate nucleus of the thalamus, which communicates with the visual cortex. **162**

2. Lateral inhibition is a mechanism by which stimulation in any area of the retina suppresses the responses in neighboring areas, thereby enhancing the contrast at light–dark borders. **163**

3. Lateral inhibition in the vertebrate retina occurs because receptors stimulate bipolar cells and also stimulate the much wider horizontal cells, which inhibit both the stimulated bipolar cells and those to the sides. **163**

4. Each neuron in the visual system has a receptive field, an area of the visual field to which it is connected. Light in the receptive field excites or inhibits a neuron depending on the light's location, wavelength, and movement. **164**

5. The mammalian vertebrate visual system has a partial division of labor. In general, the parvocellular system is specialized for perception of color and fine details; the magnocellular system is specialized for perception of depth, movement, and overall patterns. **165**

6. After damage to area V1, people report no vision, even in dreams. However, some kinds of response to light (blindsight) can occur after damage to V1 despite the lack of conscious perception. **166**

7. Within the primary visual cortex, neuroscientists distinguish simple cells with fixed excitatory and inhibitory fields, and complex cells that respond to a light pattern of a particular shape regardless of its exact location. **167**

8. Neurons within a column of the primary visual cortex have similar properties, such as responding to lines in the same orientation. **168**

9. Understanding what you see requires much more than just adding up points and lines. Vision is an active process based partly on expectations. **169**

10. During infancy, the cells of the visual cortex have nearly normal properties. However, experience is necessary to maintain and fine-tune vision. Abnormal visual experience can change the properties of visual cells, especially if the experience occurs early in life. **171**

11. Cortical neurons become unresponsive to axons from an inactive eye because of competition with the active eye. If both eyes are closed, each cortical cell remains somewhat responsive to axons from one eye or the other, although that response becomes sluggish and unselective as the weeks of deprivation continue. **171**

12. To develop good stereoscopic depth perception, a kitten or human child must have experience seeing the same object with corresponding portions of the two eyes early in life. Otherwise, each neuron in the visual cortex becomes responsive to input from just one eye. **171**

13. If a kitten sees only horizontal or vertical lines during its sensitive period, most of the neurons in its visual cortex become responsive to such lines only. For the same reason, a child with astigmatism may have decreased responsiveness to one kind of line or another. **172**

14. Some people have cataracts removed after years of cloudy vision. Vision, useless at first, improves with practice but remains imperfect in several ways. **173**

Key Terms

Terms are defined in the module on the page number indicated. They're also presented in alphabetical order with definitions in the book's Subject Index/Glossary, which begins on page 589. Interactive flash cards, audio reviews, and crossword puzzles are among the online resources available to help you learn these terms and the concepts they represent.

astigmatism **172**
blindsight **166**
complex cells **168**

end-stopped (or hypercomplex)
cells **168**
feature detectors **169**

horizontal cells **162**
koniocellular neurons **165**
lateral geniculate nucleus **162**

Thought Questions

1. After a receptor cell is stimulated, the bipolar cell receiving input from it shows an immediate strong response. A fraction of a second later, the bipolar's response decreases, even though the stimulation from the receptor cell remains constant. How can you account for that decrease? (Hint: What does the horizontal cell do?)

2. A rabbit's eyes are on the sides of its head instead of in front. Would you expect rabbits to have many cells with binocular receptive fields—that is, cells that respond to both eyes? Why or why not?

Module 5.2 | End of Module Quiz

1. What do horizontal cells in the retina do?
   - A. They inhibit neighboring receptors.
   - B. They inhibit bipolar cells.
   - C. They inhibit ganglion cells.
   - D. They stimulate ganglion cells.

2. In humans, what crosses to the contralateral hemisphere at the optic chiasm?
   - A. Half of each optic nerve, the part representing the nasal half of the retina
   - B. Half of each optic nerve, the part representing the temporal half of the retina
   - C. Half of each optic nerve, originating from random parts of the retina
   - D. All of each optic nerve

3. What is the function of lateral inhibition in the retina?
   - A. To sharpen borders
   - B. To enhance colors
   - C. To recognize objects
   - D. To increase attention

4. Suppose light strikes the retina in a circle, surrounded by dark. Which bipolar cells will show the greatest response, and which will show the least?
   - A. Bipolars connected to receptors in the center of the circle respond the most. Those connected to receptors farthest from the circle respond the least.
   - B. Bipolars connected to the receptors just outside the circumference of the circle respond most. Those connected to receptors just inside the circumference respond least.
   - C. Bipolars connected to the receptors just inside the circumference of the circle respond most. Those connected to receptors just outside the circumference respond least.
   - D. All bipolars within the circle respond equally, and those outside the circle do not respond at all.

5. What is the shape of a receptive field of a ganglion cell?
   - A. Either a bar or an edge, in a fixed position
   - B. Either a bar or an edge, anywhere within a large area of the retina
   - C. Either a bar or an edge, with a strong inhibitory field at one end
   - D. A circle, with a surround that responds in the opposite way

6. What is the shape of a receptive field of a simple cell in the primary visual cortex?
   - A. Either a bar or an edge, in a fixed position
   - B. Either a bar or an edge, anywhere within a large area of the retina
   - C. Either a bar or an edge, with a strong inhibitory field at one end
   - D. A circle, with a surround that responds in the opposite way

7. In contrast to parvocellular neurons, magnocellular neurons are more sensitive to ____.
   - A. color
   - B. small details
   - C. movement
   - D. the fovea

8. If you were in a darkened room and researchers wanted to know whether you were having visual fantasies (without asking you), they could measure activity in which brain area?

A. The retina

B. The lateral geniculate nucleus of the thalamus

C. The primary visual cortex

D. The parietal cortex

9. In most cases, blindsight apparently depends on what connection?

A. From the thalamus to the temporal cortex

B. From the occipital cortex to the temporal cortex

C. From the thalamus to the frontal cortex

D. From the occipital cortex to the frontal cortex

10. What evidence suggests that certain types of feature detectors operate in the human visual cortex?

A. When you examine Mooney faces, at first you see only meaningless blobs, but with time and effort you start to perceive faces.

B. After you stare at a waterfall or other steadily moving display, you see stationary objects as moving in the opposite direction.

C. An electrode traveling through a section of the cortex may encounter one neuron after another with receptive fields in the same orientation.

D. Children who are deprived of input in one eye become attentive only to the other eye.

11. If a kitten has one eye shut for its first few weeks of life, its visual cortex becomes insensitive to that eye. Why?

A. The receptors die.

B. Any axon that is not used for that long becomes unable to respond.

C. Activity from the active eye inhibits synapses from the inactive eye.

D. The visual cortex becomes responsive to sounds instead of light.

12. What early experience, if any, is necessary to maintain binocular input to the neurons of the visual cortex?

A. Cortical cells will always maintain binocular responsiveness, regardless of their experience.

B. Cortical cells must receive some input to each eye every day.

C. Cortical cells must receive an equal amount of input from the two eyes.

D. Cortical cells must usually receive simultaneous input from the two eyes.

13. If someone is born with dense cataracts on both eyes, and the cataracts are removed years later, what happens?

A. The person remains permanently blind.

B. The person gradually recovers all aspects of vision.

C. The person gains some vision, but remains impaired on object recognition, motion vision, and depth perception.

D. The person gains almost all aspects of vision, but remains greatly impaired on color perception.

Answers: 1B, 2A, 3A, 4C, 5D, 6A, 7C, 8C, 9A, 10B, 11C, 12D, 13C.

Parallel Processing in the Visual Cortex

If you were working on an important project for some business or government, you might receive information on a "need-to-know" basis. For example, if you were told to carry a particular package, you would need to know how heavy it is and whether it is fragile, but you might not need to know anything else. Someone else who is keeping track of the finances would need to know how much the object costs and whether it needs insurance. A third person might open the package and check to make sure the color matched the specifications.

Similarly, different parts of the brain's visual system get information on a need-to-know basis. Cells that help your hand muscles reach out to an object need to know the size and location of the object, but they don't need to know about color. They need to know a little about shape, but not in great detail. Cells that help you recognize people's faces need to be extremely sensitive to details of shape, but they can pay less attention to location.

It is natural to assume that anyone who sees an object sees everything about it—the shape, color, location, and movement. However, one part of your brain sees its shape, another sees color, another detects location, and another perceives movement (Livingstone, 1988; Livingstone & Hubel, 1988; Zeki & Shipp, 1988). Consequently, after localized brain damage, it is possible to see certain aspects of an object and not others. Centuries ago, people found it difficult to imagine how someone could see an object without seeing what color it is. Even today, you might find it surprising to learn about people who see an object without seeing where it is, or see it without seeing whether it is moving.

The Ventral and Dorsal Paths

The primary visual cortex (V1) sends information to the **secondary visual cortex (area V2)**, which processes the information further and transmits it to additional areas, as shown in Figure 5.27. The connections in the visual cortex are reciprocal. For example, V1 sends information to V2, and V2 returns information to V1. From V2, the information branches out in several directions for specialized processing.

Researchers distinguish between the ventral stream and the dorsal stream. They call the **ventral stream** through the temporal cortex the perception pathway or the "what"

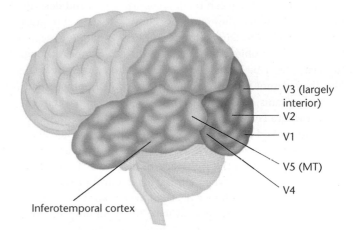

Figure 5.27 Approximate Locations of Some Major Visual Areas in Human Cortex
Information passes from V1 to V2 and from there to other areas. The other areas also receive some information directly from the thalamus.

pathway, because of its importance for identifying and recognizing objects. The **dorsal stream** through the parietal cortex is the action pathway or the "how" pathway, because of its importance for visually guided movements.

The distinction is based partly on animal studies, and partly on MRI and fMRI studies (Milner, 2012), but mostly on observations of a few patients with brain damage. A woman known as patient DF was exposed to carbon monoxide, causing damage mainly to the ventral stream—that is, the temporal cortex and its connections with the primary visual cortex (Bridge et al., 2013). She cannot name the objects she sees, cannot recognize faces, and cannot even distinguish a square from a rectangle. When she was shown a slot in the wall, she could not say whether it was horizontal or vertical. Nevertheless, when she was asked to put an envelope through the slot, she aimed it correctly at once. When asked to guess the size of an object she sees, she performs at chance levels. However, when asked to pick up the object, she reaches out correctly, adjusting her thumb and finger before touching the object (Whitwell, Milner, & Goodale, 2014). Several other patients with temporal lobe damage have similar problems. One man could not say where objects were in his room, but he could take a walk, accurately avoiding obstacles in his way. He could reach out to grab objects, and he could reach out to shake hands (Karnath, Rüter, Mandler, & Himmelbach, 2009). Another patient had such trouble recognizing objects by sight that she attached distinctive colored tapes to the important objects she needed to find in her house. However, she had no trouble reaching out to pick up any of the objects, once she had found them (Plant, James-Galton, & Wilkinson, 2015). In short, people with temporal lobe damage can use vision to guide their actions, but they cannot identify what the objects are.

People with damage to the dorsal stream (parietal cortex) have somewhat the opposite problem: They see objects but they don't integrate their vision well with their arm and leg movements. They can read, recognize faces, and describe objects in detail but they cannot accurately reach out to grasp an object. While walking, they can describe what they see, but they bump into objects, oblivious to their location. Although they can describe from memory what their furniture looks like, they cannot remember where it is located in their house (Kosslyn, Ganis, & Thompson, 2001). Often they seem uncertain where certain parts of their body are (Schenk, 2006). One patient had dorsal stream damage only in his left hemisphere. He showed low accuracy at aiming his right arm or leg toward an object on the right side of his body. However, his accuracy was normal when aiming his left arm or leg toward either side, or when aiming his right arm toward the left side (Cavina-Pratesi, Connolly, & Milner, 2013). So his problem is not with attention, and not exactly vision either. It is specifically a problem of using vision to control certain arm and leg movements.

Although the distinction between ventral and dorsal pathways is useful, we should not overstate it. Ordinarily you use both systems in coordination with each other (Farivar, 2009).

✅ STOP & CHECK ▰▰▰▰▰▰▰▰

27. Suppose someone can describe an object in detail but stumbles and fumbles when trying to walk toward it and pick it up. Which is probably damaged, the dorsal path or the ventral path?

ANSWER

27. The inability to guide movement based on vision implies damage to the dorsal path.

Detailed Analysis of Shape

In Module 5.2, we encountered simple and complex cells of the primary visual cortex (V1). As visual information goes from the simple cells to the complex cells and then to other brain areas, the receptive fields become larger and more specialized. In the secondary visual cortex (V2), just anterior to V1 in the occipital cortex, most cells are similar to V1 cells in responding to lines, edges, or sine wave gratings, except that V2 receptive fields are more elongated (Liu et al., 2016). Also,

some V2 cells respond best to corners, textures, or complex shapes (Freeman, Ziemba, Heeger, Simoncelli, & Movshon, 2013). Areas V2 and V3 (see Figure 5.27) have some cells highly responsive to color, and other cells highly responsive to the disparity between what the left and right eyes see—critical information for stereoscopic depth perception (Nasr, Polimeni, & Tootell, 2016). In later parts of the visual system, receptive properties become still more complex.

The Inferior Temporal Cortex

Cells in the **inferior temporal cortex** (see Figure 5.27) learn to recognize meaningful objects. A cell that responds to the sight of some object initially responds mainly when it sees that object from the same angle, but after a bit of experience it learns to respond almost equally to that object from other viewpoints. It is responding to the object, regardless of major changes in the pattern that reaches the retina (Murty & Arun, 2015). Similarly, in Figure 5.28, cells in a monkey's inferior temporal cortex that responded strongly to the original profile responded about the same way to its mirror image or contrast reversal, but not to a figure–ground reversal (Baylis & Driver, 2001). In terms of the actual pattern of light and dark, the figure–ground reversal is much like the original, but most people (and evidently monkeys also) see it as a white object on a black background, rather than a face.

Another study considered the phenomenon of object permanence. Children as young as age 3½ months show evidence of understanding that an object continues to exist after it goes

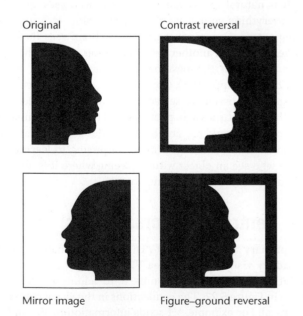

Original   Contrast reversal

Mirror image   Figure–ground reversal

Figure 5.28 Transformations of a drawing
In the inferior temporal cortex, cells that respond strongly to the original respond about the same to the contrast reversal and mirror image but not to the figure–ground reversal. Note that the figure–ground reversal resembles the original in terms of the pattern of light and darkness, but it is not perceived as the same object.
(Source: Based on Baylis & Driver, 2001)

behind an object that prevents a child from seeing it (Baillargeon, 1987). Studies of the inferotemporal cortex show a possible basis. A monkey saw an object, and then saw some other object move in front and occlude the first object. When the occluder moved away, either the original object reappeared, or a new object appeared in its place. Some cells in the inferotemporal cortex responded strongly whenever an original object reappeared, and some responded strongly whenever a new, "surprising" object appeared (Puneeth & Arun, 2016).

As we might expect, damage to the ventral pathway of the cortex leads to specialized deficits. **Visual agnosia** (meaning "visual lack of knowledge") is an inability to recognize objects despite otherwise satisfactory vision. It is a common result from damage in the temporal cortex. Someone might be able to point to visual objects and slowly describe them but fail to recognize what they are. For example, one patient, when shown a key, said, "I don't know what that is. Perhaps a file or a tool of some sort." When shown a stethoscope, he said that it was "a long cord with a round thing at the end." When he could not identify a smoker's pipe, the examiner told him what it was. He then replied, "Yes, I can see it now," and pointed out the stem and bowl of the pipe. Then the examiner asked, "Suppose I told you that the last object was not really a pipe?" The patient replied, "I would take your word for it. Perhaps it's not really a pipe" (Rubens & Benson, 1971).

Within the brain areas specialized for perceiving shape, are there further specializations for particular types of shapes? According to fMRI studies as people viewed pictures, most objects do not activate one brain area more than another. That is, the brain does not have a specialized area for seeing flowers, fish, birds, clothes, food, or rocks. However, three types of objects do produce specific responses. One part of the parahippocampal cortex (next to the hippocampus) responds strongly to pictures of places, and not so strongly to anything else. Part of the **fusiform gyrus** of the inferior temporal cortex, especially in the right hemisphere (see Figure 5.29), responds more

strongly to faces than to anything else. And an area close to this face area responds more strongly to bodies than to anything else (Downing, Chan, Peelen, Dodds, & Kanwisher, 2005; Kanwisher, 2010). The brain is amazingly adept at detecting biological motion—the kinds of motion produced by people and animals. If you attach glow-in-the-dark dots to someone's elbows, knees, hips, shoulders, and a few other places, then when that person moves in an otherwise dark room, you perceive a moving person, even though you are actually watching only a few spots of light. You can view a wonderful demonstration by doing an Internet search for Biomotion Lab and then clicking on Demos.

Recognizing Faces

Face recognition is an important skill for humans. For civilization to succeed, we have to know whom to trust and whom to distrust, and that distinction requires us to recognize people that we haven't seen in months or years. Someday you may attend a high school or college reunion and reunite with people you haven't seen in decades. You will recognize many of them, even though they have gained weight, become bald, or dyed their hair (Bruck, Cavanagh, & Ceci, 1991). Computer programmers who have tried to build machines to recognize faces have discovered the difficulty of this task that seems so easy for people.

Human newborns come into the world predisposed to pay more attention to faces than other stationary displays (see Figure 5.30). That tendency supports the idea of a built-in face recognition module. However, the infant's concept of face is not like an adult's. Experimenters recorded infants' times of gazing at one face or the other, as shown in Figure 5.31. Newborns showed a strong preference for a right-side-up face over an upside-down face, regardless of whether the face was realistic (left pair) or distorted (central pair). When confronted with two right-side-up faces (right pair), they showed no significant

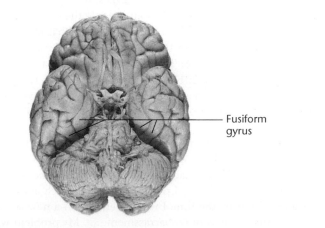

Figure 5.29 The fusiform gyrus
Many cells here are especially active during recognition of faces.
(Source: Courtesy of Dr. Dana Copeland)

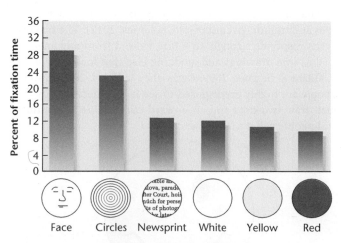

Figure 5.30 Amount of time infants spend looking at patterns
Even in the first 2 days after birth, infants look more at faces than at most other stimuli. *(Source: Based on Fantz, 1963)*

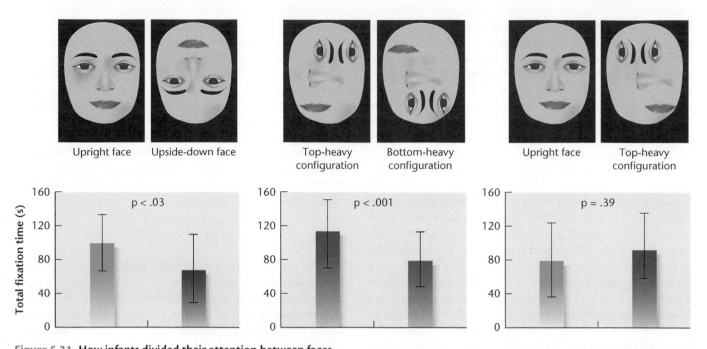

| Upright face | Upside-down face | Top-heavy configuration | Bottom-heavy configuration | Upright face | Top-heavy configuration |

Figure 5.31 How infants divided their attention between faces
A right-side-up face drew more attention than an upside-down one, regardless of whether the faces were realistic (left pair) or distorted (central pair). Infants divided their attention about equally between two right-side-up faces (right pair), even though one was realistic and the other was distorted. *(Source: From "Can a nonspecific bias toward top-heavy patterns explain newborns' face preference?" by V. M. Cassia, C. Turati, & F. Simion, 2004. Psychological Science, 15, 379–383.)*

preference between a realistic one and a distorted one (Cassia, Turati, & Simion, 2004). Evidently, a newborn's concept of face requires the eyes to be on top, but the face does not have to be realistic.

According to fMRI data, young children activate more of their brain than adults do, when trying to recognize a face (Haist, Adamo, Wazny, Lee, & Stiles, 2013). Their accuracy is also lower than that of adults. Through childhood and the early teenage years, connections strengthen between the fusiform gyrus (Figure 5.29), especially in the right hemisphere, and part of the inferior occipital cortex known as the occipital face area (Song, Zhu, Li, Wang, & Liu, 2015). The occipital face area responds strongly to parts of a face, such as the eyes and mouth (Arcurio, Gold, & James, 2012). The fusiform gyrus responds strongly to a face viewed from any angle, as well as line drawings and anything else that looks like a face (Caldara & Seghier, 2009; Kanwisher & Yovel, 2006). In fact, people are highly predisposed to see faces wherever possible. Just draw two dots and an upward curved line below them, and people call it a "smiley face."

In several cases, physicians electrically stimulated the fusiform gyrus during exploratory surgery. Varying with the intensity and duration of stimulation, the result was either a difficulty in perceiving faces (Chong et al., 2013) or a vivid distortion of faces. One patient exclaimed, "You just turned into somebody else. Your face metamorphosed" (Parvizi et al., 2012, p. 14918).

People vary considerably in their ability to recognize faces, and the reason is not just that some people don't care or don't pay attention. People with severe problems are said to have **prosopagnosia** (PROSS-oh-pag-NOH-see-ah), meaning impaired ability to recognize faces. That problem can result from damage to the fusiform gyrus, or from a failure of that gyrus to develop fully. In some people the right fusiform gyrus is significantly smaller than average and has fewer than normal connections with the occipital cortex (Grueter et al., 2007; Lohse et al., 2016; Thomas et al., 2009; Zhang, Liu, & Xu, 2015; Zhu et al., 2011). In contrast, if you can recognize faces more easily than average, it may be that you have richer than average connections between fusiform gyrus and occipital cortex.

Oliver Sacks, famous for writing about other people's neurological problems, suffered from prosopagnosia himself. In his words, "I have had difficulty recognizing faces for as long as I can remember. I did not think too much about this as a child, but by the time I was a teenager, in a new school, it was often a cause of embarrassment. . . . My problem with recognizing faces extends not only to my nearest and dearest but also to myself. Thus, on several occasions I have apologized for almost bumping into a large bearded man, only to realize that the large bearded man was myself in a mirror. The opposite situation once occurred at a restaurant. Sitting at a sidewalk table, I turned toward the restaurant window and began grooming my beard, as I often do. I then realized that what I had taken to be my reflection was not grooming himself but looking at me oddly" (Sacks, 2010, p. 37).

People with prosopagnosia can read, so visual acuity is not the problem. They recognize people's voices, so their problem is not memory (Farah, Wilson, Drain, & Tanaka, 1998). Furthermore, if they feel clay models of faces, they are worse than other people at determining whether two clay models are the same or different (Kilgour, de Gelder, & Lederman, 2004). Their problem is not vision, but something that relates specifically to faces.

When people with prosopagnosia look at a face, they can describe each element of a face, such as brown eyes, big ears, a small nose, and so forth, but they do not recognize the face as a whole. You would have a similar difficulty if you viewed faces quickly, upside down. One patient was shown 34 photographs of famous people and had a choice of two identifications for each. By chance alone, he should have identified 17 correctly; in fact, he got 18. He remarked that he seldom enjoyed watching movies or television programs because he had trouble keeping track of the characters. Curiously, his favorite movie was *Batman*, in which the main characters wore masks much of the time (Laeng & Caviness, 2001).

Did we really evolve a brain module devoted to faces? Or does the fusiform gyrus serve for all types of detailed visual recognition, for which faces are just a good example? Children with an intense interest in Pokemon cards show strong response in the fusiform gyrus when they look at Pokemon characters (James & James, 2013). Chess experts show a response there when they look at a chessboard (Bilalic, Langner, Ulrich, & Grodd, 2011). One study found that children who devoted at least an hour a day to some special interest, such as watching soccer or looking at pictures of space travel, showed fusiform gyrus responses to images related to that interest. The response was even greater for children with autism spectrum disorder, who pay less than usual attention to faces (Foss-Feig et al., 2016). As people learn to read, the fusiform gyrus becomes more responsive to words and (in the left hemisphere) less responsive to faces (Dehaene et al., 2010).

Evidently the fusiform gyrus participates in many types of detailed visual recognition. However, even in people with extreme levels of expertise, many cells in the fusiform gyrus respond more vigorously to faces than to anything else (Kanwisher & Yovel, 2006).

Motion Perception

Moving objects often merit immediate attention. A moving object might be a possible mate, something you could hunt and eat, or something that wants to eat you. If you are going to respond, you need to identify what the object is, where it is going, and how fast. The brain is set up to make those calculations quickly and efficiently.

28. The brain has no specialized areas for perceiving flowers, clothes, or food. For what items does it have specialized areas?
29. The ability to recognize faces correlates with the strength of connections between which brain areas?

ANSWERS

28. The temporal cortex has specialized areas for perceiving places, faces, and bodies, including bodies in motion. 29. Ability to recognize faces correlates with the strength of connections between the occipital face area and the fusiform gyrus.

The Middle Temporal Cortex

Two areas especially important for motion perception are area **MT** (for middle temporal cortex), also known as area **V5** (see Figure 5.27), and an adjacent region, area **MST** (medial superior temporal cortex). These areas receive input mostly from the magnocellular path (Nassi & Callaway, 2006), which detects overall patterns, including movement over large areas of the visual field. Given that the magnocellular path is color insensitive, MT is also color insensitive.

Most cells in area MT respond selectively when something moves at a particular speed in a particular direction (Perrone & Thiele, 2001). MT cells detect acceleration or deceleration as well as the absolute speed (Schlack, Krekelberg, & Albright, 2007), and they respond to motion in all three dimensions (Rokers, Cormack, & Huk, 2009). Area MT also responds to photographs that imply movement, such as a photo of people running (Kourtzi & Kanwisher, 2000). People who had electrical stimulation of area MT (while they were undergoing exploratory studies to find the cause of their severe epilepsy) report seeing vibrations or other hallucinated movements during the stimulation (Rauschecker et al., 2011). They also become temporarily impaired at seeing something that really is moving (Becker, Haarmeier, Tatagiba, & Gharabaghi, 2013). In short, MT activity is apparently central to the experience of seeing motion. Cells in the dorsal part of area MST respond best to more complex stimuli, such as the expansion, contraction, or rotation of a large visual scene, as illustrated in Figure 5.32. That kind of experience occurs when you move forward or backward or tilt your head.

When you move your head or eyes from left to right, everything in your visual field moves across your retina as if the world itself had moved right to left. (Go ahead and try it.) Yet the world seems stationary, because nothing moved relative to anything else. Neurons in areas MT and the ventral part of MST respond briskly if something moves relative to the background, but they show little response if the object and the background both move in the same direction and speed (Takemura, Ashida, Amano, Kitaoka, & Murakami, 2012). In short, MT and MST neurons enable you to distinguish between the result of eye movements and the result of object movements.

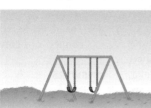

Expansion

Rotation

Figure 5.32 Stimuli that excite the dorsal part of area MST
Cells here respond if a whole scene expands, contracts, or rotates. That is, they respond if the observer moves forward or backward or tilts his or her head.

Motion Blindness

Given that areas MT and MST respond strongly to moving objects, and only to moving objects, what would happen after damage to these areas? The result is **motion blindness**, being able to see objects but unable to see whether they are moving or, if so, which direction and how fast (Marcar, Zihl, & Cowey, 1997). People with motion blindness are better at reaching for a moving object than at describing its motion (Schenk, Mai, Ditterich, & Zihl, 2000), but in all aspects of dealing with visual motion, they are far behind other people.

Motion blindness in the absence of other dysfunction is a rare condition. The best described case, "LM," reported that she felt uncomfortable when people walked around because they "were suddenly here or there but I have not seen them moving." People would seem to appear or disappear suddenly, even when she was trying to keep track of them. Someone who was walking would appear to her as "restless," but she would not know which direction the person was going. She would find it so unsettling that she would stop her own walking until the other person was gone. She could not cross a street without help, because she could not tell which cars were moving, or how fast. Pouring coffee became difficult. The flowing liquid appeared to be frozen and unmoving, so she did not stop pouring until the cup overfilled (Zihl, von Cramon, & Mai, 1983; Zihl & Heywood, 2015).

People with full color vision can imagine what it would be like to be color deficient, but it is difficult to imagine being motion blind. If something is moving, and you see it, how could you fail to see that it is moving? Because this experience seems so odd, neurologists for many years resisted the idea of motion blindness. Several patients were reported who apparently became motion blind as a result of brain damage, but most scientists ignored or disbelieved those reports. After the

discovery of area MT from monkey research, researchers saw a mechanism whereby motion blindness could (and should) occur, and the report about patient LM was acceptable.

You wonder what it would be like to be motion blind. Try this demonstration: Look at yourself in a mirror and focus on your left eye. Then shift your focus to your right eye. (*Please do this now.*) Did you see your eyes move? No, you did not. (*Oh, please try the demonstration!*)

TRY IT YOURSELF

Why didn't you see your eyes move? Your first impulse is to say that the movement was too small or too fast. Wrong. Try looking at someone else's eyes while he or she focuses first on your one eye and then the other. You *do* see the other person's eyes move, even though they moved the same distance and the same speed as your own. So an eye movement is neither too small nor too fast for you to see.

You do not see your own eyes move because area MT and parts of the parietal cortex decrease their activity during voluntary eye movements, known as **saccades** (Bremmer, Kubischik, Hoffmann, & Krekelberg, 2009). (Activity does not decrease while your eyes are following a moving object.) The brain areas that monitor saccades tell area MT and the parietal cortex, "We're about to move the eye muscles, so take a rest for the next split second." Neural activity and blood flow in MT and part of the parietal cortex begin to decrease 75 milliseconds (ms) before the eye movement and remain suppressed during the movement (Burr, Morrone, & Ross, 1994; Paus, Marrett, Worsley, & Evans, 1995; Vallines & Greenlee, 2006). In short, during a voluntary eye movement, you become motion blind, but just for a split second. Perhaps now you understand a little better what people with motion blindness experience all the time.

The opposite of motion blindness also occurs: Some people are blind *except* for the ability to detect which direction something is moving. How could someone see movement without seeing the object that is moving? Area MT gets some input directly from the lateral geniculate nucleus of the thalamus. Therefore, even after extensive damage to area V1 (enough to produce blindness), area MT still has enough input to permit motion detection (Sincich, Park, Wohlgemuth, & Horton, 2004). Again, we try to imagine this person's experience. What would it be like to see motion without seeing the objects that are moving? (Their answers don't help. When they say which direction something is moving, they insist they are just guessing.) The general point is that different areas of your brain process different kinds of visual information, and it is possible to develop many kinds of disability.

STOP & CHECK

30. When you move your eyes, why does it not seem as if the world is moving?
31. Under what circumstance does someone with an intact brain become motion blind, and what accounts for the motion blindness?

ANSWERS 30. Neurons in areas MT and MST respond strongly when an object moves relative to the background, and not when the object and background move in the same direction and speed. 31. People become motion blind shortly before and during a saccade (voluntary eye movement), because of suppressed activity in area MT.

Module 5.3 | In Closing
Aspects of Vision

Anatomists have identified at least nearly a hundred brain areas that contribute to vision in various ways. We have discussed areas responsible for detecting location, shape, faces, and movement. Why do we have so many visual areas? We can only infer that the brain, like a human society, benefits from specialization. Life works better if some people become experts at repairing cars, some at baking cakes, some at delivering babies, some at moving pianos, and so forth, than if each of us had to do everything for ourselves. Similarly, your visual system works better because visual areas specialize in a particular task without trying to do everything.

A related question: How do we put it all together? When you watch a bird fly by, you perceive its shape, color, location, and movement all at once. So it seems, anyway. How do you do that? This is the binding problem, as discussed in Chapter 3. Answering that question remains a major challenge.

Summary

1. Researchers distinguish between the ventral visual stream, responsible for perceiving objects, and the dorsal stream, responsible for visual guidance of movements. **177**
2. The inferior temporal cortex detects objects and recognizes them despite changes in position, size, and so forth. **178**
3. A circuit including the fusiform gyrus of the temporal cortex is specialized for recognizing faces. People with impairments in this circuit experience prosopagnosia, a difficulty in recognizing faces despite nearly normal vision in other regards. **179**
4. Although the fusiform gyrus is important for recognizing faces, it also contributes to other types of visual expertise. **181**
5. The middle temporal cortex (including areas MT and MST) is specialized for detecting the direction and speed of a moving object. People with damage in this area experience motion blindness, an impairment in their ability to perceive movement. **181**
6. Even people with an intact brain experience a brief period of motion blindness beginning about 75 ms before a voluntary eye movement and continuing during the eye movement. **182**

Key Terms

Terms are defined in the module on the page number indicated. They're also presented in alphabetical order with definitions in the book's Subject Index/Glossary, which begins on page 589. Interactive flash cards, audio reviews, and crossword puzzles are among the online resources available to help you learn these terms and the concepts they represent.

dorsal stream **177**
fusiform gyrus **179**
inferior temporal cortex **178**
motion blindness **182**
MST **181**
MT (or area V5) **181**
prosopagnosia **180**
saccade **182**
secondary visual cortex **177**
ventral stream **177**
visual agnosia **179**

Thought Questions

1. The visual system has specialized areas for perceiving faces, bodies, and places, but not other kinds of objects. Why might we have evolved specialized areas for these functions but not others?

2. Why is it advantageous to become motion blind during voluntary eye movements? That is, why might we have evolved this mechanism?

Module 5.3 | End of Module Quiz

1. The ventral stream of the visual system is specialized for which of these?
   A. Identifying locations
   B. Coordinating vision with movement
   C. Peripheral vision and vision under poor lighting
   D. Detailed identification of objects

2. If someone can identify objects, but does not seem to know where they are, what location of brain damage is likely?
   A. Primary visual cortex (V1)
   B. Middle temporal cortex (MT or V5)
   C. Secondary visual cortex (V2)
   D. Parietal cortex

3. What is distinctive about visual perception in the inferior temporal cortex?
   A. Cells respond only to objects that are symmetrical.
   B. Cells respond in proportion to the brightness of light.
   C. Cells respond only to objects that are moving at a particular speed.
   D. Cells respond to an object regardless of the angle of view.

4. The fusiform gyrus is specialized for which of the following?
   A. Recognizing faces and other highly familiar objects
   B. Maintaining color recognition despite changes in room lighting
   C. Identifying the direction and speed of a visual object
   D. Coordinating vision with hearing and other senses

5. If someone has trouble recognizing faces, what pathway in the nervous system is probably deficient?
   A. Connections between the primary visual cortex and area MT (V5)
   B. Connections between the fusiform gyrus and part of the occipital cortex
   C. Connections between the temporal cortex and the parietal cortex
   D. Connections between the occipital cortex and the primary motor cortex

6. What happens after damage limited to area MT?
   A. Motion blindness
   B. Face blindness
   C. Color blindness
   D. Night blindness

7. Why is it difficult to watch your own eyes move when looking in the mirror?
   A. The eye movements are too fast to see.
   B. The eye movements are too small to see.
   C. During a saccadic eye movement, the eyes do not move relative to the background of the rest of the face.
   D. During saccadic eye movements, activity decreases in area MT.

Answers: 1D, 2D, 3D, 4A, 5B, 6A, 7D.

Suggestions for Further Reading

Purves, D., & Lotto, R. B. (2003). *Why we see what we do: An empirical theory of vision.* Sunderland, MA: Sinauer Associates.

This presents a discussion of how our perception of color, size, and other visual qualities depends on our previous experience with objects and not just on the light striking the retina.

Sacks, O. (2010). *Mind's eye.* New York: Alfred Knopf.

This book includes case histories of people with brain damage who lost the ability to recognize faces, the ability to read, the ability to find their way around, and other specific visual abilities.

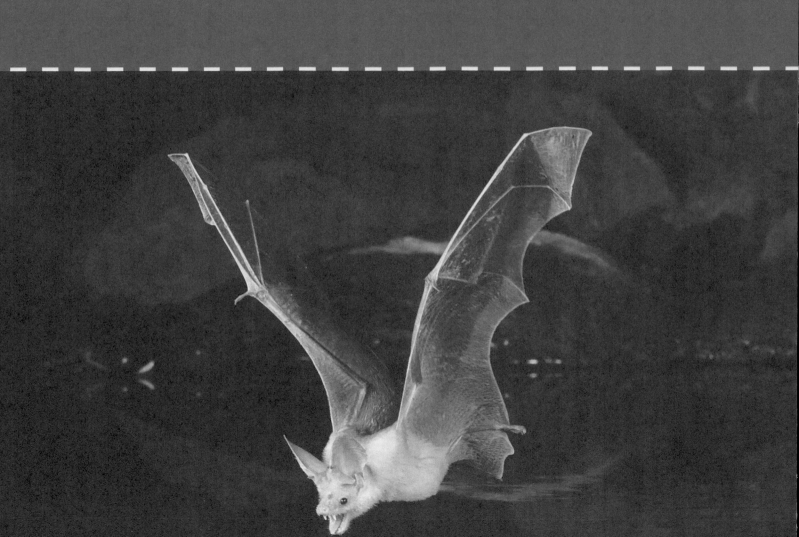

Other Sensory Systems

According to a Native American saying, "A pine needle fell. The eagle saw it. The deer heard it. The bear smelled it" (Herrero, 1985). Each species responds to the most useful kinds of information. Some birds have receptors to detect magnetic fields, useful information when orienting north and south during migration (Wu & Dickman, 2012). The ears of the green tree frog, *Hyla cinerea,* are most sensitive to sounds at the frequencies prominent in the adult male's mating call (Moss & Simmons, 1986). Mosquitoes evolved a special receptor that detects the odor of human sweat—and therefore helps them find us and bite us (McBride et al., 2014). Bats locate insects by emitting sonar waves at 20,000 to 100,000 hertz (Hz, cycles per second), well above the range of adult human hearing (Griffin, Webster, & Michael, 1960), and then locating the insects from the echoes. Bats hear the calls they use for localizing things better than they hear any other sounds (Wohlgemuth & Moss, 2016). Curiously, some moths jam the signals by emitting similar high-frequency calls of their own (Corcoran, Barber, & Conner, 2009).

Humans, too, have important sensory specializations. Our sense of taste alerts us to the bitterness of poisons (Richter, 1950; Schiffman & Erickson, 1971) but does not respond to substances such as cellulose that neither help nor harm us. Our olfactory systems are unresponsive to gases that we don't need to detect (e.g., nitrogen) but highly responsive to the smell of rotting meat. This chapter concerns how our sensory systems process biologically useful information.

Learning Objectives

After studying this chapter, you should be able to:

1. Describe the receptors for hearing, vestibular sensation, the somatic senses, and the chemical senses.
2. Explain the mechanisms of pitch perception and sound localization.
3. Compare physical and emotional pain.
4. Describe methods of relieving pain.
5. Discuss individual differences in taste and olfaction.
6. Define and describe synesthesia.

Opposite:
The sensory world of bats—which find insects by echolocation—must be very different from that of humans. (Danita Delimont/Getty Images)

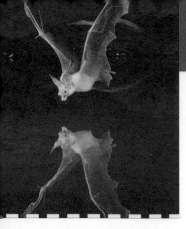

Audition

Evolution has been described as "thrifty." After it has solved one problem, it modifies that solution for other problems instead of starting from scratch. For example, imagine a gene for visual receptors in an early vertebrate. Make a duplicate of that gene, modify it slightly, and presto: The new gene makes receptors that respond to different wavelengths of light, and color vision becomes possible. In this chapter, you will see more examples of that principle. Various sensory systems have their specializations, but they also have much in common.

Sound and the Ear

Under optimum conditions, human hearing is sensitive to sounds that vibrate the eardrum by less than one-tenth the diameter of an atom, and we can detect a difference between two sounds as little as 1/30 the interval between two piano notes (Hudspeth, 2014). Ordinarily, however, we attend to hearing in order to extract useful information. If you hear footsteps in your home or a snapped twig in the forest, you know you are not alone. If you hear breathing, you know some person or animal is close. Then you hear the sound of a familiar friendly voice, and you know that all is well.

Physics and Psychology of Sound

Sound waves are periodic compressions of air, water, or other media. When a tree falls, the tree and the ground vibrate, setting up sound waves in the air that strike the ears. Sound waves vary in amplitude and frequency. The **amplitude** of a sound wave is its intensity. In general, sounds of greater amplitude seem louder, but exceptions occur. For example, a rapidly talking person seems louder than slow music of the same physical amplitude.

The **frequency** of a sound is the number of compressions per second, measured in hertz (Hz, cycles per second). **Pitch** is the related aspect of perception. Sounds higher in frequency are higher in pitch. Figure 6.1 illustrates the amplitude and frequency of sounds. The height of each wave corresponds to amplitude, and the number of waves per second corresponds to frequency.

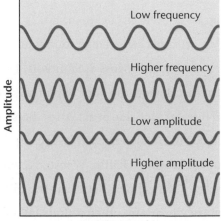
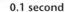

Figure 6.1 Four sound waves
The top line represents five sound waves in 0.1 second, or 50 Hz—a low-frequency sound that we experience as a low pitch. The other three lines represent 100 Hz. The vertical extent of each line represents its amplitude, which we experience as loudness.

Most adult humans hear sounds starting at about 15 to 20 Hz and ranging up to almost 20,000 Hz. Children hear higher frequencies than adults, because the ability to perceive high frequencies decreases with age and exposure to loud noises (Schneider, Trehub, Morrongiello, & Thorpe, 1986). As a rule, larger animals like elephants hear best at lower pitches, and small animals like mice hear higher pitches, including a range well above what humans hear.

In addition to amplitude and pitch, the third aspect of sound is **timbre** (TAM-ber), meaning tone quality or tone complexity. Two musical instruments playing the same note at the same loudness sound different, as do two people singing the same note at the same loudness. For example, any instrument playing a note at 256 Hz will simultaneously produce sound at 128 Hz, 512 Hz, and so forth, known as harmonics of the principal note. The amount of each harmonic differs among instruments.

People communicate emotion by alterations in pitch, loudness, and timbre. For example, the way you say "that was interesting" could indicate approval (it really was interesting), sarcasm (it really was boring), or suspicion (you think someone was hinting something). Conveying emotional information by tone of voice is known as *prosody*.

Structures of the Ear

Rube Goldberg (1883–1970) drew cartoons of complicated, far-fetched inventions. For example, a person's tread on the front doorstep might pull a string that raised a cat's tail, awakening the cat, which then chases a bird that had been

resting on a balance, which swings up to strike a doorbell. The functioning of the ear is complex enough to resemble a Rube Goldberg device, but unlike Goldberg's inventions, the ear actually works.

Anatomists distinguish the outer ear, the middle ear, and the inner ear (see Figure 6.2). The outer ear includes the **pinna**, the familiar structure of flesh and cartilage attached to each side of the head. By altering the reflections of sound waves, the pinna helps us locate the source of a sound. We have to learn to use that information because each person's pinna is shaped differently from anyone else's (Van Wanrooij

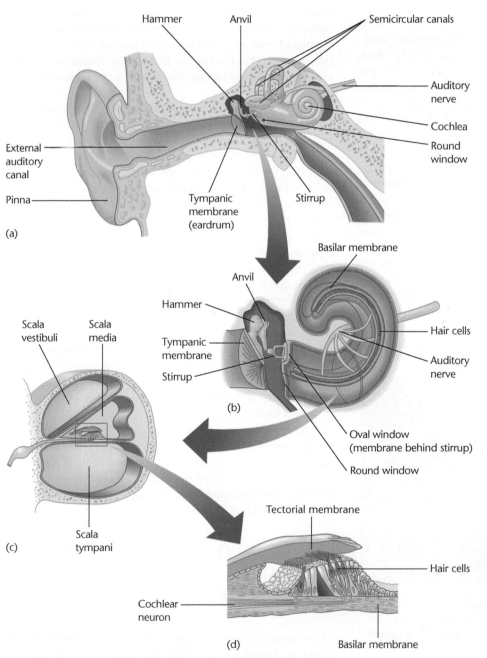

Figure 6.2 Structures of the ear
When sound waves strike the tympanic membrane in **(a)**, they vibrate three tiny bones—the hammer, anvil, and stirrup—that convert the sound waves into stronger vibrations in the fluid-filled cochlea **(b)**. Those vibrations displace the hair cells along the basilar membrane in the cochlea. **(c)** A cross section through the cochlea. **(d)** A close-up of the hair cells.

& Van Opstal, 2005). Rabbits' large movable pinnas enable them to localize sound sources even more precisely.

After sound waves pass through the auditory canal (see Figure 6.2), they enter the middle ear, a structure that had to evolve when ancient fish evolved into land animals. Because animal tissues respond to water vibrations almost the same way that water itself does, fish hearing receptors can be relatively simple. But because the same receptors would not respond well to vibrations in the air, early land animals would have heard only low-frequency sounds that were loud enough to vibrate the whole head (Christensen, Christensen-Dalsgaard, & Madsen, 2015). To develop effective hearing on land, animals needed to evolve a way to amplify sound vibrations. The structures of the middle ear and inner ear accomplish that.

When sound waves reach the middle ear, they vibrate the **tympanic membrane,** or eardrum. The tympanic membrane connects to three tiny bones that transmit the vibrations to the **oval window,** a membrane of the inner ear. These bones, the smallest bones in the body, are sometimes known by their English names (hammer, anvil, and stirrup) and sometimes by their Latin names (malleus, incus, and stapes). The tympanic membrane is about 20 times larger than the footplate of the stirrup, which connects to the oval window. As in a hydraulic pump, the vibrations of the tympanic membrane amplify into more forceful vibrations of the smaller stirrup. The net effect converts the sound waves into waves of greater pressure on the small oval window.

When the stirrup vibrates the oval window, it sets into motion the fluid in the **cochlea** (KOCK-lee-uh), the snail-shaped structure of the inner ear. Figure 6.2c shows a cross section through the cochlea and its tunnels. The auditory receptors, known as **hair cells**, lie between the basilar membrane of the cochlea on one side and the tectorial membrane on the other (see Figure 6.2d). Vibrations in the fluid of the cochlea displace the hair cells, thereby opening ion channels in its membrane. Figure 6.3

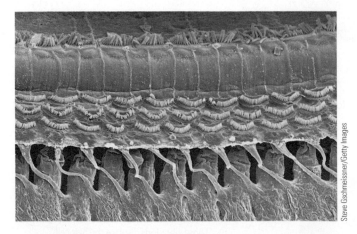

Steve Gschmeissner/Getty Images

Figure 6.3 Hair cells from a human cochlea
This artificially colored electron micrograph shows stereocilia (the crescent-shaped structures across the center of the photo) atop hair cells. As a sound wave moves the fluid across the stereocilia, it bends them, triggering responses by the hair cells.

shows an electron micrograph of human hair cells. The hair cells stimulate the cells of the auditory nerve, which is part of the eighth cranial nerve.

Pitch Perception

Your ability to understand speech or enjoy music depends on your ability to differentiate among sounds of different frequencies. How do you do it?

According to the **place theory,** the basilar membrane resembles the strings of a piano, with each area along the membrane tuned to a specific frequency. If you sound a note with a tuning fork near a piano, you vibrate the piano string tuned to that note. According to this theory, each frequency activates the hair cells at only one place along the basilar membrane, and the nervous system distinguishes among frequencies based on which neurons respond. The downfall of this theory is that the various parts of the basilar membrane are bound together too tightly for any part to resonate like a piano string.

According to the **frequency theory,** the entire basilar membrane vibrates in synchrony with a sound, causing auditory nerve axons to produce action potentials at the same frequency. For example, a sound at 50 Hz would cause 50 action potentials per second in the auditory nerve. The downfall of this theory in its simplest form is that the refractory period of a neuron, though variable among neurons, is typically about $1/_{1,000}$ second, so the maximum firing rate of a neuron is about 1000 Hz, far short of the highest frequencies we hear.

The current theory is a modification of both theories. For low-frequency sounds (up to about 100 Hz—more than an octave below middle C in music, which is 264 Hz), the basilar membrane vibrates in synchrony with the sound waves, in accordance with the frequency theory, and the auditory nerve axons generate one action potential per wave. Soft sounds activate fewer neurons, and stronger sounds activate more. Thus, at low frequencies, the frequency of impulses identifies the pitch, and the number of firing cells identifies loudness.

As sounds exceed 100 Hz, it becomes harder for any neuron to continue firing in synchrony with the sound waves. At higher frequencies, a neuron might fire on some of the waves and not others. Its action potentials are phase-locked to the peaks of the sound waves (i.e., they occur at the same phase in the sound wave), as illustrated here:

Sound wave (about 1000 Hz)

Action potentials from one auditory neuron

Other auditory neurons also produce action potentials that are phase-locked with peaks of the sound wave, but they can be out of phase with one another:

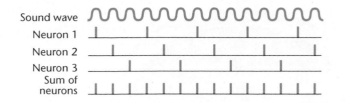

Each wave of a high-frequency tone excites at least a few auditory neurons. According to the **volley principle** of pitch discrimination, the auditory nerve as a whole produces volleys of impulses for sounds up to about 4000 per second, even though no individual axon approaches that frequency (Rose, Brugge, Anderson, & Hind, 1967). However, beyond about 4000 Hz, even staggered volleys of impulses cannot keep pace with the sound waves.

Most human hearing takes place below 4000 Hz, the approximate limit of the volley principle. For comparison, the highest key on a piano is 4224 Hz. When we hear still higher frequencies, we use a mechanism similar to the place theory. The basilar membrane varies from stiff at its base, where the stirrup meets the cochlea, to floppy at the other end of the cochlea, the apex (see Figure 6.4). A high-pitched sound sets up a traveling wave that peaks at some point along the basilar membrane, and then stops. The point at which it peaks identifies the frequency of the sound (Hudspeth, 2014). The highest frequency sounds

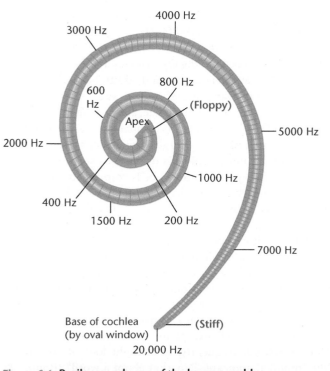

Figure 6.4 Basilar membrane of the human cochlea
High-frequency sounds excite hair cells near the base. Low-frequency sounds excite cells near the apex.

vibrate hair cells near the base, and lower frequency sounds vibrate hair cells farther along the membrane (Warren, 1999).

STOP & CHECK

1. Through which mechanism do we perceive low-frequency sounds (up to about 100 Hz)?
2. How do we perceive middle-frequency sounds (100 to 4000 Hz)?
3. How do we perceive high-frequency sounds (above 4000 Hz)?

ANSWERS 1. At low frequencies, the basilar membrane vibrates in synchrony with the sound waves, and each responding axon in the auditory nerve sends one action potential per sound wave. 2. At intermediate frequencies, no single axon fires an action potential for each sound wave, but different axons fire for different waves, and so a volley (group) of axons fires for each wave. 3. At high frequencies, the sound causes maximum vibration for the hair cells at one location along the basilar membrane.

The Auditory Cortex

As information from the auditory system passes through subcortical areas, axons cross over in the midbrain to enable each hemisphere of the forebrain to get most of its input from the opposite ear (Glendenning, Baker, Hutson, & Masterton, 1992). The information ultimately reaches the **primary auditory cortex (area A1)** in the superior temporal cortex, as shown in Figure 6.5.

The organization of the auditory cortex parallels that of the visual cortex (Poremba et al., 2003). For example, just as the visual system has separate pathways for identifying objects and acting upon them, the auditory system has a pathway in the anterior temporal cortex specialized for identifying sounds, and a pathway in the posterior temporal cortex and the parietal cortex specialized for locating sounds (Lomber & Malhotra, 2008). Just as patients with damage in area MT become motion blind, patients with damage in parts of the superior temporal cortex become motion deaf. They hear sounds, but they do not detect that a source of a sound is moving (Ducommun et al., 2004).

Just as the visual cortex is active during visual imagery, area A1 responds to imagined sounds as well as real ones. It becomes active when people view short silent videos that suggest sound—such as someone playing a piano, or a glass vase shattering on the ground (Meyer et al., 2010). In one study, people listened to several familiar and unfamiliar songs. At various points, parts of each song were replaced by 3- to 5-second gaps. When people were listening to familiar songs, they reported that they heard "in their heads" the notes or words that belonged in the gaps. That experience was accompanied by activity in area A1. During similar gaps in the unfamiliar songs, they did not hear anything in their heads, and area A1 showed no response (Kraemer, Macrae, Green, & Kelley, 2005).

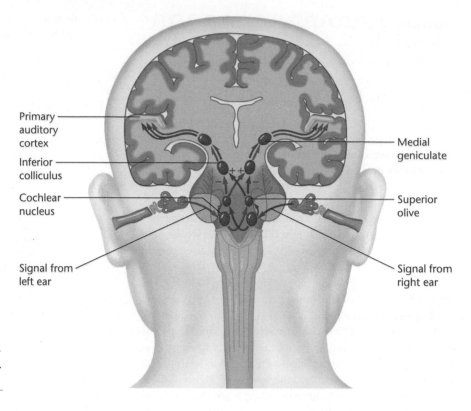

Primary auditory cortex

Inferior colliculus

Cochlear nucleus

Signal from left ear

Medial geniculate

Superior olive

Signal from right ear

Figure 6.5 Route of auditory impulses from the receptors in the ear to the auditory cortex The cochlear nucleus receives input from the ipsilateral ear only (the one on the same side of the head). All later stages have input from both ears.

Also like the visual system, development of the auditory system depends on experience. Just as rearing an animal in the dark impairs visual development, rearing one in constant noise impairs auditory development (Chang & Merzenich, 2003). (In constant noise, it is difficult to identify and learn about individual sounds.)

However, the visual and auditory systems differ in this respect: Whereas damage to the primary visual cortex (area V1) leaves someone blind, damage to the primary auditory cortex does not produce deafness. People with damage to the primary auditory cortex have trouble with speech and music, but they can identify and localize single sounds (Tanaka, Kamo, Yoshida, & Yamadori, 1991). Evidently, the cortex is not necessary for hearing, but for processing the information.

When researchers record from cells in the primary auditory cortex while playing pure tones, they find that most cells have a preferred tone. The auditory cortex provides what researchers call a *tonotopic* map of sounds, as shown in Figure 6.6. Note that cells responsive to similar frequencies tend to group together. The tonotopic map differs in detail from one person to another (Leaver & Rauschecker, 2016).

Although some cells in the auditory cortex respond well to a single tone, most cells respond best to a complex sound, such as a dominant tone and several harmonics

(Barbour & Wang, 2003; Griffiths, Uppenkamp, Johnsrude, Josephs, & Patterson, 2001; Penagos, Melcher, & Oxenham, 2004; Wessinger et al., 2001). For example, for a tone of 400 Hz, the harmonics are 800 Hz, 1200 Hz, and so forth. We experience a tone with harmonics as richer than one without them. Surrounding the primary auditory cortex are the secondary auditory cortex and additional areas that respond best to relevant natural sounds, such as animal calls, birdsong, machinery noises, music, and speech (Theunissen & Elie, 2014). While people were undergoing an exploratory procedure preliminary to surgery for epilepsy, researchers recorded from individual cells in the area surrounding the primary auditory cortex. Some cells responded strongly to particular speech sounds, such as all the vowels or all the nasal sounds (m, n, and ñ) (Mesgarani, Cheung, Johnson, & Chang, 2014).

The auditory cortex is important not just for hearing, but also for thinking about concepts related to hearing. People were asked to look at letter arrays and press a button to indicate whether each one was or was not a real word. The task was easy enough that most people were almost always correct. People with damage to the auditory cortex performed normally, except for words relating to sounds. Not always, but frequently, they might look at something like "thunder" indicate, "No, that is not a word" (Bonner & Grossman, 2012). That study is significant, as it supports

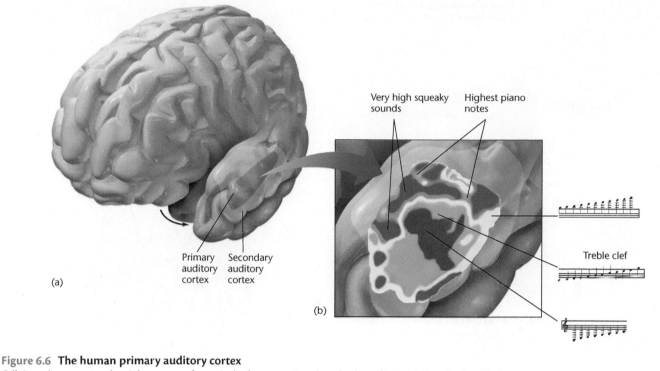

Figure 6.6 The human primary auditory cortex
Cells in each area respond mainly to tones of a particular frequency. Based on the data of Leaver & Rauschecker, 2016.

the theory that human concepts rely on associations with the sensations or actions that initially established them. If you cannot imagine a sound, then a word relating to sound seems meaningless.

STOP & CHECK

4. How is the auditory cortex like the visual cortex?
5. What is one way in which the auditory and visual cortices differ?
6. What evidence suggests that human concepts rely on activation of the relevant sensory or motor areas of the cortex?

Sound Localization

You are walking alone when suddenly you hear a loud noise. You want to know what produced it (friend or foe), but equally, you want to know where it came from. Sound localization is less accurate than visual localization, but nevertheless impressive. Owls localize sounds well enough to capture mice in the dark.

Determining the direction and distance of a sound requires comparing the responses of the two ears. One method is the difference in *time of arrival* at the two ears. A sound coming directly from one side reaches your closer ear about 600 microseconds (μs) before the other. A smaller difference in arrival times indicates a sound source nearer to your midline. Time of arrival is useful for localizing sounds with a sudden onset. Most birds' alarm calls increase gradually in loudness, making them difficult for a predator to localize.

Another cue for location is the difference in intensity between the ears. For high-frequency sounds, with a wavelength shorter than the width of the head, the head creates a *sound shadow* (see Figure 6.7), making the sound louder for the closer ear. In adult humans, this mechanism produces accurate sound localization for frequencies above 2000 to 3000 Hz and less accurate localizations for lower frequencies.

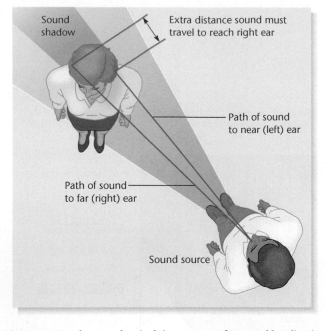

Figure 6.7 Loudness and arrival times as cues for sound localization
Sounds reaching the closer ear arrive sooner as well as louder because the head produces a "sound shadow."
(Source: Based on Lindsay & Norman, 1972)

A third cue is the *phase difference* between the ears. Every sound wave has phases with peaks 360 degrees apart. Figure 6.8 shows sound waves that are in phase or out of phase. If a sound originates to the side of the head, the sound wave strikes the two ears out of phase, as shown in Figure 6.9. How much out of phase depends on the frequency of the sound, the size of the head, and the direction of the sound. Phase differences provide information that is useful for localizing sounds with frequencies up to about 1500 Hz in humans. Speech sounds and music are well within this range.

If your head is under water, you will have trouble localizing low- and medium-frequency sounds. The reason is that sounds travel faster in water than in air, so a sound arrives at the two ears almost simultaneously and the phase differences are small, also.

In short, humans localize low frequencies by phase differences, and high frequencies by loudness differences. We can localize a sudden sound of any frequency by the times of onset. All of these methods require learning, because as your head grows, the distance between your ears increases, and you need to recalibrate how you localize sounds (Kumpik, Kacelnik, & King, 2010).

What would happen if you became deaf in one ear? At first, as you would expect, all sounds would seem to come directly from the side of the intact ear. (That ear hears a sound louder and sooner than the other ear because the other ear doesn't hear it at all.) Eventually, however, people learn to interpret loudness cues when they hear familiar sounds in a familiar location. They infer that louder sounds come from the side of the intact ear and softer sounds come from the opposite side. Their accuracy does not match that of people with two ears, but it becomes helpful under some conditions (Van Wanrooij & Van Opstal, 2004).

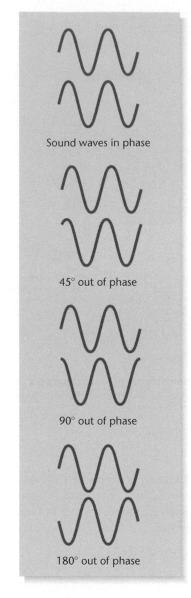

Figure 6.8 Sound waves in phase or out of phase
Sound waves that reach the two ears in phase are perceived as coming from directly in front of (or behind) the hearer. The more out of phase the waves, the farther the sound source is from the body's midline.

✅ STOP & CHECK

7. Which method of sound localization is more effective for an animal with a small head? Which is more effective for an animal with a large head? Why?

ANSWER

7. An animal with a small head localizes sounds mainly by differences in loudness because the ears are not far enough apart for differences in onset time to be useful. An animal with a large head localizes sounds mainly by differences in onset time because its ears are far apart and well suited to noticing differences in phase or onset time.

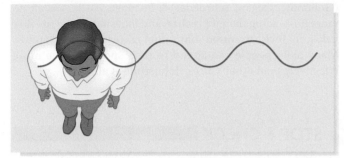

Figure 6.9 Phase differences as a cue for sound localization A sound coming from anywhere other than straight ahead or straight behind reaches the two ears at different phases of the sound wave. The difference in phase is a signal to the sound's direction. With high-frequency sounds, the phases become ambiguous.

Individual Differences

An estimated 4 percent of people have *amusia,* commonly called "tone deafness" (Hyde & Peretz, 2004). Although not really unable to detect differences in tones, they generally do not detect a change less than about the difference between C and C-sharp (Loui, Alsop, & Schlaug, 2009). Furthermore, they have trouble recognizing tunes, cannot tell whether someone is singing off-key, and do not detect a "wrong" note in a melody. They also have trouble gauging people's mood, such as happy or sad, from tone of voice (Thompson, Marin, & Stewart, 2012).

For people with amusia, the auditory cortex appears to be approximately normal, but it has fewer than average connections to the frontal cortex (Hyde et al., 2007; Loui et al., 2009; Norman-Haignere et al., 2016). That is, the deficit is evidently not in hearing itself. Rather, these people have poor memory for pitch (Tillman, Leveque, Fornoni, Abouy, & Caclin, 2016), and perhaps poor attention to pitch. Transcranial alternating current applied to the scalp is a noninvasive way to stimulate the underlying area of the brain. When this procedure was applied to part of the right prefrontal cortex of people with amusia, their ability to remember pitch improved to almost normal levels (Schaal, Pfeifer, Krause, & Pollok, 2015). The implication is that amusia results from either an impairment of the prefrontal cortex, or input to it from the auditory cortex.

Absolute pitch (or "perfect pitch") is the ability to hear a note and identify it—for example, "That's a B-flat." Genetic predisposition contributes (Theusch, Basu, & Gitschier, 2009), but early musical training is also important. Not everyone with musical training develops absolute pitch, but almost everyone with absolute pitch had early musical training (Athos et al., 2007). Absolute pitch is also more common among people who speak tonal languages, such as Vietnamese and Mandarin Chinese (Deutsch, Henthorn, Marvin, & Xu, 2006). In those languages, the meaning of a sound depends on its pitch, and therefore, people learn from infancy to pay close attention to slight changes of pitch.

In the traditional manner of testing for absolute pitch, a researcher plays a pure note and asks someone to name it. By that method, only about one person in 10,000 qualifies, and we are tempted to think of absolute pitch as a "superpower." However, by other methods of testing, the ability seems more common. For example, many professional violinists cannot name the pitch of a pure note but become much more accurate if they hear a violin note with its harmonics. Similar results apply to pianists and presumably people who play other instruments (Wong & Wong, 2014). Nonmusicians cannot name a note, but if they listen to the theme song from a familiar television show, most can tell whether it was played in its usual key or a different one (Schellenberg & Trehub, 2003). Evidently the ability to recognize a pitch is common, even if the ability to name it is not.

Deafness

Although few people are totally unable to hear, many people have enough impairment to prevent speech comprehension. The two categories of hearing loss are conductive deafness and nerve deafness.

Diseases, infections, or tumorous bone growth can prevent the middle ear from transmitting sound waves properly to the cochlea. The result, **conductive deafness** or **middle-ear deafness**, is sometimes temporary. If it persists, it can be corrected by surgery or by hearing aids that amplify sounds. Because people with conductive deafness have a normal cochlea and auditory nerve, they readily hear their own voices, conducted through the bones of the skull directly to the cochlea, bypassing the middle ear. Because they hear themselves clearly, they may accuse others of mumbling or talking too softly.

Nerve deafness, or **inner-ear deafness,** results from damage to the cochlea, the hair cells, or the auditory nerve. If it is confined to one part of the cochlea, it impairs hearing of certain frequencies and not others. Nerve deafness can be inherited, it can result from disease, or it can result from exposure to loud noises. For example, many soldiers, construction workers, and fans of loud rock music expose themselves to noise levels that damage the synapses and neurons of the auditory system. Gradually they begin to notice ringing in the ears or impaired hearing (Kujawa & Liberman, 2009).

Tinnitus (tin-EYE-tus) is frequent or constant ringing in the ears. In some cases, tinnitus may be due to a phenomenon similar to phantom limb, discussed in Chapter 4. Damage to part of the cochlea is like an amputation: If the brain no longer gets its normal input, axons representing other parts of the body may invade part of the brain area that usually responds to sounds. In many cases, people who have lost their hearing in a particular range report ringing in the ears in the same range, suggesting that some other input is activating part of the auditory cortex. However, many people have tinnitus without hearing loss or reorganization of the cortex (Elgoyhen, Langguth, De Ridder, & Vanneste, 2015). Evidently tinnitus can result from more than one cause.

Hearing, Attention, and Old Age

Many older people have hearing problems despite wearing hearing aids. The hearing aids make the sounds loud enough, but people still have trouble understanding speech, especially in a noisy room or if someone speaks rapidly.

Part of the explanation is that the brain areas responsible for language comprehension have become less active (Peelle, Troiani, Grossman, & Wingfield, 2011). This trend might be just a natural deterioration, or it might be a reaction to prolonged degradation of auditory input. That is, if someone delays getting hearing aids, the language cortex doesn't get its normal input and it begins to become less responsive.

The rest of the explanation relates to attention. Frequently you want to listen to one person in a noisy room. To hear what you care about, you need to filter out all the other sounds (Mesgarani & Chang, 2013). Healthy young people can filter out irrelevant sounds highly effectively (Molloy, Griffiths, Chait, & Lavie, 2015).

Many older people have a loss of inhibitory neurotransmitters in the auditory portions of the brain. As a result, they have trouble suppressing irrelevant sounds. Also, because of decreased inhibitory transmission, the auditory cortex has gradual, spread-out responses to each sound instead of a quick, crisp response to each one. Therefore, the response to one sound partly overlaps the response to another (Anderson, Parbery-Clark, White-Schwoch, & Kraus, 2012). Attention improves if the listener watches the speaker's face (Golumbic, Cogan, Schroeder, & Poeppel, 2013). We all do more lip-reading than we realize, and focusing on the speaker helps to lock attention onto the corresponding sounds. Many older people can attend to their spouse's voice more effectively than other voices (Johnsrude et al., 2013).

STOP & CHECK

8. What evidence suggests that absolute pitch depends on special experiences?
9. Which type of hearing loss—conductive deafness or nerve deafness—would be more common among members of rock bands and why?
10. Why do many older people have trouble hearing speech in spite of wearing hearing aids?

ANSWERS

8. Absolute pitch occurs almost entirely among people who had early musical training and is also more common among people who speak tonal languages, which require greater attention to pitch. 9. Nerve deafness is common among rock band members because their frequent exposure to loud noises causes damage to the cells of the ear. 10. In some cases the language areas of the cortex have become less responsive. Also, auditory areas of the brain have decreased levels of inhibitory neurotransmitters, and the result is decreased ability to focus attention on one speaker in a noisy environment.

Module 6.1 | In Closing

Functions of Hearing

We spend much of our day listening to language, and we sometimes forget that the original, primary function of hearing has to do with simpler but extremely important issues: What do I hear? Where is it? Is it coming closer? Is it a potential mate, a potential enemy, potential food, or something irrelevant? The organization of the auditory system is well suited to answering these questions.

Summary

1. Sound waves vibrate the tympanic membrane. Three tiny bones convert these vibrations into more forceful vibrations of the smaller oval window, setting in motion the fluid inside the cochlea. Waves of fluid inside the cochlea stimulate the hair cells that send messages to the brain. **188**

2. We detect the pitch of low-frequency sounds by the frequency of action potentials in the auditory system. At intermediate frequencies, we detect volleys of responses across many receptors. We detect the pitch of the highest-frequency sounds by the area of greatest response along the basilar membrane. **190**

3. The auditory cortex resembles the visual cortex in many ways. Both have one system specialized for identifying stimuli and one system for localizing them. Both are important for imagining sensory stimuli. Both have specialized areas for detecting motion. **191**

4. Each cell in the primary auditory cortex responds best to a particular frequency of tones, although many respond better to complex tones than to a single frequency. **192**

5. Areas bordering the primary auditory cortex respond to more complex sounds and analyze their meaning. The auditory cortex contributes to understanding the meaning of words related to sound. **192**

6. We localize high-frequency sounds according to differences in loudness between the ears. We localize low-frequency sounds by differences in phase. If a sound occurs suddenly, we localize it by the times of onset in the two ears. **193**

7. People vary in their attention to sounds and their ability to process them. Some people are impaired at detecting or remembering differences in sounds. Some people can listen to a tone and identify it, such as C-sharp. **195**

8. Deafness may result from damage to the nerve cells or to the bones that conduct sounds to the nerve cells. **195**

9. Many older people have trouble attending to relevant information and filtering out the distractions, largely because of the loss of inhibitory neurotransmitters in auditory areas of the brain. **196**

Key Terms

Terms are defined in the module on the page number indicated. They're also presented in alphabetical order with definitions in the book's Subject Index/Glossary, which begins on page 589. Interactive flash cards, audio reviews, and crossword puzzles are among the online resources available to help you learn these terms and the concepts they represent.

amplitude **188**
cochlea **190**
conductive deafness (middle-ear deafness) **195**
frequency **188**
frequency theory **190**
hair cells **190**

nerve deafness (inner-ear deafness) **195**
oval window **190**
pinna **189**
pitch **188**
place theory **190**

primary auditory cortex (area A1) **191**
timbre **188**
tinnitus **195**
tympanic membrane **190**
volley principle **191**

Thought Questions

1. Why do you suppose that the human auditory system evolved sensitivity to sounds in the range of 20 to 20,000 Hz instead of some other range of frequencies?

2. The text explains how we might distinguish loudness for low-frequency sounds. How might we distinguish loudness for a high-frequency tone?

Module 6.1 | End of Module Quiz

1. When ancient fish evolved into land animals, why did they need to evolve the elaborate mechanisms of the middle ear and inner ear?

   A. To amplify sounds
   B. To localize sounds

   C. To remember sounds
   D. To distinguish among pitches

2. Where are the auditory receptors, known as hair cells?

   A. In the auditory nerve
   B. Along the basilar membrane of the cochlea

   C. Between the incus and the stapes
   D. In the pinna

3. How do we identify a low-pitched sound?

   A. Low frequencies cause only weak vibrations of the basilar membrane.
   B. Each frequency produces a peak response at one point along the basilar membrane.

   C. The whole basilar membrane vibrates in synchrony with the sound frequency.
   D. Each frequency vibrates a different part of the pinna.

4. How do we identify a high-pitched sound?

   A. High frequencies cause only weak vibrations of the basilar membrane.
   B. Each frequency produces a peak response at one point along the basilar membrane.

   C. The whole basilar membrane vibrates in synchrony with the sound frequency.
   D. Each frequency vibrates a different part of the pinna.

5. What is one way in which the auditory cortex is not analogous to the visual cortex?

A. The auditory cortex does not have separate pathways for identifying and localizing stimuli.

B. Damage to the primary auditory cortex does not cause deafness.

C. Just imagining a sound does not activate the auditory cortex.

D. Variations in early experience do not modify the auditory cortex.

6. What is meant by a "tonotopic map"?

A. Each location in the auditory cortex responds to a preferred tone.

B. The auditory cortex has axons back and forth to every other part of the cortex.

C. Each neuron in the auditory cortex responds differently depending on the location of the source of sound in space.

D. Each cell in the auditory cortex has a "partner" cell in the visual cortex.

7. What type of sound do we localize by comparing the time of arrival at the two ears?

A. Slow-onset sounds

B. Sudden sounds

C. High-frequency sounds

D. Low-frequency sounds

8. Absolute pitch is more common among what type of people?

A. People who had a period of auditory deprivation during early childhood

B. People with extensive musical training beginning in early childhood

C. People who learned two languages beginning in early childhood

D. People with many older brothers and sisters

9. Why do many older people have trouble understanding speech despite using hearing aids?

A. Lack of inhibitory transmission in the auditory cortex

B. Gradual shrinkage of the cochlea

C. Decrease in social responsiveness

D. Inability to remember the meanings of common words

Answers: 1A, 2B, 3C, 4B, 5B, 6A, 7B, 8B, 9A.

The Mechanical Senses

If you place your hand on the surface of your radio, you feel the vibrations that you hear. If you practiced enough, could you learn to "hear" the vibrations with your fingers? Sorry, that won't work. If an earless species had enough time, might its vibration detectors evolve into sound detectors? Yes! In fact, our ears did evolve in that way. Much of evolution consists of taking something that evolved for one purpose and modifying it for another purpose.

The *mechanical senses* respond to pressure, bending, or other distortions of a receptor. They include touch, pain, and other body sensations, as well as vestibular sensation, which detects the position and movement of the head. Audition is also a mechanical sense because the hair cells are modified touch receptors. We considered it separately because of its complexity and importance.

Vestibular Sensation

Try to read a page while you jiggle your head up and down or back and forth. You will find that you can read it fairly easily, unless you jiggle your head too fast. Now hold your head steady and jiggle the page up and down, back and forth. In that case, you can hardly read it at all. Why?

TRY IT YOURSELF

When you move your head, the vestibular organ adjacent to the cochlea monitors movements and directs compensatory movements of your eyes. When your head moves left, your eyes move right; when your head moves right, your eyes move left. Effortlessly, you keep your eyes focused on what you want to see (Brandt, 1991). When you quickly move the page back and forth, however, the vestibular organ cannot keep your eyes on target.

Sensations from the vestibular organ detect the direction of tilt and the amount of acceleration of the head. You use that information automatically for guiding eye movements and maintaining balance. Mice with an impairment of vestibular sensation frequently lose their balance and fall down. They cannot swim or float because they are often upside down (Mariño et al., 2010). Similarly, people with impairments of the vestibular system stagger and fall.

The vestibular organ, shown in Figure 6.10, consists of the *saccule, utricle,* and three semicircular canals. Like the hearing receptors, the vestibular receptors are modified touch receptors.

Calcium carbonate particles called *otoliths* lie next to the hair cells. When the head tilts in different directions, the otoliths push against different sets of hair cells and excite them (Hess, 2001). The otoliths tell the brain which direction you are moving, but they also record which direction the head tilts when you are at rest.

The three **semicircular canals,** oriented in perpendicular planes, are filled with a fluid and lined with hair cells. Acceleration of the head at any angle causes the fluid in one of these canals to move, just as the water in a bucket will splash if you jerk the bucket from side to side. The fluid then pushes against the hair cells in the semicircular canals, setting up action potentials. Unlike the saccule and utricle, the semicircular canals record only the amount of acceleration, not the position of the head at rest. They are also insensitive to sustained motion. If you start forward on a bicycle, car, or airplane, the semicircular canals respond as you accelerate, but as you continue at a steady pace, the receptors stop responding.

The vestibular organ is nearly the same size for all mammalian species. Whales are 10 million times as massive as mice, but their vestibular organ is only 5 times as large (Squires, 2004). Evidently a small vestibular organ provides all the information we need. For analogy, small thermometers can be nearly as accurate as larger ones.

⊘ STOP & CHECK

11. People with damage to the vestibular system have trouble reading street signs while walking. Why?

ANSWER
11. The vestibular system enables the brain to shift eye movements to compensate for changes in head position. Without feedback about head position, a person would not be able to correct the eye movements, and the experience would be like watching a jiggling book page.

Somatosensation

The **somatosensory system**, the sensation of the body and its movements, is not one sense but many, including discriminative touch (which identifies the shape of an object), deep pressure, cold, warmth, pain, itch, tickle, and the position and movement of joints.

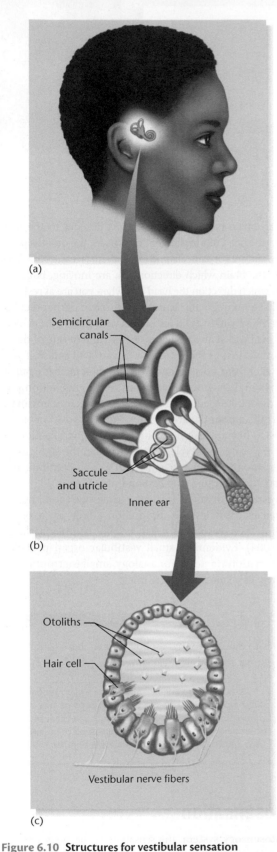

(a)

(b)

(c)

Semicircular
canals

Saccule
and utricle

Inner ear

Otoliths

Hair cell

Vestibular nerve fibers

Figure 6.10 Structures for vestibular sensation
(a) Location of the vestibular organs. (b) Structures of the vestibular organs. (c) Cross section through a utricle. Calcium carbonate particles, called otoliths, press against different hair cells depending on the tilt and acceleration of the head.

Somatosensory Receptors

Table 6.1 describes somatosensory receptors, including those shown in Figure 6.11 (Iggo & Andres, 1982; Zimmerman, Bai, & Ginty, 2014). Other receptors not in the table respond to joint movement or muscle movements.

Consider the **Pacinian corpuscle,** which detects vibrations or sudden displacements on the skin (see Figure 6.12). At the center is the neuron membrane. The onion-like outer structure provides mechanical support that resists gradual or constant pressure. It thereby insulates the neuron against most touch stimuli. However, a sudden or vibrating stimulus bends the membrane, enabling sodium ions to enter, depolarizing the membrane (Loewenstein, 1960).

Merkel disks respond to light touch, such as when you feel an object. Suppose you feel objects with thin grooves like these, without looking at them, and try to feel whether the grooves go left to right or up and down:

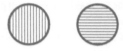

The experimenter varies the width of the grooves to find the narrowest grooves you can discern. On average, women can detect grooves about 1.4 mm apart, whereas men need the grooves to be about 1.6 mm apart. Your first question might be, "Who cares?" but if you get past that question, your second question might be *why* men and women differ. Unlike many sex differences, this one is easy to explain. It reflects the fact that on the average, women have smaller fingers. Apparently women have the same number of Merkel disks as men, but compacted into a smaller area. If you compare men and women who have the same finger size, their touch sensitivity is the same (Peters, Hackeman, & Goldreich, 2009).

The body has specialized receptors to detect temperature, a critical variable to monitor, given that overheating or

Table 6.1 | Somatosensory Receptors and Probable Functions

Receptor	Location	Responds to:
Free nerve ending	Any skin area	Pain and temperature
Hair-follicle receptors	Hair-covered skin	Movement of hairs
Meissner's corpuscles	Hairless areas	Movement across the skin
Pacinian corpuscles	Any skin area	Vibration or sudden touch
Merkel's disks	Any skin area	Static touch
Ruffini endings	Any skin area	Skin stretch
Krause end bulbs	Mostly hairless areas	Uncertain

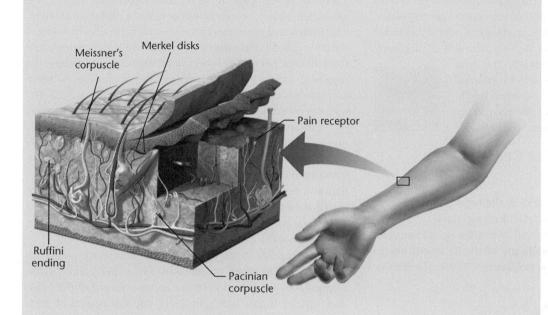

Figure 6.11 **Sensory receptors in the skin**
The receptors respond to several types of skin sensation, as described in Table 6.1.

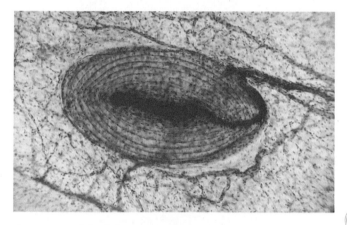

Figure 6.12 A Pacinian corpuscle
Pacinian corpuscles are receptors that respond best to sudden displacement of the skin or to high-frequency vibrations. The onion-like outer structure provides a mechanical support to the neuron inside it so that a sudden stimulus can bend it but a sustained stimulus cannot.
(Source: Ed Reschke)

Our temperature receptors also respond to certain chemical stimuli. **Capsaicin,** a chemical found in hot peppers such as jalapeños, stimulates the receptors for painful heat. Capsaicin can produce burning or stinging sensations on many parts of your body, as you may have experienced if you ever touched the insides of hot peppers and then rubbed your eyes. Szechuan peppers stimulate the heat receptors, and in addition stimulate certain touch receptors that give a tingling sensation (Bautista et al., 2008). Menthol and mint stimulate the coolness receptor (McKemy, Neuhausser, & Julius, 2002). So advertisements mentioning "the cool taste of menthol" are literally correct.

STOP & CHECK

12. How do jalapeños produce a hot sensation?

ANSWER

12. Jalapeños and other hot peppers contain capsaicin, which stimulates receptors that are sensitive to painful heat.

Tickle

The sensation of tickle is interesting but poorly understood. Why does it exist at all? Why do you laugh if someone fingers your armpit, neck, or the soles of your feet? Chimpanzees respond to similar sensations with bursts of panting that resemble laughter. And yet tickling is unlike humor. We love humor, but most people don't like being tickled, at least not for long. Laughing at a joke makes you more likely to laugh at the next joke. But being tickled doesn't change your likelihood of laughing at a joke (Harris, 1999).

Why can't you tickle yourself? It is for the same reason that you cannot surprise yourself. When you touch yourself, your brain compares the resulting stimulation to the "expected"

overcooling the body can be fatal. The systems for cooling and heating show an interesting asymmetry: Cold-sensitive neurons in the spinal cord respond to a drop in temperature. For example, a cell that responds to a drop from 39° C to 33° C would also respond to a drop from 33° C to 27° C. Thus, on a very hot day, you might detect a breeze as "cool," even though the air in the breeze is fairly warm. Cold-sensitive neurons adapt quickly, and show little response to a constant low temperature. In contrast, heat-sensitive neurons in the spinal cord respond to the absolute temperature, and they do not adapt. A cell that responds to 44° C will respond the same way regardless of whether the skin was hotter, cooler, or the same temperature a minute or two ago (Ran, Hoon, & Chen, 2016).

stimulation and generates a weaker somatosensory response than you would experience from an unexpected touch (Blakemore, Wolpert, & Frith, 1998). Actually, some people can tickle themselves—a little—if they tickle the right side of the body with the left hand or the left side with the right hand. Also, you might be able to tickle yourself as soon as you wake up, before your brain is fully aroused. See whether you can remember to try that some time when you awaken.

Somatosensation in the Central Nervous System

Information from touch receptors in the head enters the central nervous system (CNS) through the cranial nerves. Information from receptors below the head enters the spinal cord and passes toward the brain through any of the 31 spinal nerves (see Figure 6.13), including 8 cervical nerves, 12 thoracic nerves,

5 lumbar nerves, 5 sacral nerves, and 1 coccygeal nerve. Each spinal nerve has a sensory component and a motor component.

Each spinal nerve *innervates* (connects to) a limited area of the body called a **dermatome** (see Figure 6.14). For example, the third thoracic nerve (T3) innervates a strip of skin just above the nipples as well as the underarm area. But the borders between dermatomes are less distinct than Figure 6.14 implies. Each dermatome overlaps one-third to one-half of the next dermatome.

Various types of somatosensory information—such as touch, pressure, and pain—travel through the spinal cord in separate pathways toward the thalamus, which then sends impulses to different areas of the primary somatosensory cortex, located in the parietal lobe. Information about skin sensations also goes to areas such as the anterior portion of the cingulate gyrus (see Figure 3.10) and insular cortex, which respond only to the pleasantness of the sensation, not the sensation itself (Case et al., 2016).

Two parallel strips along the somatosensory cortex respond mostly to touch on the skin. Two other parallel strips respond mostly to deep pressure and movement of the joints and muscles (Kaas, 1983). In short, various aspects of body

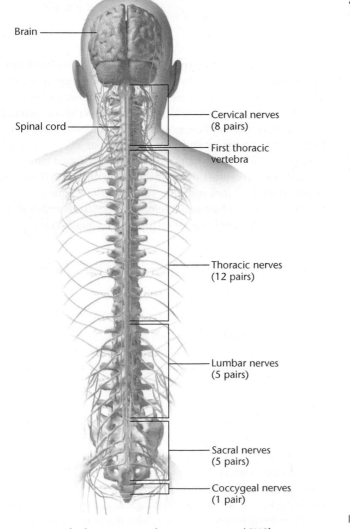

Figure 6.13 The human central nervous system (CNS)
Spinal nerves from each segment of the spinal cord exit through the correspondingly numbered opening between vertebrae.
(© Argosy Publishing Inc.)

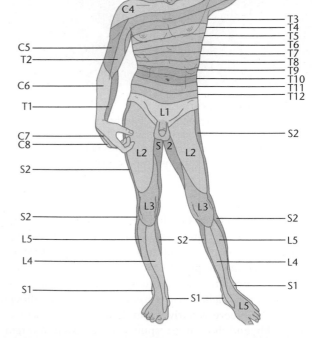

Figure 6.14 Dermatomes innervated by the 31 sensory spinal nerves
Areas I, II, and III of the face are not innervated by the spinal nerves but instead by three branches of the fifth cranial nerve. Although this figure shows distinct borders, the dermatomes actually overlap one another by about one-third to one-half of their width.

sensation remain mostly separate all the way to the cortex. Along each strip of somatosensory cortex, each subarea responds to a particular area of the body, as shown in Figure 3.23.

The primary somatosensory cortex is essential for touch experiences. When weak, brief stimuli are applied to the fingers, people are conscious of only those that produce a certain level of arousal in the primary somatosensory cortex (Palva, Linkenkaer-Hansen, Näätänen, & Palva, 2005). If someone touches you quickly on two nearby points on the hand, you will probably have an illusory experience of a single touch midway between those two points. When that happens, the activity in the primary somatosensory cortex corresponds to that midway point (Chen, Friedman, & Roe, 2003). In other words, the activity corresponds to what you experience, not what has actually stimulated your receptors.

Damage to the somatosensory cortex impairs body perceptions. A patient who had damage in the somatosensory cortex had trouble putting her clothes on correctly. Also she could not point correctly in response to such directions as "show me your elbow," although she pointed correctly to objects in the room. When told to touch her elbow, her most frequent response was to feel her wrist and arm and suggest that the elbow was probably around there, somewhere (Sirigu, Grafman, Bressler, & Sunderland, 1991).

One patient had an illness that destroyed all the myelinated somatosensory axons from below his nose but spared his unmyelinated axons. He still felt temperature, pain, and itch, because they depend on the unmyelinated axons. However, he had no conscious perception of touch, which depends on myelinated axons. Curiously, if someone lightly stroked his skin, he experienced a vague sense of pleasure. Recordings from his brain indicated no arousal of his primary somatosensory cortex but increased activity in the insular cortex, which responds to light touch and other pleasant emotional experiences (Björnsdotter, Löken, Olausson, Vallbo, & Wessberg, 2009). Evidently, unmyelinated axons conveyed enough activity to the insular cortex to produce the emotional aspect of touch even though he had no conscious sensation of the touch itself.

STOP & CHECK

13. In what way is somatosensation several senses instead of one?
14. What evidence suggests that the somatosensory cortex is essential for the conscious perception of touch?
15. How do the responses to skin sensations differ between the somatosensory cortex and the insular cortex or the anterior cingulate cortex?

ANSWERS 13. We have several types of receptors, sensitive to touch, heat, and so forth, and different parts of the somatosensory cortex respond to different kinds of skin stimulation. 14. People are conscious of only those touch stimuli that produce sufficient arousal in the primary somatosensory cortex. Also, cells in the somatosensory cortex respond to what someone experiences, even if it is an illusion. 15. The somatosensory cortex is necessary for conscious perception of the location and type of skin sensation. The insular cortex and anterior cingulate cortex respond to the pleasantness.

Pain

Many sensations sometimes evoke strong emotions, but pain is unique among senses because it *always* evokes an emotion, an unpleasant one. Pain and depression are closely linked. People in pain are likely to become depressed and unmotivated (Schwartz et al., 2014). People who are depressed become more sensitive to pain. Economic insecurity leads to depression and makes a pain feel worse (Chou, Parmar, & Galinsky, 2016). Even a signal that suggests possible danger increases pain (Harvie et al., 2015). Some languages do not have a separate word for depressed; they describe a depressed state of mind as "sick" or "pained." Also, pain and depression are both sensitive to placebo effects. But more about that issue later.

Have you ever wondered why morphine decreases pain after surgery but not during the surgery itself? Or why some people seem to tolerate pain so much better than others? Or why even the slightest touch on sunburned skin is so painful? Research on pain addresses these and other questions.

Stimuli and Spinal Cord Paths

Pain sensation begins with the least specialized of all receptors, a bare nerve ending (see Figure 6.11). Because the axons carrying pain information have little or no myelin, they conduct impulses relatively slowly, in the range of 2 to 20 meters per second (m/s). The thicker and faster axons convey sharp pain. The thinner ones convey duller pain, such as postsurgical pain. Mild pain releases the neurotransmitter glutamate, whereas stronger pain releases glutamate but also certain neuropeptides including substance P and CGRP (calcitonin gene-related peptide).

The pain-sensitive cells in the spinal cord relay information to several sites in the brain. One path extends to the ventral posterior nucleus of the thalamus and then to the somatosensory cortex. The spinal paths for pain and touch are parallel, but with one important difference, as illustrated in Figure 6.15: The pain pathway crosses immediately from receptors on one side of the body to a tract ascending the contralateral side of the spinal cord. Touch information travels up the ipsilateral side of the spinal cord to the medulla, and then crosses to the contralateral side. Consider what happens to pain and touch if someone receives a cut that goes halfway through the spinal cord. You can reason out the answer in the next Stop & Check question.

STOP & CHECK

16. Suppose you suffer a cut through the spinal cord on the right side only. For the part of the body below that cut, will you lose pain sensation on the left side or the right side? Will you lose touch sensation on the left side or the right side?

ANSWER 16. You will lose pain sensation on the left side of the body because pain information crosses the spinal cord at once. You will lose touch sensation on the right side because touch pathways remain on the ipsilateral side until they reach the medulla.

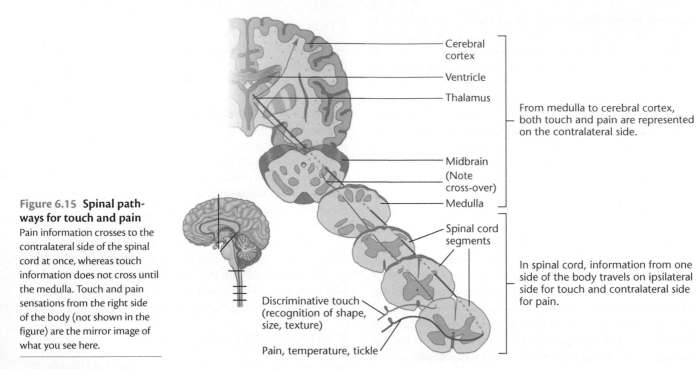

Figure 6.15 Spinal pathways for touch and pain
Pain information crosses to the contralateral side of the spinal cord at once, whereas touch information does not cross until the medulla. Touch and pain sensations from the right side of the body (not shown in the figure) are the mirror image of what you see here.

Cerebral cortex

Ventricle

Thalamus

From medulla to cerebral cortex, both touch and pain are represented on the contralateral side.

Midbrain (Note cross-over)

Medulla

Spinal cord segments

In spinal cord, information from one side of the body travels on ipsilateral side for touch and contralateral side for pain.

Discriminative touch (recognition of shape, size, texture)

Pain, temperature, tickle

Emotional Pain

In addition to the somatosensory cortex, painful stimuli also activate a path that goes through the medulla, and then to the thalamus, and then to the amygdala, hippocampus, prefrontal cortex, and anterior cingulate cortex (see Figure 6.16). These areas react not to the sensation itself but to its emotional aspect (Hunt & Mantyh, 2001). If you watch someone—especially

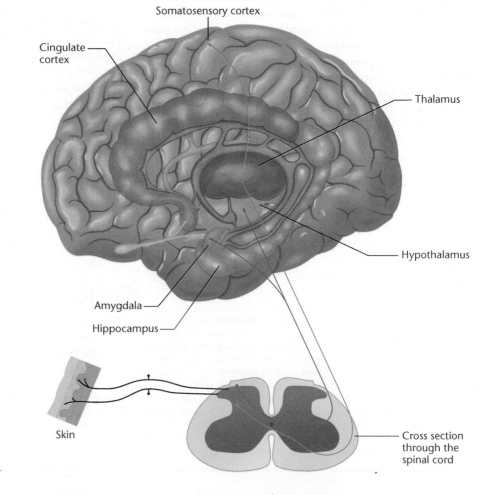

Somatosensory cortex

Cingulate cortex

Thalamus

Hypothalamus

Amygdala

Hippocampus

Skin

Cross section through the spinal cord

Figure 6.16 Pain messages in the human brain
A pathway to the thalamus, and from there to the somatosensory cortex, conveys the sensory aspects of pain. A separate pathway to the hypothalamus, amygdala, and cingulate cortex produces the emotional aspects.
(Source: Hunt & Mantyh, 2001)

someone you care about—experiencing pain, you experience sympathetic pain that shows up as activity in your cingulate cortex and other cortical areas (Corradi-Dell'Acqua, Hofstetter, & Vuilleumier, 2011; Singer et al., 2004). A hypnotic suggestion to feel no pain decreases the responses in the cingulate cortex without much effect on the somatosensory cortex (Rainville, Duncan, Price, Carrier, & Bushnell, 1997). That is, someone responding to a hypnotic sensation feels the painful sensation almost normally but reacts with emotional indifference. People with damage to the cingulate gyrus still feel pain, but it no longer distresses them (Foltz & White, 1962).

Sometimes you might say that someone hurt your feelings. After a romantic breakup, you might say you feel emotional pain. Is it just an expression, or is emotional distress really like pain?

Hurt feelings do resemble physical pain in several regards. Imagine yourself in this experiment: You sit in front of a computer screen, playing a virtual ball-tossing game with two people your own age. You "catch" a ball and then "throw" it to one of the others, who then tosses it back to someone. Unbeknownst to you, the other two have been paid to play certain roles. At first they throw it to you a fair share of times, but before long they start passing it back and forth between the two of them, leaving you out. Not much is at stake here, but the experience reminds you of all those times when people left you out of a conversation, times when people didn't invite you to their parties, and so forth since early childhood. It hurts. Experimenters monitored people's brain activity during this virtual ball-throwing task and found significantly increased activity in the cingulate cortex, an area responsive to the emotional aspects of pain (Eisenberger, Lieberman, & Williams, 2003).

What happens with more intense hurt feelings? Experimenters measured brain activity while young adults remembered a recent romantic breakup, made more intense by looking at a photo of the ex-boyfriend or ex-girlfriend. In this case, the hurt feelings showed up as activity in both the emotional areas (especially the cingulate cortex) and the sensory areas responsive to physical pain (Kross, Berman, Mischel, Smith, & Wager, 2011).

Hurt feelings are like real pain in another way: You can relieve hurt feelings with pain-relieving drugs such as acetaminophen (Tylenol®)! Researchers repeated the virtual ball-tossing study, but gave some people acetaminophen and the others a placebo. Those taking acetaminophen showed much less response in the cingulate cortex and other emotionally responsive areas. The researchers also asked college students to keep daily records about hurt feelings and social pain, while some took daily acetaminophen pills and others took a placebo. Those taking acetaminophen reported fewer cases of hurt feelings, and the frequency of hurt feelings declined over days as they continued taking the pills (De Wall et al., 2010). In short, hurt feelings are a great deal like physical hurt. (The next time someone says you hurt their feelings, just tell them to quit complaining and take a Tylenol!) However, there is a price to pay: People taking acetaminophen also decrease their evaluations of positive experiences (Durso, Luttrell, & Way, 2015). Under the influence of that pill, the bad experiences are not as bad, and the good experiences are not as good.

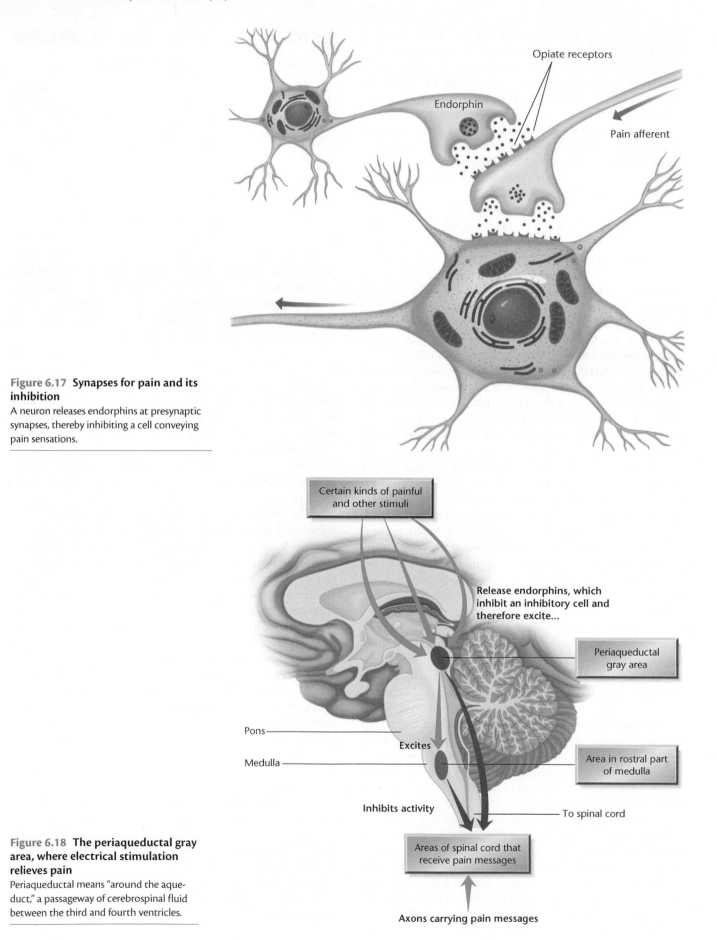

Figure 6.17 Synapses for pain and its inhibition
A neuron releases endorphins at presynaptic synapses, thereby inhibiting a cell conveying pain sensations.

Opiate receptors

Endorphin

Pain afferent

Certain kinds of painful and other stimuli

Release endorphins, which inhibit an inhibitory cell and therefore excite...

Periaqueductal gray area

Pons

Excites

Medulla

Area in rostral part of medulla

Inhibits activity

To spinal cord

Areas of spinal cord that receive pain messages

Axons carrying pain messages

Figure 6.18 The periaqueductal gray area, where electrical stimulation relieves pain
Periaqueductal means "around the aqueduct," a passageway of cerebrospinal fluid between the third and fourth ventricles.

pain receptors also receive input from touch receptors and from axons descending from the brain. These other inputs can close the "gates" for the pain messages—and they do so at least partly by releasing endorphins. You have no doubt noticed that when you have an injury, you can decrease the pain by gently rubbing the skin around it or by concentrating on something else.

Morphine does not affect large-diameter axons that convey sharp pain. For that reason, morphine is ineffective against the sharp pain of a surgeon's knife. However, morphine does block messages from thinner axons that convey slower, duller pain such as postsurgical pain (Taddese, Nah, & McCleskey, 1995).

Cannabinoids and Capsaicin

Morphine and other opiates are effective pain reducers, but they have limitations. For example, prolonged treatment of pain with morphine activates parts of the immune system, with results that include an *increase* in sensitivity to pain (Grace et al., 2016). Thus, researchers search for other ways to relieve pain. Cannabinoids—chemicals derived from or similar to marijuana—block certain kinds of pain. However, cannabinoids can produce problems of their own, including memory impairment (Viñals et al., 2015), and research on cannabinoids for pain relief has not been extensive.

Unlike opiates, cannabinoids act mainly in the periphery of the body rather than the CNS. Researchers found that if they deleted the cannabinoid receptors in the peripheral nervous system of laboratory animals while leaving the receptors intact in the CNS, cannabinoids lost most of their ability to decrease pain (Agarwal et al., 2007).

Another approach uses capsaicin, a chemical in jalapeños and similar peppers that stimulates receptors for heat. Capsaicin rubbed onto a sore shoulder, an arthritic joint, or other painful area produces a temporary burning sensation followed by a longer period of decreased pain. When applied in high doses, or at lower doses for a prolonged period, capsaicin causes an excessive buildup of calcium in heat receptors, and damages the mitochondria in those receptors, rendering the cell nonfunctional for a substantial time (Anand & Bley, 2011).

Do not try eating hot peppers to reduce pain in, say, your legs. The capsaicin you eat passes through the digestive system without entering the blood. Therefore, eating it will not relieve your pain—unless the pain is in your tongue (Karrer & Bartoshuk, 1991).

Placebos

In much medical research, an experimental group receives a potentially active treatment and the control group receives a **placebo,** a drug or other procedure with no pharmacological effects. Placebos have little influence on most conditions, but they often relieve pain, depression, and anxiety (Hróbjartsson & Gøtzsche, 2001; Wager & Atlas, 2015). People who receive placebos do not just *say* the pain decreased; scans of the brain and spinal cord also show a decreased response (Eippert, Finsterbusch, Binget, & Büchel, 2009). Conversely, if someone is told to expect pain to increase, the nervous system increases its response (Geuter & Büchel, 2013; Koban & Wager, 2016). Placebos reduce pain but they produce an even greater effect on the

emotional response to pain, as recorded in the cingulate cortex (Petrovic, Kalso, Petersson, & Ingvar, 2002; Wager, Scott, & Zubieta, 2007). They also reduce the emotional response to watching someone else in pain (Rütgen, Seidel, Riecansky, & Lamm, 2015). Oddly, placebos can reduce pain even when people know they are receiving a placebo. The physician can say that this is just a placebo but many people respond well to a placebo, and sure enough, that is the result (Rosenzweig, 2016).

Although placebos decrease pain partly by relaxation, that is not the whole explanation. In one study, people were given painful injections into both hands and both feet. They were also given a placebo cream on one hand or foot and told that it was a powerful painkiller. People reported decreased pain in the area that got the placebo but normal pain on the other three extremities (Benedetti, Arduino, & Amanzio, 1999). If placebos were simply producing relaxation, the relaxation should have affected all four extremities. Distraction is not the whole explanation, either. Distraction plus placebo relieves pain more than distraction alone does (Buhle, Stevens, Friedman, & Wager, 2012). A placebo increases activity in parts of the prefrontal cortex, suggesting that a placebo exerts its effects by top-down control of sensations and emotions (Meyer et al., 2015).

STOP & CHECK

18. Why do opiates relieve dull pain but not sharp pain?
19. How do the pain-relieving effects of cannabinoids differ from those of opiates?
20. Which aspect of pain is most responsive to relief by placebos?

ANSWERS

18. Endorphins block messages from the thinnest pain fibers, conveying dull pain, but not from thicker fibers, carrying sharp pain. 19. Unlike opiates, cannabinoids exert most of their pain-relieving effects in the peripheral nervous system, not the CNS. 20. Placebos primarily relieve the emotional aspect of pain.

Sensitization of Pain

If you have ever been sunburned, you remember how even a light touch on that sunburned skin became dreadfully painful. Damaged or inflamed tissue, such as sunburned skin, releases histamine, nerve growth factor, and other chemicals that help repair the damage but also magnify the responses of nearby heat and pain receptors (Chuang et al., 2001; Devor, 1996; Tominaga et al., 1998). Nonsteroidal anti-inflammatory drugs, such as ibuprofen, relieve pain by reducing the release of chemicals from damaged tissues (Hunt & Mantyh, 2001).

Some people suffer chronic pain long after an injury has healed. As we shall see in the chapter on memory, a barrage of stimulation to a neuron can potentiate its synaptic receptors so that they respond more vigorously to the same input in the future. That mechanism is central to learning and memory, but unfortunately, pain activates the same mechanism. A barrage of painful stimuli potentiates the cells responsive to pain so that they respond more vigorously to similar stimulation in the future (Bliss, Collingridge, Kaang, & Zhuo, 2016). In effect, the brain learns how to feel pain, and it gets better at it.

Therefore, to prevent chronic pain, it helps to limit pain from the start. Suppose you are about to undergo major surgery. Which approach is best?

1. Take medication to relieve pain before the surgery.
2. Begin medication soon after awakening from surgery.
3. Postpone the medication as long as possible and take as little as possible.

Perhaps surprisingly, the research supports answer 1: Take a pain-relieving treatment before the surgery (Coderre, Katz, Vaccarino, & Melzack, 1993). Allowing pain messages to bombard the brain during and after the surgery increases the sensitivity of the pain nerves and their receptors (Malmberg, Chen, Tonagawa, & Basbaum, 1997). People who begin taking morphine or other medications before surgery need less help afterward.

STOP & CHECK

21. How do ibuprofen and other nonsteroidal anti-inflammatory drugs decrease pain?
22. In what way is chronic pain like memory?

ANSWERS

21. Anti-inflammatory drugs block the release of chemicals from damaged tissues, which would otherwise magnify the effects of pain receptors. 22. One mechanism for memory is that repeated stimulation at a synapse increases its later response to the same type of stimulation. Similarly, repeated pain messages increase a synapse's response to similar stimuli, and therefore the result is chronic pain.

Itch

Have you ever wondered, "What is itch, anyway? Is it a kind of pain? A kind of touch? Or something else altogether?" The answer is, itch is a separate sensation. Researchers have identified special receptors for itch (Y.-G. Sun et al., 2009) and two spinal cord paths conveying itch (Bourane et al., 2015).

You have two kinds of itch that feel about the same, although their causes are different. First, when you have mild tissue damage, such as when your skin is healing after a cut, your skin releases histamines that dilate blood vessels and produce an itching sensation. Second, contact with certain plants, especially

cowhage (a tropical plant with barbed hairs), also produces itch. Antihistamines block the itch that histamines cause but not the itch that cowhage causes. Conversely, rubbing the skin with capsaicin relieves the itch that cowhage causes, but it has little effect on the itch that histamine causes (Johanek et al., 2007).

The itch receptors are slow to respond, and when they do, their axons transmit impulses at the unusually slow velocity of only half a meter per second. At that rate, an action potential from your foot needs 3 or 4 seconds to reach your head. Imagine the delay for a giraffe or an elephant. You might try lightly rubbing some rough leaves against your ankle. Note how soon you feel the touch sensation and how much more slowly you notice the itch.

Itch is useful because it directs you to scratch the itchy area and remove whatever is irritating your skin. Vigorous scratching produces mild pain, and pain inhibits itch (Davidson, Zhang, Khasabov, Simone, & Giesler, 2009). Opiates, which decrease pain, increase itch (Andrew & Craig, 2001; Y. Liu et al., 2010; Moser & Giesler, 2013). This inhibitory relationship between pain and itch is clear evidence that itch is not a type of pain. Further evidence is the demonstration that blocking itch fibers does not reduce pain (Roberson et al., 2013).

This research helps explain an experience that you may have noticed. When a dentist gives you Novocain before drilling a tooth, part of your face becomes numb. An hour or more later, as the drug's effects start to wear off, you may feel an itchy sensation in the numb portion of your face. But when you try to scratch it, you feel nothing because the touch and pain sensations are still numb. Evidently, the effects of Novocain wear off faster for itch than for touch and pain. The fact that you can feel itch at this time is evidence that it is not just a form of touch or pain. It is interesting that scratching the partly numb skin does not relieve the itch. Evidently, scratching has to produce some pain to decrease the itch.

STOP & CHECK

23. Do opiates increase or decrease itch sensations?
24. Suppose someone suffers from constant itching. What kinds of drugs might help relieve it?

ANSWERS

23. Opiates increase itch by blocking pain sensations. (Pain decreases itch.) 24. Two kinds of drugs might help—histamines or capsaicin—depending on the source of the itch.

The Mechanical Senses

The mechanical senses alert you to important information, from heat to cold and from pain to gentle, pleasant touch. The system consists of many receptors, spinal paths, and

brain areas. Yet we perceive all this information together—for instance, when you feel the shape and temperature of an object.

You also integrate touch with other senses. For example, suppose someone touches you so lightly that you don't feel it. If at the same time you see a picture of someone touching you in just that way, facilitation by what you see enables you to feel the touch (Serino, Pizzoferrato, & Làdavas, 2008). All the senses combine to give a unified experience.

Summary

1. The vestibular system detects the position and acceleration of the head and adjusts body posture and eye movements accordingly. **199**

2. The somatosensory system has receptors that detect several kinds of stimulation of the skin and internal tissues. **199**

3. The brain maintains several parallel somatosensory representations of the body. **202**

4. Activity in the primary somatosensory cortex corresponds to what someone is experiencing, even if it is illusory. **203**

5. Injurious stimuli excite pain receptors, which are bare nerve endings. **203**

6. Painful information takes two routes to the brain. A route leading to the somatosensory cortex conveys the sensory information, including location in the body. A route to the anterior cingulate cortex conveys the emotional aspect. **204**

7. Hurt feelings are like pain. They activate the cingulate cortex, as physical pain does, and acetaminophen relieves both hurt feelings and physical pain. **205**

8. Opiate drugs attach to the brain's endorphin receptors. Endorphins decrease pain by blocking activity of pain neurons. Both pleasant and unpleasant experiences release endorphins. **205**

9. A harmful stimulus may give rise to a greater or lesser degree of pain depending on other current and recent stimuli. According to the gate theory of pain, other stimuli close gates in the spinal cord and block the transmission of pain. **205**

10. Placebos decrease pain, especially the emotional aspect of pain. They do so by top-down control from the prefrontal cortex. **207**

11. Chronic pain bombards pain synapses with repetitive input, and increases their responsiveness to later stimuli through a process like learning. Morphine is most effective as a painkiller if it is used promptly. Allowing the nervous system to be bombarded with prolonged pain messages increases the later sensitivity to pain. **207**

12. Itch is relayed to the brain by spinal cord pathways separate from pain and touch. The axons for itch transmit impulses more slowly than other sensations. They can be inhibited by pain messages. **208**

Key Terms

Terms are defined in the module on the page number indicated. They're also presented in alphabetical order with definitions in the book's Subject Index/Glossary, which begins on page 589. Interactive flash cards, audio reviews, and crossword puzzles are among the online resources available to help you learn these terms and the concepts they represent.

capsaicin **201**
dermatome **202**
endorphins **205**
gate theory **205**

opioid mechanisms **205**
Pacinian corpuscle **200**
periaqueductal gray area **205**
placebo **207**

semicircular canals **199**
somatosensory system **199**

Thought Question

How could you determine whether hypnosis releases endorphins?

Module 6.2 | End of Module Quiz

1. The vestibular system is responsible for which of these observations about behavior?
   A. Foods have stronger taste while they are hot than while the same foods are cold.
   B. You can localize sounds well in the air, but poorly when you are under water.
   C. You can describe the positions of your hands and feet without looking at them.
   D. You can read a page better while shaking your head than while shaking the page.

2. Under which of these circumstances would the semicircular canals respond most vigorously?

   A. When you are lying in an unusual, uncomfortable position

   B. When you are moving at a slow, steady speed

   C. When you are moving at a rapid, steady speed

   D. When you are moving and changing speed

3. To what extent does the nervous system maintain separate representations of touch, heat, pain, and other aspects of somatic sensation?

   A. Not at all. A single kind of receptor responds to all kinds of somatic sensation.

   B. The receptors vary, but all kinds of sensation merge in the spinal cord.

   C. The spinal cord maintains separate representations, but the various types merge in the cerebral cortex.

   D. Different types of sensation remain separate even in the cerebral cortex.

4. In which of these ways do coldness receptors differ from heat receptors?

   A. Coldness receptors respond to a change in temperature, not to the absolute temperature.

   B. The response of a coldness receptor grows stronger and stronger until you find a warmer place.

   C. Coldness receptors also respond to certain chemicals, whereas heat receptors do not.

   D. Coldness receptors respond only to life-threatening levels of cold.

5. What does the anterior cingulate cortex contribute to both the sense of touch and the sense of pain?

   A. It responds to an increase or decrease of the sensation, not the absolute level.

   B. It responds to the emotional aspect of the sensation.

   C. It stores a memory of the sensation.

   D. It compares touch or pain to visual and auditory sensations.

6. Suppose you suffer a cut through the spinal cord on the left side only. For the part of the body below that cut, you will lose pain sensation on the right side of the body and touch sensation on the left side. Why?

   A. The left side of the body is more sensitive to pain than the right side is.

   B. The right side of the body is more sensitive to pain than the left side is.

   C. Pain axons cross the spinal cord at once, but touch fibers do not.

   D. Pain axons regrow after injury, but touch axons do not.

7. Certain drugs that relieve pain also relieve which of the following?

   A. Itch

   B. Attention deficit disorder

   C. Hurt feelings

   D. Narcolepsy

8. In what way does pain relief by cannabinoids differ from pain relief by opiates?

   A. Cannabinoids act on the periphery, not the brain.

   B. Cannabinoids produce no unwanted side effects.

   C. The benefits of cannabinoids are mostly placebo effects.

   D. Cannabinoids act mainly by effects on the medulla.

9. Do placebos relieve pain just by relaxation? And what is the evidence?

   A. Yes. People who are already relaxed gain no benefits from placebos.

   B. Yes. Placebos are effective only for people who are high in neuroticism.

   C. No. A placebo can relieve pain in one body part without affecting another.

   D. No. People who take a placebo become even more nervous than before.

10. Why do many people suffer chronic pain long after an injury has healed?

    A. The brain has learned to increase its pain perception.

    B. The skin exhausts its supply of histamine.

    C. They took morphine too soon after a surgical operation.

    D. The blood flow to the injured area did not increase.

11. Which type of sensation inhibits itch sensations?

    A. Olfaction

    B. Taste

    C. Pain

    D. Hearing

Answers: 1D, 2D, 3D, 4A, 5B, 6C, 7C, 8A, 9C, 10A, 11C.

The Chemical Senses

Suppose you had the godlike power to create a new species of animal, but you could equip it with only one sensory system. Which sense would you give it?

Your first impulse might be to choose vision or hearing because of their importance to humans. But an animal with only one sensory system is not going to be much like humans, is it? And if you had only vision, and never tasted anything or felt pain or touch, would you have any idea what those visual stimuli meant? To have any chance of survival, your animal will have to be small, slow, and maybe even one-celled. What sense will be most useful to such an animal?

Theorists believe that the first sensory system of the earliest animals was a chemical sensitivity (Parker, 1922). A chemical sense enables a small animal to find food, avoid certain kinds of danger, and even locate mates.

Now imagine that you have to choose one of your senses to lose. Which one will it be? Most of us would not choose to lose vision, hearing, or touch. Losing pain sensitivity can be dangerous. You might choose to sacrifice your smell or taste.

Curious, isn't it? If an animal is going to survive with only one sense, it almost has to be a chemical sense, and yet to humans, with many other well-developed senses, the chemical senses seem dispensable. Perhaps we underestimate their importance.

Taste

Vision, hearing, and touch provide information useful for many purposes, but taste is useful for just one function, telling us whether to swallow something or spit it out. That function is more important for some species than for others. Dolphins have almost no taste receptors (Jiang et al., 2012). Because they eat only fish, and swallow them whole, they have little need for the sense of taste. Cats, hyenas, seals, and sea lions have no sweetness receptors (Jiang et al., 2012). Being carnivores (meat eaters), they never choose their food by sweetness. If you see a cat lapping up milk, it is going for the proteins or fats, not the sweetness.

Taste results from stimulation of the **taste buds,** the receptors on the tongue. When we talk about the taste of food, we generally mean flavor, which is a combination of taste and smell. Whereas other senses remain separate throughout the cortex, taste and smell axons converge onto many of the same cells in an area called the endopiriform cortex (Fu, Sugai, Yoshimura, & Onoda, 2004). That convergence enables taste and smell to combine their influences on food selection.

Taste Receptors

The receptors for taste are not true neurons but modified skin cells. Like neurons, taste receptors have excitable membranes and release neurotransmitters to excite neighboring neurons, which in turn transmit information to the brain. Like skin cells, however, taste receptors are gradually sloughed off and replaced, each one lasting about 10 to 14 days (Kinnamon, 1987).

Mammalian taste receptors are in taste buds located in **papillae** on the surface of the tongue (see Figure 6.19). A given papilla may contain up to 10 or more taste buds (Arvidson & Friberg, 1980), and each taste bud contains about 50 receptor cells.

In adult humans, taste buds lie mainly along the edge of the tongue. You can demonstrate this principle as follows: Soak a small cotton swab in sugar water, salt water, or vinegar. Then touch it lightly on the center of your tongue, not too far toward the back. If you get the position right, you will experience little or no taste. Then try it again on the edge of your tongue and notice the taste.

TRY IT YOURSELF

Now change the procedure a bit. Wash your mouth out with water and prepare a cotton swab as before. Touch the soaked portion to one edge of your tongue and then slowly stroke it to the center of your tongue. It will seem as if you are moving the taste to the center of your tongue. In fact, you are getting only a touch sensation from the center of your tongue. You attribute the taste you had on the side of your tongue to every other spot you stroke (Bartoshuk, 1991).

How Many Kinds of Taste Receptors?

Traditionally, people in Western society have described tastes in terms of sweet, sour, salty, and bitter. However, some tastes defy categorization in terms of these four labels (Schiffman & Erickson, 1980; Schiffman, McElroy, & Erickson, 1980). How could we determine how many kinds of taste we have?

One way to identify taste receptor types is to find procedures that alter one receptor but not others. For example,

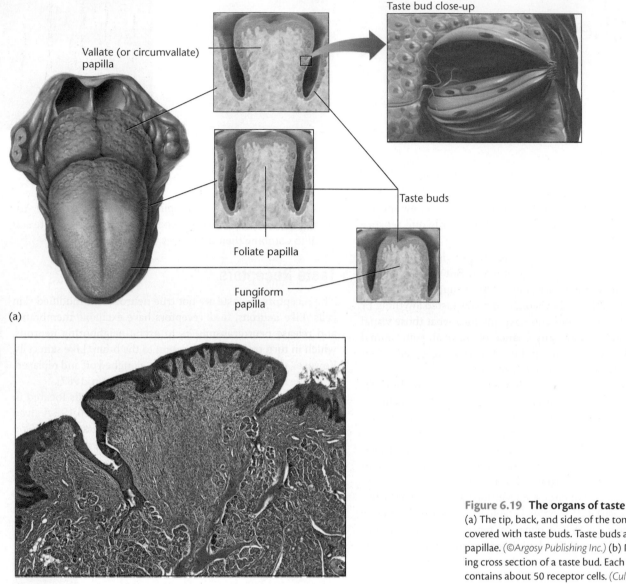

(a)

(b)

Figure 6.19 The organs of taste
(a) The tip, back, and sides of the tongue are covered with taste buds. Taste buds are located in papillae. *(©Argosy Publishing Inc.)* (b) Photo showing cross section of a taste bud. Each taste bud contains about 50 receptor cells. *(Cultura Science/ Alvin Telser, PhD/Oxford Scientific/Getty Images)*

chewing a miracle berry (native to West Africa) gives little taste itself but temporarily changes sweet receptors. Miracle berries contain a protein—miraculin—that modifies sweet receptors, enabling acids to stimulate them (Bartoshuk, Gentile, Moskowitz, & Meiselman, 1974). If you try miracle berry extracts (available via the Internet), anything acidic will taste sweet in addition to its usual sour taste for the next half hour. Some people use these extracts as diet aids, so they can get sweet tastes without the calories.

But don't overdo it. A colleague and I once spent an evening experimenting with miracle berries. We drank straight lemon juice, sauerkraut juice, even vinegar. All tasted extremely sweet, but we awoke the next day with mouths full of ulcers. Those things are still acids, even when they taste sweet.

Have you ever drunk orange juice just after brushing your teeth? How could something so wonderful suddenly taste so bad? Most toothpastes contain sodium lauryl sulfate, a chemical that intensifies bitter tastes and weakens sweet ones, apparently by coating the sweet receptors and preventing anything from reaching them (DeSimone, Heck, & Bartoshuk, 1980; Schiffman, 1983).

Another taste-modifying substance is an extract from the plant *Gymnema sylvestre* (Frank, Mize, Kennedy, de los Santos, & Green, 1992). Some health food and herbal remedy stores sell dried leaves of *Gymnema sylvestre*, from which you can brew a tea. (*Gymnema sylvestre* pills won't work for this demonstration.) Soak your tongue in the tea for about 30 seconds and then try tasting various substances. Salty, sour, and bitter substances taste the same as usual, but sugar becomes tasteless. Candies taste sour, bitter, or salty. (Those tastes were already present, but you barely noticed them because of the sweetness.) Curiously, the artificial sweetener aspartame (NutraSweet®) loses only some, not all, of its sweetness, implying that it stimulates an additional receptor besides the sugar receptor (Schroeder & Flannery-Schroeder, 2005). Note: This demonstration is probably risky for anyone with diabetes, because *Gymnema sylvestre* also alters sugar absorption in the intestines. Also note: One side effect of this demonstration is greenish bowel movements for the next few days. Don't panic if you notice that little souvenir of your experience. The overall point of these demonstrations is that we do have receptors that are sensitive to one taste or another.

Further evidence for separate types of taste receptors comes from studies of the following type: Soak your tongue for 15 seconds in a sour solution, such as unsweetened lemon juice. Then try tasting some other sour solution, such as dilute vinegar. You will find that the second solution tastes less sour than usual, and perhaps not sour at all. This phenomenon, called **adaptation,** reflects the fatigue of receptors sensitive to sour tastes. Now try tasting something salty, sweet, or bitter. These substances taste about the same as usual. In short, you fail to show **cross-adaptation**—reduced response to one taste after exposure to another (McBurney & Bartoshuk, 1973). Evidently, the sour receptors are different from the other taste receptors. Similarly, you can show that salt receptors are different from the others and so forth.

Although we have long known that people have at least four kinds of taste receptors, several types of evidence suggest a fifth, glutamate, as in monosodium glutamate (MSG). The tongue has a glutamate receptor that resembles the receptors for glutamate as a neurotransmitter (Chaudhari, Landin, & Roper, 2000). Recall the idea that evolution is "thrifty": After something evolves for one purpose, it can be modified for other purposes. Glutamate tastes somewhat like unsalted chicken broth. The English language had no word for this taste, so English-speaking researchers adopted the Japanese word *umami*.

Perhaps we have a sixth type of taste also, the taste of fats. When people taste long-chain fatty acids, they say the taste is not sweet, sour, salty, nor bitter, and only slightly resembles umami. Researchers did their best to make sure people were responding to a taste experience, and not just a texture. They suggested the term *oleogustus* for the taste of fats (Running, Craig, & Mattes, 2015). We shall see whether that term becomes popular.

In addition to the fact that different chemicals excite different receptors, they produce different rhythms of action potentials. For other senses we assume—rightly or wrongly—that what matters is the number of action potentials per unit of time. In taste, the temporal pattern is also important, perhaps more important. Figure 6.20 shows the responses of a brain neuron to five-second presentations of sucrose (sweet), NaCl (salty), HCl (sour), and quinine (bitter). This neuron responded to all four, but with different patterns over time. For example, its response to NaCl faded rapidly, whereas the response to sucrose took longer to start and then remained

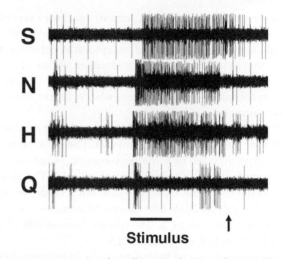

Figure 6.20 Responses of a cell in a rat brain to four tastes
Each taste was presented for 5 seconds, marked by the Stimulus line at the bottom. Responses persisted until the tongue was washed with water, at the point marked by the arrow. The four lines represent S = sucrose (sweet); N = NaCl, table salt (salty); H = HCl, hydrochloric acid (sour); and Q = quinine (bitter).
(*Source: From "Quality time: Representation of a multidimensional sensory domain through temporal coding," by P. M. Di Lorenzo, J.-Y. Chen, & J. D. Victor, 2009, Journal of Neuroscience, 29, pp. 9227–9238.*)

steady (Di Lorenzo, Chen, & Victor, 2009). Do these patterns actually code taste experiences? Yes. Researchers stimulated rats' brain cells responsive to taste with an electrical pattern matching that for quinine. The rats backed away from whatever they were drinking at the time, reacting as if they were tasting something bitter (Di Lorenzo, Leshchinsky, Moroney, & Ozdoba, 2009). Electrical stimulation at other temporal patterns did not cause this reaction.

Jalapeños and other hot peppers produce a hot mouth sensation that is not considered a taste. The evolution of hot peppers is an interesting story. Most plants produce chemicals that discourage animals from eating them. The capsaicin in hot peppers discourages mammals, but not birds, because birds' heat receptor does not respond to capsaicin. A bird that eats a jalapeño eventually excretes its seeds, undigested, along with the other components of bird poop that serve as fertilizer. That is, birds spread the seeds and nourish their growth. Mammals, in contrast, chew any seeds that they eat, rendering them inactive. In short, jalapeños and similar plants gain an advantage by discouraging mammals but permitting birds to eat them.

Mechanisms of Taste Receptors

The saltiness receptor is simple. Recall that a neuron produces an action potential when sodium ions cross its membrane. A saltiness receptor, which detects the presence of sodium, simply permits sodium ions on the tongue to cross its membrane. Chemicals that prevent sodium from crossing the membrane weaken salty tastes (DeSimone, Heck, Mierson, & DeSimone, 1984; Schiffman, Lockhead, & Maes, 1983). Sour receptors detect the presence of acids (Huang et al., 2006).

Sweetness, bitterness, and umami receptors resemble the metabotropic synapses discussed in Chapter 2. After a molecule binds to one of these receptors, it activates a G protein that releases a second messenger within the cell. People have two types of sweetness receptors and two types of umami receptors, each with somewhat different sensitivities (Barretto et al., 2015).

Bitter taste used to be a puzzle because bitter substances include a long list of dissimilar chemicals. Their only common factor is that they are to some degree toxic. What receptor could identify such a diverse set of chemicals? The answer is that we have not one bitter receptor but a family of 30 or more (Barretto et al., 2015; Matsunami, Montmayeur, & Buck, 2000). Each responds to a few related compounds (Born, Levit, Niv, Meyerhof, & Belvens, 2013).

One consequence of having so many bitter receptors is that we detect a great variety of dangerous chemicals. The other is that because each type of bitter receptor is present in small numbers, we don't detect very low concentrations of bitter substances.

Many bitter chemicals also trigger receptors in the nose, provoking coughing and sneezing if you happen to inhale them (Tizzano et al., 2010). That is, bitter chemicals are toxic, and the body does anything it can to expel them.

✓ STOP & CHECK ▅▅▅▅▅▅▅▅▅

25. Suppose you find a new, unusual-tasting food. How could you determine whether we have a special receptor for that food or whether we taste it with a combination of the other known taste receptors?

26. If someone injected into your tongue a chemical that blocks the release of second messengers, how would it affect your taste experiences?

────────────────────────────────

ANSWERS **25.** You could test for cross-adaptation. If the new taste cross-adapts with others, then it uses the same receptors. If it does not cross-adapt, it may have a receptor of its own. Another possibility would be to find some procedure that blocks this taste without blocking other tastes. **26.** The chemical would block your experiences of sweet, bitter, and umami but should not prevent you from tasting salty and sour.

────────────────────────────────

Taste Coding in the Brain

Information from the receptors in the anterior two-thirds of the tongue travels to the brain along the chorda tympani, a branch of the seventh cranial nerve (the facial nerve). Taste information from the posterior tongue and the throat travels along branches of the ninth and tenth cranial nerves. What do you suppose would happen if someone anesthetized your chorda tympani? You would no longer taste anything in the anterior part of your tongue, but you probably would not notice, because you would still taste with the posterior part. However, the probability is

about 40 percent that you would experience taste "phantoms," analogous to the phantom limb experience discussed in Chapter 4 (Yanagisawa, Bartoshuk, Catalanotto, Karrer, & Kveton, 1998). That is, you might experience taste even when nothing was on your tongue. Evidently, the inputs from the anterior and posterior parts of your tongue interact in complex ways.

The taste nerves project to the **nucleus of the tractus solitarius (NTS),** a structure in the medulla (Travers, Pfaffmann, & Norgren, 1986). From the NTS, information branches out, reaching the pons, the lateral hypothalamus, the amygdala, the ventral-posterior thalamus, and two areas of the cerebral cortex (Pritchard, Hamilton, Morse, & Norgren, 1986; Yamamoto, 1984). One of these areas, the somatosensory cortex, responds to the touch aspects of tongue stimulation. The other area, known as the insula, is the primary taste cortex. The insula in each hemisphere of the cortex receives input from both sides of the tongue (Stevenson, Miller, & McGrillen, 2013). A few of the major connections are illustrated in Figure 6.21. Certain areas of the insula are dominated by cells responding mainly to sweet tastes, whereas other areas are dominated by cells responding to bitter (Peng et al., 2015).

Variations in Taste Sensitivity

It is easy to assume that foods taste the same to someone else as they do to you. And if we ask people to describe how strong various foods taste, they agree on which foods have bland, strong, or very strong flavors. However, when you rate some food as tasting "very strong," you mean that it is strong compared to your other taste experiences, which might be stronger or weaker than someone else's. In fact, some people have three times as many taste buds as other people do on the *fungiform papillae* near the tip of the tongue (Hayes, Bartoshuk, Kidd, & Duffy, 2008). (See Figure 6.22.) That anatomical difference depends partly on genetics but also on age, hormones, and other influences. Women's taste sensitivity varies with their hormones and reaches its maximum during early pregnancy, when estradiol levels are high (Prutkin et al., 2000). That tendency is probably adaptive: During pregnancy, a woman needs to be more careful than usual to avoid harmful foods.

People with more taste buds, known as **supertasters**, tend to dislike strongly flavored foods, especially foods that taste very bitter to them, but only mildly bitter to other people. People at the opposite end, having the fewest taste buds, tolerate many somewhat bitter foods. A demonstration sometimes used in biology laboratory classes is to taste phenylthiocarbamide (PTC) or 6-*n*-propylthiouracil (PROP). Most people taste low concentrations as bitter, but people with the fewest taste buds—misleadingly known as *nontasters*—taste it only at high concentrations. One gene controls most of the variance, although other genes contribute as well (Kim et al., 2003).

Researchers have collected extensive data about the percentage of nontasters in different populations, as shown in Figure 6.23 (Guo & Reed, 2001). The figure shows no obvious

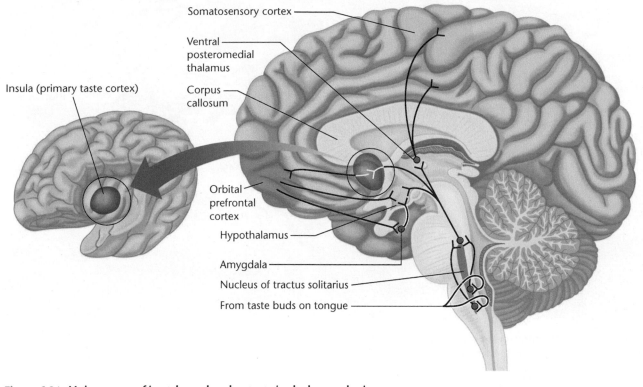

Figure 6.21 Major routes of impulses related to taste in the human brain
The thalamus and cerebral cortex receive impulses from both the left and the right sides of the tongue.
(*Source: Based on Rolls, 1995*)

relationship between tasting PTC and cuisine. For example, nontasters are common in India, where the food is spicy, and also in Britain, where it is relatively bland.

Although most supertasters avoid strong-tasting or spicy foods, you cannot confidently identify yourself as supertaster, taster, or nontaster based on just your food preferences. Culture and familiarity exert large effects on people's food preferences, in addition to the role of the taste buds.

If you would like to classify yourself as a taster, nontaster, or supertaster, follow the instructions in Table 6.2.

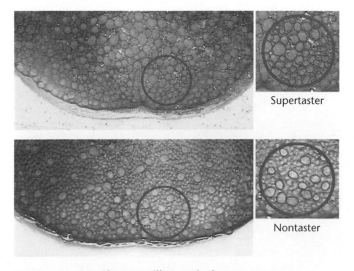

Figure 6.22 Fungiform papillae on the human tongue
People with a greater density of papillae (top) are supertasters, with strong reactions to intense tastes. People with fewer papillae are tasters or non-tasters (bottom). (*Source: Linda Bartoshuk*)

Table 6.2 | Are You a Supertaster, Taster, or Nontaster?

Equipment: ¼-inch hole punch, small piece of wax paper, cotton swab, blue food coloring, flashlight, and magnifying glass

Make a ¼-inch hole with a standard hole punch in a piece of wax paper. Dip the cotton swab in blue food coloring. Place the wax paper on the tip of your tongue, just right of the center. Rub the cotton swab over the hole in the wax paper to dye a small part of your tongue. With the flashlight and magnifying glass, have someone count the number of pink, unstained circles in the blue area. They are your fungiform papillae. Compare your results to the following averages:

Supertasters:	25 papillae
Tasters:	17 papillae
Nontasters:	10 papillae

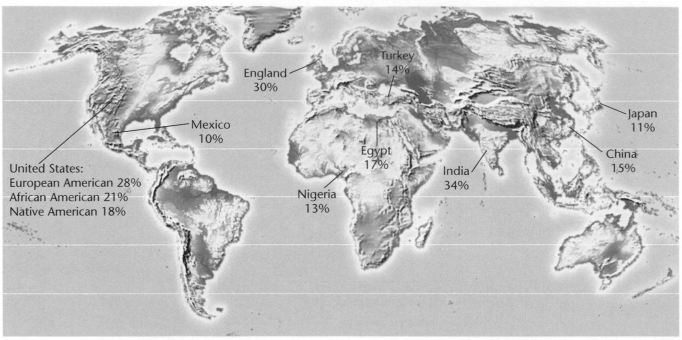

Linda Bartoshuk

Figure 6.23 Percentage of nontasters in several human populations
Most of the percentages are based on large samples, including more than 31,000 in Japan and 35,000 in India.
(*Source: Based on Guo & Reed, 2001*)

✓ **STOP & CHECK** ▬▬▬▬▬▬▬

27. Why are supertasters more sensitive to tastes than other
people are?

ANSWER   ˙spnq ǝʇsɐʇ ǝɹoɯ ǝʌɐɥ ʎǝɥ⊥ **˙**Ɫ̄Z

Olfaction

Olfaction, the sense of smell, is the response to chemicals that contact the membranes inside the nose. For most
mammals, olfaction is critical for finding food and mates
and for avoiding dangers. For example, rats and mice show
an immediate, unlearned avoidance of the smells of cats,
foxes, and other predators. Those smells also cause them
to release stress hormones (Kondoh et al., 2016). Mice that
lack the relevant olfactory receptors fail to avoid, as illustrated in Figure 6.24 (Kobayakawa et al., 2007). People with
certain diseases have a characteristic, unpleasant odor, and
people who avoid that odor decrease the risk of contagion
(Olsson et al., 2014).

Consider also the star-nosed mole and water shrew,
two species that forage along the bottom of ponds and
streams for worms, shellfish, and other invertebrates. We
might assume that olfaction would be useless under water.
However, these animals exhale tiny air bubbles onto the
ground and then inhale them again. By doing so, they can
follow an underwater trail well enough to track their prey
(Catania, 2006).

We marvel at feats like this and at the ability of a blood-
hound to find someone by following an olfactory trail through
a forest. We assume that we could never do anything like that.
Of course we cannot follow an olfactory trail while standing upright, with our noses far above the ground! But what if
you got down on your hands and knees and put your nose to

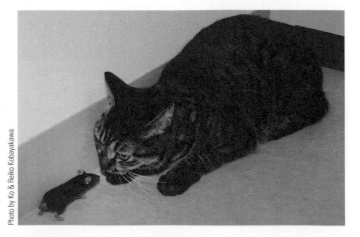

Photo by Ko & Reiko Kobayakawa

Figure 6.24 The result of losing one type of olfactory receptor
Normal mice innately avoid the smell of cats, foxes, and other predators.
This cat had just finished a large meal.
(*Source: Kobayakawa et al., 2007*)

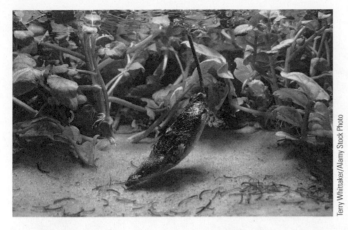

A water shrew

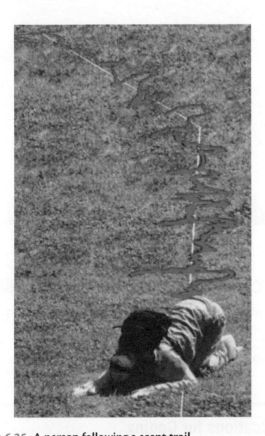

Figure 6.25 A person following a scent trail
Most people successfully followed a trail with only their nose to guide them.
(*Source: Reprinted by permission from Macmillan Publishers Ltd. From: Nature Neuroscience, 10, 27–29, Mechanisms of scent-tracking in humans; J. Porter et. al, 2007.*)

the ground? Researchers blindfolded 32 young adults, made them wear gloves, and then asked them to try to follow a scent trail across a field. The scent was chocolate oil. (They decided to use something that people care about.) Most of the participants succeeded and improved their performance with practice. Figure 6.25 shows one example (Porter et al., 2007).

So our olfaction is better than we might guess, if we give it a fair chance (even though bloodhounds are still much better).

Olfaction is especially important for our food selection. Much of the flavor of a food is really based on its odor. Try holding your nose while you eat, and notice how much flavor you lose.

Olfaction also plays an important role in social behavior. You may have heard the expression "smell of fear," and research supports that idea. Experimenters collected sweat from young men's armpits while the men watched videos that evoked fear, disgust, or no emotion. Later the researchers recorded facial expressions by young women who sniffed the samples. Women smelling the fear samples showed a mild fear expression and those who smelled the disgust samples looked disgusted. Those smelling the neutral samples showed little or no expression (de Groot, Smeets, Kaldewaij, Duijndam, & Semin, 2012). Evidently smells give us a clue to how someone else is feeling.

If you were exposed to the smells of other people (with no other information about them), and you rated their desirability as a potential romantic partner, you would probably prefer people who smell a little different from yourself and your family members (Havlicek & Roberts, 2009). Avoiding a mate who smells like your brother or sister reduces the chance of inbreeding. It also increases the probability that your children will have a good variety of immunities, because chemicals from the immune system contribute to body odors. Curiously, when women start taking contraceptive pills, their preference for a different-smelling mate decreases (Roberts, Gosling, Carter, & Petrie, 2008). One speculation is that the risk of inbreeding is unimportant for women who cannot become pregnant at that moment.

Olfactory Receptors

Researchers estimate that people can distinguish among more than a trillion olfactory stimuli. Yes, "estimate." Don't imagine some participant facing a trillion vials of odorous chemicals. On each trial, the researchers offered two vials that were the same and one that was different, and the task was to pick the one that was different. The two identical vials might have a mixture of 30 chemicals, whereas the different one had 20 of those same chemicals plus 10 other ones. From people's ability to pick out the different vial, the researchers calculated that more than a trillion distinctions are possible (Bushdid, Magnasco, Vosshall, & Keller, 2014).

The neurons responsible for smell are the **olfactory cells** that line the olfactory epithelium in the rear of the nasal air passages (see Figure 6.26). In mammals, each olfactory cell has cilia (threadlike dendrites) that extend from the cell body into the mucous surface of the nasal passage. Olfactory receptors are located on the cilia.

How many kinds of olfactory receptors do we have? Researchers answered the analogous question for color vision in the 1800s but took much longer for olfaction. Linda Buck and Richard Axel (1991) identified a family of

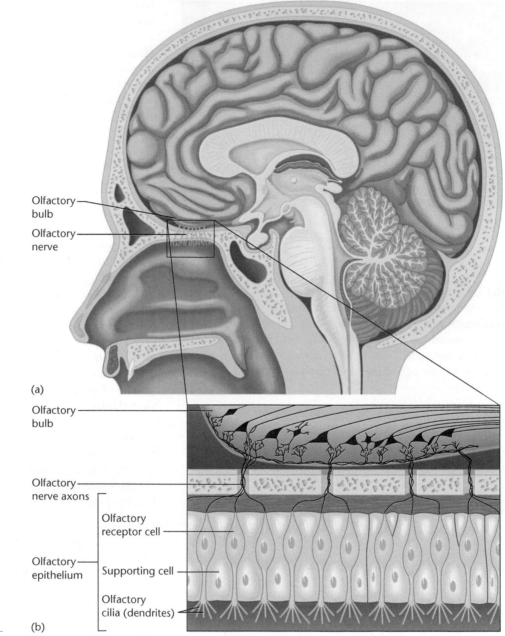

Olfactory bulb

Olfactory nerve

(a)

Olfactory bulb

Olfactory nerve axons

Olfactory epithelium

Olfactory receptor cell

Supporting cell

Olfactory cilia (dendrites)

(b)

Figure 6.26 Olfactory receptors
(a) Location of receptors in nasal cavity.
(b) Close-up of olfactory cells.

proteins in olfactory receptors, as shown in Figure 6.27. Like metabotropic neurotransmitter receptors, each of these proteins traverses the cell membrane seven times and responds to a chemical outside the cell (here an odorant molecule instead of a neurotransmitter) by triggering changes in a G protein inside the cell. The G protein then provokes chemical activities that lead to an action potential. The best estimate is that humans have several hundred olfactory receptor proteins, whereas rats and mice have about a thousand types (Zhang & Firestein, 2002). Correspondingly, rats can distinguish among odors that seem the same to humans (Rubin & Katz, 2001). Each olfactory neuron has only one of the possible olfactory receptor proteins (Hanchate et al., 2015).

STOP & CHECK

28. In what way do olfactory receptors resemble metabotropic neurotransmitter receptors?

ANSWER

28. Like metabotropic neurotransmitter receptors, an olfactory receptor acts through a G protein that triggers further events within the cell.

Implications for Coding

We have only three kinds of cones and five kinds of taste receptors, so researchers were surprised to find so many kinds of olfactory receptors. That diversity makes possible narrow

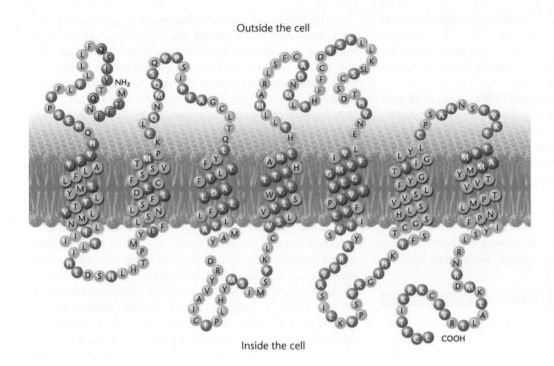

Outside the cell

Inside the cell

Figure 6.27 One of the olfactory receptor proteins This protein resembles the synaptic receptor protein in Figure 2.16. It responds to a chemical outside the cell and triggers activity of a G protein inside the cell. Different olfactory receptors differ slightly in their structure. Each little circle in this diagram represents one amino acid of the protein. The light green circles represent amino acids that are the same in most of the olfactory receptor proteins. The dark green circles represent amino acids that vary. (*Source: Based on Buck & Axel, 1991*)

specialization of functions. To illustrate, because we have only three kinds of cones, each cone contributes to every color perception. Each olfactory receptor responds to only a few stimuli. The response of one receptor might mean, "a fatty acid with a straight chain of three to five carbon atoms." The response of another might mean, "either a fatty acid or an aldehyde with a straight chain of five to seven carbon atoms" (Araneda, Kini, & Firestein, 2000; Imamura, Mataga, & Mori, 1992; Mori, Mataga, & Imamura, 1992). The combined activity of those two receptors identifies a chemical precisely.

The question may have occurred to you, "Why did evolution go to the bother of designing so many olfactory receptor types? After all, color vision gets by with just three types of cones." The main reason is that light energy can be arranged along a single dimension, wavelength. Olfaction processes airborne chemicals that do not range along a single continuum.

Messages to the Brain

When an olfactory receptor is stimulated, its axon carries an impulse to the olfactory bulb (see Figure 3.12). Although the receptors sensitive to a particular chemical are scattered haphazardly in the nose, their axons find their way to the same target cells in the olfactory bulb, such that chemicals of similar smell excite neighboring areas, and chemicals of different smell excite more separated areas (Horowitz, Saraiva, Kuang, Yoon, & Buck, 2014).

The olfactory bulb sends axons to the olfactory area of the cerebral cortex. A complex substance such as a food activates a scattered population of cells (Lin, Shea, & Katz, 2006; Rennaker, Chen, Ruyle, Sloan, & Wilson, 2007). Many cells respond strongly to a particular kind of food, such as berries or melons (Yoshida & Mori, 2007). As in the olfactory bulb,

chemicals that smell similar to us evoke activity in neighboring cells (Howard, Plailly, Grueschow, Haynes, & Gottfried, 2009).

Olfactory receptors are vulnerable to damage because they are exposed to the air. Unlike your receptors for vision and hearing, which remain with you for a lifetime, an olfactory receptor has an average survival time of just over a month. At that point, a stem cell matures into a new olfactory cell in the same location as the first and expresses the same receptor protein (Nef, 1998). Its axon then has to find its way to the correct target in the olfactory bulb. Each olfactory neuron axon contains copies of its olfactory receptor protein, which it uses like an identification card to find its correct partner (Barnea et al., 2004; Strotmann, Levai, Fleischer, Schwarzenbacher, & Breer, 2004). However, if the entire olfactory surface is damaged at once by a blast of toxic fumes so that the system has to replace all the receptors at the same time, many of them fail to make the correct connections, and olfactory experience does not fully recover (Iwema, Fang, Kurtz, Youngentob, & Schwob, 2004).

Individual Differences

People vary in their sense of smell more than you might guess. Most of the genes controlling olfactory receptors have variant forms, and on average, two people chosen at random probably differ in about 30 percent of their olfactory receptor genes (Mainland et al., 2014). Compared to anyone else you know, you probably experience some smells as stronger, some as weaker, some as more pleasant, and some as less pleasant.

In addition to individual differences based on genes, odor sensitivity declines with age. The decline varies among odors. For example, sensitivity to mushroom odor apparently remains constant as people age, sensitivity to onion odor declines moderately, and sensitivity to rose odor declines greatly (Seow, Ong, & Huang, 2016). A sharp decline in odor sensitivity is often an early symptom of Alzheimer's disease or Parkinson's disease (Doty & Kamath, 2014).

Women detect odors more readily than men, at all ages and in all cultures that researchers have tested (Doty, Applebaum, Zusho, & Settle, 1985; Saxton et al., 2014; Yousem et al., 1999). In addition, young adult women gradually become more and more sensitive to a faint odor they repeatedly attend to, until they can detect it in concentrations one ten-thousandth of what they could at the start (Dalton, Doolittle, & Breslin, 2002). Men, girls before puberty, and women after menopause do not show that effect, so it apparently depends on female hormones. We can only speculate on why we evolved a connection between female hormones and odor sensitization.

STOP & CHECK

29. What is the mean life span of an olfactory receptor?
30. What factors contribute to individual differences in olfactory sensitivity?

ANSWERS

29. Most olfactory receptors survive a little more than a month before dying and being replaced. 30. People differ in olfactory sensitivity because of genetics, age, and gender.

Pheromones

An additional sense is important for most mammals, although less so for humans. The **vomeronasal organ (VNO)** is a set of receptors located near, but separate from, the olfactory receptors. Unlike olfactory receptors, the VNO receptors respond only to **pheromones,** chemicals released by an animal that affect the behavior of other members of the same species. For example, if you have ever had a female dog that wasn't neutered, whenever she was in her fertile (estrus) period, even though you kept her indoors, your yard attracted every male dog in the neighborhood that was free to roam.

Each VNO receptor responds to just one pheromone, in concentrations as low as one part in a hundred billion (Leinders-Zufall et al., 2000). Furthermore, the receptor does not adapt to a repeated stimulus. Have you ever been in a room that seems smelly at first but not a few minutes later? Your olfactory receptors respond to a new odor but not to a continuing one. VNO receptors, however, continue responding even after prolonged stimulation (Holy, Dulac, & Meister, 2000).

In adult humans, the VNO is tiny and has no receptors (Keverne, 1999; Monti-Bloch, Jennings-White, Dolberg, & Berliner, 1994). It is vestigial—that is, a leftover from our evolutionary past. Nevertheless, part of the human olfactory mucosa contains receptors that resemble other species' pheromone receptors (Liberles & Buck, 2006; Rodriguez, Greer, Mok, & Mombaerts, 2000).

The behavioral effects of pheromones apparently occur unconsciously. That is, people react to certain chemicals in human skin even when they describe them as odorless. The smell of a sweaty woman increases a man's testosterone secretions, especially if the woman was near her time of ovulation (Miller & Maner, 2010). This effect is stronger for heterosexual men than for homosexual men (Savic, Berglund, & Lindström, 2005). The smell of a sweaty man does not increase sexual arousal in women. Instead, it increases release of cortisol, a stress hormone (Wyart et al., 2007). Evidently a man reacts to a sweaty woman as a sex signal, and a woman reacts to a sweaty man as a potential danger signal.

The best-documented effect of a human pheromone relates to the timing of women's menstrual cycles. According to several (but not all) reports, women who spend much time together find that their menstrual cycles become more synchronized, unless they are taking birth control pills (McClintock, 1971; Weller, Weller, Koresh-Kamin, & Ben-Shoshan, 1999; Weller, Weller, & Roizman, 1999). To test whether pheromones are responsible for the synchronization, researchers exposed young volunteer women to the underarm secretions of a donor woman. In two studies, most of the women exposed to the secretions became synchronized to the donor's menstrual cycle (Preti, Cutler, Garcia, Huggins, & Lawley, 1986; Russell, Switz, & Thompson, 1980).

Another study dealt with the phenomenon that a woman in an intimate relationship with a man tends to have more regular menstrual periods than women not in an intimate relationship. According to one hypothesis, the man's pheromones promote this regularity. In the study, young women who were not sexually active were exposed daily to a man's underarm secretions. (Getting women to volunteer for this study wasn't easy.) Gradually, over 14 weeks, most of these women's menstrual periods became more regular than before (Cutler et al., 1986). In short, human body secretions probably do act as pheromones, although the effects are more subtle than in most other mammals.

STOP & CHECK

31. What is a major difference between olfactory receptors and those of the vomeronasal organ?

ANSWER

31. Olfactory receptors adapt quickly to a continuous odor, whereas receptors of the vomeronasal organ continue to respond. Also, vomeronasal sensations are apparently capable of influencing behavior even without being consciously perceived.

Synesthesia

Finally, let's consider something that is not one sense but a combination: **Synesthesia** is the experience some people have in which stimulation of one sense evokes a perception of that sense and another one also. For example, someone might perceive the letter J as green or say that each taste feels like a particular shape on the tongue (Barnett et al., 2008). In the words of one person, "To me, the taste of beef is dark blue. The smell of almonds is pale orange. And when tenor saxophones play, the music looks like a floating, suspended coiling snake-ball of lit-up purple neon tubes" (Day, 2005, p. 11).

Various studies attest to the reality of synesthesia. People reporting synesthesia have increased amounts of gray matter in certain brain areas and altered connections to other areas (Jäncke, Beeli, Eulig, & Hänggi, 2009; Rouw & Scholte, 2007; Weiss & Fink, 2009). People who perceive colors in letters and numbers have increased connections between the brain areas responding to colors and those responding to letters and numbers (Tomson, Narayan, Allen, & Eagleman, 2013). They also show behavioral characteristics that would be hard to pretend. Try to find the 2 among the 5s in each of the following displays:

```
555555555555    555555555555    555555555555
555555555555    555555555555    552555555555
555555525555    555555555555    555555555555
555555555555    555555555525    555555555555
```

One person with synesthesia was able to find the 2 consistently faster than other people, explaining that he just looked for a patch of orange! However, he was slower than other people to find an 8 among 6s because both 8 and 6 look blue to him (Blake, Palmeri, Marois, & Kim, 2005). Another person had trouble finding an A among 4s because both look red but could easily find an A among 0s because 0 looks black (Laeng, Svartdal, & Oelmann, 2004). Oddly, however, someone who sees the letter P as yellow had no trouble finding it when it was printed in black ink on a yellow page. In some way, he sees the letter both in its real color (black) *and* its synesthetic color (Blake et al., 2005).

What causes synesthesia? It clusters in families, suggesting a genetic predisposition (Barnett et al., 2008), and it frequently occurs in the same families as people with absolute pitch, suggesting that the two conditions share a genetic predisposition (Gregerson et al., 2013). However, obviously people are not born with a letter-to-color or number-to-color synesthesia. (No one is born knowing the letters of the alphabet.) In some cases, we see where people learned their associations. Researchers found 10 people with synesthesia whose associations matched or nearly matched the colors of Fisher-Price refrigerator magnets

they had used as children, such as red A, yellow C, and green D (Witthoft & Winawer, 2013). Only a small percentage of children who play with these magnets develop synesthesia, and most people with synesthesia have other associations, so the toys represent only one part of the explanation.

When people misperceive a stimulus—as in an illusion—the synesthetic experience corresponds to what the person *thought* the stimulus was, not what it actually was (Bargary, Barnett, Mitchell, & Newell, 2009). This result implies that the phenomenon occurs in the cerebral cortex, not in the receptors or their first connections to the nervous system. Furthermore, for some people, the idea of a word triggers a synesthetic experience before they have thought of the word itself. One person who could not think of "castanets" said it was on the tip of the tongue . . . not sure what the word was, but it tasted like tuna (Simner & Ward, 2006). One man with color vision deficiency reports synesthetic colors that he does not see in real life. He calls them "Martian colors" (Ramachandran, 2003). Evidently, his brain can see all the colors, even though his cones cannot send the messages.

One hypothesis is that axons from one cortical area branch into another cortical area. This explanation does apply to at least some cases. One woman suffered damage to the somatosensory area of her right thalamus. Initially she was, as expected, insensitive to touch in her left arm and hand. Over a year and a half, she gradually recovered part of her touch sensation. However, during that period, the somatosensory area of her right cortex was receiving little input. Some axons from her auditory system invaded the somatosensory cortex. As a result, she developed an unusual auditory-to-touch synesthesia. Many sounds cause her to feel an intense tingling sensation in her left arm and hand (Beauchamp & Ro, 2008; Naumer & van den Bosch, 2009).

✔ STOP & CHECK

32. What evidence indicates that people learn their synesthetic associations, at least in some cases?
33. If someone reports seeing a particular letter in color, in what way is it different from a real color?

ANSWERS

32. Some people have letter-color synesthesia that matches the colors of refrigerator magnets they played with in childhood. 33. Someone who perceives a letter as yellow (when it is actually in black ink) can nevertheless see it on a yellow page.

Module 6.3 | In Closing

Senses as Ways of Knowing the World

Ask the average person to describe the current environment, and you will probably get a description of what he or she sees and hears. If nonhumans could talk, most species would start by describing what they smell. A human, a dog, a bat, and a

snail may be in the same place, but the environments they perceive are very different. Our senses are adapted to provide us with information useful to our way of life.

We sometimes underestimate the importance of taste and smell. People who lose their sense of taste say they no longer enjoy eating and find it difficult to swallow (Cowart, 2005). Many people who lose the sense of smell feel permanently depressed. Taste and smell cannot compete with vision and hearing for telling us about what is happening in the distance, but they are essential for telling us about what is right next to us or about to enter our bodies. They are also important for our enjoyment of life.

Summary

1. Taste receptors are modified skin cells inside taste buds in papillae on the tongue. **211**

2. We have receptors sensitive to the tastes of sweet, sour, salty, bitter, umami (glutamate), and possibly fat. Taste is coded by the relative activity of different kinds of cells but also by the rhythm of responses within a given cell. **211**

3. Salty receptors respond simply to sodium ions crossing the membrane. Sour receptors detect the presence of acids. Sweet, bitter, and umami receptors act by a second messenger within the cell, similar to the way a metabotropic neurotransmitter receptor operates. **213**

4. Mammals have 30 or more kinds of bitter receptors, enabling them to detect many types of harmful substances. **214**

5. Part of the seventh cranial nerve conveys information from the anterior two-thirds of the tongue. Parts of the ninth and tenth cranial nerves convey information from the posterior tongue and the throat. The two nerves interact in complex ways. **214**

6. People vary in their sensitivity to tastes, especially bitter tastes, because of variations in their number of taste buds. **214**

7. Olfactory receptors are proteins, each of them highly responsive to a few related chemicals and unresponsive to others. Vertebrates have hundreds of olfactory receptors, each contributing to the detection of a few related odors. **217**

8. Olfactory neurons in the cerebral cortex respond to complex patterns, such as those of a food. **219**

9. Olfactory neurons survive only a month or so. The new cells that replace them become sensitive to the same chemicals as the ones they replace, and they send their axons to the same targets. **219**

10. People vary in their sensitivity to odors, because of differences in genetics, age, and gender. **219**

11. In most mammals, each vomeronasal organ (VNO) receptor is sensitive to only one chemical, a pheromone. A pheromone is a social signal. Humans also respond somewhat to pheromones, although our receptors are in the olfactory mucosa, not the VNO. **220**

12. Some people experience synesthesia, a sensation in one modality after stimulation in another one. For example, someone might see purple neon tubes while listening to saxophones. In some cases, the explanation is that axons from one sense have invaded brain areas responsible for a different sense. **220**

Key Terms

Terms are defined in the module on the page number indicated. They're also presented in alphabetical order with definitions in the book's Subject Index/Glossary, which begins on page 589. Interactive flash cards, audio reviews, and crossword puzzles are among the online resources available to help you learn these terms and the concepts they represent.

adaptation **213**
cross-adaptation **213**
nucleus of the tractus solitarius (NTS) **214**
olfaction **215**
olfactory cells **217**
papillae **211**
pheromones **220**
supertasters **214**
synesthesia **220**
taste bud **211**
vomeronasal organ (VNO) **220**

Thought Question

Suppose a chemist synthesizes a new chemical that turns out to have an odor. Presumably, we do not have a specialized receptor for that chemical. Explain how our receptors detect it.

Module 6.3 | End of Module Quiz

1. What type of cell is a taste receptor?
   A. A modified neuron
   B. A modified skin cell
   C. A modified gland cell
   D. A modified muscle cell

2. Which of these observations provides evidence that we have several types of taste receptor?

A. Certain chemicals can modify one taste without affecting others.

B. People from different cultures tend to have different taste preferences.

C. Increasing the temperature of a food enhances its flavors.

D. Taste receptors are replaced after lasting two weeks or less.

3. The receptors for sweet, bitter, and umami tastes all resemble which of these?

A. Metabotropic synaptic receptors

B. The rods in the retina

C. The hair cells of the auditory system

D. Endocrine glands

4. Why is it possible for us to taste a wide variety of chemicals as bitter?

A. All bitter substances are chemically similar.

B. We have 30 or more types of bitter receptors.

C. We have a bitter receptor that is versatile enough to detect many types of chemicals.

D. Sweet and sour receptors can detect bitter substances.

5. Why are some people more sensitive than others are to low concentrations of taste or smell?

A. People with more activity in their prefrontal cortex pay more attention to sensations.

B. People who know more words for taste or smell can remember and report them better.

C. Some people have faster axons between the tongue and the brain.

D. Some people have more taste receptors or odor receptors than others do.

6. How do we manage to smell a wide variety of chemicals?

A. An olfactory receptor varies the amplitude and velocity of its action potentials to indicate the type of odor.

B. The difference in response between the left nostril and the right nostril identifies the odor.

C. The ratio of firing among three types of olfactory receptors identifies the odor.

D. We have hundreds of types of olfactory receptors.

7. When a new olfactory receptor forms to replace one that died, does it connect to the same site in the olfactory bulb as the previous receptor? If so, how?

A. No, it connects at random with a site in the olfactory bulb.

B. It connects to the correct site because only one neuron in the olfactory bulb has a vacancy.

C. It finds the correct site by chemical attraction.

D. Each axon connects to the nearest neuron in the olfactory bulb.

8. The vomeronasal organ responds to what stimuli?

A. Pheromones

B. Pain and temperature

C. Tilt and acceleration of the head

D. Taste

9. What is the best-documented example of an effect of pheromones on humans?

A. The smell of a sweaty man increases a woman's sexual arousal.

B. People tend to be sexually attracted to someone who smells like members of their own family.

C. Women who spend much time together tend to synchronize their menstrual cycles.

D. Men can detect a woman's sexual interest by pheromones she secretes.

10. What behavioral evidence indicates that synesthesia is real, and not just something that people claim to experience?

A. Some people's associations match the colors of refrigerator magnets they played with in childhood.

B. Most people change their synesthetic associations from one year to the next.

C. People with synesthesia can find a 2 among 5s, or a 6 among 8s, faster than usual if they have different synesthetic colors, and slower if they have the same color.

D. It is easy to teach someone to develop a synesthesia.

Answers: 1B, 2A, 3A, 4B, 5D, 6D, 7C, 8A, 9C, 10C.

Suggestions for Further Reading

Henshaw, J. M. (2012). *A tour of the senses.* Baltimore: Johns Hopkins University Press. Excellent explanation of the physics of hearing and other senses.

Horowitz, S. S. (2012). *The universal sense: How hearing shapes the mind.* New York: Bloomsbury. Entertaining description of sound, music, and the role of hearing in the lives of humans and other species.

Thernstrom, M. (2010). *The pain chronicles.* New York: Farrar, Straus and Giroux. Why can some people withstand terrible injuries with little apparent pain? Why do others suffer endlessly? This book explores these and other questions about pain.

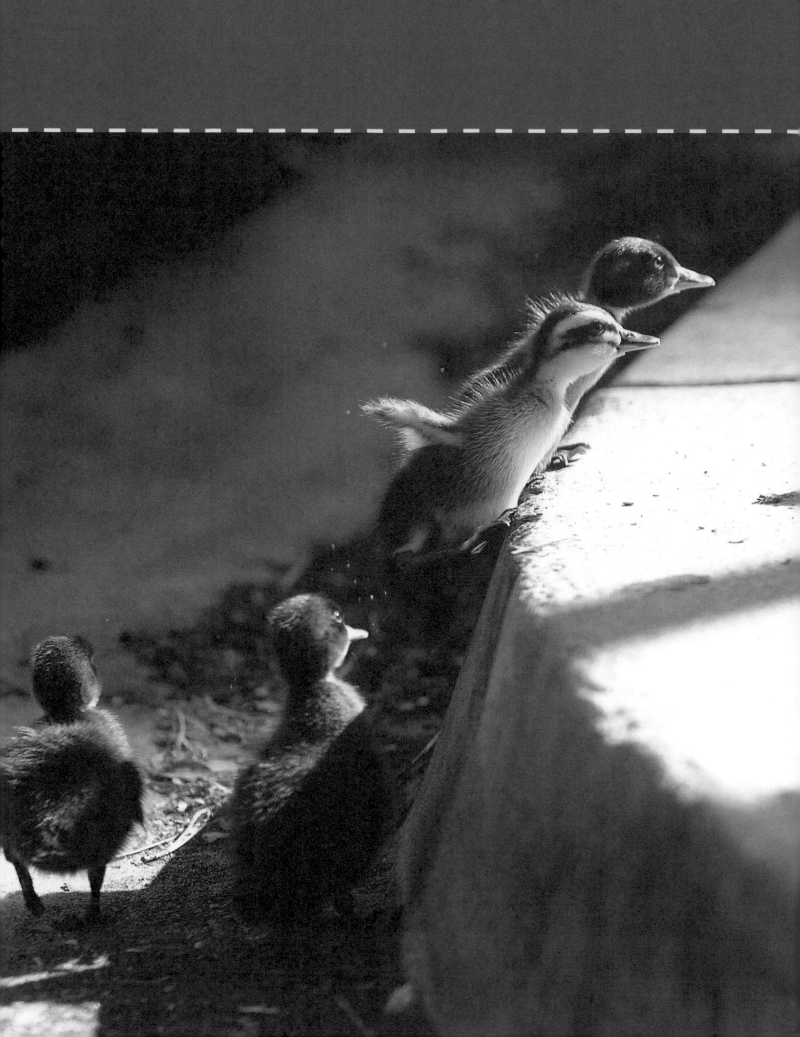

Movement

Before we get started, please try this: Get out a pencil and a sheet of paper, and put the pencil in your nondominant hand. For example, if you are right-handed, put it in your left hand. Now, with that hand, draw a face in profile—that is, facing one direction or the other but not straight ahead. *Please do this now before reading further.*

TRY IT YOURSELF

If you tried the demonstration, you probably notice that your drawing is more childlike than usual. It is as if part of your brain stored the way you used to draw as a young child. Now, if you are right-handed and therefore drew the face with your left hand, why did you draw it facing to the right? At least I assume you did, because more than two-thirds of right-handers drawing with their left hand draw the profile facing right. They revert to the pattern shown by young children. Up to about age 5 or 6, children drawing with the right hand almost always draw people and animals facing left, but when using the left hand, they almost always draw them facing right. But *why*? They say, "it's easier that way," but *why* is it easier that way? We have much to learn about the control of movement and how it relates to perception, motivation, and other functions.

Learning Objectives

After studying this chapter, you should be able to:

1. List the types of muscles and the proprioceptors that control them.
2. Describe the cortical mechanisms that control movement and its inhibition.
3. Contrast the anatomy and functions of the lateral and medial corticospinal tracts.
4. Describe the functions of the cerebellum and basal ganglia.
5. Evaluate the evidence regarding the role of consciousness in planning a movement.
6. Discuss the causes of Parkinson's disease and Huntington's disease.

Opposite:
Ultimately, what brain activity accomplishes is the control of movement—a far more complex process than it might seem.

(ZUMA Press Inc./Alamy Stock Photo)

Module 7.1

The Control of Movement

Why do we have a brain? Plants survive just fine without one. So do sponges, which are animals, even if they don't act like them. But plants don't move, and neither do sponges. A sea squirt (a marine invertebrate) has a brain during its infant stage, when it swims, but when it transforms into an adult, it attaches to a surface, becomes a stationary filter feeder, and digests its own brain, as if to say, "Now that I've stopped traveling, I won't need this brain thing anymore." Ultimately, the purpose of a brain is to control behaviors, and behaviors are movements.

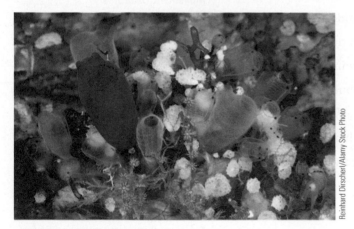

Adult sea squirts attach to a surface, never move again, and digest their own brains.

"But wait," you might reply. "We need a brain for other things, too, don't we? Like seeing, hearing, understanding speech . . ."

Well, what would be the value of seeing and hearing if you couldn't do anything? Understanding speech wouldn't do you much good unless you could do something about it. A great brain without muscles would be like a computer without a monitor, printer, or other output. No matter how powerful the internal processing, it would be useless.

Muscles and Their Movements

All animal movement depends on muscle contractions. Vertebrate muscles fall into three categories (see Figure 7.1): **smooth muscles** that control the digestive system and other organs, **skeletal** or **striated muscles** that control movement of

the body in relation to the environment, and **cardiac muscles** that control the heart.

Each muscle is composed of many fibers, as Figure 7.2 illustrates. Although each muscle fiber receives information from only one axon, a given axon may innervate more than one muscle fiber. For example, the eye muscles have a ratio of about one axon per three muscle fibers, and the biceps muscles of the arm have a ratio of one axon to more than a hundred fibers (Evarts, 1979). This difference allows the eye to move more precisely than the biceps.

A **neuromuscular junction** is a synapse between a motor neuron axon and a muscle fiber. In skeletal muscles, every axon releases acetylcholine at the neuromuscular junction, and acetylcholine always excites the muscle to contract. A deficit of acetylcholine or its receptors impairs movement. Each muscle makes just one movement, a contraction. There is no message to cause relaxation; the muscle relaxes when it receives no message to contract. There is also no message to move a muscle in the opposite direction. Moving a leg or arm back and forth requires opposing sets of muscles, called **antagonistic muscles**. At your elbow, for example, your **flexor** muscle brings your hand toward your shoulder and your **extensor** muscle straightens the arm (see Figure 7.3).

✓ STOP & CHECK

1. Why do we move the eye muscles with greater precision than the biceps muscles?
2. Which transmitter causes a skeletal muscle to contract?

ANSWERS
1. Each axon to the biceps muscles innervates about a hundred fibers; therefore, it is not possible to change the movement by a small amount. In contrast, an axon to the eye muscles innervates only about three fibers. 2. Acetylcholine. And remember that a muscle's only movement is to contract.

Fast and Slow Muscles

Imagine you are a small fish. Your only defense against bigger fish, diving birds, and other predators is your ability to swim away (see Figure 7.4). Your temperature is the same as

226

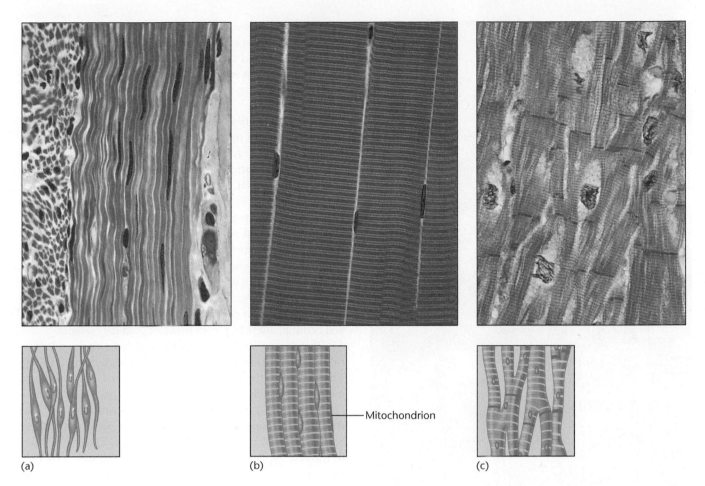

Figure 7.1 Vertebrate muscles
(a) Smooth muscle, found in the intestines and other organs, consists of long, thin cells. **(b)** Skeletal, or striated, muscle consists of long cylindrical fibers with stripes. **(c)** Cardiac muscle, found in the heart, consists of fibers that fuse together at various points. Because of these fusions, cardiac muscles contract together, not independently.
(Illustrations after Starr & Taggart, 1989) All © Ed Reschke

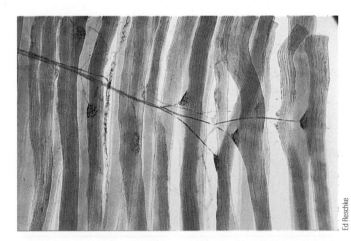

Figure 7.2 An axon branching to innervate several muscle fibers
Movements can be more precise where each axon innervates only a few fibers, as with eye muscles, than where it innervates many fibers, as with biceps muscles.

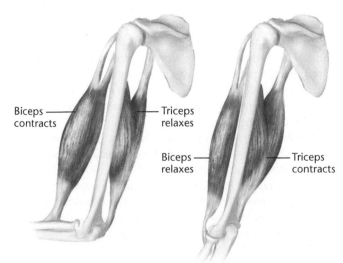

Figure 7.3 Antagonistic muscles
The biceps of the arm is a flexor. The triceps is an extensor.
(Source: Starr & Taggart, 1989)

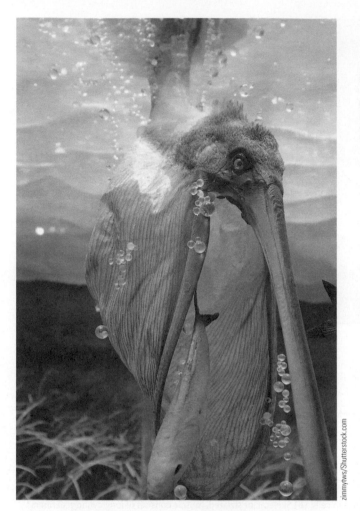

zimmytws/Shutterstock.com

Figure 7.4 Temperature and movement
Fish are "cold blooded," but many of their predators, such as this pelican, are not. At cold temperatures, each fish muscle contracts more slowly than usual, but a fish compensates by using more muscles.

We rely on our slow-twitch and intermediate fibers, similar to a fish's red muscles, for the least strenuous activities. For example, you could talk for hours without fatiguing your lip muscles. You might walk for a long time, too. But if you run up a steep hill at full speed, you switch to fast-twitch fibers that fatigue rapidly.

Slow-twitch fibers do not fatigue because they are **aerobic**—they use oxygen during their movements. You can think of them as "pay as you go." Prolonged use of fast-twitch fibers results in fatigue because the process is **anaerobic**—using reactions that do not require oxygen at the time but need oxygen for recovery. Using them builds up an *oxygen debt.* Imagine yourself bicycling. At first your activity is aerobic, using your slow-twitch fibers. However, your muscles use glucose, and after a while your glucose supplies begin to dwindle. Low glucose activates a gene that inhibits the muscles from using glucose, thereby saving glucose for the brain's use (Booth & Neufer, 2005). You start relying more on the fast-twitch muscles that depend on anaerobic use of fatty acids. As you continue bicycling, your muscles gradually fatigue.

People vary in their percentages of fast-twitch and slow-twitch fibers, for reasons based on both genetics and training. The Swedish ultramarathon runner Bertil Järlaker built up so many slow-twitch fibers in his legs that he once ran 2,188 mi (3,521 km) in 50 days (an average of 1.7 marathons per day) with only minimal signs of pain or fatigue (Sjöström, Friden, & Ekblom, 1987). Contestants in the Primal Quest race have to traverse approximately 500 kilometers (310 miles) by running, mountain climbing, mountain biking, river rafting, and ocean kayaking over 6 to 10 days in summer heat. To endure this ordeal, contestants need many adaptations of their muscles and metabolism (Pearson, 2006). In contrast, competitive sprinters have more fast-twitch fibers and other adaptations for speed instead of endurance (Andersen, Klitgaard, & Saltin, 1994; Canepari et al., 2005).

the water around you, and because muscle contractions are chemical processes, they slow down in the cold. So when the water gets cold, presumably you will move more slowly, right? Strangely, you will not. You will have to use more muscles than before, but you will swim at about the same speed (Rome, Loughna, & Goldspink, 1984).

A fish has three kinds of muscles: red, pink, and white. Red muscles produce the slowest movements, but they do not fatigue. White muscles produce the fastest movements, but they fatigue rapidly. Pink muscles are intermediate in speed and rate of fatigue. At high temperatures, a fish relies mostly on red and pink muscles. At colder temperatures, the fish relies more and more on white muscles, maintaining its speed but fatiguing faster.

All right, you can stop imagining you are a fish. Human and other mammalian muscles have various kinds of muscle fibers mixed together, not in separate bundles as in fish. Our muscle types range from **fast-twitch fibers** with fast contractions and rapid fatigue to **slow-twitch fibers** with less vigorous contractions and no fatigue (Hennig & Lømo, 1985).

STOP & CHECK

3. In what way are fish movements impaired in cold water?
4. Duck breast muscles are red ("dark meat"), whereas chicken breast muscles are white. Which species probably can fly for a longer time before fatiguing?

ANSWERS

3. Although a fish can move rapidly in cold water, it fatigues easily. 4. Ducks can fly great distances, as they often do during migration. The white muscle of a chicken breast has the power necessary to get a heavy body off the ground, but it fatigues rapidly. Chickens seldom fly far.

Muscle Control by Proprioceptors

As you are walking along on a bumpy road, you occasionally set your foot down a little too hard or not quite hard enough. You adjust your posture and maintain your balance without even thinking about it. How do you do that?

A baby is lying on its back. You playfully tug its foot and then let go. At once, the leg bounces back to its original position. How and why?

In both cases, proprioceptors control the movement (see Figure 7.5). A **proprioceptor** (from the Latin *proprius,* meaning "one's own") is a receptor that detects the position or movement of a part of the body—in these cases, a muscle. Muscle proprioceptors detect the stretch and tension of a muscle and send messages that enable the spinal cord to adjust its signals. When a muscle is stretched, the spinal cord sends a signal to contract it reflexively. This **stretch reflex** is *caused* by a stretch; it does not *produce* one.

One kind of proprioceptor is the **muscle spindle,** a receptor parallel to the muscle that responds to a stretch. Whenever the muscle is stretched more than the antagonistic muscle, the muscle spindle sends a message to a motor neuron in the spinal cord, which in turn sends a message back to the muscle, causing a contraction (Dimitriou, 2014). Note that this reflex provides for negative feedback: When a muscle and its spindle

are stretched, the spindle sends a message that results in a muscle contraction that opposes the stretch.

When you set your foot down on a bump on the road, your knee bends a bit, stretching the extensor muscles of that leg. The sensory nerves of the spindles send action potentials to the motor neuron in the spinal cord, and the motor neuron sends action potentials to the extensor muscle. Contracting the extensor muscle straightens the leg, adjusting for the bump on the road.

A physician who asks you to cross your legs and then taps just below the knee is testing your stretch reflexes (see Figure 7.6). The tap stretches the extensor muscles and their spindles, resulting in a message that jerks the lower leg upward. A leg that jerks excessively or not at all may indicate a neurological problem.

Golgi tendon organs, also proprioceptors, respond to increases in muscle tension. Located in the tendons at opposite ends of a muscle, they act as a brake against an excessively vigorous contraction. Some muscles are so strong that they could damage themselves if too many fibers contracted at once. Golgi tendon organs detect the tension that results during a muscle contraction. Their impulses travel to the spinal cord, where they excite interneurons that inhibit the motor neurons. In short, a vigorous muscle contraction inhibits further contraction by activating the Golgi tendon organs.

TRY IT YOURSELF

The proprioceptors not only control important reflexes but also provide the brain with information. Here is an illusion that you can try: Find a small, dense object and a larger, less dense object that weighs the same as the small one. For example, you might try a golf ball and a large

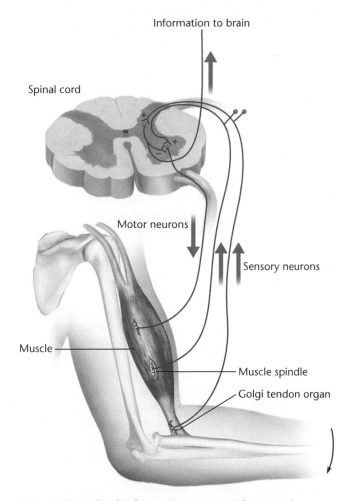

Figure 7.5 Two kinds of proprioceptors regulate muscle contractions
When a muscle is stretched, nerves from the muscle spindles transmit impulses that lead to contraction of the muscle. Contraction of the muscle stimulates the Golgi tendon organ, which acts as a brake or shock absorber to prevent a contraction that is too quick or extreme.

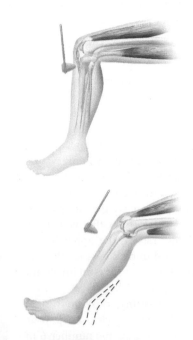

Figure 7.6 The knee-jerk reflex
This is one example of a stretch reflex.

plastic model of a golf ball. Drop one of the objects onto someone's hand while he or she is watching. (Watching is essential.) Then remove it and drop the other object onto the same hand. Most people report that the small one felt heavier. The reason is that with the larger object, people set themselves up with an expectation of a heavier weight. The actual weight displaces their proprioceptors less than expected and therefore yields the perception of a lighter object. You can get a similar result by asking someone to lift a small, heavy box and a larger box that weighs the same, or even a bit more. The smaller box will seem heavier. A general principle is that the brain reacts to sensations that differ from its expectations or predictions (Barrett & Simmons, 2015).

STOP & CHECK

5. If you hold your arm straight out and someone pulls it down slightly, it quickly bounces back. Which proprioceptor is responsible?
6. What is the function of Golgi tendon organs?

ANSWERS

5. The muscle spindle 6. Golgi tendon organs respond to muscle tension and thereby prevent excessively strong muscle contractions.

Units of Movement

Movements include speaking, walking, threading a needle, and throwing a basketball while off balance and evading two defenders. Different kinds of movement need different kinds of control by the nervous system.

Voluntary and Involuntary Movements

Reflexes are consistent automatic responses to stimuli. We generally think of reflexes as *involuntary* because they are insensitive to reinforcements, punishments, and motivations. The stretch reflex is one example. Another is the constriction of the pupil in response to bright light.

Few behaviors are purely voluntary or involuntary, reflexive or nonreflexive. Walking, which we think of as voluntary, includes involuntary components. When you walk, you automatically compensate for the bumps and irregularities in the road. The knee-jerk reflex that your physician tests contributes to walking; raising the upper leg reflexively moves the lower leg forward in readiness for the next step. You also swing your arms automatically as an involuntary consequence of walking.

Try this: While sitting, raise your right foot and make clockwise circles. Keep your foot moving while you draw the number 6 in the air with your right hand. Or just move your right hand in counterclockwise circles. You

TRY IT YOURSELF

will probably reverse the direction of your foot movement. It is difficult to make "voluntary" clockwise and counterclockwise movements on the same side of the body at the same time. However, it is not at all difficult to move your left hand in one direction while moving the right foot in the opposite direction.

Movements Varying in Sensitivity to Feedback

The military distinguishes ballistic missiles from guided missiles. A ballistic missile is launched like a thrown ball: Once it is launched, no one can change its aim. A guided missile detects the target and adjusts its trajectory to correct its aim.

Similarly, some movements are ballistic, and others are corrected by feedback. A **ballistic movement**, such as a reflex, is executed as a whole: Once initiated, it cannot be altered. However, most behaviors are subject to feedback correction. For example, when you thread a needle, you make a slight movement, check your aim, and then readjust. Similarly, a singer who holds a single note hears any wavering of the pitch and corrects it.

Sequences of Behaviors

Many rapid sequences of behaviors depend on **central pattern generators**, neural mechanisms in the spinal cord that generate rhythmic patterns of motor output. Examples include the mechanisms that generate wing flapping in birds, fin movements in fish, and the "wet dog shake." The stimulus that activates a central pattern generator does not control the frequency of the alternating movements. For example, a cat scratches itself at a rate of three to four strokes per second, regardless of what caused it to start scratching. Cells in the lumbar segments of the spinal cord generate this rhythm, and they continue doing so even if they are isolated from the brain or if the muscles are paralyzed (Deliagina, Orlovsky, & Pavlova, 1983). Researchers have identified the neural mechanisms of excitation and inhibition that produce these rhythms (Hägglund et al., 2013).

A fixed sequence of movements is called a **motor program**. For example, a mouse periodically grooms itself by sitting up, licking its paws, wiping them over its face, closing its eyes as the paws pass over them, licking the paws again, and so forth (Fentress, 1973). Once begun, the sequence is fixed from beginning to end. By comparing species, we see that a motor program can be gained or lost through evolution. For example, if you hold a chicken above the ground and drop it, its wings extend and flap. Chickens with featherless wings make the same movements, even though they fail to break their fall (Provine, 1979, 1981). Chickens, of course, still have the genetic programming to fly. On the other hand, ostriches, emus, and rheas, which have not used their wings for flight for millions of generations, have lost

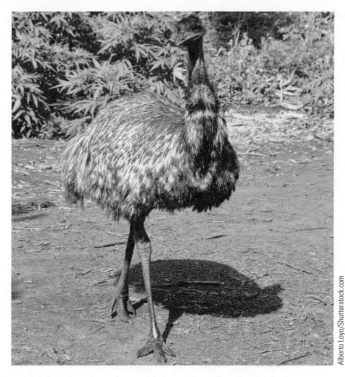

Nearly all birds reflexively spread their wings when dropped. However, emus—which lost the ability to fly through evolutionary time—do not spread their wings.

the genes for flight movements and do not flap their wings when dropped (Provine, 1984). (You might pause to think about the researcher who found a way to drop these huge birds to test the hypothesis.)

Do humans have any built-in motor programs? Yawning is one example (Provine, 1986). A yawn includes a prolonged open-mouth inhalation, often accompanied by stretching, and a shorter exhalation. Yawns are consistent in duration, with a mean of just under 6 seconds. Certain facial expressions are also programmed, such as smiles, frowns, and the raised-eyebrow greeting. Hugging is not a built-in motor program, but it is interesting to note that the average nonromantic hug lasts 3 seconds for people throughout the world (Nagy, 2011). That is, even our voluntary behaviors have a surprising degree of regularity and predictability.

Module 7.1 | In Closing

Categories of Movement

Charles Sherrington described a motor neuron in the spinal cord as "the final common path." He meant that regardless of what sensory and motivational processes occupy the brain, the final result is either a muscle contraction or the delay of a muscle contraction. A motor neuron and its associated muscle participate in a great many kinds of movements, and we need many brain areas to control them.

Summary

1. Vertebrates have smooth, skeletal, and cardiac muscles. **226**

2. All nerve–muscle junctions rely on acetylcholine as their neurotransmitter. **226**

3. Skeletal muscles range from slow muscles that do not fatigue to fast muscles that fatigue quickly. We rely on the slow muscles most of the time, but we recruit the fast muscles for brief periods of strenuous activity. **228**

4. Proprioceptors are receptors sensitive to the position and movement of a part of the body. Two kinds of proprioceptors, muscle spindles and Golgi tendon organs, help regulate muscle movements. **229**

5. Some movements, especially reflexes, proceed as a unit, with little if any guidance from sensory feedback. Other movements, such as threading a needle, are guided and redirected by sensory feedback. **230**

6. Central pattern generators produce fixed sequences of behaviors with a fixed rhythm. **230**

Key Terms

Terms are defined in the module on the page number indicated. They're also presented in alphabetical order with definitions in the book's Subject Index/Glossary, which begins on page 589. Interactive flash cards, audio reviews, and crossword puzzles are among the online resources available to help you learn these terms and the concepts they represent.

Thought Question

Would you expect jaguars, cheetahs, and other great cats to have mostly slow-twitch, nonfatiguing muscles in their legs or mostly fast-twitch, quickly fatiguing muscles? What kinds of animals might have mostly the opposite kind of muscles?

Module 7.1 | End of Module Quiz

1. After acetylcholine causes a flexor muscle to move your hand toward your shoulder, what would move it the other direction?
   A. A different transmitter causes the muscle to relax.
   B. A different transmitter causes the muscle to move the other direction.
   C. Acetylcholine causes the extensor muscle to contract.
   D. A different transmitter causes the extensor muscle to contract.

2. What happens to a fish's movement speed in colder water?
   A. The fish swims more slowly.
   B. The fish swims at the same speed by making each muscle contract more strongly.
   C. The fish swims at the same speed by recruiting more muscle fibers.
   D. The fish swims faster.

3. Which of the following is true of mammals' slow-twitch muscle fibers?
   A. Because they are aerobic, they are subject to rapid fatigue.
   B. Because they are anaerobic, they are subject to rapid fatigue.
   C. Because they are aerobic, they do not fatigue rapidly.
   D. Because they are anaerobic, they do not fatigue rapidly.

4. Which of the following describes a stretch reflex?
   A. The receptor detects that a muscle is stretched, and sends a signal to contract it reflexively.
   B. The receptor detects that a muscle is contracted, and sends a signal to stretch it reflexively.

5. A muscle spindle and a Golgi tendon organ are both described as what?
   A. Optic receptors
   B. Metabolic receptors
   C. Proprioceptors
   D. Chemoreceptors

6. What determines the rhythm of a cat's scratching movements, or the wet dog shakes?
   A. The rhythm of activity produced by the stimulus itself
   B. The structure of the muscles
   C. Commands from the prefrontal cortex
   D. A set of neurons in the spinal cord

Answers: 1C, 2C, 3C, 4A, 5C, 6D.

Brain Mechanisms of Movement

Why do we care how the brain controls movement? One goal is to help people who have spinal cord damage or limb amputations. Suppose we could listen in on their brain messages and decode what movements they would like to make. Then biomedical engineers might route those messages to muscle stimulators or robotic limbs. Sound like science fiction? Not really. Researchers implanted an array of microelectrodes into the motor cortex of a woman who was paralyzed from the neck down. Then they connected electrodes in her primary motor cortex to a robotic arm, enabling her to make simple reaching and grasping movements, as shown in Figure 7.7 (Hochberg et al., 2012). A man who became quadriplegic after a diving accident gradually learned to use his brain activity to control a device that stimulated muscles in his arm. For example, he learned to pick up a bottle and pour it into a cup (Bouton et al., 2016). Further progress will depend on both the technology and advances in understanding the brain mechanisms of movement.

Controlling movement depends on many brain areas, as illustrated in Figure 7.8. Don't get too bogged down in details

of the figure at this point. We shall attend to each area in due course.

The Cerebral Cortex

Since the pioneering work of Gustav Fritsch and Eduard Hitzig (1870), neuroscientists have known that direct electrical stimulation of the **primary motor cortex**—the precentral gyrus of the frontal cortex, just anterior to the central sulcus (see Figure 7.9)—elicits movements. The motor cortex does not send messages directly to the muscles. Its axons extend to the brainstem and spinal cord, which generate the impulses that control the muscles. In most mammals, axons from the cerebral cortex connect only to interneurons of the brainstem or spinal cord, which in turn control motor neurons. In humans and other primates, some axons go directly from the cerebral cortex to motor neurons, presumably giving us greater dexterity (Kinoshita et al., 2012).

The cerebral cortex is particularly important for complex actions such as talking or writing. It has much less control over coughing, sneezing, gagging, laughing, or crying (Rinn, 1984). Perhaps the lack of cerebral control explains why it is hard to perform those actions voluntarily. The primary motor cortex is also active when you imagine movements, remember movements, or understand verbs related to movements (Tomasino & Gremese, 2016).

Figure 7.10 (which repeats parts of Figure 3.23) shows which areas of the somatosensory cortex feel which parts of the body, and which areas of the motor cortex control muscles in which parts of the body. A key point is the similarity between the two. The motor cortex is just anterior to the somatosensory cortex, and the two match up nicely. The brain area that controls the left hand is near the area that feels the left hand, the area that controls the left foot is near the area that feels the left foot, and so forth. You need to feel a body part to control its movement accurately.

Don't read Figure 7.10 as implying that each spot in the motor cortex controls a single muscle. The region responsible for any finger overlaps the regions responsible for other fingers (Sanes, Donoghue, Thangaraj, Edelman, & Warach, 1995). Furthermore, the output of a given neuron influences movements of the hand, wrist, and arm, and not just a single muscle (Vargas-Irwin et al., 2010).

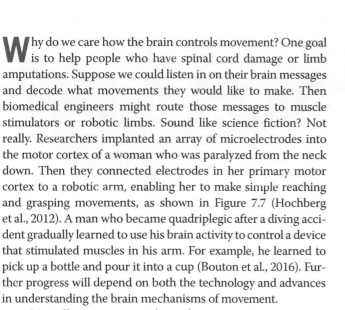
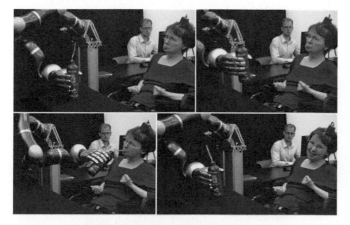

Figure 7.7 Recordings from the brain control a robotic arm
After a stroke in this woman's midbrain cut off connections from her cortex to the spinal cord, she lost all control of her arm and leg muscles. A neural decoder connected cells in her motor primary motor cortex to a robotic arm, enabling her to pick up a coffee cup, drink from it, and put it back.
Source: From Reach and grasp by people with tetraplegia using aneurally controlled robotic arm, by L. R. J. Vogel et al., 2012, Nature, 485, pp. 372–375.

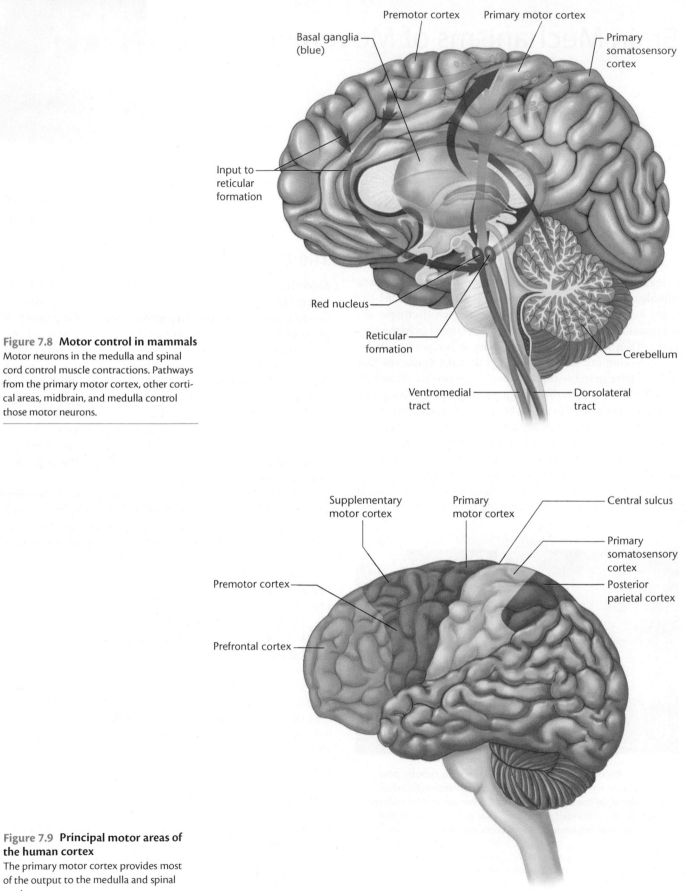

Figure 7.8 Motor control in mammals
Motor neurons in the medulla and spinal cord control muscle contractions. Pathways from the primary motor cortex, other cortical areas, midbrain, and medulla control those motor neurons.

Figure 7.9 Principal motor areas of the human cortex
The primary motor cortex provides most of the output to the medulla and spinal cord.

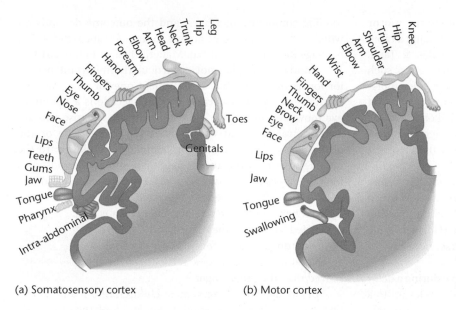

Figure 7.10 Coronal section through the primary somatosensory cortex and primary motor cortex
The motor cortex lies just anterior to the somatosensory cortex. The motor area responsible for moving a certain body part is aligned with the somatosensory area responsible for feeling that body part. Communication between sensing and moving is essential. (*Adapted from Penfield & Rasmussen, 1950*)

For many years, researchers studied the motor cortex in laboratory animals by stimulating neurons with brief electrical pulses, usually less than 50 milliseconds (ms) in duration. The results were brief muscle twitches. Later researchers found different results when they lengthened the pulses to half a second. Instead of twitches, they elicited complex movement patterns. For example, stimulation of one spot caused a monkey to make a grasping movement with its hand, move its hand to just in front of the mouth, and open its mouth—as if it were picking up something and getting ready to eat it (Graziano, Taylor, & Moore, 2002). Repeated stimulation of this same spot elicited the same result each time, regardless of the initial position of the monkey's hand. That is, the stimulation produced a certain *outcome*, not a particular *muscle movement*. The motor cortex orders an outcome and leaves it to the spinal cord and other areas to find the right combination of muscles (Scott, 2004).

STOP & CHECK

7. What aspect of brain anatomy facilitates communication between body sensations and body movements?
8. What evidence indicates that cortical activity represents the "idea" of the movement and not just the muscle contractions?

ANSWERS

7. The motor cortex and the somatosensory cortex are adjacent, and the area of motor cortex devoted to a particular body structure is aligned with the somatosensory cortex area responsive to the same structure. 8. Activity in the motor cortex leads to a particular outcome, such as movement of the hand to the mouth, regardless of what muscle contractions are necessary given the hand's current location.

Planning a Movement

One of the first areas to become active in planning a movement is the **posterior parietal cortex** (see Figure 7.9), which monitors the position of the body relative to the world (Snyder, Grieve, Brotchie, & Andersen, 1998). This part of the cortex is proportionately larger in humans than in most other primates, reflecting its enhanced role in selecting appropriate actions (Kaas & Stepniewska, 2016). People with posterior parietal damage have trouble finding objects in space, even after describing their appearance accurately. When walking, they frequently bump into obstacles (Goodale, 1996; Goodale, Milner, Jakobson, & Carey, 1991).

Brain surgery is sometimes conducted on people who are awake and alert, with only the skin of their scalp anesthetized. (The brain itself has no pain receptors.) During the course of such surgery, physicians can briefly stimulate certain brain areas and record the results. When they stimulate parts of the posterior parietal cortex, people frequently report an *intention* to move—such as an intention to move the left hand. After more intense stimulation at the same locations, people report that they believe they *did* make the movement—although, in fact, they did not (Desmurget et al., 2009).

Several studies used fMRI to measure brain responses while people were preparing to move. The details vary, but the general idea is that people see a first signal that tells them what they are supposed to do, and then they have to wait a few seconds for a second signal that says to make the movement now. Or people see a first signal with partial information about what they will or will not have to do, and then after a short delay a second signal that tells them more precisely what to do. In each of these cases, the posterior parietal cortex is active throughout the delay, evidently preparing for the movement (Hesse, Thiel, Stephan, & Fink, 2006; Lindner, Iyer, Kagan, & Andersen, 2010).

The prefrontal cortex and the **supplementary motor cortex** are also important for planning and organizing a rapid sequence of movements (Shima, Isoda, Mushiake, & Tanji, 2007; Tanji & Shima, 1994). If you have a habitual action, such as turning left when you get to a certain corner, the supplementary motor cortex is essential for inhibiting that habit when you need to do something else (Isoda & Hikosaka, 2007). The supplementary motor cortex also becomes active after an error in movement, developing ways to inhibit the incorrect movement the next time (Bonini et al., 2014).

The **premotor cortex** is most active immediately before a movement. It receives information about the target to which the body is directing its movement, as well as information about the body's current position and posture (Hoshi & Tanji, 2000). Both kinds of information are, of course, necessary to direct a movement toward a target.

The **prefrontal cortex**, which is also active during a delay before a movement, stores sensory information relevant to a movement. It is also important for considering the probable outcomes of possible movements (Tucker, Luu, & Pribram, 1995). If you had damage to this area, many of your movements would be disorganized, such as showering with your clothes on or pouring water on the tube of toothpaste instead of the toothbrush (Schwartz, 1995). Interestingly, this area is inactive during dreams, and the actions we dream about doing are often as illogical as those of people with prefrontal cortex damage (Braun et al., 1998; Maquet et al., 1996). If you do something absentminded first thing in the morning, it may be that your prefrontal cortex is not fully awake.

✓ STOP & CHECK

9. How does the posterior parietal cortex contribute to movement? The premotor cortex? The supplementary motor cortex? The prefrontal cortex?

ANSWER

9. The posterior parietal cortex is important for perceiving the location of objects and the position of the body relative to the environment. It is also active for planning of a movement. The premotor cortex and supplementary motor cortex are also active in preparing a movement shortly before it occurs. The supplementary motor cortex inhibits a habitual action when it is inappropriate. The prefrontal cortex stores sensory information relevant to a movement and considers possible outcomes of a movement.

Inhibiting a Movement

Next, consider the situation in which you need to restrain yourself from following some impulse. The traffic light changes from red to green, but just as you are about to drive forward, you hear an ambulance siren telling you to get out of the way. Or you start to swing at a tennis ball in a doubles match when your partner shouts, "let it go," because it will land out of bounds. In cases like these, two brain areas are

sending competing messages, and the outcome depends on whether the stop message arrives in time to cancel the action message (Schmidt, Leventhal, Mallet, Chen, & Berke, 2013).

Another example—not a particularly important behavior for its own sake, but a convenient one for psychologists to study—is the **antisaccade task**. A saccade is a voluntary eye movement from one target to another. Suppose you are staring straight ahead when something to one side or the other moves. You have a strong tendency to look toward the moving object. In the antisaccade task, you are supposed to look the *opposite* direction. You can try it yourself: Hold one hand to the left of someone's head and the other hand to the right. When you wiggle a finger, the person is instructed to look at the *other* hand. Or have someone do the same for you. Most people agree that it is easier to look at the finger that moved than the other finger.

Before age 5 to 7 years, most children find it almost impossible to ignore the wiggling finger and look the other way. Ability to perform this task gradually improves as the prefrontal cortex slowly matures, reaching peak levels in young adulthood (Bucci & Seessau, 2012). Performance deteriorates in old age, because the prefrontal cortex is highly vulnerable to damage (Sweeney, Rosano, Berman, & Luna, 2001). Performing the antisaccade task requires sustained activity in parts of the prefrontal cortex and basal ganglia *before* seeing the wiggling finger (Velanova, Wheeler, & Luna, 2009; Watanabe & Munoz, 2010). That is, the brain prepares to inhibit the unwanted action and substitute a different one. Many adults who have neurological or psychiatric disorders affecting the prefrontal cortex or basal ganglia have trouble on this task (Munoz & Everling, 2004). As you might guess, people with attention deficit/hyperactivity disorder (ADHD), who tend to be impulsive in other ways, also have difficulty with the antisaccade task (Lee, Lee, Chang, & Kwak, 2015; Loe, Feldman, Yasui, & Luna, 2009).

Mirror Neurons

Of discoveries in neuroscience, one of the most exciting to psychologists has been **mirror neurons**, which are active both during preparation for a movement and while watching someone else perform the same or a similar movement (Rizzolatti & Sinigaglia, 2010). Mirror neurons were first reported in the premotor cortex of monkeys (Gallese, Fadiga, Fogassi, & Rizzolatti, 1996) and later in other areas and other species, including humans (Dinstein, Hasson, Rubin, & Heeger, 2007; Kilner, Neal, Weiskopf, Friston, & Frith, 2009). These neurons became theoretically exciting because of the idea that they may be important for understanding other people, identifying with them, and imitating them. For example, mirror neurons in part of the frontal cortex become active when people smile or see someone else smile, and they respond especially strongly in people who report identifying strongly with other people (Montgomery, Seeherman, & Haxby, 2009). Many people have speculated that a lack of mirror neurons might be responsible for autism or schizophrenia, disorders associated with deficient social relationships. However, several studies found evidence of normal mirror neurons in both of these conditions (e.g., Andrews, Enticott, Hoy, Thomson & Fitzgerald, 2015; Dinstein et al., 2010).

Mirror neurons are activated not only by seeing an action, but also by any reminder of the action. Certain cells respond to hearing an action as well as seeing or doing it (Kohler et al., 2002; Ricciardi et al., 2009). Other cells respond to either doing an action or reading about it (Foroni & Semin, 2009; Speer, Reynolds, Swallow, & Zacks, 2009).

The possibilities are exciting, but before we speculate too far, we need to address an important question: Do mirror neurons *cause* imitation and social behavior, or do they *result from* them? Put another way, are we born with neurons that respond to the sight of a movement and also facilitate the same movement? If so, they could be important for social learning. Or do we learn which visible movements correspond to movements of our own, and then develop the connections that produce mirror neurons? In the latter case, mirror neurons are not responsible for imitation or socialization (Heyes, 2010).

The best, perhaps only, evidence for inborn mirror neurons came from reports that some newborn infants imitate tongue protrusion and other expressions, as shown in Figure 7.11. That result suggests built-in mirror neurons that connect the sight of a movement to the movement itself (Meltzoff & Moore, 1977). However, later results have cast doubt on that conclusion. Newborns react to many types of excitement by protruding the tongue, and what appears to be imitation can be coincidental. An extensive study found that infants' expressions and gestures do not match what they see more often than we would expect by chance (Oostenbroek et al., 2016).

Several types of evidence suggest that mirror neurons develop their properties by learning. In both monkey and human infants, many mirror neurons do not respond to observations of others' movements until after the infants have practiced making those movements themselves (Shaw & Czekóová, 2013). Also, researchers identified mirror neurons that responded both when people moved a certain finger, such as the index finger, and when they watched someone else move the same finger. Then they asked people to watch a display on the screen and move their index finger whenever the hand on the screen moved the little finger. They were to move their little finger whenever the hand on the screen moved the index finger. After some practice, these "mirror" neurons turned into "counter-mirror" neurons that responded to movements of one finger by that person and the sight of a different finger on the screen (Catmur, Walsh, & Heyes, 2007). In other words, many mirror neurons modify their properties by learning, and probably developed their original properties by learning also.

✓ **STOP & CHECK**

10. When expert pianists listen to familiar, well-practiced music, they imagine the finger movements, and the finger area of their motor cortex becomes active, even if they are not moving their fingers (Haueisen & Knösche, 2001). If we regard those neurons as another kind of mirror neuron, what do these results imply about the origin of mirror neurons?

ANSWER

10. These neurons must have acquired these properties through experience. That is, they did not enable pianists to copy what they hear. They developed as pianists learned to copy what they hear.

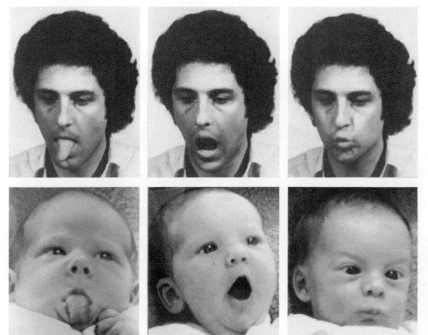

Figure 7.11 Infants appear to imitate certain facial expressions

What appears to be imitation may be coincidence. Infants' expressions sometimes match what they see, but not always.

(Source: From A.N. Meltzoff & M.K. Moore, "Imitation of facial and manual gestures by human neonates." Science, 1977, 198, pp. 75–78.)

Table 7.1 | Disorders of the Spinal Cord

Disorder	Description	Cause
Paralysis	Inability for voluntary movement in part of the body	Damage to motor neurons or their axons in the spinal cord
Paraplegia	Loss of sensation and voluntary muscle control in the legs (Despite the lack of sensations from the genitals, stimulation of the genitals can produce orgasm.)	A cut through the spinal cord in the thoracic region or lower
Quadriplegia (or **tetraplegia**)	Loss of sensation and voluntary muscle control in both arms and legs	Cut through the spinal cord in the cervical (neck) region (or cortical damage)
Hemiplegia	Loss of sensation and voluntary muscle control in the arm and leg of either the right or left side	Cut halfway through the spinal cord or damage to one hemisphere of the cerebral cortex
Tabes dorsalis	Impaired sensations and muscle control in the legs and pelvic region, including bowel and bladder control	Damage to the dorsal roots of the spinal cord from the late stage of syphilis
Poliomyelitis	Paralysis	A virus that damages motor neurons in the spinal cord
Amyotrophic lateral sclerosis	Gradual weakness and paralysis, starting with the arms and spreading to the legs	Unknown. Traced to genetic mutations in some cases, and to exposure to toxins in other cases

Connections from the Brain to the Spinal Cord

Messages from the brain must reach the medulla and spinal cord, which control the muscles. Diseases of the spinal cord impair the control of movement in various ways, as listed in Table 7.1. Paths from the cerebral cortex to the spinal cord are called the **corticospinal tracts**. We have two such tracts, the lateral and medial corticospinal tracts. Both tracts contribute in some way to nearly all movements, but certain movements rely on one tract more than the other.

The **lateral corticospinal tract** is a pathway of axons from the primary motor cortex, surrounding areas of the cortex, and from the **red nucleus,** a midbrain area that controls certain aspects of movement (see Figure 7.12). Axons of the lateral tract extend directly from the motor cortex to their target neurons in the spinal cord. In bulges of the medulla called *pyramids,* the lateral tract crosses to the contralateral

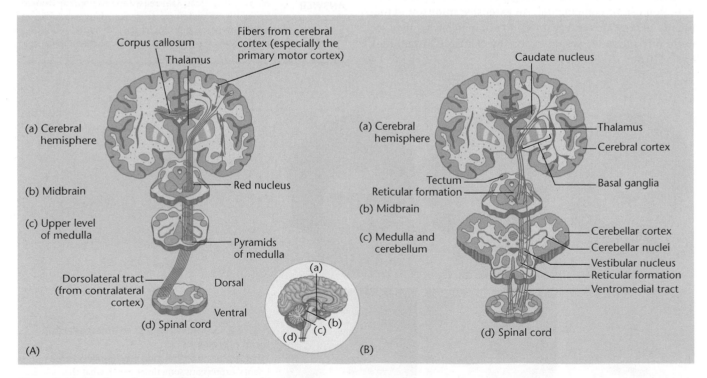

Figure 7.12 The lateral and medial corticospinal tracts
The lateral tract **(a)** crosses from one side of the brain to the opposite side of the spinal cord and controls precise and discrete movements of the extremities, such as hands, fingers, and feet. The medial tract **(b)** controls trunk muscles for postural adjustments and bilateral movements such as standing, bending, turning, and walking.

(opposite) side of the spinal cord. (For that reason, the lateral tract is also called the pyramidal tract.) It controls movements in peripheral areas, especially the hands and feet.

The **medial corticospinal tract** includes axons from many parts of the cerebral cortex, not just the primary motor cortex and its surrounding areas. The medial path also includes axons from the midbrain tectum, the reticular formation, and the **vestibular nucleus**, a brain area that receives input from the vestibular system (see Figure 7.12). Axons of the medial tract go to *both* sides of the spinal cord, not just to the contralateral side. The medial tract controls mainly the muscles of the neck, shoulders, and trunk and therefore bilateral movements as walking, turning, bending, standing up, and sitting down (Kuypers, 1989). You can move your fingers on just one side of the body, but a movement such as standing up or sitting down must include both sides.

The functions of the lateral and medial tracts should be easy to remember: The lateral tract controls muscles in the lateral parts of the body, such as hands and feet. The medial tract controls muscles in the medial parts of the body, including trunk and neck.

Figure 7.12 compares the lateral and medial corticospinal tracts. Figure 7.13 compares the lateral tract to the spinal pathway bringing touch information to the cortex. Note that both paths cross in the medulla and that the touch information arrives at brain areas side by side with those areas responsible for motor control. Touch is obviously essential for

movement. You have to know what your hands are doing now to control their next action.

Suppose someone suffers a stroke that damages the primary motor cortex of the left hemisphere. The result is a loss of the lateral tract from that hemisphere and a loss of movement control on the right side of the body. Eventually, depending on the location and amount of damage, the person may regain some muscle control from spared axons in the lateral tract. If not, using the medial tract can approximate the intended movement. For example, someone with no direct control of the hand muscles might move the shoulders, trunk, and hips in a way that repositions the hand.

✓ STOP & CHECK

11. What kinds of movements does the lateral tract control? The medial tract?

ANSWER   11. The lateral tract controls detailed movements in the periphery on the contralateral side of the body. For example, the lateral tract from the left hemisphere controls the right side of the body. The medial tract controls trunk movements bilaterally.

The Cerebellum

The term *cerebellum* is Latin for "little brain." Decades ago, most texts described the function of the cerebellum as "balance and coordination." Well, yes, people with cerebellar damage do lose balance and coordination, but that description understates the importance of this structure. The cerebellum contains more neurons than the rest of the brain combined (Williams & Herrup, 1988) and a huge number of synapses.

The cerebellum contributes to many aspects of brain functioning, especially anything that relates to aim or timing. People with cerebellar damage have trouble tapping a rhythm, clapping hands, pointing at a moving object, speaking, writing, typing, or playing a musical instrument. They are impaired at almost all athletic activities, except ones like weight lifting that do not require aim or timing. Researchers have found enlarged cerebellums in college basketball players (Park et al., 2009), competitive speed skaters (Park et al., 2012), and world-class mountain climbers (Di Paola, Caltagirone, & Petrosini, 2013). However, we do not know whether the enlargement is the cause or the result of skillful activity.

Cerebellar damage does not impair *continuous* motor activity (Spencer, Zelaznik, Diedrichsen, & Ivry, 2003). For example, people with such damage can draw continuous circles like the ones shown here, which do not require starting or stopping an action.

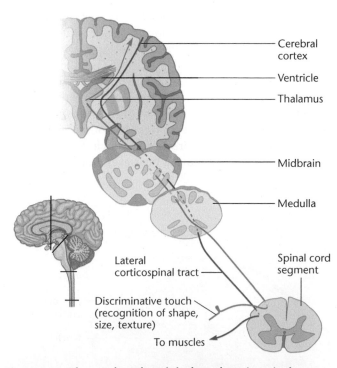

Figure 7.13 The touch path and the lateral corticospinal tract
Both paths cross in the medulla so that each hemisphere has access to the opposite side of the body. The touch path goes from touch receptors toward the brain; the corticospinal path goes from the brain to the muscles.

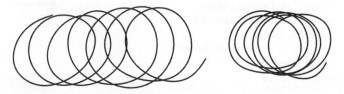

Here is a quick way to test the cerebellum: Ask someone to look at one spot and then to move the eyes quickly to focus on another spot. Saccades (sa-KAHDS), voluntary eye movements from one fixation point to another, depend on impulses from the cerebellum and the frontal cortex to the cranial nerves. Someone with cerebellar damage has difficulty programming the angle and distance of eye movements (Dichgans, 1984). The eyes make many short movements until, by trial and error, they eventually find the intended spot.

In the *finger-to-nose test,* the person is instructed to hold one arm straight out and then, at command, to touch his or her nose as quickly as possible. A normal person does so in three steps. First, the finger moves ballistically to a point just in front of the nose. This *move* function depends on the cerebellar cortex (the surface of the cerebellum), which sends messages to the deep nuclei (clusters of cell bodies) in the interior of the cerebellum (see Figure 7.14). Second, the finger remains steady at that spot for a fraction of a second. This *hold* function depends on the nuclei alone (Kornhuber, 1974). Finally, the finger moves to the nose by a slower movement that does not depend on the cerebellum.

Someone with damage to the cerebellar cortex has trouble with the initial rapid movement. The finger misses the nose, stops too soon, or goes too far. Someone with damage to the cerebellar nuclei has difficulty with the hold segment: The finger reaches a point in front of the nose and then wavers.

The symptoms of cerebellar damage resemble those of alcohol intoxication: clumsiness, slurred speech, and inaccurate eye movements. A police officer testing someone for drunkenness may use the finger-to-nose test or similar tests because the cerebellum is one of the first brain areas that alcohol affects.

Functions Other than Movement

The cerebellum is not only a motor structure, and it becomes active in many situations when the individual is not moving. In one study, functional MRI measured cerebellar activity while people performed several tasks (Gao et al., 1996). When they simply lifted objects, the cerebellum showed little activity. When they felt things with both hands to decide whether they were the same or different, the cerebellum was much more active. The cerebellum responded even when the experimenter rubbed an object across an unmoving hand. That is, the cerebellum responds to sensory stimuli even in the absence of movement. The cerebellum also responds to violations of sensory expectations. If you reach out your hand expecting to feel something and then don't feel it, or feel something when you didn't expect to, your cerebellum reacts strongly (Schlerf, Ivry, & Diedrichsen, 2012).

Richard Ivry and his colleagues have emphasized the importance of the cerebellum for behaviors that depend on precise timing of short intervals (from about a millisecond to 1.5 seconds). For example, people with cerebellar damage can accurately judge the loudness of a sound, but not its duration. Consider a classical conditioning procedure in which a sound predicts a puff of air to your eyes to occur one second later. Someone with cerebellar damage learns the connection, but does not time the eyeblink to the appropriate time. Timing is also important for aim. If you have trouble timing a moving object, such as a ball thrown toward you, you will not be able to anticipate its trajectory, and you will fail to catch it. In short, when cerebellar damage impairs movement, the reason may be that the damage impaired the perception of timed stimuli related to the movement (Baumann et al., 2015).

People who are accurate at one kind of timed movement, such as tapping a rhythm with a finger, tend also to be good at other timed movements, such as tapping a rhythm with a foot, and at judging which visual stimulus moved faster and which delay between tones was longer. People with cerebellar damage are impaired at all of these tasks (Ivry & Diener, 1991; Keele & Ivry, 1990).

The cerebellum also appears critical for certain aspects of attention. In one study, people were told to keep their eyes fixated on a central point. At various times, they would see the letter E on either the left or right half of the screen, and they were to indicate the direction in which it was oriented (E, Ǝ, ⱻ, or ⱷ) without moving their eyes. Sometimes, they

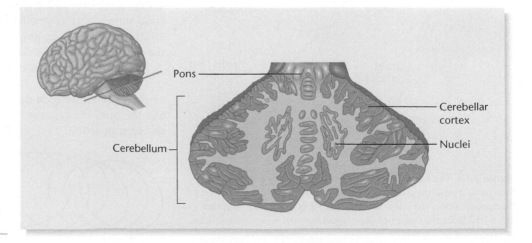

Figure 7.14 Location of the cerebellar nuclei relative to the cerebellar cortex
In the inset at the upper left, the line indicates the plane shown in detail at the lower right.

saw a signal telling where the letter would be on the screen. For most people, that signal improved their performance even if it appeared just 100 ms before the letter. For people with cerebellar damage, the signal had to appear nearly a second before the letter to be helpful. Evidently, people with cerebellar damage need longer to shift their attention (Townsend et al., 1999).

✔️ **STOP & CHECK** ▬▬▬▬▬▬▬

12. What kind of perceptual task would be most impaired by damage to the cerebellum?

ANSWER

12. Damage to the cerebellum impairs perceptual tasks that depend on accurate timing.

Cellular Organization

The cerebellum receives input from the spinal cord, from the sensory systems by way of the cranial nerve nuclei, and from the cerebral cortex. That information eventually reaches the **cerebellar cortex**, the surface of the cerebellum (see Figure 7.14).

Figure 7.15 shows the types and arrangements of neurons in the cerebellar cortex. The figure is complex, but concentrate on these main points:

- The neurons are arranged in a precise geometrical pattern, with multiple repetitions of the same units.
- The **Purkinje** (pur-KIN-jee) **cells** are flat (two-dimensional) cells in sequential planes, parallel to one another.
- The **parallel fibers** are axons parallel to one another and perpendicular to the planes of the Purkinje cells.
- Action potentials in parallel fibers excite one Purkinje cell after another. Each Purkinje cell then transmits an inhibitory message to cells in the **nuclei of the cerebellum** (clusters of cell bodies in the interior of the cerebellum) and the vestibular nuclei in the brainstem, which in turn send information to the midbrain and the thalamus.
- Depending on which and how many parallel fibers are active, they might stimulate only the first few Purkinje cells or a long series of them. Because the parallel fibers' messages reach Purkinje cells one after another, the greater the number of excited Purkinje cells, the greater their collective *duration* of response. That is, if the parallel fibers stimulate only the first few Purkinje cells, the result is a brief message to the target cells; if they stimulate more Purkinje cells, the message lasts longer. The sequence of Purkinje cells controls the timing of the output, including both its onset and offset (Thier, Dicke, Haas, & Barash, 2000).

✔️ **STOP & CHECK** ▬▬▬▬▬▬▬

13. How are the parallel fibers arranged relative to one another and to the Purkinje cells?
14. If a larger number of parallel fibers are active, what is the effect on the collective output of the Purkinje cells?

ANSWERS

13. The parallel fibers are parallel to one another and perpendicular to the planes of the Purkinje cells. 14. As a larger number of parallel fibers become active, the Purkinje cells increase their duration of response.

The Basal Ganglia

The term **basal ganglia** applies collectively to a group of large subcortical structures in the forebrain (see Figure 7.16). (*Ganglia* is the plural of *ganglion*.) Various authorities differ in which structures they include as part of the basal ganglia, but everyone includes at least the **caudate nucleus**, the **putamen** (pyuh-TAY-men), and the **globus pallidus**. The caudate nucleus and putamen together are known as the **striatum** or **dorsal striatum**. The striatum receives input from the cerebral cortex and substantia nigra and sends its output to the globus pallidus, which then sends output to the thalamus and frontal cortex (Saunders et al., 2015). Figure 7.17 shows two pathways, known as the direct and indirect pathways. The direct pathway from the striatum inhibits the globus pallidus, which inhibits part of the thalamus. By inhibiting an inhibitor, the net effect is excitation. Neuroscientists long believed that the direct pathway stimulates movements whereas the indirect pathway inhibits them. However, later evidence found that both pathways are active before a movement and neither is active when the animal is at rest (Calabresi, Picconi, Tozzi, Ghiglieri, & Di Filippo, 2014; Cui et al., 2013). Probably the direct pathway enhances the selected movement, whereas the indirect pathway inhibits inappropriate competing movements (Kravitz, Tye, & Kreitzer, 2012). The indirect pathway is essential for learned performance. Researchers found that impairing the indirect pathway greatly slowed rats' ability to learn to press one lever or another depending on what tone they heard (Nishizawa et al., 2012).

The basal ganglia are particularly important for spontaneous, self-initiated behaviors. For example, a monkey in one study was trained to move one hand to the left or right to receive food. On trials when it heard a signal indicating exactly when to move, the basal ganglia showed little activity. However, on other trials the monkey saw a light indicating that it should start its movement in not less than 1.5 seconds and finish in not more than 3 seconds. Therefore, the monkey had to choose its own starting time. Under those conditions, the basal ganglia were highly active (Turner & Anderson, 2005).

In another study, people used a computer mouse to draw lines on a screen while researchers used PET scans to examine brain activity. Activity in the basal ganglia increased when

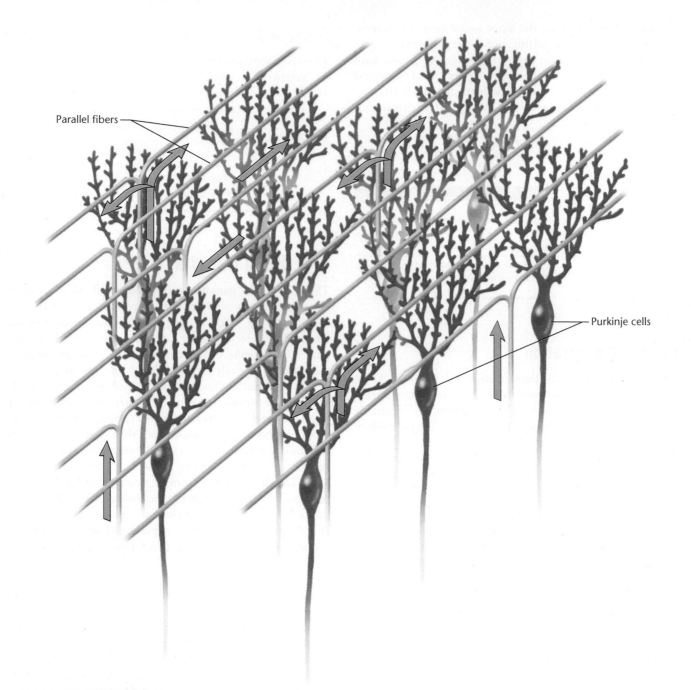

Parallel fibers

Purkinje cells

Figure 7.15 Cellular organization of the cerebellum
Parallel fibers (yellow) activate one Purkinje cell after another. Purkinje cells (red) inhibit a target cell in one of the nuclei of the cerebellum (not shown, but toward the bottom of the illustration). The more Purkinje cells that respond, the longer the target cell is inhibited. In this way, the cerebellum controls the duration of a movement.

people drew a new line but not when they traced a line already on the screen (Jueptner & Weiller, 1998). Again, the basal ganglia seem critical for self-initiated actions, and not for stimulus-elicited actions. In general, self-initiated behaviors have a slower onset than those in response to a stimulus. For example, if you are driving your car and you decide you need to change lanes to make a turn, you react slowly. Imagine how much faster you react if a deer charges in front of you. Another example: When you raise your hand to ask a question

in class, ordinarily you ponder it for a while, eventually decide to ask the question, and slowly raise your hand. But if the professor asks how many would like to postpone Friday's test, you raise your hand at once.

The difference between stimulus-initiated and self-initiated behaviors has an interesting consequence. Many old Western movies included a gunfight between the hero and the villain. Always the villain drew his gun first, but the hero was faster, and even though he started later, he won the draw.

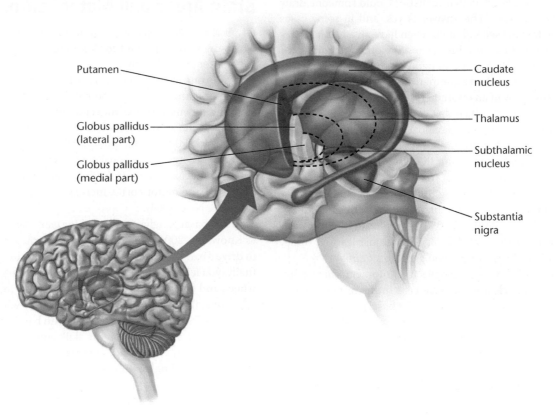

Figure 7.16 Location of the basal ganglia
The basal ganglia surround the thalamus and are surrounded by the cerebral cortex.

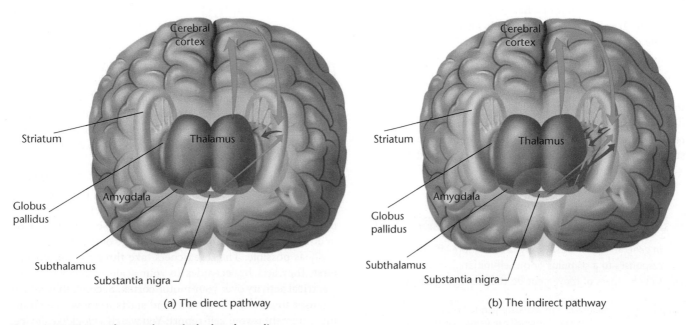

(a) The direct pathway

(b) The indirect pathway

Figure 7.17 Two pathways through the basal ganglia
The indirect pathway has extra connections within the globus pallidus and back and forth to the subthalamus.

Researchers wondered, is that realistic? Could someone draw second and still win? The answer is yes, and in some cases the person drawing second might even have an advantage, because a reaction to a stimulus (seeing the other person go for his gun) is faster than a spontaneous movement. In one experiment, two people had a competition. While watching each other, they had to wait an unpredictable period of time—if they acted too soon, the results didn't count—and then press three buttons in a particular order (analogous to drawing a gun and shooting). So, each person sometimes initiated the action and sometimes reacted after seeing the other person act, but the one who completed the action first was the winner. On average, when people were reacting to the other person's act, they made the movements 9 percent faster (Welchman, Stanley, Schomers, Miall, & Bülthoff, 2010). A replication found similar results (La Delfa et al., 2013). So, you just learned something useful for the next time you get into a gunfight.

The role of the basal ganglia in movement control has gradually become clearer. Because cells in the primary motor cortex become active before those in the basal ganglia, the basal ganglia must not be responsible for selecting which movement to make. Rather, their role is to regulate the vigor of the movement (Turner & Desmurget, 2010). Many cells in the basal ganglia cells respond strongly to signals indicating that a response will probably lead to reward (Ikemoto, Yan, & Tan, 2015). Stimulating dopamine type 1 receptors (D1) in the direct pathway of the striatum produces the same behavioral effects that an increase in reward does (Tai, Lee, Benavidez, Bonci, & Wilbrecht, 2012). Activity in the indirect pathway makes responses slower and less vigorous (Yttri & Dudman, 2016).

After damage to the striatum, animals still learn to choose the response that produces the larger reward, but they don't respond more vigorously for the larger reward (Wang, Miura, & Uchida, 2013). Describing the role of the basal ganglia in these terms makes sense of what we see in patients with damage to the basal ganglia, as in Parkinson's disease. They are capable of strong movements, and sometimes they do move strongly, in response to immediate signals. (Remember, the basal ganglia control mainly self-initiated movements.) However, their spontaneous movements are slow and weak, as if they felt little motivation to move. We consider Parkinson's disease in more detail in the next module. Also consider the relevance to depression: When the dopamine pathway to the striatum becomes less active, the result is depressed mood and a lack of motivation.

STOP & CHECK

15. In general, do the basal ganglia have more effect on responses to a stimulus or on self-initiated movements?
16. Which aspect of movement do the basal ganglia control?

ANSWERS 15. The basal ganglia have more influence on self-initiated movements, which are generally slower. 16. The basal ganglia control the vigor of movements.

Brain Areas and Motor Learning

Of all the brain areas responsible for control of movement, which ones are important for learning new skills? The apparent answer is all of them.

Neurons in the motor cortex adjust their responses as a person or animal learns a motor skill. At first, movements are slow and inconsistent. As movements become faster, relevant neurons in the motor cortex increase their firing rates (Cohen & Nicolelis, 2004). After prolonged training, the movement patterns become more consistent from trial to trial, and so do the patterns of activity in the motor cortex. In engineering terms, the motor cortex increases its signal-to-noise ratio (Kargo & Nitz, 2004).

The basal ganglia are critical for learning new habits (Yin & Knowlton, 2006). For example, when you are first learning to drive a car, you have to think about everything you do. Eventually, you learn to signal for a left turn, change gears, turn the wheel, and change speed all at once. You also inhibit many irrelevant actions. If you try to explain exactly what you do, you will probably find it difficult. People with basal ganglia damage are impaired at learning motor skills and at converting new movements into smooth, "automatic" responses (Poldrack et al., 2005; Willingham, Koroshetz, & Peterson, 1996).

STOP & CHECK

17. What kind of learning depends most heavily on the basal ganglia?

ANSWER 17. The basal ganglia are essential for learning motor habits that are difficult to describe in words.

Conscious Decisions and Movement

Where does conscious decision come into all of this? Each of us has the feeling, "I consciously decide to do something, and then I do it." That sequence seems so obvious that we might not even question it, but research casts doubt on this assumption.

Imagine yourself in the following study (Libet, Gleason, Wright, & Pearl, 1983). You are instructed to flex your wrist whenever you choose. You don't choose which movement to make, but you choose the time freely. You should not decide in advance when to move but let the urge occur as spontaneously as possible. The researchers take three measurements. First, they attach electrodes to your scalp to record evoked electrical activity over your motor cortex. Second, they attach a sensor to record when your hand starts to move. The third measurement is your self-report: You watch a clocklike device, as shown in Figure 7.18, in which a spot of light moves around the circle every 2.56 seconds. You are to watch that clock.

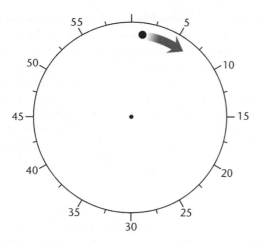

Figure 7.18 Procedure for Libet's study of conscious decision and movement
The participant was to make a spontaneous decision to move the wrist and remember where the light was at the time of that decision.
(Source: From "Time of conscious intention to act in relation to onset of cerebral activities (readiness potential): The unconscious initiation of a freely voluntary act," by B. Libet et al., in Brain, 106, pp. 623–42. Reprinted by permission of Oxford University Press.)

Do not decide in advance that you will flex your wrist when the spot on the clock gets to a certain point. However, when you do decide to move, note where the spot of light is at the moment when you decide, and remember it so you can report it later.

The procedure starts. You think, "Not yet . . . not yet . . . not yet . . . NOW!" You note where the spot was at that critical instant and report, "I made my decision when the light was at the 25 position." The researchers compare your report to their records of your brain activity and your wrist movement. On the average, people report that their decision to move occurred about 200 ms before the actual movement. (The

decision occurred then. People *report* the decision later.) For example, if you reported that your decision to move occurred at position 25, your decision came 200 ms before the movement that began at position 30. (Remember, the light moves around the circle in 2.56 seconds.) However, your motor cortex produces a kind of activity called a **readiness potential** before any voluntary movement, and on the average, the readiness potential begins at least 500 ms before the movement. In this example, it would start when the light was at position 18, as illustrated in Figure 7.19.

The results varied among individuals, but most were similar. The key point is that the brain activity responsible for the movement apparently began *before* the person's conscious decision! The results seem to indicate that your conscious decision does not cause your action. Rather, you become conscious of the decision after the process leading to action has already been underway for about 300 milliseconds.

As you can imagine, this experiment has sparked much discussion among philosophers as well as psychologists. The research has been replicated in several laboratories, so the results are solid (e.g., Lau, Rogers, Haggard, & Passingham, 2004; Trevena & Miller, 2002). One objection is that people cannot accurately report the time they become conscious of something. However, when people are asked to report the time of a sensory stimulus, or the time that they made a movement (instead of the decision to move), their estimates are usually within 30 to 50 ms of the correct time (Lau et al., 2004; Libet et al., 1983). That is, they cannot report the exact time when something happens, but they are close.

Nevertheless, we are probably less accurate at reporting the time of a conscious decision than the time of a sensory stimulus. After all, we often need to know when something happened, but we seldom need to know exactly when we made a decision. Furthermore, Libet's method asks someone

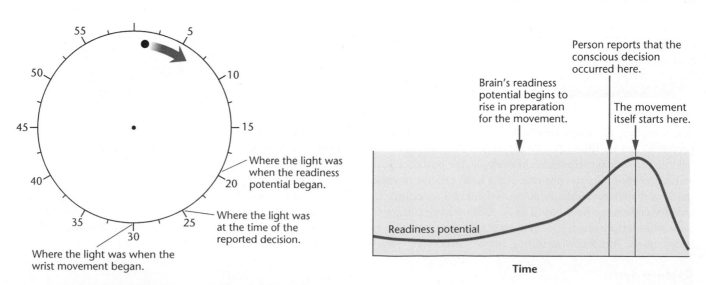

Figure 7.19 Results from study of conscious decision and movement
On average, the brain's readiness potential began at least 300 ms before the reported decision, which occurred 200 ms before the movement.
(Source: From "Time of conscious intention to act in relation to onset of cerebral activities (readiness potential): The unconscious initiation of a freely voluntary act," by B. Libet et al., in Brain, 106, pp. 623–42. Reprinted by permission of Oxford University Press.)

to identify the instant when he or she decided to flex the wrist, as if the decision happened instantaneously. In fact, such a decision builds up gradually (Guggisberg & Mottaz, 2013). The movement is a spontaneous, self-initiated movement, the type that depends on the basal ganglia, the type of movement that has a slow onset. Reporting when you decided to make a voluntary movement is like reporting when you fell in love with someone: You can report the time when you were sure of it, but the process developed gradually long before that.

When people report the time of their decision, maybe they are just guessing. Suppose we repeat Libet's experiment with one change: When you make your movement, you will hear a sound, which you naturally assume is simultaneous with your movement. Sometimes it is, but sometimes it is delayed by a fraction of a second after your movement. On occasions when it is delayed, your reported time of making a conscious decision is also delayed! Apparently your report of when you made your decision depends on when you think the movement occurred (Banks & Isham, 2009; Rigoni, Brass, & Sartori, 2010). If your report of when you decided is little more than a guess, then Libet's results don't tell us as much as we thought they did.

Let's consider one more experiment: You watch a screen that displays letters of the alphabet, one at a time, changing every half-second. In this case you choose not just when to act, but which of two acts to do. You should decide at some point whether to press a button on the left or one on the right. When you make that decision, press the button immediately, and remember what letter was on the screen at the moment when you decided which button to press. Meanwhile, the researchers record activity from your cortex. The result: People usually report a letter they saw within one second of making the response. Remember, the letters changed only twice a second, so it wasn't possible to determine the time of decision with great accuracy. However, it wasn't necessary, because parts of the frontal and parietal cortices showed activity specific to the left

or right hand *7 to 10 seconds* before the response (Soon, Brass, Heinze, & Haynes, 2008). That is, someone monitoring your cortex could, in this situation, predict which choice you were going to make a few seconds before you were aware of making the decision. Evidently a decision to move develops more slowly than we might have guessed, and we are conscious of the decision only toward the end of the process.

None of these results deny that you make a *voluntary* decision. The implication, however, is that what we identify as a conscious decision is the perception of a gradual brain process. It probably begins with unconscious processes that build up to a certain level before they become conscious.

Does brain activity always start 7 to 10 seconds before a movement? Of course not. If you see or hear something that calls for an action—such as a pedestrian darting into the road while you are driving—you respond within a split second. Again you see the importance of the distinction between stimulus-triggered movements and self-initiated movements.

STOP & CHECK

18. Explain the evidence suggesting that a conscious decision to move does not cause the movement.
19. Why are some researchers skeptical of this evidence?

ANSWERS
18. Researchers recorded responses in people's cortex that predicted the upcoming response. Those brain responses occurred earlier than the time people reported as "when they made the decision." 19. The studies assume that people accurately report the times of their intentions. However, people's reports are influenced by events after the movement, and therefore we cannot be confident of their accuracy. Furthermore, a decision to make a voluntary movement is a gradual process that cannot be pinpointed to a single instant.

Module 7.2 | In Closing
Movement Control and Cognition

It is tempting to describe behavior in three steps—first we perceive, then we think, and finally we act. Brain areas do not fall into those neat categories. For example, the posterior parietal cortex monitors the position of the body relative to visual space and thereby helps guide movement. Its functions are sensory, cognitive, and motor. The cerebellum has traditionally been considered a major part of the motor system, but it is now known to be important in timing sensory processes. People

with basal ganglia damage are slow to start or select a movement. They are also often described as cognitively slow; that is, they hesitate longer than usual before making any kind of choice. In short, organizing a movement is not something we tack on at the end of our thinking. It is intimately intertwined with all of our sensory and cognitive processes. The study of movement is not just the study of muscles. It is the study of how we decide what to do.

Summary

1. The primary motor cortex is the main source of brain input to the spinal cord. The spinal cord contains central pattern generators that actually control the muscles. **233**

2. Each area of the motor cortex is closely aligned with a portion of the somatosensory cortex that pertains to the same body part. **233**

3. The primary motor cortex produces patterns representing the intended outcome, not just the muscle contractions. **235**

4. Areas near the primary motor cortex—including the prefrontal, premotor, and supplementary motor cortices—are active in detecting stimuli for movement and preparing for a movement. **236**

5. The ability to inhibit an inappropriate behavior develops gradually in children and adolescents, depending on maturation of the prefrontal cortex and basal ganglia. **236**

6. Mirror neurons in various brain areas respond to both a self-produced movement and an observation of a similar movement by another individual. Their role in imitation and social behavior is uncertain. In many, possibly all, cases they develop their properties by learning, and they may be a result of imitation more than a cause of it. **236**

7. The lateral tract, which controls movements in the periphery of the body, has axons that cross from one side of the brain to the opposite side of the spinal cord. The medial tract controls bilateral movements near the midline of the body. **238**

8. The cerebellum is critical for movements that require accurate aim and timing. **239**

9. The cerebellum has multiple roles in behavior, including sensory functions related to perception of the timing or rhythm of stimuli. **240**

10. The cells of the cerebellum are arranged in a regular pattern that enables them to produce outputs of precisely controlled duration. **241**

11. The basal ganglia are a group of large subcortical structures that are important for self-initiated behaviors. The basal ganglia process information about probable rewards and thereby regulate the vigor of responses. **241**

12. The learning of a motor skill depends on changes occurring in both the cerebral cortex and the basal ganglia. **244**

13. When people identify the instant when they formed a conscious intention to move, their time precedes the actual movement by about 200 ms but follows the start of motor cortex activity by about 300 ms. However, it is not clear how accurately people can report the time of a conscious decision. A voluntary decision to move develops gradually, not suddenly. **244**

Key Terms

Terms are defined in the module on the page number indicated. They're also presented in alphabetical order with definitions in the book's Subject Index/Glossary, which begins on page 589. Interactive flash cards, audio reviews, and crossword puzzles are among the online resources available to help you learn these terms and the concepts they represent.

antisaccade task **236**
basal ganglia **241**
caudate nucleus **241**
cerebellar cortex **241**
corticospinal tracts **238**
globus pallidus **241**
lateral corticospinal tract **238**
medial corticospinal tract **239**

mirror neurons **236**
nuclei of the cerebellum **241**
parallel fibers **241**
posterior parietal cortex **235**
prefrontal cortex **236**
premotor cortex **236**
primary motor cortex **233**
Purkinje cells **241**

putamen **241**
readiness potential **245**
red nucleus **238**
striatum or dorsal striatum **241**
supplementary motor cortex **236**
vestibular nucleus **239**

Thought Question

Human infants are at first limited to gross movements of the trunk, arms, and legs. The ability to move one finger at a time matures gradually over at least the first year. What hypothesis would you suggest about which brain areas controlling movement mature early and which areas mature later?

Module 7.2 | End of Module Quiz

1. What is the route from the motor cortex to the muscles?
   A. Axons from the motor cortex go directly to the muscles.
   B. Axons from the motor cortex go to the thalamus, which has axons to the muscles.
   C. Axons from the motor cortex go to the cerebellum, which has axons to the muscles.
   D. Axons from the motor cortex go to the brainstem and spinal cord, which have axons to the muscles.

2. A half-second stimulation in the motor cortex produces what kind of result?
   A. Isolated muscle twitches
   B. Contraction of a particular combination of muscles
   C. Contraction of whatever muscles are necessary to produce a particular outcome
   D. Contractions of different muscles that vary unpredictably from one trial to another

3. When a movement occurs, which of the following brain areas is the last one to reach its peak of activity?

A. The primary motor cortex

B. The posterior parietal cortex

C. The premotor cortex

D. The prefrontal cortex

4. What does the antisaccade task measure?

A. The ability to inhibit a movement

B. The ability to vary the strength of a movement

C. The ability to control the speed of a movement

D. The ability to alternate between antagonistic muscles

5. Before we conclude that mirror neurons help people imitate, which of the following should research demonstrate?

A. Mirror neurons respond to both seeing and hearing someone else's movement.

B. Mirror neurons occur in the same brain areas of humans as in monkeys.

C. Mirror neurons have different properties for people from different cultures.

D. Mirror neurons develop their properties before children start to imitate.

6. What does the medial corticospinal tract control?

A. Bilateral movements of the trunk of the body

B. Contralateral movements of the trunk of the body

C. Bilateral movements of the arms, hands, and feet

D. Contralateral movements of the arms, hands, and feet

7. What does the finger-to-nose test measure?

A. Possible dysfunction of the basal ganglia

B. Possible dysfunction of the cerebellum

C. Possible dysfunction of the prefrontal cortex

D. Possible dysfunction of the primary motor cortex

8. The cerebellum is most important for which aspect of movement?

A. Strength

B. Timing

C. Direction

D. Inhibition

9. How are the parallel fibers arranged relative to the Purkinje cells?

A. They are parallel to them.

B. They are perpendicular to them.

C. They are arranged at random angles.

D. They circle around each Purkinje cell.

10. Which of the following characterizes the movements that depend heavily on the basal ganglia?

A. Stimulus-triggered, and generally faster than self-initiated movements

B. Stimulus-triggered, and generally slower than self-initiated movements

C. Self-initiated, and generally faster than responses that a stimulus triggers

D. Self-initiated, and generally slower than responses that a stimulus triggers

11. In what way, if at all, does basal ganglia activity relate to motivation?

A. The basal ganglia increase vigor of response depending on expected reward value.

B. The basal ganglia help to maintain constant behavior even when motivation is low.

C. The basal ganglia become active only when you are competing against someone else.

D. Basal ganglia activity has nothing to do with motivation.

12. What kind of learning depends most heavily on the basal ganglia?

A. Learned movements that depend on precise timing

B. Motor habits that are difficult to describe in words

C. Learning to recall specific life events

D. Learning what foods to eat

13. According to Libet's study, what is the order of events in a voluntary movement?

A. People form an intention, then activity begins in the premotor cortex, and finally the movement starts.

B. People form an intention at the same time that activity begins in the premotor cortex, and a bit later, the movement starts.

C. Activity begins in the premotor cortex, and a bit later, people are aware of forming an intention, and finally the movement starts.

D. Activity begins in the premotor cortex, and a bit later, people are aware of forming an intention, and simultaneously the movement starts.

Answers: 1D, 2C, 3A, 4A, 5D, 6A, 7B, 8B, 9B, 10D, 11A, 12B, 13C.

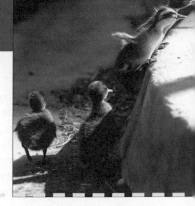

Movement Disorders

If you have damage in your spinal cord, peripheral nerves, or muscles, you cannot move, but cognitively you are the same as ever. In contrast, brain disorders that impair movement also impair mood, memory, and cognition. We consider two examples: Parkinson's disease and Huntington's disease.

Parkinson's Disease

Parkinson's disease (also known as *Parkinson disease*), which strikes 1 to 2 percent of people over age 65, results from the gradual loss of dopamine-releasing axons from the substantia nigra to the striatum (part of the basal ganglia). With the loss of this input, the striatum decreases its inhibition of the globus pallidus, which therefore increases its inhibitory input to the thalamus, as shown in Figure 7.20. The primary results are rigidity, muscle tremors, slow movements, and difficulty initiating voluntary activity. People with Parkinson's disease are still capable of movement, and sometimes they move normally in response to signals or instructions, such as when following a parade (Teitelbaum, Pellis, & Pellis, 1991). However, their spontaneous movements are slow and weak. The movement problems include both a difficulty activating a movement and a difficulty inhibiting inappropriate movements (Jahanshahi, Obeso, Rothwell, & Obeso, 2015). Another common symptom is a lack of motivation and pleasure (Martínez-Horta et al., 2014). Many but not all Parkinson's patients have cognitive deficits, which may include problems with attention, language, or memory (Miller, Neargarder, Risi, & Cronin-Golomb, 2013).

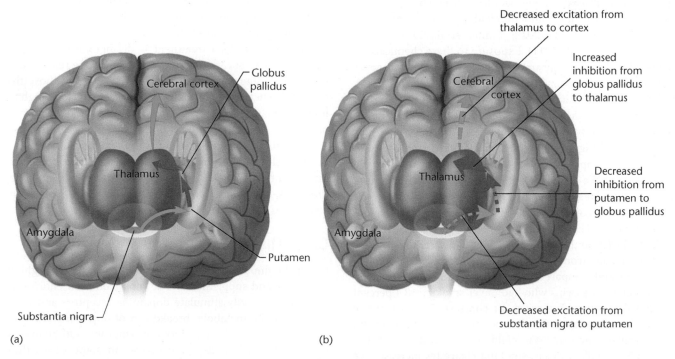

Figure 7.20 Connections from the substantia nigra: (a) normal and (b) in Parkinson's disease
Excitatory paths are shown in green; inhibitory are in red. Decreased excitation from the substantia nigra decreases inhibition from the striatum, leading to increased inhibition from the globus pallidus. The net result is decreased excitation from the thalamus to the cortex.
(Source: Based on Yin & Knowlton, 2006)

Causes

The problem starts in the substantia nigra, but what causes the damage to the substantia nigra? Researchers have identified at least 28 gene variants that increase the risk of Parkinson's disease (Nalls et al., 2014). None of those genes by itself has a major effect, but having several of them produces a cumulative effect. Still, no one can examine your chromosomes and predict with much accuracy whether or not you will develop the disease (Darweesh et al., 2016).

An accidental discovery implicated exposure to toxins as another factor in Parkinson's disease (Ballard, Tetrud, & Langston, 1985). In northern California in 1982, several young adults developed symptoms of Parkinson's disease after using a drug similar to heroin. Before the investigators could alert the community to the danger, many other users had developed symptoms ranging from mild to fatal (Tetrud, Langston, Garbe, & Ruttenber, 1989). The substance responsible for the symptoms was **MPTP**, a chemical that the body converts to **MPP+**, which accumulates in, and then destroys, neurons that release dopamine, partly by impairing the transport of mitochondria from the cell body to the synapse[1] (Kim-Han, Antenor-Dorsey, & O'Malley, 2011; Nicklas, Saporito, Basma, Geller, & Heikkila, 1992).

No one supposes that Parkinson's disease often results from using illegal drugs. A more likely hypothesis is that people are sometimes exposed to hazardous environmental chemicals that damage cells of the substantia nigra. Many studies, though not all, have shown a somewhat increased risk of Parkinson's disease among people with much exposure to insecticides, herbicides, and fungicides (Freire & Koifman, 2012; Pezzoli & Cereda, 2013; Tanner et al., 2011; Wan & Lin, 2016; Wang et al., 2011). Exposure to these chemicals increases the risk especially among people with any of the genes that predispose to Parkinson's (Cannon & Greenamyre, 2013). If someone also had a traumatic head injury, the risk goes up even more (Lee, Bordelon, Bronstein, & Ritz, 2012). In short, most cases result from a combination of influences.

What else might influence the risk of Parkinson's disease? Researchers compared the lifestyles of people who did and didn't develop the disease. One factor that stands out consistently is cigarette smoking and coffee drinking: People who smoke cigarettes or drink coffee have less chance of developing Parkinson's disease (Li, Li, Liu, Shen, & Tang, 2015; Ritz et al., 2007). (Read that sentence again.) One study took questionnaire results from more than a thousand pairs of young adult twins and compared the results to medical records decades later. Of the twins who had never smoked, 18.4 percent developed Parkinson's disease. In contrast, 13.8 percent of the smokers developed the disease, as did only 11.6 percent of the heaviest smokers (Wirdefeldt, Gatz, Pawitan, & Pedersen, 2005). Needless to say, smoking cigarettes increases the risk of lung cancer and other diseases more than it decreases the risk of Parkinson's disease. One study focusing on coffee

found that people who drank 10 or more cups of coffee per day had only one-fourth the risk of Parkinson's disease that other people had (Sääksjärvi, Knekt, Rissanen, Laaksonen, Reunanen, & Männistö, 2008). However, correlation does not mean causation. People who drink that much coffee may differ from other people in other ways as well.

STOP & CHECK

20. How does MPTP exposure influence the likelihood of Parkinson's disease? What are the effects of cigarette smoking?

ANSWER 20. Exposure to MPTP can induce symptoms of Parkinson's disease. Cigarette smoking is correlated with decreased risk of the disease.

L-Dopa Treatment

Because Parkinson's disease results from a dopamine deficiency, a logical goal is to restore the missing dopamine. A dopamine pill would be ineffective because dopamine does not cross the blood–brain barrier. Physicians in the 1950s and 1960s reasoned that **L-dopa**, a precursor to dopamine that does cross the barrier, might be a good treatment. In contrast to all the medicines that were discovered by trial and error, this was the first drug in psychiatry or neurology, and one of the first in all of medicine, to emerge from a plausible theory. Taken as a daily pill, L-dopa reaches the brain, where neurons convert it to dopamine. L-dopa is still the most common treatment for Parkinson's disease.

However, L-dopa treatment is disappointing in several ways (Obeso et al., 2008). It increases dopamine release in all axons, including those that had deteriorated and those that were still functioning normally. It produces spurts of high release alternating with lower release. Even if it adequately replaces lost dopamine, it does not replace other transmitters that are also depleted (Tritsch, Ding, & Sabatinni, 2012). It does not slow the continuing loss of neurons. And it produces unpleasant side effects such as nausea, restlessness, sleep problems, low blood pressure, repetitive movements, and sometimes hallucinations and delusions.

Other Therapies

Given the limitations of L-dopa, researchers have sought alternatives and supplements. The most common choices are drugs that directly stimulate dopamine receptors and drugs that block the metabolic breakdown of dopamine. To varying degrees, these drugs reduce the symptoms, although none of them halt the underlying disease. In some cases, these drugs provoke impulsive or compulsive behaviors (Wylie et al., 2012). In advanced cases, physicians sometimes implant electrodes to stimulate areas deep in the brain (de Hemptinne et al., 2015). Exactly why that procedure helps is uncertain. One hypothesis is that people with Parkinson's disease have

[1]The full names of these chemicals are 1-methyl-4 phenyl-1,2,3,6-tetrahydropyridine and 1-methyl-4-phenylpyridinium ion. (Let's hear it for abbreviations.)

excessive synchrony of firing in the basal ganglia, and the stimulation breaks up unhealthy rhythms.

A potentially exciting strategy has been "in the experimental stage" since the 1980s. In a pioneering study, M. J. Perlow and colleagues (1979) injected the chemical 6-OHDA (6-hydroxydopamine, a chemical modification of dopamine) into rats to damage the substantia nigra of one hemisphere, producing Parkinson's-type symptoms on the opposite side of the body. After the movement abnormalities stabilized, the experimenters transplanted substantia nigra tissue from rat fetuses into the damaged brains. Most recipients recovered much of their normal movement within four weeks. Control animals that suffered the same brain damage without receiving grafts showed little or no recovery. This is only a partial brain transplant, but still, the Frankensteinian implications are striking.

If such surgery works for rats, might it also for humans? Ordinarily, scientists test any experimental procedure extensively with laboratory animals before trying it on humans, but with Parkinson's disease, the temptation was too great. People in the late stages have little to lose and are willing to try almost anything. The obvious problem is where to get the donor tissue. Several early studies used tissue from the patients' own adrenal gland. Although that tissue is not composed of neurons, it does produce dopamine. Unfortunately, the adrenal gland transplants seldom produced much benefit (Backlund et al., 1985).

Another possibility is to transplant brain tissue from aborted fetuses. Fetal neurons transplanted into the brain of patients with Parkinson's sometimes survive for years and make synapses with the patients' own cells. However, the operation is expensive and difficult, requiring brain tissue from four to eight aborted fetuses. For years, the benefits to the patients were small at best (Freed et al., 2001; Olanow et al., 2003). Results improved when physicians aided survival of the graft by giving drugs to suppress the immune reaction. Occasionally the procedure has been reasonably successful. One 59-year-old man received a transplant from four human embryos into the putamen on the right side of his brain. His condition improved dramatically, and for the next 10 years he had only minor symptoms, while remaining on a low dose of L-dopa. After that, he gradually deteriorated. Still, when he died 24 years after the operation, a postmortem analysis revealed that thousands of the transplanted cells still survived, with intact synapses (Li et al., 2016). So, the procedure can work, although it is still far from ideal. The effectiveness depends on the age and health of the patients, the number and placement of transplanted cells, the immune response, and other factors (Wenker, Leal, Farías, Zeng, & Pitossi, 2016).

A related approach is to take **stem cells**—immature cells that are capable of differentiating into other cell types—guide their development so that they produce large quantities of L-dopa, and then transplant them into the brain. The idea sounds promising, but researchers will need to overcome several difficulties before this might become an effective treatment (Bjorklund & Kordower, 2013).

The research on brain transplants has suggested yet another possibility for treatment. In several experiments, the transplanted tissue failed to survive, but the recipient showed behavioral recovery anyway (Redmond et al., 2007). Presumably, the transplanted tissue released neurotrophins that stimulated axon and dendrite growth in the recipient's own brain. Work with mice has shown promising results for a neurotrophin to repair Parkinson-like damage (Airavaara et al., 2012). Applying that procedure to humans would still require surgery to deliver the neurotrophin, as neurotrophins do not cross the blood–brain barrier.

✅ **STOP & CHECK** ▬▬▬▬▬▬▬

21. How does L-dopa relieve the symptoms of Parkinson's disease?
22. In what ways is L-dopa treatment disappointing?
23. What procedure has improved the effectiveness of brain grafts for treatment of Parkinson's disease?

ANSWERS   21. L-dopa enters the brain, where neurons convert it to dopamine, thus increasing the supply of a depleted neurotransmitter. 22. L-dopa increases dopamine activity in spurts and in all neurons, not steadily and not just in those that need help. It does not stop the loss of neurons. It has unpleasant side effects. 23. Results improved somewhat after physicians began giving drugs to suppress the immune response.

Huntington's Disease

Huntington's disease (also known as *Huntington disease* or *Huntington's chorea*) is a severe neurological disorder. The prevalence varies geographically and ethnically. The condition affects about 17 per 100,000 Americans of European ancestry, less than half that many Europeans within Europe itself, probably fewer Africans—although the data for Africa are sparse—and very few Asians (Rawlins et al., 2016).

Motor symptoms usually begin with arm jerks and facial twitches. Then tremors spread to other parts of the body and develop into writhing (M. A. Smith, Brandt, & Shadmehr, 2000). (*Chorea* comes from the same root as *choreography*. The rhythmic writhing of chorea resembles dancing.) Gradually, the tremors interfere more and more with walking, speech, and other voluntary movements. People lose the ability to develop motor skills (Willingham et al., 1996). The disorder is associated with gradual, extensive brain damage, especially in the basal ganglia but also in the cerebral cortex (Tabrizi et al., 1999) (see Figure 7.21). Because the output from the basal ganglia is inhibitory to the thalamus, damage to the basal ganglia leads to increased activity in motor areas of the thalamus. That increase produces the involuntary jerky movements.

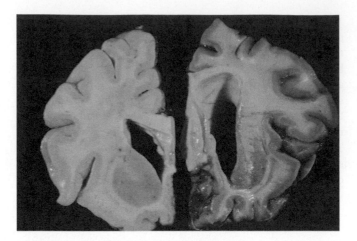

Figure 7.21 Brain of a normal person (left) and a person with Huntington's disease (right)
The angle of cut through the normal brain makes the lateral ventricle look larger in this photo than it actually is. Even so, note how much larger it is in the patient with Huntington's disease. The ventricles expand because of the loss of neurons.
(Robert E. Schmidt, Washington University)

People with Huntington's disease also suffer psychological disorders including apathy, depression, sleeplessness, memory impairment, anxiety, hallucinations and delusions, poor judgment, alcoholism, drug abuse, and sexual disorders ranging from complete unresponsiveness to indiscriminate promiscuity (Shoulson, 1990). In many cases the psychological problems, especially apathy, become apparent up to 10 years before the motor symptoms lead to a diagnosis (Martinez-Horta et al., 2016).

Huntington's disease can occur at any age, but most often between the ages of 30 and 50. Once the symptoms emerge, both the psychological and motor symptoms grow progressively worse and culminate in death.

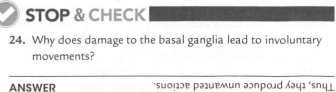

STOP & CHECK

24. Why does damage to the basal ganglia lead to involuntary movements?

ANSWER

24. Output from the basal ganglia to the thalamus is inhibitory. After damage to the basal ganglia, the thalamus, and therefore the cortex, receive less inhibition. Thus, they produce unwanted actions.

Heredity and Presymptomatic Testing

For every other disorder we consider in this text, a genetic contribution is present, but no one gene produces a major effect. Huntington's disease is an exception to that rule. One gene—an autosomal dominant gene (i.e., one not on the X or Y chromosome)—is responsible. As a rule, a mutant gene that causes the loss of a function is recessive. The fact that

the Huntington's gene is dominant implies that it produces the gain of some undesirable function.

Imagine that as a young adult you learn that your mother or father has Huntington's disease. In addition to your grief about your parent, you know that you have a 50 percent chance of getting the disease yourself. Would you want to know in advance whether or not you were going to get the disease? Knowing the answer might help you decide whether to have children, whether to enter a career that required many years of education, and so forth. However, getting bad news might not be easy to handle.

In 1993, researchers located the gene for Huntington's disease on chromosome number 4, a spectacular accomplishment for the technology available at the time (Huntington's Disease Collaborative Research Group, 1993). Now an examination of your chromosomes can reveal with almost perfect accuracy whether or not you will get Huntington's disease.

The critical area of the gene includes a sequence of bases C-A-G (cytosine, adenine, guanine), which is repeated 11 to 24 times in most people. That repetition produces a string of 11 to 24 glutamines in the resulting protein. People with up to 35 C-A-G repetitions are considered safe from Huntington's disease. Those with 36 to 38, possibly even 39 or 40, might not get the disease, and if they do, it probably will not manifest until old age (Kay et al., 2016). People with more repetitions are nearly certain to get the disease, unless they die of other causes earlier. The more C-A-G repetitions someone has, the earlier the probable onset of the disease, as shown in Figure 7.22 (U.S.–Venezuela Collaborative Research Project, 2004). In short, a chromosomal examination predicts not only

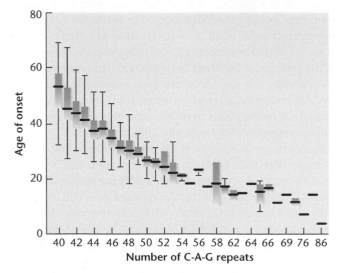

Figure 7.22 Relationship between C-A-G repeats and age of onset of Huntington's disease
For each number of C-A-G repeats, the graph shows the age of onset. The green bars show the range that includes the middle 50 percent of observations, from the 75th percentile to the 25th percentile. The vertical lines show the full range of observations.
(Source: From the U.S.-Venezuela Collaborative Research Project (2004). Proceedings of the National Academy of Sciences, USA, 101, pp. 3498–3503.)

whether someone will get Huntington's disease but also approximately when. The graph shows a considerable amount of variation in age of onset, especially for those with fewer C-A-G repeats. Evidently other factors besides genes also influence the age of onset, such as stressful experiences, drug or alcohol abuse, and perhaps diet and exercise (Byars, Beglinger, Moser, Gonzalez-Alegre, & Nopoulos, 2012).

Figure 7.23 shows comparable data for Huntington's disease and seven other neurological disorders. Each of them relates to an extended sequence of C-A-G repeats in a gene. An extended sequence of repeats also increases the risk of several other conditions not shown in the figure, including fragile X syndrome and amyotrophic lateral sclerosis (Nelson, Orr, & Warren, 2013). In each case, people with the greatest number of repeats have the earliest onset of disease (Gusella & Mac-Donald, 2000). Those with a smaller number will be older, if they get the disease at all. As a rule, heritability is greater for early-onset disorders than for those with later onset. We also see that pattern for Parkinson's disease, Alzheimer's disease, alcoholism, depression, and schizophrenia.

Identification of the gene for Huntington's disease led to the discovery of the protein that it codes, which has been designated **huntingtin**. Huntingtin occurs throughout the human body, although its mutant form produces no known harm outside the brain. The mutant form impairs neurons and glia in several ways, including effects on mitochondria and potassium channels (Tong et al., 2014; Yano et al., 2014).

In the early stages of the disease, it increases neurotransmitter release, sometimes causing overstimulation of the target cells (Romero et al., 2007). Later, the protein forms clusters that impair the neuron's mitochondria (Panov et al., 2002). It also impairs the transport of chemicals down the axon (Morfini et al., 2009).

Identifying the abnormal huntingtin protein and its cellular functions has enabled investigators to search for drugs that might be helpful. One promising approach is to develop drugs that partially suppress the expression of the gene for huntingtin. Research with animal models has shown favorable results for this possibility (Keiser, Kordasiewicz, & McBride, 2016).

⊘ STOP & CHECK ▬▬▬▬▬

25. What procedure enables physicians to predict who will or will not get Huntington's disease and to estimate the age of onset?

ANSWER

25. Physicians can count the number of consecutive repeats of the combination C-A-G on one gene on chromosome 4. If the number is fewer than 36, the person will not develop Huntington's disease. For repeats of 36 or more, the larger the number, the more certain the person is to develop the disease and the earlier the probable age of onset.

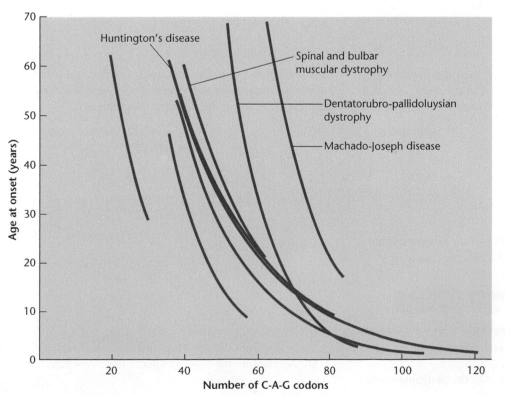

Figure 7.23 Relationship between C-A-G repeats and age of onset of eight diseases
The *x* axis shows the number of C-A-G repeats; the *y* axis shows the mean age at onset of disease. The various lines represent Huntington's disease and seven others. The four unlabeled lines are for four types of spinocerebellar ataxia. The key point is that for each disease, the greater the number of repeats, the earlier the probable onset of symptoms.
(Reproduced with permission from "Molecular genetics: Unmasking polyglutamine triggers in neurogenerative disease," by J. F. Gusella and M. E. MacDonald, Figure.1, p. 111 in Neuroscience, 1, pp. 109–115, copyright 2000 Macmillan Magazines, Ltd.)

Module 7.3 | In Closing

Movement Disorders Affect More than Movement

Parkinson's disease and Huntington's disease emphasize the point that control of movement is closely related to cognition. People with either condition are likely to suffer apathy, cognitive deficits, and a lack of pleasure and motivation. The

psychological problems often develop before any noticeable motor problems. In short, the mechanisms of movement are also the mechanisms of thought.

Summary

1. Parkinson's disease and Huntington's disease both result from brain deterioration that includes the basal ganglia. **249, 251**

2. Parkinson's disease is characterized by impaired initiation of activity, slow and inaccurate movements, tremor, rigidity, depression, and cognitive deficits. **249**

3. Parkinson's disease is associated with the degeneration of dopamine-containing axons from the substantia nigra to the caudate nucleus and putamen. **249**

4. Researchers have identified many gene variants that increase the risk of Parkinson's disease, although none of them by itself has a major effect. **250**

5. The chemical MPTP selectively damages neurons in the substantia nigra and leads to the symptoms of Parkinson's disease. Some cases of Parkinson's disease may result in part from exposure to toxins. **250**

6. The most common treatment for Parkinson's disease is L-dopa, which crosses the blood–brain barrier and enters neurons that convert it into dopamine. However, the

effectiveness of L-dopa varies, and it produces unwelcome side effects. **250**

7. Many other treatments are in use or in the experimental stage, including the transfer of immature neurons into a damaged brain area. **250**

8. Huntington's disease is a hereditary condition marked by deterioration of motor control as well as apathy, depression, memory impairment, and other cognitive disorders. **251**

9. By examining a gene on chromosome 4, physicians can determine whether someone is likely to develop Huntington's disease later in life. The more C-A-G repeats in the gene, the earlier the likely onset of symptoms. **252**

10. The gene responsible for Huntington's disease alters the structure of a protein, known as huntingtin. Inhibiting the production of that protein is a theoretically possible treatment. **253**

Key Terms

Terms are defined in the module on the page number indicated. They're also presented in alphabetical order with definitions in the book's Subject Index/Glossary, which begins on page 589. Interactive flash cards, audio reviews, and crossword puzzles are among the online resources available to help you learn these terms and the concepts they represent.

huntingtin **253**
Huntington's disease **251**
L-dopa **250**

MPP+ **250**
MPTP **250**

Parkinson's disease **249**
stem cells **251**

Thought Question

Haloperidol is a drug that blocks dopamine synapses. What effect would it probably have for Parkinson's disease?

Module 7.3 | End of Module Quiz

1. Deterioration of which axons leads to Parkinson's disease?
   A. Axons from the primary motor cortex to the spinal cord
   B. Axons from the basal forebrain to the prefrontal cortex
   C. Axons from the substantia nigra to the striatum
   D. Axons from the basal ganglia to the cerebellum

2. People with Parkinson's disease show the greatest impairment with which type of movement?

   A. Reflexes
   B. Spontaneous voluntary movements
   C. Movements in response to a stimulus
   D. Movements when other people are around

3. Which of these chemicals damages the brain in a way that resembles Parkinson's disease?

   A. Capsaicin
   B. L-dopa
   C. Cannabinol
   D. MPTP

4. In what way is L-dopa treatment for Parkinson's disease unusual?

   A. It produces behavioral benefits without entering the brain.
   B. Unlike most drugs, it produces no unpleasant side effects.
   C. The treatment becomes more and more effective over time.
   D. It was based on a theory instead of trial and error.

5. What is the most common age of onset for Huntington's disease?

   A. Early childhood (3 to 7 years old)
   B. The teenage years (13 to 19)
   C. Middle age (30 to 50)
   D. Old age (65 to 80)

6. Why does damage to the basal ganglia lead to involuntary movements in Huntington's disease?

   A. The damage interrupts inhibitory axons from the primary motor cortex to the spinal cord.
   B. The cerebellum takes over the functions of the basal ganglia, and overcompensates.
   C. The person voluntarily tries to overcome the lack of coordination.
   D. Basal ganglia damage reduces inhibition of the thalamus.

7. An examination of C-A-G repeats on one gene enables physicians to predict who will develop Huntington's disease. What else does it help them predict?

   A. What other diseases the person will get
   B. The individual's personality
   C. The effectiveness of treatment
   D. The age of onset of symptoms

Answers: 1C, 2B, 3D, 4D, 5C, 6D, 7D.

Suggestions for Further Reading

Klawans, H. L. (1996). *Why Michael couldn't hit.* New York: Freeman. A collection of fascinating sports examples related to the brain and its disorders.

Lashley, K. S. (1951). The problem of serial order in behavior. In L. A. Jeffress (Ed.), *Cerebral mechanisms in behavior* (pp. 112–136). New York: Wiley. This classic article in psychology is a thought-provoking appraisal of what a theory of movement should explain.

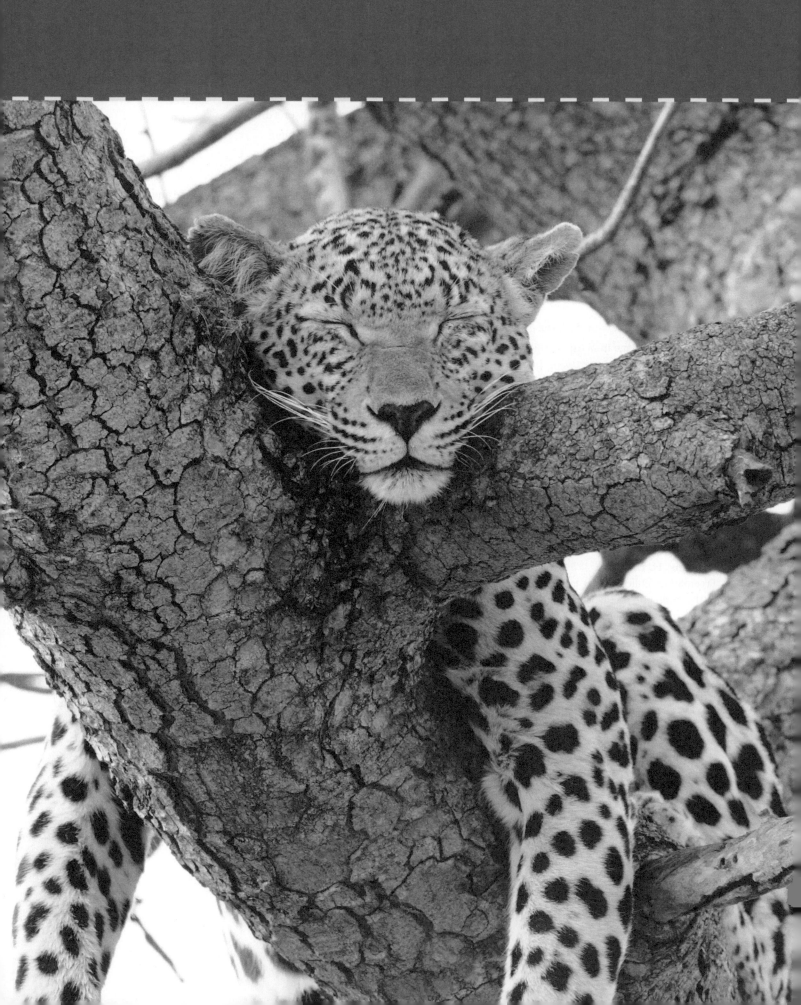

Wakefulness and Sleep

Chapter 8

Anyone deprived of sleep suffers. But if life evolved on another planet with different conditions, could animals evolve life without a need for sleep? Imagine a planet that doesn't rotate on its axis. Some animals evolve adaptations to live in the light area, others in the dark area, and still others in the twilight zone separating light from dark. There would be no need for any animal to alternate active periods with inactive periods on any fixed schedule and perhaps no need for prolonged inactive periods. If you were the astronaut who discovered these sleepless animals, you might be surprised.

Now imagine that astronauts from that planet set out on their first voyage to Earth. Imagine *their* surprise to discover animals like us with long inactive periods resembling death. To someone who hadn't seen sleep before, it would seem mysterious indeed. For the purposes of this chapter, let's adopt their perspective and ask why animals as active as we are spend a third of our lives doing so little.

Learning Objectives

After studying this chapter, you should be able to:

1. Define and describe endogenous rhythms.
2. Explain the mechanisms that set and reset the biological clock.
3. List and characterize the stages of sleep.
4. Describe the brain mechanisms of waking and sleeping.
5. Discuss several consequences of thinking of sleep as a localized phenomenon.
6. List several sleep disorders with their causes.
7. Evaluate possible explanations of the functions of sleep.
8. Describe possible explanations of dreaming.

Opposite:

Sleep is an important part of life for nearly all animals.

(Hoberman Collection/Getty Images)

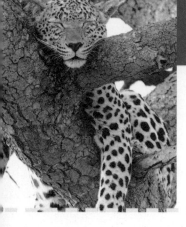

Rhythms of Waking and Sleeping

You are probably not amazed to learn that your body spontaneously generates its own rhythm of wakefulness and sleep. Psychologists of an earlier era strongly resisted that idea. When radical behaviorism dominated experimental psychology during the mid-1900s, many psychologists believed that every behavior could be traced to external stimuli. Therefore, they believed, alternation between wakefulness and sleep must depend on something in the outside world, such as changes in light or temperature. Research as early as that of Curt Richter (1922) implied that the body generates its own cycles of activity and inactivity, but it took decades of research to convince the skeptics. The idea of self-generated rhythms was a major step toward viewing animals as active producers of behaviors.

Endogenous Rhythms

An animal that produced its behavior entirely in response to current stimuli would be at a serious disadvantage. Animals often need to anticipate changes in the environment. For example, migratory birds start flying toward their winter homes before their summer territory becomes too cold. A small bird that waited for the first frost would probably die. Similarly, squirrels begin storing nuts and putting on extra layers of fat in preparation for winter long before food becomes scarce.

Animals' readiness for a change in seasons comes partly from internal mechanisms. Changes in the light–dark pattern of the day tell a migratory bird when to fly south for the winter, but what tells it when to fly back north? In the tropics, the temperature and amount of daylight are nearly the same throughout the year. Nevertheless, migratory birds fly north at the right time. Even if they are kept in a cage with no clues to the season, they become restless in the spring, and if they are released, they fly north (Gwinner, 1986). Evidently, birds generate a rhythm that prepares them for seasonal changes. We refer to that rhythm as an **endogenous circannual rhythm**. (*Endogenous* means "generated from within." *Circannual* comes from the Latin words *circum*, for "about," and *annum*, for "year.")

Animals also produce **endogenous circadian rhythms** that last about a day. (*Circadian* comes from the Latin *circum*, for "about," and *dies*, for "day.") If you go without

sleep all night—as most college students do, sooner or later—you feel sleepier and sleepier as the night goes on, but as morning arrives, you feel more alert, not less. Especially in the posterior areas of the cerebral cortex, activity correlates mainly with your circadian rhythm, and only secondarily with how long you have been awake (Muto et al., 2016).

Figure 8.1 represents the activity of a flying squirrel kept in total darkness for 25 days. Each horizontal line represents one 24-hour day. A thickening in the line represents a period of activity. Even in this unchanging environment, the animal generates a consistent rhythm of activity and sleep. Depending on the individual and the details of the procedure, the self-generated cycle may be slightly shorter than 24 hours, as in Figure 8.1, or slightly longer (Carpenter & Grossberg, 1984).

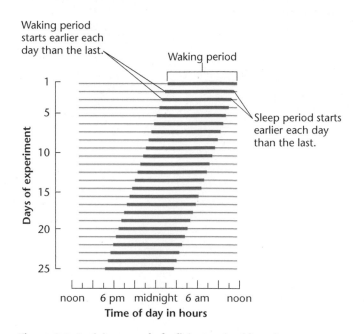

Figure 8.1 Activity record of a flying squirrel kept in constant darkness

The thickened segments indicate periods of activity as measured by a running wheel. Note that this free-running activity cycle lasts slightly less than 24 hours.

(Source: From "Phase control of activity in a rodent," by P. J. DeCoursey, 1960, Cold Spring Harbor Symposia on Quantitative Biology, 25, pp. 49–55. Reprinted by permission of Cold Spring Harbor and P. J. DeCoursey.)

Humans also generate 24-hour wake–sleep rhythms, which we can modify only a little. If we ever send astronauts to Mars, they will have to adjust to the Martian day, which lasts about 24 hours and 39 minutes of Earth time. Engineers who were monitoring the Phoenix robot mission on Mars had to live on the Martian schedule, starting work 39 minutes later each day. Most ($\frac{13}{15}$ who were studied) managed to synchronize their biological rhythms to the Martian schedule, although they did not sleep as much as usual, and some of them suffered a loss of alertness (Barger et al., 2012).

Our circadian rhythm does not easily adjust to more severe departures from a 24-hour schedule. Naval personnel on submarines are cut off from sunlight for months at a time, living under faint artificial light. In many cases, they live on a schedule of 6 hours of work, 6 hours of recreation, and 6 hours of sleep. Even though they try to sleep on this 18-hour schedule, their bodies generate rhythms of alertness and body chemistry that average about 24.3 to 24.4 hours (Kelly et al., 1999).

Circadian rhythms affect much more than just waking and sleeping. We have circadian rhythms in our eating and drinking, urination, hormone secretion, metabolism, sensitivity to drugs, and other variables. For example, although we ordinarily think of human body temperature as 37°C, our temperature fluctuates over the course of a day from a low near 36.7°C during the night to almost 37.2°C in late afternoon (see Figure 8.2). We also have circadian rhythms in mood. In one study, young adults recorded their mood throughout the day. Most showed increases in positive mood (happiness) from waking until late afternoon, and then a slight decline until bedtime. In a follow-up study, the same investigators kept young adults awake for 30 consecutive hours, starting at either 10 A.M. or 5 P.M., in a laboratory setting with constant levels of light and temperature.

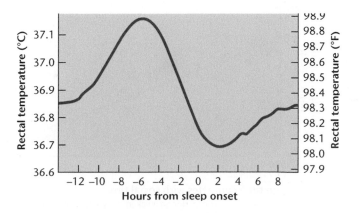

Figure 8.2 Mean rectal temperatures for nine adults
Body temperature reaches its low for the day about 2 hours after sleep onset; it reaches its peak about 6 hours before sleep onset.
(*Source: From "Sleep-onset insomniacs have delayed temperature rhythms," by M. Morris, L. Lack, and D. Dawson, 1990, Sleep, 13, pp. 1–14. Reprinted by permission.*)

Regardless of whether people started this procedure at 10 A.M. or 5 P.M., most reported their most pleasant mood around 5 P.M. and their least pleasant mood at around 5 A.M. (Murray et al., 2009). These results suggest a biologically driven circadian rhythm in our emotional well-being (see Figure 8.3).

STOP & CHECK

1. What evidence indicates that humans have an internal biological clock?

ANSWER

1. People who have lived in an environment with a light–dark schedule much different from 24 hours fail to follow that schedule and instead become wakeful and sleepy on about a 24-hour basis.

Setting and Resetting the Biological Clock

Our circadian rhythms generate a period close to 24 hours, but they are not perfect. We readjust our internal workings daily to stay in phase with the world. Sometimes, we misadjust them. On weekends, when most of us are freer to set our own schedules, we expose ourselves to lights, noises, and activity at night and then awaken late the next morning. By Monday morning, when the clock on your table indicates 7 A.M., your biological clock may say 5 A.M., and you stagger off to work or school without much pep (Moore-Ede, Czeisler, & Richardson, 1983).

Although circadian rhythms persist without light, your rhythm is not perfect. Unless something resets it from time to time, it would gradually drift away from the correct time. The stimulus that resets the circadian rhythm is referred to by the German term **zeitgeber** (TSITE-gay-ber), meaning "time-giver." Light is by far the dominant zeitgeber for land animals (Rusak & Zucker, 1979), whereas the tides are important for some marine animals. In addition to light, other zeitgebers include exercise (Eastman, Hoese, Youngstedt, & Liu, 1995), arousal of any kind (Gritton, Sutton, Martinez, Sarter, & Lee, 2009), meals, and the temperature of the environment (Refinetti, 2000). Social stimuli—that is, the effects of other people—are ineffective as zeitgebers, unless they induce exercise or other vigorous activity (Mistlberger & Skene, 2004). Although these additional zeitgebers modify the effects of light, they have only weak effects on their own. For example, people who are working in Antarctica during the constant darkness of an Antarctic winter try to maintain a 24-hour rhythm, but they drift away from it. Different people generate slightly different rhythms, until they find it more and more difficult to work together (Kennaway & Van Dorp, 1991). Astronauts in orbit face a special problem: As they orbit the Earth, a 45-minute period of daylight alternates

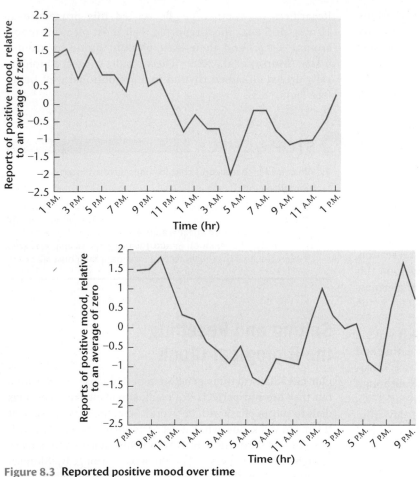

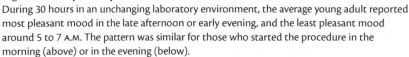

Figure 8.3 Reported positive mood over time

During 30 hours in an unchanging laboratory environment, the average young adult reported most pleasant mood in the late afternoon or early evening, and the least pleasant mood around 5 to 7 A.M. The pattern was similar for those who started the procedure in the morning (above) or in the evening (below).

(Source: From "Nature's clocks and human mood: The circadian system modulates reward motivation," by G. Murray, C. L. Nicholas, J. Kleiman, R. Dwyer, M. J. Carrington, N. B. Allen, et al., 2009, Emotion, 9, pp. 705–716.)

Particularly impressive evidence for the importance of sunlight comes from a study in Germany. Sunrise occurs at the eastern end of Germany about half an hour earlier than at the western end, even though all people set their clocks to the same time. Researchers asked adults for their preferred times of awakening and going to sleep and determined for each person the midpoint of those values. For example, if on weekends and holidays you prefer to go to bed at 12:30 A.M. and awaken at 8:30 A.M., your sleep midpoint is 4:30 A.M. Figure 8.4 shows the results. People at the eastern edge have a sleep midpoint about 30 minutes earlier than those at the west, corresponding to the fact that the sun rises earlier at the eastern edge (Roenneberg, Kumar, & Merrow, 2007). Other researchers reported similar results for Turkey and South Africa (Masal et al., 2015; Shawa & Roden, 2016).

What about blind people, who need to set their circadian rhythms by zeitgebers other than light? The results vary. Some do set their circadian rhythms by noise, temperature, meals, and activity. However, others who are not sufficiently sensitive to these secondary zeitgebers produce circadian rhythms that are a little longer than 24 hours. When their cycles are in phase with the clock, all is well, but when they drift out of phase, they experience insomnia at night and sleepiness during the day (Sack & Lewy, 2001). More than half of all blind people report frequent sleep problems (Warman et al., 2011).

with 45 minutes of darkness. If they retreat from the flight deck to elsewhere in the spacecraft, they have constant dim light. As a result, they are not fully alert during their wakeful periods or deeply asleep during rest periods (Dijk et al., 2001). On long assignments, many of them experience depression and impaired performance (Mallis & DeRoshia, 2005).

Even when we try to set our wake–sleep cycles by the clock, sunlight has its influence. Consider what happens when we shift to daylight saving time in spring. You set your clock to an hour later, and when it shows your usual bedtime, you dutifully go to bed, even though it seems an hour too early. The next morning, when the clock says it is 7 A.M. and time to get ready for work, your brain registers 6 A.M. Most people remain ill rested for days after the shift to daylight saving time. The adjustment is especially difficult for people who were already sleep deprived, including most college students (Lahti et al., 2006; Monk & Aplin, 1980). In fall, when daylight saving time ends, some people have sleep problems then, too (Harrison, 2013).

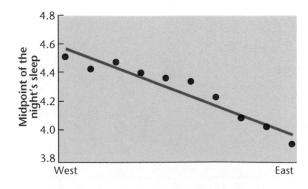

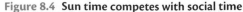

Figure 8.4 Sun time competes with social time

On days when people have no obligation to awaken at a particular time, they awaken about half an hour earlier at the eastern edge of Germany than at the western edge. Points along the *y* axis represent the midpoint between the preferred bedtime and the preferred waking time. Data are for people living in towns and cities with populations less than 300,000.

(Source: From "The human circadian clock entrains to sun time," by T. Roenneberg, C. J. Kumar, and M. Merrow, 2007, Current Biology, 17, pp. R44–R45. Reprinted by permission of the Copyright Clearance Center.)

2. Why do people at the eastern edge of a time zone awaken earlier than those at the western edge on their weekends and holidays?

ANSWER

2. *The sun rises earlier at the eastern edge than at the western edge. Evidently, the sun controls waking–sleeping schedules even when people follow the same clock time for their work schedule.*

Jet Lag

A disruption of circadian rhythms due to crossing time zones is known as **jet lag.** Travelers complain of sleepiness during the day, sleeplessness at night, depression, and impaired concentration. All these problems stem from the mismatch between internal circadian clock and external time (Haimov & Arendt, 1999). Most people find it easier to adjust to crossing time zones going west than east. Going west, we stay awake later at night and then awaken late the next morning, already partly adjusted to the new schedule. We *phase-delay* our circadian rhythms. Going east, we *phase-advance* to sleep earlier and awaken earlier (see Figure 8.5). Most people find it difficult to go to sleep before their body's usual time and difficult to wake up early the next day.

Adjusting to jet lag is often stressful. Stress elevates blood levels of the adrenal hormone *cortisol,* and many studies have shown that prolonged elevations of cortisol damage neurons in the hippocampus, a brain area important for memory. One study examined flight attendants who had spent the previous 5 years making flights across seven or more time zones—such as Chicago to Italy—with mostly short breaks (fewer than 6 days) between trips. On the average, the flight attendants had smaller than average volumes of the hippocampus and surrounding structures, and they showed memory impairments (Cho, 2001). These results suggest a danger from repeated adjustments of the circadian rhythm, although the problem here could be air travel itself. A good control group would have been flight attendants who flew long north–south routes.

Shift Work

People who sleep irregularly—such as pilots, medical interns, and shift workers in factories—find that their duration of sleep depends on when they go to sleep. When they have to sleep in the morning or early afternoon, they sleep only briefly, even if they have been awake for many hours (Frese & Harwich, 1984; Winfree, 1983). People who have done shift work for years tend to perform worse than average on cognitive tests, although because the measures are correlational, we cannot be sure of cause and effect (Marquié, Tucker, Folkard, Gentil, & Ansiau, 2015).

People who work on a night shift, such as midnight to 8 A.M., sleep during the day. At least they try to. Even after months or years on such a schedule, many workers adjust incompletely. They continue to feel groggy on the job, they sleep poorly during the day, and their body temperature continues to peak when they are sleeping in the day instead of while they are working at night. In general, night-shift workers have more accidents than day-shift workers.

People who work at night have great difficulty adjusting their circadian rhythm, because most buildings use artificial lighting in the range of 150 to 180 lux, which is only moderately effective in resetting the rhythm (Boivin, Duffy, Kronauer, & Czeisler, 1996). People adjust best to night work if they sleep in a very dark room during the day and work under very bright lights at night, comparable to the noonday sun (Czeisler et al., 1990). Short-wavelength (bluish) light helps to reset the circadian rhythm better than long-wavelength light does (Czeisler, 2013).

Morning People and Evening People

Circadian rhythms differ among individuals. Some people ("morning people," or "larks") awaken early, reach their peak of productivity early, and become less alert later in the day. Others ("evening people," or "owls") warm up more slowly, both literally and figuratively, reaching their peak in the late

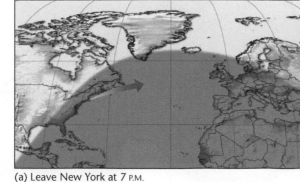

(a) Leave New York at 7 P.M.

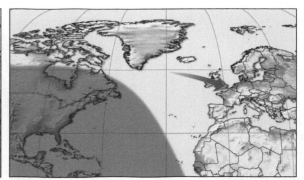

(b) Arrive in London at 7 A.M., which is 2 A.M. in New York

Figure 8.5 Jet lag
Eastern time is later than western time. People who travel five time zones east fall asleep on the plane and then must awaken when it is morning at their destination but night back home.

afternoon or evening. They tolerate staying up all night better than morning people do (Taillard, Philip, Coste, Sagaspe, & Bioulac, 2003). Among shift workers, morning people are most impaired when working the night shift and evening people are most impaired when working the morning shift (Juda, Vetter, & Roenneberg, 2013). Many people are, of course, intermediate between the two extremes.

A convenient way to classify people is to ask, "On holidays and vacations when you have no obligations, what time is the middle of your sleep?" For example, if you sleep from 1 A.M. until 9 A.M. on those days, your middle is 5 A.M. As Figure 8.6 shows, people differ by age. As a child, you almost certainly went to bed early and woke up early. As you entered adolescence, you started staying up later and waking up later, when you had the opportunity. The mean preferred time of going to sleep gets later and later until about age 20 and then gradually reverses (Roenneberg et al., 2004). The tendency to stay up later and awaken later during adolescence occurs in every culture that researchers have studied throughout the world (Gradisar, Gardner, & Dohnt, 2011). The same trend also occurs in rats, monkeys, and other species (Hagenauer & Lee, 2012; Winocur & Hasher, 1999, 2004), apparently resulting from increased levels of sex hormones (Hagenauer & Lee, 2012; Randler et al., 2012). From a functional standpoint, we can only speculate as to why staying up late and waking up late might be more advantageous for adolescents than for children or adults.

So, being a morning person or an evening person depends partly on age. It also depends on genetics and several environmental factors, including artificial light. In low-tech societies without electric lights, people go to sleep about three hours after sunset, seldom awaken during the night, and wake up at sunrise.

In similar societies after gaining electric lights, people stay awake later and get less sleep (de la Iglesia et al., 2015; Yetish et al., 2015). People who live in a big city, surrounded by bright lights, are more likely to stay up late than are people in rural areas.

The tendency for most young people to be evening types causes problems. In the United States and many other countries, high school classes start at 8:00 A.M. or earlier. Most teenagers are at least a bit drowsy at that time, some more than others. Those who are strongly evening types tend to get lower than average test scores, especially in their morning classes, even if they have average or above-average intelligence (Preckel, Lipnevich, Anastasiya, Schneider, & Roberts, 2011; Preckel et al., 2013; van der Vinne et al., 2015). Possibly as a result of school frustration, or perhaps just as a result of staying up late, they are more likely than others to use alcohol, overeat, and engage in other risky behaviors (Hasler & Clark, 2013; Roenneberg, Allebrandt, Merrow, & Vetter, 2012). Even beyond the teenage years, morning people report being happier than evening people, on average, possibly because their biological rhythms are more in tune with their 9-to-5 work schedule (Biss & Hasher, 2012). The morning type versus evening type distinction affects other aspects of behavior also. One study found that morning type people tend to be more moral and honest in the morning, whereas evening type people tend to be more moral and honest in the evening (Gunia, Barnes, & Sah, 2014).

Mechanisms of the Biological Clock

How does the body generate a circadian rhythm? Curt Richter (1967) introduced the concept that the brain generates its own rhythms—a biological clock—and he reported that the

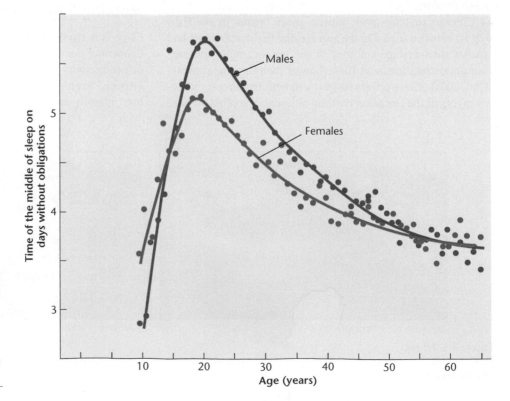

Figure 8.6 Age differences in circadian rhythms
People reported the time of the middle of their sleep, such as 3 A.M. or 5 A.M., on days when they had no obligations.
(Source: Reprinted from "A marker for the end of adolescence," by T. Roenneberg et al., Current Biology, 14, pp. R1038–R1039, Figure 1, copyright 2004, with permission from Elsevier.)

biological clock is insensitive to most forms of interference. Blind or deaf animals generate circadian rhythms, although they slowly drift out of phase with the external world. The circadian rhythm remains surprisingly steady despite food or water deprivation, X-rays, tranquilizers, alcohol, anesthesia, lack of oxygen, most kinds of brain damage, or the removal of endocrine organs. Even an hour or more of induced hibernation often fails to reset the biological clock (Gibbs, 1983; Richter, 1975). Evidently, the biological clock is a hardy, robust mechanism.

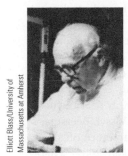

Curt P. Richter
(1894–1988)
I enjoy research more than eating. (Richter, personal communication)

The Suprachiasmatic Nucleus (SCN)

Although cells throughout the body generate circadian rhythms, the main driver of rhythms for sleep and body temperature is the **suprachiasmatic** (soo-pruh-kie-as-MAT-ik) **nucleus**, or **SCN**, a part of the hypothalamus (Refinetti & Menaker, 1992). It gets its name from its location just above ("supra") the optic chiasm (see Figure 8.7). After damage to the SCN, the body's rhythms become erratic.

The SCN generates circadian rhythms itself in a genetically controlled manner. If SCN neurons are disconnected from the rest of the brain or removed from the body and maintained in tissue culture, they continue to produce a circadian rhythm of action potentials (Earnest, Liang, Ratcliff, & Cassone, 1999; Inouye & Kawamura, 1979). Even a single isolated SCN cell can maintain a circadian rhythm, although interactions among cells sharpen the accuracy of the rhythm (Long, Jutras, Connors, & Burwell, 2005; Yamaguchi et al., 2003).

A mutation in one gene causes hamsters' SCN to produce a 20-hour instead of 24-hour rhythm (Ralph & Menaker, 1988).

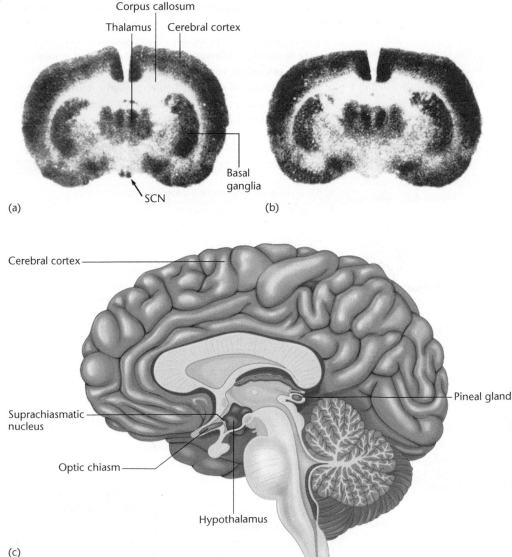

Figure 8.7 The suprachiasmatic nucleus (SCN) of rats and humans
The SCN is at the base of the brain, as seen in these coronal sections through the plane of the anterior hypothalamus. Each rat was injected with radioactive 2-deoxyglucose, which is absorbed by the most active neurons. A high level of absorption of this chemical produces a dark appearance on the slide. Note the greater activity in SCN neurons of a rat injected during the day (a), than in one injected at night (b). *(Source: From "Suprachiasmatic nucleus: Use of 14C-labeled deoxyglucose uptake as a functional marker," by W. J. Schwartz and H. Gainer, 1977, Science, 197, pp. 1089–1091. Reprinted by permission from AAAS/American Association for the Advancement of Science.)* (c) A sagittal section through a human brain showing the location of the SCN and the pineal gland.

Researchers surgically removed the SCN from adult hamsters and transplanted SCN tissue from hamster fetuses into the adults. When they transplanted SCN tissue from fetuses with a 20-hour rhythm, the recipients produced a 20-hour rhythm. When they transplanted tissue from fetuses with a 24-hour rhythm, the recipients produced a 24-hour rhythm (Ralph, Foster, Davis, & Menaker, 1990). That is, the rhythm followed the pace of the donors, not the recipients. Again, the results show that the rhythms come from the SCN itself.

✓ STOP & CHECK

3. What evidence strongly indicates that the SCN produces the circadian rhythm itself?

ANSWER

3. SCN cells produce a circadian rhythm of activity even if they are kept in cell culture isolated from the rest of the body. Also, when hamsters received transplanted SCN neurons, their circadian rhythm followed the pattern of the donor animals.

How Light Resets the SCN

Figure 8.7 shows the position of the SCN in the human brain, just above the optic chiasm. A small branch of the optic nerve, known as the *retinohypothalamic path,* from the retina to the SCN, alters the SCN's settings.

Most of the input to that path, however, does not come from normal retinal receptors. Mice with genetic defects that destroy nearly all their rods and cones nevertheless reset their biological clocks in synchrony with the light (Freedman et al., 1999; Lucas, Freedman, Muñoz, Garcia-Fernández, & Foster, 1999). Also, consider blind mole rats (see Figure 8.8), whose

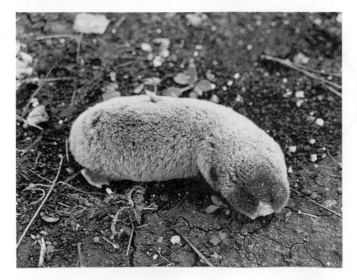

Figure 8.8 A blind mole rat
Although blind mole rats are blind in other regards, they reset their circadian rhythms in response to light.
(Source: Courtesy of Eviatar Nevo)

eyes are covered with folds of skin and fur. They are evolutionarily adapted to spend most of their lives underground. They have fewer than 900 optic nerve axons compared with 100,000 in hamsters. Even a bright flash of light evokes no startle response and no measurable change in brain activity. Nevertheless, light resets their circadian rhythms, enabling them to be awake only at night (de Jong, Hendriks, Sanyal, & Nevo, 1990).

The surprising explanation is that the retinohypothalamic path to the SCN comes from a special population of retinal ganglion cells that have their own photopigment, called *melanopsin,* unlike the ones found in rods and cones (Hannibal, Hindersson, Knudsen, Georg, & Fahrenkrug, 2001; Lucas, Douglas, & Foster, 2001). These special ganglion cells receive some input from rods and cones (Gooley et al., 2010; Güler et al., 2008), but even if they do not receive that input, they respond directly to light (Berson, Dunn, & Takao, 2002). These special ganglion cells are located mainly near the nose, from which they see toward the periphery (Visser, Beersma, & Daan, 1999). They respond to light slowly and turn off slowly when the light ceases (Berson, Dunn, & Takao, 2002). Therefore, they respond to the overall average amount of light, not to instantaneous changes in light. The average intensity over a period of time is, of course, exactly the information the SCN needs to gauge the time of day. These ganglion cells respond mainly to short-wavelength (blue) light. For that reason, exposure to television, video games, computers, and so forth, all of which emit mostly short-wavelength light, tends to phase-delay the circadian rhythm and make it difficult to fall asleep at the usual time (Czeisler, 2013).

✓ STOP & CHECK

4. How does light reset the biological clock?
5. People who are blind because of cortical damage can still synchronize their circadian rhythm to the local pattern of day and night. Why?

ANSWERS

4. A branch of the optic nerve, the retinohypothalamic path, conveys information about light to the SCN. The axons comprising that path originate from special ganglion cells that respond to light by themselves, even if they do not receive input from rods or cones. 5. If the retina is intact, melanopsin-containing ganglion cells can still send messages to the SCN, resetting its rhythm.

The Biochemistry of the Circadian Rhythm

The suprachiasmatic nucleus produces the circadian rhythm, but how? Research on production of the circadian rhythm began with insects. Studies on the fruit fly *Drosophila* found several genes responsible for a circadian rhythm (X. Liu et al., 1992; Sehgal, Ousley, Yang, Chen, & Schotland, 1999). Two of these genes, known as *period* (abbreviated *PER*) and *timeless* (*TIM*), produce the proteins PER and TIM. The concentration of these two proteins, which promote sleep and inactivity,

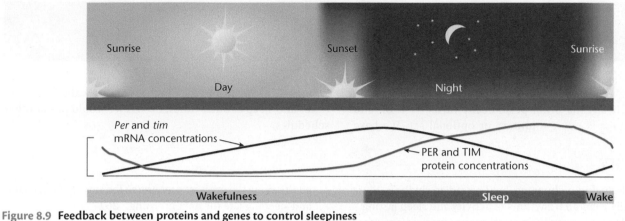

Figure 8.9 Feedback between proteins and genes to control sleepiness
In fruit flies (*Drosophila*), the concentrations of the mRNA levels for PER and TIM oscillate over a day, and so do the proteins that they produce.

oscillates over a day, based on feedback interactions among neurons. Early in the morning, the messenger RNA levels responsible for producing PER and TIM start at low concentrations. As they increase during the day, they increase synthesis of the proteins, but the process takes time, and so the protein concentrations lag hours behind, as shown in Figure 8.9. As the PER and TIM protein concentrations increase, they feed back to inhibit the genes that produce the messenger RNA molecules. Thus, during the night, the PER and TIM concentrations are high, but the messenger RNA concentrations are declining (Nitabach & Taghert, 2008). By the next morning, PER and TIM protein levels are low, the flies awaken, and the cycle is ready to start again. Because the feedback cycle takes about 24 hours, the flies generate a circadian rhythm even in an unchanging environment. However, in addition to the automatic feedback, light activates a chemical that breaks down the TIM protein, thereby increasing wakefulness and synchronizing the internal clock to the external world (Ashmore & Sehgal, 2003).

Why do we care about flies? The reason is that analyzing the mechanism in flies told researchers what to look for in humans and other mammals. Mammals have three versions of the PER protein and several proteins closely related to TIM and the others found in flies (Reick, Garcia, Dudley, & McKnight, 2001; Zheng et al., 1999). Mutations in the genes producing PER proteins lead to alterations of sleep schedules. People with certain PER mutations have been found to have a circadian rhythm shorter than 24 hours, as if they were moving about a time zone east every day (Chong, Ptácek, & Fu, 2012; Jones et al., 1999; Zhang et al., 2016). They consistently get sleepy early in the evening and awaken early in the morning. Most people look forward to days when they can stay up late. People with an altered PER gene look forward to times when they can go to bed early. Most people with this sleep abnormality suffer from depression (Xu et al., 2005). As we see again in Chapter 14, sleep impairments and depression are closely linked. Other known mutations shorten the amount of sleep needed per day or impair people's ability to rebound from temporary sleep deprivation (Dijk & Archer, 2010; Jones, Huang, Ptácek, & Fu, 2013).

✅ **STOP & CHECK**

6. How do the proteins TIM and PER relate to sleepiness in *Drosophila*?

ANSWER   6. The proteins TIM and PER remain low during most of the day and begin to increase toward evening. They reach high levels at night, promoting sleep. They also feed back to inhibit the genes that produce them, so that their level declines toward morning.

Melatonin

The SCN regulates waking and sleeping by controlling activity levels in other brain areas, including the **pineal gland** (PIN-ee-al; see Figure 8.7), an endocrine gland located just posterior to the thalamus (Aston-Jones, Chen, Zhu, & Oshinsky, 2001; von Gall et al., 2002). The pineal gland releases the hormone **melatonin**. Melatonin is a widespread chemical, found in nearly all animals—sponges are the only known exception—as well as in plants and bacteria. In all cases, it is released mostly at night. In diurnal animals like humans, it increases sleepiness. In nocturnal animals, it increases wakefulness, even in such a remote example as the larval form of a marine worm (Tosches, Bucher, Vopalensky, & Arendt, 2014). People who have pineal gland tumors sometimes stay awake for days at a time (Haimov & Lavie, 1996). In addition to regulating sleep and wakefulness, melatonin also helps control the onset of puberty and bodily adjustments to changes of season (such as hibernation).

Melatonin secretion starts to increase about 2 or 3 hours before bedtime. Taking a melatonin pill in the evening has little effect on sleepiness because the pineal gland produces melatonin at that time anyway. However, people who take melatonin earlier start to become sleepy (Crowley & Eastman, 2013). In the process, it shifts the circadian rhythm such that the person starts to become sleepy earlier than usual the next day also. Melatonin pills are sometimes helpful for people who travel across time zones and need to sleep at an unaccustomed time.

Module 8.1 | In Closing

Sleep–Wake Cycles

Unlike an electric appliance that stays on until some-one turns it off, the brain periodically turns itself on and off. Sleepiness is not a voluntary or optional act. We have biological mechanisms that prepare us to wake at certain times and sleep at other times, even if we would prefer other schedules.

Summary

1. Animals, including humans, have circadian rhythms—internally generated rhythms of activity and sleep lasting about 24 hours, even in an unchanging environment. It is difficult to adjust to a sleep schedule much different from 24 hours. **258**

2. Although the biological clock continues to operate in constant light or constant darkness, the onset of light resets the clock. Even when people set their waking and sleeping times by the clock, the timing of sunrise strongly influences their circadian rhythm. **259**

3. It is easier for most people to follow a cycle slightly longer than 24 hours (as when traveling west) than to follow a cycle shorter than 24 hours (as when traveling east). **261**

4. If people wish to work at night and sleep during the day, the best way to shift the circadian rhythm is to have bright lights at night and darkness during the day. **261**

5. Some people are most alert early in the morning, and others become more alert later in the day. On average, young adults show the greatest preference for staying awake late and sleeping late the next morning. **261**

6. The suprachiasmatic nucleus (SCN), a part of the hypothalamus, generates the body's circadian rhythms for sleep and temperature. **263**

7. Light resets the biological clock partly by a branch of the optic nerve that extends to the SCN. Those axons originate from a special population of ganglion cells that respond directly to light in addition to receiving some input from rods and cones. **264**

8. The genes controlling the circadian rhythm are almost the same in mammals as in insects. Circadian rhythms result from a feedback cycle based on genes that produce the proteins PER and TIM, and the ability of those proteins to inhibit the genes that produce them. **264**

9. The SCN controls the body's rhythm partly by directing the release of melatonin by the pineal gland. The hormone melatonin increases sleepiness; if given at certain times of the day, it can also reset the circadian rhythm. **265**

Key Terms

Terms are defined in the module on the page number indicated. They're also presented in alphabetical order with definitions in the book's Subject Index/Glossary, which begins on page 589. Interactive flash cards, audio reviews, and crossword puzzles are among the online resources available to help you learn these terms and the concepts they represent.

endogenous circadian rhythms **258**
endogenous circannual rhythm **258**
jet lag **261**

melatonin **265**
pineal gland **265**
suprachiasmatic nucleus (SCN) **263**

zeitgeber **259**

Thought Question

Why would evolution have enabled blind mole rats to synchronize their SCN activity to light, even though they cannot see well enough to make any use of the light?

Module 8.1 | End of Module Quiz

1. Workers on certain submarines work 6 hours, relax 6 hours, and then sleep 6 hours. After weeks on this schedule, what happens to their circadian rhythm?

    A. It adjusts to produce an 18-hour rhythm.
    B. It continues producing the usual 24-hour rhythm.

    C. It produces a rhythm intermediate between 18 and 24 hours.
    D. It stops producing any rhythm at all.

2. Why do people in Antarctica during the winter often find it difficult to work together?

    A. Their work schedules keep them so busy that they cannot sleep enough.

    B. Their circadian rhythms drift out of phase with one another.

    C. After living together in close quarters for so long, they start to irritate one another.

    D. They get homesick.

3. For most young adults, what happens to mood as a function of time of day?

    A. Mood tends to be most pleasant early in the morning.

    B. Mood tends to be most pleasant around noon.

    C. Mood tends to be most pleasant in late afternoon or early evening.

    D. Mood fluctuates, but on average is about the same for one time as for another.

4. Why do people in eastern Germany awaken earlier, on average, than those in western Germany?

    A. The sun rises earlier in eastern Germany.

    B. Eastern Germany is in a different time zone.

    C. A gene that inactivates melatonin is more common in eastern Germany.

    D. A gene that inactivates melatonin is more common in western Germany.

5. Why do many high school students get worse test grades in the morning than in the afternoon?

    A. Most schools schedule the math and science courses mainly in the morning.

    B. Teenagers tend to stay up late and awaken late.

    C. Many teenagers do not eat a healthy breakfast.

    D. Many high schools are not adequately heated during the morning.

6. What evidence most strongly indicates that the SCN produces the circadian rhythm itself?

    A. Damage to the SCN disrupts the circadian rhythm.

    B. SCN cells isolated from the body continue to produce a circadian rhythm.

    C. Animals with a faster circadian rhythm have a larger SCN.

    D. The SCN increases its activity during wakeful periods and decreases it during sleep.

7. Light can reset the SCN's rhythm even after damage to all rods and cones. Why?

    A. The SCN itself responds to light.

    B. The SCN receives input from the pineal gland.

    C. The SCN receives input from skin cells that respond to light.

    D. The SCN receives input from ganglion cells that respond to light.

8. If you want to get to sleep on time, what should you avoid?

    A. Long-wavelength light late in the evening

    B. Short-wavelength light late in the evening

    C. Long-wavelength light early in the morning

    D. Short-wavelength light early in the morning

9. After the proteins TIM and PER reach a high level during the day, what causes their level to decrease at night?

    A. High levels of the proteins inhibit the genes that produce these proteins.

    B. The genes that produce these proteins become less active when temperature drops.

    C. Rapid production of the proteins depleted the supply of the amino acids needed to make them.

    D. Decreased light stimulation decreases excitatory transmission throughout the nervous system.

10. When is melatonin mostly released?

    A. At night, for all species

    B. During the day, for all species

    C. At night for species active at night; during the day for species active during the day

    D. At night for species active during the day; during the day for species active at night

Answers: 1B, 2B, 3C, 4A, 5B, 6B, 7D, 8B, 9A, 10A.

Stages of Sleep and Brain Mechanisms

Suppose you buy a new battery-powered toy. After you play with it for 4 hours, it suddenly stops. You wonder whether the batteries are dead or whether the toy needs repair. Later, you discover that this toy always stops after playing for 4 hours but it operates again a few hours later even without repairs or a battery change. You begin to suspect that the manufacturer designed it to prevent you from playing with it all day. Now you try to find the device that turns it off. You are asking a new question. If you thought that the toy stopped because it needed repairs or new batteries, you would not ask which device turned it off.

Similarly, if we think of sleep as something like wearing out a machine, we do not ask which part of the brain produces it. But if we think of sleep as a specialized state evolved to serve particular functions, we look for the mechanisms that regulate it.

Sleep and Other Interruptions of Consciousness

Let's start with some distinctions. Sleep is a state that the brain actively produces, characterized by decreased activity and decreased response to stimuli. In contrast, **coma** (KOH-muh) is an extended period of unconsciousness caused by head trauma, stroke, or disease. Someone in a coma has a low level of brain activity and little or no response to stimuli. A strong pinch or a loud noise can awaken a sleeping person but not someone in a coma. Typically, someone in a coma either dies or begins to recover within a few weeks.

Someone in a **vegetative state** alternates between periods of sleep and moderate arousal, although even during the more aroused state, the person shows no awareness of surroundings and no purposeful behavior. Breathing is more regular, and a painful stimulus produces at least the autonomic responses of increased heart rate, breathing, and sweating. A **minimally conscious state** is one stage higher, with brief periods of purposeful actions and a limited amount of speech comprehension. A vegetative or minimally conscious state can last for months or years.

Brain death is a condition with no sign of brain activity and no response to any stimulus. Physicians usually wait until someone has shown no sign of brain activity for 24 hours before pronouncing brain death, at which point most people believe it is ethical to remove life support.

The Stages of Sleep

Nearly every scientific advance comes from new or improved measurements. Researchers did not even suspect that sleep has stages until they accidentally measured them. The electroencephalograph (EEG), as described in Chapter 3, records an average of the electrical potentials of the cells and fibers in the brain areas nearest to each electrode on the scalp (see Figure 8.10). If half the cells in some area increase their electrical potentials while the other half decrease, they cancel out. The EEG record rises or falls when most cells do the same thing at the same time. You might compare it to a record of the noise in a sports stadium: It shows only slight fluctuations until some event gets everyone yelling at once. The EEG enables brain researchers to monitor brain activity during sleep.

Figure 8.11 shows data from a **polysomnograph,** a combination of EEG and eye-movement records, for a college student during various stages of sleep. Figure 8.11a presents a period of relaxed wakefulness for comparison. Note the steady series of **alpha waves** at a frequency of 8 to 12 per second. Alpha waves are characteristic of relaxation, not of all wakefulness.

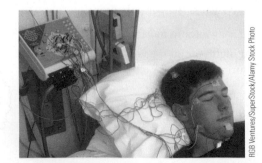

Figure 8.10 Sleeping person with electrodes in place on the scalp for recording brain activity

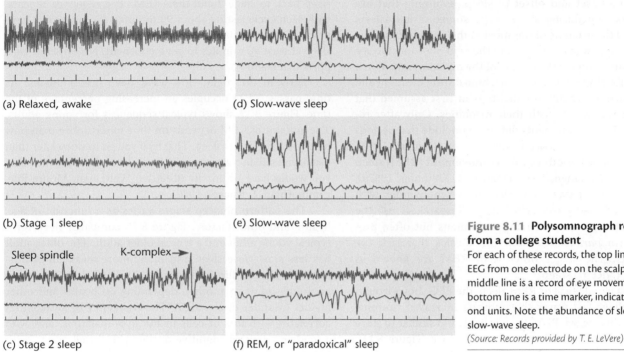

(a) Relaxed, awake

(b) Stage 1 sleep

Sleep spindle K-complex →

(c) Stage 2 sleep

(d) Slow-wave sleep

(e) Slow-wave sleep

(f) REM, or "paradoxical" sleep

Figure 8.11 Polysomnograph records from a college student
For each of these records, the top line is the EEG from one electrode on the scalp. The middle line is a record of eye movements. The bottom line is a time marker, indicating 1-second units. Note the abundance of slow waves in slow-wave sleep.
(*Source: Records provided by T. E. LeVere*)

In Figure 8.11b, sleep has just begun. During this period, called stage 1 sleep, the EEG is dominated by irregular, jagged, low-voltage waves. Brain activity is less than in relaxed wakefulness but higher than in other sleep stages. As Figure 8.11c shows, the prominent characteristics of stage 2 are K-complexes and sleep spindles. A **K-complex** is a sharp wave associated with temporary inhibition of neuronal firing (Cash et al., 2009). A **sleep spindle** is a burst of 12- to 14-Hz waves for at least half a second. Sleep spindles result from oscillating interactions between cells in the thalamus and the cortex. Sleep spindles increase in number after new learning, and the number of sleep spindles correlates positively with improvements in certain types of memory (Eschenko, Mölle, Born, & Sara, 2006; Mednick et al., 2013; Hennies, Ralph, Kempkes, Cousins, & Lewis, 2016). Evidently the sleep spindles represent activity related to the consolidation of memory. Most people are fairly consistent in their amount of spindle activity from one night to another, and the amount of spindle activity correlates more than 0.7 with nonverbal tests of IQ (Fogel, Nader, Cote, & Smith, 2007). Who would have guessed that brain waves during sleep could predict IQ scores?

During **slow-wave sleep**, heart rate, breathing rate, and brain activity decrease, whereas slow, large-amplitude waves become more common (see Figures 8.11d and e). Older sources distinguished between stage 3 sleep (Figure 8.11d) with fewer slow waves, and stage 4 (Figure 8.11e) with more of them.

Slow waves indicate that neuronal activity is highly synchronized. In stage 1 and in wakefulness, the cortex continues substantial activity. Because most neurons are out of phase with one another, the EEG is full of short, rapid, choppy waves. During slow-wave sleep, input to the cerebral cortex is greatly inhibited, and most cells synchronize their activity.

STOP & CHECK

7. What do large, slow waves on an EEG indicate?

ANSWER 7. Large, slow waves indicate a low level of activity, with much synchrony of response among neurons.

Paradoxical or REM Sleep

Many discoveries occur when researchers stumble upon something by accident. In the 1950s, the French scientist Michel Jouvet was trying to test the learning abilities of cats after removal of the cerebral cortex. Because, as you can imagine, decorticate mammals don't do much, Jouvet recorded slight movements of the muscles and EEGs from the hindbrain. He noticed that during certain periods of apparent sleep, the cats' brain activity was relatively high, but their neck muscles were completely relaxed. Jouvet (1960) then recorded the same phenomenon in normal, intact cats and named it **paradoxical sleep** because it is deep sleep in some ways and light in others. (The term *paradoxical* means "apparently self-contradictory.")

Meanwhile, in the United States, Nathaniel Kleitman and Eugene Aserinsky were observing eye movements to measure the onset and offset of sleep, assuming that eye movements stop during sleep. After someone fell asleep, they turned the machine off for most of the night because the recording paper was expensive and they did not expect to see anything interesting in the middle of the night anyway. When they occasionally turned on the machine during the night and saw evidence of eye movements, they at first assumed that something was wrong with their machines. Only after repeated careful measurements did they conclude that periods of rapid eye movements occur during sleep (Dement, 1990). They called these periods **rapid eye movement (REM) sleep** (Aserinsky & Kleitman, 1955; Dement & Kleitman, 1957a), and soon realized that REM sleep was synonymous with what Jouvet called *paradoxical sleep*. Researchers use the term *REM sleep* when referring to humans but often prefer the term *paradoxical sleep* for species that lack eye movements. The stages other than REM are known as **non-REM (NREM) sleep.**

During paradoxical or REM sleep, the EEG shows irregular, low-voltage fast waves that indicate increased neuronal activity. In this regard, REM sleep is light, and similar to stage 1 except for the eye movements, as shown in Figure 8.11f. However, the postural muscles of the body, including those that support the head, are more relaxed during REM than in other stages. In this regard, REM is deep sleep. REM is also associated with erections in males and vaginal moistening in females. Heart rate, blood pressure, breathing rate, and facial twitches fluctuate during REM more than in other stages. In short, REM sleep combines aspects of deep sleep, light sleep, and features that are difficult to classify as deep or light.

When you fall asleep, you start in stage 1 and slowly progress to stage 2 and then into slow-wave sleep, although loud noises or other intrusions can interrupt the progress. After about an hour of sleep, you begin to cycle from slow-wave sleep back to stage 2 and then REM. The sequence repeats, with each cycle lasting about 90 minutes. (Some people have inferred that because a cycle lasts 90 minutes, you need to sleep at least 90 minutes to get any benefit. No evidence supports that claim.)

Early in the night, slow-wave sleep predominates. As time passes, REM occupies an increasing percentage of the time. Figure 8.12 shows typical sequences for young adults. The amount of REM depends on time of day more than how long you have been asleep. That is, if you go to sleep later than usual, you still increase your REM at about the same time that you would have ordinarily (Czeisler, Weitzman, Moore-Ede, Zimmerman, & Knauer, 1980).

The pattern of sleep stages varies as a function of age, health, and other factors. Figure 8.13 compares sleep for a typical young adult and a typical older adult. The older adult has less slow-wave sleep and many more awakenings during the night (Scullin & Bliwise, 2015). The results vary from one older adult to another, depending on health and other factors (Mander et al., 2015). The frequency of awakenings correlates with loss of cells in the hypothalamus, and with a tendency toward cognitive decline (Blackwell et al., 2014; Lim et al., 2014).

Shortly after the discovery of REM, researchers believed it was almost synonymous with dreaming. William Dement and Nathaniel Kleitman (1957b) found that people who were awakened during REM reported dreams 80 percent to 90 percent of the time. Later research, however, found that people awakened during non-REM sleep sometimes report dreams also. REM dreams are more likely than NREM dreams to include visual imagery and complicated plots, but not always. Some people continue to report dreams despite an apparent lack of REM (Solms, 1997). In short, REM is not the same thing as dreaming.

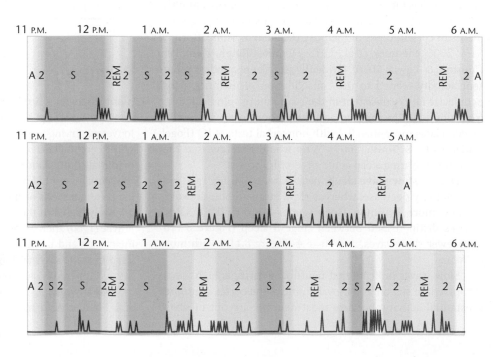

Figure 8.12 Sleep stages on three nights
Columns indicate awake, stage 2, slow-wave sleep, and REM. Deflections in the line at the bottom of each chart indicate shifts in body position. Note that slow-wave sleep occurs mostly in the early part of the night's sleep, whereas REM sleep becomes more prevalent later.
(Based on Dement & Kleitman, 1957a)

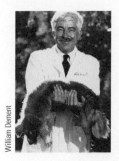

William Dement

William Dement

The average person would not, at first blush, pick watching people sleep as the most apparent theme for a spine-tingling scientific adventure thriller. However, there is a subtle sense of awe and mystery surrounding the "short death" we call sleep. (Dement, 1972, p. xi)

✔ STOP & CHECK

8. How can an investigator determine whether a sleeper is in REM sleep?
9. During which part of a night's sleep is REM most common?

ANSWERS

8. Examine EEG pattern and eye movements. 9. REM becomes most common toward the end of the night's sleep.

Brain Mechanisms of Wakefulness, Arousal, and Sleep

Any animal needs to regulate its level of alertness carefully. Maintaining maximum alertness at all times would waste energy. Becoming completely unresponsive would be risky. Many brain areas participate in the control of sleep and wakefulness.

Brain Structures of Arousal and Attention

After a cut through the midbrain separates the forebrain and part of the midbrain from all the lower structures, an animal enters a prolonged state of sleep for the next few days. Even after weeks of recovery, the wakeful periods are brief. We might suppose a simple explanation: The cut isolated the brain from the sensory stimuli that come up from the medulla and spinal cord. However, if a researcher cuts each individual tract that enters the medulla and spinal cord, thus depriving the brain of the sensory input, the animal still has normal periods of wakefulness and sleep. Evidently, the midbrain does more than just relay sensory information. It has its own mechanisms to promote wakefulness.

A cut through the midbrain decreases arousal by damaging the **reticular formation**, a structure that extends from the medulla into the forebrain. Some neurons of the reticular formation have axons ascending into the brain, and some have axons descending into the spinal cord. Those with axons descending into the spinal cord form part of the medial tract of motor control, as discussed in Chapter 7. In 1949, Giuseppe Moruzzi and H. W. Magoun proposed that the reticular formation neurons with ascending axons are well suited to regulate arousal. The term *reticular* (based on the Latin word *rete*, meaning "net") describes the widespread connections among neurons in this system. One part of the reticular formation that contributes to cortical arousal is known as the **pontomesencephalon** (Woolf, 1996). (The term derives from *pons* and *mesencephalon*, or "midbrain.") These neurons receive input from many sensory systems and also generate activity of their own, varying with the circadian rhythm. Their axons extend into the forebrain, as shown in Figure 8.14. Axons from some of the cells release GABA, which inhibits or interrupts behavior and promotes slow-wave sleep (Anaclet et al., 2014; Giber et al., 2015). Axons from other cells release acetylcholine, glutamate, or dopamine, producing arousal in the hypothalamus, thalamus, and basal forebrain. These transmitters produce wakefulness partly by regulating the levels of potassium and other ions that produce a constant state of arousal. After the ions are in a state that supports arousal, they tend to remain at a stable concentration. For that reason, waking up is generally faster than falling asleep (Ding et al., 2016).

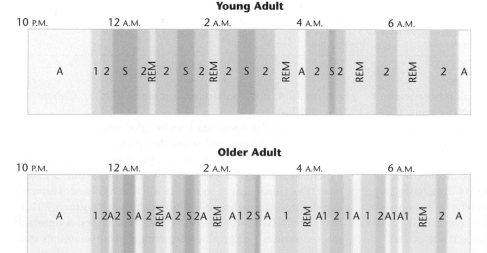

Figure 8.13 Typical sleep stages for a young adult and an older adult
Columns indicate awake, stage 1, stage 2, slow-wave sleep, and REM. Note that the older adult has less slow-wave sleep and more frequent awakenings. Based on data from Scullin & Bliwise (2015).

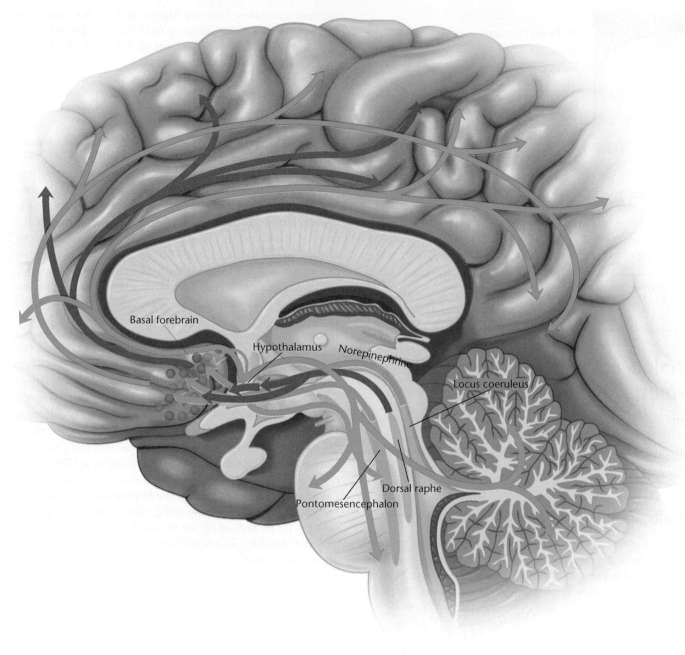

Figure 8.14 Brain mechanisms of sleeping and waking
Green arrows indicate excitatory connections. Red arrows indicate inhibitory connections.
(Source: Based on J.-S. Lin, Hou, Sakai, & Jouvet, 1996; Robbins & Everitt, 1995; Szymusiak, 1995.)

The **locus coeruleus** (LOW-kus ser-ROO-lee-us; literally, "dark blue place"), a small structure in the pons, is usually inactive, especially during sleep, but it emits bursts of impulses in response to meaningful events, especially those that produce emotional arousal (Sterpenich et al., 2006). Axons from the locus coeruleus release norepinephrine widely throughout the cortex, so this tiny area has a huge influence. Output from the locus coeruleus increases what engineers call "gain." That is, it increases the activity of the most active neurons and decreases the activity of less active neurons. The result is enhanced attention to important information and enhanced memory (Eldar, Cohen, & Niv, 2013).

The hypothalamus has intermingled neurons, some that promote wakefulness and some that promote sleep (Konadhode, Pelluru, & Shiromani, 2015). One axon pathway from the hypothalamus releases the excitatory neurotransmitter *histamine* (Lin, Hou, Sakai, & Jouvet, 1996), which enhances arousal and alertness throughout the brain (Panula & Nuutinen, 2013). Many antihistamine drugs, often used for allergies, counteract this transmitter and produce drowsiness. Antihistamines that do not cross the blood–brain barrier avoid that side effect.

Another pathway from the hypothalamus, mainly from the lateral and posterior nuclei of the hypothalamus, releases a peptide neurotransmitter called either **orexin** or **hypocretin**. The reason for two names is that two research teams discovered this chemical almost simultaneously in 1998, and gave it different names. For simplicity, this text will stick to the term *orexin*, but if you find the term *hypocretin* elsewhere, it means the same thing. The axons releasing orexin extend from the hypothalamus to the basal forebrain and many other areas, enhancing wakefulness and activity (Sakurai, 2007). Orexin is not necessary for waking up, but it is for *staying* awake. That is, most adult humans stay awake for roughly 16 to 17 hours at a time, even when nothing much is happening. Staying awake depends on orexin, especially toward the end of the day (Lee, Hassani, & Jones, 2005). Mice lacking orexin alternate between waking and sleeping, even during an activity that usually sustains arousal, such as running in a running wheel (Anaclet et al., 2009). Optogenetic inhibition of orexin neurons causes mice to go quickly into slow-wave sleep (Tsunematsu, Kilduff, Boyden, Takahashi, & Yamanaka, 2011).

Drugs that block orexin receptors help people go to sleep (Kukkonen, 2013; Uslaner et al., 2013). The United States Food and Drug Administration has approved one such drug, suvorexant.

Other pathways from the lateral hypothalamus regulate cells in the **basal forebrain** (an area just anterior and dorsal to the hypothalamus). Basal forebrain cells provide axons that extend throughout the thalamus and cerebral cortex, some of them increasing wakefulness and others inhibiting it (Xu et al., 2015) (see Figure 8.14). Acetylcholine stimulates the basal forebrain cells that promote wakefulness, although those cells release other transmitters to the cortex (Zant et al., 2016).

STOP & CHECK

10. Why do most antihistamines make people drowsy?
11. What would happen to the sleep–wake schedule of someone who lacked orexin?

ANSWERS

10. A pathway from the hypothalamus uses histamine as its neurotransmitter to increase arousal. Antihistamines that cross the blood-brain barrier block those synapses. 11. Someone without orexin would alternate between brief periods of waking and sleeping.

Sleep and the Inhibition of Brain Activity

Sleep depends partly on decreased sensory input to the cerebral cortex. During sleep, neurons in the thalamus become hyperpolarized, decreasing their readiness to respond to stimuli and decreasing the information they transmit to the cortex (Coenen, 1995). However, although responsiveness decreases, a moderate amount remains. For example, parents usually awaken quickly at the sound of a crying infant. During the lighter stages of non-REM sleep, the brain responds to any meaningful speech

(Andrillon, Poulsen, Hansen, Léger, & Kouider, 2016). During any stage, an intense enough stimulus produces arousal.

During sleep, spontaneously active neurons continue firing at only slightly less than their usual rate. How, then, do we remain unconscious in spite of sustained neuronal activity? The answer is inhibition. During sleep, axons that release the inhibitory neurotransmitter GABA increase their activity, interfering with the spread of information from one neuron to another (Massimini et al., 2005). Connections from one brain area to another become weaker (Boly et al., 2012; Esser, Hill, & Tononi, 2009). When stimulation doesn't spread through the brain, you don't become conscious of it. (This point arises again in the module about consciousness.)

Because sleep depends on GABA-mediated inhibition, sleep can be local within the brain (Krueger et al., 2008). That is, you might have substantial inhibition in one brain area and not so much in another. Ordinarily, all brain areas wake up or go to sleep at nearly the same time, but not always. Thinking of sleep as a local phenomenon helps make sense of some otherwise puzzling phenomena. Consider sleepwalking, also known by the fancier term *somnambulism*. Sleepwalkers are asleep in much of the brain, but awake in the motor cortex and a few other areas (Terzaghi et al., 2012). They generally have their eyes open, they orient to the world enough to find their way around, and they often remember some of what they did while sleepwalking. Nevertheless, they are confused and vulnerable to hurting themselves or others, because most of the brain is not alert enough to process information and make reasonable decisions (Zadra, Desautels, Petit, & Montplaisir, 2013).

Another example is lucid dreaming. During lucid dreaming, someone is dreaming but aware of being asleep and dreaming. Although most of the brain is asleep, much activity around 40 Hz (cycles per second) occurs in the frontal and temporal cortex (Voss et al., 2014). Evidently that activity enables conscious monitoring of dreams that the rest of the brain is generating. Someone having a lucid dream can control the content of the dream to some extent, as well as eye movements. In one study, young adults who had frequent lucid dreams learned to use their eye movements to signal the onset of a lucid dream. When they had lucid dreams about moving their hands, activity increased in the areas of motor cortex responsible for preparing for an actual hand movement (Dresler et al., 2011).

Another example: Have you ever had the experience of waking up but finding that you cannot move your arms or legs? During REM sleep, cells in the pons and medulla send messages that inhibit the spinal neurons that control the body's large muscles (Brooks & Peever, 2012). A cat with damage to those cells moves around awkwardly during REM sleep, as if it were acting out its dreams (Morrison, Sanford, Ball, Mann, & Ross, 1995; see Figure 8.15). Ordinarily, when you awaken from a REM period, those cells in the pons shut off quickly and you regain muscle control. But occasionally, most of the brain wakes up while the pons remains in REM. The result is your experience of being temporarily paralyzed—a disturbing experience, if you don't understand it (Cheyne & Pennycook, 2013).

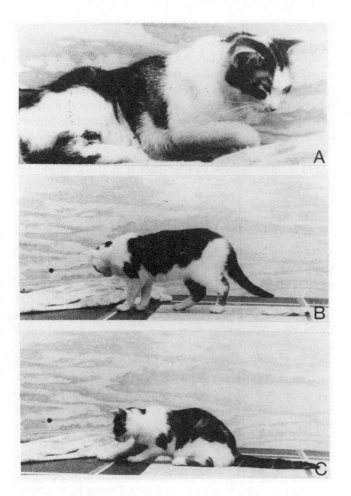

Figure 8.15 A cat with a lesion in the pons, wobbling about during REM sleep
Cells of an intact pons send inhibitory messages to the spinal cord neurons that control the large muscles.
(Source: Morrison, A. R., Sanford, L. D., Ball, W. A., Mann, G. L., & Ross, R. J., "Stimulus-elicited behavior in rapid eye movement sleep without atonia", Behavioral Neuroscience, 109, pp. 972–979, 1995. Published by APA and reprinted with permission.)

✓ STOP & CHECK

12. What would happen to sleeping and waking if you took a drug that blocked GABA?

13. Someone who has just awakened sometimes speaks in a loose, unconnected, illogical way. How could you explain this finding?

ANSWERS

12. You would remain awake, or at least somewhat conscious. (Tranquilizers put people to sleep by facilitating GABA.) 13. People often awaken from a REM period, because REM is abundant toward morning when people usually awaken. Different brain areas don't wake up all at once. Shortly after awakening, certain brain areas may still be in a REM-like state, and thinking may have an illogical, dreamlike quality.

Brain Activity in REM Sleep

Researchers interested in the mechanisms of REM decided to use a PET scan to determine which brain areas increased or decreased their activity during REM. Although that research might sound simple, PET requires injecting a radioactive chemical. Imagine trying to give sleepers an injection without awakening them. Further, a PET scan yields a clear image only if the head remains motionless during data collection. If the person tosses or turns even slightly, the blurry image is worthless.

To overcome these difficulties, researchers in two studies persuaded young people to sleep with their heads firmly attached to masks that did not permit any movement. They also inserted a cannula (plastic tube) into each person's arm so that they could inject radioactive chemicals at various times during the night. So imagine yourself in that setup. You have a cannula in your arm and your head is locked into position. Now try to sleep.

Because the researchers foresaw the difficulty of sleeping under these conditions (!), they had their participants stay awake the entire previous night. Someone who is tired enough can sleep even under trying circumstances. (Maybe.)

Now that you appreciate the heroic nature of the procedures, here are the results: During REM sleep, activity increased in the pons (which triggers the onset of REM sleep) and the limbic system (which is important for emotional responses). Activity decreased in the primary visual cortex, the motor cortex, and the dorsolateral prefrontal cortex but increased in parts of the parietal and temporal cortex (Braun et al., 1998; Maquet et al., 1996). REM sleep is associated with a distinctive pattern of high-amplitude electrical potentials known as **PGO waves**, for pons-geniculate-occipital (see Figure 8.16). Waves of neural activity are detected first in the pons, shortly afterward in the lateral geniculate nucleus of the thalamus, and then in the occipital cortex (Brooks & Bizzi, 1963; Laurent, Cespuglio, & Jouvet, 1974).

A path of axons from the ventral medulla releasing GABA promotes REM sleep. Exciting or inhibiting these axons can initiate or stop REM. Apparently these axons initiate REM by inhibiting other inhibitory neurons—a case of excitation by a double negative (Weber et al., 2015). Several other transmitters also influence REM. Injections of the drug *carbachol*, which stimulates acetylcholine synapses, quickly move a sleeper into REM sleep (Baghdoyan, Spotts, & Snyder, 1993). Note that acetylcholine is important for both wakefulness and REM sleep, states of brain arousal. Serotonin and norepinephrine interrupt REM sleep (Boutrel, Franc, Hen, Hamon, & Adrien, 1999; Singh & Mallick, 1996).

Sleep Disorders

How much sleep is enough? Individuals vary genetically in their need for sleep. Mice with one genetic mutation sleep almost four hours per day longer than other mice, and if deprived of some of that extra sleep, they react just as badly as

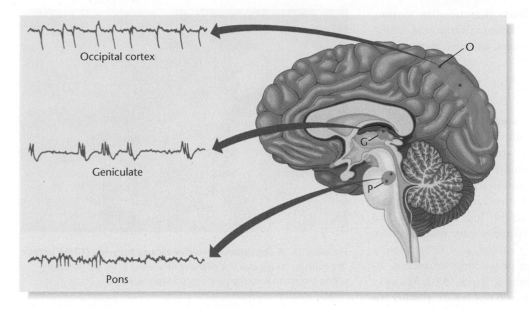

Figure 8.16 PGO waves
PGO waves start in the pons (P), and then show up in the lateral geniculate (G) and the occipital cortex (O). Each PGO wave is synchronized with an eye movement in REM sleep.

normal mice that are deprived of part of their sleep. That is, the mutant gene increases their *need* for sleep (Funato et al., 2016). The average adult human needs 7½ to 8 hours of sleep per night, but some people need more, and a few have been known to do well with as little as 3 hours per night (Jones & Oswald, 1968; Meddis, Pearson, & Langford, 1973). The best gauge of **insomnia**—inadequate sleep—is how someone feels the following day. If you feel tired during the day, you are not sleeping enough at night. Sleep deprivation impairs memory, attention, and cognition (Scullin & Bliwise, 2015). It also magnifies unpleasant emotional reactions and increases the risk of depression (Altena et al., 2016).

Causes of insomnia include noise, uncomfortable temperatures, stress, pain, diet, and medications. Insomnia can also be the result of epilepsy, Parkinson's disease, brain tumors, depression, anxiety, or other neurological or psychiatric conditions. Some children suffer insomnia because they are milk-intolerant, and their parents, not realizing the intolerance, give them milk to drink right before bedtime (Horne, 1992). One man suffered insomnia until he realized that he dreaded going to sleep because he hated waking up to go jogging. After he switched his jogging time to late afternoon, he slept without difficulty. In short, try to identify the reason for your sleep problems before you try to solve them.

Some cases of insomnia relate to shifts in circadian rhythms (MacFarlane, Cleghorn, & Brown, 1985a, 1985b). Ordinarily, people fall asleep while their temperature is declining and awaken while it is rising, as in Figure 8.17a. Someone whose rhythm is *phase delayed,* as in Figure 8.17b, has trouble falling asleep at the usual time, as if the hypothalamus thinks it isn't late enough (Morris, Lack, & Dawson, 1990). Someone whose rhythm is *phase advanced,* as in Figure 8.17c, falls asleep easily but awakens early.

Another cause of insomnia is, paradoxically, the use of sleeping pills. Frequent use causes dependence and an inability to sleep without the pills (Kales, Scharf, & Kales, 1978). For most people, drinking coffee during the evening interferes

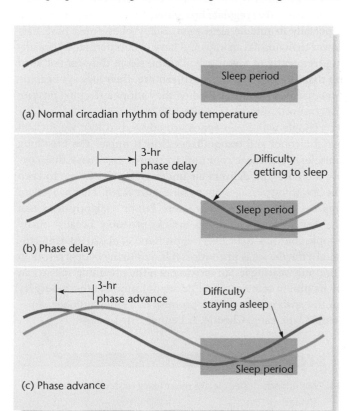

Figure 8.17 Insomnia and circadian rhythms
People with a phase delay have trouble getting to sleep. People with a phase advance have trouble staying asleep.

with sleep. Coffee also phase-delays the circadian rhythm, causing a delay in the release of melatonin (Burke et al., 2015). Ordinarily that delay causes problems, although it might help combat jet lag after traveling west.

Sleep Apnea

One type of insomnia is **sleep apnea**, impaired ability to breathe while sleeping. People with sleep apnea have breathless periods of a minute or so from which they awaken gasping for breath. They may not remember their awakenings, although they certainly notice the consequences, such as sleepiness during the day and impaired attention. People with sleep apnea are at increased risk of stroke, heart problems, and other disorders. People with sleep apnea have multiple brain areas that appear to have lost neurons, and consequently, many of them show deficiencies of learning, reasoning, attention, and impulse control (Beebe & Gozal, 2002; Macey et al., 2002). These correlational data do not tell us whether the brain abnormalities led to sleep apnea or sleep apnea led to the brain abnormalities. However, research with rodents suggests the latter: Mice that are subjected to frequent periods of low oxygen (as if they hadn't been breathing) lose some neurons and impair others, especially in areas responsible for alertness (Zhu et al., 2007).

Sleep apnea results from several causes, including genetics, hormones, and old-age deterioration of the brain mechanisms that regulate breathing. Another cause is obesity, especially in middle-aged men. Many obese men have narrower than normal airways and have to compensate by breathing frequently or vigorously. During sleep, they cannot keep up that rate of breathing. Furthermore, their airways become even narrower than usual when they adopt a sleeping posture (Mezzanotte, Tangel, & White, 1992).

People with sleep apnea are advised to lose weight and avoid alcohol and tranquilizers (which impair the breathing muscles). The most common treatment is a mask that covers the nose and delivers air under enough pressure to keep the breathing passages open (see Figure 8.18). That procedure improves sleep and blood pressure, but only slightly decreases the risk of stroke or heart attack, probably because many people continue to be overweight (Guo et al., 2016). Unfortunately, the device is uncomfortable and many people refuse to continue wearing it. Surgery to open the breathing spaces can be helpful in some cases, but disappointing in others. Surgery on the jawbone has shown promise in a small number of patients (Tsui, Yang, Cheung, & Leung, 2016).

✓ STOP & CHECK

14. What kinds of people are most likely to develop sleep apnea?

ANSWER

14. Sleep apnea is most common among people with a genetic predisposition, old people, and overweight middle-aged men.

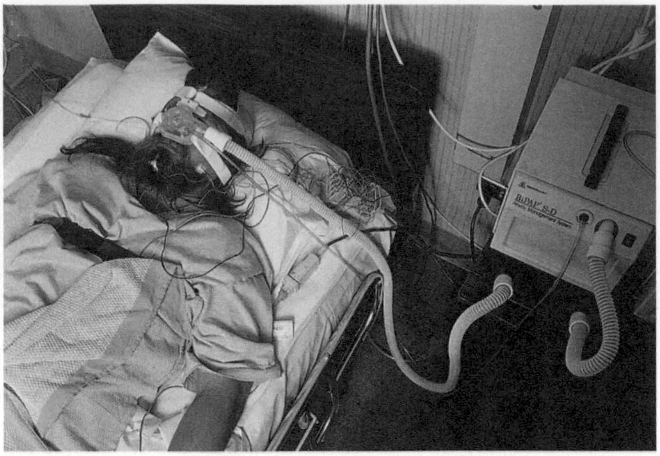

Figure 8.18 A continuous positive airway pressure (CPAP) mask The mask fits snugly over the nose and delivers air at a fixed pressure, strong enough to keep the breathing passages open. (*Russell Curtis/Science Source*)

Narcolepsy

Narcolepsy, a condition characterized by frequent periods of sleepiness during the day, strikes about 1 person in 1,000. It sometimes runs in families, but most cases emerge in people with no affected relatives. The H1N1 flu virus in 2009–2010 caused many cases of narcolepsy (Tesoriero et al., 2016). Narcolepsy has four main symptoms, although not every patient has all four. Each of these symptoms can be interpreted as an intrusion of a REM-like state into wakefulness:

1. Attacks of sleepiness during the day.
2. Occasional cataplexy—an attack of muscle weakness while the person remains awake. Cataplexy is often triggered by strong emotions, such as anger or great excitement. (One man suddenly collapsed during his wedding ceremony.)
3. Sleep paralysis—an inability to move while falling asleep or waking up. Many people have experienced sleep paralysis at least once or twice, but people with narcolepsy experience it frequently.
4. Hypnagogic hallucinations—dreamlike experiences that the person has trouble distinguishing from reality, often occurring at the onset of sleep.

The cause relates to the neurotransmitter orexin. People with narcolepsy lack the hypothalamic cells that produce and release orexin (Thannickal et al., 2000). Why they lack them is unknown, but the most likely possibility is an autoimmune reaction, in which the immune system attacks part of the body—in this case, cells with orexin (Hallmayer et al., 2009). Recall that orexin is important for maintaining wakefulness. Consequently, people lacking orexin alternate between short waking periods and short sleepy periods, instead of staying awake throughout the day. Dogs that lack the gene for orexin receptors have symptoms much like human narcolepsy, with frequent alternations between wakefulness and sleep (Lin et al., 1999). The same is true for mice that lack orexin (Hara, 2001; Mochizuki et al., 2004).

As discussed in Chapter 7, people with Huntington's disease have widespread damage in the basal ganglia. In addition, most lose neurons in the hypothalamus, including the neurons that make orexin. As a result, they have problems staying awake during the day and difficulty staying asleep at night (Morton et al., 2005).

So far no one has developed a drug that specifically activates orexin receptors. Administering orexin itself is not a good option, because it does not readily cross the blood–brain barrier. The most common treatment is stimulant drugs such as methylphenidate (Ritalin), which enhance dopamine and norepinephrine activity.

⊘ **STOP & CHECK** ▬▬▬▬▬▬

15. What is the relationship between orexin and narcolepsy?

ANSWER

15. Orexin is important for staying awake. Therefore, people or animals lacking either orexin or the receptors for orexin develop narcolepsy, characterized by bouts of sleepiness during the day.

Periodic Limb Movement Disorder

Another sleep disorder is **periodic limb movement disorder**, characterized by repeated involuntary movement of the legs and sometimes the arms during sleep. It is distinct from restless leg syndrome, in which people often feel an urge to kick a leg even while awake.

Many people, perhaps most, experience an occasional involuntary kick, especially when starting to fall asleep. Leg movements are not a problem unless they become persistent. In people with periodic limb movement disorder, mostly middle-aged and older, the legs kick once every 20 to 30 seconds for minutes or hours, mostly during NREM sleep.

REM Behavior Disorder

For most people, the major postural muscles are relaxed and inactive during REM sleep. However, people with **REM behavior disorder** move around vigorously during their REM periods, apparently acting out their dreams. They frequently dream about defending themselves against attack, and they may punch, kick, and leap about. They often injure themselves or other people and damage property (Olson, Boeve, & Silber, 2000).

Mice deficient in GABA and other inhibitory neurotransmitters show running, jerking, and chewing movements during REM sleep, and overall disrupted sleep. Because of these similarities to human cases, the results suggest that inadequate inhibitory transmission may be responsible for REM behavior disorder (Brooks & Peever, 2011).

Night Terrors and Sleepwalking

Night terrors are experiences of intense anxiety from which a person awakens screaming in terror. A night terror is more severe than a nightmare, which is simply an unpleasant dream. Night terrors occur during NREM sleep and are more common in children than adults. Dream content, if any, is usually simple, such as a single image.

Sleepwalking runs in families and occurs mostly in children. Most people who sleepwalk, and many of their relatives, have one or more additional sleep difficulties such as chronic snoring, disordered sleep breathing, bed-wetting, and night terrors (Cao & Guilleminault, 2010). The causes of sleepwalking are not well understood, but it is more common when people are sleep deprived or under unusual stress (Zadra & Pilon, 2008). It is most common during slow-wave sleep early in the night and usually not accompanied by dreaming. (It does not occur during REM sleep, when the large muscles are completely relaxed.) Sleepwalking is usually harmless but not always. One teenage girl walked out of her house, climbed a crane, and went back to sleep on a support beam. Fortunately, a pedestrian saw her and called the police. Sleepwalkers have been known to eat, rearrange furniture, fall off balconies, and drive cars—while disregarding lanes and traffic lights. Unlike wakeful actions, the deeds of sleepwalkers are poorly planned and usually not remembered. Evidently, some parts of the brain are awake and other parts are asleep (Gunn & Gunn, 2007). Incidentally, contrary to common sayings, it is not dangerous to awaken a sleepwalker. It is not particularly helpful either, but it is not dangerous.

An analogous condition is sleep sex or "sexsomnia," in which sleeping people engage in sexual behavior, either with a partner or by masturbation, and do not remember it afterward. Some cases occur when someone with sleep apnea suddenly awakens partially and confused during non-REM sleep. One case resulted from a peculiar, apparently unprecedented side effect of an antidepressant drug. Many people with sexsomnia were sleepwalkers as children. Overall, the condition is not well understood (Schenck, 2015).

Sexsomnia poses a threat to romances and marriages. As one woman said, "After getting married a few years ago, my husband told me I was masturbating in my sleep. I was mortified, thinking back to all the slumber parties as a girl, and then when I was older and my little sister stayed the night at my house! How many others might have witnessed and not said anything? My new marriage is on the rocks, since I'm having such good sex in my sleep, I have NO desire while I'm awake. This is killing my relationship with my husband" (Mangan, 2004, p. 290).

Stages of Sleep

Chemists divide the world into elements, biologists divide life into species, and physicians distinguish one disease from another. Similarly, psychologists try to recognize the most natural or useful distinctions among types of behavior or experience. The discovery of stages of sleep was a major landmark in psychology because researchers found a previously unrecognized distinction that is both biologically and psychologically important. It also demonstrated that external measurements—in this case, EEG recordings—can be used to identify internal experiences. We now take it largely for granted that an electrical or magnetic recording from the brain can tell us something about a person's experience, but it is worth pausing to note what a surprising discovery that was in its time.

Summary

1. During sleep, brain activity decreases, but a stimulus can awaken the person. Someone in a coma cannot be awakened. A vegetative state or minimally conscious state can last months or years, during which the person shows only limited responses. Brain death is a condition without brain activity or responsiveness of any kind. **268**

2. Over the course of about 90 minutes, a sleeper goes through stages 1, 2, and slow-wave sleep and then returns through stage 2 to a stage called REM (rapid eye movement sleep). **268**

3. REM sleep or paradoxical sleep is a condition marked by rapid eye movements, more cortical activity than other sleep, relaxation of the body's postural muscles, and an increased probability of vivid dreams. **269**

4. The brain has multiple systems for arousal. The pontomesencephalon, hypothalamus, and basal forebrain include some neurons that promote wakefulness and others that promote sleep. **271**

5. The locus coeruleus is active in response to meaningful events. It facilitates attention and new learning. **272**

6. Orexin is a peptide that maintains wakefulness. Cells in the lateral and posterior nuclei of the hypothalamus release this peptide. **273**

7. During sleep, enhanced release of GABA limits neuronal activity and blocks the spread of activation. Sometimes this suppression is stronger in one brain area than another. Therefore, it is possible for part of the brain to be more awake than another is. **273**

8. REM sleep is associated with activity in a number of brain areas, including the pons, limbic system, and parts of the parietal and temporal cortex. Activity decreases in the prefrontal cortex, the motor cortex, and the primary visual cortex. **274**

9. REM sleep begins with PGO waves, which are waves of brain activity transmitted from the pons to the lateral geniculate to the occipital lobe. **274**

10. People with sleep apnea have long periods without breathing while they sleep. So far, none of the treatments is fully satisfactory. **276**

11. People with narcolepsy have attacks of sleepiness during the day. Narcolepsy is associated with a deficiency of the neurotransmitter orexin. **276**

12. Sleepwalking and sexsomnia are cases of somewhat purposeful, somewhat confused behaviors during partial arousal from sleep. The person is unlikely to remember the episode later. **277**

Key Terms

Terms are defined in the module on the page number indicated. They're also presented in alphabetical order with definitions in the book's Subject Index/Glossary, which begins on page 589. Interactive flash cards, audio reviews, and crossword puzzles are among the online resources available to help you learn these terms and the concepts they represent.

alpha waves **268**
basal forebrain **273**
brain death **268**
coma **268**
insomnia **275**
K-complex **269**
locus coeruleus **272**
minimally conscious state **268**
narcolepsy **276**

night terrors **277**
non-REM (NREM) sleep **270**
orexin (or hypocretin) **273**
paradoxical sleep **269**
periodic limb movement disorder **277**
PGO waves **274**
polysomnograph **268**
pontomesencephalon **271**

rapid eye movement (REM) sleep **270**
REM behavior disorder **277**
reticular formation **271**
sleep apnea **276**
sleep spindle **269**
slow-wave sleep (SWS) **269**
vegetative state **268**

Thought Question

Unlike adults, infants alternate between short waking periods and short naps. What can we infer about their neurotransmitters?

Module 8.2 | End of Module Quiz

1. Of the following, which shows the LEAST brain activity?

   A. Slow-wave sleep
   B. Coma

   C. Vegetative state
   D. Minimally conscious state

2. Sleep spindles in stage 2 sleep appear to be important for which of the following?

   A. Consolidation of memory
   B. Inhibition of impulses

   C. Defense mechanisms against anxiety
   D. Control of body temperature

3. What do the high-amplitude slow waves of slow-wave sleep indicate?

   A. An increased level of brain activity
   B. Synchrony among neurons

   C. Muscle contractions
   D. Responses to sensory stimulation

4. Why is REM sleep also known as paradoxical sleep?

   A. Activity in the left hemisphere does not match the activity in the right hemisphere.
   B. We did not know it existed until its discovery in the 1950s.

   C. It is deep sleep in some ways and light in others.
   D. Because a pair of docs discovered it.

5. At which time, if any, is slow-wave sleep most common?

   A. Immediately after falling asleep
   B. Not immediately, but during the early part of the night's sleep

   C. Near the end of the night's sleep
   D. During all parts equally

6. What tends to activate the locus coeruleus?

   A. Stomach contractions
   B. Conflict between emotions

   C. Meaningful information
   D. Sexual desire

7. What is the role of orexin with regard to wakefulness and sleep?

   A. It stimulates REM sleep.
   B. It inhibits the spread of brain activity while someone is asleep.

   C. It helps someone stay awake.
   D. It is active during switches back and forth between wakefulness and sleep.

8. Why are people unconscious during slow-wave sleep?

   A. Inhibitory transmitters block the spread of activity in the cortex.
   B. The sensory receptors become unresponsive to nearly all input.

   C. Spontaneous activity ceases in the neurons of the cortex.
   D. Circulating hormones block the sodium gates in axon membranes.

9. If you awaken but find you temporarily cannot move your arms or legs, what is happening?

   A. You are probably developing a severe neurological disease.
   B. You are probably just being lazy.

   C. You need more time to get the blood flowing to your muscles.
   D. Most of your brain is awake, but part of your pons and medulla remain in REM sleep.

10. Of the following, which one is *not* associated with an increased probability of sleep apnea?

    A. Having a relative with sleep apnea
    B. Being female

    C. Being overweight
    D. Being middle-aged

11. Narcolepsy is linked to a deficit of which neurotransmitter?

    A. Dopamine
    B. GABA

    C. Orexin
    D. Acetylcholine

Why Sleep? Why REM? Why Dreams?

Why do you sleep? "That's easy," you reply. "I sleep because I get tired." Well, yes, but you are not tired in the sense of muscle fatigue. You need almost as much sleep after a day of sitting around the house as after a day of intense physical or mental activity (Horne & Minard, 1985; Shapiro, Bortz, Mitchell, Bartel, & Jooste, 1981). Furthermore, you could rest your muscles just as well while awake as while asleep. (In fact, if your muscles ache after strenuous exercise, you probably find it difficult to sleep.)

You feel tired at the end of the day because inhibitory processes in your brain force you to become less aroused and less alert. That is, we evolved mechanisms to cause sleep. Why?

Functions of Sleep

Sleep serves many functions. During sleep, we rest our muscles, decrease metabolism, perform cellular maintenance in neurons (Vyadyslav & Harris, 2013), reorganize synapses, and strengthen memories. People who don't get enough sleep react more severely than average to stressful events (Minkel et al., 2012). They may develop symptoms of mental illness or may aggravate symptoms they already had (van der Kloet, Merckelbach, Giesbrecht, & Lynn, 2012). Inadequate sleep is a major cause of accidents by workers and poor performance by college students. Driving while sleep deprived is comparable to driving under the influence of alcohol (Falleti, Maruff, Collie, Darby, & McStephen, 2003). Even one night of sleeplessness activates the immune system (Matsumoto et al., 2001). That is, you react to sleep deprivation as if you were ill. Clearly, we need to sleep. Is there, however, a primary or original reason?

Sleep and Energy Conservation

Even if we identified what seems to be the most important function of sleep for humans today, it might not be the function for which sleep originally evolved. By analogy, what is the main function of computers? You might use a computer to write papers, send email, search the Internet, play video games, store and display photographs, play music, or find a date. All of those are valuable functions, but the original purpose was to do mathematical calculations. Similarly, sleep probably started with a simple function to which evolution added others later. Even bacteria have circadian rhythms of activity and inactivity (Mihalcescu, Hsing, & Leibler, 2004). What benefit of sleep applies to all species, even those with little or no nervous system?

A likely hypothesis is that sleep's original function—and still an important one—is to save energy (Kleitman, 1963; Siegel, 2009, 2012). Nearly every species is more efficient at some times of day than at others. Those with good vision are more efficient in the day. Those that rely on other senses instead of vision are more efficient at night, when their predators cannot see them. Sleep conserves energy during the inefficient times, when activity would be wasteful and possibly dangerous. NASA's Rover spacecraft, built to explore Mars, had a mechanism to make it "sleep" at night to conserve its batteries. During sleep, a mammal's body temperature decreases by 1° or 2°C, enough to save a significant amount of energy. Muscle activity decreases, saving more energy. Animals increase their sleep duration during food shortages, when energy conservation is especially important (Berger & Phillips, 1995).

Sleep is therefore in some ways analogous to hibernation. Hibernation is a true need. A ground squirrel that is prevented from hibernating becomes as disturbed as a person who is prevented from sleeping. However, the function of hibernation is simply to conserve energy while food is scarce.

Analogous to Sleep: Hibernation

Hibernating animals decrease their body temperature to only slightly above that of the environment, but not low enough for their blood to freeze. Heart rate drops to almost nothing, brain activity drops to almost nothing, neuron cell bodies shrink, and many synapses disappear, regenerating later when body temperature increases (Peretti et al., 2015). A few curious facts about hibernation:

1. Whether or not bears hibernate is a matter of definition. Bears sleep most of the winter, lowering their body temperature a few degrees and decreasing their metabolism and heart rate (Tøien et al., 2011), but their state is not as extreme as that of smaller hibernators such as bats and ground squirrels.
2. Hamsters also hibernate, and the pet stores generally do not tell people about it. If you keep your pet hamster in

a cool, dimly lit place during the winter, and it appears to have died, make sure that it is not just hibernating before you bury it!

3. Many reptiles and amphibians become dormant, a state similar to hibernating, during the winter. They depress their metabolism and remain inactive until spring (Sanders et al., 2015).

4. Hibernating animals come out of hibernation for a few hours, either once every few days or once in a few weeks, depending on the species. However, they spend most of this nonhibernating time asleep (Barnes, 1996; Williams, Barnes, Richter, & Buck, 2012).

5. Hibernation retards or suspends the aging process. Hamsters that spend longer times hibernating have proportionately longer life expectancies than other hamsters do (Lyman, O'Brien, Greene, & Papafrangos, 1981). Fat-tailed dwarf lemurs, which hibernate, survive years longer than related species of the same size that do not hibernate (Blanco & Zehr, 2015). Hibernation is also a period of relative invulnerability to infection and trauma. Procedures that would ordinarily damage the brain, such as inserting a needle into it, produce little if any harm during hibernation (Zhou et al., 2001).

Species Differences in Sleep

If one of the main functions of sleep is to decrease activity at times of relative inefficiency, we might expect to find little or no sleep in species that are equally effective at all times of day. Indeed, evidence supports that expectation. Mexican cavefish, which you can buy at a pet store, are from a species that has one population that lives in normal waters subject to day and night, and several populations that evolved to live in caves with no light and virtually no changes in temperature. In contrast to the population in normal waters, which average more than 13 hours of sleep per day, the populations in caves vary between 2 and 4 hours of sleep per day (Duboué & Keene, 2016; Duboué, Keene, & Borowsky, 2011; Kavanau, 1998). Many animals that live near the North or South Pole greatly decrease their sleep during summer, when the sun is constantly above the horizon. For example, while male sandpipers are competing for mates above the Arctic Circle, many of them are active up to 23 hours per day for nearly three weeks, with no apparent harm to their health or alertness (Lesku et al., 2012). Many reindeer and penguins have long periods of nearly constant wakefulness, with no apparent circadian rhythm (Bloch, Barnes, Gerkema, & Helm, 2013).

Certain other species abandon or decrease their sleep under certain circumstances. After a dolphin or whale gives birth, both mother and baby stay awake 24 hours a day for the first couple of weeks while the baby is especially vulnerable. Neither shows any sign of harm from sleep deprivation (Lyamin, Pryaslova, Lance, & Siegel, 2005). Even at other times, dolphins, whales, and other aquatic mammals face a problem related to sleep: At all times of day, they need to be

alert enough to come to the surface periodically for a breath of air. To do so, they evolved the ability to sleep on one side of the brain at a time. The two hemispheres take turns sleeping, always leaving one awake enough to control swimming and breathing (Rattenborg, Amlaner, & Lima, 2000). Seals also sleep in one hemisphere at a time when they are at sea, although they sleep in both hemispheres at the same time when they are on land (Lyamin, Kosenko, Lapierre, Muikhametov, & Siegel, 2008).

Swifts are small, dark birds that chase insects. They get all the nutrition and water they need from the insects. When a baby European swift first takes off from its nest, how long would you guess its first flight lasts, until it comes to land again?

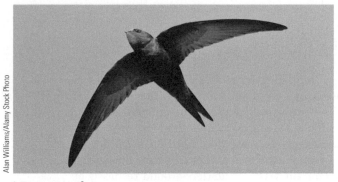

A European swift

The answer: up to 2 years. Except during treacherous storms, the bird doesn't land on solid ground until it is old enough to mate and build a nest. In the meantime, it spends both days and nights in the air. At night it heads into the wind, sticks out its wings, and glides (Bäckman & Alerstam, 2001). Does it sleep all night while flying? Does it sleep with one hemisphere at a time? Or has it abandoned sleep altogether? Answering these questions would require recording EEG from a small bird in flight, not much bigger than a house sparrow. However, measuring EEG is more feasible in a much larger bird that also spends most nights in the air. Great frigate birds fly over the ocean for weeks or months at a time, eating flying fish, flying squid (yes, there is such a thing), and anything else that comes at or above the surface. These birds never land on the water, because their feathers would become waterlogged and prevent the bird from taking flight again. So frigate birds spend the night in the air. EEG records show that they have periods of slow-wave sleep in just one hemisphere, and REM periods in both hemispheres equally. Moreover, their sleep episodes are brief, averaging just 11 seconds, and totaling less than 45 minutes per night. By contrast, when they are on land (mainly to nest and rear young), they sleep 12 or more hours per day (Rattenborg et al., 2016). A bird flying at sea needs nearly constant alertness, but a large bird sitting on a nest does not.

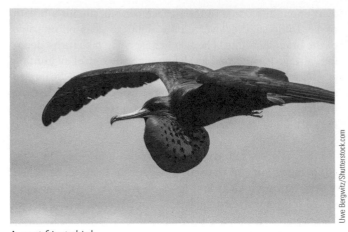

A great frigate bird

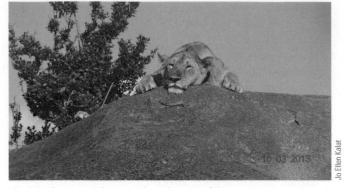

The lion sleeps tonight . . . and maybe part of the morning . . . and much of the afternoon, too.

Migrating birds face a problem: During a week or two in fall and spring, they forage for food during the day and do their migratory flying at night, leaving them little time for sleep. They apparently decrease their need for sleep during migration. If a bird is kept in a cage during the migration season, it flutters around restlessly at night, sleeping only a third its usual amount. It compensates to some extent with brief drowsy periods (less than 30 seconds each) during the day (Fuchs, Haney, Jechura, Moore, & Bingman, 2006). Still, it gets very little sleep, while remaining alert and performing normally on learning tasks. If the same bird is deprived of sleep during other seasons of the year, its performance suffers (Rattenborg et al., 2004). Exactly how a mother dolphin, great frigate bird, or migratory bird decreases its sleep need is unknown, but the fact that it is possible fits with the idea that sleep is primarily a way to conserve energy, rather than a way to fulfill a need that one could not fulfill in other ways.

Animal species vary in their sleep habits in ways that make sense if we ask how many hours the animal needs to be awake, and therefore how long it can afford to spend conserving energy (Allison & Cicchetti, 1976; Campbell & Tobler, 1984). Grazing animals that need to eat for many hours per day get less sleep than carnivores (meat eaters) that satisfy their nutritional needs with a single meal. Animals that need to be on the alert for predators get little sleep, whereas the predators themselves sleep easily. Insect-eating bats are active in the early evening, when moths and similar insects are most abundant, and then they sleep the rest of the day (see Figure 8.19).

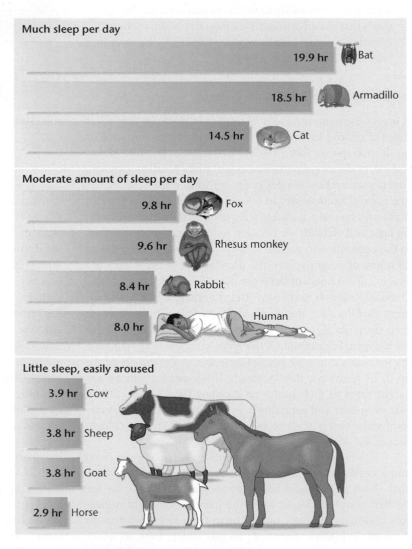

Figure 8.19 Hours of sleep per day for various species
Generally, predators and others that are safe when they sleep tend to sleep a great deal. Animals in danger of being attacked while they sleep spend less time asleep.

STOP & CHECK

16. What might one predict about the sleep of fish that live deep in the ocean?
17. What kind of animal tends to get more than the average amount of sleep?

ANSWERS

16. The deep ocean, like a cave, has no light and no difference between day and night. These fish might not need to sleep because they are equally efficient at all times of day and have no reason to conserve energy at one time more than another. 17. Predators get much sleep, and so do species that are unlikely to be attacked during their sleep (such as armadillos).

Sleep and Memory

Another function of sleep is improved memory. If you do not get a good night's sleep, your memory and cognition will suffer the next day (Appleman, Albouy, Doyon, Cronin-Golomb, & King, 2016; Yoo, Hu, Gujar, Jolesz, & Walker, 2007). In contrast, if you learn something and then go to sleep, or even take a nap, your memory solidifies and may even become better than it was before sleep (Hu, Stylos-Allan, & Walker, 2006; Korman et al., 2007; Nettersheim, Hallschmid, Born, & Diekelmann, 2015; Payne et al., 2015). In one study, students memorized a foreign vocabulary list (in Swahili) until they had said each item correctly just once. Then 12 hours later they tried again. Those who learned the list in the morning and tried again in the evening had forgotten most of the words. Those who learned in the evening, slept, and tried again in the morning did much better (Mazza et al., 2016). So, if you want to memorize something, study it before going to sleep. Better yet, study before going to sleep and then review after you awaken.

Sleep also helps people reanalyze their memories: In one study, people who had just practiced a complex task were more likely to perceive a hidden rule (an "aha" experience) after a period of sleep than after a similar period of wakefulness (Wagner, Gais, Haider, Verleger, & Born, 2004). Another study found that a nap that included REM sleep enhanced performance on certain kinds of creative problem solving (Cai, Mednick, Harrison, Kanady, & Mednick, 2009). However, an afternoon nap also leaves someone less alert than usual for the next half hour (Groeger, Lo, Burns, & Dijk, 2011). Both REM sleep and slow-wave sleep have been linked to strengthening of memories (Boyce, Glasgow, Williams, & Adamantidis, 2016; Gais, Plihal, Wagner, & Born, 2000; Plihal & Born, 1997; Wei, Krishnan, & Bazhenov, 2016).

How does sleep enhance memory? Researchers recorded activity in the hippocampus during learning, and then recorded from the same locations during sleep, using microelectrodes within cells for laboratory animals and electrodes on the scalp for humans. The results: Patterns that occurred during sleep resembled those that had occurred during learning, except that they were more rapid during sleep. Furthermore, the amount of hippocampal activity during sleep correlated highly with the subsequent improvement in performance (Derégnaucourt, Mitra, Fehér, Pytte, & Tchernichovski, 2005; Euston, Tatsuno, & McNaughton, 2007; Huber, Ghilardi, Massimini, & Tononi, 2004; Ji & Wilson, 2007; Maquet et al., 2000; Peigneux et al., 2004). As the brain replays its experiences during sleep it forms new dendritic branches and strengthens the memories (Yang et al., 2014). However, the hippocampus also replays recently learned patterns during quiet waking periods, not just during sleep (Karlsson & Frank, 2009).

One way for sleep to strengthen memory is by weeding out the less successful connections. The chapter on memory (Chapter 12) describes long-term potentiation, the ability of new experiences to strengthen synaptic connections. Suppose that every time you learn something, your brain strengthened certain synapses without making adjustments elsewhere. As you learned more and more, you would have more and more brain activity. By middle age, your brain might be burning with constant activity. To prevent runaway overactivity, your brain compensates for strengthening some synapses by weakening or removing others, mostly during sleep (Liu, Faraguna, Cirelli, Tononi, & Gao, 2010; Maret, Faraguna, Nelson, Cirelli, & Tononi, 2011; Vyazovskiy, Cirelli, Pfister-Genskow, Faraguna, & Tononi, 2008). Weakening less appropriate synapses emphasizes the ones that were strengthened during wakefulness.

STOP & CHECK

18. How does weakening synapses during sleep improve memory?

ANSWER

18. Weakening the less active synapses enables the strengthened ones to stand out by contrast.

Functions of REM Sleep

An average person spends about a third of his or her life asleep and about a fifth of sleep in REM, totaling about 600 hours of REM per year. Presumably, REM serves a biological function. But what is it?

One way to approach this question is to compare the people or animals with more REM to those with less. REM sleep is widespread in mammals and birds, indicating that it is part of our ancient evolutionary heritage. Some species, however, have far more than others. As a rule, the species with the most total sleep hours also have the highest percentage of REM sleep (Siegel, 1995). Cats spend up to 16 hours a day sleeping, much or most of it in REM sleep. Rabbits, guinea pigs, and sheep sleep less and spend little time in REM.

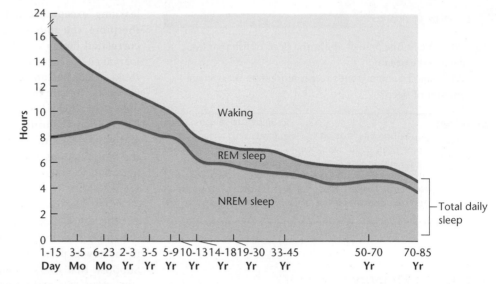

Figure 8.20 Sleep patterns for people of various ages
REM sleep occupies about 8 hours a day in newborns but less than 2 hours in most adults. The sleep of infants is not quite like that of adults, however, and the criteria for identifying REM sleep are not the same.
(Source: From "Ontogenetic development of human sleep-dream cycle," by H. P. Roffwarg, J. N. Muzio, and W. C. Dement, 1966, Science, 152, pp. 604–609. Copyright 1966 AAAS. Reprinted by permission.)

Figure 8.20 illustrates the relationship between age and REM sleep for humans. The trend is the same for other mammalian species. Infants get more REM and more total sleep than adults do, confirming the pattern that more total sleep predicts a higher percentage of REM sleep. Among adult humans, those who sleep 9 or more hours per night have the highest percentage of REM sleep, and those who sleep 5 or fewer hours have the least percentage. This pattern implies that although REM is no doubt important, NREM is more tightly regulated. The amount of NREM varies less among individuals and among species.

One hypothesis is that REM is important for strengthening memory (Crick & Mitchison, 1983). Although memory consolidation does occur during REM, many people take antidepressant drugs that severely decrease REM sleep but cause no memory problems (Rasch, Pommer, Diekelmann, & Born, 2009). Research on laboratory animals indicates that antidepressant drugs sometimes even enhance memory (Parent, Habib, & Baker, 1999).

Another hypothesis sounds odd because we tend to imagine a glamorous role for REM sleep: David Maurice (1998) proposed that REM just shakes the eyeballs back and forth enough to get sufficient oxygen to the corneas of the eyes. The corneas, unlike the rest of the body, get oxygen directly from the surrounding air. During sleep, because they are shielded from the air, they deteriorate slightly (Hoffmann & Curio, 2003). They do get some oxygen from the fluid behind them (see Figure 5.1), but when the eyes are motionless, that fluid becomes stagnant. Moving the eyes increases the oxygen supply to the corneas. According to this view, REM is a way of arousing a sleeper just enough to shake the eyes back and forth, and the other manifestations of REM are just by-products. This idea makes sense of the fact that REM occurs mostly toward the end of the night's sleep, when the fluid behind the eyes would be the most stagnant. It also makes sense of the fact that individuals who spend more hours asleep devote a greater percentage of sleep to REM. (If you

don't sleep long, you have less need to shake up the stagnant fluid.) However, as mentioned, many people take antidepressants that restrict REM sleep. They are not known to suffer damage to the cornea.

✓ **STOP & CHECK** ▬▬▬▬▬

19. What kinds of individuals get more REM sleep than others? (Think in terms of age, species, and long versus short sleepers.)

ANSWER
19. Much REM sleep is more typical of the young than the old, and of those who get much sleep than those who get little.

Biological Perspectives on Dreaming

Dream research faces a special problem: All we know about dreams comes from people's self-reports, and researchers have no way to check the accuracy of those reports. In fact, we forget most dreams, and even when we do remember them, the details fade quickly.

The Activation-Synthesis Hypothesis

According to the **activation-synthesis hypothesis**, a dream represents the brain's effort to make sense of sparse and distorted information. Dreams begin with periodic bursts of spontaneous activity in the pons—the PGO waves previously described—that activate some parts of the cortex but not others. The cortex combines this haphazard input with whatever other activity was already occurring and does its best to synthesize a story that makes sense of the information (Hobson & McCarley, 1977; Hobson, Pace-Schott, & Stickgold, 2000; McCarley & Hoffman, 1981).

Consider how this theory handles a couple of common dreams. Most people have had occasional dreams of falling or flying. While you are asleep, you lie flat, unlike your posture for the rest of the day. Your brain in its partly aroused condition feels the vestibular sensation of your position and interprets it as flying or falling. Have you ever dreamed that you were trying to move but couldn't? Most people have. An interpretation based on the activation-synthesis theory is that during REM sleep (which accompanies most dreams), your motor cortex is inactive and your major postural muscles are virtually paralyzed. That is, when you are dreaming, you really *cannot* move, you feel your lack of movement, and thus, you dream of failing to move.

One criticism is that the theory's predictions are vague. If we dream about falling because of the vestibular sensations from lying down, why don't we *always* dream of falling? If we dream we cannot move because our muscles are paralyzed during REM sleep, why don't we *always* dream of being paralyzed? Furthermore, most dreams have no apparent connection to any current stimuli (Foulkes & Domhoff, 2014; Nir & Tononi, 2010).

The Neurocognitive Hypothesis

The **neurocognitive hypothesis** regards dreams as thinking that takes place under unusual conditions. It emphasizes that dreams begin with spontaneous brain activity related to recent memories (Solms, 1997, 2000).

During sleep, the brain gets relatively little information from the sense organs, and the primary visual and auditory areas of the cortex have lower than usual activity. Therefore, other brain areas are free to generate images without constraints or interference. Also, the primary motor cortex is suppressed, as are the motor neurons of the spinal cord, so arousal cannot lead to action. Activity is suppressed in the prefrontal cortex, which is important for working memory. Consequently, we not only forget most dreams after we awaken, but we also lose track of what has been happening within a

dream, and sudden scene changes are common. We also lose a sense of volition—that is, planning (Hobson, 2009). It seems that events just happen, without any intention on our part.

Meanwhile, activity is relatively high in the inferior (lower) part of the parietal cortex, an area important for visuospatial perception. Patients with damage here fail to bind body sensations with vision. They also report no dreams. Fairly high activity is also found in the areas of visual cortex other than the primary visual cortex. Those areas are presumably important for the visual imagery that accompanies most dreams. Finally, activity is high in the hypothalamus, amygdala, and other areas important for emotions and motivations (Gvilia, Turner, McGinty, & Szymusiak, 2006).

So the idea is that either internal or external stimulation activates parts of the parietal, occipital, and temporal cortex. The arousal develops into a hallucinatory perception, with no sensory input from area V1 to override it. This idea, like the activation-synthesis hypothesis, is hard to test because it does not make specific predictions about who will have what dream and when.

✓ STOP & CHECK

20. According to the neurocognitive hypothesis, why do we have visual imagery during dreams? Why do dreams sometimes make an incoherent or illogical story?

ANSWER 20. We have visual imagery because areas of the visual cortex other than the primary visual cortex become active, without any input from the eyes. Dreams are sometimes incoherent or illogical because low activity in the prefrontal cortex means poor memory for what has just happened.

Module 8.3 | In Closing
Our Limited Self-Understanding

Without minimizing how much we do understand about sleep, it is noteworthy how many basic questions remain. What is the function of REM sleep? Does dreaming have a function, or is it just an accident? Our lack of knowledge about activities that

occupy so much of our time underscores a point about the biology of behavior: We evolved tendencies to behave in certain ways that lead to survival and reproduction. The behavior can serve its function even when we do not fully understand that function.

Summary

1. One important function of sleep is to conserve energy at a time when the individual would be less efficient. Animal species vary in their sleep per day depending on their feeding habits and how much danger they face while asleep. **280**

2. In addition to saving energy, sleep serves other functions, including enhancement of memory. **283**

3. REM sleep occupies the greatest percentage of sleep in the individuals and species that sleep the most total hours. **283**

4. According to the activation-synthesis hypothesis, dreams are the brain's attempts to make sense of the information reaching it, based mostly on haphazard input originating in the pons. **284**

5. According to the neurocognitive hypothesis, dreams originate mostly from the brain's own motivations, memories, and arousal. The stimulation often produces peculiar results because it does not have to compete with normal visual input and does not get organized by the prefrontal cortex. **285**

Key Terms

Terms are defined in the module on the page number indicated. They're also presented in alphabetical order with definitions in the book's Subject Index/Glossary, which begins on page 589. Interactive flash cards, audio reviews, and crossword puzzles are among the online resources available to help you learn these terms and the concepts they represent.

activation-synthesis hypothesis **284**

neurocognitive hypothesis **285**

Thought Question

Why would it be harder to deprive someone of just NREM sleep than just REM sleep?

Module 8.3 | End of Module Quiz

1. Certain animal species have evolved to sleep very little under which of these circumstances?
   A. The animals can easily find an abundance of food.
   B. The environment is about the same 24 hours a day.
   C. The weather often changes drastically from one day to the next.
   D. Several closely related species live in the same geographical area.

2. How do whales and dolphins get oxygen at night?
   A. They absorb oxygen from the water.
   B. They sleep in just one hemisphere at a time.
   C. They lower their metabolism so that they need to breathe only a few times per night.
   D. They store oxygen in their digestive system.

3. When frigate birds spend weeks at sea, what do they do about sleep?
   A. They sleep while floating on the water.
   B. They sleep only in brief episodes, and not much overall.
   C. They go without sleep altogether.
   D. They sleep as much as usual, but while gliding.

4. If we want to predict how many hours a day some species sleeps, which of these questions would be most helpful in making that prediction?
   A. What color is the animal?
   B. Does the animal live north or south of the equator?
   C. What does the animal eat?
   D. How intelligent is the animal?

5. Sleep often improves memory. How?
   A. Synapses increase their supply of serotonin and norepinephrine.
   B. Certain synapses become weakened, enabling others to stand out by contrast.
   C. Overall brain activity increases.
   D. The brain increases its ratio of sodium ions to potassium ions.

6. Of the following groups, which one tends to spend the highest percentage of sleep in the REM stage?
   A. Infants
   B. Those who sleep only a few hours per night
   C. Prey animals, such as sheep and horses
   D. Teenagers

7. According to the neurocognitive hypothesis, what are dreams?
   A. Dreams are disguised representations of unconscious wishes.
   B. Dreams are reactions to whatever sensory stimuli are present at the time.
   C. Dreams are memories of the experiences of our ancestors.
   D. Dreams are thinking that occurs under unusual conditions.

Answers: 1B, 2B, 3B, 4C, 5B, 6A, 7D.

Suggestions for Further Reading

Dement, W. C. (1992). *The sleepwatchers.* Stanford, CA: Stanford Alumni Association.

Fascinating, entertaining account of sleep research by one of its leading pioneers.

Moorcroft, W. H. (2013). *Understanding sleep and dreaming,* 2nd ed. New York: Springer.

Excellent review of the psychology and neurology of sleep and dreams.

Refinetti, R. (2016). *Circadian physiology* (3rd ed.). Boca Raton, FL: CRC Press.

Marvelous summary of research on circadian rhythms and the relevance to human behavior.

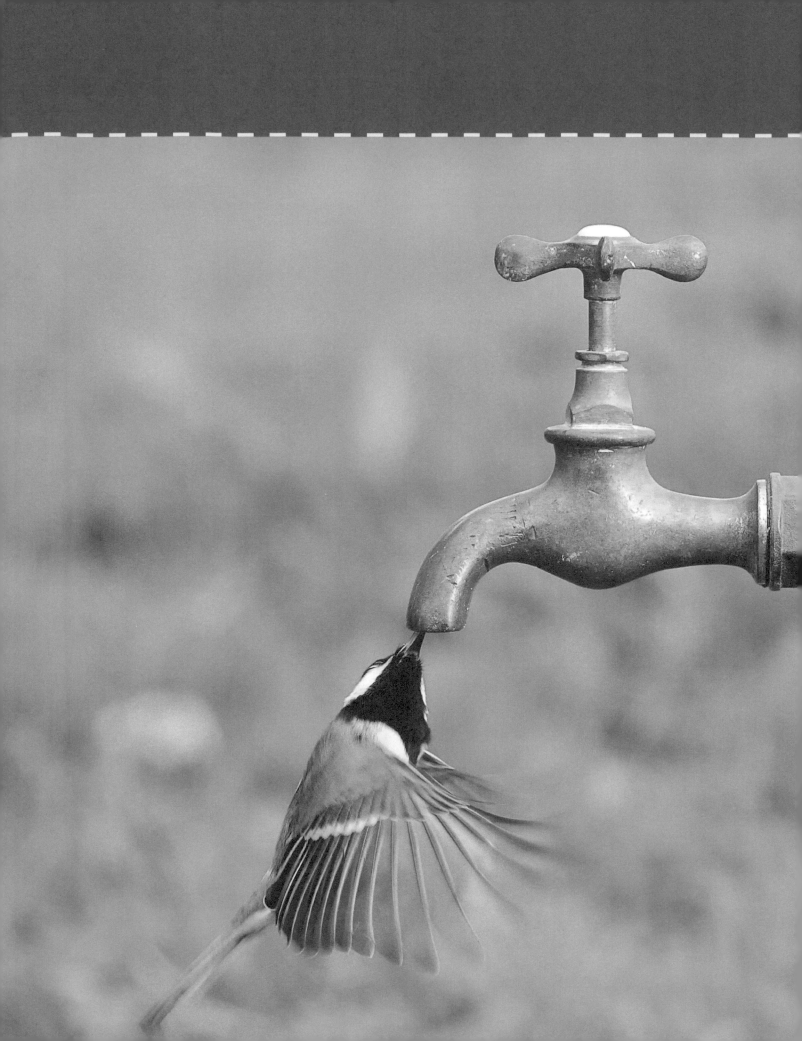

Internal Regulation

Chapter 9

What is life? You could define life in many ways depending on whether your purpose is medical, legal, philosophical, or poetic. Biologically, the necessary condition for life is *a coordinated set of chemical reactions*. Not all chemical reactions are alive, but all life has well-regulated chemical reactions.

Every chemical reaction in a living body takes place in a water solution at a rate that depends on the types of molecules, their concentration, and their temperature. Our behavior is organized to keep the right chemicals in the right proportions and at the right temperature.

Learning Objectives

After studying this chapter, you should be able to:

1. List examples of how temperature regulation contributes to behaviors.
2. Explain why a constant high body temperature is worth all the energy it costs.
3. Describe why a moderate fever is advantageous in fighting an infection.
4. Distinguish between osmotic and hypovolemic thirst, including the brain mechanisms for each.
5. Describe the physiological factors that influence hunger and satiety.

Opposite:
All life on Earth requires water, and animals drink it wherever they can find it.
(© iStock.com/StockPhotoAstur)

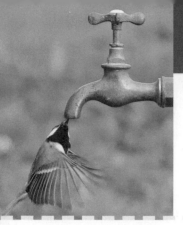

Module 9.1

Temperature Regulation

ere's an observation that puzzled biologists for years: When a small male garter snake emerges from hibernation in early spring, it emits female pheromones for the first day or two. The pheromones attract larger males that swarm all over him, trying to copulate. Presumably, the tendency to release female pheromones must have evolved to provide the small male some advantage. But what? Biologists speculated about ways in which this pseudo-mating experience might help the small male attract real females. The truth is simpler: A male that has just emerged from hibernation is so cold that it has trouble slithering out of its burrow. The larger males emerged from hibernation earlier and already had a chance to warm themselves in a sunny place. When the larger males swarm all over the smaller male, they warm him and increase his activity level (Shine, Phillips, Waye, LeMaster, & Mason, 2001).

Here are more examples that temperature regulation helps to explain:

- Have you ever noticed gulls, ducks, or other large birds standing on one leg (see Figure 9.1)? Why do they do that, when balancing on two legs would seem easier? One reason is to conserve body heat on cold days. By standing on one leg, they protect the heat in the other leg (Ehrlich, Dobkin, & Wheye, 1988).
- Vultures sometimes defecate onto their own legs. Are they just careless slobs? No. They defecate onto their legs on hot days so that the evaporating excretions will cool their legs (Ehrlich, Dobkin, & Wheye, 1988).
- For many years, biologists puzzled about the function of toucans' huge, clumsy bills (see Figure 9.2). The answer is temperature regulation (Tattersall, Andrade, & Abe, 2009). While flying on hot days, a toucan directs more blood flow to the beak, where the passing air cools it. At night the toucan tucks its bill under a wing to prevent undue loss of heat.
- Most lizards live solitary lives, but Australian thick-tailed geckos sometimes form tight huddles. Why? They live in an environment with rapid temperature fluctuations. They huddle only when the environmental temperature is falling rapidly. By huddling, they increase insulation and prevent a rapid drop in body temperature (Shah, Shine, Hudson, & Kearney, 2003).

- The Japanese giant hornet sometimes invades bee colonies, kills one or more bees, and takes them to feed to its larvae. When one of these hornets invades a hive of Japanese honeybees, the bees form a tight swarm of more than 500, surrounding the hornet in a tiny ball. Why? The combined body heat of all those bees raises the temperature to a level that is lethal to the hornet, but not to the bees (Ono, Igarashi, Ohno, & Sasaki, 1995).
- Migratory birds do most of their migratory flying at night. Why? The nights are cooler. A bird flying in midday would overheat and frequently have to stop for a drink, often in places where fresh water is difficult to find.

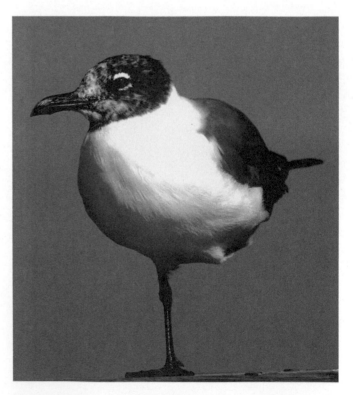

Figure 9.1 Why do birds sometimes stand on one foot?
One reason is that holding one leg next to the body keeps it warm.
(F1online digitale Bildagentur GmbH/Alamy Stock Photo)

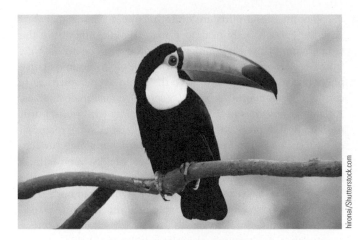

Figure 9.2 Why do toucans have such huge bills?
They use their bills to radiate heat when they need to cool the body. They cover the bill at night to decrease heat loss.

- Decades ago, psychologists reported that infant rats appeared deficient in certain aspects of learning, eating, and drinking. Later results showed that the real problem was temperature control. Researchers generally test animals at room temperature, about 20° to 23°C (68 to 73°F), which is comfortable for adult humans but dangerously cold for an isolated baby rat (see Figure 9.3). Infant rats that seem incapable of some task in a cold room do much better in a warmer room (Satinoff, 1991).
- Certain studies found that female rats learned best during their fertile period (estrus), but in other studies, they learned best a day or two before their fertile period (proestrus). The difference depended on the temperature of the room. Rats in estrus do better in a cooler environment, presumably because they are generating so much heat on their own. Rats in proestrus do better in a warmer environment (Rubinow, Arseneau, Beverly, & Juraska, 2004).

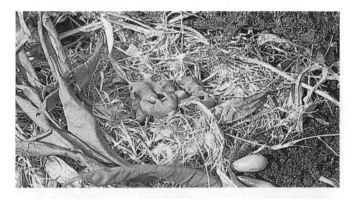

Figure 9.3 Difficulties of temperature regulation for a newborn rodent
A newborn rat has no hair, thin skin, and little body fat. If left exposed to the cold, it becomes inactive.
(A. Blank/NAS/Science Source)

The point is that temperature affects behavior in many ways that we easily overlook. The modules on thirst and hunger, later in this chapter, present further examples of how temperature control affects behavior.

Homeostasis and Allostasis

Physiologist Walter B. Cannon (1929) introduced the term **homeostasis** (HO-mee-oh-STAY-sis) to refer to temperature regulation and other biological processes that keep body variables within a fixed range. The process resembles the thermostat in a house with heating and cooling systems. Someone sets the minimum and maximum temperatures on the thermostat. When the temperature in the house drops below the minimum, the thermostat triggers the furnace to provide heat. When the temperature rises above the maximum, the thermostat turns on the air conditioner. For another example, stand and balance on one foot. Whenever your weight happens to shift left, right, forward, or backward, you quickly correct your position to maintain balance.

Homeostatic processes in animals trigger physiological and behavioral activities that keep certain variables within a set range. In many cases, the range is so narrow that we refer to it as a **set point**, a single value that the body works to maintain. For example, if calcium is deficient in your diet and its concentration in the blood begins to fall below the set point of 0.16 g/L (grams per liter), storage deposits in your bones release additional calcium into the blood. If the calcium level in the blood rises above 0.16 g/L, you store part of the excess in your bones and excrete the rest. Similar mechanisms maintain constant blood levels of water, oxygen, glucose, sodium chloride, protein, fat, and acidity (Cannon, 1929). Processes that reduce discrepancies from the set point are known as **negative feedback**. Much of motivated behavior can be described as negative feedback: Something causes a disturbance, and behavior proceeds until it relieves the disturbance.

However, the concept of homeostasis is not fully satisfactory, because the body does not maintain complete constancy. For example, your body temperature is about half a Celsius degree higher in mid-afternoon than in the middle of the night. Most animals maintain a nearly constant body weight from day to day, but add body fat in fall and decrease it in spring. (The increased fat is a good reserve in preparation for probable food shortage during the winter. It also provides insulation against the cold.) We can describe these alterations as changes in the set point, but even changes in the set point don't fully account for many observations. Much of our behavior anticipates a need before it occurs. For example, a sign of danger provokes a sudden increase in heart rate, blood pressure, and sweating, preparing the body for vigorous activity. Similarly, as the air is starting to warm up, a hiker increases thirst and decreases urine production by the kidneys, anticipating probable sweating and dehydration. (Other animals do the same.) To describe these dynamic changes, researchers use the term **allostasis** (from the Greek roots meaning "variable" and "standing"), which means the adaptive way in which the body anticipates needs depending on the situation, avoiding errors rather than just correcting them (McEwen, 2000; Sterling, 2012). We shall encounter additional examples of allostasis later in this chapter. Homeostasis and allostasis don't work perfectly, of course. If they did, we would not have problems such as obesity, high blood pressure, or diabetes.

✓ STOP & CHECK

1. How does the idea of allostasis differ from homeostasis?

ANSWER 1. Homeostasis keeps certain body variables within a fixed range by reacting to changes. Allostasis acts in advance to prevent or minimize changes.

Controlling Body Temperature

If you were to list your strongest motivations in life, you might not think to include temperature regulation, but it has a high priority biologically. An average young adult expends about 2600 kilocalories (kcal) per day. Where do you suppose all that energy goes? It is not to muscle movements or mental activity. Most of it goes to **basal metabolism,** the energy used to maintain a constant body temperature while at rest. Maintaining your body temperature uses about twice as much energy as all other activities *combined* (Burton, 1994). We produce that much heat largely by metabolism in brown adipose cells, cells that are more like muscle cells than like white fat cells. They burn fuel as muscle cells do, but release it directly as heat instead of as muscle contractions.

Amphibians, reptiles, and most fish are **ectothermic,** meaning that they depend on external sources for body heat instead of generating it themselves. A synonym is *poikilothermic,* from Greek roots meaning "varied heat." An ectothermic animal's body temperature is nearly the same as the temperature of its environment. People often call such animals "cold-blooded," but they are cold only when the environment is cold. Poikilothermic animals lack physiological mechanisms of temperature regulation such as shivering and sweating, but they can regulate their body temperature behaviorally. A desert lizard moves between sunny areas, shady areas, and burrows to maintain a fairly steady body temperature. However, behavioral methods do not enable animals to maintain the same degree of constancy that mammals and birds have.

Although nearly all fish, amphibians, and reptiles are ectothermic, a few exceptions to that rule do occur. A few large fish, including sharks and tuna, maintain their core body temperature well above that of the surrounding water most of the time (Bernal, Donley, Shadwick, & Syme, 2005). The tegu lizards of South America, about the size of a large rabbit, increase their metabolism during the mating season, raising their body temperature to sometimes 10°C above that of the environment (Tattersall et al., 2016).

Mammals and birds are **endothermic,** meaning that they generate enough body heat to remain significantly above the temperature of the environment. A synonym is *homeothermic,* from Greek roots meaning "same heat." Endothermic animals use physiological mechanisms to keep their core temperature nearly constant. Endothermy is costly, especially for small animals. An animal *generates* heat in proportion to its total mass, but it *radiates* heat in proportion to its surface area. A small mammal or bird, such as a mouse or a hummingbird, has a high surface-to-volume ratio and therefore radiates heat rapidly. Such animals need much fuel each day to maintain their body temperature.

To cool ourselves when the air is warmer than body temperature, we have only one physiological mechanism, evaporation. Humans sweat to expose water for evaporation. For species that don't sweat, the alternatives are licking themselves and panting. As water evaporates, it cools the body. However, if the air is humid as well as hot, the moisture does not evaporate. Furthermore, you endanger your health if you cannot drink enough to replace the water you lose by sweating. If you sweat without drinking, you become dehydrated (low on water). You then protect your body water by sweating less, despite the risk of overheating (Tokizawa et al., 2010).

Several physiological mechanisms increase your body heat in a cold environment. One is shivering. Any muscle contractions, such as those of shivering, generate heat. Second, decreased blood flow to the skin prevents the blood from cooling too much. The consequence is warm internal organs but cold skin. A third mechanism works well for most mammals, though not humans: When cold, they fluff out their fur to increase insulation. (We humans also fluff out our "fur" by erecting the tiny hairs on our skin—"goose bumps." That mechanism was more useful back when our remote ancestors had a fuller coat of fur.)

We also use behavioral mechanisms, just as ectothermic animals do. In fact, we prefer to rely on behavior when we can. The more we regulate our temperature behaviorally, the less energy we need to spend physiologically (Refinetti & Carlisle, 1986). Finding a cool place on a hot day is much better than sweating (see Figure 9.4). Finding a warm place on a cold day is

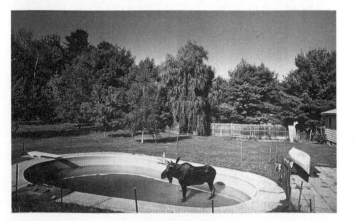

Figure 9.4 One way to cope with the heat
On a hot day, wouldn't you do the same?
(Sun-Journal/Ken Love/AP Images)

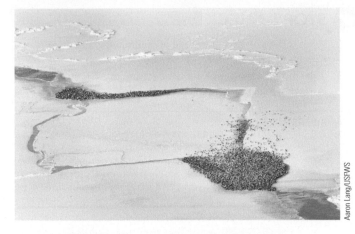

Aaron Lang/USFWS

Figure 9.5 Behavioral regulation of body temperature
Spectacled eiders pool their body heat to melt holes in the ice of the Arctic Ocean, thereby surviving the winter without migrating.

much smarter than shivering. Here are a few other behavioral mechanisms of temperature regulation:

- Put on more clothing or take it off. This human strategy accomplishes what other mammals accomplish by fluffing out or sleeking their fur.
- Become more active to get warmer or less active to avoid overheating.
- To get warm, huddle with others. If you are waiting at a bus stop on a cold day, you might feel shy about suggesting to a stranger that you hug each other to keep warm. Other species have no such inhibitions (see Figure 9.5). Emperor penguin chicks huddle together to pool their heat, increasing their insulation enough to survive an Antarctic winter. Spectacled eiders (in the duck family) spend their winters in the Arctic Ocean, which is mostly covered with ice. When more than 150,000 eiders crowd together, they not only keep warm but also melt a big hole in the ice where they can dive for fish (Weidensaul, 1999).

Surviving in Extreme Cold

If the atmospheric temperature drops below 0°C (32°F), you maintain your body temperature by shivering, shifting blood flow away from the skin, and so forth. However, an ectothermic animal, which by definition takes the temperature of its environment, is vulnerable. If its body temperature drops below the freezing point of water, ice crystals form. Because water expands when it freezes, ice crystals would tear apart blood vessels and cell membranes, killing the animal.

Many amphibians and reptiles avoid that risk by burrowing or finding other sheltered locations. However, some frogs, fish, and insects survive through winters in northern Canada where even the underground temperature approaches −40° C (which is also −40° F). How do they do it? Some insects and fish stock their blood with glycerol and other antifreeze

chemicals at the start of the winter (Liou, Tocilj, Davies, & Jia, 2000). Wood frogs actually do freeze, but they have several mechanisms to reduce the damage. They start by withdrawing most fluid from their organs and blood vessels and storing it in extracellular spaces. Therefore, ice crystals have room to expand when they form, without tearing blood vessels or cells. Also, the frogs have chemicals that cause ice crystals to form gradually, not in chunks. Finally, they have extraordinary blood-clotting capacity that quickly repairs any blood vessels that do rupture (Storey & Storey, 1999).

The Advantages of Constant High Body Temperature

As mentioned, we spend about two-thirds of our total energy maintaining body temperature (basal metabolism). An ectothermic animal, with a much lower level of basal metabolism, needs far less fuel. If we didn't maintain a constant, high body temperature, we could eat less and spend less effort finding food. Given the substantial costs of maintaining our body temperature, it must provide an important advantage, or we would not have evolved these mechanisms. What is that advantage?

For the answer, think back to the chapter on movement: As the water gets colder, a fish recruits more and more fast-twitch muscle fibers to remain active, despite the risk of rapid fatigue. The same is true for amphibians and reptiles. On a very cold day, a lizard has to change its defense strategy: If it ran away from a predator, it would either run more slowly than usual or recruit all of its fast-twitch muscles and fatigue rapidly. So, instead of running, it tries to fight the predator—an act requiring a briefer burst of activity, though it is often a losing battle (James, 2013).

Birds and mammals keep their bodies warm at all times and therefore stay constantly ready for vigorous activity, regardless of the temperature of the air. In other words, we eat a great deal to support our high metabolism so that even if the weather is cold, we can still run rapidly without great fatigue. Let's qualify this point, however: On a cold day, you divert blood away from the periphery to protect the internal organs and to avoid losing too much heat to the surrounding air. The result is that your muscles are not quite as warm as usual. A competitive athlete needs to warm up, literally, to increase the muscles' temperature on a cold day.

Why did mammals evolve a body temperature of 37°C (98°F) instead of some other value? From the standpoint of muscle activity, we gain an advantage by being as warm as possible. A warmer animal has warmer muscles and therefore runs faster with less fatigue than a cooler animal. When a reptile has a choice of environments at different temperatures, it usually chooses to warm itself to 37° to 38°C (98° to 100°F) (Wagner & Gleeson, 1997).

If warmer is better, why not heat ourselves to an even higher temperature? First, maintaining a higher temperature requires more fuel and energy. Second, and more importantly, beyond about 41°C (105°F), proteins begin to break their bonds and lose their useful properties. Birds' body temperatures are in fact about 41°C.

It is possible to evolve proteins that are stable at higher temperatures; indeed, odd microscopic animals called thermophiles survive in boiling water. However, to do so, they need many extra chemical bonds to stabilize their proteins. The enzymatic properties of a protein depend on its flexibility, so making proteins rigid enough to withstand high temperatures makes them inactive at more moderate temperatures (Feller, 2010). In short, our body temperature of 37°C is a trade-off between the advantages of high temperature for rapid movement and the disadvantages of high temperature for protein stability and energy expenditure.

Reproductive cells require a cooler environment than the rest of the body (Rommel, Pabst, & McLellan, 1998). Birds lay eggs and sit on them, instead of developing them internally, because the birds' internal temperature is too hot for an embryo. Similarly, in most male mammals, the scrotum hangs outside the body, because sperm production requires a cooler temperature than the rest of the body. (It's not just for decoration.) A man who wears his undershorts too tight keeps his testes too close to the body, overheats them, and produces fewer healthy sperm cells. Pregnant women are advised to avoid hot baths and anything else that might overheat a developing fetus.

✅ STOP & CHECK

2. What is the primary advantage of maintaining a constant high body temperature?
3. Why did mammals evolve a temperature of 37°C (98°F) instead of some other temperature?

ANSWERS

2. A constant high body temperature keeps an animal ready for rapid, prolonged muscle activity even in cold weather. 3. Animals gain an advantage in being as warm as possible and therefore as fast as possible. However, proteins lose stability at temperatures much above 37°C (98°F).

Brain Mechanisms

The physiological changes that regulate body temperature—such as shivering, sweating, and changes in blood flow to the skin—depend on areas in and near the hypothalamus (see Figure 9.6), especially the anterior hypothalamus and the preoptic area, located just anterior to the anterior hypothalamus. (It is called *preoptic* because it is near the optic chiasm, where the optic nerves cross.) Because of the close relationship between the preoptic area and the anterior

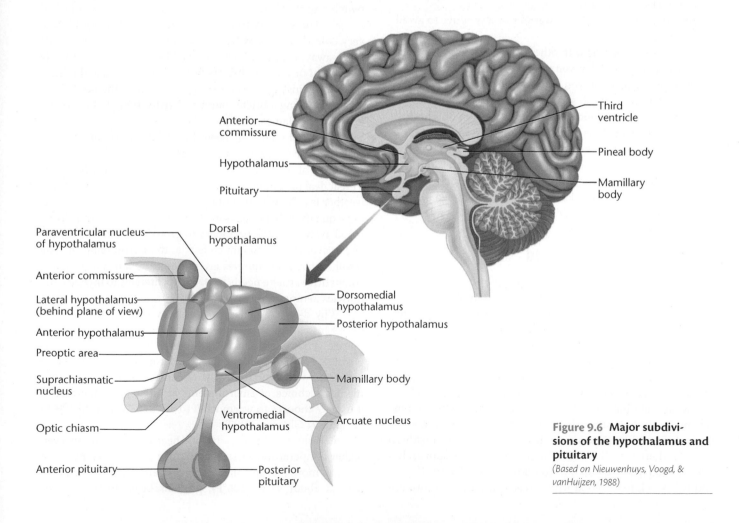

Figure 9.6 Major subdivisions of the hypothalamus and pituitary
(Based on Nieuwenhuys, Voogd, & vanHuijzen, 1988)

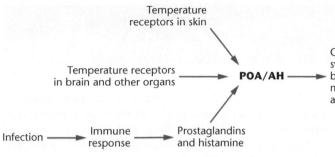

Figure 9.7 Integration of temperature information by the POA/AH
If the brain and skin are overheated, the POA/AH sends signals that lead to sweating and other methods of heat loss. If the brain and skin are cooled, or if prostaglandins and histamine indicate an infection, the POA/AH initiates shivering, increased heart rate, decreased blood flow to the skin, and increased metabolism by brown adipose tissue.

hypothalamus, researchers often treat them as a single area, the **preoptic area/anterior hypothalamus**, or **POA/AH**. The POA/AH and a couple other hypothalamic areas send output to the hindbrain's raphe nucleus, which controls the autonomic responses such as shivering, sweating, changes in heart rate and metabolism, and changes in blood flow to the skin (Morrison, 2016; Yoshida, Li, Cano, Lazarus, & Saper, 2009).

The POA/AH integrates several types of information (Nakamura, 2011). It receives input from temperature receptors in the skin, in the organs, and in the hypothalamus (Song et al., 2016). If either the skin or the hypothalamus is hot, an animal sweats or pants vigorously and seeks a cooler location. If either is cold, the animal shivers and seeks a warmer location. The animal reacts most vigorously if the skin and hypothalamus are both hot or both cold. The POA/AH also receives input from the immune system, which reacts to an infection by sending prostaglandins and histamines to the POA/AH (Ek et al., 2001; Leon, 2002; Tabarean, Sanchez-Alavez, & Sethi, 2012). Those chemicals are the cause of shivering, increased metabolism, and other processes that produce a fever. People lacking the appropriate receptors for those chemicals fail to develop a fever, even when they have pneumonia or similar diseases (Hanada et al., 2009). Figure 9.7 summarizes the role of the POA/AH.

The POA/AH is not the only brain area that detects temperature, but it is the primary area for controlling physiological mechanisms of temperature regulation such as sweating or shivering. After damage to the POA/AH, mammals can still regulate body temperature, but less efficiently. They also use the behavioral mechanisms that a lizard might use, such as seeking a warmer or colder location (Satinoff & Rutstein, 1970; Van Zoeren & Stricker, 1977).

Fever

A fever represents an increased set point for body temperature. Just as you shiver or sweat when your body temperature goes below or above its usual 37°C, when you have a fever of, say, 39°C (102°F), you shiver or sweat whenever your temperature deviates from that level. In other words, fever is not something an infection does to the body; it is something the hypothalamus directs the body to produce. Moving to a cooler room does not lower your fever. Your body just works harder to keep its temperature at the feverish level.

Because newborn rabbits have an immature hypothalamus, they do not shiver in response to infections. If they are given a choice of environments, however, they select a spot warm enough to raise their body temperature and produce a fever by behavioral means (Satinoff, McEwen, & Williams, 1976). Fish and reptiles with an infection also choose a warm enough environment, if they can find one, to produce a feverish body temperature (Kluger, 1991). Again, the point is that fever is something the animal does to fight an infection.

Does fever do any good? Certain types of bacteria grow less vigorously at high temperatures than at normal mammalian body temperatures. Also, the immune system works more vigorously at an increased temperature (Skitzki, Chen, Wang, & Evans, 2007). Other things being equal, developing a moderate fever increases an individual's chance of surviving a bacterial infection (Kluger, 1991). However, a fever above about 39°C (103°F) in humans does more harm than good, and a fever above 41°C (109°F) is life-threatening (Rommel, Pabst, & McLellan, 1998).

STOP & CHECK

4. What are the sources of input to the POA/AH?
5. If you had damage to your POA/AH, what would happen to your body temperature?

ANSWERS

4. The POA/AH receives input from temperatures in the skin, the organs, and the hypothalamus. It also receives prostaglandins and histamines when the immune system detects an infection. 5. You would be much less able to shiver, sweat, or control other physiological mechanisms that control body temperature. However, you could still try to find a place in the environment that keeps you close to your normal temperature.

STOP & CHECK

6. What evidence indicates that fever is an adaptation to fight illness?

ANSWER

6. The body will shiver or sweat to maintain its elevated temperature at a nearly constant level. Also, fish, reptiles, and immature mammals with infections use behavioral means to raise their temperature to a feverish level. Furthermore, a moderate fever inhibits bacterial growth and increases the probability of surviving a bacterial infection.

Module 9.1 | In Closing
Combining Physiological and Behavioral Mechanisms

Physiological mechanisms and behavioral mechanisms work together. Your body has physiological mechanisms to maintain constant body temperature, including shivering, sweating, and changes in blood flow. You also rely on behavioral mechanisms, such as finding a cooler or warmer place, adding or removing clothing, and so forth. Redundancy reduces your risk: If one mechanism fails, another mechanism comes to your rescue. It is not, however, a true redundancy in the sense of two mechanisms doing exactly the same thing. Each of your mechanisms of temperature regulation solves an aspect of the problem in a different way. We shall see this theme again in the discussions of thirst and hunger.

Summary

1. It is easy to overlook the importance of temperature regulation. Many seemingly odd animal behaviors make sense as ways to heat or cool the body. **290**
2. Homeostasis is a tendency to maintain a body variable near a set point. Temperature, hunger, and thirst are almost homeostatic, but the set point changes in varying circumstances. **291**
3. A high body temperature enables a mammal or bird to move rapidly without excessive fatigue even in a cold environment. **293**
4. From the standpoint of muscle activity, the higher the body temperature, the better. However, as temperatures increase, protein stability decreases, and more energy is needed to maintain body temperature. Mammalian body temperature of 37°C is a compromise between these competing considerations. **293**
5. The preoptic area and anterior hypothalamus (POA/AH) are critical for temperature control. Cells there monitor both their own temperature and that of the skin and organs. When they receive input indicating an infection, they initiate responses that produce a fever. **294**
6. All animals rely partly on behavioral mechanisms for temperature regulation. **295**
7. A moderate fever helps an animal combat an infection. **295**

Key Terms

Terms are defined in the module on the page number indicated. They are also presented in alphabetical order with definitions in the book's Subject Index/Glossary, which begins on page 589. Interactive flash cards, audio reviews, and crossword puzzles are among the online resources available to help you learn these terms and the concepts they represent.

allostasis **291**
basal metabolism **292**
ectothermic **292**

endothermic **292**
homeostasis **291**
negative feedback **291**

preoptic area/anterior hypothalamus (POA/AH) **295**
set point **291**

Thought Question

Speculate on why birds have higher body temperatures than mammals.

Module 9.1 | End of Module Quiz

1. What is meant by allostasis?
   A. Processes that react to any change to bring the body back to equilibrium
   B. Processes that anticipate future needs
   C. Random changes in the internal processes of the body
   D. The ideal levels of all body variables

2. Well over half of the human body's energy is devoted to which of the following?
   A. Basal metabolism
   B. Muscle contractions
   C. Brain activity
   D. Keeping the heart going

3. How do ectothermic animals regulate their body temperature, if at all?

   A. They move to a location with a more favorable temperature.

   B. They use physiological mechanisms such as shivering and sweating.

   C. They increase their metabolic rate.

   D. They do not regulate their body temperature at all.

4. Which of the following is an ectothermic animal?

   A. Penguin

   B. Human

   C. Mouse

   D. Snake

5. What is the primary advantage of maintaining a constant high body temperature?

   A. It saves us the energy from having to look for a comfortable temperature.

   B. It keeps the muscles ready for rapid, prolonged activity even in cold weather.

   C. It enables the digestive system to process a greater variety of nutrients.

   D. It enables us to survive in warmer climates.

6. If we inserted a probe into your POA/AH and heated it, what would happen?

   A. You would sweat.

   B. You would shiver.

   C. You would seek a warmer environment.

   D. Your skin receptors sensitive to temperature would become more sensitive.

7. When you have an infection, what causes the fever?

   A. The infective agent stimulates the heart to beat faster.

   B. The infective agent impairs the activity of the hypothalamus.

   C. The immune system delivers prostaglandins and histamine to the hypothalamus.

   D. The immune system decreases blood flow to the brain.

8. Which of the following is the most correct description of a fever?

   A. Fever is one way in which the body fights against bacteria.

   B. Fever is one way in which bacteria cause damage to the body.

   C. Fever indicates that the POA/AH is not functioning properly.

   D. Fever is a result of synchrony between the heart and the lungs.

Answers: 1B, 2A, 3A, 4D, 5B, 6A, 7C, 8A.

Module 9.2

Thirst

Water constitutes about 70 percent of the mammalian body. Because the concentration of chemicals in water determines the rate of all chemical reactions in the body, you need to maintain the water in your body within narrow limits. The body also needs enough fluid in the circulatory system to maintain normal blood pressure. You could survive for days, maybe weeks, without food, but not long without water.

Mechanisms of Water Regulation

Species differ in their strategies for maintaining water. Beavers and other animals that live in rivers or lakes drink plenty of water, eat moist foods, and excrete dilute urine. In contrast, most gerbils and other desert animals go through life without drinking at all. They gain water from their food and they have many adaptations to avoid losing water, including the ability to excrete dry feces and concentrated urine. Unable to sweat, they avoid the heat of the day by burrowing under the ground. Their highly convoluted nasal passages minimize water loss when they exhale.

We humans vary our strategy depending on circumstances. If you cannot find enough to drink or if the water tastes bad, you conserve water by excreting more concentrated urine and decreasing your sweat, somewhat like a gerbil, although not to the same extreme. Your posterior pituitary (see Figure 9.6) releases the hormone **vasopressin** that raises blood pressure by constricting blood vessels. (The term *vasopressin* comes from *vas*cular *press*ure.) The increased pressure helps compensate for the decreased blood volume. Vasopressin is also known as **antidiuretic hormone (ADH)** because it enables the kidneys to reabsorb water from urine and therefore make the urine more concentrated. (*Diuresis* means "urination.") You also increase your secretion of vasopressin while sleeping so that you can preserve your body water while you cannot drink (Trudel & Bourque, 2010). Vasopressin helps you get through the night without going to the toilet.

In most cases, our strategy is closer to that of beavers: We drink more than we need and excrete the excess. (However, if you drink extensively without eating, as many alcoholics do, you may excrete enough body salts to harm yourself.) Most of our drinking is with meals or in social situations, and most people seldom experience intense thirst.

Osmotic Thirst

We distinguish two types of thirst. Eating salty foods causes *osmotic* thirst, and losing fluid by bleeding or sweating induces *hypovolemic* thirst.

The combined concentration of all *solutes* (molecules in solution) in mammalian body fluids remains at a nearly constant level of 0.15 M (molar). (Molarity is a measure of the number of particles per unit of solution, regardless of the size of each particle. A 1.0 M solution of sugar and a 1.0 M solution of sodium chloride have the same number of molecules per liter.) This fixed concentration of solutes is a set point, similar to the set point for temperature. Any deviation activates mechanisms that restore the concentration of solutes to the set point.

Osmotic pressure is the tendency of water to flow across a semipermeable membrane from the area of low solute concentration to the area of higher concentration. A semipermeable membrane is one through which water can pass but solutes cannot. The membrane surrounding a cell is almost a semipermeable membrane because water flows across it freely and various solutes flow either slowly or not at all between the *intracellular fluid* inside the cell and the *extracellular fluid* outside it. Osmotic pressure occurs when solutes are more concentrated on one side of the membrane than on the other.

If you eat something salty, sodium ions spread through the blood and the extracellular fluid but do not cross the membranes into cells. The result is a higher concentration of solutes (including sodium) outside the cells than inside. The resulting osmotic pressure draws water from the cells into the extracellular fluid. Certain neurons detect their own loss of water and then trigger **osmotic thirst**, a drive for water that

(a) Greater concentration of solutes (green dots) outside the cell than inside.

(b) Water flows out of the cell, equalizing the solute concentration and shrinking the cell.

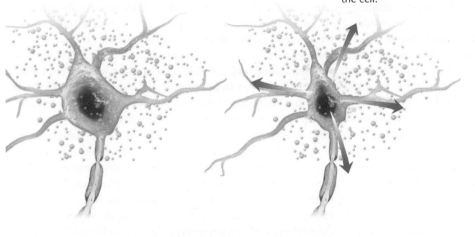

Figure 9.8 The consequence of a difference in osmotic pressure
(a) Suppose a solute such as NaCl is more concentrated outside the cell than inside. (b) Water flows by osmosis out of the cell until the concentrations are equal. Neurons in certain brain areas detect their own dehydration and trigger thirst.

helps restore the normal state (see Figure 9.8). The kidneys also excrete more concentrated urine to rid the body of excess sodium and maintain as much water as possible.

How does the brain detect osmotic pressure? It has receptors around the third ventricle, including the **OVLT** (organum vasculosum laminae terminalis) and the **subfornical organ (SFO)** (Hiyama, Watanabe, Okado, & Noda, 2004) (see Figure 9.9). Those receptors detect osmotic pressure and the sodium content of the blood (Tiruneh, Huang, & Leenen, 2013). The OVLT also receives input from receptors

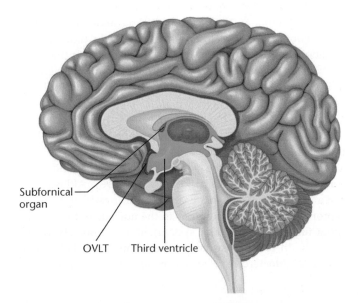

Figure 9.9 The brain's receptors for osmotic pressure and blood volume
These neurons are in areas surrounding the third ventricle of the brain, where no blood–brain barrier prevents blood-borne chemicals from entering the brain.
(Based in part on DeArmond, Fusco, & Dewey, 1974; Weindl, 1973)

in the digestive tract, enabling it to anticipate an osmotic need before the rest of the body experiences it (Bourque, 2008).

The brain areas surrounding the third ventricle are in a good position to monitor the contents of the blood, because the blood–brain barrier is weak in this area, enabling chemicals to enter that would not reach neurons elsewhere in the brain. The danger, of course, is that a weak blood–brain barrier exposes neurons to potential harm. At least in mice, new neurons form in this area, replacing ones that may have died (Hourai & Miyata, 2013). Other species have not yet been tested.

The subfornical organ has one population of neurons that increases thirst and another population that suppresses it (Abbott, Machado, Geerling, & Saper, 2016; Oka, Ye, & Zuker, 2015). Those axons combine with input from the OVLT, the stomach, and elsewhere to provide input to the hypothalamus. The **lateral preoptic area** and surrounding parts of the hypothalamus control drinking (Saad, Luiz, Camargo, Renzi, & Manani, 1996). The **supraoptic nucleus** and the **paraventricular nucleus (PVN)** control the rate at which the posterior pituitary releases vasopressin.

All of this is true, so far as it goes: When your cells start to become dehydrated, they stimulate osmotic thirst. However, remember the concept of allostasis: Your body does not just react to needs, but also it anticipates needs. For example, when you eat a meal, especially a salty meal, your cells are going to need water, but you drink at once instead of waiting until your osmotic pressure changes. Also, as a study with mice showed, shortly before time to go to sleep, the body's circadian rhythm triggers increased secretion of vasopressin, which inhibits the need to urinate and therefore helps retain water when drinking cannot occur. At the same time, vasopressin stimulates thirst (Gizowki, Zaelzer, & Bourque, 2016). That is why you often feel an urge to drink something shortly before going to sleep, even if your cells' osmotic pressure is quite normal at the time.

When you are thirsty, how do you know when to stop drinking? You do *not* continue drinking while the digestive system absorbs the water and then the circulatory system pumps it to the hypothalamus. That process takes 15 minutes or more, and if you continued drinking for that long, you would drink far more than you need. Again, allostasis to the rescue: Not only do you start when you anticipate a future need, but also you stop drinking when you anticipate that you have fulfilled a need. Researchers recording activity from mouse brains found that one minute of drinking suppressed the activity of thirst-sensitive neurons in the subfornical organ, long before water reached the blood, much less the brain (Zimmerman et al., 2016). Cooling the tongue also suppressed activity in the subfornical organ. Thus we may conclude that drinking can serve two purposes, the need for water and the need for temperature regulation.

✓ STOP & CHECK

8. Would adding salt to the body's extracellular fluids increase or decrease osmotic thirst?
9. Why are you likely to feel thirst just before bedtime? Would you feel just as thirsty if you went to sleep at an unusual time?

ANSWERS 8. Adding salt to the extracellular fluids would increase osmotic thirst because it would draw water from the cells into the extracellular spaces. 9. At bedtime, your body secretes vasopressin, which helps conserve water and also stimulates thirst. Both responses help you get through the night while you cannot drink. Your circadian rhythm triggers the increased vasopressin, so you would not feel as thirsty before going to sleep at an unusual time.

Hypovolemic Thirst and Sodium-Specific Hunger

Suppose you lose a significant amount of body fluid by bleeding, diarrhea, or sweating. Although your body's osmotic pressure stays the same, you need fluid. Your heart has trouble pumping blood to the head, and nutrients do not flow as easily as usual into your cells. Receptors in your kidneys and on your blood vessels react to the decreased blood pressure by sending messages to the brain to release vasopressin, which constricts blood vessels and conserves the fluid you still have. Also, the kidneys release the enzyme *renin*, which splits a portion off

angiotensinogen, a large protein in the blood, to form angiotensin I, which other enzymes convert to **angiotensin II**. Like vasopressin, angiotensin II constricts the blood vessels, compensating for the drop in blood pressure (see Figure 9.10).

Angiotensin II also helps trigger thirst, in conjunction with receptors that detect blood pressure in the large veins. However, this thirst is different from osmotic thirst, because you need to restore lost salts and not just water. This kind of thirst is known as **hypovolemic** (HI-po-vo-LEE-mik) **thirst**, meaning thirst based on low volume. When angiotensin II reaches the brain, it stimulates neurons in areas adjoining the third ventricle (Fitts, Starbuck, & Ruhf, 2000; Mangiapane & Simpson, 1980; Tanaka et al., 2001). Those neurons send axons to the hypothalamus, where they release angiotensin II as their neurotransmitter (Tanaka, Hori, & Nomura, 2001). That is, the neurons surrounding the third ventricle both respond to angiotensin II and release it. As in many other cases, the connection between a neurotransmitter and its function is not arbitrary. The brain uses a chemical that was already performing a related function elsewhere in the body.

Whereas an animal with osmotic thirst needs water, one with hypovolemic thirst cannot drink much pure water. Pure water would dilute its body fluids and lower the solute concentration in the blood. The animal therefore increases its preference for salty water (Stricker, 1969).

An animal that becomes deficient in sodium shows an immediate strong preference for salty tastes, known as **sodium-specific hunger** (Richter, 1936), even for extremely concentrated salt solutions that it would ordinarily reject (Robinson & Berridge, 2013). Neurons in several brain areas suddenly react much more strongly than usual to salty tastes (Tandon, Simon, & Nicolelis, 2012). You may have noticed this phenomenon yourself. A woman around the time of menstruation, or anyone who has sweated heavily, finds that salty snacks taste especially good. In contrast, specific hungers for other vitamins and minerals have to be learned by trial and error (Rozin & Kalat, 1971).

Sodium-specific hunger depends partly on hormones (Schulkin, 1991). When the body's sodium reserves are low, the adrenal glands produce **aldosterone** (al-DOSS-ter-one), a hormone that causes the kidneys, salivary glands, and sweat glands to retain salt (Verrey & Beron, 1996). Aldosterone and angiotensin II together change the properties of taste receptors on the tongue, neurons in the nucleus of the tractus solitarius (part of the taste system), and neurons elsewhere in the brain to increase salt intake (Krause & Sakal, 2007). Note that aldosterone indicates low sodium, and angiotensin

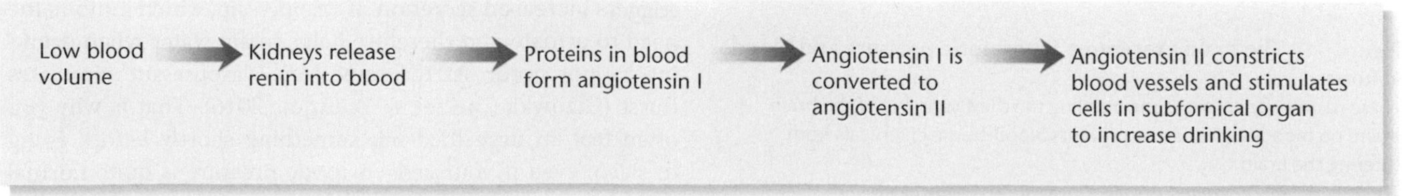

Low blood volume → Kidneys release renin into blood → Proteins in blood form angiotensin I → Angiotensin I is converted to angiotensin II → Angiotensin II constricts blood vessels and stimulates cells in subfornical organ to increase drinking

Figure 9.10 Hormonal response to hypovolemia

Table 9.1 | Osmotic and Hypovolemic Thirst

Type of Thirst	Caused by	Best Relieved by	Receptor Location
Osmotic	High solute concentration outside cells	Pure water	OVLT, subfornical organ, and digestive tract
Hypovolemic	Low blood volume	Water containing solutes, near 0.15M	Kidneys and blood vessels

II indicates low blood volume. Either one by itself produces only a small increase in salt intake, but their combined effect is substantial, sometimes producing a preference for

salt over sugar and everything else (Geerling & Loewy, 2008). Table 9.1 summarizes the differences between osmotic thirst and hypovolemic thirst.

✓ STOP & CHECK

10. Who would drink more pure water—someone with osmotic thirst or someone with hypovolemic thirst?
11. What are the contributions of angiotensin II and aldosterone?

Module 9.2 | In Closing
The Psychology and Biology of Thirst

You may have thought that temperature regulation happens automatically and that water regulation depends on your behavior. You can see now that the distinction is not entirely correct. You control your body temperature partly by automatic means, such as sweating or shivering, but also partly by behavioral means, such as choosing a warm or a cool place.

You control your body water partly by the behavior of drinking but also by hormones that alter kidney activity. If your kidneys cannot regulate your water and sodium adequately, your brain gets signals to change your drinking or sodium intake. In short, keeping your body's chemical reactions going depends on both skeletal and autonomic controls.

Summary

1. Mammalian species have evolved ways of maintaining body water, ranging from frequent drinking (beavers) to extreme conservation of fluids (gerbils). Humans alter their strategy depending on the availability of acceptable fluids. **298**
2. An increase in the osmotic pressure of the blood draws water out of cells, causing osmotic thirst. Neurons in the OVLT and subfornical organ detect changes in osmotic pressure and send information to hypothalamic areas responsible for vasopressin secretion and for drinking. **298**
3. The subfornical organ initiates thirst in anticipation of future need, such as during a meal and shortly before bedtime. It decreases thirst after drinking, long before the ingested water reaches the cells that need it. **299**
4. Loss of blood volume causes hypovolemic thirst. To satisfy hypovolemic thirst it is necessary to drink water containing solutes. **300**
5. Hypovolemic thirst is triggered by the hormone angiotensin II, which increases when blood pressure falls. **300**
6. Loss of sodium salts from the body triggers a craving for salty tastes. **300**

Key Terms

Terms are defined in the module on the page number indicated. They're also presented in alphabetical order with definitions in the book's Subject Index/Glossary, which begins on page 589. Interactive flash cards, audio reviews, and crossword puzzles are among the online resources available to help you learn these terms and the concepts they represent.

Thought Questions

1. An injection of concentrated sodium chloride triggers osmotic thirst, but an injection of equally concentrated glucose does not. Why not?

2. If all the water you drank leaked out through a tube connected to the stomach, how would your drinking change?

3. Many women crave salt during pregnancy. Why?

Module 9.2 | End of Module Quiz

1. Which of these happens after you eat something salty?

    A. The sodium-potassium pump becomes less active.

    B. The sodium-potassium pump becomes more active.

    C. Salt flows into the cells.

    D. Water flows out of the cells.

2. What would happen as a result of adding salt to the body's extracellular fluids?

    A. Increased osmotic thirst

    B. Decreased osmotic thirst

    C. Increased hypovolemic thirst

    D. Decreased hypovolemic thirst

3. What does vasopressin do?

    A. It increases both urination and thirst.

    B. It decreases both urination and thirst.

    C. It decreases urination and increases thirst.

    D. It increases urination and decreases thirst.

4. Why do you stop drinking before water reaches the cells that need it?

    A. Your throat is no longer dry.

    B. Your stomach is full.

    C. Drinking inhibits neurons responsible for thirst.

    D. Drinking stimulates vasopressin release.

5. What is the most effective way to satisfy hypovolemic thirst?

    A. Drink pure water slowly.

    B. Drink pure water rapidly.

    C. Drink water containing some salt or other solutes.

    D. Alternate between drinking water and drinking alcohol.

Answers: 1D, 2A, 3C, 4C, 5C.

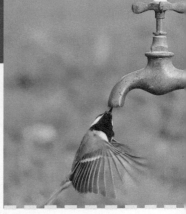

Module 9.3

Hunger

Species differ in their eating strategies. A snake or crocodile might devour a huge meal and then eat nothing more for months (see Figure 9.11). As a rule, predators have large digestive systems capable of handling infrequent but huge meals (Armstrong & Schindler, 2011). Bears eat as much as they can whenever they can. It is a sensible strategy because bears' main foods—fruits and nuts—are available in large quantities for only short times. Bears' occasional feasts tide them over through times of starvation. You might think of it as survival of the fattest. (Sorry about that one.)

A small bird, at the other extreme, eats only what it needs at the moment. The advantage of restraint is that low weight helps it fly away from predators, and even a few extra milligrams might make a difference (see Figure 9.12). However, in cold climates, a bird needs to store a substantial amount to get through the night. To survive through Alaska winters, every night, a chickadee finds a hollowed tree or other nesting site that provides as much insulation as possible. Then it lowers its body temperature into a state almost like hibernation. Still, it has to shiver throughout the night to prevent its body from freezing, and all that shivering requires energy. During Alaskan winters, a chickadee eats enough each day to increase

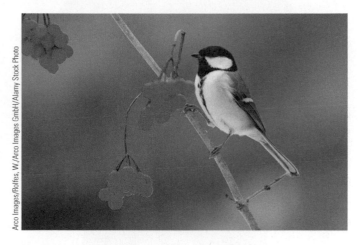

Figure 9.12 A great tit, a small European bird
Ordinarily, when food is abundant, tits eat just what they need each day and maintain minimal fat reserves. When food is harder to find, they eat more and live off fat reserves between meals. During an era when their predators were scarce, tits started putting on more fat regardless of the food supplies.

its body weight by 10 percent and then loses that amount at night (Harrison, 2008; Sharbaugh, 2001). For comparison, imagine a 50 kg (110 lb) person gaining 5 kg (11 lb) during the day and then shivering it off at night.

As a rule, people neither limit their diet as strictly as small birds do nor stuff themselves nonstop like bears. Human eating is noteworthy in that we have a relatively small digestive system for an animal of our size. A prominent speculation is that our ability to cook food (and therefore make it easier to digest) made it possible for us to evolve a smaller digestive system and nevertheless gain all the energy we need for a large brain.

Choosing which food to eat and how much to eat is an important decision. We use a wide array of learned and unlearned mechanisms to help in the process.

Digestion and Food Selection

Examine the digestive system, as diagrammed in Figure 9.13. Its function is to break food into smaller molecules that the cells can use. Digestion begins in the mouth, where enzymes in the saliva break down carbohydrates. Swallowed food travels

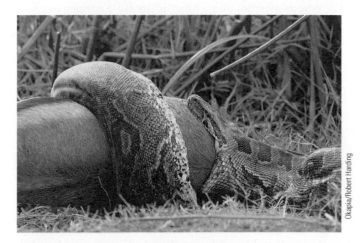

Figure 9.11 A python swallowing a gazelle
The gazelle weighed about 50 percent more than the snake. Many reptiles eat huge but infrequent meals. Their total intake over a year is far less than that of a mammal. We mammals need far more fuel because we use so much more energy, mainly for maintaining basal metabolism.

303

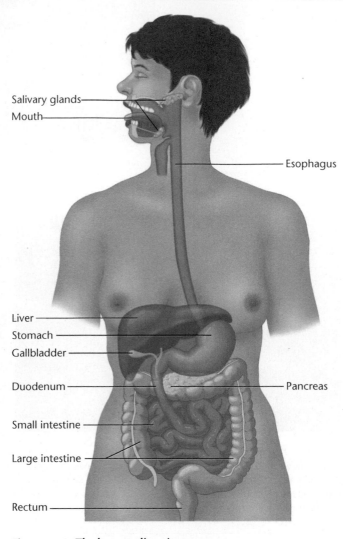

Salivary glands

Mouth

Esophagus

Liver

Stomach

Gallbladder

Duodenum

Pancreas

Small intestine

Large intestine

Rectum

Figure 9.13 The human digestive system

down the esophagus to the stomach, where it mixes with hydrochloric acid and enzymes that digest proteins. The stomach stores food for a time, and then a round sphincter muscle opens at the end of the stomach to release food to the small intestine.

The small intestine has enzymes that digest proteins, fats, and carbohydrates. It also absorbs digested materials into the blood, which carries those chemicals to body cells that either use them or store them for later use. The large intestine absorbs water and minerals and lubricates the remaining materials to excrete them.

Consumption of Dairy Products

Newborn mammals survive at first on mother's milk. As they grow older, they stop nursing for several reasons: The milk supply declines, the mother pushes them away, and they begin to eat other foods. Most mammals at about the age of weaning lose the intestinal enzyme **lactase**, which is necessary for metabolizing **lactose**, the sugar in milk. Adult mammals can drink a little milk, but consuming too much causes stomach

cramps, gas, and diarrhea (Ingram, Mulcare, Itan, Thomas, & Swallow, 2009; Rozin & Pelchat, 1988). The declining level of lactase may be an evolved mechanism to encourage weaning at the appropriate time.

Humans are a partial exception to this rule. Many adults have enough lactase levels to consume milk and other dairy products throughout life. However, the prevalence of the necessary genes varies. Nearly all the adults in China and surrounding countries are unable to metabolize lactose, as do varying numbers of people in other parts of the world (Curry, 2013; Flatz, 1987; Rozin & Pelchat, 1988). People who are lactose intolerant can consume a little milk, and larger amounts of cheese and yogurt, which are easier to digest, but they generally learn to limit their intake.

The genetic ability to metabolize lactose in adulthood is common in societies with a long history of domesticated cattle. Within Africa, the distribution of ability to digest lactose varies sharply from place to place. Whereas Europeans who can digest lactose in adulthood all have variants of the same gene, people in various parts of Africa have genes that differ from one another and from Europeans, indicating that genes for adult lactose digestion evolved independently several times as various groups began domesticating cattle (Tishkoff et al., 2007). When cow's milk became available, the selective pressure was strong in favor of genes enabling people to digest it. Figure 9.14 shows the distribution of lactose tolerance across the eastern hemisphere. About 25 percent of Native American adults can digest lactose. For other residents of the Americas, the probability of digesting lactose depends on the origins of their ancestors.

✓ STOP & CHECK

12. Why do most Southeast Asian adults avoid drinking much milk?

ANSWER   12. Most Southeast Asian adults lack the genes that help digest lactose, the main sugar in milk.

Food Selection and Behavior

Does your food selection change your behavior? Many people have unsubstantiated beliefs in this regard. For example, many people believe that eating sugar makes children hyperactive. The best way to test this claim is to have children eat snacks with sugar on randomly selected days and artificially sweetened snacks on other days, without telling them or anyone else what they received on a given day. Studies of this type have found no significant effect of sugar on children's activity level, play behaviors, or school performance (Ells et al., 2008; Milich & Pelham, 1986). The belief that sugar causes hyperactivity is apparently an illusion based on people's tendency to see what they expect to see.

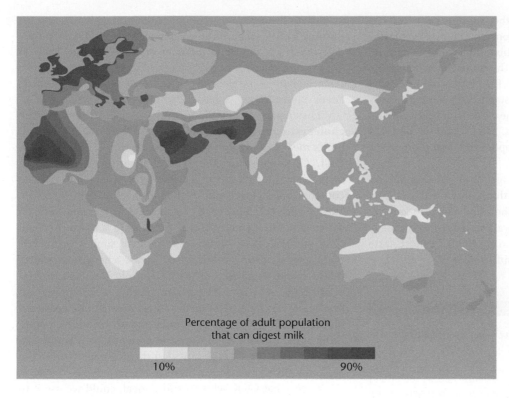

Percentage of adult population
that can digest milk

10%   90%

Figure 9.14 Percentage of adults who are lactose tolerant
People in areas with high lactose tolerance (e.g., Britain and Scandinavia) are likely to enjoy milk and other dairy products throughout their lives. Adults in areas with low tolerance (including Southeast Asia) drink less milk, if any.
(*Source: Curry, 2013*)

Another common misconception is that eating turkey causes sleepiness, supposedly because eating turkey increases the supply of tryptophan, which enables the brain to make serotonin and melatonin. That idea probably originated from the observation that many people in the United States feel sleepy after turkey dinner on Thanksgiving. However, turkey has only an average amount of tryptophan. The sleepiness on Thanksgiving afternoon results from overeating in general, not from turkey.

Nevertheless, it is true that tryptophan helps the brain produce melatonin, which aids sleepiness. Other than taking tryptophan pills, the most reliable way to increase tryptophan in the brain is to eat a diet high in carbohydrates. Here is the explanation: Tryptophan enters the brain by an active-transport protein that it shares with phenylalanine and other large amino acids. When you eat carbohydrates, your body reacts by increasing secretion of insulin, which moves sugars into storage, and also moves phenylalanine into storage (in liver cells and elsewhere). By reducing the competition from phenylalanine, this process makes it easier for tryptophan to reach the brain, inducing sleepiness (Silber & Schmitt, 2010). In short, the dessert at your big meal induces sleepiness much more than turkey does.

On the other hand, one old belief, long dismissed as nonsense, appears to be true. That belief is that fish is brain food. Many fish, especially salmon, contain oils that support brain functioning. Mothers who eat much seafood during pregnancy tend to have children who perform better on tests of cognitive ability, both in infancy and later (Julvez et al., 2016). Old people with a genetic risk of dementia show smaller than average cognitive declines if they consistently eat seafood (van de Rest et al., 2016).

Short- and Long-Term Regulation of Feeding

Eating is far too important to be entrusted to just one mechanism. Your brain gets messages from your mouth, stomach, intestines, fat cells, and elsewhere to regulate your eating.

Oral Factors

You're a busy person, right? If you could get all the nutrition you need by swallowing a pill, would you do it? Once in a while you might, but not often. People like to eat. In fact, people like to taste and chew even when they are not hungry. Figure 9.15 shows a piece of 6500-year-old chewing gum made from birch-bark tar. The small tooth marks indicate that a child or teenager chewed it. Anthropologists don't know how the ancient people removed the sap to make the gum, and they aren't sure why anyone would chew something that tasted as bad as this gum probably did (Battersby, 1997). Clearly, the urge to chew is strong.

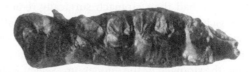

Figure 9.15 Chewing gum from about 4500 B.C.
The gum, made from birch-bark tar, has small tooth marks indicating that a child or adolescent chewed it.
(*Source: Reprinted by permission from Macmillan Publishers Ltd., "Plus c'est le meme chews," by Stephen Battersby, Nature, 1997.*)

Could you become satiated without tasting your food? In one experiment, college students consumed lunch five days a week by swallowing one end of a rubber tube and then pushing a button to pump a liquid diet into the stomach (Jordan, 1969; Spiegel, 1973). (Yes, they were paid for participating.) After a few days of practice, each person established a consistent pattern of pumping in a constant volume of the liquid each day and maintaining a constant body weight. Most found the untasted meals unsatisfying, however, and reported a desire to taste or chew something (Jordan, 1969).

Could you satisfy your hunger by taste alone? In **sham-feeding** experiments, everything an animal swallows leaks out of a tube connected to the esophagus or stomach. Sham-feeding animals eat and swallow almost continually without becoming satiated (G. P. Smith, 1998). In short, taste contributes to satiety, but it is not sufficient.

STOP & CHECK

13. What evidence indicates that taste is not sufficient for satiety?

ANSWER

13. Animals that sham-feed chew and taste their food but do not become satiated.

The Stomach and Intestines

The main signal to end a meal is distension of the stomach. The importance of stomach distension explains why sham feeding does not satisfy hunger, and why eating satisfies your hunger before the nutrition reaches any of the cells that need it. Stomach distension was always a likely hypothesis to explain satiety, but it wasn't easy to demonstrate. In a decisive experiment, researchers attached an inflatable cuff at the connection between the stomach and the small intestine (Deutsch, Young, & Kalogeris, 1978). Inflating the cuff prevented food from passing to the duodenum, and deflating it allowed it to pass again. Researchers carefully ensured that the cuff was not painful to the animal and did not interfere with feeding. The key result was that, when the cuff was inflated, an animal ate a certain amount and then stopped until the cuff was deflated. Evidently, stomach distension is sufficient to produce satiety. The **vagus nerve** (cranial nerve X) conveys information to the brain about the stretching of the stomach walls. However, people who have had their stomach surgically removed because of stomach cancer or other disease still report satiety, so mechanisms other than stomach distension can also produce satiety. Later researchers found that meals end after distension of either the stomach or the duodenum (Seeley, Kaplan, & Grill, 1995).

The **duodenum** (DYOU-oh-DEE-num or dyuh-ODD-ehn-uhm), the part of the small intestine adjoining the stomach, is a major site for absorbing nutrients. Nerves from the duodenum inform the brain not only about distension, but also about the type and amount of nutrition. How do your intestines "know" what you ate? You have taste receptors in your digestive tract, similar to the ones on your tongue. They do not provide you with a conscious experience, but they do alter brain activity to influence your sense of satiety (Cvijanovic, Feinle-Bisset, Young, & Little, 2015; van Avesaat et al., 2015).

Distension of the duodenum releases the hormone **cholecystokinin** (ko-leh-SIS-teh-KI-nehn) **(CCK)**, which limits meal size in two ways (Gibbs, Young, & Smith, 1973). First, CCK constricts the sphincter muscle between the stomach and the duodenum, causing the stomach to hold its contents and fill more quickly than usual (McHugh & Moran, 1985; Smith & Gibbs, 1998). In that way it hastens stomach distension, the primary signal for ending a meal. Second, CCK stimulates the vagus nerve to send signals to the hypothalamus, causing cells there to release a neurotransmitter that is a shorter version of the CCK molecule itself (Kobelt et al., 2006; Schwartz, 2000). The process is something like sending a fax: The CCK in the intestines cannot cross the blood–brain barrier, but it stimulates cells to release something almost like it. As in the case of angiotensin and thirst, the body uses the same chemical in the periphery and in the brain for closely related functions.

Given that CCK helps to end a meal, could we use it to help people who are trying to lose weight? Unfortunately, no. CCK produces short-term effects only. It limits the size of the meal, but an animal that has eaten a smaller than usual meal compensates by overeating at the next meal (Cummings & Overduin, 2007).

STOP & CHECK

14. What evidence shows that stomach distension is sufficient for satiety?
15. What are two mechanisms by which CCK increases satiety?

ANSWERS

14. If a cuff is attached to the junction between the stomach and duodenum so that food cannot leave the stomach, an animal becomes satiated when the stomach is full. 15. When the duodenum is distended, it releases CCK, which closes the sphincter muscle between the stomach and duodenum. CCK therefore increases the rate at which the stomach distends. Also, neural signals from the intestines cause certain cells in the hypothalamus to release CCK as a neurotransmitter, and at its receptors, it triggers decreased feeding.

Glucose, Insulin, and Glucagon

Digestion converts much of a meal into glucose, an important source of energy throughout the body and nearly the only fuel of the brain. Two pancreatic hormones, insulin and glucagon, regulate the flow of glucose into cells. Immediately before a meal (as you react to the sight and smell of the food), as well as during and after a meal, the pancreas increases release of **insulin**, which enables glucose to enter the cells. The brain cells are an exception, because glucose can enter them without need for insulin. Some of the excess glucose produced by a meal enters the liver, which converts it to glycogen and stores it. Some also enters fat cells, which convert it to fat and store it. The net effect prevents blood glucose levels from rising too sharply.

As time passes after a meal, the blood glucose level falls, insulin levels drop, glucose enters the cells more slowly, and hunger increases (Pardal & López-Barneo, 2002) (see Figure 9.16). The pancreas increases release of **glucagon**, stimulating the liver to convert some of its stored glycogen back to glucose.

If the insulin level stays constantly high, the body continues moving blood glucose into the cells, including the liver cells and fat cells, long after a meal. Before too long, blood glucose drops, because glucose is leaving the blood without any new glucose entering. The result is increased hunger. In autumn, animals that are preparing for hibernation have constantly high insulin levels. They rapidly

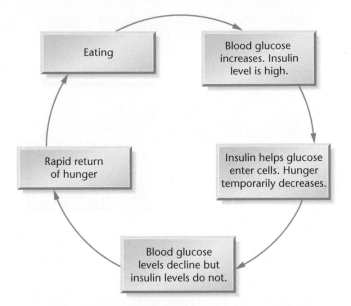

Figure 9.17 Effects of steady high insulin levels on feeding
Constantly high insulin causes blood glucose to be stored as fats and glycogen. Because it becomes difficult to mobilize the stored nutrients, hunger returns soon after each meal.

deposit much of each meal as fat and glycogen, grow hungry again, and continue gaining weight (see Figure 9.17). That weight gain is a valuable preparation for a season when the animal will have to survive off its fat reserves. Most humans also eat more in autumn than in other seasons, as shown in Figure 9.18 (de Castro, 2000). In the United States, we tend to blame our autumn weight gain on the Halloween and Thanksgiving holidays, but the real reason is probably an evolved drive to increase our reserves in preparation for winter. In ancient times, food was scarce in winter.

If the insulin level remains constantly low, as in people with type 1 diabetes, blood glucose levels may be three or more times the normal level, but little of it enters the cells

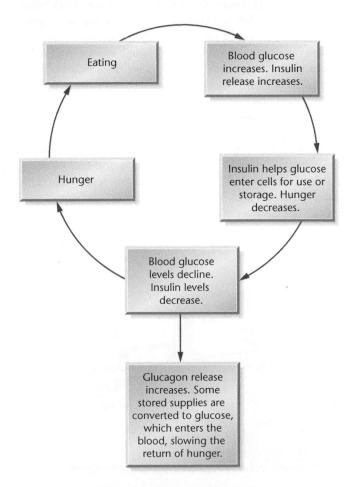

Figure 9.16 Insulin and glucagon feedback system
When glucose levels rise, the pancreas releases the hormone insulin, which helps glucose enter cells, including liver cells and fat cells that store fuel for future use. The entry of glucose into cells suppresses hunger and decreases eating, thereby lowering the glucose level.

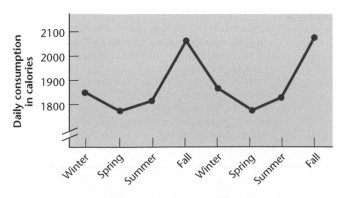

Figure 9.18 People eat more in fall than in other seasons
Mean intake increases by more than 10 percent, on the average, according to people's eating diaries.
(*Source: Modified from de Castro, J. M., 2000, Eating behavior: Lessons from the real world of humans. Nutrition, 16, 800–813.*)

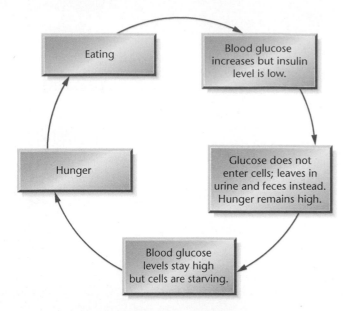

Figure 9.19 People with untreated type 1 diabetes eat much but lose weight
Because of their low insulin levels, the glucose in their blood cannot enter the cells, either to be stored or to be used. Consequently, they excrete glucose in their urine while their cells are starving.

(see Figure 9.19). People and animals with diabetes eat more food than normal because their cells are starving (Lindberg, Coburn, & Stricker, 1984), but they excrete most of their glucose, and they lose weight. Note that either prolonged high or prolonged low insulin levels increase eating, but for different reasons and with different effects on body weight.

✓ **STOP & CHECK**

16. Why do people with very low insulin levels eat so much? Why do people with constantly high levels eat so much?

17. What would happen to someone's appetite if insulin levels and glucagon levels were both high?

ANSWERS

16. Those with very low levels, as in type 1 diabetes, cannot get glucose to enter their cells, and therefore, they are constantly hungry. They pass much of their nutrition in the urine and feces. Those with constantly high levels deposit much of their glucose into fat and glycogen, so within a short time after a meal, the supply of blood glucose drops. **17.** When glucagon levels rise, stored glycogen is converted to glucose, which enters the blood. If insulin levels are high also, the glucose entering the blood is free to enter all the cells. So the result would be decreased appetite.

Leptin

Taste, stomach distension, duodenum distension, and insulin help regulate the onset and offset of a meal. However, we cannot expect those mechanisms to be completely accurate.

Imagine what would happen if you consistently ate either too little or too much. The body needs a long-term mechanism to compensate for day-to-day mistakes.

It does so by monitoring fat supplies. Researchers had long suspected some kind of fat monitoring, but they discovered the actual mechanism by accident. They found that mice of a particular genetic strain consistently become obese, as shown in Figure 9.20 (Zhang et al., 1994). After researchers identified the responsible gene, they found the peptide it makes, a previously unknown hormone that they named **leptin**, from the Greek word *leptos*, meaning "slender" (Halaas et al., 1995). Unlike insulin, which is so evolutionarily ancient that we find it throughout the animal kingdom, leptin is limited to vertebrates (Morton, Cummings, Baskin, Barsh, & Schwartz, 2006). In genetically normal mice, as well as humans and other species, the body's fat cells produce leptin: The more fat cells, the more leptin. Mice with a mutation in the *leptin* gene fail to produce leptin.

Leptin signals your brain about your fat reserves. When your fat reserves decrease, leptin levels decline, and you react by eating more and becoming less active, to save energy. When leptin levels return to normal, you eat less and become more active (Campfield, Smith, Guisez, Devos, & Burn, 1995; Elias et al., 1998). In adolescence, a certain level of leptin triggers the onset of puberty. If your fat supply is too low to provide for your own needs, you don't have enough energy to provide for a baby. On the average, thinner people enter puberty later. Leptin also activates the sympathetic nervous system and increases blood pressure (Mark, 2013).

Because a mouse with a mutation in the *leptin* gene does not make leptin, its brain reacts as if its body has no fat stores and must be starving. The mouse eats as much as possible, conserves its energy by not moving much, and fails to enter puberty. Injections of leptin reverse these symptoms: The mouse then eats less, becomes more active, and enters puberty (Pelleymounter et al., 1995).

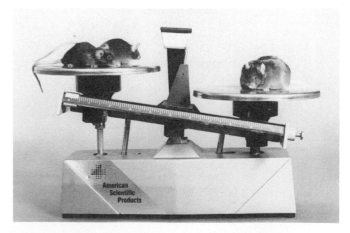

Figure 9.20 The effects of a mutation in the *leptin* gene on body weight
Mice with this gene eat more, move around less, and gain weight.
(*Source: Reprinted by permission from Macmillan Publishers Ltd: Nature, Positional cloning of the mouse obese gene and its human homologue, Zhang et al., 1994.*)

As you might imagine, news of this research inspired pharmaceutical companies to hope they could make a fortune by selling leptin. After all, the body makes leptin all the time, so it should not have unpleasant side effects. Leptin does produce important benefits for those rare people who are genetically unable to make leptin. However, the great majority of overweight people produce plenty of leptin, and giving them extra leptin produces little change in their appetite (Considine et al., 1996). At first, the interpretation was that overweight people must have developed a resistance to insulin. However, later research found that extra leptin also produces little effect on normal-weight people. Low levels of leptin trigger hunger, but beyond a certain level, additional leptin only weakly suppresses intake (Ravussin, Leibel, & Ferrante, 2014). In fact, in general the mechanisms that promote hunger are stronger and more insistent than those for satiety. Evolution has apparently prepared us to avoid starvation more vigorously than we avoid eating too much.

STOP & CHECK

18. Why are leptin injections less helpful for most overweight people than for mice with a mutation in the *leptin* gene?

ANSWER 18. Those mice fail to produce leptin. Nearly all overweight people produce enough leptin, and extra leptin only weakly suppresses appetite.

Brain Mechanisms

How does your brain decide when you should eat and how much? Hunger depends on the contents of your stomach and intestines, the availability of glucose to the cells, and your body's fat supplies, as well as your health and body temperature. Furthermore, if someone offers you a tasty treat, you might enjoy eating it even if you were not hungry. Just seeing a picture of highly appealing food increases your appetite (Harmon-Jones & Gable, 2009). People eat more on weekends than on other days, and more when eating with friends or family than when eating alone (de Castro, 2000). All these types of information converge onto several nuclei of the hypothalamus (see Figure 9.6).

As shown in Figure 9.21, many kinds of information impinge onto two kinds of cells in the arcuate nucleus of the hypothalamus, which is regarded as the master area for controlling appetite (Mendieta-Zéron, López, & Diéguez, 2008). Axons extend from the arcuate nucleus to other areas of the hypothalamus. Even though this figure leaves out some of the neurotransmitters and other complexities, it may be intimidating. Let's go through the key mechanisms step by step.

The Arcuate Nucleus and Paraventricular Hypothalamus

The **arcuate nucleus** of the hypothalamus has one set of neurons sensitive to hunger signals and a second set sensitive to satiety signals. In Figure 9.21, excitatory paths are noted in

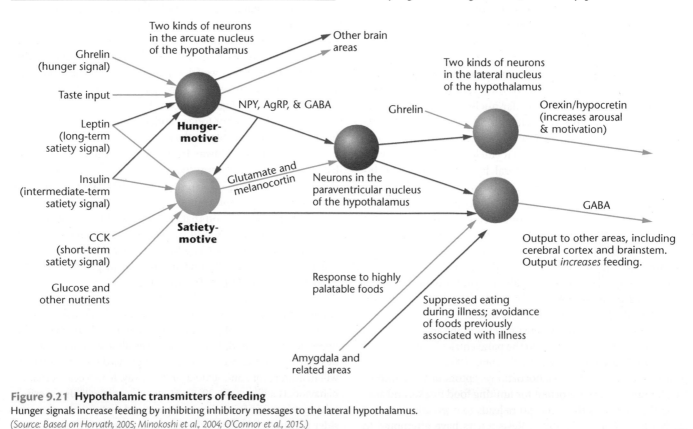

Figure 9.21 Hypothalamic transmitters of feeding
Hunger signals increase feeding by inhibiting inhibitory messages to the lateral hypothalamus.
(Source: Based on Horvath, 2005; Minokoshi et al., 2004; O'Connor et al., 2015.)

green, and inhibitory paths are in red. Most journal articles refer to one set of arcuate nucleus neurons as the "NPY/AgRP" neurons and the others as the "POMC/CART" neurons (because of some distinctive neurotransmitters that they release), but for simplicity this text will refer to them as hunger neurons and satiety neurons. The input to these cells comes from certain hormones such as insulin and leptin, but also from cells in the amygdala, basal forebrain, and thalamus (Cai, Haubensak, Anthony, & Anderson, 2014; Herman et al., 2016; Labouèbe, Boutrel, Tarussio, & Thorens, 2016).

Part of the input to the hunger-sensitive cells comes from axons releasing the neurotransmitter **ghrelin** (GRELL-in). This odd-looking word takes its name from the fact that it binds to the same receptors as growth-hormone releasing hormone (GHRH). The stomach releases ghrelin during a period of food deprivation, where it triggers stomach contractions. Ghrelin also acts on the hypothalamus to increase appetite. People who produce greater than average amounts of ghrelin respond more strongly than average to the sight of food, and they are almost twice as likely as other people to become obese (Karra et al., 2013).

The satiety-sensitive cells of the arcuate nucleus receive several types of input. Distension of the intestines triggers neurons to release the neurotransmitter CCK, a short-term signal (Fan et al., 2004). Blood glucose (a short-term signal) directly stimulates satiety cells in the arcuate nucleus (Parton et al., 2007) and prompts the pancreas to release insulin, which also stimulates the satiety cells. Body fat releases leptin, a long-term satiety signal (Diéguez, Vazquez, Romero, López, & Nogueiras, 2011). Nicotine also stimulates the satiety neurons (Mineur et al., 2011). The result is that cigarette smoking decreases appetite, and quitting smoking increases appetite, leading to weight gain.

Much of the output from the arcuate nucleus goes to the paraventricular nucleus (PVN) of the hypothalamus. Certain types of cells in the paraventricular nucleus inhibit the lateral hypothalamus, an area important for eating (Sutton et al., 2014). In Figure 9.21, notice how the hunger cells in the arcuate nucleus inhibit the paraventricular nucleus and the paraventricular nucleus inhibits the lateral hypothalamus. The inhibitory transmitters here are a combination of GABA (Tong, Jones, Elmquist, & Lowell, 2008), **neuropeptide Y (NPY)** (Stephens et al., 1995), and **agouti-related peptide (AgRP)** (Kas et al., 2004). Inhibiting an inhibitor produces net excitation, and that is how the stimuli for hunger increase eating and arousal. If the inhibition of the paraventricular nucleus is strong enough, rats eat huge meals, as tastelessly illustrated in Figure 9.22 (Billington & Levine, 1992; Leibowitz & Alexander, 1991; Morley, Levine, Grace, & Kneip, 1985).

Axons from the satiety-sensitive cells of the arcuate nucleus deliver an excitatory message to the paraventricular nucleus, releasing **melanocortins** (Ellacott & Cone, 2004) and glutamate (Fenselau et al., 2017). Melanocortin receptors in the paraventricular nucleus are important for limiting food intake, and anything that damages these receptors leads to overeating (Asai et al., 2013; Huszar et al., 1997). Researchers have attempted to

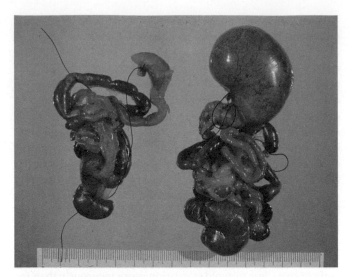

Figure 9.22 **Effects of inhibiting the paraventricular nucleus of the hypothalamus**
On the left is the digestive system of a normal rat. On the right is the digestive system of a rat that had its paraventricular hypothalamus chemically inhibited. The rat continued eating even though its stomach and intestines distended almost to the point of bursting. (Yeah, this is a little bit disgusting.)
(Source: Reprinted from "Peptide YY (PYY) a potently orexigenic agent," by J. E. Morley, A. S. Levine, M. Grace, and J. Kneip, 1985, Brain Research, 341, no. 1, pp. 200–203, with permission of Elsevier.)

find a safe drug that would stimulate melanocortin receptors as a weight-reduction treatment. However, every drug tested so far has unacceptable side effects (Krashes, Lowell, & Garfield, 2016). The amygdala and related areas send two kinds of input to the lateral hypothalamus. One path inhibits eating during illness and mediates aversion to foods previously associated with illness (Carter, Soden, Zweifel, & Palmiter, 2013). The other path stimulates eating in response to highly tasty foods (Jennings, Rizzi, Stamatakis, Ung, & Stuber, 2013). If you cannot resist eating that delicious hot fudge sundae even though you weren't hungry at all, you can blame these axons.

An additional pathway from the paraventricular nucleus leads to cells in the lateral hypothalamus that release orexin (Fu, Acuna-Goycolea, & van den Pol, 2004). We encountered these neurons in Chapter 8 because a deficiency of orexin leads to narcolepsy. In addition to its role in wakefulness, orexin has two roles in feeding. First, it increases animals' persistence in seeking food (Williams, Cai, Elliott, & Harrold, 2004). Second, orexin increases activity and motivation in general (Mahler, Moorman, Smith, James, & Aston-Jones, 2014).

Note the output from hunger-sensitive neurons in the arcuate nucleus to "other brain areas." When an animal becomes hungry to the point of possible starvation, it will do whatever is necessary to get food, but it suppresses almost all other activities. An animal that would ordinarily fight to defend its territory will instead ignore an intruder or run away. It also ceases mating behaviors (Padilla et al., 2016). Hungry people will also sacrifice other goals to get food. Researchers found that people who consider themselves honest will cheat at a game to win food when they are hungry, although they would not cheat to win something else, such as a pen (Williams, Pizarro, Ariely, & Weinberg, 2016).

As you can see, many chemicals and brain areas contribute to feeding and satiety. One consequence is that if the control of feeding goes wrong in one way, the brain has many other mechanisms to compensate for it. A closely related point is that researchers could develop drugs to control appetite by working on many routes—leptin, insulin, NPY, and so forth—but changing any one circuit might be ineffective because of compensations by the others.

✓ STOP & CHECK

19. Name three hormones that increase satiety and one that increases hunger.

20. Which neuropeptide from the arcuate nucleus to the paraventricular nucleus is most important for satiety?

ANSWERS

19. Insulin, CCK, and leptin increase satiety. Ghrelin increases hunger. 20. Melanocortin

The Lateral Hypothalamus

Output from the paraventricular nucleus acts on the **lateral hypothalamus** (see Figure 9.23), which includes so many neuron clusters and passing axons that it has been compared to a crowded train station (Leibowitz & Hoebel, 1998). The lateral hypothalamus controls insulin secretion, alters taste responsiveness, and facilitates feeding in other ways. An animal with damage in this area refuses food and water, averting its head as if the food were distasteful. The animal may starve to death unless it is force-fed, but if kept alive, it gradually recovers much of its ability to eat (see Figure 9.24).

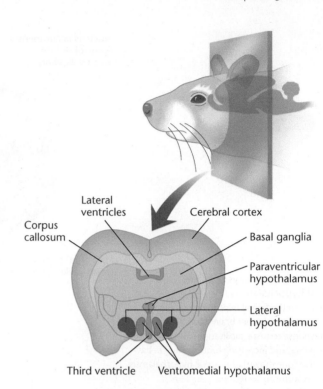

Figure 9.23 The lateral hypothalamus, ventromedial hypothalamus, and paraventricular hypothalamus
The side view above indicates the plane of the coronal section of the brain below it.
(Based on Hart, 1976)

In contrast, stimulation of the lateral hypothalamus increases the drive to eat.

Damage to the lateral hypothalamus not only kills the neurons there, but also interrupts many axons containing dopamine that pass through the area. To separate the roles of hypothalamic cells from those of passing fibers, experimenters used chemicals that damage only the cell bodies, or induced lesions in very young

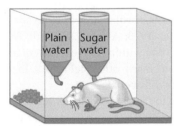

Stage 1. *Aphagia and adipsia.* Rat refuses all food and drink; must be force-fed to keep it alive.

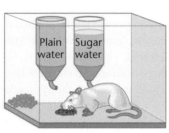

Stage 2. *Anorexia.* Rat eats a small amount of palatable foods and drinks sweetened water. It still does not eat enough to stay alive.

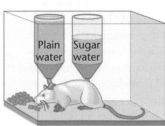

Stage 3. *Adipsia.* The rat eats enough to stay alive, though at a lower-than-normal body weight. It still refuses plain water.

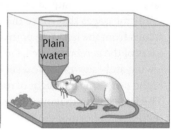

Stage 4. *Near-recovery.* The rat eats enough to stay alive, though at a lower-than-normal body weight. It drinks plain water, but only at mealtimes to wash down its food. Under slightly stressful conditions, such as in a cold room, the rat will return to an earlier stage of refusing food and water.

Figure 9.24 Recovery after damage to the lateral hypothalamus
At first, the rat refuses all food and drink. If kept alive for several weeks or months by force-feeding, it gradually recovers its ability to eat and drink enough to stay alive. However, even at the final stage of recovery, its behavior is not the same as that of normal rats.
(Based on Teitelbaum & Epstein, 1962)

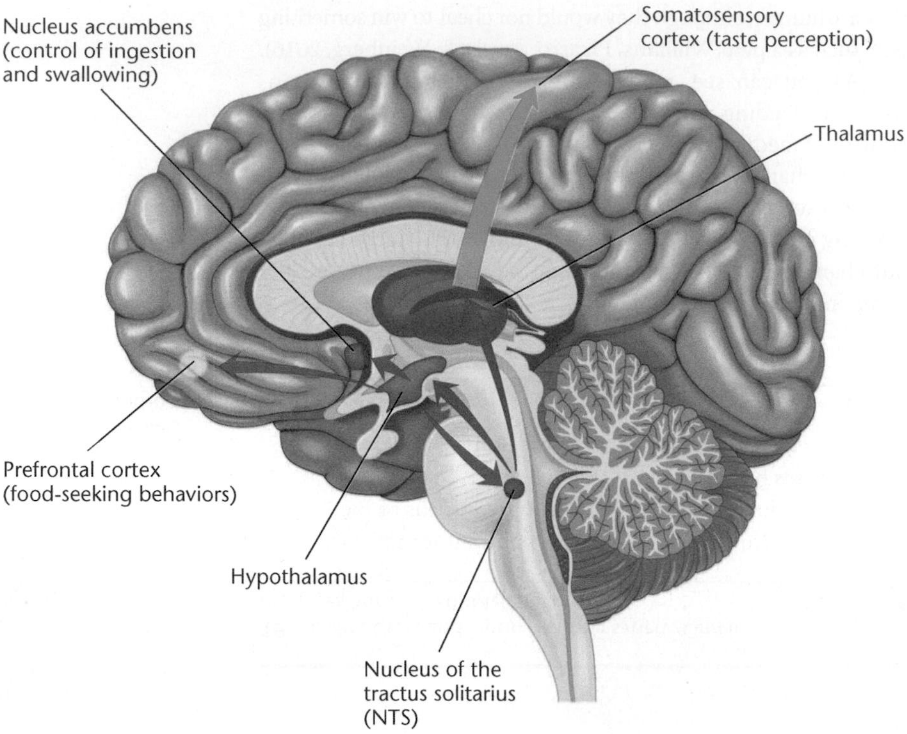

Nucleus accumbens
(control of ingestion
and swallowing)

Somatosensory
cortex (taste perception)

Thalamus

Prefrontal cortex
(food-seeking behaviors)

Hypothalamus

Nucleus of the
tractus solitarius
(NTS)

Figure 9.25 Pathways from the lateral hypothalamus
Axons from the lateral hypothalamus modify activity in several other brain areas, changing the response to taste, facilitating ingestion and swallowing, and increasing food-seeking behaviors. Also (not shown), the lateral hypothalamus controls stomach secretions.

rats, before the dopamine axons reached the lateral hypothalamus. In both cases, damaging the cell bodies produced a loss of feeding without impairing arousal or activity (Almli, Fisher, & Hill, 1979; Grossman, Dacey, Halaris, Collier, & Routtenberg, 1978; Stricker, Swerdloff, & Zigmond, 1978). In contrast, the axons passing through the lateral hypothalamus contribute to arousal, activity, and reward (Stuber & Wise, 2016). Figure 9.25 shows the ways in which the lateral hypothalamus promotes eating:

- Axons from the lateral hypothalamus to the NTS (nucleus of the tractus solitarius), part of the taste pathway, alter the taste sensation and the salivation response to the tastes. When the lateral hypothalamus detects hunger, it sends messages that make the food taste better.
- Axons from the lateral hypothalamus extend into several parts of the cerebral cortex, facilitating ingestion and swallowing and causing cortical cells to increase their response to the taste, smell, or sight of food (Critchley & Rolls, 1996).
- The lateral hypothalamus increases the pituitary gland's secretion of hormones that increase insulin secretion.
- The lateral hypothalamus sends axons to the spinal cord, controlling autonomic responses such as digestive secretions (van den Pol, 1999). An animal with damage to the lateral hypothalamus has trouble digesting foods.

✅ **STOP & CHECK**

21. In what ways does the lateral hypothalamus facilitate feeding?

ANSWER

21. Activity of the lateral hypothalamus improves taste, enhances cortical responses to food, and increases secretions of insulin and digestive juices.

Medial Areas of the Hypothalamus

Output from the **ventromedial hypothalamus (VMH)** inhibits feeding (Chee, Myers, Price, & Colmers, 2010), and therefore damage to this nucleus leads to overeating and weight gain (see Figure 9.23). Some people with a tumor in that area have gained more than 10 kg (22 lb) per month (Al-Rashid, 1971; Killeffer & Stern, 1970; Reeves & Plum, 1969). Rats with similar damage sometimes double or triple their weight (see Figure 9.26). Although these symptoms have been known as the *ventromedial hypothalamic syndrome*, damage limited to just the ventromedial hypothalamus does not consistently increase eating or body weight. To produce a large effect, the lesion must extend outside the ventromedial nucleus to invade nearby axons (Ahlskog & Hoebel, 1973; Ahlskog, Randall, & Hoebel, 1975; Gold, 1973). Neurons within the ventromedial hypothalamus itself participate in many other behaviors, including defense against attackers (Silva et al., 2016).

Recall that rats with damage to the paraventricular nucleus eat larger than average meals. In contrast, those with damage in the ventromedial area eat normal-sized meals, but they eat more frequently (Hoebel & Hernandez, 1993). One reason is that they have increased stomach motility and secretions, and their stomach empties faster than normal. The faster the stomach empties, the sooner the animal is ready for its next meal. Another reason for their frequent meals is that the damage increases insulin production (B. M. King, Smith, & Frohman, 1984), and therefore, much of each meal is stored as fat. If animals with this kind of damage are prevented from overeating, they gain weight anyway! According to Mark Friedman and Edward Stricker (1976), the problem is not that the rat gets fat from overeating. Rather, the rat overeats because it is storing so much fat. The high insulin levels

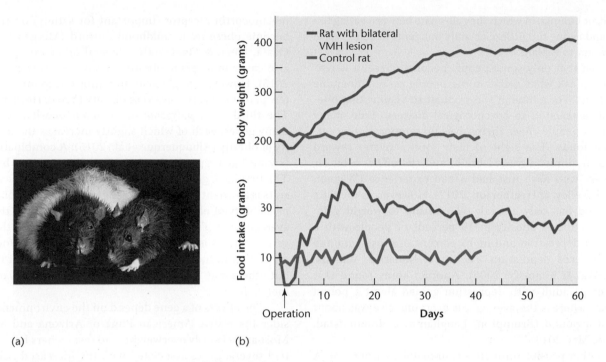

Figure 9.26 Effects of damage to the ventromedial hypothalamus

(a) On the right is a normal rat. On the left is a rat after damage to the ventromedial hypothalamus. A brain-damaged rat may weigh up to three times as much as a normal rat.

(Yoav Levy/Phototake)

(b) Weight and eating after damage to the ventromedial hypothalamus. Within a few days after the operation, the rat begins eating much more than normal.

(Reprinted by permission of the University of Nebraska Press from "Disturbances in feeding and drinking behavior after hypothalamic lesions," by P. Teitelbaum, pp. 39–69, in M. R. Jones, Ed., 1961, Nebraska Symposium on Motivation. Copyright © 1961 by the University of Nebraska Press. Copyright © renewed 1988 by the University of Nebraska Press.)

keep moving blood glucose into storage, even when the blood glucose level is low. Despite the weight gain, most of the body's cells are starving for nutrition. The result is increased hunger.

Table 9.2 summarizes the effects of lesions in several areas of the hypothalamus.

✅ STOP & CHECK

22. In what way does eating increase after damage in and around the ventromedial hypothalamus? After damage to the paraventricular nucleus?

ANSWER 22. Animals with damage to the ventromedial hypothalamus eat more frequent meals. Animals with damage to the paraventricular nucleus of the hypothalamus eat larger meals.

Eating Disorders

Insulin, leptin, glucose, CCK, and other influences provide for homeostatic control of feeding. However, the homeostatic mechanisms often fail. In particular, obesity has become a widespread problem in much of the world. Perhaps we should not be surprised. Throughout human evolution and even before that, our ancestors frequently faced food shortages, and evolution predisposed us to eat heartily whenever good food was available. If we offer rats an all-you-can-eat buffet of tasty, high-calorie foods, they respond by becoming obese (Geiger et al., 2009). Instead of asking why so many people become obese, maybe we should ask why everyone in a prosperous country does not become obese! Meanwhile, other people suffer from anorexia, in which they refuse to eat enough to

Table 9.2 | Effects of Hypothalamic Lesion

Hypothalamic Area	Effect of Lesion
Preoptic area	Deficit in physiological mechanisms of temperature regulation
Lateral preoptic area	Deficit in osmotic thirst due partly to damage to cells and partly to interruption of passing axons
Lateral hypothalamus	Undereating, weight loss, low insulin level (because of damage to cell bodies); underarousal, underresponsiveness (because of damage to passing axons)
Ventromedial hypothalamus	Increased meal frequency, weight gain, high insulin level
Paraventricular nucleus	Increased meal size, especially increased carbohydrate intake during the first meal of the active period of the day

survive, or bulimia, in which they alternate between eating too much and eating too little. Certainly hunger researchers have much to try to explain.

Given that only some people become obese, it is reasonable to ask what makes some people more vulnerable than others. For a time, it was popular to assume that obesity was a reaction to psychological distress. True, many distressed people cheer themselves up temporarily by eating rich foods. The sight of tasty food activates reward centers in almost anyone's brain, and the effect is bigger in dieters who have just had a bad experience (Wagner, Boswell, Kelley, & Heatherton, 2012). However, in the long run, mood has only a weak relationship to weight gain. One study found obesity in 19 percent of people with a history of depression and in 15 percent of those who had never suffered depression (McIntyre, Konarski, Wilkins, Soczynska, & Kennedy, 2006). Another study found that the average adult with depression gained about a pound per year, whereas the average for everyone else was about 8/10 of a pound (Brumpton, Langhammer, Romundstad, Chen, & Mai, 2013).

Another possible influence is prenatal environment. A study in rats found that if a mother consumed a high-fat diet during pregnancy, her babies developed a larger than average lateral hypothalamus and produced more than the average amount of orexin and other transmitters that facilitate increased eating (Chang, Gasinskaya, Karatayev, & Leibowitz, 2008). These changes persisted throughout life. In short, exposure to a high-fat diet before birth predisposes the offspring to increased appetite and body weight. This example illustrates epigenetic effects, as described in Chapter 4: An experience can alter the expression of the genes.

Genetics and Body Weight

You have probably noticed that most thin parents have thin children, and most heavy parents have heavy children. Studies of twins and adopted children in many countries have consistently found high heritability of body weight (Albuquerque, Stice, Rodríguez-López, Manco, & Nóbrega, 2015; Min, Chiu, & Wang, 2013; Silventoinen et al., 2016). Researchers distinguish three types of heritability for obesity. One type, *syndromal* obesity, results when a gene causes a medical problem that includes obesity. For example, Prader-Willi syndrome is marked by mild cognitive disabilities, short stature, and obesity. People with this syndrome have blood levels of ghrelin four to five times higher than average (Cummings et al., 2002). Ghrelin, you will recall, is a peptide related to food deprivation. The fact that people with Prader-Willi syndrome overeat and still produce high ghrelin levels suggests that their problem relates to an inability to turn off ghrelin release.

A second type, *monogenic* obesity, occurs when a single gene leads to obesity without other physical or mental abnormalities. People with a mutation in the gene for the melanocortin receptor (important for satiety) overeat and become obese from childhood onward (Mergen, Mergen, Ozata, Oner, & Oner, 2001). Several other rare genes can also cause monogenic obesity (van der Klaauw & Farooqi, 2015). However, single-gene mutations account for only a few percent of cases of severe obesity (Yeo & Heisler, 2012). The third type, *polygenic* or *common* obesity, relates to many genes, each of which slightly increases the probability of obesity (Albuquerque et al., 2015). A combination of a few such genes produces more effect than any one by itself. The first such gene to be demonstrated with replicable results is a variant form of the *FTO* gene that raises someone's probability of obesity to about two-thirds greater than the average level (Frayling et al., 2007). Exactly how the *FTO* gene operates is uncertain, as is the mechanism for other genes that influence weight gain. Some may affect hunger, but others may influence activity levels, digestion, or basal metabolism.

The effects of a gene depend on the environment. Consider the Native American Pima of Arizona and Mexico. Most are seriously overweight, and researchers have identified several genes associated with the increased risk (Bian et al., 2010; Muller et al., 2010). However, obesity was uncommon among them in the early 1900s, when their diet consisted mostly of desert plants that ripen in the brief rainy season. The Pima apparently evolved a strategy of eating all they could when food was available, because it would have to carry them through periods of scarcity. They also evolved a tendency to conserve energy by limiting their activity. Now, with a more typical U.S. diet that is high in calories, the strategy of overeating and inactivity is maladaptive. In short, their weight depends on the combination of genes and environment. Neither one by itself has this effect.

STOP & CHECK

23. Why did the Pima begin gaining weight in the mid-1900s?

ANSWER

23. They shifted from a diet of local plants that were seasonally available to a calorie-rich diet that is available throughout the year.

Weight Loss Techniques

In the United States, obesity is considered a disease, and never mind the fact that we don't have a clear definition of what we mean by *disease.* One positive consequence of calling it a disease is that people are relieved from thinking of themselves as morally guilty for being overweight. Another consequence is that insurance companies will now pay treatment providers to help relieve obesity. A possible negative consequence is that some may decide that they have no control and may as well quit trying to lose weight.

You will hear advocates of a particular diet plan brag that many people on their plan lost a significant amount of weight. That statement may be true, but it means little unless we know how long they kept the weight off, or how many other people tried the plan and failed to lose weight. In fact, few people on any diet lose much weight and keep it off permanently. Many psychologists now recommend small changes in diet ("eat a little less than usual") on the expectation that more people will stick to this diet (Stroebele et al., 2008). Another recommendation is to promote good health by getting good nutrition and physical exercise, regardless of what happens to weight (Mann, Tomiyama, & Ward, 2015). For exercise to be helpful, it does not need to be strenuous, but it needs to be sustained, such as brisk walking for an hour a day on most days (Wyatt, 2013).

Particularly important advice is to reduce or eliminate the intake of soft drinks. Researchers have found that people who consume at least one soft drink per day are more likely than others to be overweight, and if they are not already overweight, they are more likely than others to become overweight (Dhingra et al., 2007; Liebman et al., 2006). Around 1970, American companies began sweetening their beverages with high-fructose corn syrup instead of sugar. Fructose is somewhat sweeter than common table sugar, and the hope was that people could satisfy their craving for sweets with fewer calories. Clearly, this idea didn't work, as obesity has become more common, not less common, since then. It is possible that fructose actually increases the problem. Whereas glucose (another common sugar) stimulates release of leptin and insulin that help reduce hunger, fructose has little effect on leptin or insulin (Teff et al., 2004). Therefore, if you drink something with fructose, you gain calories without feeling satiated. Also, if you consume much fructose, the body stores most of it as fat (Bray, Nielsen, & Popkin, 2004). Laboratory studies have shown that rats that are offered drinks containing fructose develop obesity, type 2 diabetes, and high blood pressure (Tappy & Lê, 2010).

Another idea was to sweeten beverages with nonnutritive sweeteners, in hopes of satisfying a craving for sweets without any calories at all. Again, this idea has been ineffective. Since the advent of diet drinks, obesity has continued to increase in prevalence, and consumption of sugars has *increased.* That is, many people use the diet drinks but maintain or increase their sugar intake in other ways. Furthermore, consumption of artificial sweeteners increases the abundance of the types of intestinal bacteria that are associated with type 2 diabetes (Suez et al., 2014).

Apparently there is no such thing as "satisfying" a craving for sweet tastes. Eating sweet, high-calorie food increases the preference for similar foods for days afterward, and people who gain weight increase their enjoyment of sweet, high-calorie foods (Liu et al., 2016; Stice & Yokum, 2016).

When diet and exercise fail to help someone lose weight, another option is weight-loss drugs. Unfortunately, most of the drugs that help people lose weight produce unpleasant side effects, and most physicians avoid prescribing them. Still another option is gastric bypass surgery, in which part of the stomach is sewed off so that food cannot enter. Remember that stomach distension is a major contributor to satiety. By decreasing stomach size, the surgery makes it possible for a smaller meal to produce satiety. The surgery poses enough risk that it is recommended only in fairly serious cases of obesity, but in about two-thirds of cases, it does help people lose excess weight, improve their blood pressure, and decrease the risk of type 2 diabetes (Puzziferri et al., 2014).

Here is still another option, experimental and controversial: People's digestive systems have thousands of species of microorganisms that help digest the foods and perform many other functions, some helpful to us and some harmful (Cryan & Dinan, 2012). The types of microorganisms found in people with obesity differ from those in leaner people. Researchers working with mice found that transferring microorganisms from lean mice to obese mice helped the obese mice lose weight (Ridaura et al., 2013). Umm . . . to be more specific, what they did was to transplant feces from one digestive system to another. Might this work with humans?

⊘ STOP & CHECK

24. For someone who is trying to lose weight, why would it be a good idea to cut down on sweets altogether?

ANSWER

24. Sugars provide many calories. Although fructose provides fewer calories for a given amount of sweet taste, it is less effective at triggering a sense of satiety. People who try to satisfy their sweet cravings with artificial sweeteners do not generally cut down on total calories. Furthermore, artificial sweeteners promote the types of intestinal bacteria that are associated with type 2 diabetes.

Bulimia Nervosa

Bulimia nervosa is a condition in which people alternate between binges of overeating and periods of strict dieting. Many, but not all, induce themselves to vomit. In the United States, about 1.5 percent of women and 0.5 percent of men develop bulimia at some time in life. It has become more common over the years. That is, bulimia is more common among young people today than it ever was in their parents' generation and more common in their parents' generation than in their grandparents'. The increase is presumably due to the increased availability of large quantities of tasty high-calorie foods.

On average, people with bulimia show a variety of biochemical abnormalities, including increased production of ghrelin, a hormone associated with increased appetite (Monteleone, Serritella, Scognamiglio, & Maj, 2010). The biochemistry is probably a result of the binges and purges, rather than a cause.

After therapy that decreases the symptoms of bulimia, the ghrelin and other body chemicals return toward normal levels (Tanaka et al., 2006).

In important ways, bulimia resembles drug addiction (Hoebel, Rada, Mark, & Pothos, 1999). Eating tasty foods activates the same brain areas as addictive drugs, such as the nucleus accumbens. Drug addicts who cannot get drugs sometimes overeat instead, and food-deprived people or animals become more likely than others to use drugs.

Researchers examined rats that were food deprived for 12 hours a day, including the first 4 hours of their wakeful period, and then offered a very sweet, syrupy sugar solution. Over several weeks on this regimen, the rats drank more and more each day, especially during the first hour of availability each day. The intake released dopamine and opioid (opiatelike) compounds in the brain, similar to the effects of highly addicting drugs (Colantuoni et al., 2001, 2002). It also increased the levels of dopamine type 3 receptors in the brain—again, a trend resembling that of rats that receive morphine (Spangler et al., 2004). If they were then deprived of this sweet liquid, they showed withdrawal symptoms, including head shaking, teeth chattering, and tremors. An injection of morphine relieved these symptoms. In short, the rats showed clear indications of an addiction to big doses of sugar (Avena, Rada, & Hoebel, 2008). Similarly, we can regard bulimic cycles of dieting and binge eating as an addiction.

Anorexia Nervosa

Anorexia nervosa is characterized by a refusal to eat enough to maintain a healthy body weight. In some cases it becomes life threatening. Anorexia occurs in about one percent of women and one-third of a percent of men, with onset in the teenage years or early 20s and generally for a long persistence (Hudson, Hiripi, Pope, & Kessler, 2007). People with anorexia do not regard food as tasting bad. Rather, they express an exaggerated fear of growing fat. When they eat, they strongly prefer low-fat, low-calorie foods (Foerde, Steinglass, Shohamy, & Walsh, 2015). Contrary to what we might expect of people verging on starvation, those with anorexia generally engage in extensive physical activity.

Studies of the brain in people with anorexia reveal abnormalities of dopamine release and other variables, but these abnormalities are probably the result of prolonged weight loss rather than the cause (Sodersten, Bergh, Leon, & Zandian, 2016). The psychological abnormalities may be results rather than causes, also. For decades, psychologists and psychiatrists have considered anorexia as a reaction to depression. However, although many people with anorexia do show signs of depression, little or no evidence indicates that they suffered depression prior to having anorexia (Bühren et al., 2014; Zerwas et al., 2013). They generally do not have large numbers of relatives with depression, and they do not respond well to antidepressive drugs or psychotherapy.

An alternative view is that the primary problem is the weight loss itself. Imagine a ballet dancer, competitive athlete, or other young person who follows a strict diet to lose weight quickly. What might happen? We can model some—of course not all—of the symptoms of anorexia in rats. Force the rats onto a diet of eating for no more than one hour per day, keep them in a cool room, and provide a running wheel. Digesting food generates heat, but within an hour or two after eating, a rat starts to feel cold and reacts by running in the wheel, generating body heat but also burning calories. On this schedule, a rat loses a little weight each day. After losing a fair amount of weight, the rat stops eating even when food is available, and unless the experimenter intervenes, the rat can die of starvation in the presence of food. None of this happens in a warmer room (Cerrato, Carrera, Vazquez, Echevarria, & Gutiérrez, 2012). (Here is another example of temperature regulation influencing behavior in a surprising way!)

So, one hypothesis is that someone who diets to lose weight begins running or other exercise, especially on colder days (Carrera et al., 2012), and as a result loses more and more weight. A treatment based on this idea starts by keeping the person warm, either by wearing a jacket or staying in a warm room. Physical exercise is strictly limited. Then, to overcome the person's fear of overeating and becoming fat, food is put on a special plate connected to a computer that monitors food intake. The person tries to eat at the normal, average pace, with feedback like a video game. Six European clinics tried this approach with 571 patients. Within 13 months, three-fourths were fully recovered, and none had died (Bergh et al., 2013). That success rate is far better than what any other treatment can claim. Certainly, more research is necessary. So far, this approach is not well known in North America.

⊘ **STOP & CHECK** ▬▬▬▬▬▬▬

25. What evidence from rats suggests that bulimia resembles an addiction?

26. If rats are limited to eating for one hour a day, what determines whether or not they will lose weight?

ANSWERS

25. Rats that alternate between food deprivation and a very sweet diet gradually eat more and more, and they react to deprivation of the sweet diet with head shaking and teeth chattering, like the symptoms of morphine withdrawal. 26. If the room is cool and the rats have access to a running wheel, they will exercise enough to keep warm, which is also enough to force them to lose weight.

The Multiple Controls of Hunger

The brain areas that control eating monitor taste, blood glucose, stomach distension, duodenal contents, body weight, fat cells, hormones, social influences, and more. Because the system is so complex, it can produce errors in many ways. However, the complexity of the system also provides a kind of security: If one part of the system makes a mistake, another part can counteract it. We notice people who choose a poor diet or eat the wrong amount, but perhaps we should be even more impressed by how many people eat appropriately. The regulation of eating succeeds not in spite of its complexity but because of it.

Summary

1. The ability to digest a food is one major determinant of preference for that food. For example, people who cannot digest lactose generally do not like to eat dairy products. **304**

2. Widespread beliefs that sugar causes hyperactivity and that turkey causes sleepiness are unfounded. However, research does support the idea that eating fish is good for brain functioning. **304**

3. People and animals eat partly for the sake of taste. However, a sham-feeding animal, which tastes its foods but does not absorb them, eats far more than normal. Taste is not sufficient to satisfy hunger. **305**

4. In addition to taste, other factors controlling hunger include distension of the stomach and intestines, secretion of CCK by the duodenum, and the availability of glucose and other nutrients to the cells. **306**

5. Appetite depends partly on the availability of glucose and other nutrients to the cells. The hormone insulin increases the entry of glucose to the cells, including cells that store nutrients for future use. Glucagon mobilizes stored fuel and converts it to glucose in the blood. Thus, the combined influence of insulin and glucagon determines how much glucose is available at any time. **306**

6. Fat cells produce a peptide called leptin, which provides the brain with a signal about weight loss or gain and therefore corrects day-to-day errors in the amount of feeding. Low levels of leptin increase hunger more effectively than high levels decrease it. **308**

7. The arcuate nucleus of the hypothalamus receives signals of both hunger and satiety. Good-tasting foods and the transmitter ghrelin stimulate neurons that promote hunger. Glucose, insulin, leptin, and CCK stimulate neurons that promote satiety. **309**

8. Axons from the two kinds of neurons in the arcuate nucleus send competing messages to the paraventricular nucleus, releasing neuropeptides that are specific to the feeding system. Cells in the paraventricular nucleus inhibit the lateral nucleus of the hypothalamus. Hunger signals increase feeding by decreasing the inhibition from the paraventricular nucleus. **310**

9. The lateral nucleus of the hypothalamus facilitates feeding by axons that enhance taste responses elsewhere in the brain and increase the release of insulin and digestive juices. **311**

10. The ventromedial nucleus of the hypothalamus and the axons passing by it influence eating by regulating stomach emptying time and insulin secretion. Animals with damage in this area eat more frequently than normal because they store much of each meal as fat and then fail to mobilize their stored fats for current use. **312**

11. Obesity is partly under genetic control. Syndromal obesity occurs if a gene leads to both obesity and other medical problems. Monogenic obesity results from a single gene that does not impair other body functions. Common obesity is influenced by many genes, as well as environmental factors. **314**

12. Dieting is seldom an effective means of long-term weight loss. Reducing consumption of soft drinks is highly recommended. Stomach bypass surgery is an option for relatively severe cases of obesity. **315**

13. Bulimia nervosa is characterized by alternation between undereating and overeating. It has been compared to addictive behaviors. **315**

14. Anorexia nervosa is characterized by refusal to eat enough to maintain a healthy weight. Antidepressant treatments are seldom effective. The increased physical activity associated with anorexia may be motivated by temperature regulation. **316**

Key Terms

Terms are defined in the module on the page number indicated. They're also presented in alphabetical order with definitions in the book's Subject Index/Glossary, which begins on page 589. Interactive flash cards, audio reviews, and crossword puzzles are among the online resources available to help you learn these terms and the concepts they represent.

agouti-related peptide (AgRP) **310**
anorexia nervosa **316**
arcuate nucleus **309**
bulimia nervosa **315**
cholecystokinin (CCK) **306**
duodenum **306**

ghrelin **310**
glucagon **307**
insulin **307**
lactase **304**
lactose **304**
lateral hypothalamus **311**

leptin **308**
melanocortin **310**
neuropeptide Y (NPY) **310**
sham-feeding **306**
vagus nerve **306**
ventromedial hypothalamus (VMH) **312**

Thought Question

For most people, insulin levels tend to be higher during the day than at night. Use this fact to explain why people grow hungry a few hours after a daytime meal but not so quickly at night.

Module 9.3 | End of Module Quiz

1. If someone lacks the gene for digesting lactose, which of these outcomes is likely?
   A. Bulimia nervosa
   B. Increased craving for sweet tastes
   C. Delay in the onset of puberty
   D. Discomfort after drinking milk

2. Which of the following is true?
   A. High intake of sugar leads to hyperactive behavior.
   B. Turkey contains large amounts of chemicals that lead to sleepiness.
   C. Artificial sweeteners help to satisfy a craving for sweet tastes.
   D. Fish oils are beneficial for brain functioning.

3. Which part of the body secretes CCK?
   A. The duodenum
   B. The fat cells
   C. The stomach
   D. The liver

4. When food distends the duodenum, the duodenum releases the hormone CCK. By what *peripheral* mechanism (outside the brain) does it increase satiety?
   A. CCK increases stomach contractions.
   B. CCK tightens the sphincter muscle between the stomach and the duodenum.
   C. CCK increases the ability of nutrients to enter cells.
   D. Cells in the hypothalamus release CCK as a neurotransmitter.

5. Which of these does insulin do?
   A. It helps the intestines digest glucose.
   B. It helps glucose enter cells.
   C. It converts glucose into glutamate.
   D. It converts stored fats into glucose.

6. Which part of the body secretes leptin?
   A. The duodenum
   B. The fat cells
   C. The stomach
   D. The liver

7. Which part of the brain is generally considered the master area for control of appetite?
   A. The hippocampus
   B. The prefrontal cortex
   C. The caudate nucleus
   D. The arcuate nucleus

8. Which part of the body secretes ghrelin?

   A. The duodenum
   B. The fat cells

   C. The stomach
   D. The liver

9. How do taste and ghrelin promote eating and arousal?

   A. They increase excitation from the paraventricular nucleus to the arcuate nucleus, an area that excites the lateral hypothalamus.
   B. They increase inhibition from the paraventricular nucleus to the arcuate nucleus, an area that inhibits the lateral hypothalamus.

   C. They increase excitation from the arcuate nucleus to the paraventricular nucleus, an area that excites the lateral hypothalamus.
   D. They increase inhibition from the arcuate nucleus to the paraventricular nucleus, an area that inhibits the lateral hypothalamus.

10. If researchers could find a safe drug that stimulates melanocortin receptors, what would be the probable benefit?

    A. Improving memory
    B. Helping people go to sleep

    C. Combatting anorexia nervosa
    D. Helping people lose weight

11. Cell bodies in the lateral hypothalamus are most important for which of the following?

    A. Temperature regulation
    B. Sleep

    C. Eating
    D. Satiety

12. How has the prevalence of obesity changed since the availability of high-fructose corn syrup and artificially sweetened diet beverages?

    A. Each of them helped lower the prevalence of obesity.
    B. High-fructose corn syrup helped lower obesity rates, but diet drinks did not.

    C. Diet drinks helped lower obesity rates, but high-fructose corn syrup did not.
    D. The prevalence of obesity has increased after the availability of both of these.

13. Bulimia nervosa has been compared to which of the following?

    A. Borderline personality disorder
    B. Paranoid schizophrenia

    C. Drug addiction
    D. Fear of heights

14. Temperature regulation is a likely explanation for which aspect of anorexia?

    A. Higher prevalence in women than men
    B. Increased exercise

    C. Fear of becoming fat
    D. Age of onset

Answers: 1D, 2D, 3A, 4B, 5B, 6B, 7D, 8C, 9D, 10D, 11C, 12D, 13C, 14B.

Suggestions for Further Reading

Allen, J. S. (2012). *The omnivorous mind: Our evolving relationship with food.* Cambridge, MA: Harvard University Press. A discussion of all the ways eating affects our lives.

Gisolfi, C. V., & Mora, F. (2000). *The hot brain: Survival, temperature, and the human body.* Cambridge, MA: MIT Press. Discusses research on temperature regulation.

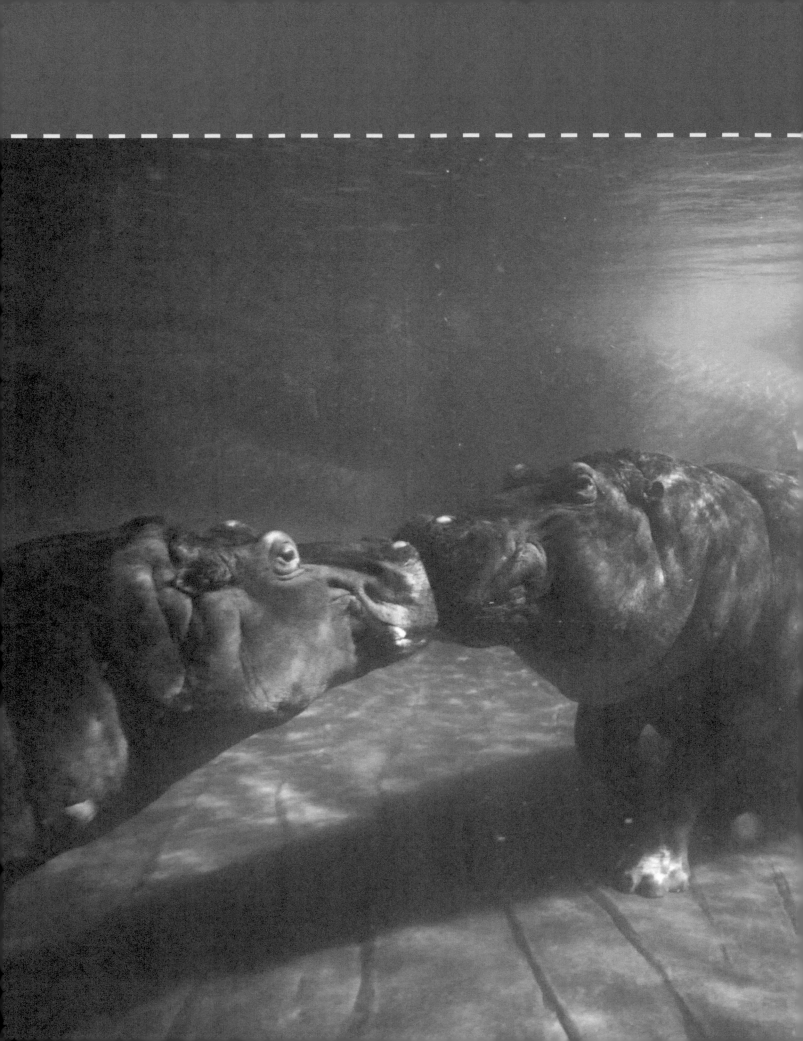

Reproductive Behaviors   Chapter 10

What good is sex? Well, yes, of course: We enjoy it. Presumably we evolved to enjoy it because sexual activity sometimes leads to reproduction, which passes on genes. You evolved from a long line of ancestors who engaged in sexual activity at least once.

But why did we evolve to reproduce sexually instead of individually? In some species of reptiles, a female sometimes reproduces *asexually*—that is, using only her own genes and none from a male (Booth, Johnson, Moore, Schal, & Vargo, 2011). Asexual reproduction would produce offspring exactly like yourself, instead of only half like yourself. What advantage does sex provide?

You might suggest the advantage of having a partner while you rear children. In humans, that kind of cooperation is usually helpful. However, many species reproduce sexually even though the male doesn't help at all with the young, and in some fish species, *neither* sex cares for the young—they just release their sperm and eggs in the same place and then depart.

Biologists' explanation is that sexual reproduction increases variation and thereby enables quick evolutionary adaptations to changes in the environment, especially new viruses and parasites (Morran, Schmidt, Gelarden, Parrish, & Lively, 2011). Certain invertebrates reproduce sexually when they live in a complex and changing environment, but reproduce without sex when they live in a constant environment (Becks & Agrawal, 2010).

Sex also avoids spreading disadvantageous genes. Suppose you have a new helpful mutation and a harmful mutation. If you reproduced asexually, all your offspring would have both the good and the bad mutation. But with sexual reproduction, some will get the good without the bad (McDonald, Rice, & Desai, 2016). Also, if you have a disadvantageous mutation in one gene and your mate has a disadvantageous mutation in a different gene, your children might have a normal copy of both genes (Lumley et al., 2015).

In this chapter, we consider many questions about sexual reproduction that we often ignore or take for granted. We also consider some of the ways in which being biologically male or female influences our behavior.

Learning Objectives

After studying this chapter, you should be able to:

1. Describe the role of the SRY gene in mammalian sexual development.
2. Distinguish between organizing and activating effects of hormones.
3. Explain the role of testosterone in the development of genital anatomy.
4. Explain why brain anatomy differs on average between males and females, and why the degree of masculinization or feminization may vary among brain areas for a given individual.
5. List some examples of activating effects on the behavior of males and females.
6. Describe the roles of hormones and experiences in parental behavior.
7. Discuss and evaluate possible evolutionary explanations of men's and women's sexual behaviors.
8. Explain the relevance of intersexes for understanding the role of hormones in the development of sex-typed behaviors.
9. Discuss possible biological influences on the development of sexual orientation.

Opposite:

Humans may be the only species that plans parenthood, but all species have a strong biological drive that leads to parenthood. (Kevin Schafer/Getty Images)

Sex and Hormones

Being male or female influences many aspects of your life. For humans and other mammals, it all begins with your genes. Females have two X chromosomes, whereas males have an X and a Y chromosome. (The mechanism of sex determination is different for birds, reptiles, and fish.) Biologists used to believe that the chromosomes determine sexual differentiation entirely through hormones. Let's examine that story, and then see how it is incomplete.

Male and female mammals start with the same anatomy during an early stage of prenatal development. Both have a set of **Müllerian ducts** (precursors to female internal structures) and a set of **Wolffian ducts** (precursors to male internal structures), as well as undifferentiated gonads. If you examine an embryo at an early stage of development, you cannot tell whether it is male or female. A little later, a gene on the male's Y chromosome, the **SRY gene** (sex-determining region on the Y chromosome), causes those undifferentiated gonads to develop into **testes,** the sperm-producing organs. The testes produce **androgens** (hormones that are more abundant in males) that increase the growth of the testes, causing them to produce more androgens

and so forth. That positive feedback cannot go on forever, but it continues during early development. Androgens also cause the Wolffian ducts to develop into *seminal vesicles* (saclike structures that store semen) and the *vas deferens* (a duct from the testis into the penis). The testes also produce *Müllerian-inhibiting hormone (MIH)* that causes the Müllerian ducts to degenerate. The final result is the development of a penis and scrotum. Because females do not have the SRY gene, their gonads develop into **ovaries** instead of testes, and their Wolffian ducts degenerate. Because their ovaries do not produce MIH, females' Müllerian ducts develop and mature into oviducts, uterus, and the upper vagina. Figure 10.1 shows how the primitive unisex structures develop into male or female external genitals.

From then on, the males' testes produce more androgens than **estrogens** (hormones that are more abundant in females), whereas the females' ovaries produce more estrogens than androgens. The adrenal glands also produce both androgens and estrogens. These two types of hormones have similar effects in some ways and opposing effects in others. They are **steroid hormones,** containing four carbon rings, as in Figure 10.2.

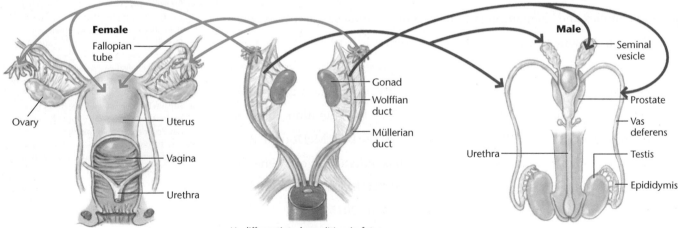

Figure 10.1 Differentiation of human genitals
We begin life with undifferentiated structures, as shown in the center. The gonad of the fetus, shown in blue, develops into either the ovaries, as shown on the left, or the testes, as shown on the right. The Müllerian ducts of the fetus develop into a female's uterus, oviducts, and the upper part of the vagina. The Wolffian ducts of the fetus develop into a male's seminal vesicles (which store semen) and vas deferens, a duct from the testis into the penis. The Müllerian ducts degenerate in males, and the Wolffian ducts degenerate in females.
(Source: Based on Netter, 1983)

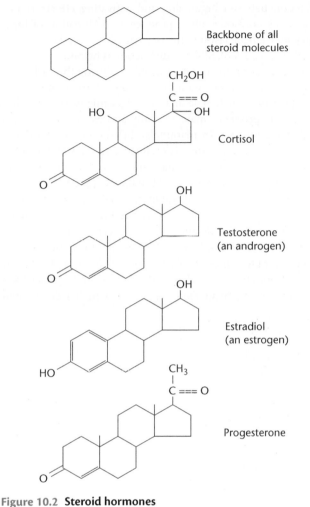

Figure 10.2 **Steroid hormones**
Note the chemical similarity between testosterone and estradiol.

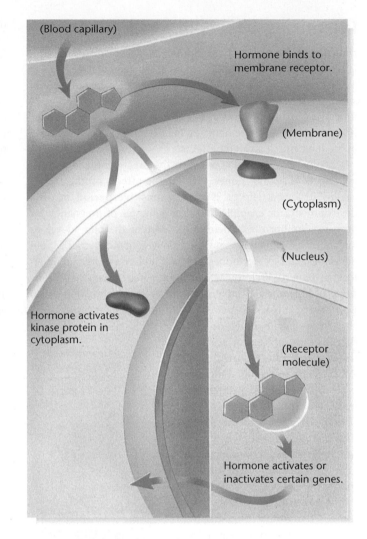

Figure 10.3 **Routes of action for steroid hormones**
Steroid hormones such as estrogens and androgens bind to membrane receptors, activate proteins in the cytoplasm, and activate or inactivate certain genes.
(*Source: Revised from Starr & Taggart, 1989*)

Steroids exert their effects in three ways (Nadal, Díaz, & Valverde, 2001). First, they bind to membrane receptors, like neurotransmitters, exerting rapid effects. Second, they enter cells and activate certain kinds of proteins in the cytoplasm. Third, they bind to receptors that bind to chromosomes, where they activate or inactivate certain genes (see Figure 10.3).

Androgens and estrogens are categories of chemicals; neither androgen nor estrogen is a specific chemical itself. The most widely known androgen is **testosterone.** The most prominent type of estrogen is **estradiol. Progesterone,** another predominantly female hormone, prepares the uterus for the implantation of a fertilized ovum and promotes the maintenance of pregnancy.

For many years, biologists assumed that hormones account for all the biological differences between males and females. Later research demonstrated that the X and Y chromosomes control some differences independently of hormones (Arnold, 2009). At least three genes on the Y chromosome (found only in men) are active in specific brain areas, and at least one gene on the X chromosome is active only in the female brain (Arnold, 2004; Carruth, Reisert, & Arnold, 2002; Vawter et al., 2004). In both humans and nonhumans,

the Y chromosome has many sites that alter the expression of genes on other chromosomes (Lemos, Araripe, & Hartl, 2008). In short, genes on the X and Y chromosomes produce effects beyond those that we can trace to androgens and estrogens.

STOP & CHECK

1. What does the SRY gene do?
2. How do sex hormones affect neurons?

ANSWERS

1. The SRY gene (sex-determining region on the Y chromosome) causes the undifferentiated gonad of a mammal to develop into a testis, which then produces testosterone and MIH to direct development toward the male pattern. 2. Sex hormones, which are steroids, bind to receptors on the membrane, activate certain proteins in the cell's cytoplasm, and activate or inactivate particular genes.

Organizing Effects of Sex Hormones

If we injected estrogens into adult males and androgens into adult females, could we make males act like females or females act like males? The results vary among species, but in general short-term exposure produces no apparent effect and prolonged exposure produces only limited changes in behavior (Henley, Nunez, & Clemens, 2011). Hormones injected early in life have much stronger effects.

Biologists distinguish between the organizing and activating effects of sex hormones. **Organizing effects** produce long-lasting structural effects. During a **sensitive period** in early development, for example, the first trimester of pregnancy for humans, sex hormones determine whether the body develops female or male genitals, and they alter certain aspects of brain development. Sex hormones produce additional organizing effects at puberty (Schulz, Molenda-Figueira, & Sisk, 2009). The surge of hormones at puberty produces breast development in women, facial hair and penis growth in men, changes in voice, and male–female differences in the anatomy of certain parts of the hypothalamus (Ahmed et al., 2008). Some of the differences in brain anatomy between males and females increase during this time (Chung, de Vries, & Swaab, 2002). The changes developing at puberty persist throughout life, even after the concentration of sex hormones declines.

Activating effects are more temporary, continuing only while a hormone is present or shortly beyond. For example, current hormone levels influence the degree of sex drive. The burst of hormones during pregnancy produces temporary effects on emotional arousal, aggressive behavior, learning, and cognition (Agrati, Fernández-Guasti, Ferreño, & Ferreira, 2011; Workman, Barha, & Galea, 2012). Some women experience mood changes over the menstrual cycle (Kiesner, Mendle, Eisenlohr-Moul, & Pastore, 2016). We shall encounter other examples of activating effects later in this chapter. The organizing effects set the stage for activating effects. For example, organizing effects set up the female hypothalamus such that later hormones can activate the menstrual cycle. The

distinction between organizing and activating effects is not absolute, as hormones often produce a combination of temporary and longer-lasting effects (Arnold & Breedlove, 1985; C. L. Williams, 1986). Still, the distinction is helpful.

Let's focus on the organizing effects during the early sensitive period, when hormones determine whether an embryo develops a male or female anatomy. You might imagine that testosterone produces male anatomy and estradiol produces female anatomy. No. In mammals, differentiation of the external genitals depends mainly on testosterone. A high level of testosterone causes the external genitals to develop the male pattern, and a low level leads to the female pattern. Estradiol and certain genes highly activated in females are essential for proper development of a female's uterus and other internal organs, but they have little effect on the external genitals.

The human sensitive period for genital formation occurs during the first trimester of pregnancy (Money & Ehrhardt, 1972). At first, the external genitals of males and females look the same, as shown in Figure 10.4. As a male's developing

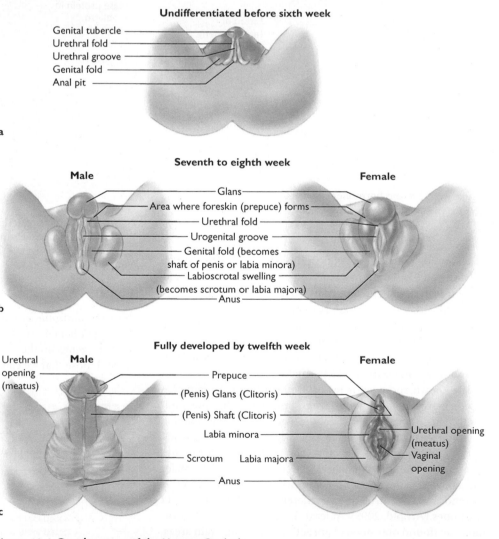

Figure 10.4 Development of the Human Genitals
The initial appearance is the same for all. Depending on the level of testosterone and its metabolite, dihydrotestosterone, the embryo develops either the male pattern or the female pattern.

testes secrete testosterone, certain enzymes convert it to di-hydrotestosterone, which is far more effective at promoting growth of the penis. If levels of dihydrotestosterone are high enough, the tiny genital tubercle grows and develops into a penis. If the levels are low, the tubercle develops into a clitoris. Similarly, depending on levels of testosterone and dihydrotes-tosterone, the embryo develops either a scrotum, characteris-tic of males, or labia, characteristic of females.

Much of the research exploring sexual development has been in rodents. In rats, testosterone begins masculinizing the external genitals during the last several days of pregnancy and first few days after birth and then continues masculin-izing them at a declining rate for the next month (Bloch & Mills, 1995; Bloch, Mills, & Gale, 1995; Davis, Shryne, & Gorski, 1995; Rhees, Shryne, & Gorski, 1990). A female rat that is injected with testosterone during this period is partly masculinized, just as if her own body had produced the tes-tosterone (Ward & Ward, 1985). Her clitoris grows larger than normal, and her behavior is partly masculinized. She approaches sexually receptive females (Woodson & Balleine, 2002), mounts them, and makes copulatory thrusting move-ments rather than arching her back and allowing males to mount her. In short, early testosterone promotes the male pattern and inhibits the female pattern (Gorski, 1985; Wilson, George, & Griffin, 1981).

Injecting a genetic male with estrogens produces little ef-fect on his external anatomy. However, if he lacks androgens or androgen receptors, he develops the female-typical pattern of anatomy and behavior. That outcome could result from castration (removal of the testes), a genetic deficiency of an-drogen receptors, or prenatal exposure to drugs that interfere with androgen response, such as alcohol, marijuana, haloperi-dol (an antipsychotic drug), phthalates (chemicals common in many manufactured products), and cocaine (Ahmed, Shryne, Gorski, Branch, & Taylor, 1991; Dalterio & Bartke, 1979; Hull, Nishita, Bitran, & Dalterio, 1984; Raum, McGivern, Peterson, Shryne, & Gorski, 1990; Swan et al., 2010). Obviously, the amount of interference depends on the type of drug and the amount of exposure. To a slight extent, even aspirin interferes with the male pattern of development (Amateau & McCarthy, 2004). Although estradiol does not significantly alter a male's external anatomy, estradiol and several related compounds do produce abnormalities of the prostate gland—the gland that produces a fluid that accompanies and protects sperm cells when ejaculated during intercourse. Some of those estradiol-like compounds are now prevalent in the linings of plastic bot-tles and cans, so almost everyone is exposed to them (Timms, Howdeshell, Barton, Richter, & vom Saal, 2005). In short, male development is vulnerable to many sources of interference.

Researchers used to say that nature's default setting is to make every mammal a female unless told to do otherwise. Add early testosterone and the individual becomes a male; without testosterone, it develops as a female. That generalization is an overstatement. A genetic female that lacks estradiol during early life develops approximately normal female external anat-omy but does not develop normal sexual behavior or normal

internal anatomy. Even if she is given estradiol injections as an adult, she shows little sexual response toward either male or female partners (Bakker, Honda, Harada, & Balthazart, 2002; Brock, Baum, & Bakker, 2011). So estradiol is essential for fe-male development, including certain aspects of brain differen-tiation, even if it is not important for external anatomy.

STOP & CHECK

3. What would be the external genital appearance of a mammal exposed to high levels of both androgens and estrogens during early development? What if it were exposed to low levels of both?

4. From the standpoint of protecting a male fetus's sexual development, what are some drugs that a pregnant woman should avoid?

ANSWERS

3. A mammal exposed to high levels of both male and female hormones will appear male. One exposed to low levels of both will appear female. External genital devel-opment depends mostly on the presence or absence of androgens, and is nearly independent of estradiol levels. 4. Pregnant women should avoid alcohol, marijuana, haloperidol, phthalates, and cocaine because these drugs interfere with male sexual development. Even aspi-rin and the chemicals lining bottles and cans produce mild abnormalities. Obviously, the results depend on both quantities and timing of exposure to these chemicals.

Sex Differences in the Brain

On average, male and female brains differ in many ways. Sev-eral brain areas form a larger percentage of the male than fe-male brain, whereas other areas constitute a larger portion of the female brain, as Figure 10.5 shows (Cahill, 2006). Most of the brain areas highlighted in that figure have no direct con-nection to reproductive behavior. The brain differences are not simply a result of the fact that men are larger. When re-searchers compare men and women who have the same over-all brain volume, many of the patterns shown in Figure 10.5 still emerge (Luders, Gaser, Narr, & Toga, 2009). In addition to the cortical areas shown in Figure 10.5, males and females differ on average in the hypothalamus, pituitary gland, parts of the spinal cord, and elsewhere. For example, parts of the female hypothalamus generate a cyclic pattern of hormone release, as in the human menstrual cycle, whereas the male hypothalamus releases hormones more steadily.

What causes all these differences? Research, much of it by Margaret McCarthy and her colleagues, has found that the mechanisms differ from one brain area to another. Within the hypothalamus, the differences trace back to sex hormones, but the hormones act in different ways for different areas. Most of the research has used rats, where the sex hormones act in a surprising way. During early development (shortly before birth and the first few days afterward), the blood contains high levels of **alpha-fetoprotein** that binds to circulating estradiol

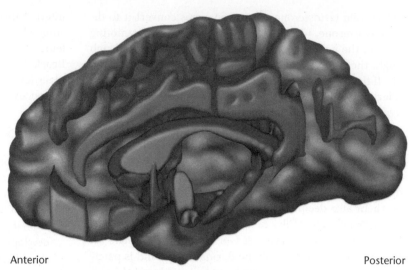

Figure 10.5 Men's and women's brains
Areas in pink are, on the average, larger in women relative to the total mass of the brain. Areas in blue are, on the average, larger in men relative to the total mass.
(*Source: From Cahill, L. (2006). Why sex matters for neuroscience. Nature Reviews Neuroscience, 7, 477–484. Reprinted by permission of Macmillan Publishing Ltd.*)

Anterior   Posterior

and prevents it from entering cells (Gorski, 1980; MacLusky & Naftolin, 1981). Therefore the female brain is not exposed to estradiol at this time. The male's testosterone is free to enter the hypothalamus, where an enzyme converts much of it to estradiol, and the estradiol exerts *masculinizing* effects at this time. That is, for early development in rodents, testosterone is a way of getting estradiol into the hypothalamus. (You're right, that is confusing.)

At any rate, the estradiol acts by different routes in different parts of the hypothalamus. In the medial preoptic area, both testosterone itself and estradiol increase the production of a chemical called prostaglandin E_2, which leads to an increase in microglia, dendritic spines, and synapses (Lenz, Nugent, Haliyur, & McCarthy, 2013; Nugent et al., 2015). These expansions make later male sexual behavior possible. In part of the ventromedial hypothalamus, estradiol activates an enzyme called PI3 kinase that increases the release of glutamate from presynaptic neurons, and therefore causes postsynaptic neurons to increase their dendritic branching (Schwarz, Liang, Thompson, & McCarthy, 2008). The ventromedial hypothalamus contributes to aggressive and sexual behavior as well as feeding. In the arcuate nucleus and the anteroventral periventricular nucleus, estradiol increases GABA production, which acts on astrocytes to *decrease* dendritic spines. The result for males is shrinkage of these areas that are important for female sexual behavior. These areas remain larger in females because of *low* levels of estradiol early in life (McCarthy, 2010; McCarthy & Arnold, 2011). Table 10.1 summarizes these

mechanisms. In humans and other primates, testosterone acts on the hypothalamus directly instead of by conversion to estradiol. However, the final mechanism in terms of prostaglandins, PI3 kinase, and so forth appear to be the same as in rodents.

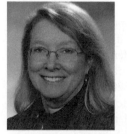

Margaret McCarthy

In the past two decades, the range of neurobiological, psychological, and psychiatric endpoints found to differ between males and females has expanded beyond reproduction into every aspect of the healthy and diseased brain, and thereby demands our attention. (*McCarthy, 2016*)

Now, why is all this important? Because the mechanisms differ from one hypothalamic area to another, it is possible for one area to become more masculinized or more feminized than another. The same is certainly true for the other brain areas, as shown in Figure 10.5. For most brain areas, the male–female differences are less well understood than they are for the hypothalamus, but researchers have established that the mechanisms include not only testosterone and estradiol, but also close to a hundred genes that are more active in one sex or the other (Reinius et al., 2008). Because genes vary, and so do factors that cause epigenetic changes, the "average" brain

Table 10.1 | **Sexual differentiation of the hypothalamus**

Hypothalamic Area	Male–Female Difference	Caused by
Medial preoptic area	More dendritic spines and synapses in males	Testosterone and estradiol increase production of prostaglandin E_2.
Ventromedial nucleus	More widely branched dendrites in males	Estradiol activates PI3 kinase, which increases glutamate release.
Arcuate nucleus and anteroventral periventricular nucleus	More dendritic spines and synapses in females	Estradiol increases GABA production, which acts on astrocytes to decrease dendritic branching.

structure does not apply to any individual. Very few people have a brain that is male-typical or female-typical in all regards. Instead, almost anyone's brain is a mosaic of male-typical, female-typical, and approximately neutral areas (Joel et al., 2015). How all this relates to behavior is mostly uncertain. You may hear someone remark that some difference between male and female brains "explains" why men and women behave differently in some regard. In most cases, the relationship between the brain differences and the behavioral differences is mere speculation (de Vries & Södersten, 2009). Nevertheless, it is certainly true that just as most brains are a mosaic of male-typical and female-typical areas, most people have a mixture of male-typical, female-typical, and neutral interests, attitudes, and activities.

✔ STOP & CHECK

5. How would the external genitals appear on a genetic female rat that lacked alpha-fetoprotein?
6. Why is any individual's brain more masculinized or feminized in some areas than others?

ANSWERS

5. A female that lacked alpha-fetoprotein would be masculinized by her own estradiol, as researchers have in fact demonstrated (Bakker et al., 2006). 6. The mechanisms for sexual differentiation vary from one brain area to another. People vary in the genes, as well as the epigenetic influences, that modify brain development in different brain areas.

Sex Differences in Play

What aspects of behavior might prenatal hormones influence? In the second module of this chapter, we shall consider influences on sexual behavior and sexual orientation, but at this point let's consider possible influences on childhood play.

Typically, many boys play mostly with toy cars and trains, balls, guns, and roughhouse activities. Girls are more likely than boys to spend time with dolls and calmer, cooperative play. Preferences tend to be consistent over time. Children who show the greatest preference for boy-typical activities at age 3 usually show the greatest amount of boy-typical activities at age 13, and those with the greatest preference for

girl-typical activities at 3 usually show the greatest preference for girl-typical activities at age 13 (Golombok, Rust, Zervoulis, Golding, & Hines, 2012).

Much of this pattern results from socialization, as most parents give their sons and daughters different sets of toys. However, socialization need not be the whole story. Indeed, it may be that parents give those toys because previous generations found that boys and girls often differ in their interests from the start. In one study, infants 3 to 8 months old (too young to walk, crawl, or do much with a toy) sat in front of pairs of toys, where researchers could monitor eye movements. The girls looked at dolls more than they looked at toy trucks. The boys looked at both about equally (Alexander, Wilcox, & Woods, 2009). (Note that the children had not seen the trucks move, so at this point the trucks were simply unknown objects.) This study suggests a predisposition for boys and girls to prefer different types of toys, although we should consider an alternative explanation: Girls mature faster than boys, and perhaps it was harder for boys at this age to show a preference, whatever that preference may have been.

In two studies male monkeys played with balls and toy cars more than female monkeys did, whereas the females played more with dolls (Alexander & Hines, 2002; Hassett, Siebert, & Wallen, 2008). Figure 10.6 summarizes the results from one of those studies. Monkeys' preferences were not as strong as most children's, but it is noteworthy that the sexes differed at all in their first encounters with these toys. Other studies found that prenatal injections of testosterone to female monkey fetuses led to increased masculine-type play after they were born. In those cases the focus was on spontaneous, rough-and-tumble play rather than playing with toys, but the idea is similar (Wallen, 2005).

Two studies correlated chemicals in the mother's blood during pregnancy with their children's choices of toys years later. Researchers took blood samples from pregnant women, measuring testosterone, some of which would enter the fetus. When the daughters reached age 3½, researchers observed their toy play. The girls who had been exposed to higher testosterone levels in prenatal life showed slightly elevated preferences for boys' toys (Hines et al., 2002). These girls were anatomically normal, and we have no reason to believe that the parents treated girls differently based on how much testosterone had been present in prenatal life. Another study measured testosterone levels in infants over the first 6 months and

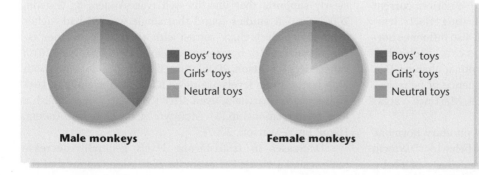

Male monkeys   **Female monkeys**

- Boys' toys
- Girls' toys
- Neutral toys

Figure 10.6 Toy choices by male and female monkeys
Male monkeys spent more time than female monkeys did with "boys' toys."
(*Source: Based on data from "Sex differences in response to children's toys in nonhuman primates (Cercopithecus aethiops sabaeus)," by G. M. Alexander & M. Hines, 2002, Evolution and Human Behavior, 23, 467–479.*)

compared results to their toy choices at age 14 months. Girls with higher testosterone levels in early infancy spent more time than average playing with toy trains, compared to other girls. Boys with higher testosterone levels spent less time than other boys did playing with dolls (Lamminmäki et al., 2012).

In another study, researchers measured phthalate levels in pregnant women. Phthalates inhibit testosterone production. U.S. law bans phthalates from children's toys, but pregnant women are exposed to phthalates from other sources, including perfumes, hair spray, food packaging, and others. Researchers measured phthalate levels in pregnant women's urine samples and compared results to the sons' toy use at ages 3 to 6. On average, sons of women with high phthalate levels showed less interest in typical boys' toys, and more interest in typical girls' toys (Swan et al., 2010). In summary, these studies suggest that prenatal hormones, especially testosterone, alter the brain in ways that influence differences between boys and girls in their activities and interests.

Do these studies imply that prenatal hormones determine toy preferences, regardless of rearing? No. In fact, prenatal hormones and rearing interact in an interesting way. It is possible for girls to develop a condition called *congenital adrenal hyperplasia* (discussed in the next module) as a result of very high testosterone levels before birth. Compared to other girls, they are less likely to imitate what a woman or young girl does, and less likely to be influenced by information that certain things are intended for girls (Hines et al., 2016). That is, the prenatal hormones weaken their tendency to be socialized the way most other girls are.

⊘ STOP & CHECK

7. What evidence most directly links children's toy play to prenatal hormones?
8. What are the effects of phthalates on sexual development?

ANSWERS

7. Girls whose mothers had higher testosterone levels during pregnancy tend to play with boys' toys more than the average for other girls. 8. Phthalates inhibit testosterone production. Boys whose mothers had higher phthalate exposure tend to play with boys' toys less than the average for other boys.

Activating Effects of Sex Hormones

At any time in life, not just during a sensitive period, current levels of testosterone or estradiol exert activating effects, temporarily modifying behavior. Behaviors can also influence hormonal secretions. For example, when doves court each other, each stage of their behavior initiates hormonal changes that alter the birds' readiness for the next sequence of behaviors (Erickson & Lehrman, 1964; Lehrman, 1964; Martinez-Vargas & Erickson, 1973).

In addition to the sex hormones, the pituitary hormone **oxytocin** is also important for reproductive behavior. Oxytocin stimulates contractions of the uterus during delivery of a baby,

and it stimulates the mammary gland to release milk. Sexual pleasure also releases oxytocin, especially at orgasm (Murphy, Checkley, Seckl, & Lightman, 1990). People typically experience a state of relaxation shortly after orgasm as a result of oxytocin release. Oxytocin is apparently responsible for the calmness and lack of anxiety after orgasm (Waldherr & Neumann, 2007).

Males

Testosterone, essential for male sexual arousal, acts partly by increasing touch sensitivity in the penis (Etgen, Chu, Fiber, Karkanias, & Morales, 1999). Sex hormones also bind to receptors that increase responses in parts of the hypothalamus, including the ventromedial nucleus, the medial preoptic area (MPOA), and the anterior hypothalamus.

Testosterone primes the MPOA and several other brain areas to release dopamine. MPOA neurons release dopamine strongly during sexual arousal, and the more dopamine they release, the more likely the male is to copulate (Putnam, Du, Sato, & Hull, 2001). Castrated male rats produce normal amounts of dopamine in the MPOA, but they do not release it in the presence of a receptive female, and they do not attempt to copulate (Hull, Du, Lorrain, & Matuszewich, 1997).

In moderate concentrations, dopamine stimulates mostly type D_1 and D_5 receptors, which facilitate erection of the penis in the male (Hull et al., 1992) and sexually receptive postures in the female (Apostolakis et al., 1996). In higher concentrations, dopamine stimulates type D_2 receptors, which lead to orgasm (Giuliani & Ferrari, 1996; Hull et al., 1992). Whereas dopamine stimulates sexual activity, the neurotransmitter serotonin inhibits it by blocking dopamine release (Hull et al., 1999). Many antidepressant drugs increase serotonin activity, and one of their side effects is decreased sexual arousal.

Levels of testosterone correlate positively with men's sexual arousal and their drive to seek sexual partners. Researchers found that, on average, married men and men living with a woman in a committed relationship have lower testosterone levels than single, unpaired men of the same age (M. McIntyre et al., 2006). Two interpretations are possible: One is that marriage decreases testosterone levels, because of decreased need to compete for a sexual partner. Consistent with this idea, one study found increased testosterone levels around the time of a divorce (Mazur & Michalek, 1998). The other interpretation is that men with lower testosterone levels are more likely than others to marry and remain faithfully married, and research clearly supports that idea as well (van Anders & Watson, 2006). Similar studies found that single women had higher testosterone levels than women with a long-term partner, either homosexual or heterosexual (van Anders & Goldey, 2010; van Anders & Watson, 2006). Also, both men and women with high testosterone levels are more likely than average to seek additional sex partners, even after they marry or establish a long-term relationship (M. McIntyre et al., 2006; van Anders, Hamilton, & Watson, 2007).

Decreases in testosterone levels generally decrease male sexual activity. For example, castration (removal of the testes) generally decreases a man's sexual interest and activity. Anti-androgen drugs can help sex offenders reduce their sexual impulsiveness (Winder et al., 2014). However, low testosterone is not the usual basis for **impotence,** the inability to have an erection. The most common cause is impaired blood circulation, especially in older men. The drug sildenafil (Viagra) increases male sexual ability by prolonging the effects of nitric oxide, which increases blood flow to the penis. (As mentioned in Chapter 2, nitric oxide also increases blood flow in the brain.)

✓ STOP & CHECK

9. By what mechanism does testosterone affect the hypothalamic areas responsible for sexual behavior?

10. What are two explanations for why married men tend to have lower testosterone levels than single men?

ANSWERS

9. Testosterone primes hypothalamic cells to be ready to release dopamine. **10.** First, marriage decreases the need to seek sexual partners and therefore may lower the testosterone level. Second, men with lower testosterone levels are more likely to marry and remain married.

Females

A woman's hypothalamus and pituitary interact with the ovaries to produce the **menstrual cycle,** a periodic variation in hormones and fertility over the course of about 28 days (see Figure 10.7). After the end of a menstrual period, the anterior pituitary releases **follicle-stimulating hormone (FSH),** which promotes the growth of a follicle in the ovary. The follicle nurtures the *ovum* (egg cell) and produces several types of estrogen, including estradiol. Toward the middle of the menstrual cycle, the follicle builds up more and more receptors to FSH, so even though the actual concentration of FSH in the blood is decreasing, its effects on the follicle increase. As a result, the follicle produces increasing amounts of estradiol. The increased release of estradiol causes an increased release of FSH as well as a sudden surge in the release of **luteinizing hormone (LH)** from the anterior pituitary (see the top graph in Figure 10.7). FSH and LH combine to cause the follicle to release an ovum.

The remnant of the follicle (now called the *corpus luteum*) releases the hormone progesterone, which prepares the uterus for the implantation of a fertilized ovum. Progesterone also inhibits the further release of LH. If the woman is pregnant, estradiol and progesterone levels continue to increase. If she is not pregnant, both hormones decline (as shown in Figure 10.7), the lining of the uterus is cast off (menstruation), and the cycle begins again.

One consequence of high estradiol and progesterone levels during pregnancy is fluctuating activity at the serotonin 3 ($5HT_3$) receptor, which is responsible for nausea (Rupprecht

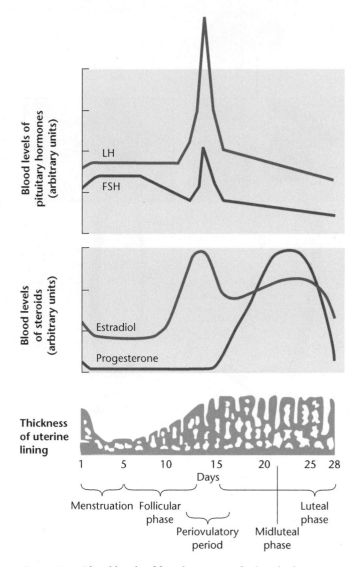

Figure 10.7 Blood levels of four hormones during the human menstrual cycle
Note that estrogen and progesterone are both at high levels during the midluteal phase but drop sharply at menstruation.

et al., 2001). Pregnant women often experience nausea because of the heightened activity of that receptor. Figure 10.8 summarizes the interactions between the pituitary and the ovary. Increased sensitivity to nausea may be an evolved adaptation to minimize the risk of eating something harmful to the fetus.

Birth control pills prevent pregnancy by interfering with the usual feedback cycle between the ovaries and the pituitary. The most widely used birth control pill, the *combination pill,* containing estrogen and progesterone, prevents the surge of FSH and LH that would otherwise release an ovum. The estrogen–progesterone combination also thickens the mucus of the cervix, making it harder for a sperm to reach the egg, and prevents an ovum, if released, from implanting in the uterus. Thus, the pill prevents pregnancy in a combination of

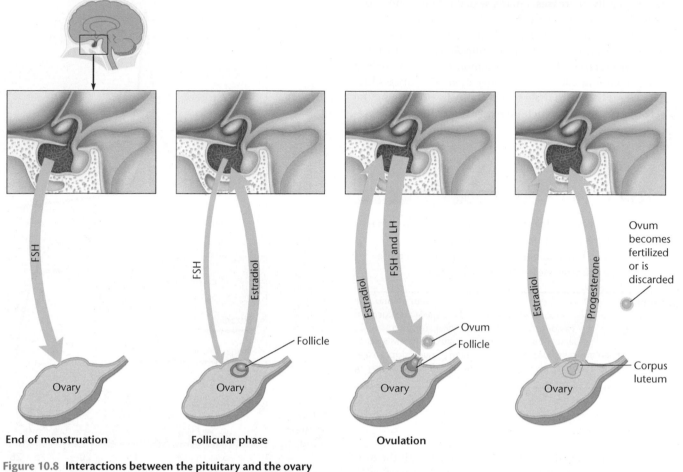

End of menstruation   **Follicular phase**   **Ovulation**

Figure 10.8 Interactions between the pituitary and the ovary
FSH from the pituitary stimulates a follicle of the ovary to develop and produce estradiol, releasing a burst of FSH and LH from the pituitary. Those hormones cause the follicle to release its ovum and become a corpus luteum. The corpus luteum releases progesterone while the ovary releases estradiol.

ways. Note, however, that it does not protect against sexually transmitted diseases such as AIDS or syphilis. "Safe sex" must go beyond the prevention of pregnancy.

In female rats, a combination of estradiol and progesterone is the most effective combination for enhancing sexual behavior (Matuszewich, Lorrain, & Hull, 2000). Estradiol increases the sensitivity of the *pudendal nerve,* which transmits tactile stimulation from the vagina and cervix to the brain (Komisaruk, Adler, & Hutchison, 1972). Estradiol also appears to be essential to female sexual behavior in all the other mammals that have been tested.

Nevertheless, the idea arose that human female sexual desire might depend on testosterone. Much evidence now argues against that idea. Most women report a decrease in sexual desire after menopause, which decreases estradiol levels, or after surgical removal of the ovaries, which also reduces estradiol levels (Graziottin, Koochaki, Rodenberg, & Dennerstein, 2009). Administering enough estradiol to return it to normal levels increases sexual desire. Administering testosterone can increase a woman's sexual desire, but only if administered at levels far above what a woman would experience naturally (Cappelletti & Wallen, 2016). Furthermore, a study comparing women's increases and decreases of sexual interest

from day to day across one or two months found that sexual desire correlated strongly with changes in levels of estradiol, not testosterone (Roney & Simmons, 2013).

One reason why earlier researchers suspected that testosterone was important was that a woman's estradiol levels peak sharply during the **periovulatory period,** the days around the middle of the menstrual cycle, when fertility is highest, but her probability of sexual intercourse does not increase sharply at that time. Testosterone levels, which remain somewhat more stable across the month, might therefore be responsible for desire. However, a woman's probability of sexual intercourse on a given day depends on her partner's desires at least as much as her own. According to two studies, women not taking birth control pills *initiate* sexual activity more often during the periovulatory period than at other times of the month (Adams, Gold, & Burt, 1978; Udry & Morris, 1968) (see Figure 10.9). Also, unmarried women flirt with an appealing man more during this period than at other times (Cantú et al., 2014; Durante & Li, 2009). On average, women during the periovulatory period become more likely than usual to wear red or pink, colors that most men consider sexy (Beall & Tracy, 2013; Eisenbruch, Simmons, & Roney, 2015). In the presence of an attractive man, they are more likely than usual to walk slowly, with a gait

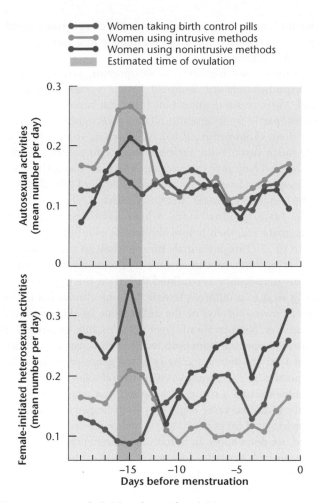

Figure 10.9 Female-initiated sexual activities
The top graph shows autosexual activities (masturbation and sexual fantasies); the bottom graph shows female-initiated activities with a male partner. "Intrusive" birth control methods are diaphragm, foam, and condom; "nonintrusive" methods are IUD and vasectomy. Women other than pill users initiate sex more often when their estrogen levels peak.
(*Source: Adams, Gold, & Burt, 1978*)

Another study used a method that is, shall we say, not common among laboratory researchers. The researchers studied erotic lap dancers, who earn tips by dancing between a man's legs, rubbing up against his groin, while wearing, in most cases, just a bikini bottom. Lap dancers recorded the times of their menstrual periods and the amount of tip income they received each night. Lap dancers who were taking contraceptive pills (which keep hormone levels nearly constant) earned about the same amount from one day to another. Those not taking contraceptive pills received the largest tips during the periovulatory period (Miller, Tybur, & Jordan, 2007). Presumably the women felt and acted sexier at this time.

Effects of Sex Hormones on Nonsexual Characteristics

Men and women differ in many ways other than their sexual behavior. Nearly all those differences vary at least somewhat according to culture, and it is easy to exaggerate the extent of difference (as in "Women are from Venus, Men are from Mars"). Still, a few trends are moderately consistent.

One well-documented gender difference in behavior is that women tend to be better than men at recognizing facial expressions of emotion. Might sex hormones contribute to this difference? One way to approach the question experimentally is to administer extra testosterone to women. In one study, women's task was to examine photos of faces and try to identify the expressed emotions among six choices: anger, disgust, fear, happiness, sadness, and surprise. The photos were morphed from 0 percent (neutral expression) to 100 percent expression of an emotion. Figure 10.10 shows the example for anger. After women received testosterone, most became temporarily less accurate at recognizing facial expressions of anger (van Honk & Schutter, 2007). The implication is that testosterone interferes with attention to emotional expressions. Other studies found that testosterone decreased women's ability to infer people's mood from watching their eyes, whereas estradiol increased men's emotional responses to seeing a person in distress (Olsson, Kopsida, Sorjonen, & Savic, 2016; van Honk et al., 2011).

that men consider sexy (Fink, Hugill, & Lange, 2012; Guéguen, 2012). In short, sexual interest peaks at the periovulatory period and influences behavior in many ways, generally without the woman's conscious recognition of the effect.

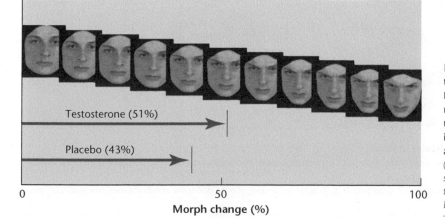

Figure 10.10 Stimuli to measure people's ability to identify emotion
For each of six emotions, researchers prepared views ranging from 0 percent to 100 percent expression of the emotion. In this case, the emotion is anger. Women identified the expression more quickly, on average, after a placebo injection than after a testosterone injection.
(*Source: From "Testosterone reduces conscious detection of signals serving social correction," by J. van Honk & D. J. L. G. Schutter, Psychological Science, 18, 663–667. Used by permission of Blackwell Publishing.*)

✓ STOP & CHECK

11. At what time in a woman's menstrual cycle do her estradiol levels increase? When are they lowest?

12. When is a woman most likely to act sexy and initiate sexual activity?

ANSWERS

11. Estradiol levels increase during the days leading up to the middle of the menstrual cycle. They are lowest during and just after menstruation. 12. During the periovulatory period.

Parental Behavior

Hormonal changes during pregnancy prepare a female mammal to provide milk, and also prepare her to care for the young. Her behavior changes in many ways when she becomes a mother. In addition to nursing and caring for the young, she eats and drinks more than usual, and becomes less fearful and more aggressive, especially in defense of her young. When a mammalian mother delivers her babies, she increases her secretion of oxytocin and prolactin, which promote milk production and several aspects of maternal behavior (Rilling & Young, 2014). Prolactin also inhibits sensitivity to leptin, enabling the mother to eat more than usual.

In addition to secreting hormones, the female changes her pattern of hormone receptors. Late in pregnancy, sensitivity to estradiol increases in the brain areas important for maternal behavior and attention to the young (Rosenblatt, Olufowobi, & Siegel, 1998), including the medial preoptic area, anterior hypothalamus, and nucleus accumbens (Brown, Ye, Bronson, Dikkes, & Greenberg, 1996; Pereira & Ferreira, 2016) (see Figure 10.11). We have already encountered the preoptic area/anterior hypothalamus, or POA/AH, because of its importance for temperature regulation, thirst, and sexual

behavior. The nucleus accumbens plays a central role in feeding. In short, most brain areas participate in a variety of behavioral functions.

Another key hormone is vasopressin, synthesized by the hypothalamus and secreted by the posterior pituitary gland. Vasopressin is important for social behavior in many species, partly by facilitating olfactory recognition of other individuals (Tobin et al., 2010). Male prairie voles, which secrete much vasopressin, establish long-term pair bonds with females and help rear their young. The males with the highest vasopressin levels show the highest level of sexual fidelity to their mates (Okhovat, Berrio, Wallace, Ophir, & Phelps, 2015). Male meadow voles, which have low vasopressin levels, mate and then ignore the female and her young (see Figure 10.12). Imagine a male meadow vole in a long, narrow cage. At one end, he can sit next to a female with which he has just mated. (She is confined there.) At the other end, he can sit next to a different female. Will he choose his recent mate (showing loyalty) or the new female (seeking variety)? The answer: Neither. He sits right in the middle, by himself, as far away as possible from both females. However, researchers found a way to increase activity of the genes responsible for vasopressin in the meadow voles' hypothalamus. Suddenly, the voles showed a strong attachment to a recent mate and, if placed into the same cage, they even helped her take care of her babies (Lim et al., 2004). Whether the female was surprised, we don't know. In humans, researchers have reported that men with genes for less-active forms of the vasopressin receptor are less likely to marry, more likely to have marital conflicts or threat of divorce, and in general less likely to show altruistic behavior toward others (Walum et al., 2008; Wang et al., 2016). Women with the less-active form of the receptor were less attentive to their young children (Avinun, Ebstein, & Knafo, 2012).

Ordinarily, female rats ignore or avoid baby rats, mainly because of an aversion to their odor. When a female gives

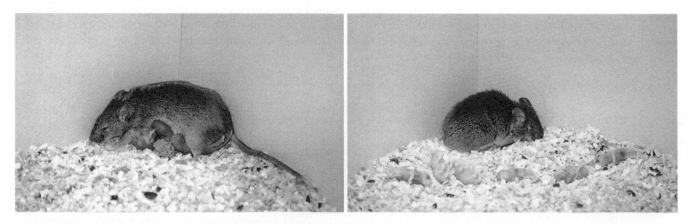

Figure 10.11 Brain development and maternal behavior in mice

The mouse on the left shows normal maternal behavior. The one on the right has a genetic mutation that impairs the development of the preoptic area and anterior hypothalamus.

(Source: Reprinted from Cell, 86/2, Brown, J. R., Ye, H., Bronson, R. T., Dikkes, P., & Greenberg, M. E., "A defect in nurturing in mice lacking the immediate early gene fosB," 297–309, 1996, with permission of Elsevier.)

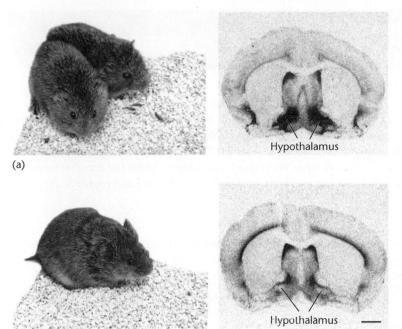

(a)

(b)

Hypothalamus

Hypothalamus

Figure 10.12 **Effects of vasopressin on social and mating behaviors**
Prairie voles (top) form long-term pair bonds. Staining of their brain shows much expression of the hormone vasopressin in the hypothalamus. A closely related species, meadow voles (bottom), show no social attachments. Their brains have lower vasopressin levels, as indicated by less staining in the hypothalamus.
(Source: Reprinted with permission from "Enhanced partner preference in a promiscuous species by manipulating the expression of a single gene," by Lim, M. M., Wang, Z., Olazabal, D. E., Ren, X., Terwillinger, E. F., & Young, L. J., Nature, 429, 754–757. Copyright 2004 Nature Publishing Group/Macmillan Magazines Ltd.)

birth, the delivery causes a change in her brain that makes the infants' odor more appealing (Lévy, Keller, & Poindron, 2004). However, suppose an experimenter leaves a female rat that has never been pregnant with some baby rats. Because they cannot survive without the care that she fails to provide, the experimenter periodically replaces them with new, healthy babies. Over a few days, the female gradually becomes more attentive, builds a nest, assembles the babies in the nest, licks them, and does everything else that normal mothers do, except nurse them. (Without giving birth, she does not secrete the prolactin and oxytocin necessary for milk production.) This experience-dependent behavior does not require hormonal changes and occurs even in females that had their ovaries removed (Mayer & Rosenblatt, 1979; Rosenblatt, 1967). It occurs even in males, despite the fact that male rats ordinarily do not participate in care for the young. In nature, they would not remain close enough to the mother or her young to develop this effect. You might think this process is just a laboratory curiosity, but it is important in nature. Although hormonal changes trigger the early stage of maternal care, the hormones start to decline a few days later. By that time, the experience of being with the young triggers the same types of maternal behavior, and the same types of brain activity, that the early hormones did (Rosenblatt, 1970; Stolzenberg & Champagne, 2016).

In humans, the hormonal changes during pregnancy and delivery enable a mother to produce milk. Brain scans also show growth of several areas in her brain from early to late pregnancy and then delivery, especially in areas responsible for reward and motivation. The amount of expansion in those areas correlates with the positive emotions a woman expresses about having a baby (Kim, Strathearn, & Swain, 2016). Overall,

however, human parental behavior is experience-dependent more than hormone-dependent.

Several studies show a correlation between fathers' hormones and their behavior toward their infants and toddlers. On average, a man's testosterone level declines and his prolactin level increases when a baby is born, but only if the man has a close relationship with the mother, and only in societies where men contribute to infant care (Edelstein et al., 2015; Storey & Ziegler, 2016). On average, men with lower testosterone levels and higher prolactin levels spend more time playing with and caring for their children (Gordon, Zagoory-Sharon, Leckman, & Feldman, 2010; Mascaro, Hackett, & Rilling, 2013). Because these are correlational data, we do not know to what extent the hormones are the cause of the men's behavior, and to what extent they are the result.

✅ STOP & CHECK

13. What factors are responsible for maternal behavior shortly after rats give birth? What factors become more important in later days?

ANSWER

13. The early stage of rats' maternal behavior depends on a surge in the release of the hormones prolactin and estradiol. A few days later, her experience with the young decreases the responses that would tend to make her reject them. Experience with the young maintains maternal behavior after the hormone levels begin to drop.

Module 10.1 | In Closing

Reproductive Behaviors and Motivations

A mother rat licks her babies all over shortly after their birth, and that stimulation is essential for their survival. Why does she do it? Presumably, she does not understand that licking will help them. She licks because they are covered with a salty fluid that tastes good to her. If she has access to other salty fluids, she stops licking her young (Gubernick & Alberts, 1983).

Analogously, sexual behavior in general serves the function of passing on our genes, but we engage in sexual behavior just because it feels good. We evolved a tendency to enjoy the sex act. The same principle holds for hunger, thirst, and other motivations: We evolved tendencies to enjoy the acts that increased our ancestors' probability of surviving and reproducing.

Summary

1. Male and female behaviors differ because of sex hormones that activate particular genes. Also, certain genes on the X and Y chromosomes exert direct effects on brain development. **322**

2. Organizing effects of a hormone, exerted during a sensitive period, produce relatively permanent alterations in anatomy and physiology. **324**

3. In the absence of sex hormones, an infant mammal develops female-looking external genitals. The addition of testosterone shifts development toward the male pattern. Extra estradiol, within normal limits, does not determine whether the individual looks male or female. However, estradiol is essential for normal development of a female's internal anatomy. **324**

4. Many brain areas differ on average between males and females. The mechanisms behind these differences vary from one area to another. Consequently a given individual's brain areas have a mosaic of male-typical, female-typical, and neutral anatomy. **325**

5. In adulthood, sex hormones activate sex behaviors, partly by facilitating activity in the medial preoptic area and anterior hypothalamus. **328**

6. A woman's menstrual cycle depends on a feedback cycle that controls the release of several hormones. Although women can respond sexually at any time in their cycle, on average, their sexual desire is greatest during the fertile period of the menstrual cycle, when estradiol levels are high. **329**

7. Sex hormones also influence behaviors not directly related to sexual reproduction, such as the ability to recognize emotional expressions. **331**

8. Hormones released around the time of giving birth facilitate maternal behavior in females of many mammalian species. Prolonged exposure to young also induces parental behavior. In humans, the hormonal changes during pregnancy and delivery enable a woman to produce milk. Testosterone levels decline around the time of birth for many fathers, and those with lower testosterone levels tend to participate more in infant care. **332**

Key Terms

Terms are defined in the module on the page number indicated. They're also presented in alphabetical order with definitions in the book's Subject Index/Glossary, which begins on page 589. Interactive flash cards, audio reviews, and crossword puzzles are among the online resources available to help you learn these terms and the concepts they represent.

activating effects **324**

alpha-fetoprotein **325**

androgens **322**

estradiol **323**

estrogens **322**

follicle-stimulating hormone (FSH) **329**

impotence **329**

luteinizing hormone (LH) **329**

menstrual cycle **329**

Müllerian ducts **322**

organizing effects **324**

ovaries **322**

oxytocin **328**

periovulatory period **330**

progesterone **323**

sensitive period **324**

SRY gene **322**

steroid hormones **322**

testes **322**

testosterone **323**

Wolffian ducts **322**

Thought Questions

1. The pill RU-486 produces abortions by blocking the effects of progesterone. Why would blocking progesterone interfere with pregnancy?

2. The presence or absence of testosterone determines whether a mammal will differentiate as a male or a female. In birds, the story is the opposite: The presence

or absence of estrogen is critical (Adkins & Adler, 1972). What problems would sex determination by estrogen create if that were the mechanism for mammals? Why do those problems not arise in birds? (Hint: Think about the difference between live birth and hatching from an egg.)

3. Antipsychotic drugs, such as haloperidol and chlorpromazine, block activity at dopamine synapses. What side effects might they have on sexual behavior?

Module 10.1 | End of Module Quiz

1. What does the *SRY* gene do?
   A. It increases mammalian parental behavior.
   B. It controls the production of prolactin.
   C. It causes a mammalian embryo to develop into a female.
   D. It causes a mammalian embryo to develop into a male.

2. Why is it impossible to have both a penis and a clitoris?
   A. Either one develops from the same embryonic structure.
   B. The production of testosterone interferes with production of estradiol.
   C. Forming a clitoris requires having two X chromosomes.
   D. The developing embryo would not have enough fuel to develop both structures.

3. What is the main difference between organizing effects and activating effects of hormones?
   A. Organizing effects are long-lasting, whereas activating effects are temporary.
   B. Organizing effects alter brain activity, whereas activating effects alter other parts of the body.
   C. Organizing effects are excitatory, whereas activating effects are inhibitory.
   D. Organizing effects depend on estrogens, whereas activating effects depend on androgens.

4. What causes an embryo to develop female external genitals?
   A. A high ratio of estradiol to testosterone
   B. A high level of estradiol, regardless of testosterone
   C. A high level of both estradiol and testosterone
   D. A low level of testosterone, regardless of estradiol

5. How does sexual differentiation of the brain differ between rodents and primates?
   A. In rodents it depends on the level of testosterone. In primates it depends on the level of estradiol.
   B. In rodents it depends on the level of estradiol. In primates it depends on oxytocin.
   C. In rodents, testosterone must be aromatized to estradiol before it affects developing neurons.
   D. In primates, testosterone must be aromatized to estradiol before it affects developing neurons.

6. Which of these is true about sex differences in brain anatomy?
   A. On average, males and females have the same anatomy for all brain areas.
   B. Wherever males and females differ in brain anatomy, testosterone is responsible.
   C. Wherever males and females differ in brain anatomy, a gene on the Y chromosome is responsible.
   D. The mechanisms of sexual differentiation vary from one area to another.

7. Prenatal exposure to higher than average levels of testosterone produces what effect, if any, on girls?
   A. It leads to earlier than average onset of puberty.
   B. It leads to lower than average intelligence.
   C. It leads to higher than average interest in boys' toys and activities.
   D. It produces no noticeable effect.

8. When an antidepressant drug increases serotonin levels, which inhibits dopamine release, what happens to sexual behavior?
   A. Indiscriminate approach to both male and female partners
   B. Increased sexual arousal
   C. Decreased sexual arousal
   D. Prolonged orgasm

9. Compared to other men, what are the testosterone levels of married men?
   A. Lower than average
   B. About the same as average
   C. Higher than average

10. What does the combination pill for birth control contain?

   A. Estradiol and testosterone
   B. Testosterone and insulin

   C. Estradiol and progesterone
   D. Oxytocin and vasopressin

11. Female sex drive depends on which hormone or hormones?

   A. Estradiol
   B. Testosterone

   C. Estradiol and testosterone equally
   D. Oxytocin

12. Vasopressin increases male mammals' probability of which behavior?

   A. Homosexuality
   B. Sleep

   C. Care for young
   D. Attack

Answers: 1D, 2A, 3A, 4D, 5C, 6D, 7C, 8C, 9A, 10C, 11A, 12C.

Variations in Sexual Behavior

People vary in their frequency of sexual activity, preferred types of sexual activity, and sexual orientation. In this module, we explore some of that diversity, but first we consider a few differences between men and women in general. Do men's and women's mating behaviors make biological sense? If so, should we interpret these behaviors as products of evolution? These questions are difficult and controversial.

Evolutionary Interpretations of Mating Behavior

Part of Charles Darwin's theory of evolution by natural selection was that individuals whose genes help them survive will produce more offspring, and therefore the next generation will resemble those with these favorable genes. A second part of his theory, not so widely accepted at first, was **sexual selection**: Genes that make an individual more appealing to the other sex will increase the probability of reproduction, and therefore the next generation will resemble those with such genes.

Sexual selection can go only so far, however, if it starts to interfere with survival. A male deer with large antlers attracts females, but being impressive wouldn't help if the weight interfered with his movement. A bird's bright colors attract potential mates, but they also run the risk of attracting a predator's attention. In many bird species, the male is brightly colored, but the female is not, presumably because she sits on the nest and needs to be less conspicuous. In a few species, such as phalaropes, the female is more brightly colored, but in those species, the female lays the egg and deserts it, leaving the dull-colored male to sit on the nest. In species where the male and female share the nesting duties, such as pigeons and doves, the male and female look alike, and neither is especially gaudy.

In humans, too, some of the differences between men and women may be results of sexual selection. That is, to some extent women evolved based on what appeals to men, and men evolved based on what appeals to women. Certain aspects of behavior may also reflect evolutionary pressures for men and women. Evolutionary psychologists cite several possible examples, although each has been controversial (Buss, 2000). Let's examine examples.

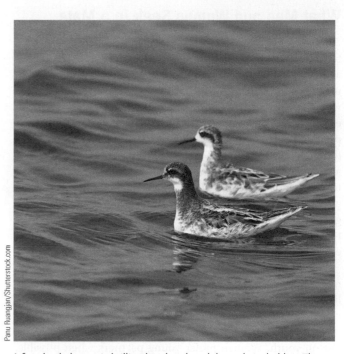

A female phalarope is brilliantly colored, and the male is drabber. The female lays eggs and deserts the nest, leaving the male to attend to it.

Interest in Multiple Mates

Across cultures, more men than women seek opportunities for casual sexual relationships with many partners. Why? From the evolutionary standpoint of spreading one's genes, men can succeed by either of two strategies (Gangestad & Simpson, 2000): Be loyal to one woman and devote your energies to helping her and her babies, or mate with many women and hope that some of them can raise your babies without your help. No one needs to be conscious of these strategies, of course. The idea is that men in the past who acted in either of these ways propagated their genes, and today's men have inherited genes that promote these behaviors. In contrast, a woman can have no more than one pregnancy per 9 months, regardless of her number of sex partners. So evolution may have predisposed men, or at least some men, to be more interested in multiple mates than women are.

337

One objection is that a woman does sometimes gain from having multiple sex partners (Hrdy, 2000). If her husband is infertile, then mating with another man could be her only way of reproducing. Also, another sexual partner may provide aid of various sorts to her and her children. In addition, she has the possibility of "trading up," abandoning her first mate for a better one. So the prospect of multiple mates may be more appealing to men, but it has advantages for women, too.

Another objection is that researchers have no direct evidence that genes influence people's preferences for one mate or many. We shall return to this issue later.

What Men and Women Seek in a Mate

Almost all people prefer a romantic partner who is healthy, intelligent, honest, and physically attractive. Often, women have additional interests that are less common for men. In particular, women are more likely than men are to prefer a mate who is likely to be a good provider (Buss, 2000). According to evolutionary theorists, the reason is this: While a woman is pregnant or taking care of a small child, she needs help getting food and other requirements. Evolution would have favored any gene that caused women to seek good providers. Related to this tendency, most women tend to be cautious during courtship. Even if a man seems interested in her, a woman is generally slow to conclude that he has a strong commitment to her (Buss, 2001). She would not want a man who acts interested and then leaves when she needs him.

Men tend to have a stronger preference for a young partner. An evolutionary explanation is that young women are likely to remain fertile longer than older women are, so a man can have more children by pairing with a young woman. Men remain fertile into old age, so a woman has less need to insist on youth. Women prefer young partners when possible, but in many societies, only older men have enough financial resources.

Are these preferences rooted in genetics? Perhaps, but the variation from culture to culture suggests a strong learned component. In countries where women have good educational, economic, and employment opportunities, a woman is more likely to choose a partner close to her own age, and less likely to choose based on wealth (Zentner & Mitura, 2012).

Differences in Jealousy

Traditionally, in nearly all cultures, men have been more jealous of a wife's possible infidelity than women have been of a husband's infidelity. From an evolutionary standpoint, why? If a man is to pass on his genes—the key point in evolution—he needs to be sure that the children he supports are his own. An unfaithful wife threatens that certainty. A woman knows that any children she bears are her own, so she does not have the same worry. (She might, however, worry that her husband might start supporting some other woman's children, instead of her own children.) The degree of jealousy varies among cultures. Some cultures tolerate sexual infidelity by husbands, and some do not, and the intensity of prohibition against

wives' infidelity varies. However, no known society considers infidelity more acceptable for women than for men.

Which would upset you more: if your partner had a brief sexual affair with someone else, or if he or she became emotionally close to someone else? In general, men tend to be more jealous about sexual infidelity than women are, whereas women tend to be more jealous about emotional infidelity. However, these differences are small, and they vary depending on the procedure and the population tested (Carpenter, 2012; Sagarin et al., 2012). Both men and women are upset about either sexual or emotional infidelity.

Evolved or Learned?

In many species of mammals and birds, a male defends his sexual access to one or more females and attacks any other approaching male. Meanwhile, the female shows little or no response if her male sexually approaches some other female. In such cases an interpretation in terms of evolutionary selection is generally noncontroversial. However, the interpretation is less clear for our own species. One reason is that when someone argues that evolutionary selection led men to be interested in multiple sex partners or to be more jealous than women are, it may sound like a justification for men to act that way. (It is not. Even if we have a biological predisposition to act a certain way, it does not force us to do so. Civilization requires us to override many selfish impulses.) But even if we leave aside the ethical implications, the scientific data are not conclusive on how much of our sexual behavior is evolutionarily guided and how much is learned. Mating customs show some similarities across cultures, but also important differences. Yes, of course our behavioral tendencies are a product of evolution. But it is not clear that evolution micromanages our behavior, down to such details as whether to look for a mate with high earning potential or how jealous to be of an unfaithful mate.

STOP & CHECK

14. What evolutionary advantage is suggested for why women are more interested in men's wealth and success than men are interested in women's wealth?

ANSWER

14. During pregnancy and early child care, a female is limited in her ability to get food and therefore prefers a male partner who can provide for her. A healthy male is not similarly dependent on a female.

Gender Identity and Gender-Differentiated Behaviors

Many fish can change between male and female. For fish, sexual identity is more fluid than it is for us. (Please excuse the bad pun.) In the animated film *Finding Nemo*, after Nemo's mother died, in reality the clown fish father would have changed into a female at that point. However, the biologist who advised the film producers agreed that scientific accuracy on this point would have been more confusing to children than helpful (Cressey, 2016)!

People do not have the same flexibility as fish, but we do have variations in sexual development. Let us specify from the start: "Different" does not mean "wrong." People differ naturally in their sexual development just as they do in anything else.

Gender identity is what we consider ourselves to be. The biological differences between males and females are *sex differences*, whereas the differences that result from people's regarding themselves as male or female are *gender differences.* To maintain this useful distinction, we should resist the trend to speak of the "gender" of fish, fruit flies, and so forth. Gender identity is a human characteristic.

Most people accept the gender identity that matches their external appearance, which also matches the way they were reared, but some do not. Psychologists used to assume that gender identity depends mainly or entirely on the way people rear their children. However, several kinds of evidence suggest that biological factors, especially prenatal hormones, are important also.

Intersexes

A **hermaphrodite** (from Hermes and Aphrodite in Greek mythology) has anatomy intermediate between male and female, or shows a mixture of male and female anatomies (Haqq & Donahoe, 1998). A *true hermaphrodite* has some testicular tissue and some ovarian tissue. One way for this to happen is for a woman to release two ova, each fertilized by a different sperm, which then fuse instead of becoming twins. If one of the fertilized ova had an XX chromosome pattern and the other had XY, the resulting child has some XX cells and some XY cells. True hermaphrodites are rare for humans, and except for those rare cases, the term should be avoided.

More commonly, some people develop an intermediate appearance because of an atypical hormone pattern. Recall that testosterone masculinizes the genitals and the hypothalamus during early development. A genetic male with low levels of testosterone or a deficiency of testosterone receptors may develop a female or intermediate appearance (Misrahi et al., 1997). A genetic female who is exposed to more testosterone than the average female can be partly masculinized.

The most common cause of this condition is **congenital adrenal hyperplasia (CAH)**, meaning overdevelopment of the adrenal glands from birth. Ordinarily, the adrenal gland has a negative feedback relationship with the pituitary gland. The pituitary secretes adrenocorticotropic hormone (ACTH), which stimulates the adrenal gland. Cortisol, one of the hormones from the adrenal gland, feeds back to decrease the release of ACTH. Some people have a genetic limitation in their ability to produce cortisol. Because the pituitary fails to receive much cortisol as a feedback signal, it continues secreting more ACTH, causing the

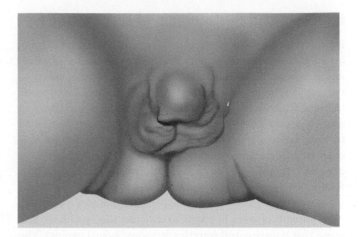

Figure 10.13 External genitals of a genetic female, age 3 months
The genitals were masculinized by excess androgens from the adrenal gland before birth.

adrenal gland to secrete more and more of its other hormones, including testosterone. In a genetic male, the extra testosterone causes little effect. However, genetic females with this condition develop various degrees of masculinization of their external genitals. (The ovaries and other internal organs are less affected.) Figure 10.13 shows an example. After birth, these children are given medical treatments to bring their adrenal hormones within normal levels. Some are also given surgery to alter their external genital appearance, as we shall discuss later.

A person whose sexual development is intermediate, as in Figure 10.13, is called an **intersex.** An alternative is to use the term *differences of sexual development.* How common are intersexes? An estimated 1 child in 100 in the United States is born with some degree of genital ambiguity, and 1 in 2000 has enough ambiguity to make its male or female status uncertain (Blackless et al., 2000). However, the accuracy of these estimates is doubtful, as hospitals and families keep the information private. Maintaining confidentiality is of course important, but an unfortunate consequence is that intersexed people have trouble finding others like themselves. For more information, consult the website of the Intersex Society of North America (ISNA).

⊘ **STOP & CHECK** ▬▬▬▬▬

15. What is a common cause for a genetic female (XX) to develop a partly masculinized anatomy?

ANSWER

15. If a genetic female is genetically deficient in her ability to produce cortisol, the pituitary gland does not receive negative feedback signals and therefore continues stimulating the adrenal gland. The adrenal gland then produces large amounts of its other hormones, including testosterone, which masculinizes development.

Interests and Preferences of Girls with CAH

For many years, the policy was to raise most intersexes as girls, on the assumption that surgery could make them look like normal girls, and they would develop behaviors corresponding to the way they were reared. However, their brains were exposed to higher than normal testosterone levels during prenatal and early postnatal life compared to other girls. What happened to their behavior? As discussed in the first module of this chapter, prenatal levels of testosterone correlate with girls' toy choices. The same idea applies here. In several studies, girls with CAH were observed in a room full of toys—including some that were girl typical (dolls, plates and dishes, cosmetics kits), some that were boy typical (toy car, tool set, gun), and some that were neutral (puzzles, crayons, board games). The girls with CAH played with boys' toys more than most other girls did, but less than the average for boys (Pasterski et al., 2005, 2011). When the children tested with a parent present, again the girls with CAH were intermediate between the other two groups. Other studies found that the girls exposed to the largest amount of testosterone in early development showed the largest preference for boys' toys (Berenbaum, Duck, & Bryk, 2000; Nordenström, Servin, Bohlin, Larsson, & Wedell, 2002). You might wonder whether the parents, knowing that these girls had been partly masculinized in appearance, might have encouraged tomboyish activities. Observations of the parents showed that they generally encouraged the girls to play with whatever they wanted to play with (Wong, Pasterski, Hindmarsh, Geffner, & Hines, 2013). On average, girls with CAH also perform slightly better than most other girls on spatial and mechanical skills, on which boys generally do better than girls (Berenbaum, Bryk, & Beltz, 2012; Hampson & Rovet, 2015). It is uncertain how much the variation in these skills reflects abilities and how much it reflects interests (Feng, Spence, & Pratt, 2007; Tarampi, Heydari, & Hegarty, 2016).

A study of girls with CAH in adolescence found that, on average, their interests are intermediate between those of typical male and female adolescents. For example, they read more sports magazines and fewer style and glamour magazines than the average for other teenage girls (Berenbaum, 1999). In adulthood, they show more physical aggression than most other women do, and less interest in infants (Mathews, Fane, Conway, Brook, & Hines, 2009). They are more interested in rough sports and more likely than average to be in heavily male-dominated occupations such as auto mechanic and truck driver (Frisén et al., 2009). Nevertheless, most continue to identify as female (Meyer-Bahlburg et al., 2016). Together, the results imply that prenatal and early postnatal hormones influence people's interests as well as their physical development.

Testicular Feminization

Certain individuals with an XY chromosome pattern produce normal amounts of androgens, including testosterone, but lack the receptor that enables those chemicals to activate genes in a cell's nucleus. Consequently, the cells do not respond to androgens. This condition, known as **androgen insensitivity** or **testicular feminization**, occurs in various degrees resulting in anatomy that ranges from a smaller than average penis to genitals like those of a typical female, in which case no one has any reason to suspect the person is anything other than female, until puberty. Then, although her breasts develop and hips broaden, she does not menstruate, because her body has internal testes instead of ovaries and a uterus. The vagina is short and leads to nothing but skin. Also, pubic hair is sparse or absent, because it depends on androgens in females as well as males. Psychologically, she develops as a typical female.

STOP & CHECK

16. If a genetic female is exposed to extra testosterone during prenatal development, what behavioral effect is likely?
17. What would cause a genetic male (XY) to develop a partly feminized external anatomy?

ANSWERS

16. A girl who is exposed to extra testosterone during prenatal development is more likely than most other girls to prefer boy-typical activities. 17. A genetic male with a gene that prevents testosterone from binding to its receptors will develop an appearance that partly or completely resembles a female.

Issues of Gender Assignment and Rearing

Girls with CAH and related conditions are born with appearances ranging from almost typical female to something intermediate between female and male. Some genetic males are born with a very small penis because of a condition called *cloacal exstrophy*, a defect of pelvis development (Reiner & Gearhart, 2004). Despite their genital anatomy, they had typical male levels of testosterone in prenatal development.

How should children with either of these conditions be reared? Beginning in the 1950s, medical doctors began recommending that anyone with an intermediate or ambiguous genital appearance should be reared as a girl, using surgery if necessary to make the genitals look more feminine (Dreger, 1998). The reason was that it is easier to reduce an enlarged clitoris to normal female size than expand it to penis size. If necessary, surgeons can build an artificial vagina or lengthen a short one. After the surgery, the child looks female. Physicians and psychologists assumed that any child who was consistently reared as a girl would fully accept that identity.

And she lives happily ever after, right? Not necessarily. Of the males with cloacal exstrophy who are reared as girls, all develop typical male interests, many or most eventually demand reassignment as males, and nearly all develop sexual attraction toward women, not men (Reiner & Gearhart, 2004).

Girls with the CAH history also have a difficult sexual adjustment, especially if they were subjected to clitoris-reduction surgery. A surgically created or lengthened vagina may be satisfactory to a male partner, but it provides no sensation to the woman and requires frequent attention to prevent it from scarring over. Many such women have urinary incontinence and significant sexual difficulties, including lack of orgasm. Many report no sexual partner ever and little pleasure in sex (Frisén et al., 2009; Meyer-Bahlburg, Dolezal, Baker, & New, 2008; Minto, Liao, Woodhouse, Ransley, & Creighton, 2003; Nordenström et al., 2010; van der Zwan et al., 2013; Zucker et al., 1996). In one study, 25 percent said they had never had a love relationship of any type (Jürgensen et al., 2013).

Many intersexes wish they had their original enlarged clitoris instead of the mutilated, insensitive structure left to them by a surgeon. Moreover, intersexes resent being deceived. Historian Alice Dreger (1998) describes the case of one intersex:

> As a young person, [she] was told she had "twisted ovaries" that had to be removed; in fact, her testes were removed. At the age of twenty, "alone and scared in the stacks of a [medical] library," she discovered the truth of her condition. Then "the pieces finally fit together. But what fell apart was my relationship with both my family and physicians. It was not learning about chromosomes or testes that caused enduring trauma, it was discovering that I had been told lies. I avoided all medical care for the next 18 years. . . . [The] greatest source of anxiety is not our gonads or karyotype. It is shame and fear resulting from an environment in which our condition is so unacceptable that caretakers lie." (p. 192)

How *should* such a child be reared? A growing number of specialists follow these recommendations:

- Be completely honest with the intersexed person and the family, and do nothing without their informed consent.
- Identify the child as male or female based mainly on the predominant external appearance. That is, there should be no bias toward calling every intersex a female. Those born with masculinized external genitals seldom make a successful adaptation to a female gender assignment (Houk & Lee, 2010).
- Rear the child as consistently as possible, but be prepared that the person might later be sexually oriented toward males, females, both, or neither.
- Do *not* perform genital surgery on a child. Such surgery impairs the person's erotic sensation and is at best premature, as no one knows how the child's sexual orientation will develop. If the intersexed person makes an informed request for such surgery in adulthood, then it is appropriate, but otherwise it should be avoided. (Diamond & Sigmundson, 1997)

Discrepancies of Sexual Appearance

To resolve the roles of rearing and hormones in determining gender identity, the most decisive observation would come from rearing a normal male baby as a female or rearing a normal female baby as a male. If the resulting adult fully accepts the assigned role, we would know that upbringing determines gender identity. Although no one would perform such an experiment intentionally, we can learn from accidental events. In some cases, someone was exposed to a more-or-less normal pattern of male hormones before and shortly after birth but then reared as a girl.

One type of case was reported first in the Dominican Republic and then in other places, usually in communities with much inbreeding. In each case, certain genetic males fail to produce 5α-*reductase 2,* an enzyme that converts testosterone to *dihydrotestosterone.* Dihydrotestosterone is more effective than testosterone for masculinizing the external genitals. At birth, these individuals appear to be female, although some have a swollen clitoris and somewhat "lumpy" labia. Although they are considered girls and reared as such, their brains had been exposed to male levels of testosterone during early development. At puberty, the testosterone levels increase sharply, and even without conversion to dihydrotestosterone, the result is growth of a penis and scrotum, enough to be clearly male.

Women: Imagine that at about age 12 years, your external genitals suddenly changed from female to male. Would you say, "Okay, I guess I'm a boy now"? Most of these people reacted exactly that way. The girl-turned-boy developed a male gender identity and directed his sexual interest toward females (Cohen-Kettenis, 2005; Imperato-McGinley, Guerrero, Gautier, & Peterson, 1974). Remember, these were not typical girls. Their brains had been exposed to male levels of testosterone from prenatal life onward.

A particularly disturbing case concerns one infant boy whose penis foreskin would not retract enough for easy urination. His parents took him to a physician to circumcise the foreskin, but the physician, using an electrical procedure, set the current too high and accidentally burned off the entire penis. On the advice of respected authorities, the parents elected to rear the child as a female, with the appropriate surgery. What makes this case especially interesting is that the child had a twin brother (whom the parents did not let the physician try to circumcise). If both twins developed satisfactory gender identities, one as a girl and the other as a boy, the results would say that rearing was decisive in gender identity.

Initial reports claimed that the child reared as a girl had a female gender identity, though she also had strong tomboyish tendencies (Money & Schwartz, 1978). However, by about age 10, she had figured out that something was wrong and that "she" was really a boy. She had preferred boys' activities and played only with boys' toys. She even tried urinating in a standing position, despite always making a mess. By age 14, she insisted that she wanted to live as a boy. At that time, her (now his) father tearfully explained the earlier events. The child changed names and became known as a boy. At age 25, he married a somewhat older woman and adopted her children. Clearly, a biological predisposition had won out over the family's attempts to rear the child as a girl (Colapinto, 1997; Diamond & Sigmundson, 1997). A few years later, the story ended tragically with this man's suicide.

We should not draw universal conclusions from a single case. However, the point is that it was a mistake to impose surgery and hormonal treatments to try to force this child to become female. When the prenatal hormone pattern of the brain is in conflict with a child's appearance, no one can be sure how that child will develop psychologically. Hormones don't have complete control, but rearing patterns don't, either.

⊘ **STOP & CHECK** ▌▌▌▌▌▌▌▌

18. When children who had been reared as girls reached puberty and grew a penis and scrotum, what happened to their gender identity?

ANSWER

18. Most changed their gender identity from female to male.

Sexual Orientation

Contrary to what biologists once assumed, same-sex genital contact occurs in many animal species, and not just in captive animals, those that cannot find a member of the opposite sex, or those with hormonal abnormalities (Bagemihl, 1999). If "natural" means "occurs in nature," then homosexuality is natural. Nevertheless, exclusive, lifelong homosexual orientation has been demonstrated in only two species—humans and sheep (Bailey et al., 2016).

People *discover* their sexual orientation. They can choose their actions, but not their desires or orientation, any more than people choose whether to be left-handed or right-handed. Whereas most men discover their sexual orientation early, many women are slower. Boys' feminine-type behaviors in childhood and adolescence correlate strongly with homosexual orientation in adulthood (Cardoso, 2009; Alanko et al., 2010), but girls' masculine-type behaviors are poor predictors of later sexual orientation (Alanko et al., 2010; Udry & Chantala, 2006).

Although the results vary from one survey to another, the mean estimate is that about 3.5 percent of adults in the United States identify as gay or lesbian (Gates, 2011). The percentage varies depending on how the question is worded (Bailey et al., 2016). The percentage also varies somewhat among countries, although we do not know how much of the apparent difference is due to secrecy or inaccurate reporting. In addition, a few percent of people who identify as straight have had at least one homosexual experience, or acknowledge occasional same-sex attraction (Norris, Marcus, & Green, 2015). *Transgender* people—those who have switched their gender identity—constitute perhaps 0.3 percent of the American population, although researchers have less confidence in the accuracy of this number.

Bisexuality is considerably more common in women than in men, and more common in younger people than in older

people (Ward, Dahlhamer, Galinsky, & Joestl, 2014). Relatively few men are bisexual, although some are "mostly straight" or "mostly gay" (Savin-Willliams, 2016). Even though a man may have had both homosexual and heterosexual experiences, his preference and fantasies almost always lean strongly one way than the other, rather than being equal (Norris, Marcus, & Green, 2015; Rieger, Chivers, & Bailey, 2005). Some women switch between homosexual and heterosexual orientations, possibly more than once (Diamond, 2007). Men rarely switch orientations.

Behavioral and Anatomical Differences

Homosexual and heterosexual people differ anatomically in several ways. On average, the shape of the nose and the shape of the forehead differ between homosexual and heterosexual men, and also between homosexual and heterosexual women (Skorska, Geniole, Vrysen, McCormick, & Bogaert, 2015). On average, heterosexual men are slightly taller and heavier than homosexual men (Bogaert, 2010). However, let's emphasize the terms "on average" and "slightly": The difference on average is only 1.5 cm (about half an inch). Contrary to the stereotype, some homosexual men are tall, athletic, and masculine in appearance.

On average, people who differ in sexual orientation also differ in certain behaviors that are not directly related to sex. For example, gay men are more likely than average to choose "female-typical" careers such as florist or hairdresser. That tendency has been documented in Samoa as well as in American and European cultures (Semenyna & Vasey, 2016). Also, whereas heterosexual men usually give directions in terms of distances and north, south, east, or west, women and homosexual men are more likely to describe landmarks (Hassan & Rahman, 2007).

Genetics

Early studies of the genetics of human sexual orientation began by advertising in gay or lesbian publications for homosexual people with twins. When someone responded, the researchers contacted the other twin to fill out a questionnaire that included sexual orientation. The results showed a stronger concordance (agreement) for monozygotic than dizygotic twins (Bailey et al., 2016). Note, this does *not* say that monozygotic twins are more likely to be homosexual than dizygotic twins are. It says that monozygotic twins are more likely to have the *same* sexual orientation.

However, the kind of person who answers an ad in a gay or lesbian magazine is probably not typical of others. A later study examined the data from all the twins in Sweden between ages 20 and 47 (Långström, Rahman, Carlström, & Lichtenstein, 2010). The Swedish study differed not only in the breadth of the sample, but also in the behavioral criterion. Instead of asking about sexual orientation, the researchers asked whether someone had ever had a same-sex partner. Figure 10.14 compares the data from the two studies. The

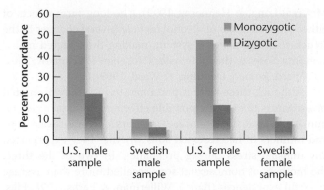

Figure 10.14 Twin concordance for homosexuality
The concordance for homosexual orientation (U.S. study) or homosexual activity (Swedish study) was higher for monozygotic twins than for dizygotic twins.
(Source: Based on the data of Bailey & Pillard, 1991; Bailey, Pillard, Neale, & Agyei, 1993; Långström, Rahman, Carlström, & Lichtenstein, 2010.)

results do not indicate number of people with homosexual activity or orientation. Rather, they indicate concordance—the probability of homosexual activity or orientation in one twin, given that the other twin had already indicated such activity. Although both sets of results show a higher concordance for monozygotic than dizygotic twins, note the huge difference between the studies. Other studies of twins in several countries also found higher concordance for sexual orientation in monozygotic than dizygotic twins, but the magnitude of the effect has varied considerably (Alanko et al., 2010; Burri, Cherkas, Spector, & Rahman, 2011).

Modern methods also enable researchers to compare chromosomes. The results have identified a couple of sites where one form of a gene is somewhat more common in homosexual than heterosexual men (Sanders et al., 2015). Two studies reported a higher incidence of homosexuality among the maternal than paternal relatives of homosexual men (Camperio-Ciani, Corna, & Capiluppi, 2004; Hamer, Hu, Magnuson, Hu, & Pattatucci, 1993). For example, they reported that uncles and cousins on the mother's side were more likely to be homosexual than uncles and cousins on the father's side. These results suggested a gene on the X chromosome, which a man necessarily receives from his mother. However, other studies have found no difference between relatives on the mother's and father's side (Bailey et al., 1999; Rice, Anderson, Risch, & Ebers, 1999; VanderLaan, Forrester, Petterson, & Vasey, 2013), and one study found more homosexual relatives on the father's side (Schwartz, Kim, Kolundzija, Rieger, & Sanders, 2010). Consequently, it seems doubtful that any gene on the X chromosome plays a major role.

An Evolutionary Question

A common estimate is that the average homosexual man has one-fifth as many children as the average heterosexual man. If a homosexual orientation has a genetic basis, why hasn't

evolution selected strongly against those genes? Several possibilities are worth considering. One is that genes for homosexuality are maintained by kin selection, as discussed in Chapter 4. That is, even if homosexual people do not have children themselves, they might do a wonderful job of helping their brothers and sisters rear children. Survey data in the United States indicate that homosexual men are no more likely, and perhaps less likely, than heterosexuals to help support their relatives (Bobrow & Bailey, 2001). However, observations in Samoa found that homosexual men are more helpful than average toward their nephews and nieces (Vasey & VanderLaan, 2010). It is difficult to know what might have been the usual pattern through human existence.

According to a second hypothesis, genes that produce male homosexuality might produce advantageous effects in their relatives, increasing their probability of reproducing and spreading the genes. What those advantages might be is a matter for speculation. A couple of studies have reported that relatives of gay men have a somewhat greater than average number of children (Camperio-Ciani, Corna, & Capiluppi, 2004; Schwartz et al., 2010). To evaluate this possibility more seriously, it would be best to study societies that do not practice family planning.

A third idea is that homosexuality relates to epigenetics rather than changes in DNA sequence (Rice, Friberg, & Gavrilets, 2012). As mentioned in Chapter 4, it is possible for environmental events to attach an acetyl group or a methyl group (CH_3) to activate or inactivate a gene. Some epigenetic changes persist from one generation to the next. Perhaps epigenetic changes affect certain genes often enough to produce the observed prevalence of homosexuality.

✓ **STOP & CHECK** ▬▬▬▬▬▬

19. For which kind of twin pair is the concordance for sexual orientation greatest?

20. It seems difficult to explain how a gene could remain at a moderately high frequency in the population if most men with the gene do not reproduce. How would the hypothesis about epigenetics help with the explanation?

ANSWERS

19. Monozygotic twins have higher concordance than dizygotic twins. Be sure to state this point correctly: Do not say that homosexuality is more common in monozygotic than dizygotic twins. It is the *concordance* that is greater—that is, the probability that both twins have the *same* sexual orientation. 20. According to this hypothesis, some unidentified event in the environment can attach an acetyl group or a methyl group to some gene, increasing or decreasing its activity. That gene modification could be passed to the next generation, producing evidence for a hereditary effect, even though there is no "gene for homosexuality." If events like this happen often enough, the result could be a moderately high prevalence of homosexuality, even if men with the inactivated gene seldom reproduce.

Prenatal Influences

Adult hormone levels do *not* explain sexual orientation. On average, homosexual and heterosexual men have nearly the same hormone levels, and most lesbian women have about the same hormone levels as heterosexual women. However, it is possible that sexual orientation depends on testosterone levels during a sensitive period of brain development (Ellis & Ames, 1987). Animal studies have shown that prenatal or early postnatal hormones can produce organizing effects on both external anatomy and brain development. External anatomy develops at a different time from the brain, and so it is possible for early hormones to alter the brain without changing external anatomy.

The mother's immune system may exert prenatal effects. Studies in several countries report that the probability of a homosexual orientation is slightly higher among men who have older brothers, regardless of the number of sisters and younger brothers (Blanchard, 2008; Bogaert, 2003b; Bozkurt, Bozkurt, & Sonmez, 2015; Purcell, Blanchard, & Zucker, 2000; Schwartz et al., 2010). Furthermore, what matters is the number of *biological* older brothers. Growing up with older stepbrothers or adopted brothers has no apparent influence. Having a biological older brother has an influence, even if the brothers were reared separately (Bogaert, 2006). In short, the influence does not stem from social experiences. The key is how many previous times the mother gave birth to a son. The most prominent hypothesis is that a mother's immune system sometimes reacts against a protein in a son and then attacks subsequent sons enough to alter their development. That hypothesis fits with the observation that later-born homosexual men tend to be shorter than average (Bogaert, 2003a).

Another possible influence of prenatal environment relates to stress on the mother during pregnancy. Research has shown that prenatal stress alters sexual development in laboratory animals. In several experiments, rats in the final week of pregnancy had the stressful experience of confinement in tight Plexiglas tubes for more than 2 hours each day under bright lights. In some cases, they were given alcohol as well. These rats' daughters looked and acted approximately normal. The sons, however, had normal male anatomy but, in adulthood, often responded to the presence of another male by arching their backs in the typical rat female posture for sex (I. L. Ward, Ward, Winn, & Bielawski, 1994). Most males that were subjected to either prenatal stress or alcohol developed male sexual behavior in addition to these female sexual behaviors, but those that were subjected to both stress and alcohol had decreased male sexual behaviors (I. L. Ward, Bennett, Ward, Hendricks, & French, 1999).

Prenatal stress and alcohol may alter brain development through several routes. Stress releases endorphins, which can antagonize the effects of testosterone on the hypothalamus (O. B. Ward, Monaghan, & Ward, 1986). Stress also elevates levels of certain adrenal hormones (corticosterone in rats, cortisol in human) that decrease testosterone release (O. B. Ward, Ward, Denning, French, & Hendricks, 2002; M. T. Williams, Davis,

McCrea, Long, & Hennessy, 1999). The long-term effects of either prenatal stress or alcohol include several changes in the structure of the nervous system, making the affected males' anatomy closer to that of females (Nosenko & Reznikov, 2001; I. L. Ward, Romeo, Denning, & Ward, 1999).

Although these studies pertained to rats, they prompted investigators to examine possible effects of prenatal stress on humans. Three surveys asked mothers of homosexual sons and mothers of heterosexual sons whether they experienced any unusual stress during pregnancy. In two of the three, the mothers of homosexual sons recalled more than average stressful experiences (Bailey, Willerman, & Parks, 1991; Ellis, Ames, Peckham, & Burke, 1988; Ellis & Cole-Harding, 2001). However, these studies relied on women's memories of pregnancies more than 20 years earlier. A better but more difficult procedure would be to measure stress during pregnancy and examine the sexual orientation of the sons many years later.

So, what explains the differences in sexual orientation? The answer is probably not the same in all instances. Genetic or epigenetic factors contribute, as well as prenatal environment. Later experiences probably contribute too, although we know little about the types of experience that would be decisive.

⊘ **STOP & CHECK** ▬▬▬▬

21. By what route might having an older brother increase the probability of male homosexuality?
22. How might stress to a pregnant rat alter the sexual orientation of her male offspring?

ANSWERS

21. Having an older brother might increase the probability of male homosexuality by altering the mother's immune system in the prenatal environment. The effect of the older brother does not depend on growing up in the same home. 22. Evidently, the stress increases the release of endorphins in the hypothalamus, and very high endorphin levels can block the effects of testosterone.

Brain Anatomy

Do brains also differ as a function of sexual orientation? The results are complex. On average, homosexual men are shifted partly in the female-typical direction for some brain structures but not others. Similarly, on average, homosexual women's brains are slightly shifted in the male direction in some ways but not others (Rahman & Wilson, 2003). Several of the reported differences have no clear relationship to sexuality itself, although they may relate to other behavioral differences between heterosexual and homosexual people.

On average, the left and right hemispheres of the cerebral cortex are of nearly equal size in heterosexual females, whereas the right hemisphere is a few percent larger in heterosexual males. Homosexual males resemble heterosexual females in

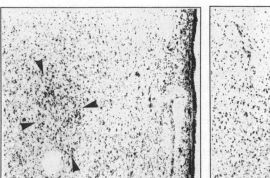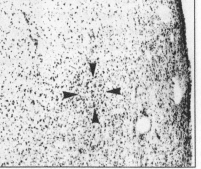

Figure 10.15 Typical sizes of interstitial nucleus 3 of the anterior hypothalamus
On the average, the volume of this structure was more than twice as large in a sample of heterosexual men (left) than in a sample of homosexual men (right), for whom it was about the same size as in women. *(Source: From "A difference in hypothalamic structure between heterosexual and homosexual men," by S. LeVay, Science, 253, pp. 1034–1037. Copyright 1991. Reprinted with permission from AAAS.)*

this regard, and homosexual females are intermediate between heterosexual females and males. Also, in heterosexual females, the left amygdala has more widespread connections than the right amygdala, whereas in heterosexual males, the right amygdala has more widespread connections. Again, homosexual males resemble heterosexual females in this regard, and homosexual females are intermediate (Savic & Lindström, 2008). The anterior commissure (see Figure 3.13) is, on average, larger in heterosexual women than in heterosexual men. In homosexual men, it is at least as large as in women, perhaps even slightly larger (Gorski & Allen, 1992). The suprachiasmatic nucleus (SCN) is also larger in homosexual men than in heterosexual men (Swaab & Hofman, 1990). However, when interpreting these and other reported differences, we should remember two cautions (Kaiser, Haller, Schmitz, & Nitsch, 2009): First, we don't know whether these brain differences are causes or effects of sexual orientation. Brain differences can predispose to different behaviors, but it is also true that persistent behaviors can change brain anatomy. Second, it is relatively easy to publish results showing a difference between two groups, such as homosexual and heterosexual people, even if the difference was unpredicted, small, and hard to explain. It is less easy to publish results showing no difference. Thus it is likely that the published papers overstate certain anatomical differences.

The most widely cited research concerns the third interstitial nucleus of the anterior hypothalamus (INAH-3), which is generally more than twice as large in heterosexual men as in women. This area has more cells with androgen receptors in men than in women (Shah et al., 2004), and probably plays a role in male sexual behavior, although the exact role is uncertain and probably varies among animal species. In other species it is known as the *sexually dimorphic nucleus*, although calling it a "nucleus" is a bit of an overstatement. It is a subdivision of a subdivision of the preoptic hypothalamus.

Simon LeVay (1991) examined INAH-3 in 41 people who had died between the ages of 26 and 59. Of these, 16 were heterosexual men, 6 were heterosexual women, and 19 were homosexual men. All of the homosexual men, 6 of the 16 heterosexual men, and 1 of the 6 women had died of AIDS. LeVay found that the mean volume of INAH-3 was larger in heterosexual men than in heterosexual women or homosexual men,

who were about equal in this regard. Figure 10.15 shows typical cross sections for a heterosexual man and a homosexual man. Figure 10.16 shows the distribution of volumes for the three groups. Note that the difference between heterosexual men and the other two groups is fairly large, on average, and that the cause of death (AIDS versus other) has no clear relationship to the results. LeVay (1993) later examined the hypothalamus of a homosexual man who died of lung cancer; he had a small INAH-3, like the homosexual men who died of AIDS. In Figure 10.16, note also the substantial amount of variation among individuals. If you could examine some man's INAH-3, you could make a reasonable guess about sexual orientation, but you could not be confident.

A later study partly replicated these trends. Researchers found that the INAH-3 nucleus of homosexual men was intermediate between those of heterosexual men and heterosexual

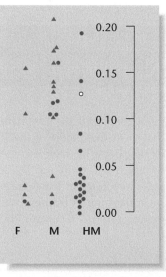

Figure 10.16 Volumes of the interstitial nucleus 3 of the anterior hypothalamus (INAH-3)
Samples are females (F), heterosexual males (M), and homosexual males (HM). Each filled circle represents a person who died of AIDS, and each triangle represents a person who died from other causes. The one open circle represents a bisexual man who died of AIDS.
(Source: Reprinted with permission from "A difference in hypothalamic structure between heterosexual and homosexual men," by S. LeVay, Science, 253, pp. 1034–1037. Copyright © 1991 American Association for the Advancement of Science.)

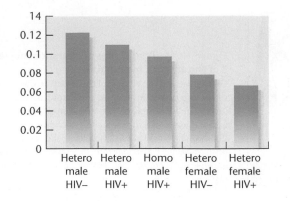

Figure 10.17 Another comparison of INAH-3
In this study, the mean volume for homosexual men was larger than that of heterosexual women but smaller than that of heterosexual men.
(Source: Based on data of Byne et al., 2001)

women. Also, the volume was smaller in HIV-positive than HIV-negative individuals (Byne et al., 2001). Figure 10.17 displays the means for five groups. On microscopic examination of the INAH-3, researchers found that heterosexual men had larger neurons than homosexual men but about the same number. Neither this study nor LeVay's earlier study included homosexual females. Still another study found INAH-3 to be larger in heterosexual males than in male-to-female transsexuals—that is, people born as males who changed their identities to female (Garcia-Falgueras & Swaab, 2008).

The meaning of these results is not clear. Do differences in the hypothalamus influence sexual orientation, or does sexual activity influence the size of hypothalamic neurons? Some brain areas do grow or shrink in adults because of hormones or behavioral activities (Cooke, Tabibnia, & Breedlove, 1999). A nonhuman study offers suggestive results. About 8 percent of rams (male sheep) direct their sexual behavior toward other males. One area of the anterior hypothalamus is larger in female-oriented rams than in male-oriented rams and larger in male-oriented rams than in females (Roselli, Larkin, Resko, Stellflug, & Stormshak, 2004). (Whether this area corresponds to human INAH-3 is uncertain.) This area becomes larger in male than female sheep before birth as a result of prenatal testosterone levels (Roselli, Stadelman, Reeve, Bishop, & Stormshak, 2007). In sheep, at least, an anatomical difference appears before any sexual behavior, and so it is more likely a cause than a result. The same may or may not be true in humans.

✓ **STOP & CHECK**

23. In LeVay's study, what evidence argues against the idea that INAH-3 volume depends on AIDS rather than sexual orientation?

ANSWER
23. In his study, the average size of INAH-3 was about the same for heterosexual men who died of AIDS and those who died of other causes. One homosexual man who died of other causes had about the same size INAH-3 as homosexual men who died of AIDS.

Module 10.2 | In Closing

We Are Not All the Same

When Alfred Kinsey conducted the first massive surveys of human sexual behavior in the middle of the 20th century, he found that most of the people he interviewed considered their own behavior "normal," whatever it was. Many believed that sexual activity much more frequent than their own was abnormal and might even lead to insanity (Kinsey, Pomeroy, & Martin, 1948; Kinsey, Pomeroy, Martin, & Gebhard, 1953).

How far have we come since then? People today are more aware and generally more accepting of sexual diversity than they were in Kinsey's time. Still, intolerance remains common. Biological research will not tell us how to treat one another, but it can help us understand how we come to be so different.

Summary

1. In many species, males and females evolve different appearances and behaviors because of sexual selection. That is, they evolve in ways that make them more appealing to the other sex. **337**

2. Many of the mating habits of people can be interpreted in terms of increasing the probability of passing on our genes. However, it is hard to know to what extent the differences between men and women are evolutionary adaptations and to what extent they are learned. **337**

3. People can develop ambiguous genitals or genitals that don't match their chromosomal sex for several reasons. The most common is congenital adrenal hyperplasia, in which a genetic defect in cortisol production leads to overstimulation of the adrenal gland and therefore extra testosterone production. When that condition occurs in a female fetus, she becomes partly masculinized. **339**

4. On the average, girls with a history of congenital adrenal hyperplasia show more interest in boy-typical toys than

other girls do, and during adolescence and young adulthood, they continue to show partly masculinized interests. **340**

5. Testicular feminization, or androgen insensitivity, is a condition in which someone with an XY chromosome pattern is partly or fully insensitive to androgens and therefore develops a female external appearance. **340**

6. People born with intermediate or ambiguous genitals are called intersexes. For many years, physicians recommended surgery to make these people look more feminine. However, many intersexes do not develop an unambiguous female identity, and many protest against the imposed surgery. **340**

7. Some children have a gene that decreases their early production of dihydrotestosterone. Such a child looks female at birth and is considered a girl but develops a penis at adolescence. Most of these people then accept a male gender identity. **341**

8. On average, homosexual people differ from heterosexual people in several anatomical and physiological regards, although the averages do not apply to every individual. **342**

9. Plausible biological explanations for homosexual orientation include genetics, prenatal hormones, and (in males) reactions to the mother's immune system. Hormone levels in adulthood are within the normal range. **342**

10. Several hypotheses have been offered for how genes promoting homosexuality could remain at moderate frequencies in the population although homosexual people are less likely than average to have children. **343**

11. On the average, certain aspects of brain anatomy differ between homosexual and heterosexual men, although it is not certain whether these differences are causes or effects of the behavior. **344**

Key Terms

Terms are defined in the module on the page number indicated. They're also presented in alphabetical order with definitions in the book's Subject Index/Glossary, which begins on page 589. Interactive flash cards, audio reviews, and crossword puzzles are among the online resources available to help you learn these terms and the concepts they represent.

androgen insensitivity **340**
congenital adrenal
  hyperplasia **339**

gender identity **339**
hermaphrodite **339**
intersex **339**

sexual selection **337**
testicular feminization **340**

Thought Questions

1. On average, intersexes have IQ scores in the 110 to 125 range, well above the mean for the population (Dalton, 1968; Ehrhardt & Money, 1967; Lewis, Money, & Epstein, 1968). One possible interpretation is that a hormonal pattern intermediate between male and female promotes great intellectual development. Another possibility is that intersexuality may be more common in intelligent families than in less intelligent ones or that the more educated families are more likely to bring their intersexed children to an investigator's attention. What kind of study would be best for deciding among these hypotheses? (For one answer, see Money & Lewis, 1966.)

2. Recall LeVay's study of brain anatomy in heterosexual and homosexual men. Certain critics have suggested that one or more of the men classified as "heterosexual" might actually have been homosexual or bisexual. If so, would that fact strengthen or weaken the overall conclusions?

Module 10.2 | End of Module Quiz

1. What is meant by the term "sexual selection"?
   A. Having an XX or XY chromosome pattern determines whether one develops as a female or a male.
   B. Hormones during a sensitive period produce long-lasting effects on anatomy and behavior.
   C. Some people choose to switch from one gender identity to another.
   D. Evolution favors characteristics that make an individual more appealing to the opposite sex.

2. Evolutionary psychologists try to explain which of the following phenomena?
   A. On average, men are more interested in multiple sex partners than women are.
   B. The mechanisms controlling sex differences in the brain vary among brain areas.
   C. Sex drive depends on testosterone in males and estradiol in females.
   D. Dopamine and serotonin have largely opposite effects on sexual arousal.

3. Congenital adrenal hypertrophy results from a genetic disability to produce normal amounts of which hormone?

   A. Testosterone

   B. Estradiol

   C. Vasopressin

   D. Cortisol

4. A girl's interest in boys' toys correlates positively with which of the following?

   A. The size of her hippocampus

   B. Exposure to testosterone before birth

   C. Exposure to cortisol before birth

   D. Exposure to oxytocin before birth

5. What causes testicular feminization, in which a genetic male looks female?

   A. High levels of estradiol during an early sensitive period

   B. Lack of receptors for testosterone

   C. A mutation in the *SRY* gene

   D. A genetic disability to produce cortisol

6. When genetic males appeared to be female at birth, but developed a male anatomy at puberty, what happened to their gender identity?

   A. They continued to have a female identity.

   B. They switched to a male identity.

   C. They alternated frequently between male and female identities.

   D. They simultaneously maintained both male and female identities.

7. The conclusion that sexual orientation is partly heritable depends mainly on what evidence?

   A. Identification of a particular gene strongly linked to sexual orientation

   B. Comparisons of sexual orientation in many cultures

   C. Comparisons of monozygotic and dizygotic twins

   D. Comparisons of male homosexuals with female homosexuals

8. Which of the following would increase the probability that a boy will develop a homosexual orientation?

   A. Living in a family with one or more older sisters

   B. Living in a family with an older, adopted brother

   C. Having a biological older brother, even if he did not live in the same house

   D. Having either an adopted or biological younger brother

9. In what way was INAH-3 distinctive for most of the homosexual men, in comparison to heterosexual men, in LeVay's study and the follow-up research?

   A. This nucleus had fewer than average neurons but only in men who died of AIDS.

   B. This nucleus had fewer than average neurons regardless of the cause of death.

   C. This nucleus had neurons with smaller than average volume.

   D. This nucleus had fewer neurons, but each of them had a larger than average volume.

Answers: 1D, 2A, 3D, 4B, 5B, 6B, 7C, 8C, 9C.

Suggestions for Further Reading

Bailey, J. M., Vasey, P. L., Diamond, L. M., Breedlove, S. M., Vilain, E., & Epprecht, M. (2016). Sexual orientation, controversy, and science. *Psychological Science in the Public Interest*, *17*, 45–101. An article that thoroughly and objectively reviews research on sexual orientation.

Colapinto, J. (2000). *As nature made him: The boy who was raised as a girl.* New York: HarperCollins. Describes the boy whose penis was accidentally removed, as presented on page **341**.

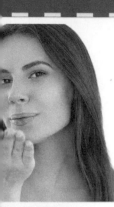
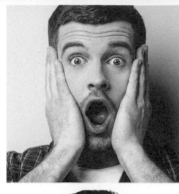
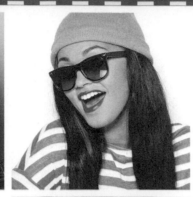
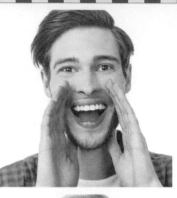
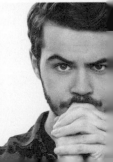

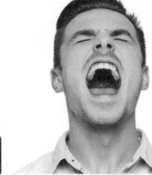
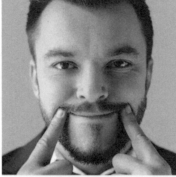
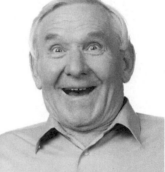
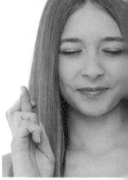

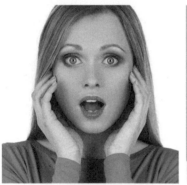
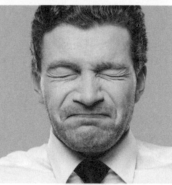
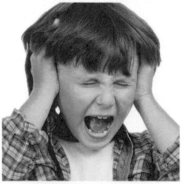

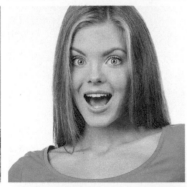
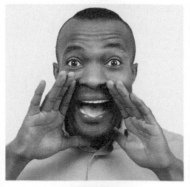
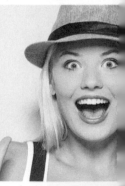

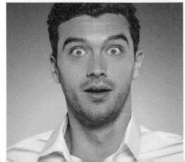
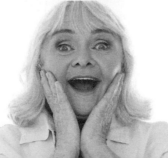

Emotional Behaviors   Chapter 11

Unfortunately, one of the most significant things ever said about emotion may be that every-one knows what it is until they are asked to define it.

Joseph LeDoux (1996, p. 23)

Suppose researchers have discovered a new species—let's call it species X—and psychologists begin testing its abilities. They place food behind a green card and nothing behind a red card and find that after a few trials, X always goes to the green card. So we conclude that X shows learning, memory, and hunger. Then researchers offer X a green card and a variety of gray cards; X still goes to the green, so it must have color vision and not just brightness discrimination. Next they let X touch a blue triangle that is extremely hot. X makes a loud sound and backs away. Someone picks up the blue triangle (with padded gloves) and starts moving with it rapidly toward X. As soon as X sees this happening, it makes the same sound, turns, and starts moving rapidly away. Shall we conclude that it feels fear?

If you said yes, now let me add: I said this was a new species, and so it is, but it's a new species of robot, not animal. Do you still think X feels fear? Most people are willing to talk about artificial learning, memory, intelligence, or motivation, but not emotion.

If such behavior isn't adequate evidence for emotion in a robot, is it adequate evidence for an animal? When a dog runs away from a threat, you probably infer that it is afraid, but what about an insect that escapes as you approach? Was it afraid? If you disturb a beehive and the bees attack you, are they angry? How could you be sure, one way or the other? Emotion is a difficult topic because it implies conscious feelings that we cannot observe. Biological researchers therefore talk mostly about emotional *behaviors*, which are observable, even if the emotional feelings are not. Still, most of us hope eventually to understand the emotional experiences themselves.

Learning Objectives

After studying this chapter, you should be able to:

1. Discuss the role of the autonomic nervous system in emotional feelings.
2. Explain reasons to be skeptical of the idea of a few basic emotions.
3. Discuss the role of emotions in moral reasoning.
4. Describe what is known about the genetics of aggression and anxiety.
5. Discuss the role of the amygdala in emotional processing.
6. Comment on methods of relief from anxiety.
7. Define the general adaptation syndrome.
8. Describe the effects of stress on the immune system.

Opposite:
People express emotion by facial expressions, gestures, and postures. (g-stockstudio/Shutterstock.com)

What Is Emotion?

By one definition, emotion includes "cognitive evaluations, subjective changes, autonomic and neural arousal, and impulses to action" (Plutchik, 1982, p. 551). That sounds okay, but by that definition, don't hunger and thirst count as emotions? One definition of motivation is "an internal process that modifies the way an organism responds to a certain class of external stimuli" (Numan & Woodside, 2010). By that definition, don't happiness, sadness, fear, and anger count as motivations? Distinguishing between motivation and emotion is difficult, and maybe there is no real difference.

Regardless of how we define emotion, psychologists generally agree that emotion has components including cognitions ("This is a dangerous situation"), feelings ("I feel frightened"), actions ("Run away now"), and physiological changes (increased heart rate and breathing rate). How do the components relate to one another?

Emotions and Autonomic Arousal

Emotional situations arouse the two branches of the autonomic nervous system—the sympathetic and the parasympathetic. Figure 11.1 reviews the anatomy. Researchers had long recognized that the sympathetic nervous system stimulates certain organs, such as the heart, while inhibiting others, such as the stomach and intestines. Walter Cannon (1945) was the first to recognize the pattern: It stimulates organs important

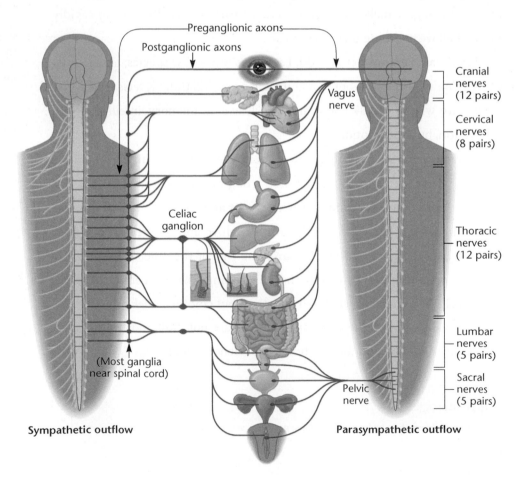

Figure 11.1 The sympathetic and parasympathetic nervous systems Review Chapter 3 for more information.

for vigorous "fight-or-flight" activities while inhibiting vegetative activities that can wait until later. The parasympathetic nervous system increases digestion and other processes that save energy and prepare for later events.

Nevertheless, most situations evoke a combination of sympathetic and parasympathetic arousal (Wolf, 1995). For example, nausea is associated with sympathetic stimulation of the stomach (decreasing its contractions and secretions) and parasympathetic stimulation of the intestines and salivary glands. We think of danger as something that would elicit sympathetic activity, but often it does not. If a small animal sees a potential predator at a great distance, it becomes alert, but inactive. (The predator is less likely to notice an immobile animal.) The little animal's heart rate *decreases*, by parasympathetic input. Only when the threat approaches within attacking distance does the sympathetic nervous system take over. Similarly, humans become alert and inactive with decreased heart rate when they are aware of a danger remote in either location or time (Löw, Weymar, & Hamm, 2015).

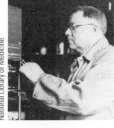

Walter B. Cannon (1871–1945)

As a matter of routine I have long trusted unconscious processes to serve me.... [One] example I may cite was the interpretation of the significance of bodily changes which occur in great emotional excitement, such as fear and rage. These changes—the more rapid pulse, the deeper breathing, the increase of sugar in the blood, the secretion from the adrenal glands—were very diverse and seemed unrelated. Then, one wakeful night, after a considerable collection of these changes had been disclosed, the idea flashed through my mind that they could be nicely integrated if conceived as bodily preparations for supreme effort in flight or in fighting.

How does the autonomic nervous system relate to emotions? Common sense holds that you feel an emotion that changes your heart rate and prompts other responses. In contrast, according to the **James-Lange theory** (James, 1884), the autonomic arousal and skeletal actions come first. What you experience as an emotion is the label you give to your responses: You feel afraid *because* you run away, and you feel angry *because* you attack.

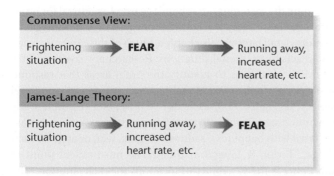

You might object, "How would I know to run away before I was scared?" In a later paper, William James (1894) clarified his position. An emotion includes cognitions, actions, and feelings. The cognitive aspect comes first. You quickly appraise something as good, bad, frightening, or whatever. Your appraisal of the situation leads to an appropriate action, such as running away, attacking, or sitting motionless with your heart racing. When James said that arousal and actions lead to emotions, he meant they lead to the *feeling* aspect of an emotion. That is,

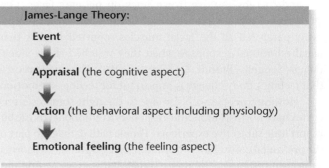

If we think of "feeling" in its narrow sense of being a sensation, the theory seems almost self-evident. Where else would sensations come from, except from something going on in the body? Still, the James-Lange theory leads to two predictions: People with weak autonomic or skeletal responses should feel less emotion, and causing or increasing someone's responses should enhance an emotion. Let's consider the evidence.

Is Physiological Arousal Necessary for Emotional Feelings?

People with damage to the spinal cord have no sensations or voluntary movements from the level of the damage downward. (Reflexes remain.) Nevertheless, they generally report experiencing emotions about the same as before their injury (Cobos, Sánchez, Pérez, & Vila, 2004; Deady, North, Allan, Smith, & O'Carroll, 2010). That result might suggest that emotions don't depend on feedback from movement, but these people continue to have facial expressions and changes in heart rate, which they can detect. So although they are cut off from some of the sensation usually associated with an emotion, they continue to feel important aspects.

In people with an uncommon condition called **pure autonomic failure,** output from the autonomic nervous system to the body fails, either completely or almost completely. Heart beat and other organ activities continue, but the nervous system no longer regulates them. Someone with this condition does not react to stressful experiences with changes in heart rate, blood pressure, or sweating. According to the James-Lange theory, we would expect such people to report no emotions. In fact, they report having the same emotions as anyone else, and they have little difficulty identifying what emotion a character in a story would probably experience

(Heims, Critchley, Dolan, Mathias, & Cipolotti, 2004). However, they say they feel their emotions much less intensely than before (Critchley, Mathias, & Dolan, 2001). Presumably, when they report that they experience emotions, they refer to the cognitive aspect: "Yes, I'm angry, because this is a situation that calls for anger." But if they *feel* the anger, they feel it weakly. Their decreased emotional feeling is consistent with predictions from the James-Lange theory.

Here is another example: Botulinum toxin ("BOTOX") blocks transmission at synapses and nerve–muscle junctions. Physicians sometimes use it to paralyze the muscles for frowning and thereby remove frown lines on people's faces. One study found that people with BOTOX injections that temporarily paralyzed all the facial muscles reported weaker than usual emotional responses when they watched short videos (Davis, Senghas, Brandt, & Ochsner, 2010). The implication is that feeling a body change is important for feeling an emotion.

However, people with damage to the right somatosensory cortex have normal autonomic responses to emotional music but report little subjective experience. People with damage to part of the prefrontal cortex have weak autonomic responses but normal subjective responses (Johnsen, Tranel, Lutgendorf, & Adolphs, 2009). These results suggest that autonomic responses and subjective experience are not always connected to each other.

Is Physiological Arousal Sufficient for Emotions?

According to the James-Lange theory, emotional feelings result from the body's actions. If your heart started racing and you started sweating and breathing rapidly, would you feel an emotion? Not necessarily. You might have those reactions from vigorous exercise, or they might accompany an illness with fever. However, if you had sudden intense arousal of the sympathetic nervous system without knowing the reason, you might experience it as an emotion. Such is the case with a **panic attack**, when people gasp for breath, worry that they are suffocating, and experience great anxiety (Klein, 1993).

Although physiological responses are seldom sufficient to produce emotional feelings, they increase the feelings. Increases in heart rate intensify ratings of both pleasant and unpleasant emotions, especially in people who are most sensitive to their internal state (Dunn et al., 2010). For example, if you watched a horror movie in a cold room, where the temperature caused you to shiver, you might rate the movie as scarier than you would have in a warmer room (Sugamura & Higuchi, 2015). It is easier to feel angry while standing (and therefore in a position to attack) than while lying in a more helpless position (Harmon-Jones & Peterson, 2009). Because perceptions of your body's actions contribute to your emotional feelings, many psychologists describe emotions as "embodied"—that is, they depend on responses of the body.

Nevertheless, many psychologists from the start have been dissatisfied with the James-Lange theory. Walter Cannon (1927) objected that feedback from the viscera is neither necessary nor sufficient for emotion, that it does not distinguish one emotion from another, and that it is too slow to account for how fast we identify an event as happy, sad, or frightening. He and others have proposed additional theories, and no consensus has emerged (Moors, 2009). So here we are, well over a hundred years after William James proposed one of the first theories in psychology, and we still haven't decided whether it is correct. Shouldn't psychologists be embarrassed?

The problem may be that different theorists are talking about different questions, even when they use the same words. When James's defenders talk about "emotional feelings," they mean literally feelings—that is, sensations—and sensations come only from sense organs, such as those that detect body actions. Other theorists are talking about the complete emotional experience. Moreover, the debate about theories of emotion may be ultimately fruitless. Except for inspiring some interesting research studies of the types just described, theories of emotion don't have much application. In fact, several influential modern theorists question whether our whole concept of emotion is misguided.

Is Emotion a Useful Concept?

To talk about "an" emotion, such as anger or fear, implies that it is a coherent whole. Nearly all definitions of emotion say that it includes several aspects, such as cognition, feeling, and action. However, those aspects do not always stick together. Sometimes you suddenly feel nervous (a feeling), but you don't know why (no cognition), and you do nothing about it (no action). Is your nervous feeling an emotion? You could also have the cognition "this is flu season," and take action (a vaccination), without feeling any sensation of nervousness or fear. Does that combination constitute emotion, part of an emotion, or no emotion? In short, the various aspects of emotion do not always stick together.

Furthermore, although emotional feelings correlate strongly with arousal of the autonomic nervous system, no particular emotion is consistently associated with a distinctive pattern of autonomic activity (Lang, 2014). For example, heart rate and breathing rate increase with the intensity of an emotion, but they do not distinguish fear from anger. Mild activation of the parasympathetic nervous system facilitates compassion toward others (Kogan et al., 2014; Stellar, Cohen, Oveis, & Keltner, 2015), but it occurs in other situations as well. You could not confidently identify someone's emotion by measuring heart rate, breathing rate, or any other autonomic response.

Traditionally, the **limbic system**—the forebrain areas surrounding the thalamus—has been regarded as critical for emotion (see Figure 11.2). We consider one part of it, the amygdala, in more detail later in this chapter. Much of the cerebral cortex also reacts to emotional situations. Researchers have used PET or fMRI techniques to identify the brain areas that respond while people look at emotional pictures or listen to emotional stories. In Figure 11.3, each dot represents a research study that found significant activation of a particular cortical area associated with happiness, sadness, disgust, fear, or anger (Phan, Wager, Taylor, & Liberzon, 2002). The most salient point of this figure is the variability of locations for each emotion. The

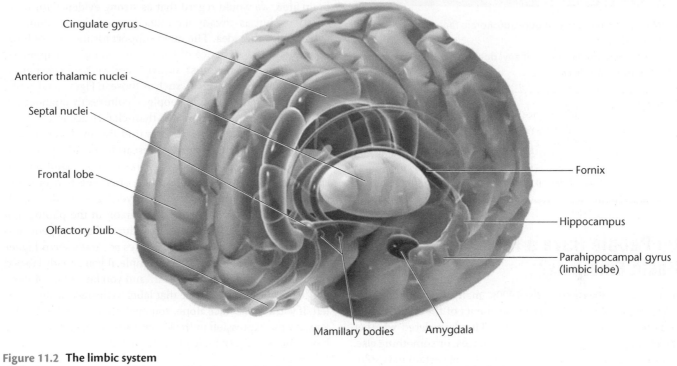

Cingulate gyrus

Anterior thalamic nuclei

Septal nuclei

Frontal lobe

Olfactory bulb

Mamillary bodies

Amygdala

Fornix

Hippocampus

Parahippocampal gyrus (limbic lobe)

Figure 11.2 The limbic system
The limbic system is a group of structures in the interior of the brain. Here you see them as if the exterior of the brain were transparent.
(*Source: Based on MacLean, 1949*)

results apparently depend more on the details of procedure than on which emotion was targeted. Researchers have identified neurons in the amygdala that appear to be specific for *perceiving* a particular emotion in someone's expression (S. Wang et al., 2014), but with the possible exception of happiness, no brain area appears to be specific for *experiencing* any particular emotion (Heller et al., 2013; Lindquist, Wager, Kober, Bliss-Moreau, & Barrett, 2012; Mueller et al., 2015).

The lack of any consistent link between emotional feelings and physiological responses suggests that emotion may not be a coherent category. Lisa Feldman Barrett (2012) has argued that emotions are a real category only in the same sense that weeds are a real category. Nothing in nature makes weeds different from flowers. They differ only because people favor certain plants ("flowers") and disfavor other plants ("weeds"). Similarly, emotion is a socially constructed category that serves our purposes.

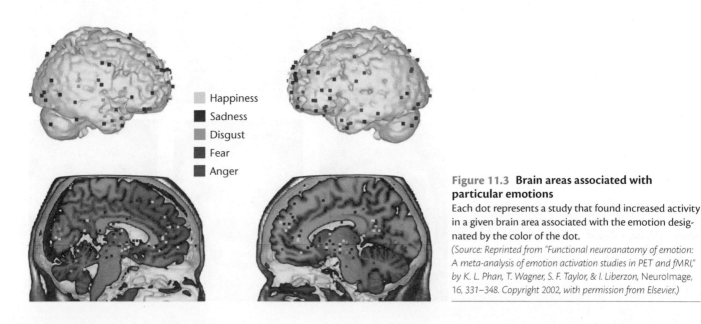

Happiness
Sadness
Disgust
Fear
Anger

Figure 11.3 Brain areas associated with particular emotions
Each dot represents a study that found increased activity in a given brain area associated with the emotion designated by the color of the dot.
(*Source: Reprinted from "Functional neuroanatomy of emotion: A meta-analysis of emotion activation studies in PET and fMRI," by K. L. Phan, T. Wagner, S. F. Taylor, & I. Liberzon, NeuroImage, 16, 331–348. Copyright 2002, with permission from Elsevier.*)

1. What is the relevance of pure autonomic failure to the study of emotions?
2. In what physiological way, if any, does one type of emotion differ from another?

ANSWERS

1. People with pure autonomic failure do not react to events with changes in heart rate or other autonomic functions. They report still having emotional experiences but they do not feel them as strongly. 2. No type of emotion has a unique pattern of physiological activity, either in the autonomic nervous system or in the brain.

Do People Have a Few Basic Emotions?

In the late 1800s and early 1900s, many psychological researchers hoped to identify the elements of the mind, analogous to the elements of chemistry. They wondered whether the elements were thoughts, ideas, images, or something else. Before long, that quest seemed futile. Later, certain psychologists hoped to find the elements of motivation, offering lists of the basic motivations. That pursuit led to fascinating questions such as whether breathing counts as just one motivation or two (inhaling and exhaling). Today, emotion is the only area in which many researchers still hope to identify elements of experience, to list a few "basic" emotions.

If we found that each emotion was identified with its own brain area, we would regard that as strong evidence for basic emotions, but as already mentioned, research has found no evidence for that idea. The main support for the idea of basic emotions is the existence of facial expressions for happiness, sadness, fear, anger, disgust, surprise, and perhaps other emotions. If shown a set of faces, such as those in Figure 11.4, and a list of emotion terms, most people in cultures throughout the world pair them up with greater-than-chance accuracy.

However, many psychologists find this evidence unconvincing. The faces used in most research, including those in Figure 11.4, were posed to try to maximize recognition. For spontaneous expressions, observers often see two or more emotions in a single face, and observers' guesses do not always match the self-report by the person in the photograph (Kayyal & Russell, 2013). The procedure of asking people to match the six faces to six labels makes accuracy seem higher than it would be otherwise. For example, if you already labeled the face at the lower right as "fear," and you know one of them has to be "surprise," you give that label to the face at the lower left. If you saw that face alone, you might have called it "fear." If you saw the expression in the lower center by itself, you might have called it anger instead of disgust (Pochedly, Widen, & Russell, 2012).

Another problem: People recognize expressions from their own culture better than those from other cultures (Gendron, Roberson, van der Vyver, & Barrett, 2014). Young people in two cultures largely isolated from Western influences were able to recognize the expression for happiness at better than 50 percent accuracy, but they had low accuracy on

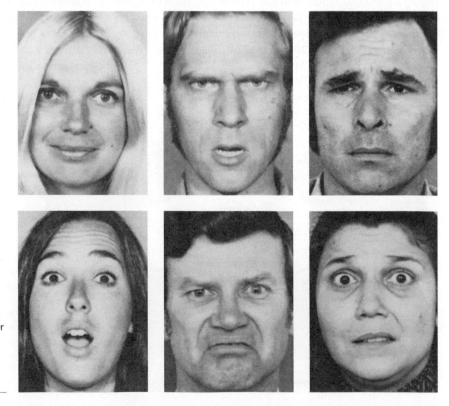

Figure 11.4 Facial expressions of emotion
Can you identify which face corresponds to happiness, sadness, fear, anger, disgust, and surprise? Check answer A on page **360**.
(Source: Reprinted from Unmasking the face *(2nd ed.), by P. Ekman & W. V. Friesen, 1984. Palo Alto, CA: Consulting Psychologists Press.)*

other expressions, especially the expression intended to show anger (Crivelli, Jarillo, Russell, & Fernández-Dols, 2016).

Furthermore, we rarely identify someone's emotion from facial expression alone. Participants in one study viewed photos of pro tennis players who had just won or lost a point in a difficult, high-stakes match (see Figure 11.5). From photos of body posture, the observers could usually guess whether the player was happy (having won the last point) or sad (having just lost it). But from facial expression alone, the observers could do no better than chance guessing (Aviezer, Trope, & Todorov, 2012). Another study also found that for both children and adults, the expressions of intense pleasure look similar to those for intense pain (Wenzler, Levine, van Dick, Oertel-Knöckel, & Aviezer, 2016).

An alternative to the idea of basic emotions is that emotional feelings vary along two or more continuous dimensions, such as weak versus strong, or pleasant versus unpleasant. Physiological evidence fits this idea (Wilson-Mendenhall, Barrett, & Barsalou, 2013). For example, activation versus inhibition is an important dimension.

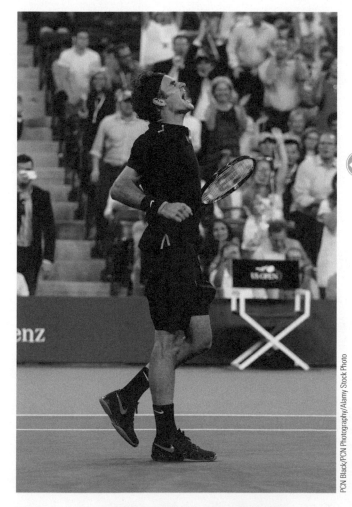

Figure 11.5 Emotional expressions in posture and face
Can you identify whether the player had just won or lost? Check answer B on page **360**.

Activity of the left hemisphere, especially its frontal and temporal lobes, relates to what Jeffrey Gray (1970) called the **behavioral activation system (BAS),** marked by low to moderate autonomic arousal and a tendency to approach, which could characterize happiness or anger. Increased activity of the frontal and temporal lobes of the right hemisphere is associated with the **behavioral inhibition system (BIS),** which increases attention and arousal, inhibits action, and stimulates emotions such as fear and disgust (Davidson & Fox, 1982; Davidson & Henriques, 2000; Murphy, Nimmo-Smith, & Lawrence, 2003; Reuter-Lorenz & Davidson, 1981).

People in one experiment viewed pictures flashed on one side or the other of the visual field, to prime one hemisphere or the other to process the information. People were quicker and more accurate at identifying happy faces when the information went to the left hemisphere. They had an advantage in processing sad or frightened information when the information went to the right hemisphere (Najt, Bayer, & Hausmann, 2013). Such results support an association between left hemisphere and approach, and between the right hemisphere and inhibition of action.

The difference between the hemispheres relates to personality: On the average, people with greater activity in the frontal cortex of the left hemisphere tend to be happier, more outgoing, and more fun-loving. People with greater right-hemisphere activity tend to be socially withdrawn, less satisfied with life, and prone to unpleasant emotions (Knyazev, Slobodskaya, & Wilson, 2002; Schmidt, 1999; Shackman, McMenamin, Maxwell, Greischar, & Davidson, 2009; Urry et al., 2004).

STOP & CHECK

3. What evidence challenges the idea that we identify people's emotions by their facial expressions?

ANSWER

3. Given a photo of a spontaneous facial expression, people usually see more than one emotion and often don't see the emotion described by the person whose face was shown. People recognize expressions from their own culture better than those from other cultures. Also, in everyday life we identify someone's emotion by a combination of cues, including posture, context, gestures, and tone of voice.

The Functions of Emotion

If we evolved the capacity to experience and express emotions, emotions must have been adaptive for our ancestors, and probably for us as well. What good do emotions do?

For certain emotions, the answer is clear. Fear alerts us to escape from danger. Anger directs us to attack an intruder. Disgust tells us to avoid something that might cause illness. The adaptive value of happiness, sadness, embarrassment, and other emotions is less obvious, although researchers have suggested plausible possibilities. Emotional expressions help us communicate our needs to others and understand other people's needs and probable actions. Also, emotions provide a useful guide when we need to make a quick decision.

Emotions and Moral Decisions

When we make important decisions, we pay much attention to how we think an outcome will make us feel. Consider the following moral dilemmas, of which Figure 11.6 illustrates three:

The Trolley Dilemma. A runaway trolley is headed toward five people on a track. The only way you can prevent their death is to switch the trolley onto another track, where it will kill one person. Would it be right to pull the switch?

The Footbridge Dilemma. You are standing on a footbridge overlooking a trolley track. A runaway trolley is headed toward five people on a track. The only way you can

prevent their death is to push a heavy-set stranger off the footbridge and onto the track so that he will block the trolley. Would it be right to push him?

The Lifeboat Dilemma. You and six other people are on a lifeboat in icy waters, but it is overcrowded and starting to sink. If you push one of the people off the boat, the boat will stop sinking and the rest of you will survive. Would it be right to push someone off?

The Hospital Dilemma. You are a surgeon, and five of your patients will die soon unless they get organ transplants. Each needs the transplant of a different organ, and you haven't been able to find organ donors for any of them. A nurse bursts into your office: "Good news! A visitor to the hospital has just arrived, who has exactly the same tissue type as all five of your patients! We can kill this visitor and use the organs to save the five others!" Would it be right to do so?

In each of these dilemmas, you can save five people (including yourself in the lifeboat case) by killing one person.

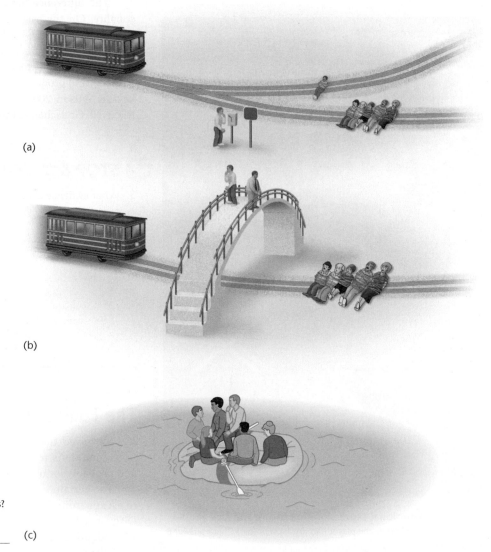

Figure 11.6 Three moral dilemmas
(a) Would you divert a runaway train so it kills one person instead of five? **(b)** Would you push someone off a footbridge so a runaway train kills him instead of five others? **(c)** Would you push someone off a sinking lifeboat to save yourself and four others?

However, although that may be true logically, the decisions do not feel the same. Most people say (hesitantly) that it is right to pull the switch in the trolley dilemma, fewer say yes in the footbridge and lifeboat dilemmas, and almost no one endorses killing one person to save five others in the hospital dilemma. Brain scans show that contemplating the footbridge or lifeboat dilemma activates brain areas known to respond to emotions, including parts of the prefrontal cortex and cingulate gyrus (Greene, Sommerville, Nystrom, Darley, & Cohen, 2001). When you contemplate these situations, you react emotionally because you identify with the person whose suffering and death you might cause by your action, and that feeling is especially intense if you imagine putting your hands on someone rather than just flipping a switch. People with the strongest autonomic arousal are the least likely to make the "logical" decision to kill one and save five others (Cushman, Gray, Gaffey, & Mendes, 2012; Navarrete, McDonald, Mott, & Asher, 2012).

When you make a moral decision, you compare the utilitarian aspect (for example, five people die versus one person dies) and the emotional aspect (how you would feel about what you did). According to fMRI studies, certain brain areas become active when people contemplate just the utilitarian aspect, other areas become active when they contemplate just the emotional aspect, and the ventromedial part of the prefrontal cortex becomes active when they compare the utilitarian and emotional aspects to make a decision (Hutcherson, Montaser-Kouhsari, Woodward, & Rangel, 2015; Shenhav & Greene, 2014). What would happen after damage to the ventromedial prefrontal cortex? In many situations, people with such damage pay little attention to events that elicit strong emotions in most of us (Sánchez-Navarro et al., 2014). When confronted with the moral dilemmas we just discussed, they are more likely than average to choose the utilitarian option of killing one to save five (Ciaramelli, Muccioli, Làdavas, & di Pellegrino, 2007; Koenigs et al., 2007). Would you flip the switch to kill one and save five if the one to be killed was a close relative, such as your mother or daughter? Almost everyone shudders and says of course not, but some people with damage to the ventromedial prefrontal cortex calmly say it would be okay to do so (Thomas, Croft, & Tranel, 2011). If you thought you could kill someone you hated and get away with it, would you do it? Some people with ventromedial prefrontal cortex damage say yes, especially if their damage occurred early in life (Taber-Thomas et al., 2014). So evidently they not only do not imagine feeling sad after the death of a loved one, but also do not imagine feeling guilty after committing murder. For further evidence of that tendency, consider two economic games: In the one-shot Dictator game, you are the Dictator, and you are given some money to divide between yourself and someone else, whatever way you choose. Most people split it evenly or almost evenly. People with ventromedial prefrontal damage keep about 90 percent, on average. In the Trust game, one person gets some money and has

the option of giving some of it to a Trustee. If so, the amount given triples in value, and the Trustee can return any amount of it, such as half, to the first person. People with ventromedial prefrontal damage give less to the Trustee, showing decreased trust. If they are in the position of Trustee, they keep all or nearly all of the money instead of returning part of it (Krajbich, Adolphs, Tranel, Denburg, & Camerer, 2009). In short, they show very little concern for others.

The most famous case of prefrontal damage is that of Phineas Gage. In 1848, an explosion sent an iron rod through Gage's prefrontal cortex. Amazingly, he survived. During the next few months, he showed impulsive behavior and poor decision making, two common symptoms of prefrontal damage. However, the reports about his behavior provide little detail. Over the years, with multiple retellings, people exaggerated the meager facts available (Kotowicz, 2007).

We know more about a modern case. Antonio Damasio (1994) examined a man with prefrontal cortex damage who expressed almost no anger, sadness, or pleasure. Contrary to the idea that unemotional means logical, he made bad decisions that cost him his job, his marriage, and his savings. When tested in the laboratory, he successfully predicted the probable outcomes of various decisions. For example, when asked what would happen if he cashed a check and the bank teller handed him too much money, he knew the probable consequences of returning it or walking away with it. But he admitted, "I still wouldn't know what to do" (Damasio, 1994, p. 49). He knew that one action would win him approval and another would get him in trouble, but he apparently did not anticipate that approval would feel good and trouble would feel bad. Any choice requires consideration of values and emotions—how we think one outcome or another will make us feel. In Damasio's words, "Inevitably, emotions are inseparable from the idea of good and evil" (Damasio, 1999, p. 55).

Of course, it is also true that emotions sometimes interfere with good decisions. If you were driving and suddenly started skidding on a patch of ice, what would you do? A patient with damage to his prefrontal cortex who faced this situation calmly followed the advice he had always heard: Take your foot off the accelerator and steer in the direction of the skid (Shiv, Loewenstein, Bechara, Damasio, & Damasio, 2005). Most people in this situation panic, hit the brakes, and steer away from the skid, making a bad situation worse.

✔ STOP & CHECK

4. After damage to the ventromedial prefrontal cortex, what happens to people's moral reasoning and concern for others?

ANSWER 4. Such people become more likely to endorse the utilitarian option, even in situations where most people would find it emotionally unacceptable. They show decreased concern for others.

Emotions and the Nervous System

Although we regard emotions as nebulous internal states, they are fundamentally biological. As William James observed in the early days of psychology, emotions are "embodied." An emotional feeling relates to the actions and sensations of the body.

Biological research sheds light on many of the central questions about the psychology of emotions. For example, one issue is whether people have a few basic emotions or continuous dimensions along which emotions vary. Biological research so far seems more consistent with the idea of dimensions. Studies of people with brain damage also shed light on the functions of emotion, particularly with relation to moral behavior and decision making. Far from being an impediment to intelligent behavior, emotional reactions are often a useful quick guide to appropriate actions.

Summary

1. Most attempts to define emotion include several aspects including cognition, feelings, and action. **352**

2. The sympathetic nervous system readies the body for emergency fight-or-flight activities. **352**

3. According to the James-Lange theory, the feeling aspect of an emotion results from feedback from actions of the muscles and organs. **353**

4. People with impaired autonomic responses continue to report emotional experiences, although the feeling aspect is weaker than before. **353**

5. Bodily sensations can strengthen emotional feelings. **354**

6. The various components of an emotion do not always occur together. Also, apparently no emotion corresponds to activity in a single brain area. For these and other reasons, many psychologists are uncertain that emotion is a natural category. **354**

7. People recognize others' emotions partly on the basis of facial expressions, but the recognition depends partly on culture and experience. The research on facial expressions does not conclusively demonstrate a small number of basic emotions. An alternative view is that emotions vary along two or more dimensions. **356**

8. Activation of the frontal and temporal areas of the left hemisphere is associated with approach and the behavioral activation system. The corresponding areas of the right hemisphere are associated with withdrawal, decreased activity, and the behavioral inhibition system. **357**

9. Damage to the ventromedial prefrontal cortex in many cases impairs the ability to anticipate emotional consequences, alters responses to moral dilemmas, and impairs decision making. **359**

Key Terms

Terms are defined in the module on the page number indicated. They're also presented in alphabetical order with definitions in the book's Subject Index/Glossary, which begins on page 589. Interactive flash cards, audio reviews, and crossword puzzles are among the online resources available to help you learn these terms and the concepts they represent.

behavioral activation system (BAS) **357**

behavioral inhibition system (BIS) **357**

James-Lange theory **353**

limbic system **354**

panic attack **354**

pure autonomic failure **353**

Thought Question

According to the James-Lange theory, we should expect people with pure autonomic failure to experience weaker than average emotions. What kind of people might experience stronger than average emotions?

Answers to Questions in the Text

Question A, page 356: From left to right: happiness, anger, sadness, surprise, disgust, fear.

Question B, page 357: Roger Federer had just won the match. Could you have guessed that from the facial expression alone?

Module 11.1 | End of Module Quiz

1. The parasympathetic nervous system is most active during which of the following?

   A. Fight-or-flight activities

   B. Digesting food

   C. Intense emotions

   D. Conversations

2. According to the James-Lange theory, feedback from the body's actions is responsible for which aspect of emotion?

   A. Appraisal

   B. Feeling

   C. Coping

   D. Compassion

3. When researchers looked for brain areas associated with particular emotions, what did they find?

   A. Each emotion is centered in a different brain area.

   B. Anger is easy to localize in one brain area, but other emotions are not.

   C. Happiness depends on one brain area, but other emotions do not.

   D. No brain area is responsible for one and only one emotion.

4. Several lines of evidence argue against the idea that facial expressions demonstrate the existence of six basic emotions. Which of the following is NOT one of those lines of evidence?

   A. Asking people to match six faces to six labels interferes with accuracy.

   B. People's guesses about someone's emotion do not always match what the person reported.

   C. Depending on someone's posture, a given facial expression can have several meanings.

   D. People can recognize expressions from their own culture better than those of others.

5. Which brain area is associated with the behavioral activation system and a tendency to approach?

   A. The right hemisphere

   B. The left hemisphere

   C. The amygdala

   D. The hippocampus

6. Damage to the ventromedial prefrontal cortex increases which tendency in making decisions?

   A. Greater conformity to the majority opinion

   B. Longer delays in making decisions

   C. More choices based on emotional feelings

   D. More utilitarian choices

Answers: 1B, 2B, 3D, 4A, 5B, 6D.

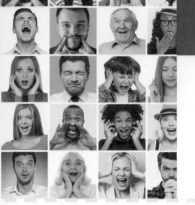

Attack and Escape Behaviors

Have you ever watched a cat play with a rat or mouse before killing it? It might kick, bat, toss, pick up, shake, and carry the rodent. Is the cat sadistically tormenting its prey? No. A cat usually goes for a quick kill if the rodent is small and inactive or if the cat has been given drugs that lower its anxiety. The same cat withdraws altogether if confronted with a large, menacing rodent. In intermediate situations, the cat bats, tosses, and otherwise interacts with a mixture of attack and escape behaviors that might look to us like play (Adamec, Stark-Adamec, & Livingston, 1980; Biben, 1979; Pellis et al., 1988).

Most of the vigorous emotional behaviors we observe in animals fall into the categories of attack and escape, and it is no coincidence that we describe the sympathetic nervous system as the fight-or-flight system. Anger and fear are closely related both behaviorally and physiologically.

Attack Behaviors

Attack behavior depends on the individual as well as the situation. If a hamster intrudes into another hamster's territory, the home hamster sniffs the intruder and eventually attacks, but usually not at once. Suppose the intruder leaves, and a little later, another hamster intrudes. The home hamster attacks faster and more vigorously than before. The first attack enhances home hamster's readiness to attack against any intruder for the next 30 minutes or more (Potegal, 1994). It is as if the first attack gets the hamster in the mood to fight. During that period, activity builds up in the corticomedial area of the amygdala (see Figure 11.7), and as it does so, it increases the hamster's probability of attacking (Potegal, Ferris, Hebert, Meyerhoff, & Skaredoff, 1996; Potegal, Hebert, DeCoster, & Meyerhoff, 1996). Something similar happens in people: If you hold a toddler's arm to prevent him or her from playing with a toy, the result is sometimes screaming and other signs of anger. If you do it again 30 seconds later, the anger is more rapid and more intense (Potegal, Robison, Anderson, Jordan, & Shapiro, 2007). (*Don't* try it yourself. It's unkind.)

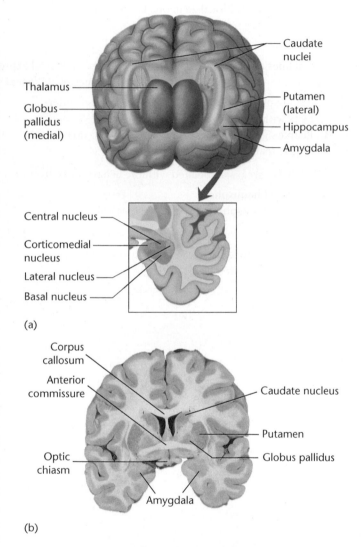

Figure 11.7 Location of amygdala in the human brain
The amygdala, located in the interior of the temporal lobe, receives input from many cortical and subcortical areas. Part **(a)** shows several nuclei of the amygdala.
(*Source: [a] Based on Hanaway, Woolsey, Gado, & Roberts, 1998; Nieuwenhuys, Voogd, & vanHuijzen, 1988; [b] Photo courtesy of Dr. Dana Copeland.*)

Heredity and Environment in Violence

As with almost anything else in psychology, individual differences in aggressive, violent, or antisocial behavior depend on both heredity and environment. Many environmental factors are easy to identify. People who were abused in childhood, people who witnessed violent abuse between their parents, and people who live in a violent neighborhood are more likely than average to express violent behavior. Another factor is exposure to lead, which is harmful to developing brains. Since the banning of lead-based paints and the rise of unleaded gasoline, the prevalence of violent crime has declined, possibly as a result of the decreased lead in the environment (Nevin, 2007).

What about heredity? Twin studies generally indicate a significant amount of heritability for aggressive behavior, but the results vary for many reasons, including how the researchers measure aggression (Veroude et al., 2016). Some studies have measured real-world criminal violence, some have measured relatively trivial "aggressive" behavior in a laboratory setting, and some have relied on answers to questionnaires. Many studies have failed to distinguish between offensive and defensive violence. Furthermore, heritability for antisocial behavior is fairly high in middle-class neighborhoods, but much lower in the most impoverished neighborhoods (Burt, Klump, Gorman-Smith, & Neiderhiser, 2016). The interpretation is that extremely bad environment can elicit antisocial behavior in almost anyone. The same behavior is less common in wealthier environments and more likely to have a genetic predisposition.

Researchers have repeatedly sought to identify individual genes linked to aggressive behavior, without notable success. Then they explored the possibility of interactions between heredity and environment. Particularly interesting is the gene controlling the enzyme *monoamine oxidase A (MAO$_A$)*. After a neuron releases serotonin, dopamine, or norepinephrine, most of it returns to the neuron via reuptake. At that point the enzyme MAO$_A$ breaks down some of it, preventing possible accumulation of an excessive amount. People vary in their genes for MAO$_A$, and the low-activity form shows a possible link to aggression. However, the effect of the gene depends on prior experience. A pioneering study reported that the low-activity form of the gene increased violent behavior *only* in people who had a seriously troubled childhood environment, such as being physically abused or watching parents fight (Caspi et al., 2002). This result is fascinating because of its apparent demonstration of an interaction between genetics and environment. Figure 11.8 illustrates this result.

Since then, most but not all studies have replicated this finding (e.g., Carver, Johnson, Joormann, Kim, & Nam, 2011; Fergusson, Boden, Horwood, Miller, & Kennedy, 2012; Gallardo-Pujol, Andrés-Pueyo, & Maydeu-Olivares, 2013; McDermott, Dawes, Prom-Wormley, Eaves, & Hatemi, 2013). The explanation is uncertain. One hypothesis is that the less active form of the gene is linked to greater emotional reactivity (Weeland, Overbeek, de Castro, & Matthus, 2015).

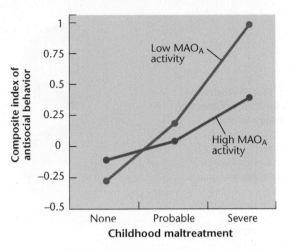

Figure 11.8 Genes, environment, and antisocial behavior in men
The *y* axis represents a complex score combining several types of measurement. Higher scores indicate more aggressive behaviors.
(*Source: From "Role of genotype in the cycle of violence in maltreated children," by A. Caspi, et al, Science, 297, 851–854. © 2002 AAAS.*)

✓ STOP & CHECK

5. What relationship did Caspi et al. (2002) report between the enzyme MAO$_A$ and antisocial behavior?

ANSWER

5. Overall, people with genes for high or low production of MAO$_A$ do not differ significantly in their probability of antisocial behavior. However, among those who suffered serious maltreatment during childhood, people with lower levels of the enzyme showed higher rates of antisocial behavior.

Hormonal Effects

Most fighting in the animal kingdom is by males competing for mates, and their aggressive behavior depends heavily on testosterone. Similarly, throughout the world, men fight more often than women, commit more violent crimes, shout more insults at one another, and so forth. Moreover, young adult men, who have the highest testosterone levels, have the highest rate of aggressive behaviors and violent crimes. Women's violent acts are in most cases less severe (Archer, 2000).

If we compare people of the same age, those with higher testosterone levels tend on average to be more aggressive. Researchers have documented that tendency for both men and women (Peterson & Harmon-Jones, 2012). However, the effects of testosterone are smaller than most people expect (Archer, Birring, & Wu, 1998; Archer, Graham-Kevan, & Davies, 2005). Figure 11.9 shows one set of results. High testosterone levels were more common among men convicted of violent crimes than for those convicted of less violent crimes, but the differences are small. One explanation is that aggressive behavior depends on a sudden burst of testosterone in

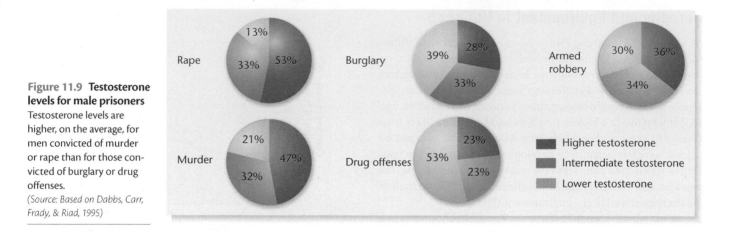

Figure 11.9 Testosterone levels for male prisoners Testosterone levels are higher, on the average, for men convicted of murder or rape than for those convicted of burglary or drug offenses.
(Source: Based on Dabbs, Carr, Frady, & Riad, 1995)

response to some event rather than the baseline level of testosterone (which is easier to measure). A study found that training disruptive children to control their violent impulses produced its benefits by decreasing the testosterone bursts that occurred after perceived insults or mistreatment (Carré, Iselin, Welker, Hariri, & Dodge, 2014).

Correlational studies are not ideal for studying testosterone effects, because people with high testosterone levels may be unusual in other regards also. A better approach is to compare the results of administering testosterone or a placebo. Two studies, one with men and one with women, found that testosterone increased behaviors that are likely to enhance someone's status or prestige (Boksem et al., 2013; Dreher et al., 2016). Fighting for status is, of course, common among men.

Several studies used the idea of temporarily increasing testosterone levels in women. Because most women start with low testosterone levels, the researchers can readily measure the effects of an increase. In one study, testosterone increased the amount of time women spent looking at angry faces (Terburg, Aarts, & van Honk, 2012). In another study, women were asked to make judgments about visual stimuli, either individually or in pairs. Testosterone did not alter accuracy of individuals' judgments, but it reduced the accuracy of pairs' decisions (Wright et al., 2012). The women became more likely to argue instead of collaborating, and one of them—not necessarily the more correct one—dominated the decision. This result fits with other research showing that committees work more harmoniously if they include a high percentage of women—presumably women who hadn't just been given testosterone (Wooley, Chabris, Pentland, Hashmi, & Malone, 2010).

✔ STOP & CHECK

6. Why did researchers test the effects of testosterone on women?

ANSWER

6. Studying the correlation between men's testosterone and their aggressive behavior does not demonstrate cause and effect. Administering testosterone to women is more likely to produce demonstrable effects because women start with a lower level.

Serotonin Synapses and Aggressive Behavior

Several lines of evidence link impulsive, aggressive behavior to low serotonin release. Let's examine some of this evidence.

Nonhuman Animals

Much of the earliest evidence came from studies on mice. Luigi Valzelli (1973) found that isolating male mice for 4 weeks increased their aggressive behavior and decreased their serotonin turnover. When neurons release serotonin, they reabsorb most of it and synthesize enough to replace the amount that washed away. Thus, the amount present in neurons remains fairly constant, but if we measure the serotonin metabolites in body fluids, we gauge the **turnover,** the amount that neurons released and replaced. Researchers measure serotonin turnover by the concentration of **5-hydroxyindoleacetic acid (5-HIAA),** serotonin's main metabolite, in the cerebrospinal fluid (CSF). Measuring the amount in the blood or urine is a simpler but less accurate alternative.

Comparing genetic strains of mice, Valzelli and his colleagues found that social isolation lowered serotonin turnover by the greatest amount in the strains that reacted with the greatest amount of fighting after social isolation (Valzelli & Bernasconi, 1979). Other methods of decreasing serotonin turnover also increase aggressive behavior (Audero et al., 2013). Serotonin activity is lower in juvenile rodents than in adults, and fighting is more frequent in the juveniles (Taravosh-Lahn, Bastida, & Delville, 2006).

Humans

Many early studies reported low serotonin turnover in people with a history of violent behavior, including people convicted of arson and other violent crimes (Virkkunen, Nuutila, Goodwin, & Linnoila, 1987) and people who attempt suicide by violent means, as illustrated in Figure 11.10 (Brown et al., 1982; Edman, Åsberg, Levander, & Schalling, 1986; Mann, Arango, & Underwood, 1990; Pandey et al., 1995; Roy, DeJong, & Linnoila, 1989; Sher et al., 2006; Spreux-Varoquaux et al., 2001). Follow-up studies on people released from prison found

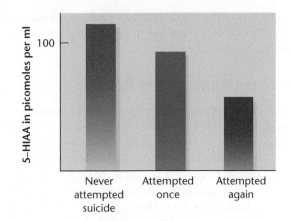

Figure 11.10 Levels of 5-HIAA in the CSF of people with depression
Measurements for the suicide-attempting groups were taken after the first attempt. Low levels of 5-HIAA indicate low serotonin turnover.
(Source: Based on results of Roy, DeJong, & Linnoila, 1989)

that those with lower serotonin turnover had a greater probability of further convictions for violent crimes (Virkkunen, DeJong, Bartko, Goodwin, & Linnoila, 1989; Virkkunen, Eggert, Rawlings, & Linnoila, 1996).

More recent studies have found less consistent effects. Part of the reason is that the early studies measured actual behavior, whereas many of the more recent studies measured aggression or hostility by answers to questionnaires (Duke, Bègue, Bell, & Eisenlohr-Moul, 2013). Overall, low serotonin turnover does appear to correlate with human aggressive behavior, but the correlation is weak, certainly not high enough to use it for making any predictions about an individual's behavior.

Testosterone, Serotonin, and Cortisol

According to a growing consensus, aggressive behavior does not correlate strongly with any one chemical because it depends on a combination. Testosterone, especially a sudden burst of testosterone, facilitates aggressive, assertive, dominant behavior. Serotonin tends to inhibit impulsive behaviors. Even more strongly, the hormone cortisol inhibits aggression. The adrenal gland secretes cortisol during periods of stress and anxiety, and cortisol leads to cautious behavior that conserves energy.

Whereas anxiety increases cortisol levels, anger decreases it (Kazén, Kuenne, Frankenberg, & Quirin, 2012). Studies with both males and females of several ages have found that a combination of high testosterone and low cortisol increases aggressive and risky behaviors (Mehta, Welker, Zilioli, & Carré, 2015; Montoya, Terburg, Bos, & van Honk, 2012; Platje et al., 2015). The general interpretation is that low cortisol means decreased fear of harmful consequences, whereas testosterone increases the expected pleasure or gain. Yes, the opportunity for attack is often perceived as rewarding (Falkner, Grosenick, Davidson, Deisseroth, & Lin, 2016).

Still, even a combined measure of testosterone, cortisol, and serotonin provides only a modest relationship to aggressive behavior. Several medications for restraining anxiety are effective enough to justify their use in some cases. No pill is likely to be effective in controlling violence. If we want to limit violent behavior, we shall need to seek behavioral means.

STOP & CHECK

7. If we want to know how much serotonin the brain has been releasing, what should we measure?
8. What is the relationship between cortisol and aggressive behavior?

ANSWERS

7. We can measure the concentration of 5-HIAA, a serotonin metabolite, in the cerebrospinal fluid or other body fluids. The more 5-HIAA, the more serotonin has been released and presumably resynthesized. **8.** Cortisol tends to inhibit impulsive behaviors, including aggression.

Fear and Anxiety

Do we have any built-in, unlearned fears? Yes, at least one: A sudden loud noise causes a newborn to arch the back, briefly extend the arms and legs, and cry. This reaction is called the *Moro reflex.* You might argue that it does not demonstrate fear, but only distress. Oh, well, suit yourself. It looks like fear to most people. After infancy, a loud noise elicits the closely related **startle reflex**: Auditory information goes first to the cochlear nucleus in the medulla and from there directly to an area in the pons that commands tensing the muscles, especially the neck muscles. Tensing the neck muscles is important because the neck is so vulnerable to injury. Information reaches the pons within 3 to 8 ms after a loud noise, and the full startle reflex occurs in less than two-tenths of a second (Yeomans & Frankland, 1996).

Although you don't have to learn to fear loud noises, your current mood or situation modifies your reaction. Your startle reflex is more vigorous if you are already tense. People with post-traumatic stress disorder show an enhanced startle reflex (Grillon, Morgan, Davis, & Southwick, 1998). So do people who report much anxiety, even if they don't qualify for a psychiatric diagnosis (McMillan, Asmundson, Zvolensky, & Carleton, 2012). In short, variations in the startle reflex correlate well enough with anxiety that we can measure the startle reflex to measure anxiety. Don't underestimate the power of that statement. Research on other types of emotion is hampered by the difficulty of measurement. For happiness, researchers rely almost entirely on self-reports, which are of questionable accuracy. Smiles are even less valid indicators of happiness, as people often smile without being happy or feel happy without smiling. We have no acceptable way to measure happiness in nonhuman animals. Researchers sometimes observe fighting to measure anger, but you could fight without being angry, or you could be angry without fighting. Again, facial expressions are only moderately valid measures of anger.

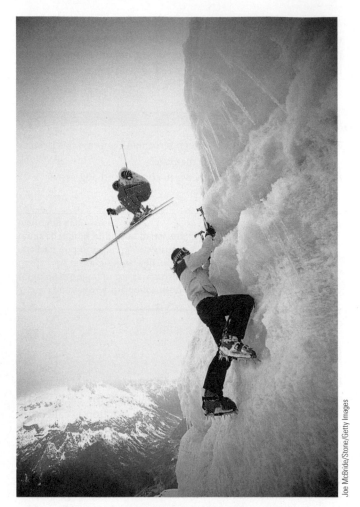

People's choices of activities depend in part on how easily they develop anxiety.

The suitability of the startle reflex as a behavioral measure of anxiety means that we can use it with laboratory animals to explore the brain mechanisms.

Role of the Amygdala in Rodents

Research with rodents has demonstrated the importance of the amygdala for fear and anxiety. The research with rodents has a good chance of applying to humans as well, because the anatomy and connections of the amygdala are nearly the same from one species to another (Janak & Tye, 2015). In research with nonhumans, psychologists first measure the startle response to a loud noise. Then they repeatedly pair a stimulus, such as a light or sound, with shock. Finally, they present the new stimulus just before the loud noise and determine how much it increases the startle response. A control group is tested with a stimulus that has not been paired with shock. Results of such studies consistently show that after rats or mice have learned to associate a stimulus with shock, that stimulus becomes a fear signal, and presenting that signal just before a sudden loud noise enhances the startle response. Conversely, a stimulus previously associated with pleasant stimuli or the absence of danger becomes a safety signal that decreases the startle reflex (Schmid, Koch, & Schnitzler, 1995).

Investigators determined that the amygdala (see Figures 11.7 and 11.11) is important for enhancing the startle reflex, and for learned fears in general. A rat with damage to the amygdala still shows a normal startle reflex, but signals of danger or safety do not modify the reflex. In one study, rats were repeatedly exposed to a light followed by shock and then tested for their responses to a loud noise. Intact rats showed a moderate startle reflex ordinarily, but showed an enhanced response if the light preceded the noise. In contrast,

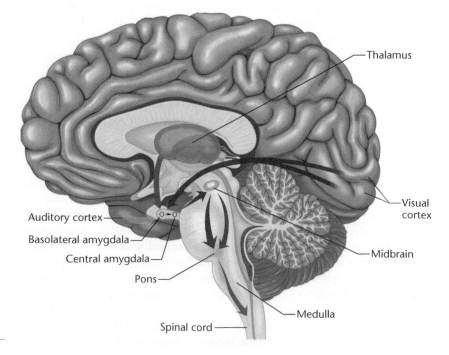

Figure 11.11 Amygdala and learned fears
The central amygdala receives sensory input from the lateral and basolateral amygdala. It sends output to the central gray area of the midbrain, which relays information to a nucleus in the pons responsible for the startle reflex. Damage anywhere along the route from the amygdala to the pons interferes with learned fears that modify the startle reflex.

rats with damage in the path from the amygdala to the hindbrain showed the same startle reflex regardless of the light (Hitchcock & Davis, 1991).

An odd parasite has evolved a way to exploit the consequences of amygdala damage (Berdoy, Webster, & Macdonald, 2000). *Toxoplasma gondii* is a protozoan that infects many mammals but reproduces only in cats. Cats excrete the parasite's eggs in their feces, thereby releasing them into the ground. Rats or mice that burrow in the ground can become infected with the parasite. When the parasite enters a rodent, in many cases (about 50 percent) it migrates to the brain where it damages the amygdala. The rodent then fearlessly approaches a cat, guaranteeing that the cat will eat the rat and that the parasite will find its way back into a cat!

Researchers have worked out many of the connections responsible for the amygdala's effects. Much input from sensory systems including vision and hearing goes to the lateral and basolateral areas of the amygdala, which relay the information to the central amygdala, which combines it with pain and stress information that it received from the thalamus (Penzo et al., 2015). Learning a fear strengthens synapses at several of the connections along this route (Herry & Johansen, 2014). A strain of mice with stronger connections between the lateral and central amygdala is characterized by heightened anxiety in many situations (Abrabos et al., 2013). Perhaps that connection is important for human differences in fears and anxieties also.

By stimulating or damaging parts of laboratory animals' amygdala, researchers have found that one path through the amygdala is responsible for fear of pain, another path for fear of predators, and yet another for fear of aggressive members of your own species (Gross & Canteras, 2012). Also, one part of the amygdala controls changes in breathing, another controls avoidance of potentially unsafe places, and another controls learning which particular places are safest (Kim et al., 2013). The path from the amygdala responsible for freezing in the presence of danger is separate from the path controlling changes in heart rate (Tovote et al., 2016; Viviani et al., 2011). These findings are relevant to psychological theories about emotion, because they demonstrate that what we call fear is a conglomerate of separate aspects, not a single indivisible state.

The amygdala is important for learning to fear a particular stimulus, but that is not the only type of fear conditioning. If a rat has received shocks after a particular stimulus in a particular cage, it learns to fear the stimulus (by changes in the amygdala) but it also learns to fear the cage . . . and new cages . . . and new situations. The same is true for humans. If you have been attacked, you fear anything associated with that attack, but also you become more fearful in general, in a variety of situations. It is as if your brain has decided, "This is a dangerous world. I need to be alert for new threats." This long-term, generalized emotional arousal depends on a brain area called the **bed nucleus of the stria terminalis** (Duvarci, Bauer, & Paré, 2009; Toufexis, 2007). The stria terminalis is a set of axons that connect the bed nucleus to the amygdala, as shown in Figure 11.12.

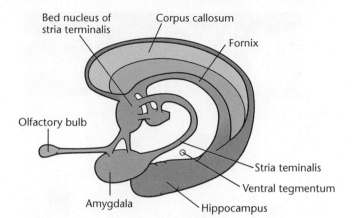

Figure 11.12 The bed nucleus of the stria terminalis
The bed nucleus is critical for long-term adjustments of anxiety, whereas the amygdala is responsible for fear of individual items. The stria terminalis is a set of axons connecting its bed nucleus to the amygdala.

STOP & CHECK

9. What brain mechanism enables the startle reflex to be so fast?
10. How could a researcher use the startle reflex to determine whether some stimulus causes fear?

ANSWERS

9. Loud noises activate a path from the cochlea to cells in the pons that trigger a tensing of neck muscles. 10. Present the stimulus before giving a loud noise. If the stimulus increases the startle reflex beyond its usual level, then the stimulus produced fear.

Studies of the Amygdala in Monkeys

The effect of amygdala damage in monkeys was described in classic studies early in the 1900s and is known as the *Klüver-Bucy syndrome,* from the names of the primary investigators. Monkeys showing this syndrome are tame and placid. They attempt to pick up lighted matches and other objects that they ordinarily avoid. They display less than the normal fear of snakes or of larger, more dominant monkeys (Kalin, Shelton, Davidson, & Kelley, 2001). They have impaired social behaviors, largely because they don't seem to learn which monkeys to approach with caution. Like rats with amygdala damage, monkeys with such damage are impaired at learning what to fear (Kazama, Heuer, Davis, & Bachevalier, 2012). Among intact monkeys, those with a more vigorously reactive amygdala tend to show the greatest fear in response to a noise or an intruder (Oler et al., 2010).

Response of the Human Amygdala to Visual Stimuli

Studies using fMRI show that the human amygdala responds strongly when people look at photos that arouse fear or at photos of faces showing fear or anger (Mattavelli et al., 2014).

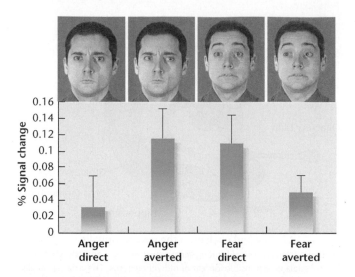

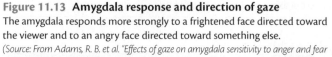

Figure 11.13 **Amygdala response and direction of gaze**
The amygdala responds more strongly to a frightened face directed toward the viewer and to an angry face directed toward something else.
(Source: From Adams, R. B. et al. "Effects of gaze on amygdala sensitivity to anger and fear faces," Science, 2003, 300:1536. Reprinted with permission from AAAS/Science Magazine.)

It can also respond to pleasant stimuli, but only when a task requires attention to pleasant stimuli, and even then the response is never as great as it is to unpleasant stimuli (Stillman, Van Bavel, & Cunningham, 2015). The amygdala's response to a frightened face emerges in the remarkably fast time of just 74 milliseconds (ms) after presentation of the photo (Méndez-Bértolo et al., 2016), faster than the response by the fusiform gyrus and other areas responsible for facial recognition. That is, you respond to the fear in someone's face before you recognize whose face it is.

Contrary to what we might guess, the amygdala responds most strongly when a facial expression is a bit more difficult to interpret. Consider angry and frightened faces. As a rule, it is easy to interpret an angry face looking straight at you, but a fearful face looking straight at you is more puzzling. Frightened people almost always stare at whatever is frightening them, and so the only time someone stares at you with a fearful expression is when the person is afraid of *you!* Although you more easily recognize a fearful expression directed to the side, your amygdala responds more strongly if the fearful expression is directed toward you. The opposite results apply to an angry face (Adams, Gordon, Baird, Ambady, & Kleck, 2003; Adams & Kleck, 2005) (see Figure 11.13). That is, the amygdala responds more strongly to the expression that is harder to interpret.

✔ STOP & CHECK ▰▰▰▰▰▰▰▰▰

11. Given that the amygdala becomes more active when an expression is harder to interpret, can you explain why it does not respond strongly to happy faces?

ANSWER　　　　　11. Smiling faces are easy to interpret!

Individual Differences in Amygdala Response and Anxiety

Most people's tendency toward anxiety generally remains fairly consistent over time. Most infants with an "inhibited" temperament develop into shy, fearful children and then into shy adults who show an enhanced amygdala response to the sight of any unfamiliar face (Beaton et al., 2008; Schwartz, Wright, Shin, Kagan, & Rauch, 2003). Part of the variance in anxiety relates to genes (Disner et al., 2013; Li et al., 2015; Miu, Vulturar, Chis, Ungureanu, & Gross, 2013; Volman et al., 2013), and part relates to epigenetic changes caused by experiences, especially experiences early in life (Nikolova et al., 2014; Silvers et al., 2016).

Individual differences in anxiety correlate strongly with amygdala activity. In one study, college students carried a device that beeped at unpredictable times each day for 28 days, asking the students to record their emotional state at the moment. A year later the students came into a laboratory for the second part of the study, in which an fMRI recorded their amygdala response to very brief presentations of frightening pictures. The amygdala responses correlated highly with the number of unpleasant emotions they had recorded the previous year (Barrett, Bliss-Moreau, Duncan, Rauch, & Wright, 2007). Presumably they recorded so many unpleasant emotions because they were biologically predisposed to react strongly.

In a study of Israeli soldiers, researchers first measured their amygdala responses to briefly flashed unpleasant photos, at the time of the soldiers' induction into the army. Later they measured the soldiers' responses to combat stress. Those with the greatest amygdala response at the start reported the greatest amount of combat stress (Admon et al., 2009). Again, it appears that amygdala response is closely related to fear reactivity.

However, anxiety depends on more than just the amygdala. It also depends on cortical areas that help people cope with threatening information. An effective way to cope is *reappraisal*—reinterpreting a situation as less threatening. For example, if you lose your job, you might tell yourself, "This will prompt me to look for a new job. It might turn out for the best." Or you hear what might be a gunshot, but you decide it might have been a car backfiring. Reappraisal and similar methods of suppressing anxiety depend on top-down influences from the prefrontal cortex to inhibit activity in the amygdala (Marek, Strobel, Bredy, & Sah, 2013; Moscarello & LeDoux, 2013). People with stronger connections between the prefrontal cortex and the amygdala tend to make more use of reappraisal and tend to feel less anxiety (Eden et al., 2015).

Anxiety reactivity affects much of life—even, according to one study, political attitudes. People were asked a series of questions about their support for use of military force, police powers, the death penalty, gun ownership, and so forth. Researchers also measured each person's responses to sudden loud noises, repeated numerous times. As shown in Figure 11.14, those showing high support for military and

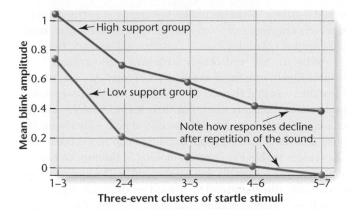

Figure 11.14 **Fear responses and political attitudes**
On the average, people who show a stronger startle response to loud noises tend to favor greater reliance on military and police powers.
(*Source: From "Political attitudes vary with physiological traits," by D. R. Oxley, K. B. Smith, J. R. Alford, M. V. Hibbing, J. L. Miller, M. Scalora, et al., 2008, Science, 321, 1667–1670. Reprinted by permission from the American Association for the Advancement of Science.*)

police action showed a greater startle response to the loud noises (Oxley et al., 2008). The interpretation is that people with a highly reactive amygdala react strongly to real or perceived dangers, and therefore support strong protection against those dangers. This relationship, of course, says nothing about whether the high support or low support group is correct. It just indicates that when we are arguing about policy, variants in brain physiology influence how we interpret uncertain types of evidence.

STOP & CHECK

12. If you wanted to predict which soldiers might have the greatest difficulty dealing with combat stress, what brain measurement might be worth trying?

ANSWER

12. Examine amygdala responses to disturbing pictures. In one study, soldiers with the greatest amygdala responses were the most likely to report great combat stress. Determining the strength of connections between prefrontal cortex and amygdala might be helpful also.

Damage to the Human Amygdala

With laboratory animals, researchers can intentionally damage the amygdala to see the effects. With humans, they have to rely on damage that occurs spontaneously. When people suffer a stroke that damages the amygdala and surrounding areas, at least in one hemisphere, they are impaired in certain ways. They can classify photos as pleasant versus unpleasant about as well as anyone else, but they experience little arousal from viewing unpleasant pictures (Berntson, Bechara, Damasio, Tranel, & Cacioppo, 2007). That is, they have no problem with the cognitive aspect of unpleasant emotions, but they lack much of the feeling aspect.

People with the rare genetic disorder *Urbach-Wiethe disease* accumulate calcium in the amygdala until it wastes away. Thus they have extensive damage to the amygdala without much damage to surrounding structures. Like the monkeys with Klüver-Bucy syndrome, they are impaired at processing emotional information and learning what to fear. Much of the research on this condition deals with a woman known by her initials, SM, who describes herself as fearless, and certainly acts that way. When she viewed 10 clips from the scariest movies the researchers could find, she reported feeling only excitement, no fear. Researchers took her to an exotic pet store. In spite of insisting that she hates snakes and spiders, she was happy to hold a snake (see Figure 11.15), and the staff repeatedly had to restrain her from touching or poking the tarantulas and venomous snakes. When the researchers took her to a "haunted house," she led the way without hesitation, venturing down dark hallways. When people dressed as monsters jumped out, other people in the group screamed, but SM laughed, curiously poked one of the monsters, and scared the monster! Her fearlessness is dangerous to her. She has been held up at gunpoint and knifepoint and has been physically assaulted repeatedly. Evidently she plunges into dangerous situations without the caution other people would show. When she describes these events, she remembers feeling angry, but not afraid (Feinstein, Adolphs, Damasio, & Tranel, 2011).

Here is another example of her fearlessness: Suppose someone you don't know approaches you, face to face. How close could that person come before you began to feel uncomfortable? Most Americans stand about 2 feet (0.7 m) away from another person, but SM's preferred distance is about half that. When a man unknown to her followed the experimenters' instruction to approach her so close that their noses touched, she showed and reported no discomfort (Kennedy, Gläscher, Tyszka, & Adolphs, 2009). (She did say she wondered whether they were "up to something.")

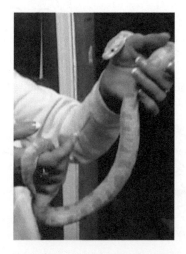

Figure 11.15 **SM, a woman with amygdala damage, holds a snake at an exotic pet store**
Although she said she hates snakes, she was curious to hold this one and wanted to touch the others, including venomous ones.
(*Source: From Feinstein, J. S., Adolphs, R., Damasio, A., & Tranel, D. (2011). The human amygdala and the induction and experience of fear. Current Biology, 21, 34–38 with permission from Elsevier.*)

The only event known to trigger her fear is breathing 35 percent carbon dioxide, which leaves a person gasping for breath. She and two others with Urbach-Wiethe disease reacted to concentrated CO_2 with a panic attack. The difference from other fear stimuli is that carbon dioxide affects the body directly, rather than by visual or auditory signals that the amygdala would have to interpret. However, although all three people said it was a terrible experience and they thought they were going to die, they all agreed to go through the experience again the following week, and did not think about the upcoming experience again during that delay (Feinstein et al., 2013). Apparently the amygdala is important for imagining the fear or thinking about the danger.

SM and other people with Urbach-Wiethe disease often fail to recognize the emotional expressions in faces, especially expressions of fear or disgust (Boucsein, Weniger, Mursch, Steinhoff, & Irle, 2001). When SM was asked to draw faces showing certain emotions (see Figure 11.16), she made good drawings of most expressions but had trouble drawing a fearful expression, saying that she did not know what such a face

would look like. When the researcher urged her to try, she drew someone crawling away with hair on end, as cartoonists often indicate fear (Adolphs, Tranel, Damasio, & Damasio, 1995).

Why do SM and others with amygdala damage have trouble identifying facial expressions of fear? At first, the assumption was that they do not feel fear and therefore cannot understand the expression. But then Ralph Adolphs and his colleagues observed that SM focuses almost entirely on the nose and mouth of each photograph. Also in everyday life, she seldom makes eye contact, looking at the mouth instead (Spezio, Huang, Castelli, & Adolphs, 2007). The amygdala automatically directs attention toward emotionally significant stimuli, even without your awareness (Amting, Greening, & Mitchell, 2010; Burra et al., 2013; Peck, Lau, & Salzman, 2013; Pishnamazi et al., 2016), but someone lacking an amygdala doesn't have this automatic tendency. Suppose you are looking at a computer screen, and a face is flashed briefly on the screen. Almost instantaneously, you would move your gaze to focus on the eyes, especially if the face was showing fear (Gamer & Büchel, 2009). SM is willing to make eye contact, but someone's eyes simply don't attract her attention as they do for other people (Kennedy & Adolphs, 2010). When researchers asked her to look at the eyes, she quickly recognized fearful expressions (Adolphs, Tranel, & Buchanan, 2005). Seeing the eyes is particularly important for recognizing fear. People express happiness with the mouth, but they express fear mainly with the eyes (Morris, deBonis, & Dolan, 2002; Vuilleumier, 2005). Figure 11.17 shows only the whites of the eyes of people expressing fear (left) and happiness (right). Most people recognize the fear expression, but not the happy expression, from the eyes alone (Whalen et al., 2004).

These observations suggest an alternative interpretation of the function of the amygdala. Instead of being responsible for *feeling* fear or other emotions, evidently it is responsible for detecting emotional information and directing attention to it.

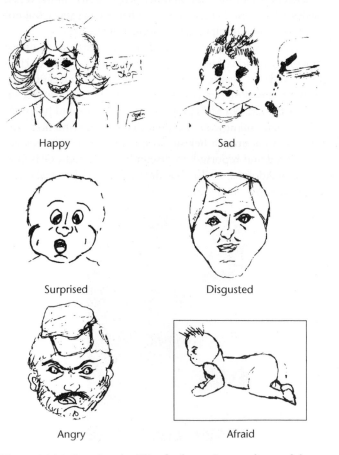

Happy

Sad

Surprised

Disgusted

Angry

Afraid

Figure 11.16 Drawings by SM, who has a damaged amygdala
She at first declined to draw a fearful expression because, she said, she could not imagine it. When urged to try, she remembered that cartoons depict frightened people with their hair on end.
(Source: From "Fear and the human amygdala," by R. Adolphs, D. Tranel, H. Damasio, and A. Damasio, Journal of Neuroscience, 15, 5879–5891. Copyright © 1995 by Oxford University Press. Reprinted by permission.)

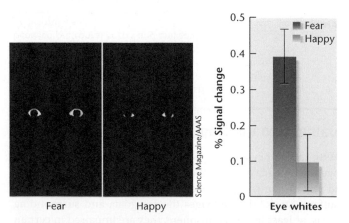

Fear   Happy

Figure 11.17 Eye expressions for fear and happiness
The eye whites alone enable most people to guess that the person on the left was feeling afraid. The right part of the figure shows the amygdala responses of typical adults to the two expressions.
(Source: From "Human amygdala responsivity to masked fearful eye whites," by P. J. Whalen et al., Science, 2004, 306, 2061. Reprinted by permission from AAAS/Science magazine.)

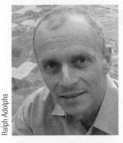

Ralph Adolphs

Will a better understanding of the social brain lead to a better understanding of social behavior? And can such knowledge ultimately be used to help our species negotiate and survive in the vastly complex social world it has helped create? To approach such questions, social neuroscientists will need to establish dialogues with other disciplines in the social and behavioral sciences, and to be highly sensitive to the public consequences of the data they generate. (*Adolphs, personal communication*)

Ralph Adolphs

✓ STOP & CHECK ▰▰▰▰▰

13. Why do people with amygdala damage have trouble recognizing expressions of fear?

ANSWER

13. They focus their vision on the nose and mouth. Expressions of fear depend almost entirely on the eyes.

Anxiety Disorders

What is the "right" amount of anxiety? It depends. Your life circumstances might justify great anxiety, or much less. Researchers can model that trend in laboratory rats. Suppose tone #1 predicts a mild shock and tone #2 predicts no shock. A rat learns to respond to tone #1 by freezing in place, and many neurons in its amygdala respond only to #1. As Figure 11.18 shows, if tone #1 predicts a strong shock, a greatly increased percentage of neurons respond to both tones (and presumably other tones that the researchers did not test). The dangers are great, and the rat is not taking any chances (Ghosh & Chattarji, 2015).

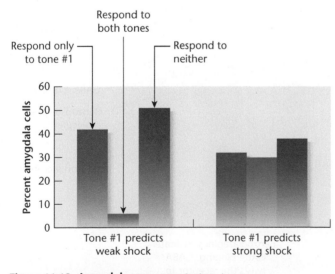

Figure 11.18　Amygdala responses to two tones
After a tone predicted a mild shock, amygdala cells responded only to that tone. If it predicted a strong shock, many amygdala cells responded unselectively to all tones.
(*Source: Based on results of Ghosh & Chattarji, 2015*)

For humans, too, widespread, generalized anxiety makes sense if you live in a war zone or if you have recently been attacked. Anxiety disorders are conditions in which someone's anxiety seems excessive for the circumstances. **Panic disorder** is characterized by frequent periods of anxiety and occasional attacks of rapid breathing, increased heart rate, sweating, and trembling—in other words, extreme arousal of the sympathetic nervous system. An important part of the disorder is frequent fear of the next panic attack. The fear of fear itself can become incapacitating. Panic disorder is more common in women than in men and far more common in adolescents and young adults than in older adults (Shen et al., 2007; Swoboda, Amering, Windhaber, & Katschnig, 2003).

What causes some people to be prone to anxiety? Twin studies suggest a genetic predisposition, although no single gene has been identified (Shimada-Sugimoto, Otowa, & Hettema, 2015). Early-life experiences can also increase susceptibility. Curiously, panic disorder occurs in about 15 percent of people with *joint laxity,* commonly known as being "double-jointed" (able to bend the fingers backward farther than usual). Even when people with joint laxity do not have panic disorder, they tend to have stronger than average fears (Bulbena et al., 2004; Bulbena, Gago, Sperry, & Bergé, 2006).

The research so far links panic disorder to abnormalities in the hypothalamus, and not necessarily the amygdala. Panic disorder is associated with decreased activity of the neurotransmitter GABA and increased levels of orexin. Orexin, as discussed in other chapters, is associated with maintaining wakefulness and activity. We might not have guessed that it would also be associated with anxiety, but apparently it is, and drugs that block orexin receptors block panic responses (Johnson et al., 2015).

People have long recognized that many soldiers returning from battle are prone to continuing anxieties and distress. Long ago, people called the condition *battle fatigue* or *shell shock.* Today, we call it **post-traumatic stress disorder (PTSD)**, marked by frequent distressing recollections (flashbacks) and nightmares about the traumatic event, avoidance of reminders of it, and vigorous reactions to noises and other stimuli (Yehuda, 2002). PTSD also occurs after other miserable experiences, such as being raped or watching someone get killed. When someone survives a traumatic experience, raising the anxiety level at least temporarily is understandable. We presumably evolved mechanisms to adjust our anxiety level up or down depending on the level of danger. However, not everyone who endures a trauma develops PTSD, and we cannot predict who will get PTSD based on the severity of the trauma or the intensity of the person's initial reaction (Harvey & Bryant, 2002; Shalev et al., 2000).

The humor publication *The Onion* once published an article about "pretraumatic stress disorder" that people developed by watching the news on television. Although this was intended as humor, psychologists later found that something like it actually happens: Some soldiers develop mild symptoms similar to post-traumatic stress disorder during *preparation* for deployment, and these soldiers are more likely than average to develop serious symptoms after actual war experiences (Berntsen & Rubin, 2015).

The increased risk relates to brain anatomy. Most victims of PTSD have a smaller than average hippocampus (Stein, Hanna, Koverola, Torchia, & McClarty, 1997). Is that difference a result of PTSD, or does it show a predisposition by people who already had a smaller hippocampus? Probably both are true. Studies on both humans and laboratory animals show that severe stress can impair function in the hippocampus and sometimes cause shrinkage (Kim, Pellman, & Kim, 2015). In addition, people who have a smaller hippocampus tend to rate their experiences as more stressful (Lindgren, Bergdahl, & Nyberg, 2016). In one study, investigators examined men who developed PTSD during war. First, they confirmed earlier reports that most of the victims of PTSD had a smaller than average hippocampus. Then they found cases in which the victim had a monozygotic twin who had not been in battle and who did not have PTSD. The results showed that the twin without PTSD *also* had a smaller than average hippocampus (Gilbertson et al., 2002). Presumably, both twins had a smaller than average hippocampus from the start, which increased the susceptibility to PTSD. Two other studies found that recovery from PTSD did not increase the size of the hippocampus, but people with the smallest hippocampus were the least likely to recover quickly (Rubin et al., 2016; van Rooij et al., 2015).

One further point about PTSD: A study compared Vietnam War veterans who suffered injuries that produced various kinds of brain damage. Of those whose damage included the amygdala, *none* suffered PTSD. Of those with damage elsewhere in the brain, 40 percent suffered PTSD (Koenigs et al., 2008). Apparently, the amygdala, which is so important for emotional processing, is essential for the extreme emotional impact that produces PTSD.

✅ STOP & CHECK

14. What evidence indicates that a smaller than average hippocampus makes people more vulnerable to PTSD?

ANSWER

14. For victims of PTSD who have a monozygotic twin, the twin also has a smaller than average hippocampus, even if he or she does not have PTSD. Also, people with a smaller hippocampus are less likely to recover easily from PTSD.

Relief from Anxiety

People have many ways to cope with anxiety—social support, reappraisal of the situation, exercise, distraction, gaining a sense of control over the situation, and so forth. Here we consider the options for biological interventions.

Pharmacological Relief

People with excessive anxiety sometimes seek relief through medications. The most common *anxiolytic* (anti-anxiety) drugs are the **benzodiazepines** (BEN-zo-die-AZ-uh-peens), such as diazepam (trade name Valium), chlordiazepoxide (Librium), and alprazolam (Xanax). Benzodiazepines bind to the **GABA$_A$ receptor,** which includes a site that binds GABA as well as sites that modify the sensitivity of the GABA site (see Figure 11.19). The brain also has other kinds of GABA receptors, such as GABA$_B$, with different behavioral effects.

At the center of the GABA$_A$ receptor is a chloride channel. When open, it permits chloride ions (Cl$^-$) to cross the membrane into the neuron, hyperpolarizing the cell or at least

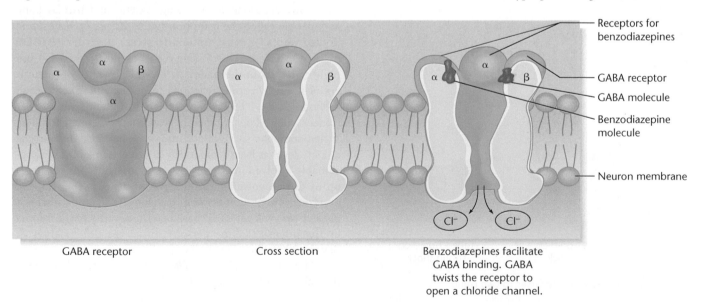

GABA receptor   Cross section   Benzodiazepines facilitate GABA binding. GABA twists the receptor to open a chloride channel.

Receptors for benzodiazepines
GABA receptor
GABA molecule
Benzodiazepine molecule
Neuron membrane

Figure 11.19 The GABA$_A$ receptor complex
Of its four receptor sites sensitive to GABA, the three alpha sites are also sensitive to benzodiazepines.
(Source: Based on Guidotti, Ferrero, Fujimoto, Santi, & Costa, 1986)

counteracting any sodium entering the cell through excitatory synapses. That is, the GABA synapse is inhibitory. Surrounding the chloride channel are four units, each containing one or more sites sensitive to GABA. Benzodiazepines bind to sites on three of those four units (labeled α in Figure 11.19). When a benzodiazepine molecule attaches, it neither opens nor closes the chloride channel but twists the receptor so that the GABA binds more easily (Macdonald, Weddle, & Gross, 1986). Benzodiazepines thus facilitate the effects of GABA.

Benzodiazepines exert their anti-anxiety effects in the amygdala, hypothalamus, midbrain, and several other areas. A minute amount of benzodiazepines injected directly into a rat's amygdala decreases learned shock-avoidance behaviors (Pesold & Treit, 1995), relaxes the muscles, and increases social approaches to other rats (Sanders & Shekhar, 1995). Benzodiazepines have other effects, including the possibility of addiction after prolonged use. Nevertheless, they provide relief from anxiety disorders, generally with fewer undesirable effects than antidepressant drugs, which are also sometimes prescribed (Offidani, Guidi, Tomba, & Fava, 2013).

An unfortunate aspect of benzodiazepines is that they are extremely stable chemically. Typically they pass through the urine intact, pass through the waste treatment plant intact, and accumulate in lakes and rivers, where they alter the eating and social behavior of resident fish (Brodin, Fick, Jonsson, & Klaminder, 2013).

Alcohol and Anxiety

Alcohol also reduces anxiety through effects on GABA receptors. Alcohol promotes the flow of chloride ions through the $GABA_A$ receptor complex by binding strongly at a special site found on only certain $GABA_A$ receptors (Glykys et al., 2007). One experimental drug, known as Ro15-4513, is particularly effective in blocking the effects of alcohol on GABA receptors (Suzdak et al., 1986). Ro15-4513 blocks the effects of alcohol on motor coordination, its depressant action on the brain, and its ability to reduce anxiety (Becker, 1988; Hoffman, Tabakoff, Szabó, Suzdak, & Paul, 1987; Ticku & Kulkarni, 1988) (see Figure 11.20).

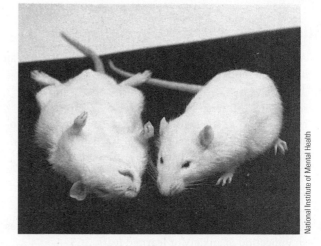

Figure 11.20 Two rats that were given the same amount of alcohol
The rat on the right was later given the experimental drug Ro15-4513. Within 2 minutes, its performance and coordination improved significantly.

Could Ro15-4513 be useful as a "sobering-up" pill or as a treatment to help people who want to stop drinking alcohol? Hoffmann-La Roche, the company that discovered the drug, concluded that it would be too risky. People who relied on the pill might think they were sober enough to drive home when they were not. Also, giving such a pill to people with alcoholism would probably backfire. Because people with alcoholism drink to get drunk, a pill that decreased their feeling of intoxication would probably lead them to drink even more.

✓ STOP & CHECK

15. What would be the effect of benzodiazepines on someone who had no GABA?

ANSWER

15. Benzodiazepines facilitate the effects of GABA, so a person without GABA would not respond to benzodiazepines.

Module 11.2 | In Closing

Doing Something about Emotions

It is hard to foresee future developments, but suppose researchers make sudden advances in linking emotional behaviors to physiological measurements. Imagine if we could take a blood sample, an fMRI scan, and a few other measurements and then predict which people will commit violent crime. How accurate would those predictions have to be before we considered using them? In what way, if any, would we use them?

And what about anxiety? Suppose research enables us to modulate people's anxiety precisely without undesirable side effects. What would be the consequences of chemically controlling everyone's anxiety? Future research will give us new options and opportunities. Deciding what to do with them is another matter.

Summary

1. An experience that gradually provokes an attack leaves an individual more ready than usual to attack again. **362**

2. Aggressive behavior relates to both genetic and environmental influences. Most evidence supports the hypothesis that a gene decreasing the activity of monoamine oxidase A increases aggressive behavior mainly among people who had abusive experiences in childhood. **363**

3. Testosterone increases the probability of aggressive or assertive behavior, and cortisol decreases it. **363**

4. Researchers measure enhancement of the startle reflex as an indication of anxiety or learned fears. **365**

5. The amygdala is critical for increasing or decreasing the startle reflex. It also mediates learned fears. **366**

6. According to studies using fMRI, the human amygdala responds strongly to fear stimuli and other stimuli that evoke strong emotional processing. It responds most strongly when the processing is effortful. **367**

7. People with damage to the amygdala fail to focus their attention on stimuli with important emotional content. **369**

8. Damage to the amygdala impairs recognition of fear expressions largely because of lack of attention to the eyes. **370**

9. Both genetics and experience can predispose people to anxiety disorders. **371**

10. People with a smaller than average hippocampus have an increased probability of developing post-traumatic stress disorder. **372**

11. Anti-anxiety drugs decrease fear by facilitating the binding of the neurotransmitter GABA to the GABA$_A$ receptors. **372**

Key Terms

Terms are defined in the module on the page number indicated. They're also presented in alphabetical order with definitions in the book's Subject Index/Glossary, which begins on page 589. Interactive flash cards, audio reviews, and crossword puzzles are among the online resources available to help you learn these terms and the concepts they represent.

bed nucleus of the stria terminalis **367**

benzodiazepines **372**

GABA$_A$ receptor **372**

5-hydroxyindoleacetic acid (5-HIAA) **364**

panic disorder **371**

post-traumatic stress disorder **371**

startle reflex **365**

turnover **364**

Thought Questions

1. Much of the play behavior of a cat can be analyzed into attack and escape components. Is the same true for children's play?

2. People with amygdala damage approach other people indiscriminately instead of trying to choose people who look friendly and trustworthy. What might be a possible explanation?

Module 11.2 | End of Module Quiz

1. Heritability of a tendency toward antisocial behavior is *lowest* for which of the following?

    A. Males
    B. Females
    C. People in impoverished neighborhoods
    D. People in middle-class neighborhoods

2. How does the gene for the less active form of the enzyme MAO$_A$ affect the probability for aggressive behavior?

    A. Increased probability, regardless of environment
    B. Decreased probability, regardless of environment
    C. Increased probability for someone who was abused in childhood
    D. Increased probability for someone who lived in a middle-class neighborhood

3. Aggressive behavior correlates with low turnover of which neurotransmitter?

    A. Serotonin
    B. Norepinephrine
    C. Dopamine
    D. Glutamate

4. Which of the following hormones tends to inhibit aggressive behavior?

   A. Cortisol

   B. Testosterone

   C. Estradiol

   D. Insulin

5. Why do we know more about the brain mechanisms of fear and anxiety than we do about other emotions?

   A. Clinical psychologists have greater interest in anxiety than in other emotions.

   B. Anxiety depends on brain areas that are easier to reach surgically.

   C. Unlike other emotions, anxiety depends on only a single neurotransmitter.

   D. Researchers can more satisfactorily measure anxiety than other emotions in laboratory animals.

6. After damage to the amygdala, what happens to the startle reflex?

   A. It becomes stronger than before.

   B. It becomes weaker than before.

   C. It disappears altogether.

   D. It becomes more consistent from one time or situation to another.

7. Suppose a researcher wants to determine whether someone is afraid of cats. Of the following, which would be the most reasonable approach?

   A. Present a photo of a cat and see whether it elicits a startle reflex.

   B. Present a photo of a cat and then a loud sound. See whether the photo enhances the usual startle reflex.

   C. Present a loud sound and then show a photo of a cat. See whether the photo calms the person after the startle reflex.

   D. Present a loud sound to both a person and a cat and see which one shows the greater startle reflex.

8. Research on the amygdala supports which of these psychological conclusions?

   A. People who experience great fear also tend to experience a great amount of anger.

   B. Sigmund Freud's insights provide the best method for treating anxiety disorders.

   C. What we call fear is a combination of several components, not an indivisible entity.

   D. People have six basic types of emotion.

9. What role does the bed nucleus of the stria terminalis play in fear or anxiety?

   A. It affects fear of the environment in general.

   B. It mediates reappraisal that reduces the response of the amygdala.

   C. It relays information from the amygdala to the midbrain.

   D. It is responsible for the extinction of learned fears.

10. The amygdala responds most strongly to which type of facial expressions?

    A. Expressions by infants and children

    B. Expressions that require some effort to understand

    C. Expressions that are directed away from the viewer

    D. Expressions of sadness

11. What, if anything, can we predict from measuring the strength of amygdala response to frightening stimuli or faces showing fear?

    A. We can predict changes in personality, as measured by questionnaires.

    B. We can predict probability of criminal behavior.

    C. We can predict probability of strong emotional responses to stressful experiences.

    D. We cannot predict anything.

12. After Urbach-Wiethe disease damaged their amygdala, two people showed no fear under most circumstances. Which of the following did, nevertheless, evoke fear?

    A. Breathing concentrated carbon dioxide

    B. Holding a snake

    C. Standing too close to a stranger

    D. Watching a horror movie

13. Which of the following types of people would be more likely than average to develop PTSD?

    A. People who have suffered damage to the amygdala

    B. People with higher than average levels of serotonin turnover

    C. People with lower than average levels of cortisol

    D. People with a smaller than average hippocampus

14. What do benzodiazepines do?

    A. They decrease cortisol secretion.

    B. They increase secretion of orexin.

    C. They facilitate GABA synapses.

    D. They inhibit serotonin synapses.

Answers: 1C, 2C, 3A, 4A, 5D, 6D, 7B, 8C, 9A, 10B, 11C, 12A, 13D, 14C.

Stress and Health

Stress is not an emotion, but it is a result of emotion, and a cause of much else. In the early days of scientific medicine, physicians made little allowance for the relation of emotions to health and disease. Today, we accept the idea that emotions and other experiences influence people's illnesses and patterns of recovery. **Behavioral medicine** emphasizes the effects of stressful experiences, diet, smoking, exercise, and other behaviors.

Stress and the General Adaptation Syndrome

Hans Selye (1979) popularized the concept of **stress**, defining it as the nonspecific response of the body to any demand made upon it. When Selye was in medical school, he noticed that patients with a wide variety of illnesses had much in common: They develop a fever, they lose their appetite, they become inactive, they are sleepy most of the day, their sex drive declines, and their immune systems become more active. Later, when doing laboratory research, he found that rats exposed to an injection of anything, as well as heat, cold, pain, confinement, or the sight of a cat responded with increased heart rate, breathing rate, and adrenal secretions. Selye inferred that any threat to the body, in addition to its specific effects, activated a generalized response to stress, which he called the **general adaptation syndrome**, due mainly to activity of the adrenal glands. In the initial stage, which he called *alarm,* the adrenal glands release the hormone epinephrine, thereby stimulating the sympathetic nervous system to ready the body for brief emergency activity. The adrenal glands also release the hormone **cortisol**, which increases blood glucose, providing the body with extra energy, and the hormone *aldosterone,* important for maintaining blood salt and blood volume. To maintain energy for emergency activity, the body temporarily suppresses less urgent activities, such as sexual arousal.

During the second stage, *resistance,* the sympathetic response declines, but the adrenal glands continue secreting cortisol and other hormones that enable the body to maintain prolonged alertness. The body adapts to the prolonged situation in whatever way it can, such as by decreasing activity to save energy. The body also has ways of adapting to prolonged cold or heat, low oxygen, and so forth.

After intense, prolonged stress, the body enters the third stage, *exhaustion.* During this stage, the individual is tired, inactive, and vulnerable because the nervous and immune systems no longer have the energy to sustain their responses.

Stress-related illnesses and psychiatric problems are widespread in industrial societies, possibly because of changes in the type of stresses we face. In our evolutionary past, the alarm stage readied our ancestors for fight or flight. Today, as Robert Sapolsky (1998) has argued, many of our crises are prolonged, such as working under a domineering boss, paying bills with inadequate income, or caring for a relative with a chronic health problem. Prolonged activation of the general adaptation syndrome can lead to exhaustion.

Selye's concept of stress specified any *change* in one's life, including both favorable and unfavorable events. Bruce McEwen (2000, p. 173) proposed an alternative definition that is better for most purposes: "events that are interpreted as threatening to an individual and which elicit physiological and behavioral responses." Although this definition differs from Selye's, the idea remains that many kinds of events can be stressful, and the body reacts to all kinds of stress in similar ways. Still, as Jerome Kagan (2016) has argued, psychologists have been willing to define stress in broad, vague terms that range from life-threatening events to brief matters of inconvenience. Consequently, research studies on stress sometimes reach contradictory conclusions about the effects on sympathetic nervous system arousal, alertness, memory, immune responses, or health.

✅ STOP & CHECK

16. What function does cortisol play in the initial response to stress?
17. How does McEwen's definition of stress differ from Selye's?

ANSWERS
16. Cortisol increases blood levels of glucose and therefore makes more energy available. 17. Selye's definition treated favorable and unfavorable changes as equally stressful. McEwen's definition focuses on events that an individual considers threatening.

Stress and the Hypothalamus-Pituitary-Adrenal Cortex Axis

Stress activates two body systems. One is the sympathetic nervous system, which prepares the body for brief fight-or-flight emergency responses. The other is the **HPA axis,** consisting of the hypothalamus, pituitary gland, and adrenal cortex. Activation of the human hypothalamus induces the anterior pituitary gland to secrete **adrenocorticotropic hormone (ACTH),** which in turn stimulates the adrenal cortex to secrete cortisol, which enhances metabolic activity, elevates blood levels of sugar, and increases alertness (see Figure 11.21). Many researchers refer to cortisol as a "stress hormone" and use measurements of cortisol level as an indication of someone's recent stress level. Compared to the autonomic nervous system, the HPA axis reacts more slowly, but it dominates the response to prolonged stressors such as living with an abusive parent or spouse.

Stress that releases cortisol mobilizes the body's energy to fight a difficult situation, but the results depend on amount and duration. Brief or moderate stress improves attention and memory formation, especially in the amygdala, which is important for learning fears (Sapolsky, 2015). It improves performance on habitual skills and relatively simple tasks, but it impairs performance that requires complex, flexible thinking (Arnsten, 2015). Stress also enhances activity of the immune

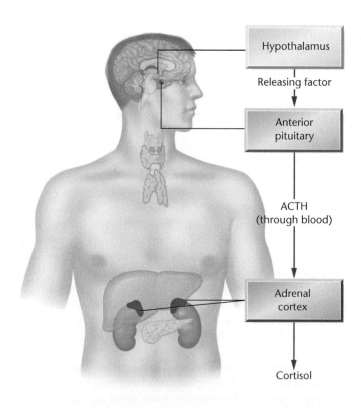

Figure 11.21 **The hypothalamus-pituitary-adrenal cortex axis** Stressful events increase secretion of the adrenal hormone cortisol, which elevates blood sugar and increases metabolism. These changes help the body sustain prolonged activity but at the expense of decreased immune system activity.

system, helping it fight illnesses (Benschop et al., 1995). However, prolonged stress impairs immune activity and memory (Mika et al., 2012). To see why, we start with an overview of the immune system.

The Immune System

The **immune system** consists of cells that protect the body against viruses, bacteria, and other intruders. The immune system is like a police force: If it is too weak, the "criminals" (viruses and bacteria) run wild and create damage. If it becomes too strong and unselective, it starts attacking "law-abiding citizens" (the body's own cells). When the immune system attacks normal cells, we call the result an *autoimmune disease*. Myasthenia gravis and rheumatoid arthritis are examples of autoimmune diseases.

Leukocytes

The primary components of the immune system are the **leukocytes,** commonly known as white blood cells. We distinguish several types of leukocytes, including B cells, T cells, and natural killer cells (see Figure 11.22):

- *B cells*, which mature mostly in the bone marrow, secrete **antibodies,** which are Y-shaped proteins that attach to particular antigens, just as a key fits a lock. Every cell has surface proteins called **antigens** (antibody-generator molecules), and you have your own unique antigens. The B cells recognize "self" antigens, but when they find an unfamiliar antigen, they attack the cell. This kind of attack defends the body against viruses and bacteria, but it also causes rejection of organ transplants from an incompatible donor, unless physicians take special steps to minimize the attack. After the body has made antibodies against a particular intruder, it "remembers" the intruder and quickly builds more of the same kind of antibody if it encounters that intruder again.
- *T cells* mature in the thymus gland. Several kinds of T cells attack intruders directly (without secreting antibodies), and some help other T cells or B cells to multiply.
- *Natural killer cells,* another kind of leukocytes, attack tumor cells and cells that are infected with viruses. Whereas each B or T cell attacks a particular kind of foreign antigen, natural killer cells attack all intruders.

In response to an infection, leukocytes and other cells produce small proteins called **cytokines** (e.g., interleukin-1, or IL-1) that combat infections. Cytokines also stimulate the vagus nerve and trigger the release of **prostaglandins** that cross the blood–brain barrier and stimulate the hypothalamus to produce fever, sleepiness, lack of energy, lack of appetite, and loss of sex drive (Maier & Watkins, 1998; Saper, Romanovsky, & Scammell, 2012). Recall Selye's observation that most illnesses produce similar symptoms, such as fever, loss of energy, and so forth. Here we see the explanation. Aspirin and ibuprofen decrease fever and other signs of illness by inhibiting prostaglandins.

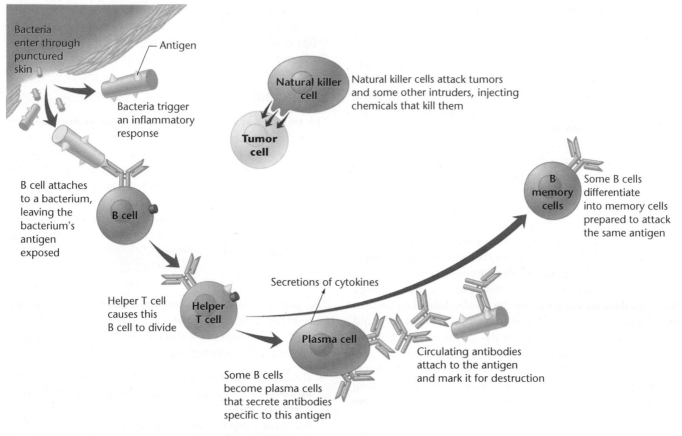

Figure 11.22 Immune system responses to a bacterial infection
B cells bind to bacteria and produce antibodies against the bacteria. When a helper T cell attaches to the B cell, it stimulates the B cell to generate copies of itself, called B memory cells, that immunize the body against future invasions by the same kind of bacteria.

Note that these symptoms of illness are actually part of the body's way of fighting the illness. Most people think of fever and sleepiness as something the illness did to them, but in fact, fever and sleepiness are strategies that evolved for fighting the illness. As discussed in Chapter 9, a moderate fever helps fight many infections. Sleep and inactivity are ways of conserving energy so that the body can devote more energy to its immune attack against the intruders. Decreased appetite may be helpful by decreasing the need for activity, and by reducing blood glucose, the preferred fuel for many microorganisms (Saper et al., 2012).

 STOP & CHECK ▐▬▬▬▬▬▬

18. What kind of cell releases cytokines?
19. What changes do prostaglandins stimulate?

ANSWERS

19. Prostaglandins stimulate the hypothalamus to produce fever, decrease hunger, decrease sex drive, and increase sleepiness.
18. Leukocytes (white blood cells) release cytokines.

Effects of Stress on the Immune System

The nervous system has more control than we might have guessed over the immune system. The study of this relationship, called **psychoneuroimmunology,** deals with how experiences alter the immune system and how the immune system in turn influences the central nervous system.

In response to a brief stressful experience, the nervous system activates the immune system to increase its production of natural killer cells and the secretion of cytokines. The elevated cytokine levels help combat infections, but they also trigger prostaglandins that reach the hypothalamus. Rats subjected to inescapable shocks show symptoms resembling illness, including sleepiness, decreased appetite, and elevated body temperature. The same is true for people who are under great stress (Maier & Watkins, 1998). Even viewing extremely disgusting images can activate the immune system and raise body temperature (Stevenson et al., 2012). In short, if you have been under much stress and start to feel lethargy or other symptoms of illness, one possibility is that your symptoms are reactions to the stress, acting through the immune system.

A prolonged stress response produces symptoms similar to depression and weakens the immune system (Lim, Huang,

Grueter, Rothwell, & Malenka, 2012; Segerstrom & Miller, 2004). A likely hypothesis is that prolonged increase of cortisol directs energy toward increasing metabolism and therefore detracts energy from synthesizing proteins, including the proteins of the immune system. For example, in 1979, at the Three Mile Island nuclear power plant, a major accident was barely contained. The people who continued to live in the vicinity during the next year had lower than normal levels of B cells, T cells, and natural killer cells. They also complained of emotional distress and showed impaired performance on a proofreading task (Baum, Gatchel, & Schaeffer, 1983; McKinnon, Weisse, Reynolds, Bowles, & Baum, 1989). A study of research scientists in Antarctica found that a 9-month period of cold, darkness, and social isolation reduced T cell functioning to about half of normal levels (Tingate, Lugg, Muller, Stowe, & Pierson, 1997).

In one study, 276 volunteers filled out an extensive questionnaire about stressful life events and then received an injection of a moderate dose of common cold virus. The hypothesis was that those with the strongest immune responses could fight off the cold, but others would succumb. People who reported brief stressful experiences were at no more risk for catching a cold than were people who reported no stress. However, for people who reported stress lasting longer than a month, the longer it lasted, the greater the risk of illness (S. Cohen et al., 1998).

Prolonged stress can also harm the hippocampus. Cortisol resulting from stress increases metabolic activity in the hippocampus, making its cells more vulnerable to damage by toxic chemicals or overstimulation (Sapolsky, 1992). Rats exposed to high stress—such as being restrained in a mesh wire retainer for 6 hours a day for 3 weeks—show shrinkage of dendrites in the hippocampus and impairments in the kinds of memory that depend on the hippocampus (Kleen, Sitomer, Killeen, & Conrad, 2006).

STOP & CHECK

20. How do the effects of stress mimic the effects of illness?
21. How does prolonged stress damage the hippocampus?

ANSWERS

20. Stress increases release of cytokines, which communicate with the hypothalamus via prostaglandins. The hypothalamus reacts with the same responses it uses to combat illness, such as inactivity and loss of appetite. 21. Stress increases the release of cortisol, which enhances metabolic activity throughout the body. When neurons in the hippocampus have high metabolic activity, they become more vulnerable to damage by toxins or overstimulation.

Coping with Stress

Individuals vary in their reactions to a stressful experience as a result of genetic predispositions and previous experiences. **Resilience**—the ability to recover well from a traumatic experience—correlates with strong social support, an optimistic viewpoint, and reappraisal of difficult situations. Those factors in turn correlate with the ability to rapidly activate the stress response and then rapidly deactivate it (Horn, Charney, & Feder, 2016). Successfully coping with moderately stressful events prepares one to cope with later events, although a history of severely adverse events leaves one too exhausted to resist (Seery, Leo, Lupien, Kondrak, & Almonte, 2013).

The ways to control stress responses include special breathing routines, exercise, meditation, and distraction, as well as, of course, trying to deal with the problem that caused the stress. Social support is one of the most powerful methods of coping with stress. People who receive more frequent hugs have a lower risk of infection (Cohen, Janicki-Deverts, Turner, & Doyle, 2015). People who feel rejected have an increased risk (Murphy, Slavich, Chen, & Miller, 2015). After death of a spouse, older people have a greatly increased risk of heart attack or stroke for the next several months (Carey et al., 2014). In one study, happily married women were given moderately painful shocks to their ankles. On various trials, they held the hand of their husband, a man they did not know, or no one. Holding the husband's hand reduced the response indicated by fMRI in several brain areas, including the prefrontal cortex. Holding the hand of an unknown man reduced the response a little, on the average, but not as much as holding the husband's hand (Coan, Schaefer, & Davidson, 2006). As expected, the brain responses corresponded to people's self-reports that social support from a loved one helps reduce stress.

Resilience is not easy to investigate. Ideally, we would want to study a large number of physically and mentally healthy people before, during, and after a series of highly stressful experiences, and compare them to similar people who faced less stress. And we would want to be sure we could keep track of each person's whereabouts over several years. It sounds like an impossibly difficult task, and it would be, for anyone except for the military. In 2009, the U.S. Army began a study of healthy young people entering military service, many of whom would be exposed to serious stress over the next few years. The army is superb at keeping track of where every soldier is at all times, and it can guarantee to do follow-up studies on each participant. The preliminary results suggest that the risk factors are similar to those previously identified in civilian populations, such as feeling depressed (Ursano et al., 2016). The army is continuing the study.

Emotions and Body Reactions

Research on stress and health provides an interesting kind of closure. Decades ago, Hans Selye argued that any stressful event leads to the general adaptation syndrome, marked by fever and other signs of illness. We now see why: The body reacts to prolonged stress by activating the adrenal cortex and the immune system, and the resulting increase in cytokines produces the same reactions that an infection would. Research has also improved our understanding of the predispositions behind post-traumatic stress disorder and makes it possible to foresee a new era of advances in psychosomatic medicine. Emotional states, which once seemed too ephemeral for scientific study, are now part of mainstream biology.

Summary

1. Hans Selye introduced the idea of the general adaptation syndrome, which is the way the body responds to all kinds of illness and stress. 376

2. Stress is difficult to define. Because people apply the term to a wide range of major and minor experiences, research results about stress are highly variable. 376

3. Stress immediately activates the sympathetic nervous system and more slowly activates the hypothalamus-pituitary-adrenal cortex axis. The adrenal cortex releases cortisol, which increases metabolism. 377

4. Although brief stress enhances the immune response and facilitates memory formation, prolonged stress drains the body of the resources it needs for other purposes. 377

5. Stress activates the immune system, helping to fight viruses and bacteria. The immune system releases cytokines, which stimulate the hypothalamus by releasing prostaglandins, which cross the blood–brain barrier. The hypothalamus reacts by activities to combat illness, including sleepiness, fever, and loss of appetite and energy. 378

6. Because stress causes release of cytokines, it can also lead to lethargy and other symptoms that resemble those of illness. 378

7. The high cortisol levels associated with prolonged stress damages cells in the hippocampus, thereby impairing memory. 379

8. People vary in their resilience to stress, based on genetics, social support, and previous experiences. 379

Key Terms

Terms are defined in the module on the page number indicated. They're also presented in alphabetical order with definitions in the book's Subject Index/Glossary, which begins on page 589. Interactive flash cards, audio reviews, and crossword puzzles are among the online resources available to help you learn these terms and the concepts they represent.

adrenocorticotropic hormone (ACTH) 377
antibodies 377
antigens 377
behavioral medicine 376
cortisol 376
cytokine 377
general adaptation syndrome 376
HPA axis 377
immune system 377
leukocyte 377
prostaglandins 377
psychoneuroimmunology 378
resilience 379
stress 376

Thought Question

If someone were unable to produce cytokines, what would be the consequences?

Module 11.3 | End of Module Quiz

1. Which hormone does the alarm stage release, but the resistance stage does not?
   A. Cortisol
   B. ACTH
   C. Epinephrine
   D. Testosterone

2. How do the functions of the HPA axis compare to those of the sympathetic nervous system?

   A. The sympathetic nervous system readies the body for brief, vigorous action, and the HPA axis controls digestion and other vegetative activities.

   B. The sympathetic nervous system activates the brain, and the HPA axis activates the rest of the body.

   C. The sympathetic nervous system readies the body for brief, vigorous action, and the HPA axis prepares the body for prolonged coping with a persistent stressor.

   D. The sympathetic nervous system is active during a stressful situation, and the HPA axis becomes active at the end of the stressful situation.

3. How does McEwen's definition of stress differ from Selye's?

   A. Selye's definition applied only to severe stress.

   B. Selye's definition applied equally to favorable or unfavorable events.

   C. Selye's definition applied only to laboratory animals.

   D. Selye's definition applied only to humans.

4. Which cells of the immune system secrete antibodies?

   A. Natural killer cells only

   B. T cells only

   C. B cells only

   D. Natural killer cells, T cells, and B cells equally

5. Why do nearly all infections produce similar symptoms, such as fever, sleepiness, and loss of energy?

   A. Every infection damages the body's ability to maintain body temperature and overall activity.

   B. "Sickness behaviors" are an effective way for a sick person to gain sympathy and help.

   C. Infectious particles clog the arteries, making it difficult for other chemicals to reach their targets.

   D. The immune system sends prostaglandins to the brain, where they stimulate the hypothalamus to produce these effects.

6. What are the effects of stress on the immune system?

   A. All stressful experiences impair the immune system.

   B. Brief stress activates the immune system, but prolonged stress weakens it.

   C. Brief stress weakens the immune system, but prolonged stress strengthens it.

   D. All stressful experiences strengthen the immune system.

7. Prolonged stress is known to damage which brain area?

   A. The visual cortex

   B. The hippocampus

   C. The cerebellum

   D. The corpus callosum

8. Which of these increases resilience?

   A. Unpredictability of events

   B. Social support

   C. Previous severely stressful experiences

   D. Breathing carbon dioxide

Answers: 1C, 2C, 3B, 4C, 5D, 6B, 7B, 8B.

Suggestions for Further Reading

Damasio, A. (1999). *The feeling of what happens.* New York: Harcourt Brace. A neurologist's account of the connection between emotion and consciousness, full of interesting examples.

Frazzetto, G. B. (2013). *Joy, guilt, anger, love.* New York: Penguin Books. Insightful description of emotional experiences, with reference to relevant neurological studies.

McEwen, B. S., with Lasley, E. N. (2002). *The end of stress as we know it.* Washington, DC: Joseph Henry Press. Readable review by one of the leading researchers.

Pfaff, D. W. (2007). *The neuroscience of fair play.* New York: Dana Press. Exploration of how the physiology of emotions, especially the amygdala, relates to moral behavior.

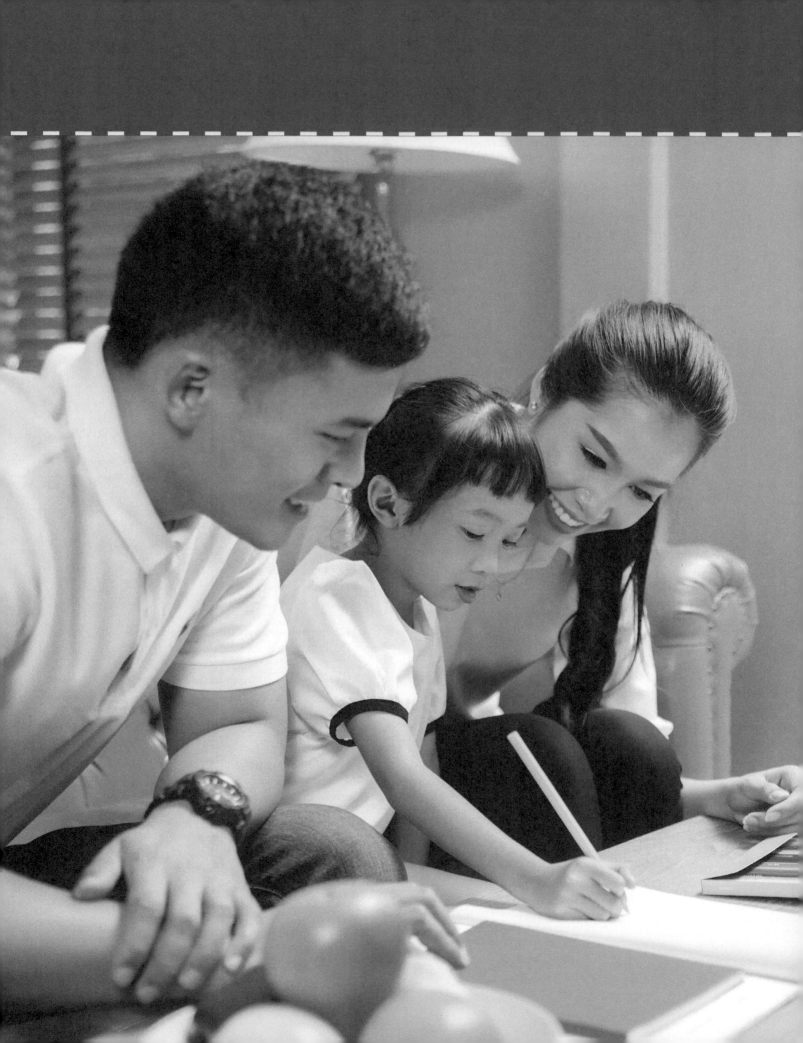

Learning, Memory, and Intelligence

Chapter 12

Suppose you type something on your computer and then save it. A year later, you come back, click the correct file name, and retrieve what you wrote. How did the computer remember what to do?

That question has two parts: First, how do the physical properties of silicon chips enable them to alter their properties when you type certain keys? Second, how does the wiring diagram take the changes in individual silicon chips and convert them into a useful activity?

Similarly, when we try to explain how you remember some experience, we deal with two questions: First, how does a pattern of sensory information alter the input–output properties of certain neurons? Second, after neurons change their properties, how does the nervous system produce the behavioral changes that we call learning or memory?

In the first two modules of this chapter we consider how the various brain areas interact to produce learning and memory. In the third module, we turn to the detailed physiology of how experience changes neurons and synapses. In the final module, we consider the elusive concept of intelligence and how it relates to brain mechanisms.

Learning Objectives

After studying this chapter, you should be able to:

1. Distinguish among types of memory.
2. Define *engram,* and describe research to localize an engram.
3. Discuss types of amnesia.
4. Contrast the functions of the hippocampus and the striatum.
5. Define Hebbian synapses.
6. Explain the mechanism of long-term potentiation.
7. Discuss the relationships among brain anatomy, genetics, and intelligence.

Opposite:
Learning produces amazingly complex behaviors.
(VectorLifestylepic/Shutterstock.com)

Learning, Memory, and Memory Loss

Suppose you lost your ability to form memories. You are aware of the present but you forget your experience from even a moment ago. You feel as if you just awakened from a deep sleep. So you write on a sheet of paper, "Just now, for the first time, I have suddenly become conscious!" A little later, you forget this experience, too. As far as you can tell, you have just now emerged into consciousness after a long sleeplike period. You look at this sheet of paper on which you wrote about becoming conscious, but you don't remember writing it. How odd! You must have written it when in fact you were not conscious! Irritated, you cross off that statement and write anew, "*NOW* I am for the first time conscious!" And a minute later, you cross that one off and write it again. Eventually, someone finds this sheet of paper on which you have repeatedly written and crossed out statements about suddenly feeling conscious for the first time.

Sound far-fetched? It really happened to a patient who developed severe memory impairments after encephalitis damaged his temporal cortex (Wilson, Baddeley, & Kapur, 1995). Life without memory means no sense of existing across time. Your memory is almost synonymous with your sense of self.

Localized Representations of Memory

Psychologists have traditionally distinguished two categories of learning, classical and instrumental conditioning. The Russian physiologist Ivan Pavlov pioneered the investigation of what we now call **classical conditioning** (see Figure 12.1a), in which pairing two stimuli changes the response to one of them (Pavlov, 1927). The experimenter starts by presenting a **conditioned stimulus (CS),** which initially elicits no response of note, and then presents the **unconditioned stimulus (UCS),** which automatically elicits the **unconditioned response (UCR).** After some pairings of the CS and the UCS (perhaps just one or two, perhaps many), the individual begins making a new, learned response to the CS, called a **conditioned response (CR).** In his original experiments, Pavlov presented a dog with a sound (CS) followed by meat (UCS), which stimulated the dog to salivate (UCR). After many such pairings, the sound alone (CS) stimulated the dog to salivate (CR). In that case and many others, the CR resembles the UCR, but in some cases, it does not. For example, if a rat experiences a CS paired with shock, the shock elicits screaming and jumping, but the CS elicits a freezing response.

In **instrumental conditioning** (also known as operant conditioning), a response leads to a reinforcer or punishment (see Figure 12.1b). A **reinforcer** is any event that increases the future probability of the response. A **punishment** is an event that suppresses the frequency of the response. For example, when a rat enters one arm of a maze and finds Froot Loops cereal (a treat that rats seem to love), the rat increases its probability of entering that arm at future opportunities. If it receives a shock instead, the probability decreases. The primary difference between classical and instrumental conditioning is that in instrumental conditioning the individual's response determines the outcome (reinforcer or punishment), whereas in classical conditioning the CS and UCS occur at certain times regardless of the individual's behavior. The behavior is useful, however, in preparing for the UCS.

Some cases of learning are difficult to label as classical or instrumental. For example, after a male songbird hears the song of his own species during his first few months, he imitates it the following year. The song that he heard was not paired with any other stimulus, so it doesn't look like classical conditioning. He learned the song without reinforcers or punishments, so we cannot call it instrumental conditioning either. That is, animals have specialized methods of learning other than classical and instrumental conditioning. Also, the way animals (including people) learn varies from one situation to another. In most situations, learning occurs only if the CS and UCS, or response and reinforcer, occur close together in time. But if you eat something, especially something unfamiliar, and get sick later, you learn a strong aversion to the taste of that food, even if taste and illness are separated by hours (Rozin & Kalat, 1971; Rozin & Schull, 1988).

Lashley's Search for the Engram

What happens in the brain when you learn something? Pavlov proposed the simple hypothesis that classical conditioning reflects a strengthened connection between a CS center and a UCS center in the brain. That strengthened connection lets any excitation of the CS center flow to the UCS center,

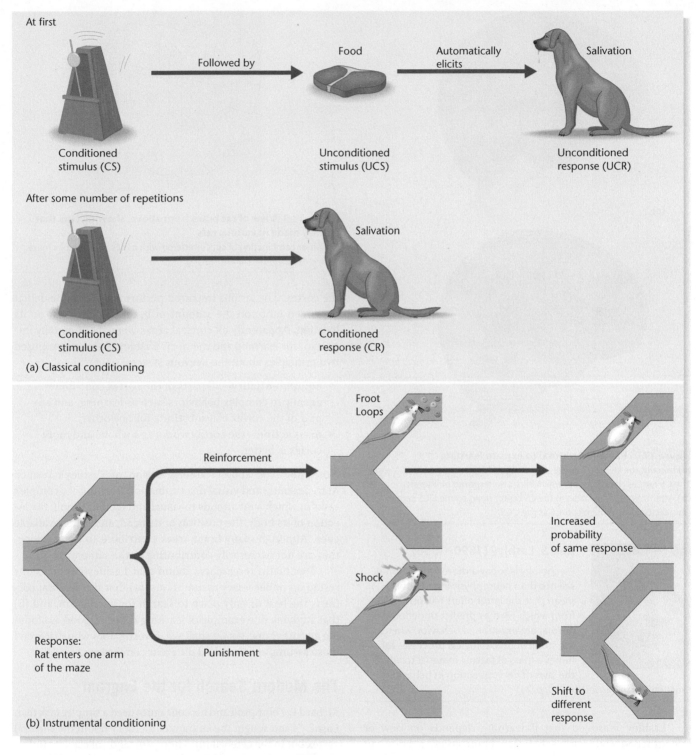

Figure 12.1 Classical conditioning and instrumental conditioning
(a) In classical conditioning, two stimuli (CS and UCS) are presented at certain times regardless of what the learner does. (b) In instrumental conditioning, the learner's behavior controls the presentation of reinforcer or punishment.

evoking a response just like the unconditioned response (see Figure 12.2). We now know that this hypothesis does not fit all behavioral observations. As mentioned, if a signal predicts shock, a rat does not react to the signal as if it were a shock. However, psychologists of an earlier era were unaware of such observations and considered Pavlov's hypothesis plausible. Karl Lashley set out to test it. Lashley was searching for the **engram**—the physical representation of what has been learned. A connection between two brain areas would be a possible example of an engram.

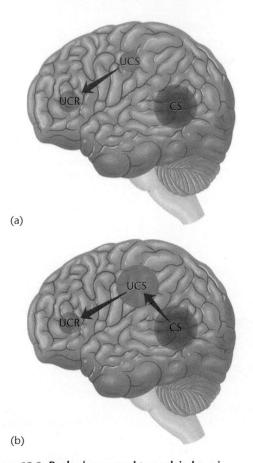

(a)

(b)

Figure 12.2 Pavlov's proposal to explain learning
(a) Initially, the UCS excites the UCS center, which excites the UCR center. The CS excites the CS center, which elicits no response of interest.
(b) After training, excitation in the CS center flows to the UCS center, thus eliciting the same response as the UCS.

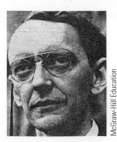

Karl S. Lashley (1890–1958)

Psychology is today a more fundamental science than neurophysiology. By this I mean that the latter offers few principles from which we may predict or define the normal organization of behavior, whereas the study of psychological processes furnishes a mass of factual material to which the laws of nervous action in behavior must conform. (*Lashley, 1930, p. 24*)

Lashley reasoned that if learning depends on new or strengthened connections between brain areas, a knife cut somewhere in the brain should interrupt that connection and abolish the learned response. He trained rats on mazes and a brightness discrimination task and then made deep cuts in varying locations in their cerebral cortices (Lashley, 1929, 1950) (see Figure 12.3). However, no knife cut significantly impaired the rats' performances. Evidently, the types of learning that he studied did not depend on connections across the cortex.

Lashley also tested whether any portion of the cerebral cortex is more important than others for learning. He trained rats on mazes before or after he removed large portions of

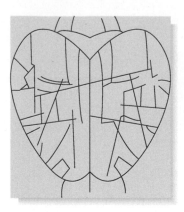

Figure 12.3 View of rat brain from above, showing cuts that Lashley made in various rats
No cut or combination of cuts interfered with a rat's memory of a maze. (*Source: Adapted from Lashley, 1950*)

the cortex. The lesions impaired performance, but the deficit depended more on the amount of brain damage than on its location. Apparently all cortical areas were about equally important for learning and memory. Lashley therefore proposed two principles about the nervous system:

- **equipotentiality**—all parts of the cortex contribute equally to complex behaviors such as learning, and any part of the cortex can substitute for any other.
- **mass action**—the cortex works as a whole, and more cortex is better.

Note, however, another interpretation of Lashley's results: Maze learning and visual discrimination learning are complex tasks in which a rat attends to visual and tactile stimuli, the location of its body, the position of its head, and other available cues. Although many brain areas contribute to the learning, they are not necessarily contributing in the same way.

Eventually, researchers found that Lashley's conclusions rested on unnecessary assumptions: (a) that the cerebral cortex is the best or only place to search for an engram, and (b) that studying one example of learning is just as good as studying any other one. As we shall see, investigators who discarded these assumptions reached different conclusions.

The Modern Search for the Engram

Richard F. Thompson and his colleagues used a simpler task than Lashley's and sought the engram of memory not in the cerebral cortex but in the cerebellum. Thompson and colleagues studied classical conditioning of eyelid responses in rabbits. They presented first a tone (CS) and then a puff of air (UCS) to the cornea of the rabbit's eye. At first, a rabbit closed its eye in response to the air puff but not to the tone. After repeated pairings, classical conditioning occurred and the rabbit blinked at the tone also. Investigators recorded the activity in various brain cells to determine which ones changed their responses during learning.

Thompson set out to determine the location of learning. Imagine a sequence of brain areas from the sensory receptors to the motor neurons controlling the muscles:

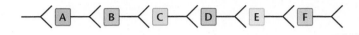

If we damage any one of those areas, learning will be impaired, but we cannot be sure that learning occurred in the damaged area. For example, if the learning occurs in area D, damage in A, B, or C will prevent learning by blocking the input to D. Damage in E or F will prevent learning by blocking the output from D. Thompson and colleagues reasoned as follows: Suppose the learning occurs in D. If so, then D has to be active at the time of the learning, and so do all the areas leading up to D (A, B, and C). However, learning should not require areas E and beyond. If area E were temporarily blocked, nothing would relay information to the muscles, so we would see no response, but learning could occur nevertheless, and we could see evidence of it later.

Thompson's research identified one nucleus of the cerebellum, the **lateral interpositus nucleus (LIP)**, as essential for learning. At the start of training, those cells showed little response to the tone, but as learning proceeded, their responses increased (Thompson, 1986). When the investigators temporarily suppressed that nucleus in an untrained rabbit, either by cooling the nucleus or by injecting a drug into it, and then presented the CSs and UCSs, the rabbit showed no responses during the training. Then they waited for the LIP to recover and continued training. At that point, the rabbit began to learn, but it learned *at the same speed* as animals that had received no previous training. Evidently, while the LIP was suppressed, the training had no effect.

But does learning actually occur *in* the LIP, or does this area just relay the information to a later area where learning occurs? In the next experiments, investigators suppressed activity in the red nucleus, a midbrain motor area that receives input from the cerebellum. When the red nucleus was suppressed, the rabbits again showed no responses during training. However, as soon as the red nucleus had recovered from the cooling or drugs, the rabbits immediately showed strong learned responses to the tone (Clark & Lavond, 1993; Krupa, Thompson, & Thompson, 1993). In other words, suppressing the red nucleus temporarily prevented the response but did not prevent learning. Evidently, learning did not require activity in the red nucleus or any area after it. Thompson and his colleagues concluded that the learning occurred in the LIP. How did they know that learning didn't depend on some area *before* the LIP? If it did, then suppressing the LIP would not have prevented learning. Figure 12.4 summarizes these experiments. This research made it possible for other researchers to explore the mechanisms in more detail, identifying the cells and neurotransmitters responsible for this particular example of an engram (Freeman, 2015).

The mechanisms for this type of conditioning are the same in many species, ranging from goldfish (Gomez et al., 2016) to humans. People who have damage in the cerebellum show either no conditioned eyeblinks (Daum et al., 1993) or only weak, inaccurately timed ones (Gerwig et al., 2005). However, they report that they know the stimulus predicts a puff of air to the eyes, and they do show a classically conditioned

change in skin conductance (Daum et al., 1993). Damage to the cerebellum impairs learning only when a discrete response needs to be made with precise timing (Poulos & Thompson, 2015). As mentioned in Chapter 7, the cerebellum is specialized for timing brief intervals.

STOP & CHECK

1. Thompson found a localized engram, whereas Lashley did not. What key differences in procedures or assumptions were probably responsible for their different results?
2. What evidence indicates that the red nucleus is necessary for performance of a conditioned response but not for learning the response?

ANSWERS

1. Thompson studied a different, simpler type of learning. Also, he looked in the cerebellum instead of the cerebral cortex. 2. If the red nucleus is inactivated during training, the animal makes no conditioned responses during the training, so the red nucleus is necessary for the response. However, as soon as the red nucleus recovers, the animal can show conditioned responses at once, without any further training, so learning occurred while the red nucleus was inactivated.

Types of Memory

Finding an engram for certain types of classical conditioning is an important accomplishment, but finding an engram for everyday memories is more challenging (Eichenbaum, 2016). For much of the 20th century, most psychologists assumed that all memory was the same. If so, they could study it with any convenient example, such as memorization of nonsense syllables, just as physicists can measure gravity by dropping any convenient object. Eventually, psychologists began to draw distinctions between one type of memory and another.

Short-Term and Long-Term Memory

Donald Hebb (1949) reasoned that no one mechanism could account for all the phenomena of learning. You can immediately repeat something you just heard, so it is clear that some memories form quickly. Old people can recall events from their childhood, so we also see that some memories last permanently. Hebb could not imagine a chemical process that is fast enough to account for immediate memory yet stable enough to provide permanent memory. He therefore proposed a distinction between **short-term memory** of events that have just occurred and **long-term memory** of events from further back. Several types of evidence supported this idea:

- Short-term memory and long-term memory differ in their capacity. If you hear a series of unrelated numbers or letters, such as DZLAUV, you can probably repeat no more than about seven of them, and with other kinds of material, your maximum is even less. You can hold a vast amount of information in long-term memory.

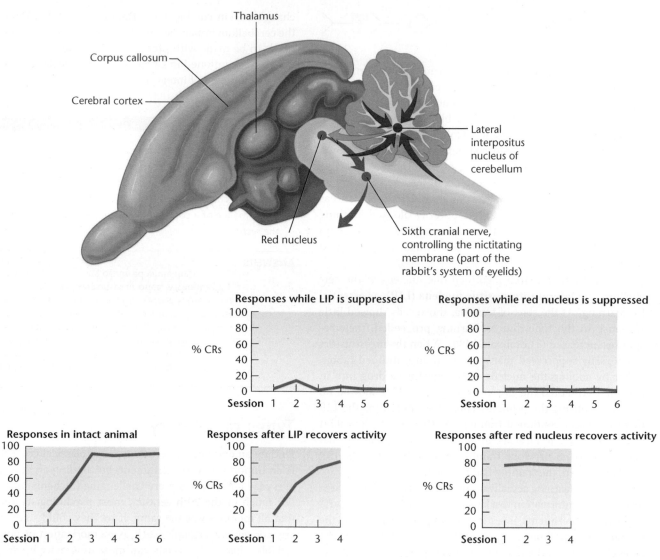

Figure 12.4 Localization of an engram
Temporarily inactivating the lateral interpositus nucleus blocked all indications of learning. After the inactivation wore off, the rabbits learned as slowly as rabbits with no previous training. Temporarily inactivating the red nucleus blocked responses during the period of inactivation, but the learned response appeared as soon as the red nucleus recovered.
(*Source: Based on the results of Clark & Lavond, 1993; Krupa, Thompson, & Thompson, 1993*)

- Short-term memory requires rehearsal. If you read the letter sequence DZLAUV and then something distracts you, your chance of repeating the letters declines rapidly (Peterson & Peterson, 1959). You can reconstruct long-term memories that you haven't thought about in years, although your recall might not be 100 percent accurate.
- Once you have forgotten something from short-term memory, it is lost. With long-term memory, a hint might help you reconstruct something you thought you had forgotten. For example, try naming all your high school teachers. After you have named all you can, you can name still more if someone shows you photos and tells you the teachers' initials.

Hebb suggested that we might store short-term memories by a reverberating circuit, in which neuron A excites neuron

B, which excites neuron C, which then reexcites neuron A. Hebb further proposed that storing something in short-term memory for a sufficient period of time made it possible for the brain to **consolidate** (strengthen) it into long-term memory, presumably by building new synapses or other structural changes. If anything interrupted the rehearsal of short-term memory before consolidation completed its course, the information was simply lost.

Our Changing Views of Consolidation

Later studies made the distinction between short-term and long-term memory increasingly problematic. First, many short-term memories are not simply temporary stores on their way to being long-term memories. When you watch a soccer or hockey match, you remember the score until it changes, perhaps an hour later. If you park your car, you remember its location until you come back to get it, perhaps hours later, maybe even days later. Holding onto a memory for a long enough time does not automatically turn it into a permanent memory.

Furthermore, consolidation isn't what we used to think it was. The original idea was that the brain held onto something in short-term memory until it could synthesize new proteins that establish a long-term memory (Canal & Gold, 2007). However, the time needed for consolidation varies enormously. If you are trying to memorize facts that you consider boring and useless, you might struggle for hours. But if someone warns you about the venomous snake that got loose in your dormitory, you won't have to repeat it over and over or write flash cards to remember it. Emotionally significant memories form quickly. In fact, if some event is extremely arousing—your first kiss, perhaps, or the moment when you heard about some tragedy—you remember not only the event itself, but those just before and after it. Psychologists call these experiences "flashbulb memories," as if a mental flashbulb illuminated everything for a moment. The physiological explanation is that highly emotional experiences arouse the locus coeruleus, which increases norepinephrine release throughout the cortex and dopamine release in the hippocampus (Takeuchi et al., 2016). Emotional experiences also increase the secretion of epinephrine and cortisol that activate the amygdala and hippocampus (Cahill & McGaugh, 1998; Murty, LaBar, & Adcock, 2012). The point is that consolidation depends on more than the time necessary to synthesize some new proteins.

Flashbulb memories have a further aspect: Suppose you are driving on a snowy day and you skid on a slippery patch. Ordinarily, you would forget this minor scare quickly. However, a minute later you skid on a second slippery patch and wreck your car. Now you form a long-term memory of not only the accident but also the earlier slip. Researchers call this the "synaptic tag-and-capture" process: Your brain tags a weak new memory for later stabilization if a similar, more important event soon follows it (Dunsmoor, Murty, Davichi, & Phelps, 2015).

Working Memory

To replace the concept of short-term memory, A. D. Baddeley and G. J. Hitch (1994) introduced the term **working memory** to refer to the way we store information while we are working with it. A common test of working memory is the **delayed response task**, in which you respond to something that you saw or heard a short while ago. Imagine that while you stare at a central fixation point, a light flashes briefly at some point toward the periphery. You stare at that central point for a few seconds until you hear a beep, and then you are supposed to look to where you remember seeing the light. This task can be modified for use with monkeys and other species. During the delay, the learner has to store a representation of the stimulus. During the delay, certain cells in the prefrontal and parietal cortex increase their activity, and different cells become active depending on the direction the eye movement will need to take (Chafee & Goldman-Rakic, 1998; Constantinidis & Klingberg, 2016).

If someone touched you on a finger and you had to remember which finger during a delay, you might simply extend that finger throughout the delay. Similarly, we might expect the brain to remember a stimulus by constant activity in one group of cells throughout the delay. However, it does not work exactly that way. Monkeys learned a task in which they saw colored squares and remembered them during a delay. When they saw squares again in the same positions, the monkeys had to respond to the one that had changed color. The initial presentation of the squares evoked bursts of gamma oscillations (45 to 100 Hz) in cells responsive to the colors and locations. During the delay, occasional gamma bursts occurred in these same cells at staggered times. No individual cell remained active during the delay. Then more frequent gamma bursts emerged at the time of the test. In short, the memory was distributed over many cells in an alternating pattern (Lundqvist et al., 2016).

STOP & CHECK

3. Why should we conclude that consolidation depends on more than just holding a short-term memory long enough for protein synthesis?

4. What mechanism causes flashbulb memories?

5. How does the cortex store a working memory during a delay?

ANSWERS

3. People can store some memories for hours or days without forming a permanent memory, whereas they form emotionally important memories quickly. 4. Emotionally exciting memories stimulate the locus coeruleus, which increases norepinephrine throughout the cortex and dopamine to the hippocampus. Emotional excitement also increases epinephrine and cortisol, which activate the amygdala and hippocampus. 5. Occasional bursts of gamma oscillations (45 to 100 Hz) occur in cells that responded to a stimulus, but the bursts alternate among cells instead of persisting throughout the delay in any one cell.

Memory Loss

In many cases, forgetting is a "feature," not a "bug" (Nørby, 2015). Forgetting the details of several similar experiences helps you abstract the important common features. Forgetting where you parked your car last week or where you met your sister for lunch last month helps you remember where you parked today and where you plan to meet for lunch tomorrow. Also, as your memory of an unpleasant event begins to fade, you start to feel better.

However, you do not want to forget important or current information. **Amnesia** is memory loss. One patient ate lunch and, 20 minutes later, ate a second lunch, apparently having forgotten the first meal. Another 20 minutes later, he started on a third lunch and ate most of it. A few minutes later, he said he would like to "go for a walk and get a good meal" (Rozin, Dow, Moscovitch, & Rajaram, 1998). Other patients with amnesia also forget that they have just eaten, although when they start to eat again, they remark on not enjoying the food as much as usual (Higgs, Williamson, Rotshtein, & Humphreys, 2008).

However, even in severe cases like these, no one loses all kinds of memory equally. People who might forget eating lunch a few minutes ago would probably still remember how to eat with a knife and fork, and which foods they like or dislike. Studies on amnesia shed light on some of the mechanisms of memory. Here we briefly consider Korsakoff's syndrome and Alzheimer's disease, and then the phenomenon of infant amnesia. The second module will consider amnesia resulting from damage to the hippocampus.

Korsakoff's Syndrome

Korsakoff's syndrome, also known as *Wernicke-Korsakoff syndrome,* is brain damage caused by prolonged thiamine deficiency. The brain needs thiamine (vitamin B_1) to metabolize glucose, its primary fuel. Severe thiamine deficiency is common among people with severe alcoholism who go for weeks at a time on a diet of nothing but alcoholic beverages, lacking in vitamins. Prolonged thiamine deficiency leads to a loss or shrinkage of neurons throughout the brain, especially in the dorsomedial thalamus, the main source of input to the prefrontal cortex. The symptoms of Korsakoff's syndrome are similar to those of people with damage to the prefrontal cortex, including apathy, confusion, and memory loss.

A distinctive symptom of Korsakoff's syndrome is **confabulation**, in which patients fill in memory gaps with guesses. (Some patients with other disorders also confabulate.) They seldom confabulate on semantic questions such as "What is the capital of Russia?" or nonsense questions such as "Who is Princess Lolita?" They confabulate mainly about their own lives, such as "What did you do last weekend?" (Borsutzky, Fujiwara, Brand, & Markowitsch, 2008; Schnider, 2003). Often, the confabulated answer was true at some time in the past but not now, such as, "I went dancing," or "I visited with my children," but sometimes the confabulation is fanciful and implausible. Occasionally, patients try to act on their spontaneous confabulations, such as trying to leave the hospital to go to work, go to the airport, or prepare dinner for guests (Nahum, Bouzerda-Wahlen, Guggisberg, Ptak, & Schnider, 2012). Most confabulated answers are more pleasant than the currently true answers (Fotopoulou, Solms, & Turnbull, 2004), perhaps merely because the patient's past life was, on the whole, more pleasant than the present.

The tendency to confabulate produces a fascinating influence on the strategies for studying. Suppose you have to learn a long list of three-word sentences such as: "Medicine cured hiccups" and "Tourist desired photograph." Would you simply reread the list many times? Or would you alternate between reading the list and testing yourself?

Medicine cured _____
Tourist desired _____.

Almost everyone learns better the second way. Completing the sentences forces you to be more active and calls your attention to the items you have not yet learned. Patients with Korsakoff's, however, learn better the first way, by reading the list over and over. The reason is, when they test themselves, they confabulate. (*"Medicine cured headache. Tourist desired passport."*) Then they remember their confabulation instead of the correct answer (Hamann & Squire, 1995).

Alzheimer's Disease

One of the most common causes of memory loss, especially in old age, is **Alzheimer's** (AHLTZ-hime-ers) **disease**. Daniel Schacter (1983) reported playing golf with an Alzheimer's patient who remembered the rules and jargon of the game correctly but kept forgetting how many strokes he took. Five times he teed off, waited for the other player to tee off, and then teed off again, having forgotten his first shot. As with other amnesic patients, patients with Alzheimer's learn procedural skills better than facts. They learn new skills but then surprise themselves with their good performance because they don't remember doing it before (Gabrieli, Corkin, Mickel, & Growdon, 1993). Their memory fluctuates from time to time, suggesting that part of their problem results from a loss of alertness or arousal (Palop, Chin, & Mucke, 2006).

Alzheimer's disease gradually progresses to more serious memory loss, confusion, depression, restlessness, hallucinations, delusions, sleeplessness, and loss of appetite. It becomes more common with age, affecting almost 5 percent of people between ages 65 and 74 and almost half of people over 85 (Evans et al., 1989). Given that more people than ever are surviving into old age, Alzheimer's is an increasing problem.

The first major clue to the cause of Alzheimer's was the fact that people with *Down syndrome* (a condition generally linked to cognitive impairments) almost invariably get Alzheimer's disease if they survive into middle age (Lott, 1982). People with Down syndrome have three copies of chromosome 21 rather than the usual two. That fact led investigators to examine chromosome 21, where they found a gene linked to many cases of early-onset Alzheimer's disease (Goate et al., 1991; Murrell, Farlow, Ghetti, & Benson, 1991). Later researchers found two more genes linked to early-onset Alzheimer's. In this case, "early" means before age 60. For the much more common late-onset condition, many genes increase or decrease the risk, but none has a large effect (Alagiakrishnan, Gill, & Fagarasanu, 2012). Many late-onset cases relate to epigenetic changes in certain genes (De Jager et al., 2014; Lunnon et al., 2014).

The genes controlling early-onset Alzheimer's disease cause a protein called **amyloid-β** to accumulate inside and outside neurons and spread from cell to cell (Riek & Eisenberg, 2016). The protein damages axons and dendrites, decreases synaptic input, and decreases plasticity (Wei, Nguyen, Kessels, Hagiwara, Sisodia, & Malinow, 2010). The damaged axons and dendrites cluster into structures called *plaques* that damage the cerebral cortex, hippocampus, and other areas, as Figures 12.5 through 12.7 show (Scheibel, 1983; Selkoe, 2000).

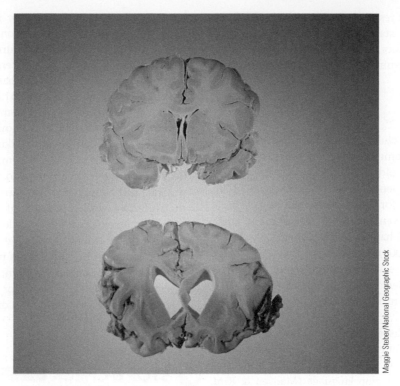

Maggie Steber/National Geographic Stock

Figure 12.5 Brain atrophy in Alzheimer's disease
A patient with Alzheimer's **(bottom)** has gyri that are clearly shrunken in comparison with those of a normal person **(top)**.

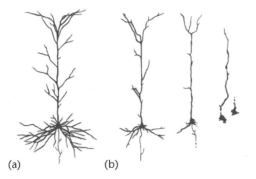

(a)   (b)

Figure 12.6 Neuronal degeneration in Alzheimer's disease
(a) A cell in the prefrontal cortex of a normal human; **(b)** cells from the same area of cortex in patients with Alzheimer's disease at various stages of deterioration.
(Source: Based on "Dendritic changes," by A. B. Scheibel, p. 70. In Alzheimer's disease, B. Reisberg, ed., 1983. Free Press.)

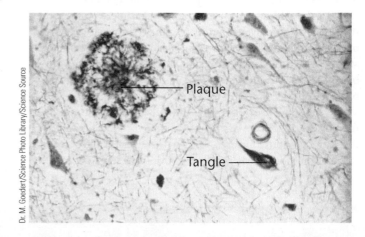

Dr. M. Goedert/Science Photo Library/Science Source

Plaque

Tangle

Figure 12.7 Cerebral cortex of a patient with Alzheimer's
Plaques and tangles result from amyloid-β and abnormal tau protein.

Nevertheless, many researchers are not convinced that amyloid-β by itself explains Alzheimer's. Many old people have high levels of amyloid-β without Alzheimer's disease, and some have Alzheimer's disease without especially high levels of amyloid-β. Of all the clinical trials of drugs that counteract amyloid-β, so far none have produced clear benefits for patients with Alzheimer's (Herrup, 2015). An alternative hypothesis relates to the **tau protein** in the intracellular support structure of axons. High levels of amyloid-β cause more phosphate groups to attach to tau proteins. The altered tau

cannot bind to its usual targets within axons, and so it starts spreading into the cell body and dendrites. The areas of cell damage in the brain correlate better with tau levels than with amyloid-β levels (Musiek & Holtzman, 2015). The altered tau is principally responsible for *tangles*, structures formed from degeneration within neurons (see Figure 12.7).

At this point, no drug is highly effective for Alzheimer's disease. A possible explanation is that by the time physicians recognize Alzheimer's disease, the damage may already be too extensive for any medication to help (Canter, Penney, &

Tsai, 2016). An important research goal is to find ways to diagnose Alzheimer's at the start, either from behavioral measures (Gamaldo, An, Allaire, Kitner-Triolo, & Zonderman, 2012) or perhaps from examination of the nerves in the retina (Frost et al., 2013).

Infant Amnesia

Infant amnesia (or early childhood amnesia) is not a disorder like Korsakoff's syndrome or Alzheimer's disease. It is the universal experience that older children and adults remember very little of what happened in their first few years of life. Young children do in fact form long-term memories. Three- and four-year-olds, and even some two-year-olds can accurately describe events that happened months ago, sometimes even years ago (Solter, 2008). However, as they grow older, they forget most of those early events (Peterson, Warren, & Short, 2011). So the proper question is not why young children fail to form long-term memories. The question is why they forget them.

Hypotheses have included the development of language or complex reasoning abilities as children grow older. However, infant amnesia can be demonstrated in rats and many other species that never develop language (Madsen & Kim, 2016). That is, rats in their first weeks of life learn easily and retain their learning for a day or more, but they do not retain it well over longer times (Brown & Freeman, 2016). Nevertheless, the early learning is not forgotten completely, because a reminder can restore an apparently lost memory. For example, after 17-day-old rats learn to avoid shock, they seem to forget the response quickly, but a return to the training site, followed by a reminder shock in a different place at a different time, restores the lost memory (Travaglia, Bisaz, Sweet, Blitzer, & Alberini, 2016). For humans, too, a reminder sometimes brings back an early memory that seemed to have been lost.

What could explain the difficulty of recalling infant memories? Research with mice points to some changes in the hippocampus, an area known to be critical for certain types of memory. Early in life, for both mice and humans, the hippocampus rapidly forms new neurons and replaces old ones with new ones. The formation of new neurons facilitates new learning, but as the new neurons and synapses displace old ones, the new learning weakens the old memories. New learning does not necessarily weaken old learning, particularly in adults (Cichon & Gan, 2015), but if both the new and old learning depended on new neurons, then a conflict arises.

In contrast to mice and humans, guinea pigs are relatively mature at birth, already walking around and eating solid food. They do not have rapid formation of new hippocampal neurons, and they do not tend to forget early memories the way rats and humans do. Furthermore, chemical procedures that interfere with formation of new neurons can impair new learning in infant mice, while also decreasing forgetting (Akers et al., 2014). Although we should be cautious about assuming that the mechanisms in mice are the same as in humans (Epp, Mera, Kohler, Josselyn, & Frankland, 2016), so far the most plausible explanation for infant amnesia is that the rapid learning in early childhood displaces memories formed in infancy.

✓ STOP & CHECK

6. On what kind of question is someone with Korsakoff's syndrome most likely to confabulate?

7. Why did researchers look for a gene on chromosome 21 as a probable cause of early-onset Alzheimer's disease?

8. What are the consequences of rapid formation of new neurons in the infant hippocampus?

ANSWERS 6. Patients with Korsakoff's syndrome most often confabulate on questions about themselves. Many confabulations are statements that were true at one time. 7. People with Down syndrome, caused by an extra copy of chromosome 21, almost always develop Alzheimer's disease in middle age. 8. Rapid formation of new neurons in the infant hippocampus facilitates new learning, but at the cost of also increasing forgetting.

Module 12.1 | In Closing

Memory and Forgetting

Decades ago, Karl Lashley supposed that the physiology of learning might be a simple matter of increasing a single pathway in the cortex. Today, we distinguish among several types of learning and memory that rely on multiple mechanisms and multiple brain areas. We learn about these mechanisms by studying forgetting as well as by studying learning.

Summary

1. Ivan Pavlov suggested that learning depends on the growth of a connection between two brain areas. Karl Lashley showed that learning does *not* depend on new connections across the cerebral cortex. **384**

2. Richard Thompson found that some instances of classical conditioning take place in small areas of the cerebellum. **386**

3. Psychologists distinguish between short-term memory and long-term memory. Short-term memory holds only

a small amount of information and retains it only briefly unless it is constantly rehearsed. **387**

4. Working memory, a modern alternative to the concept of short-term memory, stores information that one is currently using. The cortex stores a working memory by occasional bursts of high-frequency oscillations that alternate among many cells. **389**

5. Patients with Korsakoff's syndrome often fill in their memory gaps with confabulations, which they then remember as if they were true. **390**

6. Alzheimer's disease is a progressive disease, most common in old age, characterized by impaired memory and attention. Identified genes are responsible for early-onset Alzheimer's disease, but the more common late-onset condition has a variety of causes. **390**

7. Alzheimer's disease is related to deposition of amyloid-β protein in the brain, but the exact role of the protein remains uncertain. **390**

8. Not only humans but many other species also show infant amnesia, the loss of most early memories. The most promising hypothesis is that the loss is due to rapid formation of new hippocampal neurons that facilitate new learning but also displace old learning. **392**

Key Terms

Terms are defined in the module on the page number indicated. They're also presented in alphabetical order with definitions in the book's Subject Index/Glossary, which begins on page 589. Interactive flash cards, audio reviews, and crossword puzzles are among the online resources available to help you learn these terms and the concepts they represent.

Alzheimer's disease **390**
amnesia **389**
amyloid-β **390**
classical conditioning **384**
conditioned response (CR) **384**
conditioned stimulus (CS) **384**
confabulation **390**
consolidate **388**
delayed response task **389**

engram **385**
equipotentiality **386**
infant amnesia **392**
instrumental conditioning **384**
Korsakoff's syndrome **390**
lateral interpositus nucleus (LIP) **387**
long-term memory **387**
mass action **386**

punishment **384**
reinforcer **384**
short-term memory **387**
tau protein **391**
unconditioned response (UCR) **384**
unconditioned stimulus (UCS) **384**
working memory **389**

Thought Question

Lashley sought to find the engram, the physiological representation of learning. In general terms, how would you recognize an engram if you saw one? That is, what would someone have to demonstrate before you could conclude that a particular change in the nervous system was really an engram?

Module 12.1 | End of Module Quiz

1. What evidence led Lashley to draw his conclusions of equipotentiality and mass action?

   A. Learning depends on changes at synapses that use all types of neurotransmitters.
   B. Electrical stimulation of the brain can produce either reward or punishment, depending on the intensity of stimulation.
   C. EEG studies show activation throughout the brain during an experiment on learning.
   D. Impairment of learning depended on the amount of cortical damage rather than the location.

2. What assumption did Lashley make that later researchers rejected?

   A. Any convenient example of learning will reveal the mechanisms that apply to all learning.
   B. Learning requires modification of the activity at synapses.
   C. Short-term memory has to be gradually consolidated into long-term memory.
   D. Learning is distributed over many brain areas, but it depends mainly on the hippocampus.

3. Why did Thompson conclude that eyeblink conditioning depends on the lateral interpositus nucleus, instead of the red nucleus?

   A. Inactivating the red nucleus failed to suppress responses.
   B. Inactivating the red nucleus suppressed responses, and after the rabbit recovered, it had to learn the same as a rabbit that had never been trained.
   C. Inactivating the red nucleus suppressed responses to some stimuli but not others.
   D. Inactivating the red nucleus suppressed responses, but did not prevent learning.

4. What was the original concept of consolidation?

   A. The maximum time that gamma bursts can continue

   B. The time necessary to synthesize proteins

   C. The time before adrenal hormones can reach the cortex

   D. The delay at a metabotropic synapse

5. Emotional arousal facilitates consolidation by what means?

   A. Suppression of the production of new neurons in the hippocampus

   B. Occasional bursts of gamma oscillations

   C. Increased production of amyloid-β

   D. Increased release of norepinephrine, epinephrine, and cortisol

6. How does the cortex store a working memory?

   A. Suppression of the production of new neurons in the hippocampus

   B. Occasional bursts of gamma oscillations

   C. Increased production of amyloid-β

   D. Increased release of norepinephrine, epinephrine, and cortisol

7. Which of the following would probably prevent most cases of Korsakoff's syndrome?

   A. Increase the availability of free exercise facilities.

   B. Decrease the prevalence of particulate matter in air pollution.

   C. Outlaw the possession of handguns in heavily populated areas.

   D. Require all alcoholic beverages to be fortified with vitamins.

8. What type of memory do patients with Alzheimer's retain better than other types?

   A. Procedural memory better than memory of facts

   B. Memory of recent events better than memory of older events

   C. Memory of unemotional experiences better than memory of emotional experiences

   D. Working memory better than short-term memory

9. Currently, what seems the most promising explanation for infant amnesia?

   A. Increased reliance on language as children grow older

   B. More new hippocampal neurons in infants than in older individuals

   C. Inability of the infant hippocampus to store a memory

   D. Lack of gamma oscillations in the infant cortex

Answers: 1D, 2A, 3D, 4B, 5D, 6B, 7D, 8A, 9B.

The Hippocampus and the Striatum

People who suffered memory problems after localized brain damage have told us much about memory, especially about the distinctions between one type of memory and another. In this module we concentrate on two brain areas with contrasting functions in memory, the hippocampus and the striatum.

Memory Loss after Damage to the Hippocampus

In 1953, Henry Molaison, known in most research reports as H. M., was suffering about 10 minor epileptic seizures per day and a major seizure about once a week, despite trying every available antiepileptic drug. Eventually, he agreed to a desperate measure. A surgeon, William Scoville, who had experimented with various forms of lobotomy for mental illness, was familiar with two cases in which removal of much of the medial temporal lobe had relieved epilepsy. Hoping that the same might work with H. M., Scoville removed the hippocampus and nearby structures of the medial temporal cortex from both of H. M.'s hemispheres. Researchers knew almost nothing about the hippocampus at the time, and no one knew what to expect after the surgery. We now know that much of the hippocampus is active during the formation of memories and later recall (Eldridge, Engel, Zeineh, Bookheimer, & Knowlton, 2005). Although the operation reduced H. M.'s epilepsy to no more than two major seizures per year, he suffered severe memory impairment (Milner, 1959; Penfield & Milner, 1958; Scoville & Milner, 1957). Figure 12.8 shows the normal anatomy of the hippocampus and the damage in H. M.

Anterograde and Retrograde Amnesia

After the surgery, H. M.'s intellect and language abilities remained intact, and his personality remained the same except for emotional placidity (Eichenbaum, 2002). However, he suffered massive **anterograde amnesia** (inability to form memories for events that happened after brain damage). He also suffered **retrograde amnesia** (loss of memory for events that occurred before the brain damage). Initially, researchers said his retrograde amnesia was confined to 1 to 3 years before the surgery. Later, they found it was more extensive. H. M. is representative of other people who have suffered amnesia after damage to the hippocampus and surrounding structures of the medial temporal lobe. All show both anterograde and retrograde amnesia, with the retrograde amnesia being most severe for the time leading up to the damage. For example, patients with amnesia can usually tell where they lived as a child and where they lived as a teenager but might not be able to say where they lived 3 years ago (Bayley, Hopkins, & Squire, 2006).

Intact Working Memory

Despite H. M.'s huge deficits in forming long-term memories, his short-term or working memory remained intact, unless he was distracted. In one test, Brenda Milner (1959) asked him to remember the number 584. After a 15-minute delay, he recalled it correctly, explaining, "It's easy. You just remember 8. You see, 5, 8, and 4 add to 17. You remember 8, subtract it from 17, and it leaves 9. Divide 9 in half and you get 5 and 4, and there you are, 584. Easy." A moment later, after his attention had shifted to another subject, he had forgotten both the number and the complicated line of thought he had associated with it. Most other patients with severe amnesia also show normal working memory, if they avoid distraction (Shrager, Levy, Hopkins, & Squire, 2008).

Impaired Storage of Long-Term Memory

Although H. M. could recall much information that he had learned before his damage, he was severely impaired on forming new long-term memories. For several years after his operation, whenever he was asked his age and the date, he answered "27" and "1953." After a few years, he started guessing wildly, generally underestimating his age by 10 years or more and missing the date by up to 43 years (Corkin, 1984). He could read the same magazine repeatedly or work the same jigsaw puzzle repeatedly without losing interest. He could never remember that his favorite uncle had died (Corkin, 2013). Often, he told someone about a childhood incident and then, a minute or two later, told the same person the same story again (Eichenbaum, 2002). In 1980, he moved to a nursing home. Four years later, he could not say where he lived or who cared for him. Although he watched the news on television every night, he could recall only a few fragments of events since 1953. He failed to learn the meanings of new words that entered the English language, such as *Jacuzzi* and *granola* (Corkin, 2002).

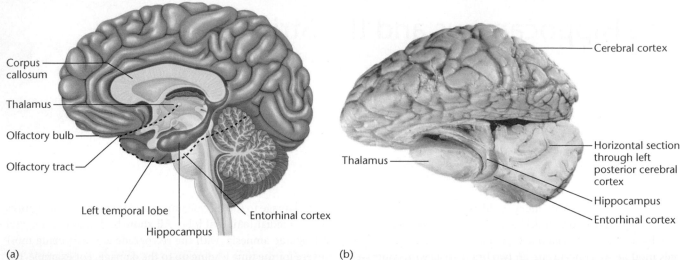

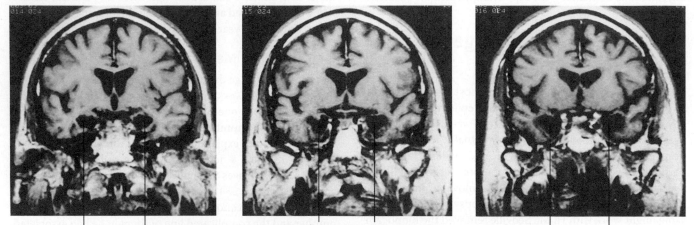

(c)

Figure 12.8 The hippocampus and its loss

(a) Location of the hippocampus in the interior of the temporal lobe. The left hippocampus is closer to the viewer than the rest of this plane; the right hippocampus is behind the plane. The dashed line marks the location of the temporal lobe, which is not visible in the midline. **(b)** Photo of a human brain from above. The top part of the left hemisphere has been cut away to show how the hippocampus loops over (dorsal to) the thalamus, posterior to it, and then below (ventral to) it. **(c)** MRI scan of H. M.'s brain, showing absence of the hippocampus. The three views show coronal planes at successive locations, anterior to posterior.

You might wonder whether he was surprised at his own appearance in a photo or mirror. Yes and no. When asked his age or whether his hair turned gray, he replied that he did not know. When shown a photo of himself with his mother, taken long after his surgery, he recognized his mother but not himself. However, when he saw himself in the mirror, he showed no surprise (Corkin, 2002). He had, of course, seen himself daily in the mirror over all these years. He also had the context of knowing that the person in the mirror must be himself, whereas the person in the photo could be anyone.

H. M. formed a few new weak **semantic memories**—that is, memories of factual information (Corkin, 2002; O'Kane, Kensinger, & Corkin, 2004). For example, when he was given first names and asked to fill in appropriate last names, his replies included some who became famous after 1953, such as these:

	H. M.'s Answer
Elvis	Presley
Martin Luther	King
Billy	Graham
Fidel	Castro
Lyndon	Johnson

He provided even more names when he was given additional information:

	H. M.'s Answer
Famous artist, born in Spain . . .	Pablo Picasso

One study found an interesting qualification to the usual rule that patients with amnesia cannot learn new information.

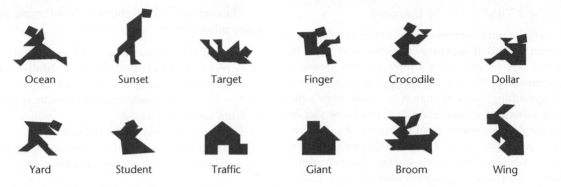

Figure 12.9 Displays for a Memory Test of Patients with Amnesia
Although they could not remember the arbitrary labels that an experimenter gave to each object (as shown), they did remember the descriptions that they devised themselves.
(*Source: From "Development of shared information in communication despite hippocampal amnesia," by M. C. Duff, J. Hengst, D. Tranel, & N. J. Cohen, 2006, Nature Neuroscience, 9, 140–146. Used by permission, Macmillan Publishing Ltd.*)

The investigators showed a series of shapes with unrelated labels, as shown in Figure 12.9. Despite many repetitions, patients with amnesia made no progress toward learning the label for each shape. Then the researchers let the patients devise their own labels. Each patient had to look at one shape at a time and describe it so that another person, who was looking at the 12 shapes unlabeled, would know which one the patient was looking at. At first, the descriptions were slow and uninformative. For the shape at the upper right of Figure 12.9, one patient said, "The next one looks almost . . . the opposite of somebody kind uh . . . slumped down, on the ground, with the same type of . . ." Eventually, he said it looked like someone sleeping with his knees bent. By the fourth trial, he quickly labeled that shape as "the siesta guy," and he continued saying the same thing from then on, even in later sessions on later days (Duff, Hengst, Tranel, & Cohen, 2006).

Severe Impairment of Episodic Memory

H. M. had severe impairment of **episodic memories**, memories of personal events. He could not describe any experience that he had after his surgery. Although he could describe facts (semantic memory) that he learned before his operation, he could describe clear memories for only two personal experiences (Corkin, 2013). Another patient, K. C., suffered widespread brain damage after a motorcycle accident, with scattered damage in the hippocampus and other locations, leading to an apparently complete loss of episodic memories. He cannot describe a single event from any time of his life, although he remembers many facts. When he looks at old family pictures in a photo album, he identifies the people and sometimes the places, but he cannot remember anything about the events that happened in the photos (Rosenbaum et al., 2005). Although his brain damage is so diffuse that we cannot be sure which part of the damage is responsible for his memory loss, the observations do tell us that the brain treats episodic memories differently from other memories.

How would memory loss affect someone's ability to imagine the future? If you try to imagine a future event, you call upon your memory of similar experiences and modify them. Studies using fMRI show that describing past events and imagining future events activate mostly the same areas, including the hippocampus (Addis, Wong, & Schacter, 2007). People with amnesia are just as impaired at imagining the future as they are at describing the past, although they have no trouble describing the present (Race, Keane, & Verfaellie, 2011). For example, here is part of one patient's attempt to imagine a future visit to a museum (Hassabis, Kumaran, Vann, & Maguire, 2007, p. 1727):

Patient: [pause] There's not a lot, as it happens.
Psychologist: So what does it look like in your imagined scene?
Patient: Well, there's big doors. The openings would be high, so the doors would be very big with brass handles, the ceiling would be made of glass, so there's plenty of light coming through. Huge room, exit on either side of the room, there's a pathway and map through the center and on either side there'd be the exhibits. [pause] I don't know what they are. There'd be people. [pause] To be honest there's not a lot coming. . . . My imagination isn't . . . well, I'm not imagining it, let's put it that way. . . . I'm not picturing anything at the moment.

The relationship between loss of episodic memory and difficulty imagining the future is theoretically interesting. Have you ever wondered what good is episodic memory? You can remember a great many events that happened to you years ago, some of them in detail. From an evolutionary standpoint, why did we evolve that ability? What good does it do to be able to remember details of an event that will never happen again? Now we see a possible answer: Remembering those details helps us imagine the future. And if we couldn't imagine the future, we couldn't plan for it.

Better Implicit Than Explicit Memory

Nearly all patients with amnesia show better *implicit* than *explicit* memory. **Explicit memory** is deliberate recall of information that one recognizes as a memory, also known as **declarative memory**. If you have an explicit or declarative memory of something, you can state it in words, draw a picture of it, or otherwise demonstrate that you know you remember it. **Implicit memory** is an influence of experience on behavior, even if you do not recognize that influence. For example, H. M. became comfortable and familiar with certain people, such as the psychologists who worked with him over the years, although he did not remember their names or where he had met them. Also, he could not say what topic a recent conversation had discussed, but he might spontaneously start talking about that same topic again (Corkin, 2013).

Another example of implicit memory: As an experiment, three hospital workers agreed to act in special ways toward a patient with amnesia (not H. M.). One worker was as pleasant as possible. The second was neutral. The third was stern, refused all requests, and made the patient perform boring tasks. After 5 days, the patient was asked to look at photos of the three workers and try to identify them or say anything he knew about them. He said he did not recognize any of them. Then he was asked which one he would approach as a possible friend or which one he would ask for help. He was asked this question repeatedly—it was possible to ask repeatedly because he never remembered being asked before—and he usually chose the photo of the "friendly" person and never chose the "unfriendly" person in spite of the fact that the unfriendly person was a beautiful woman, smiling in the photograph (Tranel & Damasio, 1993). He could not say why he chose to avoid her.

Intact Procedural Memory

Procedural memory, the development of motor skills and habits, is a special kind of implicit memory. As with other examples of implicit memory, you might not be able to describe a motor skill or habit in words, and you might not even recognize it as a memory. For example, H. M. learned to read words written backward, as they would be seen in a mirror, although he was surprised at this skill, as he did not remember having tried it before (Corkin, 2002). Patient K. C. has a part-time job at a library and has learned to use the Dewey decimal system in sorting books, although he does not remember when or where he learned it (Rosenbaum et al., 2005).

Here is another example of procedural memory: In the video game Tetris, geometrical forms such as ▭▭ and ⊕ fall from the top, and the player must move and rotate them to fill available spaces at the bottom of the screen. Normal people improve their skill over a few hours and readily describe the game and its strategy. After playing the same number of hours, patients with amnesia cannot describe the game and say they don't remember playing it. Nevertheless, they slowly improve. Moreover, when they are about to fall asleep, they report seeing images of little piles of blocks falling and rotating (Stickgold, Malia, Maguire, Roddenberry, & O'Connor, 2000). They are puzzled and wonder what these images mean!

In summary, H. M. showed the following pattern, as do many other patients with amnesia:

- Normal working memory, unless distracted
- Severe anterograde amnesia for declarative memory—that is, difficulty forming new declarative memories
- Severe loss of episodic memories, including most of those from before the damage
- Better implicit than explicit memory
- Nearly intact procedural memory, implying that procedural memory depends on other brain areas

✓ STOP & CHECK ▬▬▬▬▬

9. Which types of memory were most impaired in H. M. and people with similar amnesia?
10. Which types of memory were least impaired in H. M. and people with similar amnesia?

ANSWERS 9. H. M. had severe anterograde amnesia (difficulty forming new long-term memories) and a severe loss of episodic memories. 10. H. M. had nearly intact working memory, implicit memory, and procedural memory.

Theories of the Function of the Hippocampus

Exactly how does the hippocampus contribute to memory? Some of the research comes from patients with damage to the hippocampus, but to get better control over both the anatomy and the environment, researchers also conduct research on laboratory animals.

Larry Squire (1992) proposed that the hippocampus is critical for declarative memory, especially episodic memory. How could we test this hypothesis with nonhumans, who cannot "declare" anything? What could they do that would be the equivalent of declarative or episodic memory? Here is one possible example: A rat digs food out of five piles of sand, each with a different odor. Then it gets a choice between two of the odors and is rewarded if it goes toward the one it smelled first. Intact rats learn to respond correctly, apparently demonstrating memory of not only what they smelled but also when they smelled it. Because this task requires memory of a specific event, it seems to qualify as episodic. Rats with hippocampal damage do poorly on this task (Fortin, Agster, & Eichenbaum, 2002; Kesner, Gilbert, & Barua, 2002).

In the **delayed matching-to-sample task,** an animal sees an object (the sample) and after a delay, gets a choice between two objects, from which it must choose the one that matches the sample. In the **delayed nonmatching-to-sample task,** the procedure is the same except that the animal must choose the object that is different from the sample (see Figure 12.10). In both cases, the animal must remember which object was present on this occasion, thereby showing what we might call a declarative memory, perhaps an episodic memory. Hippocampal damage strongly impairs performance in most cases (Heuer & Bachevalier, 2011; Moore, Schettler, Killiany, Rosene, & Moss, 2012; Zola et al., 2000).

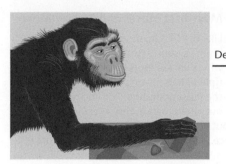
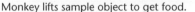
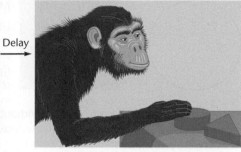

Monkey lifts sample object to get food.   Food is under the new object.

Figure 12.10 A delayed nonmatching-to-sample task

Another hypothesis relates the hippocampus to memory for context. Research with patient H. M. showed the importance of the hippocampus for episodic memory. Think about one of your own episodic memories, any one of them. Presumably it includes a context—sights, sounds, one or more locations, and a series of events. Clearly, that memory could not be stored in a single location in the brain; it has to be spread over many locations. Perhaps the hippocampus is a coordinator, a director that brings together representations from various locations, in the correct order. In short, it reconstructs the context. When people successfully retrieve an episodic memory, activity in and around the hippocampus synchronizes with activity in several parts of the cortex, consistent with the idea that the hippocampus is providing the connections that are necessary for recall (Watrous, Tandon, Conner, Pieters, & Ekstrom, 2013).

Recent episodic memories generally include much contextual detail. Some older memories do also, but in most cases the details fade and we remember only the gist of the event. Memories with much contextual detail depend on the hippocampus, but older, less detailed memories depend mainly on the cerebral cortex with less contribution from the hippocampus (Takehara-Nishiuchi & McNaughton, 2008). The same is true of rats: When rats are trained to do something, and then tested again after a short delay, they remember the response best if they are tested in the same location. That is, their memory depends on the context. As time passes, the context matters less and less, and to the extent that rats remember the response, they remember it equally well in a different location. If rats with damage to the hippocampus learn something at all, they show no difference between testing in the familiar place and some other place. Their memory doesn't depend on context, presumably because they do not remember it (Winocur, Moscovitch, & Sekeres, 2007).

✓ STOP & CHECK

11. According to the context hypothesis, why does hippocampal damage impair recent memories more than distant memories?

ANSWER

11. Recent memories include details of context, and the hippocampus is essential for memory of context. Most old memories include only the gist of the event, and the hippocampus is less important for memories of that type.

Navigation

Suppose someone blindfolds you, picks you up, and plops you down somewhere totally dark and quiet. What do you do? You want to explore, but you must be cautious. You don't know where any opportunities or dangers might be present. Now imagine waking up in your own bed. Again suppose complete darkness and quiet, but now you can walk with ease to your dresser, the door, or whatever, because you know where you are relative to everything else. Knowing where you are is a special type of memory, one that depends on the hippocampus and surrounding areas.

Several types of evidence demonstrate the importance of the hippocampus and nearby areas for spatial memory. Consider a **radial maze** with several arms—typically eight—some or all of which have a bit of food at the end (see Figure 12.11). A rat's best strategy in a radial maze is to explore each arm once and only once, remembering where it has already gone. In a variation of the task, a rat might learn that the arms with a rough floor never have food or that the arms pointing toward the window never have food. Thus, a rat can make a mistake either by entering a never-correct arm or by entering any arm twice.

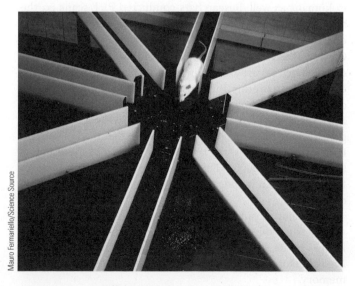

Mauro Fermariello/Science Source

Figure 12.11 A radial maze
A rat that reenters one arm before trying other arms has made an error of spatial working memory.

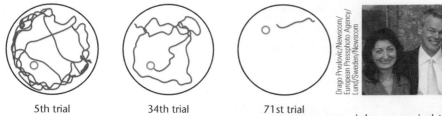

5th trial   34th trial   71st trial

Figure 12.12 The Morris water maze
An intact rat learns by trial and error. In each case the line traces the path a rat took to the platform, marked by a circle. On the fifth trial, the rat stayed mainly near the edge and never found the platform. On the 34th trial, it found the platform in 35 seconds. On the 71st trial, it went directly to the platform in 6 seconds.

(Source: From "Response learning of rats in a Morris water maze: Involvement of the medial prefrontal cortex," by J. P. C. de Bruin, W. A. M. Swinkels, & J. M. de Brabander, 1997, Behavioral Brain Research, 85, 47–55.)

Rats with damage to the hippocampus can learn to avoid the never-correct arms, but even after much training they often enter a correct arm twice. That is, they forget which arms they have already tried (Jarrard, Okaichi, Steward, & Goldschmidt, 1984; Olton & Papas, 1979; Olton, Walker, & Gage, 1978).

In the **Morris water maze,** a rat swims through murky water to find a rest platform that is just under the surface (see Figure 12.12). (Rats swim only when necessary. Humans are among the very few land mammals that swim voluntarily.) A rat with hippocampal damage slowly learns to find the platform if it always starts from the same place and can always turn the same direction to find the rest platform. However, if it has to start from a different location or if the rest platform occasionally moves from one location to another, the rat is disoriented (Eichenbaum, 2000; Liu & Bilkey, 2001). Evidently the hippocampus is essential for remembering locations.

The hippocampus is important for spatial orientation in humans as well. Researchers conducted PET scans on the brains of London taxi drivers as they answered navigation questions such as, "What's the shortest legal route from the Carlton Tower Hotel to the Sherlock Holmes Museum?" (London taxi drivers are well trained and answer with impressive accuracy.) Answering these questions activated their hippocampus much more than did answering nonspatial questions. MRI scans also revealed that the taxi drivers have a larger than average posterior hippocampus and that the longer they had been taxi drivers, the larger their posterior hippocampus (Maguire et al., 2000). This result suggests actual growth of the adult human hippocampus in response to spatial learning experiences.

A major advance in our understanding came from single-cell recordings. May-Britt Moser, Edvard Moser, and John O'Keefe shared the 2014 Nobel Prize in Physiology or Medicine for their discovery of the cells responsible for spatial memory.

The research began with the discovery of **place cells**, hippocampal neurons tuned to particular spatial locations, responding best when an animal is in a particular place and

May-Britt Moser and Edvard Moser
Like the GPS in our phones and cars, our brain's system assesses where we are and where we are heading by integrating multiple signals relating to our position and the passage of time. . . . The ability to figure out where we are and where we need to go is key to survival. Without it, we, like all animals, would be unable to find food or reproduce. Individuals—and, in fact, the entire species—would perish. (*Moser & Moser, 2016, p. 26*)

looking in a particular direction (O'Keefe & Burgess, 1996; O'Keefe & Dostrovsky, 1971). The discovery of place cells enables researchers to "read a rat's mind" to a limited degree. Suppose a rat is at a choice point in a difficult maze. It stops and looks one way and then the other a few times before proceeding. Recordings from its hippocampus show that cells become active in the proper order as if the rat were actually walking down one path or the other. That is, we can watch the brain activity as the rat imagines trying each route (Redish, 2016). People sometimes assert that humans are the only species that can imagine the future. Wrong. Even rats can, at least for the very near future. Are we sure about this? Well, we get similar results from human brains while people imagine moving from one place to another (T. I. Brown et al., 2016; Jacobs et al., 2013; J. F. Miller et al., 2013).

Many of the place cells also function as **time cells** that respond at a particular point in a sequence of time. For example, consider a rat that has to run on a treadmill for 20 seconds to receive reward. Many hippocampal cells become active at a particular time during the 20 seconds (Salz et al., 2016). Evidently rats keep track of where they are in both space and time.

The hippocampal place cells receive much of their input from the nearby entorhinal cortex (see Figure 12.8). When researchers recorded from cells in the entorhinal cortex, they found results like the ones in Figure 12.13. Each cell became active at locations separated from one another in a hexagonal grid. The cells are therefore called **grid cells**. At a given level within the entorhinal cortex, different cells respond to different sets of locations, but always in a hexagon. At each deeper level (dorsal to ventral, shown left to right in Figure 12.13), the area covered by a given cell doubles in size (Stensola et al., 2012). Many of the cells at deeper levels respond to a combination of the animal's location and the direction it is heading (Sargolini et al., 2006). Some of the cells respond to the animal's speed of locomotion instead of its location or direction (Kropff, Carmichael, Moser, & Moser, 2015). The animal determines its location and direction from a combination of inputs from several populations of cells. When an animal moves to a different environment, all the cells reorder themselves to map out the new locations.

The place cells and time cells of the hippocampus relate to the previous discussion of episodic memory. Any episodic memory refers to events that occurred in a particular place, with a particular sequence of events over time. A loss of place cells and time cells disrupts many types of memory formation.

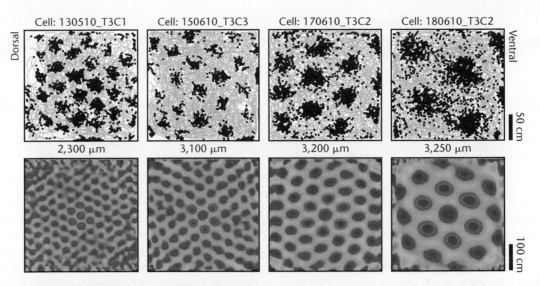

Figure 12.13　Recordings from four cells in a rat's entorhinal cortex
Each box represents one cell, and each dot within a box represents a location where that cell responded. Each cell responded to locations arranged in a hexagon. Cells at a more dorsal level in the entorhinal cortex (toward the right) had wider spacing of grids.
(Source: From "The entorhinal grid map is discretized," by H. Stensola, T. Stensola, T. Solstad, K. Frøland, M.-B. Moser, & E. I. Moser, 2012, Nature, 492, 72–78.)

✔ STOP & CHECK

12. In addition to an animal's location, what else do many place cells monitor?

13. What is the evidence that rats can imagine the future?

14. How do grid cells at ventral levels of the entorhinal cortex differ from those at dorsal levels?

ANSWERS

12. Some also respond to time or the direction the animal is heading. 13. When a rat pauses at a choice point in a maze, place cells respond in sequence as if the animal were traveling down one arm or another of the maze. 14. Moving dorsal to ventral, the grid cells respond to larger areas.

The Striatum

Episodic memory, dependent on the hippocampus, develops after a single experience. Many semantic memories also form after a single experience. That is, if someone tells you an interesting fact, you might remember it forever. Learning your spatial location can also develop quickly. However, we need a different mechanism for gradually learning habits, or learning what probably will or will not happen under certain circumstances. You take into account many types of information when you conclude that it will probably rain tomorrow, or that your mother probably wouldn't enjoy the movie you just saw, or that your favorite team will probably win its next game. You may not even be aware of all the cues you used or how you decided. Learning of this type depends on parts of the basal ganglia, specifically the caudate nucleus and the putamen, which are together known as the **striatum** (see Figure 7.16).

To illustrate, consider the following example. In each of 38 cases you have three pieces of information, here shown as blue or purple rectangles. Based on that information, guess whether it will rain tomorrow ("yes") or not ("no"). You are provided with the correct answer for the first 36. You will get the idea of the task best if you try the items one at a time. What do you guess for the final two items, and on what basis did you make that decision?

TRY IT YOURSELF

Table 12.1 | **Brain Areas for Two Types of Learning**

	Hippocampus	Striatum
Speed of learning	Can learn in a single trial	Learns gradually over many trials
Type of behavior	Flexible responses	Habits
Based on what type of feedback?	Sometimes connects information over a delay	Generally requires prompt feedback
Explicit or implicit learning?	Explicit	Implicit
What happens after damage?	Impaired declarative memory, especially episodic memory	Impaired learning of skills and habits

In this task, you could develop any of several strategies. If you simply noticed that the answer is yes more often than no (evidently you are predicting the weather in a rainy area), you could always answer yes, being correct 64 percent of the time. A better strategy is, if you see more blue than purple rectangles on a given trial, guess yes. If you see more purple than blue rectangles, guess no. That strategy is correct 83 percent. If you pay attention to just the blue versus purple rectangles in one column, your accuracy varies from 53 percent to 86 percent correct, depending on which column you choose. The best strategy is more complicated: If you see two or three blue rectangles, guess yes; if you see two or three purple rectangles, guess no; except that if it goes "blue-purple-purple," guess yes, and if it goes "blue-blue-purple," guess no. That strategy gives a correct answer 94 percent of the time with the material shown here. (So the answers for the final two items are YES, YES.)

You would not have figured out that last strategy from the small number of trials given here. But if you had the patience to continue for hundreds of trials, your accuracy would eventually, gradually climb up toward 94 percent correct. You might not be able to describe your strategy. You would just "know" somehow the right answer to guess each time. That gradual, probabilistic learning depends on the basal ganglia.

Suppose we run a test like this on people with Parkinson's disease, who have impairments of the striatum. As a rule, they perform about the same as healthy people at first, because they have an intact hippocampus and they can learn simple declarative facts such as "blue means yes and purple means no." However, even after many trials, they do not show the gradual improvement that requires the striatum. On other kinds of complex learning tasks, if they don't form an explicit, declarative memory, they don't improve at all (Moody, Chang, Vanek, & Knowlton, 2010). That is, they don't acquire nonverbal habits.

People with amnesia after hippocampal damage perform randomly on the weather task for many trials, because they form no declarative memories and they do not remember that mostly blue or mostly purple symbols would mean anything. However, if they continue for a very long time, they show gradual improvement, based on habits supported by the striatum (Bayley, Frascino, & Squire, 2005; Shohamy, Myers, Kalanithi, & Gluck, 2008). When normal people try to learn a complex task under conditions of extreme distraction, they too learn slowly, like people with a damaged hippocampus (Foerde, Knowlton, & Poldrack, 2006).

Together, these results suggest a division of labor between the striatum and other brain areas that include the hippocampus and cerebral cortex, as summarized in Table 12.1 (Balleine, Delgado, & Hikosaka, 2007; Foerde, Race, Verfaellie, & Shohamy, 2013; Foerde & Shohamy, 2011; Koralek, Jin, Long, Costa, & Carmena, 2012; Shohamy, 2011; Wan et al., 2012). However, the separation between the two systems is not complete. Nearly all learned tasks activate both systems to some extent (Albouy et al., 2008). In many cases with prolonged training, a rat's learning depends mainly on the hippocampus at the start, but comes to depend more on the striatum as the learning becomes better established (Ferbinteanu, 2016). Similarly, you know from your own experience that when you are first learning to do something—drive a car, hit a tennis ball, play a complex video game, whatever—you have to think about it step by step, but after much practice it happens almost automatically. Eventually you may even find that you have trouble explaining to someone else what you are doing.

✓ STOP & CHECK

15. Which type of memory would be easier to describe in words, memory based on the hippocampus or the striatum?

ANSWER

15. Hippocampal-based memory, being explicit, is generally easier to describe in words. The habits based on the striatum are sometimes harder to describe.

Other Brain Areas and Memory

Most of this module has focused on the hippocampus and the striatum. Chapter 11 mentioned the importance of the amygdala for fear memories. Other brain areas are important for learning and memory, too. In fact, most of the brain contributes.

Investigators asked two patients with parietal lobe damage to describe various events from their past. When tested this way, their episodic memory appeared sparse, almost devoid of details. However, the investigators asked follow-up questions, such as, "Where were you?" and "Who else was there at the time?" Then these patients answered in reasonable detail, indicating that their episodic memories were intact, as well as their speech and their willingness to cooperate.

What was lacking was their ability to elaborate on a memory spontaneously (Berryhill, Phuong, Picasso, Cabeza, & Olson, 2007). Ordinarily, when most of us recall an event, one thing reminds us of another, and we start adding one detail after another, until we have said all that we know. In people with parietal lobe damage, that process of associating one piece with another is impaired.

People with damage in the anterior temporal cortex suffer **semantic dementia,** a loss of semantic memory. One patient while riding down a road saw some sheep and asked what they were. The problem wasn't that he couldn't remember the word *sheep.* It was as if he had never seen a sheep before. When another person saw a picture of a zebra, she called it a horse but then pointed at the stripes and asked what "those funny things" were. She had lost the concept of zebra. Such patients often forget the typical color of common fruits and vegetables or the appearance of various animals. The anterior temporal cortex stores some semantic information and serves as a hub for communicating with other brain areas to bring together a full concept (Patterson, Nestor, & Rogers, 2007).

Module 12.2 | In Closing
Brain Damage and Memory

Although most psychologists of the early 20th century assumed that all learning and memory was of only one type, subject to a single set of laws, the idea of more than one type did occasionally emerge (e.g., Tolman, 1949). However, the idea did not become popular until the results of brain damage showed how someone could lose one type of memory without much loss of another. This is a clear example of neurological study contributing to psychological theory.

Summary

1. People with damage to the hippocampus have great trouble forming new long-term declarative memories, especially episodic memories. They also have trouble imagining the future. **395**

2. People with damage to the hippocampus nevertheless show implicit memory, short-term memories, and procedural memories. **395, 398**

3. Theories about the hippocampus focus on its role in declarative memory and memory for context. **398**

4. The hippocampus is especially important for remembering where one is in space and time relative to other items or events. **399**

5. The hippocampus contains place cells. Monitoring those cells shows that animals can imagine traveling in one direction or another. **399**

6. Place cells receive input from grid cells in the entorhinal cortex. Grid cells respond to a series of locations arranged in a hexagonal grid. **400**

7. Whereas the hippocampus is important for rapid storage of an event, the striatum (part of the basal ganglia) is important for gradually developing habits and for seeing complex patterns that may not be evident on a single trial. **401**

8. In some cases learning depends at first on the hippocampus and after much practice becomes dependent on the striatum. **402**

9. The parietal cortex is important for elaborating episodic memories. The anterior temporal cortex serves as a hub for semantic memories. **402**

Key Terms

Terms are defined in the module on the page number indicated. They're also presented in alphabetical order with definitions in the book's Subject Index/Glossary, which begins on page 589. Interactive flash cards, audio reviews, and crossword puzzles are among the online resources available to help you learn these terms and the concepts they represent.

anterograde amnesia **395**
declarative memory **398**
delayed matching-to-sample task **398**
delayed nonmatching-to-sample task **398**
episodic memories **397**

explicit memory **398**
grid cells **400**
implicit memory **398**
Morris water maze **400**
place cells **400**
procedural memory **398**
radial maze **399**

retrograde amnesia **395**
semantic dementia **403**
semantic memories **396**
striatum **401**
time cells **400**

Thought Question

From any observations you have made on human infants, which type of memory would you guess develops first, the hippocampal-dependent system or the striatum-dependent system?

Module 12.2 | End of Module Quiz

1. What is anterograde amnesia?
   A. Loss of factual memory
   B. Loss of memory for personal experiences
   C. Loss of memory for space and time
   D. Inability to form new memories

2. What was the status of working memory in patient H. M.?
   A. He had a complete loss of working memory.
   B. His working memory seemed normal unless he was distracted.
   C. He had reasonable working memory only for facts that he found highly interesting.
   D. Shortly after his damage, his working memory was poor, but it later recovered.

3. Which of the following was most severely impaired in patient H. M.?
   A. Episodic memory
   B. Procedural memory
   C. Implicit memory
   D. Short-term memory

4. Why is it unsurprising that H. M. had intact procedural memory?
   A. Procedural memory can develop in a single trial.
   B. Procedural memory depends on high-frequency gamma oscillations.
   C. Procedural memory does not require synaptic modifications in the brain.
   D. Procedural memory depends on the striatum, not the hippocampus.

5. What type of memory do the radial maze and Morris water maze test?
   A. Episodic memory
   B. Verbal memory
   C. Social memory
   D. Spatial memory

6. Evidence that rats can imagine the future came from recordings from what type of cell?
   A. Glia cells
   B. Place cells
   C. Face-recognition cells
   D. Visual cortex cells

7. Why are certain cells in the entorhinal cortex called grid cells?
   A. They respond to locations distributed in a hexagonal grid.
   B. They have axons that spread out in the shape of a grid.
   C. They have dendrites that spread out in the shape of a grid.
   D. They respond when an animal sees something shaped like a grid.

8. The striatum is primarily responsible for which type of learning?
   A. Gradually learning habits
   B. Acquiring and storing episodic memories
   C. Memories that people can easily describe in words
   D. Quickly adapting learned behaviors to new circumstances

9. Someone with semantic dementia has lost which of the following?
   A. Ability to understand speech
   B. Factual knowledge
   C. Ability to find the way to something
   D. Face recognition

Answers: 1D, 2B, 3A, 4D, 5D, 6B, 7A, 8A, 9B.

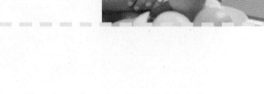

Storing Information in the Nervous System

If you walk through a field, are the footprints that you leave "memories"? How about the mud that you pick up on your shoes? If the police wanted to know who walked across that field, a forensics expert could check your footprints or your shoes to answer the question. And yet we would not call these physical traces memories in the usual sense.

Similarly, when a pattern of activity passes through the brain, it leaves a path of physical changes, but not every change is a memory. The task of finding how the brain stores memories is a challenging one, and researchers have explored many avenues that seemed promising for a while but now seem fruitless.

Blind Alleys and Abandoned Mines

Textbooks, including this one, concentrate mostly on successful research that led to our current understanding of a field. You may get the impression that science progresses smoothly, with each experiment contributing to the body of knowledge. However, if you look at old journals or textbooks, you will find discussions of many "promising" or "exciting" findings that we disregard today. Scientific research does not progress straight from ignorance to enlightenment. It explores one direction after another, a little like a rat in a complex maze, abandoning the dead ends and pursuing arms that lead further.

The problem with the maze analogy is that an investigator seldom runs into a wall that clearly identifies the end of a route. A better analogy is a prospector digging for gold, never certain whether to abandon an unprofitable spot or to keep digging just a little longer. Many previously exciting lines of research in the study of learning are now of little more than historical interest. Here are three examples:

1. Wilder Penfield sometimes performed brain surgery for severe epilepsy on conscious patients who had only scalp anesthesia. When he applied a brief, weak electrical stimulus to part of the brain, the patient could describe the experience that the stimulation evoked. Stimulation of the temporal cortex sometimes evoked vivid descriptions such as:

I feel as though I were in the bathroom at school.
I see myself at the corner of Jacob and Washington in South Bend, Indiana.

I remember myself at the railroad station in Vanceburg, Kentucky; it is winter and the wind is blowing outside, and I am waiting for a train.

Penfield (1955; Penfield & Perot, 1963) suggested that each neuron stores a particular memory, like a videotape of one's life. However, brain stimulation rarely elicited a memory of a specific event. Usually, it evoked vague sights and sounds, or recollections of common experiences such as "seeing a bed" or "hearing a choir sing 'White Christmas.'" Stimulation almost never elicited memories of doing anything—just of seeing and hearing. Also, some patients reported events that they had never actually experienced, such as being chased by a robber or seeing Christ descend from the sky. In short, the stimulation produced something more like a dream than a memory.

2. G. A. Horridge (1962) apparently demonstrated that decapitated cockroaches can learn. First he cut the connections between a cockroach's head and the rest of its body. Then he suspended the cockroach so that its legs dangled just above a surface of water. An electrical circuit was arranged as in Figure 12.14 so that the roach's leg received a shock whenever it touched the water. Each experimental roach was paired with a control roach that got a leg shock whenever the first roach did. Only the experimental roach had any control over the shock, however. This kind of experiment is known as a "yoked-control" design.

Over 5 to 10 minutes, headless roaches in the experimental group increased a response of tucking the leg under the body to avoid shocks. Those in the control group did not, on average, change their leg position as a result of the shocks. Thus, the changed response apparently qualifies as learning and not as an accidental by-product of the shocks.

These experiments initially seemed a promising way to study learning in a simple nervous system (Eisenstein & Cohen, 1965). Unfortunately, decapitated cockroaches learn slowly—wow, imagine that!—and the results vary sharply from one individual to another, limiting the usefulness of the results. After a handful of studies, interest in this line of research faded.

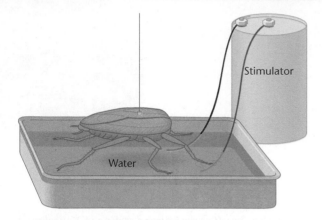

Figure 12.14 **Learning in a headless cockroach?**
The decapitated cockroach, suspended just above the water, receives a shock whenever its hind leg touches the water. A cockroach in the control group gets a shock whenever the first roach does regardless of its own behavior. According to some reports, the experimental roach learned to keep its leg out of the water.
(Source: From "Learning of leg position by the ventral nerve cord in headless insects," by G. A. Horridge, Proceedings of the Royal Society of London, B, 157, 1962, 33–52. *Copyright © 1962 The Royal Society of London. Reprinted by permission of the Royal Society of London and G. A. Horridge.)*

3. In the 1960s and early 1970s, several investigators proposed that each memory is coded as a specific molecule, probably RNA or protein. The boldest test of that hypothesis was an attempt to transfer memories chemically from one individual to another. James McConnell (1962) reported that, when planaria (flatworms) cannibalized other planaria that had been classically conditioned to respond to a light, they apparently remembered what the cannibalized planaria had learned. At least they learned the response faster than average for planaria.

   Inspired by that report, other investigators trained rats to approach a clicking sound for food (Babich, Jacobson, Bubash, & Jacobson, 1965). After the rats were well trained, the experimenters ground up their brains, extracted RNA, and injected it into untrained rats. The recipient rats learned to approach the clicking sound faster than rats in the control group did.

   That report led to a wealth of studies on the transfer of training by brain extracts. In *some* of these experiments, rats that received brain extracts from a trained group showed apparent memory of the task, whereas those that received extracts from an untrained group did not (Dyal, 1971; Fjerdingstad, 1973). The results were inconsistent and unreplicable, however, even within a single laboratory (Smith, 1975). Many laboratories failed to find any hint of a transfer effect. By the mid-1970s, most researchers saw no point in continuing this research, and funding agencies refused to consider further grants for it.

Learning and the Hebbian Synapse

Research on the physiology of learning began with Ivan Pavlov's concept of classical conditioning. Although that theory led Karl Lashley to an unsuccessful search for connections in the cerebral cortex, it also stimulated Donald Hebb to propose a mechanism for change at a synapse.

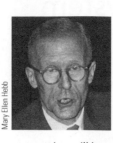

Donald O. Hebb (1904–1985)

Modern psychology takes completely for granted that behavior and neural function are perfectly correlated. . . . There is no separate soul or life force to stick a finger into the brain now and then and make neural cells do what they would not otherwise. . . . It is quite conceivable that some day the assumption will have to be rejected. But it is important also to see that we have not reached that day yet. . . . One cannot logically be a determinist in physics and chemistry and biology, and a mystic in psychology. (*Hebb, 1949, p. xiii*)

Hebb suggested that when the axon of neuron A "repeatedly or persistently takes part in firing [cell B], some growth process or metabolic change takes place in one or both cells" that increases the subsequent ability of axon A to excite cell B (Hebb, 1949, p. 62). In other words, an axon that has successfully stimulated cell B in the past becomes even more successful in the future. In still simpler words, "cells that fire together wire together." Later researchers modified this idea: Neurons that are near each other and fire together wire together (Ascoli, 2015). That saying is less catchy, but it is more accurate. The structure of the nervous system determines which connections learning can make, and how easily it can make them.

Consider how this process relates to classical conditioning. Suppose axon A initially excites cell B slightly, and axon C excites B more strongly. If A and C fire together, their combined effect on B may produce an action potential. You might think of axon A as the conditioned stimulus and axon C as the unconditioned stimulus. Pairing activity in axons A and C increases the future effect of A on B. A **Hebbian synapse** is one that can increase its effectiveness as a result of simultaneous activity in the presynaptic and postsynaptic neurons. Such synapses are essential for many kinds of associative learning.

✓ STOP & CHECK

16. How can a Hebbian synapse account for the basic phenomena of classical conditioning?

ANSWER

16. In a Hebbian synapse, pairing the activity of a weaker (CS) axon with a stronger (UCS) axon produces an action potential, and in the process strengthens the response of the cell to the CS axon. On later trials, it will produce a bigger depolarization of the postsynaptic cell, which we can regard as a conditioned response.

Single-Cell Mechanisms of Invertebrate Behavior Change

If we are going to look for a needle in a haystack, a good strategy is to look in a small haystack. Therefore, many researchers have turned to studies of invertebrates. Vertebrate and invertebrate nervous systems are organized differently, but the chemistry of the neuron, the principles of the action potential, the neurotransmitters, and their receptors are the same. If we identify the physical basis of learning and memory in an invertebrate, we have at least a hypothesis of what *might* work in vertebrates. Biologists have long used this strategy for studying genetics, embryology, and other biological processes.

Aplysia as an Experimental Animal

Aplysia, a marine invertebrate related to the slug, has been a popular animal for studies of the physiology of learning (see Figure 12.15). Compared to vertebrates, it has fewer neurons, many of which are large and easy to study. Moreover, unlike vertebrates, *Aplysia* neurons are virtually identical from one individual to another so that investigators can replicate one another's work in detail.

Much research deals with the withdrawal response: If someone touches the siphon, mantle, or gill of an *Aplysia* (see Figure 12.16), the animal vigorously withdraws the irritated structure. Investigators have traced the neural path from the touch receptors through other neurons to the motor neurons that direct the response. Using this neural pathway, investigators have studied changes in behavior as a result of experience. In 2000, Eric Kandel won a Nobel Prize for this work.

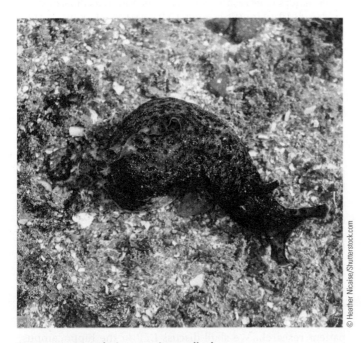

Figure 12.15 *Aplysia*, a marine mollusk
A full-grown animal is a little larger than a human hand.

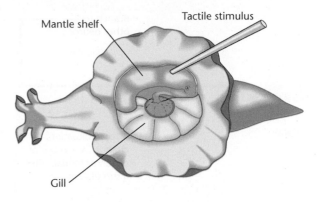

Figure 12.16 **Touching an *Aplysia* causes a withdrawal response**
The sensory and motor neurons controlling this reaction have been identified and studied.

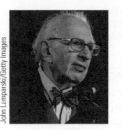

Eric R. Kandel

The questions posed by higher cognitive processes such as learning and memory are formidable, and we have only begun to explore them. Although elementary aspects of simple forms of learning have been accessible to molecular analysis in invertebrates, we are only now beginning to know a bit about the genes and proteins involved in more complex, hippocampus-based learning processes of mammals.

Habituation in *Aplysia*

Habituation is a decrease in response to a repeated stimulus that is accompanied by no change in other stimuli. For example, a sudden noise may startle you, but you respond less after repeated presentations, especially if they occur frequently or at predictable intervals. If we repeatedly stimulate an *Aplysia*'s gills with a brief jet of seawater, it withdraws at first, but after many repetitions, it stops responding. The decline in response is not due to muscle fatigue; even after habituation has occurred, direct stimulation of the motor neuron produces a full-size muscle contraction (Kupfermann, Castellucci, Pinsker, & Kandel, 1970). We can also rule out changes in the sensory neuron. The sensory neuron still gives a full, normal response to stimulation; it merely fails to excite the motor neuron as much as before (Kupfermann et al., 1970). We are therefore left with the conclusion that habituation in *Aplysia* depends on a change in the synapse between the sensory neuron and the motor neuron (see Figure 12.17).

Sensitization in *Aplysia*

If you experience an unexpected, intense pain, you temporarily react more strongly than usual to other sudden stimuli. This phenomenon is **sensitization**, an increase in response to mild stimuli as a result of exposure to more intense stimuli. Similarly, a strong stimulus almost anywhere on *Aplysia*'s skin intensifies a later withdrawal response to a touch.

Researchers traced sensitization to changes at identified synapses (Cleary, Hammer, & Byrne, 1989; Dale, Schacher,

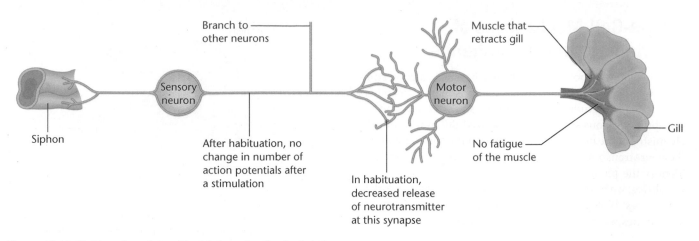

Figure 12.17 Habituation of the gill-withdrawal reflex in *Aplysia*
Touching the siphon causes gill withdrawal. After many repetitions, the response habituates (declines) because of decreased transmission at the synapse between the sensory neuron and the motor neuron.
(Redrawn from "Neuronal mechanisms of habituation and dishabituation of the gill-withdrawal reflex in aplysia," by V. Castellucci, H. Pinsker, I. Kupfermann, and E. Kandel, Science, 1970, 167, pp. 1745–1748. Copyright © 1970 by AAAS. Used by permission of AAAS and V. Castellucci.)

& Kandel, 1988; Kandel & Schwartz, 1982). Strong stimulation on the skin excites a *facilitating interneuron* that releases serotonin onto the presynaptic terminals of many sensory neurons. Serotonin blocks potassium channels in these membranes. Because potassium now flows more slowly out of the cell, the membrane repolarizes more slowly after an action potential. Therefore, the presynaptic neuron continues releasing its neurotransmitter for longer than usual. Repeating this process causes the sensory neuron to synthesize new proteins that produce long-term sensitization (Bailey, Giustetto, Huang, Hawkins, & Kandel, 2000). This research shows how it is possible to explain one example of behavioral plasticity in terms of molecular events. Later studies explored mechanisms of classical and instrumental conditioning in *Aplysia*.

⊘ **STOP & CHECK** ▬▬▬▬▬▬

17. When serotonin blocks potassium channels on the presynaptic terminal, what is the effect on transmission?

ANSWER   17. Blocking potassium channels prolongs the action potential and therefore prolongs the release of neurotransmitters, producing an increased response.

Long-Term Potentiation in Vertebrates

Since the work of Charles Sherrington and Santiago Ramón y Cajal, most neuroscientists have assumed that learning depends on changes at synapses, and the work on *Aplysia* supports that idea. The first evidence for a similar process among vertebrates came from studies of neurons in the rat hippocampus (Bliss & Lømo, 1973). The phenomenon, known as **long-term potentiation (LTP),** is this: One or more axons connected to a dendrite bombard it with a rapid series of stimuli. The burst of intense stimulation leaves some of the synapses potentiated (more responsive to new input of the same type) for minutes, days, or weeks.

LTP shows three properties that make it an attractive candidate for a cellular basis of learning and memory:

- **specificity**—If some of the synapses onto a cell have been highly active and others have not, only the active ones become strengthened. A failure of specificity is one cause of impaired learning (Ferando, Faas, & Mody, 2016).
- **cooperativity**—Nearly simultaneous stimulation by two or more axons produces LTP more strongly than does repeated stimulation by just one axon.
- **associativity**—Pairing a weak input with a strong input enhances later response to the weak input, as illustrated in Figure 12.18. In this regard, LTP matches what we would expect of Hebbian synapses. In some cases, a synapse that was almost completely inactive before LTP becomes effective afterward (Kerchner & Nicoll, 2008).

The opposite change, **long-term depression (LTD),** a prolonged decrease in response at a synapse, occurs for axons that have been less active than others, such as axon 3 in Figure 12.18 (Collingridge, Peineau, Howland, & Wang, 2010). You can think of this as a compensatory process. As one synapse strengthens, another weakens (Royer & Paré, 2003). If learning produced only a strengthening of synapses, then every time you learned something, your brain would get more and more active, constantly burning more and more fuel!

Biochemical Mechanisms

Determining how LTP or LTD occurs has been a huge research challenge because each neuron has many tiny synapses, sometimes in the tens of thousands. Isolating the chemical changes at any synapse takes an enormous amount of creative, patient research. We shall discuss LTP in the hippocampus, where it occurs most readily and where its mechanisms have been most extensively studied.

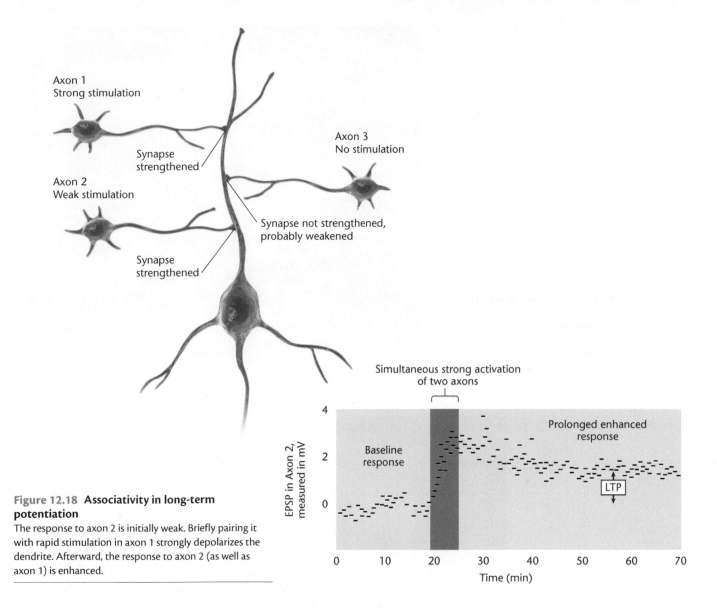

Figure 12.18 Associativity in long-term potentiation
The response to axon 2 is initially weak. Briefly pairing it with rapid stimulation in axon 1 strongly depolarizes the dendrite. Afterward, the response to axon 2 (as well as axon 1) is enhanced.

AMPA and NMDA Synapses

In a few cases, LTP depends on changes at GABA synapses (Nugent, Penick, & Kauer, 2007), but in most cases, it depends on changes at glutamate synapses. The brain has several types of receptors for glutamate, its most abundant transmitter. Neuroscientists identify types of dopamine receptors by number, such as D_1 and D_2, and GABA receptors by letter, such as $GABA_A$. They identify serotonin (5-hydroxytryptamine) synapses by both letter and number, such as $5HT_{2C}$. For glutamate, they named the receptors after certain drugs that stimulate them. Here we are interested in two types of glutamate receptors, called AMPA and NMDA. The **AMPA receptor** is excited by the neurotransmitter glutamate, but it can also respond to a drug called α-amino-3-hydroxy-5-methyl-4-isoxazolepropionic acid (abbreviated AMPA). The **NMDA receptor** is also ordinarily excited only by glutamate, but it can respond to a drug called N-methyl-D-aspartate (abbreviated NMDA).

Both are ionotropic receptors. That is, when they are stimulated, they open a channel to let ions enter the postsynaptic cell.

The AMPA receptor is a typical ionotropic receptor that opens sodium channels. However, the NMDA receptor's response to glutamate depends on the degree of polarization across the membrane. When the membrane is at its resting potential, the NMDA receptor's ion channel is usually blocked by magnesium ions. Magnesium ions, positively charged, are attracted to the negative charge inside the cells but do not fit through the NMDA channel. The NMDA channel permits ions to flow through it only if the magnesium leaves, and the surest way to detach the magnesium is to depolarize the membrane, decreasing the negative charge that attracts it (see Figure 12.19).

Suppose an axon releases glutamate repeatedly. Better yet, let's activate two axons repeatedly, side by side on the same dendrite. So many sodium ions enter through the AMPA channels that the dendrite becomes strongly depolarized. The depolarization displaces the magnesium molecules, enabling glutamate to open the NMDA channel. At that point, both sodium and calcium enter through the NMDA channel (see Figure 12.20).

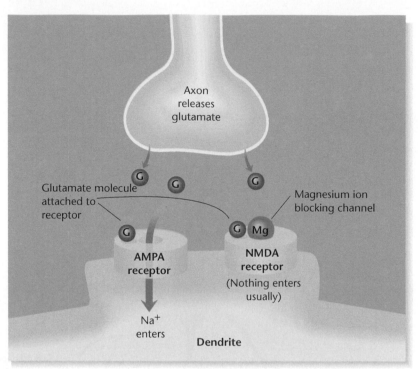

Figure 12.19 **The AMPA and NMDA receptors before LTP**
Glutamate attaches to both receptors. At the AMPA receptor, it opens a channel to let sodium ions enter. At the NMDA receptor, it binds but usually fails to open the channel, which is blocked by magnesium ions.

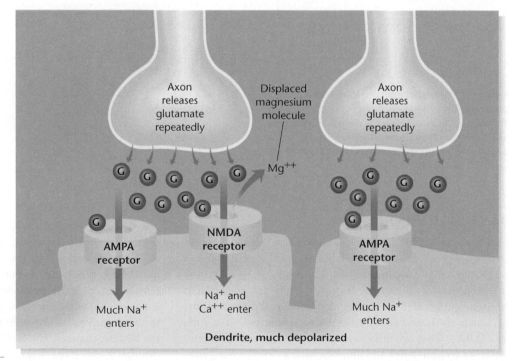

Figure 12.20 **The AMPA and NMDA receptors during LTP**
If one or more AMPA receptors have been repeatedly stimulated, enough sodium enters to largely depolarize the dendrite's membrane. Doing so displaces the magnesium ions and enables glutamate to open the NMDA receptor, through which sodium and calcium enter.

The entry of calcium is the key to producing LTP. When calcium enters through the NMDA channel, it activates a protein called CaMKII (α-calcium-calmodulin-dependent protein kinase II) (Lisman, Schulman, & Cline, 2002; Otmakhov et al., 2004). CaMKII sets in motion a series of reactions leading to release of a protein called CREB—cyclic adenosine monophosphate responsive element-binding protein. (You can see why it's almost always abbreviated.) CREB goes to the nucleus of the cell and regulates the expression of several genes. In some cases, the altered gene expression lasts for months or years, long enough to account for long-term memory (Miller et al., 2010). It is an example of an epigenetic change, depending on histone modifications (Halder et al., 2016). The effects of CaMKII are necessary for LTP and for certain types of learning. Because activated CaMKII remains at the stimulated synapse and does not diffuse elsewhere, it is responsible for the specificity aspect of LTP—the fact that only the highly activated synapses become strengthened (Lisman, Yasuda, & Raghavachari, 2012; Redondo & Morris, 2011; Wang et al., 2009).

The effects of CaMKII and CREB are magnified by **BDNF**—brain-derived neurotrophic factor, a neurotrophin similar to nerve growth factor. Persisting activity at synapses leads to action potentials that start in axons but backpropagate into the dendrites, which then release BDNF. The formation and maintenance of LTP depends on all these chemicals—CaMKII, CREB, and BDNF (Kuczewski et al., 2008; Minichiello, 2009; Silva, Zhou, Rogerson, Shobe, & Balaji, 2009), as well as others. When neurons are repeatedly activated, only those with the greatest production of these chemicals will undergo LTP (Han et al., 2007).

In some cases, LTP depends on mechanisms that increase the responsiveness of AMPA receptors (Lauterborn et al., 2016; Lisman et al., 2012). In many other cases it depends on building new branches of dendrites and synapses with either AMPA or NMDA receptors. Figure 12.21 shows an example (Zhang, Cudmore, Lin, Linden, & Huganir, 2015). Many of the new synapses that develop in the hippocampus last only weeks and are perhaps a bridge toward more permanent storage elsewhere (Attardo, Fitzgerald, & Schnitzer, 2015).

Let's summarize: When glutamate massively stimulates AMPA receptors, the resulting depolarization enables glutamate to stimulate nearby NMDA receptors also. Stimulation of the NMDA receptors lets calcium enter the cell, where it sets into motion a series of changes that build new glutamate synapses or increase response to glutamate at existing AMPA receptors. After LTP occurs, NMDA receptors revert to their original condition.

Once LTP has been established, it no longer depends on NMDA synapses. Drugs that block NMDA synapses prevent the *establishment* of LTP, but they do not interfere with the *maintenance* of LTP that was already established (Gustafsson & Wigström, 1990; Uekita & Okaichi, 2005). In other words, once LTP occurs, the AMPA receptors stay potentiated, regardless of what happens to the NMDAs.

Presynaptic Changes

The changes just described occur in the postsynaptic neuron. In many cases, LTP depends on changes in the presynaptic neuron instead or in addition. Extensive stimulation of a postsynaptic cell causes it to release a **retrograde transmitter** that travels back to the presynaptic cell to modify it. In many cases, that retrograde transmitter is nitric oxide (NO). As a result, a presynaptic neuron decreases its threshold for producing action potentials (Ganguly, Kiss, & Poo, 2000), increases its release of neurotransmitter (Zakharenko, Zablow, & Siegelbaum, 2001), expands its axon (Routtenberg, Cantallops, Zaffuto, Serrano, & Namgung, 2000), and releases its transmitter from additional sites along its axon (Reid, Dixon, Takahashi, Bliss, & Fine, 2004). When both presynaptic and postsynaptic changes contribute to LTP, the result is greater precision and stability of learning (Costa, Froemke, Sjöström, & van Rossum, 2015).

Research on LTP shows us a mechanism whereby experience can alter the input–output properties of a neuron. Many studies have shown that LTP is important for learning and that interfering with LTP interferes with learning. However, it should be clear that understanding LTP is just one step toward understanding learning. Except for the simplest cases of classical conditioning, learning requires more than just increasing the response to a stimulus. Researchers will need to continue exploring how the wiring diagram makes possible all the complexities of a learned response.

✓ STOP & CHECK

18. Before LTP: In the normal state, what is the effect of glutamate at the AMPA receptors? At the NMDA receptors?
19. During the formation of LTP, when a burst of intense stimulation releases much more glutamate than usual at two or more incoming axons, what is the effect of the glutamate at the AMPA receptors? At the NMDA receptors?
20. After the neuron has gone through LTP, what is now the effect of glutamate at the AMPA receptors? At the NMDA receptors?

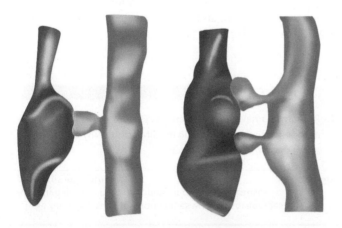

Figure 12.21 Added synapses as a result of LTP
These photos show part of one mouse dendrite before and three hours after the onset of LTP. The areas in white indicate glutamate synapses.
(*Source: From "Visualization of NMDA receptor-dependent AMPA receptor synaptic plasticity in vivo," by Y. Zhang, R. H. Cudmore, D-T. Lin, D. J. Linden, & R. L. Huganir, 2015, Nature Neuroscience, 18, 402–407.*)

ANSWERS

18. Before LTP, glutamate stimulates AMPA receptors but usually has little effect at the NMDA receptors because magnesium blocks them. **19.** During the formation of LTP, the massive glutamate input strongly stimulates the AMPA receptors, thus depolarizing the dendrite. This depolarization enables glutamate to excite the NMDA receptors also. **20.** After LTP has been established, glutamate stimulates the AMPA receptors more than before, mainly because of an increased number of AMPA receptors. At the NMDA receptors, it is again usually ineffective.

Improving Memory

One reason for studying LTP and other biological mechanisms is the hope that it might lead to practical applications. LTP depends on production of several proteins, and enhancing production of these proteins enhances memory in rodents (Routtenberg et al., 2000; Shema et al., 2011). Drugs that inhibit their production weaken memory, even if the drugs are given days after the training (Shema, Sacktor, & Dudai, 2007). Several pharmaceutical companies are investigating drugs that might improve memory by enhancing LTP, but so far nothing is available. As in the rest of medicine, many drugs that show promise in animal studies have unacceptable side effects when applied to humans.

The one type of medication that does aid memory—sometimes—is a stimulant drug such as caffeine, amphetamine, or methylphenidate (Ritalin). Although buying or selling amphetamine or methylphenidate without a prescription is illegal, many college students and some high school students have obtained the drugs and tried them at least once. The research suggests that the increased energy slightly improves memory and cognition for average or below-average students, but provides little or no benefit and maybe even harm for the best students. Little is known about the health consequences of prolonged use (Ilieva, Hook, & Farah, 2015; Smith & Farah, 2011).

Modafinil, another stimulant drug, has been approved for treating narcolepsy and other conditions that impair wakefulness, but people have also tried it (without FDA approval) for enhancing cognition and memory. The limited research so far suggests improvement on complex tasks, but the research has not yet examined the risks that long-term, repeated use might entail (Battleday & Brem, 2015).

You may have heard claims that the herb *Ginkgo biloba* improves memory. Drug companies face stiff regulation by the Food and Drug Administration before they can market a new drug, but a company marketing an herb or other naturally occurring substance does not have to demonstrate effectiveness, provided that the label or advertisement does not claim medical benefits. You may also notice that the ads for pills containing *Ginkgo biloba* leave it to your imagination what good, if any, this supplement does. Most of the research on *Ginkgo biloba* has been of low quality, and the results have been inconsistent (Yang, Wang, Sun, Zhang, & Liu, 2016). The benefits, if any, seem to be limited to people with Alzheimer's disease or similar conditions, and develop only after people have taken the herb for months (Stough & Pase, 2015).

Another herb, *Bacopa monnieri*, also known as water hyssop, has been used in India since the sixth century for several mental conditions. It works as an antioxidant and removes β-amyloids, so theoretically it seems a reasonable candidate for improving memory. The research suggests that it may help some people's memory, but again the benefits emerge only after taking the herb for months (Stough & Pase, 2015). Don't expect any help for your test next week. Flavonols are chemicals found in Chinese tea, some cocoa and chocolate, and certain fruits and vegetables. Very limited research suggests that they sometimes improve performance on certain types of memory tasks, at least in older adults (Brickman et al., 2014).

Researchers have found several ways to enhance memory in mice by altering gene expression, but each benefit comes with a cost. Mice with increased expression of a gene that enhances NMDA receptors show faster learning, but also chronic pain. Mice with another variant gene learn complex mazes faster than usual, but are worse than average at learning simple mazes. Another type of mouse learns quickly, but at the cost of learning fears quickly and failing to unlearn the fears later (Lehrer, 2009). Research with humans found that electrical stimulation to parts of the parietal or prefrontal cortex could improve certain types of memory, but always at the cost of impairing a different type of memory (Iuculano & Kadosh, 2013).

Yet another possibility, transcranial direct current stimulation, consists of applying a nonpainful 1 to 2 milliamp current to the scalp. The procedure has shown promising results for treating depression, chronic pain, Parkinson's disease, and other conditions, and possibly helps people improve attention and memory. However, the procedure sometimes improves performance on one task while impairing another. It can also be dangerous if the electrodes are improperly placed or if the duration is too long (Maslen, Douglas, Cohen Kadosh, Levy, & Savulescu, 2014).

Behavioral methods to improve memory are still the best bet. If you want to remember something later, study it well now, rehearse it later, and periodically test yourself. Consistent physical exercise also improves memory, as do good nutrition, adequate sleep, and stress management (Chapman et al., 2013; Smith & Farah, 2011).

✅ STOP & CHECK

21. Researchers have found several ways of improving memory in rodents, including genetic modification. Why do we not apply these methods to humans?

ANSWER

21. So far, every such method comes with disadvantages. Although improving functioning in one way, it causes problems in another.

Module 12.3 | In Closing

The Physiology of Memory

Why do we care about the physiology of memory? Some day our understanding may lead to practical applications. The theoretical importance is also important. Explaining memory in chemical terms underscores the idea of monism: Our experiences, our thoughts, and our memories are manifestations of chemical processes. All the researchers manipulating chemicals at tiny synapses are in a very real sense trying to help us understand human nature.

Summary

1. A Hebbian synapse becomes stronger when the presynaptic neuron releases transmitters in conjunction with an action potential in the postsynaptic neuron. **406**

2. Habituation of the gill-withdrawal reflex in *Aplysia* depends on a mechanism that decreases the release of transmitter from a particular presynaptic neuron. **407**

3. Sensitization of the gill-withdrawal reflex in *Aplysia* occurs when serotonin blocks potassium channels in a presynaptic neuron and thereby prolongs the release of transmitter from that neuron. **407**

4. Long-term potentiation (LTP) is an enhancement of response at certain synapses because of a brief but intense series of stimuli delivered to a neuron, generally by two or more axons delivering simultaneous inputs. **408**

5. If axons are active at a very slow rate, their synapses may decrease in responsiveness—a process known as long-term depression (LTD). **408**

6. LTP in hippocampal neurons occurs as follows: Repeated glutamate excitation of AMPA receptors depolarizes the membrane. The depolarization removes magnesium ions that had been blocking NMDA receptors. Glutamate is then able to excite the NMDA receptors, opening a channel for calcium ions to enter the neuron. **409**

7. When calcium enters through the NMDA-controlled channels, it activates a protein that sets in motion a series of events that increase receptor response or build additional synapses. These changes increase the later response to glutamate. **410**

8. At many synapses, LTP relates to increased release of transmitter from the presynaptic neuron, in addition to or instead of changes in the postsynaptic neuron. **411**

9. Although researchers hope to develop drugs or procedures to improve memory, at this point no procedure is clearly safe and effective for healthy people hoping to boost performance. The best way to improve memory is to learn the material well and practice it. **412**

Key Terms

Terms are defined in the module on the page number indicated. They're also presented in alphabetical order with definitions in the book's Subject Index/Glossary, which begins on page 589. Interactive flash cards, audio reviews, and crossword puzzles are among the online resources available to help you learn these terms and the concepts they represent.

AMPA receptor **409**
associativity **408**
BDNF **411**
cooperativity **408**

habituation **407**
Hebbian synapse **406**
long-term depression (LTD) **408**
long-term potentiation (LTP) **408**

NMDA receptor **409**
retrograde transmitter **411**
sensitization **407**
specificity **408**

Thought Questions

1. If a synapse has already developed LTP once, should it be easier or more difficult to get it to develop LTP again? Why?

2. The use of performance-enhancing drugs in sports is considered unethical and for most competitions illegal. Should we consider it unethical for people to use amphetamine or other performance-enhancing drugs when they are taking tests or otherwise competing academically?

Module 12.3 | End of Module Quiz

1. What is true about a Hebbian synapse?

   A. It strengthens if its activity is associated with an action potential in the postsynaptic cell.

   B. It can be either excitatory or inhibitory, depending on the activity of other nearby synapses.

   C. It includes either an AMPA site or an NMDA site.

   D. It can send messages between cells in either direction.

2. Cells that fire together wire together . . . but only if which of the following?

   A. The cells are close together.

   B. Both cells release the same neurotransmitter.

   C. Both cells are in the cerebral cortex.

   D. One cell is excitatory and the other is inhibitory.

3. Why is *Aplysia* an appealing animal for studies of the physiology of learning?

   A. Its axon is thicker than that of mammals and therefore easier to study.

   B. Unlike mammals, it uses only one neurotransmitter and two types of receptors.

   C. Compared to other invertebrates, it learns faster and remembers longer.

   D. It has relatively few neurons, and they are the same from one individual to another.

4. What is responsible for habituation in *Aplysia*?

   A. Fatigue of the muscles

   B. Decreased response by the sense organs

   C. Decreased hormonal secretions

   D. A change at a synapse

5. What is meant by the "cooperativity" of LTP?

   A. LTP is greater if two inputs are active together.

   B. LTP increases the response of many synapses, even those that were not stimulated.

   C. Pairing two stimuli leads to both habituation and sensitization.

   D. Pairing two stimuli increases the response to the stronger one.

6. What excites NMDA receptors?

   A. The transmitter norepinephrine

   B. The transmitter NMDA

   C. The transmitter glutamate, but only if other nearby synapses are silent

   D. The transmitter glutamate, but only if the membrane is depolarized

7. During the formation of LTP, which ions enter at the NMDA receptors?

   A. Calcium and magnesium

   B. Iron and magnesium

   C. Sodium and potassium

   D. Calcium and sodium

8. What does CaMKII do?

   A. It displaces magnesium and therefore permits glutamate to open calcium channels.

   B. It releases a protein that alters the expression of several genes.

   C. It diffuses from one synapse to another within the postsynaptic neuron.

   D. It sends a message back to the presynaptic neuron to alter its release of neurotransmitters.

9. How effective is *Ginkgo biloba* for improving memory?

   A. Possible benefits for older people who take the herb for months

   B. Possible benefits for people whose memory was already strong

   C. Possible benefits at first, but gradually weakening effects over time

   D. Possible benefits for classical conditioning, but not for other learning or memory

Answers: 1A, 2A, 3D, 4D, 5A, 6D, 7D, 8B, 9A.

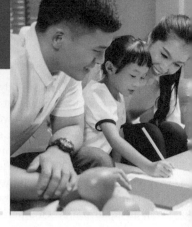

Intelligence

Intelligence, a difficult concept to define, includes learning, memory, reasoning, and problem solving. One of the first discoveries from psychological research was Charles Spearman's (1904) report that, as a rule, all measures of cognitive performance correlate positively with one another. That is, most people who are above average in math, spatial skills, language, logical reasoning, or any other cognitive skill are above average on most of the others also. Many psychologists have therefore assumed that all the skills share a single underlying factor of general intelligence, known as *g*. However, the fact that various skills correlate does not necessarily mean that they measure the same thing. Across a large number of people, the size of one brain area correlates positively with the size of any other brain area, just because health, nutrition, and other factors support the growth rate of all areas. Thus, the skills dependent on one brain area could correlate with those of another area even if they do not rely on an underlying general ability. For certain purposes we may find it convenient to talk about general intelligence, just as we talk about general athletic ability, but we should also remember that some people are intelligent in one way and not so much in another, just as people can excel in one athletic skill and not another.

Brain Size and Intelligence

People sometimes use the term *brainy* to mean intelligent. We tend to assume that bigger brains are better, but it is not that simple.

In the 1800s and early 1900s, several societies arose whose members agreed to donate their brains after death for research. No conclusion resulted. The brains of the eminent varied considerably, as did those of less eminent people. If brain anatomy were related to intellect in any way, the relation wasn't obvious (Burrell, 2004). Of course, achieving eminence depends also on opportunity, effort, and a bit of luck, not just intellectual ability. Still, the idea lingers: Even if brain size isn't strongly related to intelligence, shouldn't it have *some* relationship?

Comparing Species

All mammalian brains have the same organization, but they differ greatly in size. Does a larger brain mean greater intelligence? Long ago, Bernhard Rensch (1964) demonstrated that within a family of animals, the larger species, which have proportionately larger brains, learn faster and retain their learning better than smaller species. For example, larger rodents do better than smaller rodents, and larger species in the chicken family do better than smaller ones. However, this trend does not hold when we compare species from separate families. In particular, we humans like to think of ourselves as the most intelligent animals—after all, we get to define what intelligence means!—but whales and elephants have larger brains than we do.

Might intelligence depend on brain-to-body ratio? Figure 12.22 illustrates the relationship between logarithm of body mass and logarithm of brain mass for various vertebrates (Jerison, 1985). Note that the species we regard as most intelligent—such as, ahem, ourselves—have larger brains in proportion to body size than do the species we consider less impressive, such as frogs.

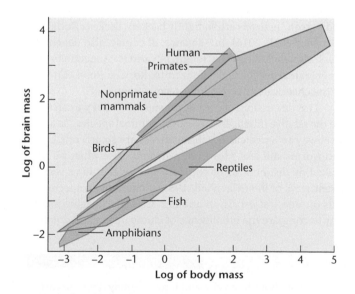

Figure 12.22 Relationship of brain mass to body mass across species
Each species is one point within one of the polygons. In general, log of body mass is a good predictor of log of brain mass. Primates in general and humans in particular have a large brain mass in proportion to body mass. *(Source: Adapted from Jerison, 1985)*

However, brain-to-body ratio has limitations also: Chihuahuas have the highest brain-to-body ratio of all dog breeds, not because they were bred for intelligence but because they were bred for small bodies (Deacon, 1997). Squirrel monkeys and marmosets have a higher brain-to-body ratio than humans. (And because of the increasing prevalence of human obesity, our brain-to-body ratio is declining!) The elephant-nose fish, which you might keep in an aquarium, has a 3 percent brain-to-body ratio compared to 2 percent for humans (Nilsson, 1999). The tiniest ants have a 15 percent brain-to-body ratio (Seid, Castillo, & Wcislo, 2011). So neither total brain mass nor brain-to-body ratio puts humans in first place.

However, humans do lead in one aspect, by a considerable margin: total number of neurons. Although whales and elephants have larger brains than humans, their neurons are larger and more spread out. Although marmosets have a greater brain-to-body ratio than humans, marmosets' bodies are much smaller, and therefore their brains and neuron number are smaller. As Figure 12.23 illustrates, humans do have the largest number of brain neurons (Herculano-Houzel, 2011a). In most animal families, the species with larger brains also have larger neurons, so that the ones with larger brains have only modestly larger numbers of neurons. In primates, however, the species with larger brains have the same size neurons as those with smaller brains, and so humans' neuron total is much elevated (Herculano-Houzel, 2012).

Thus, total number of neurons may be a reasonable correlate of intelligence. Further support for this idea comes from the observation that birds in the crow and parrot families, which have demonstrated impressive problem-solving skills, have as many neurons as a small monkey, because crows' and parrots' neurons are so tightly packed (Dicke & Roth, 2016; Olkowicz et al., 2016). Intelligence, of course, also depends on much else, including the strength of various connections in the brain (Santarnecchi, Galli, Polizzotto, Rossi, & Rossi, 2014) and all the chemicals affecting long-term potentiation.

This discussion, of course, presupposes that we can evaluate the relative intelligence of various animal species. At a gross level we can agree easily. Chimpanzees are smart, rats less so, and worms still less. However, problems arise when we try to make fine distinctions or compare species that have very different ways of life (Macphail, 1985). Sometimes a species that fails on one test excels on another. Can you imagine any fair way to compare the intelligence of chimpanzees and dolphins?

✔ STOP & CHECK ▬▬▬▬▬

22. Why are both brain size and brain-to-body ratio unsatisfactory ways of estimating animal intelligence?

ANSWER

22. If we consider ourselves to be the most intelligent species, we are confronted with the fact that we have neither the largest brains nor the highest brain-to-body ratios. Total neuron number is a more promising correlate of intelligence.

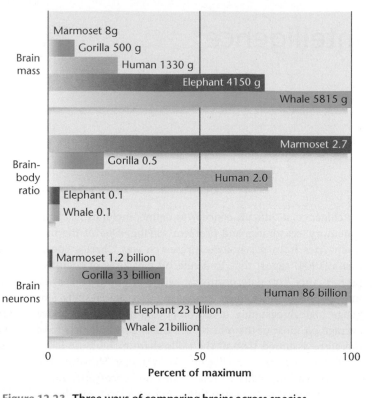

Figure 12.23 **Three ways of comparing brains across species**
Humans do not have the largest brain mass or the largest brain-to-body ratio, but we do have the largest number of brain neurons.
(*Source: Based on the best available estimates, from Herculano-Houzel, 2011a.*)

Human Data

For many years, studies of human brain size and intelligence found correlations barely above zero. However, a low correlation between two variables can mean either that they are unrelated, or that at least one of the variables was measured poorly. Most early studies measured skull size, but skull size does not correlate perfectly with brain size. (For one thing, some people are thick skulled!) Today, using more accurate measurements based on MRI, most studies find a moderate positive correlation between brain size and IQ score, averaging about 0.24 (Pietschnig, Penke, Wicherts, Zeiler, & Voracek, 2015).

Intelligence scores correlate especially with the surface area of cerebral cortex in the frontal and parietal cortex, but also with certain subcortical areas including the caudate nucleus (Basten, Hilger, & Fiebach, 2015; Colom et al., 2013; Fjell et al., 2015; Grazioplene et al., 2015; Gregory et al., 2016; Vuoksimaa et al., 2015). The surface area is the part of the brain dense with cell bodies, so this result fits with the idea that intelligence depends on the number of neurons. However, intelligence also correlates with the amount of white matter, so both neurons and the connections among neurons are important (Chiang et al., 2009; Myers et al., 2014; Narr et al., 2007; Ritchie et al., 2015; van Leeuwen et al., 2009).

So far, all this sounds reasonably clear, except for this problem: Men on average have about 10 percent larger brains than

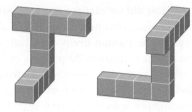

Can the set of blocks on the left be rotated to match the set at the right?

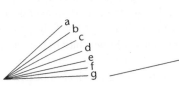

Which of the lines at the left has the same angle as the one at the right?

Figure 12.24 A spatial rotation task
People are presented with a series of pairs such as this one and asked whether the first figure could be rotated to match the second one. Here the answer is *no*. For the line-angle question, the correct answer is *e*.

women but equal IQs (Burgaleta et al., 2012; Gilmore et al., 2007; Willerman, Schultz, Rutledge, & Bigler, 1991; Witelson, Beresh, & Kigar, 2006). On average, women do somewhat better than men on certain aspects of language, including fluency, and on average men do somewhat better than women on certain spatial skills, including the items in Figure 12.24 (Jirout & Newcombe, 2015). Contrary to what many people believe, girls' grades in nearly all mathematics courses are at least as good as boys' grades from elementary school through college. Overall intelligence is equal for males and females (Hyde, Lindberg, Linn, Ellis, & Williams, 2008; Spelke, 2005).

How can we explain why men and women are equal in intellect, despite the fact that men have a larger brain? First, women average more and deeper sulci on the surface of the cortex, especially in the frontal and parietal areas (Luders et al., 2004). Consequently, the surface area of the cortex is almost equal for men and women, and therefore the number of neurons is also approximately equal (Allen, Damasio, Grabowski, Bruss, & Zhang, 2003).

Second, male and female brains are organized somewhat differently. On average, the parietal and occipital areas of the cortex are thicker in females than in males, whereas several other areas are thicker in males (Savic & Arver, 2014). Also, the pattern of connections differs between the sexes, on average, including stronger connections between the two hemispheres in females (Gong, He, & Evans, 2011; Tunc et al., 2016). Some of the anatomical differences probably relate to behavioral differences. For example, Broca's area, long associated with language production, tends to have more gray matter in female than male brains (Kurth, Jancke, & Luders, 2017). However, it is also likely that some of the brain differences have evolved to *prevent* behavioral differences! That is, female brains may be organized somewhat differently to produce the same intellectual abilities as the somewhat larger male brains (Grabowska, 2017).

The apparent link between intelligence and the number of neurons (or number of synapses, which correlates strongly) is theoretically interesting, but it takes us only so far. The correlation is certainly not high enough to justify using brain measurements to make any decisions about an individual. If you want to identify smart people, you attend to what people say and do, not their brain measurements, just as you would identify good athletes by watching their performance instead of measuring muscle size. Furthermore, a good understanding of either brain processes or psychological processes requires analysis of the more detailed ways in which each brain area contributes to specific aspects of behavior and experience.

✓ STOP & CHECK

23. Why do recent studies show a stronger relationship between brain size and IQ than older studies did?

24. How do researchers explain why males and females are equal in intelligence despite differences in brain size?

ANSWERS

23. The use of MRI greatly improves the measurement of brain size, in comparison to measurements based on the skull. **24.** Women's brains, having deeper sulci, include approximately the same number of neurons as men's brains. Also, women's brains have different patterns of connections.

Genetics and Intelligence

As with almost any important psychological variable, variations in intelligence reflect contributions from both genetic and environmental influences. Evidence for a genetic effect includes the observation that monozygotic twins resemble each other more strongly than do dizygotic twins on tests of overall intelligence, specific cognitive abilities, and brain volume (Bishop et al., 2003; Haworth et al., 2010; McGue & Bouchard, 1998; Posthuma et al., 2002). Monozygotic twins resemble each other even if they are reared in separate homes (Bouchard & McGue, 1981; Farber, 1981).

Heritability increases as people grow older, presumably because high-performing people gravitate toward educational opportunities and challenging activities that facilitate whatever genetic predispositions were present (Haworth et al., 2010; Lyons et al., 2009; Tucker-Drob & Bates, 2016). For example, the scores for monozygotic twins become more and more alike. Also, although the IQ scores of adopted children correlate moderately with those of their adoptive parents and adoptive siblings, as they grow older, the correlation with their adoptive relatives generally decreases while the correlation with their biological parents increases (Loehlin, Horn, & Willerman, 1989; Plomin, Fulker, Corley, & DeFries, 1997; Segal, McGuire, & Stohs, 2012). Nevertheless, even in young adulthood, some influence from the adoptive parents is demonstrable (Kendler, Turkheimer, Ohlsson, Sundquist, & Sundquist, 2015).

Heritability of intellectual performance is lower, however, for people who grow up in impoverished conditions and children who attend lower-quality schools (Bates, Lewis, & Weiss, 2013; Schwartz, 2015). Evidently genetic variations influence how well someone can take advantage of opportunities, but if the opportunities are sparse, a genetic advantage goes to waste.

A great many genes that are widely expressed throughout the brain contribute to intelligence. Many of these genes are described as "intolerant of variation" (M. R. Johnson et al., 2016). That is, they are the same in almost everyone, and a mutation in any of these genes leads to intellectual disabilities (Ganna et al., 2016; Gilissen et al., 2014; Lelieveld et al., 2016). For people within the normal range of intelligence, researchers have identified dozens of gene variations that correlate with measures of intelligence or academic success, but no common variant has a large effect by itself (Belsky et al., 2016; Davies et al., 2015; Okbay et al., 2016; Plomin et al., 2013). The same pattern holds for so much of psychology: Significant heritability, contributions from many genes, but no common gene with a major effect.

STOP & CHECK

25. The conclusion that genetic variation contributes to variations in human intelligence comes mainly from what type of evidence?

ANSWER

25. It is based largely on comparisons of monozygotic and dizygotic twins. Also, certain genetic mutations are known to produce intellectual disabilities, and many genetic variations are correlated with small variations of intelligence within the normal population.

Brain Evolution

Except for the specializations related to language, human brains are organized the same way as those of other mammals, especially other primates. We have the same types of neurons, the same neurotransmitters, the same types of synapses, approximately the same ratio of neurons to glia cells, the same ratio of cortex to cerebellum, and so forth (Harris & Shepherd, 2015; Herculano-Houzel, 2012). Nearly all the differences between humans and other species are quantitative. Just a few genetic differences between humans and other primates are enough to cause more rapid and more prolonged production of neurons during embryological development, leading to a larger cerebral cortex and a larger number of neurons (Bakken et al., 2016; Herculano-Houzel, 2012; Pennisi, 2015).

How did we manage to evolve such a large brain, whereas other species did not? The brain is a metabolically expensive organ. The human brain constitutes 2 percent of the body's mass, but consumes 20 percent of its fuel. The liver and digestive tract also consume a disproportionate amount of fuel. Reproduction also requires a great deal of energy. When researchers selectively bred guppies (small fish) for larger brains, they found that these guppies had less energy available for other organs and functions. In particular, the guppies produced fewer offspring than average (Kotrschal et al., 2013). In a world where most baby fish get eaten, sacrificing babies for big brains would be a bad bet, evolutionarily.

For our remote ancestors to evolve such large brains, they needed to get a great deal of nutrition, but they also needed to reduce the energy spent on other functions. Our upright walking is efficient and saves energy (Pontzer et al., 2016). At some point in our early evolutionary history, our ancestors learned to cook their food, making it easier to digest. Thus, they could evolve a smaller digestive tract than other primates, using less energy. Also, our early ancestors hunted in groups, bringing back more food than one person alone could find, and often they ate seafood, rich in nutrition. Furthermore, humans differ from chimpanzees in two genes responsible for glucose transport: We have more of the protein that transports glucose into the brain, and less of the protein that transports it into the muscles (Fedrigo et al., 2011). Thus, we devote more energy to our brains and less to physical strength. Hunting in groups and making tools for weapons made it possible to get food without using such big muscles.

Our remote ancestors also decreased the energy required for reproduction. Compared to most species, women bear fewer offspring over a lifetime, but devote enough care to increase the probability of survival. Also, human life span is unusually long, compensating for the lower frequency of births. A further essential is cooperation. Humans are inclined to cooperate. Even young children spontaneously learn to take turns, unlike chimpanzees (Melis, Grocke, Kalbitz, & Tomasello, 2016). Persisting male-female bonds, family groups, and food sharing within a community greatly reduced the burden on each mother and made it less demanding to raise an infant (Fletcher, Simpson, Campbell, & Overall, 2015; Isler & van Schaik, 2009).

STOP & CHECK

26. Why were our ancient ancestors able to evolve larger numbers of neurons than other species?

ANSWER

26. Because of cooking, cooperative breeding, and upright locomotion, they were able to decrease the energy necessary for other organs and functions.

Module 12.4 | **In Closing**

Why Are We So Intelligent?

Humans are like other mammals in many ways, but we are also unusual. We cook our food, we share food, we cooperate for raising children, and we evolved big brains. All those adaptations had to happen together. The big brains were important for cooking, sharing, and raising children. Cooking, sharing, and cooperatively raising children were essential for evolving big brains. The humans of today are the product of an amazing and very special evolutionary history.

Summary

1. Although several other species have larger brains or a larger brain-to-body ratio, the human brain has more neurons than any other species. **415**

2. Among humans, intelligence has a moderate correlation with brain size, especially with the surface area of certain parts of the cerebral cortex. **416**

3. Men and women are equal on average in their IQ scores, despite men having a larger brain. Because women have deeper sulci in the cortex, women and men have approximately the same number of neurons. **417**

4. Men's and women's brains are organized somewhat differently, either to produce differences in behavior or perhaps to prevent them. **417**

5. Both heredity and environment contribute to variations in human intelligence. **417**

6. Many genes are necessary for normal intelligence, and a mutation in any of them can lead to intellectual deficits. Within the normal range of human intelligence, many genes exert small effects. **418**

7. Ancient humans were able to evolve a larger brain and more neurons because they needed less energy than other species for locomotion, digestion, and reproduction. **418**

Key Term

Terms are defined in the module on the page number indicated. They're also presented in alphabetical order with definitions in the book's Subject Index/Glossary, which begins on page 589. Interactive flash cards, audio reviews, and crossword puzzles are among the online resources available to help you learn these terms and the concepts they represent.

g **415**

Thought Question

If we discover that another planet has intelligent life, what kind of message could we send that they might understand?

Module 12.4 | **End of Module Quiz**

1. In what way, if any, does the human brain exceed those of all other species?
   A. Humans have a larger number of neurons.
   B. Humans have the largest brain-to-body ratio.
   C. Humans have the largest brain volume.
   D. Humans do not exceed all other species in any regard.

2. Of the following, which correlates most strongly with intelligence?
   A. The ratio of excitatory to inhibitory synapses
   B. The ratio of neurons to glia cells
   C. The surface area of the cerebral cortex
   D. The strength of connections between the cerebral cortex and the cerebellum

3. In which way are men's and women's brains most similar?
   A. Total volume
   B. Number of neurons
   C. Depth of sulci in the cerebral cortex
   D. Amount of white matter

4. What happens to the heritability of intelligence, as people grow older?

   A. It decreases.
   B. It increases.

   C. It remains constant.
   D. It increases until puberty and then decreases.

5. The heritability of intelligence appears to be lowest under which of these conditions?

   A. A middle-class environment
   B. An impoverished environment

   C. An all-male population
   D. An all-female population

6. When researchers selectively bred guppies for large brains, which of these occurred?

   A. The guppies developed richer social behaviors.
   B. The guppies decreased their appetite.

   C. The guppies decreased their reproduction.
   D. The guppies increased their activity levels.

7. Which of these enabled humans to evolve a larger brain?

   A. Evolving a larger digestive tract
   B. Increased overall activity levels

   C. A vegetarian diet
   D. Learning to cook food

Answers: 1A, 2C, 3B, 4B, 5B, 6C, 7D.

Suggestions for Further Reading

Corkin, S. (2013). *Permanent present tense.* New York: Basic Books. Thorough account of the life of amnesia patient Henry Molaison and psychologists' research on his memory.

Eichenbaum, H. (2002). *The cognitive neuroscience of memory.* New York: Oxford University Press. Thoughtful treatment of both the behavioral and physiological aspects of memory.

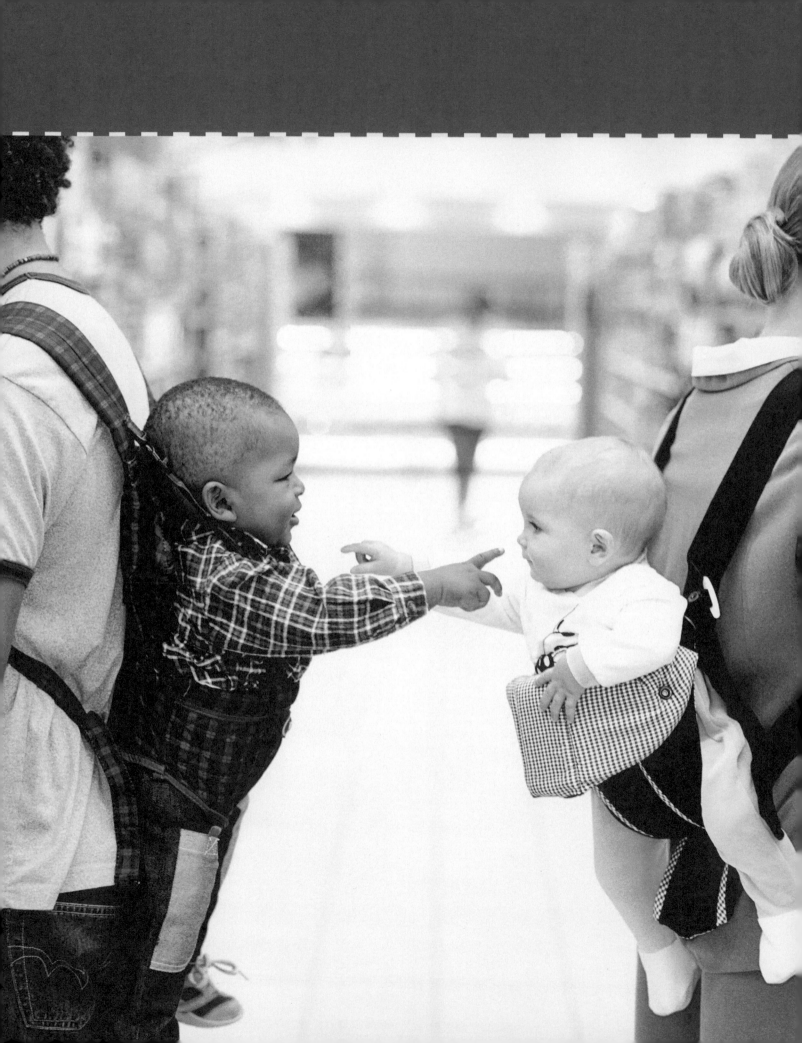

Cognitive Functions

Chapter 13

Research on the biology of vision, hearing, movement, and memory makes steady progress, because researchers can measure the stimuli and behaviors reasonably well. Language, attention, thinking, and decision making are harder to measure, and therefore harder to study. Nevertheless, many of the results are fascinating. After damage to the corpus callosum, which connects the two hemispheres, people act as if they have two fields of awareness—separate "minds," you might say. With damage to certain areas of the left hemisphere, people lose their language abilities, while remaining unimpaired in other ways. Researchers can now identify brain reactions that differ depending on whether someone is or is not conscious of a stimulus. Certain types of brain damage interfere with making good decisions or empathizing with others. We cannot yet explain cognition in much detail, but progress is occurring in areas previously regarded as unapproachable.

Learning Objectives

After studying this chapter, you should be able to:

1. Identify the primary functions of the left and right hemispheres.
2. Describe the behavioral results from split-brain surgery.
3. Describe the attempts to teach language to nonhumans.
4. Explain why increased overall intelligence does not explain how humans evolved language.
5. Contrast Broca's aphasia with Wernicke's aphasia.
6. Discuss the biological basis for dyslexia.
7. Explain why nearly all neuroscientists and philosophers favor some version of monism with regard to the mind–brain relationship.
8. Describe what brain activities differentiate between conscious and unconscious processing, and the types of research leading to these conclusions.
9. Describe research on the brain mechanisms of making decisions.
10. List some key findings about biological influences on social behavior.

Opposite:
Language may have evolved from our tendency to make gestures.
(Daly & Newton/Getty Images)

Lateralization and Language

Symmetry is common in nature. The sun, stars, and planets are nearly symmetrical, as are most animals and plants. When an atom undergoes radioactive decay, it emits identical rays in exactly opposite directions. However, the human brain is asymmetrical. The left hemisphere has somewhat different functions from the right hemisphere. Why? Presumably, assigning different functions to the two hemispheres provides some advantage. This module explores the distinctions between hemispheres, and then progresses to what we know about the biology of language.

The Left and Right Hemispheres

The left hemisphere of the cerebral cortex connects to skin receptors and muscles mainly on the right side of the body, and the right hemisphere connects to skin receptors and muscles mainly on the left side. The exception is that both hemispheres control the trunk muscles and facial muscles. The left hemisphere sees only the right half of the world, and the right hemisphere sees only the left half of the world. Each hemisphere gets auditory information from both ears but slightly stronger information from the contralateral ear. *Why* did brains evolve so that each hemisphere controls the contralateral side of the body? No one knows. Taste and smell, however, are uncrossed. Each hemisphere gets taste information from both sides of the tongue (Stevenson, Miller, & McGrillen, 2013) and smell information from the nostril on its own side (Herz, McCall, & Cahill, 1999; Homewood & Stevenson, 2001).

According to fMRI data and other methods, the left hemisphere is dominant for speech production in more than 95 percent of right-handers and nearly 80 percent of left-handers (McKeever, Seitz, Krutsch, & Van Eys, 1995). Some strongly left-handed people have right-hemisphere dominance for speech, but most left-handers have either left-hemisphere control or a mixture of left- and right-hemisphere control (Flowers & Hudson, 2013). Although the right hemisphere does not produce speech, it can understand meaningful sentences (Huth, de Heer, Griffiths, Theunissen, & Gallant, 2016). The right hemisphere has other functions, as we shall see later. Division of labor between the two hemispheres is called **lateralization**.

The left and right hemispheres exchange information through a set of axons called the **corpus callosum** and through the anterior commissure, the hippocampal commissure, and a couple of other small commissures (see Figure 13.1; see also Figures 3.10 and 3.13). If you had no corpus callosum,

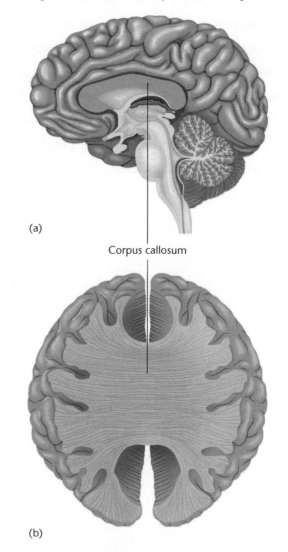

(a)

Corpus callosum

(b)

Figure 13.1 **Two views of the corpus callosum**
The corpus callosum is a large set of axons conveying information between the two hemispheres. **(a)** A sagittal section through the human brain. **(b)** A dissection (viewed from above) in which gray matter has been removed to expose the corpus callosum.

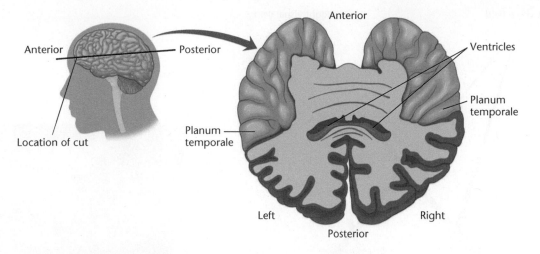

Figure 13.2 Horizontal section through a human brain
This cut, just above the surface of the temporal lobe, shows the planum temporale, an area critical for speech comprehension. It is larger in the left hemisphere than in the right hemisphere.
(Source: From "Human brain: Left-right asymmetries in temporal speech region," by N. Geschwind and W. Levitsky, 1968, Science, 161, pp. 186–187. Copyright © 1968 by AAAS and N. Geschwind. Reprinted with permission.)

your left hemisphere could react only to information from the right side of your body, and your right hemisphere could react only to information from the left. Because of the corpus callosum, however, each hemisphere receives information from both sides. Only after damage to the corpus callosum (or to one hemisphere) do we see clear evidence of lateralization.

Anatomical Differences between the Hemispheres

Norman Geschwind and Walter Levitsky (1968) found that one section of the temporal cortex, the **planum temporale** (PLAY-num tem-poh-RAH-lee), is larger in the left hemisphere for 65 percent of people (see Figure 13.2). Sandra Witelson and Wazir Pallie (1973) examined the brains of infants who died before age 3 months and found that the left planum temporale was larger in 12 of 14. Later researchers demonstrated differences even in preterm infants (Hervé, Zago, Petit, Mazoyer, & Tzourio-Mazoyer, 2013). An fMRI study showed that even 2-month-old children activate the left hemisphere more than the right when they listen to speech, though not when they listen to music (Dehaene-Lambertz et al., 2010). So the hemispheres differ from the start.

Smaller but still significant differences are found between left and right hemispheres of chimpanzees, bonobos, and gorillas (Hopkins, 2006). Many primates also show a preference for using either their right or left hand, as most humans do (Hopkins, Misiura, Pope, & Latash, 2015). Evidently, the specialization we see in the human brain built upon specializations already present in our apelike ancestors of long ago.

Visual and Auditory Connections to the Hemispheres

Before we discuss lateralization in more detail, let's consider the sensory connections to the brain. The hemispheres connect to the eyes such that each hemisphere sees the opposite half of the visual world. In rabbits and other species with eyes far to the side of the head, the left eye connects to the right hemisphere, and the right eye connects to the left. Human eyes are not connected to the brain in this way. Both of your eyes face forward, and both see both halves of the world.

In humans, each hemisphere is connected to half of each eye, as Figure 13.3 illustrates. Light from the right half of the **visual field** (what is visible at any moment) strikes the left half of each retina, which connects to the left hemisphere, which therefore sees the right visual field. Similarly, the left visual field strikes the right half of each retina, which connects to the right hemisphere. A small vertical strip down the center of each retina, covering about 5 degrees of visual arc, connects to both hemispheres (Innocenti, 1980; Lavidor & Walsh, 2004). In Figure 13.3, note how half of the axons from each eye cross to the opposite side of the brain at the **optic chiasm** (literally, the "optic cross").

> **Right visual field ⇒ left half of each retina ⇒ left hemisphere**
> **Left visual field ⇒ right half of each retina ⇒ right hemisphere**

The auditory system is organized differently. Each ear sends the information to both sides of the brain, because any brain area that contributes to localizing sounds must compare input from both ears. However, each hemisphere does pay more attention to the ear on the opposite side (Hugdahl, 1996).

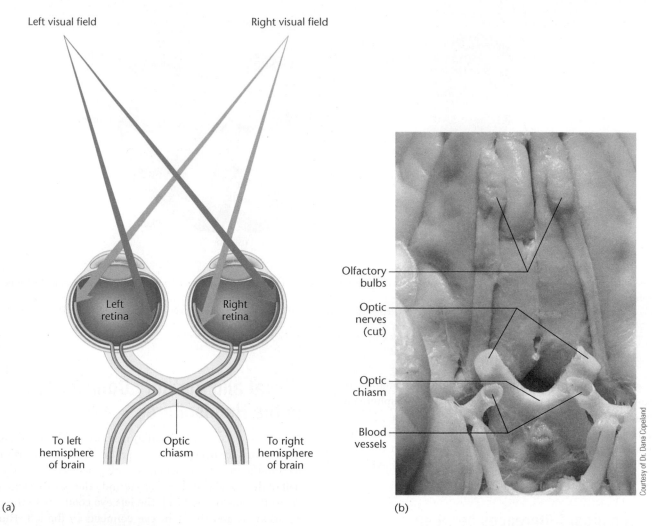

Figure 13.3 Connections from the eyes to the human brain
(a) The left hemisphere connects to the left half of each retina and thus gets visual input from the right half of the world. The opposite is true of the right hemisphere. **(b)** At the optic chiasm, axons from the right half of the left retina cross to the right hemisphere, and axons from the left half of the right retina cross to the left hemisphere.

STOP & CHECK

1. The left hemisphere of the brain is connected to the right eye in guinea pigs. In humans, the left hemisphere is connected to the left half of each retina. Explain the reason for this species difference.

2. In humans, the right half of each retina receives visual information from which side of the world and sends its output to which hemisphere?

ANSWERS

1. In guinea pigs, the right eye is far to the side of the head and sees only the right visual field. In humans, the eyes point straight ahead and half of each eye sees the right visual field. **2.** The right half of each retina receives input from the left half of the world and sends output to the right hemisphere, enabling the right hemisphere to see the left half of the world.

The Corpus Callosum and the Split-Brain Operation

Damage to the corpus callosum prevents the hemispheres from exchanging information. Occasionally, surgeons have severed the corpus callosum as a treatment for severe epilepsy, a condition characterized by repeated episodes of excessive synchronized neural activity. More than 90 percent of patients with epilepsy respond well to anti-epileptic drugs. However, if someone continues having frequent, severe seizures despite medication, physicians consider surgically removing the *focus,* the point in the brain where the seizures begin. The location of the focus varies from one person to another.

Removing the focus is not an option if someone has several foci, or if the focus is in an area considered essential for language. Therefore, in certain cases surgeons considered cutting the corpus callosum to prevent epileptic seizures from crossing from one hemisphere to the other. One benefit was that, as predicted, the person's epileptic seizures affected only half the body. (The abnormal activity could not cross the corpus callosum, so it remained within one hemisphere.) A surprising bonus was that the seizures became less frequent. Evidently, epileptic activity rebounds back and forth between the hemispheres and prolongs a seizure. If it cannot bounce back and forth across the corpus callosum, a seizure may not develop at all. Although this surgery helped a fair number of patients, it has become obsolete, as other procedures have taken its place.

How does severing the corpus callosum affect other aspects of behavior? People who have undergone surgery to the corpus callosum, referred to as **split-brain people**, maintain their intellect and motivation, they walk and talk normally, and they use their hands together on familiar tasks such as tying shoes. However, they struggle to use the hands together on tasks that they have not previously practiced (Franz, Waldie, & Smith, 2000).

Split-brain people can use the two hands independently in ways that other people cannot. For example, try drawing ∪ with your left hand while simultaneously drawing ⊃ with your right hand. Most people find this task difficult, but split-brain people do it with ease. Or try drawing circles with both hands simultaneously, but one of them just a little faster than the other (not twice as fast). Most people find this task difficult; split-brain people spontaneously draw the circles at different speeds (Kennerley, Diedrichsen, Hazeltine, Semjen, & Ivry, 2002).

Research by Roger Sperry and his students revealed behavioral effects when stimuli were limited to one side of the body (Nebes, 1974). In a typical experiment, a split-brain person stared straight ahead as the experimenter flashed words or pictures on one side of a screen, too briefly for the person to move the eyes (see Figure 13.4). Information going to one hemisphere could not cross to the other, because of the damage to the corpus callosum. The person could point with the left hand to what the right hemisphere saw, could point with the right hand to what the left hemisphere saw, and could talk about anything the left hemisphere saw. However, when the right hemisphere saw something, the person would point to it with the left hand, while saying,

"I don't know what it was. I didn't see anything." The talking left hemisphere did not know what the right hemisphere had seen.

Occasional exceptions arise to this rule. Because a small amount of information travels between the hemispheres through several smaller commissures, as shown in Figure 13.5, some split-brain people get enough information to give a partial description of what the right hemisphere saw (Berlucchi, Mangun, & Gazzaniga, 1997; Forster & Corballis, 2000).

Because the corpus callosum develops slowly, certain behaviors of young children resemble those of split-brain adults. In one study, 3- and 5-year-old children were asked to feel two fabrics, either with one hand at two times or with two hands at the same time, and say whether the materials felt the same or different. The 5-year-olds did equally well with one hand or with two. The 3-year-olds made 90 percent more errors with two hands than with one (Galin, Johnstone, Nakell, & Herron, 1979). The likely interpretation is that the corpus callosum matures sufficiently between ages 3 and 5 to facilitate the comparison of stimuli between the two hands.

Rarely, a child fails to develop a corpus callosum. One consequence is that both hemispheres are active during speech (Hinkley et al., 2016). Evidently, at birth both hemispheres are capable of developing speech, but ordinarily the left hemisphere inhibits the development of speech by the right hemisphere. If the corpus callosum is damaged, this inhibition cannot occur.

STOP & CHECK

3. What can a split-brain person do that other people cannot do?
4. Can a split-brain person name an object after feeling it with the right hand? With the left hand? Explain.

ANSWERS

3. A split-brain person can draw different things with their two hands at the same time, or move the hands at different speeds. 4. A split-brain person can describe something after feeling it with the right hand but not with the left. The right hand sends its information to the left hemisphere, which is dominant for language in most people. The left hand sends its information to the right hemisphere, which cannot speak.

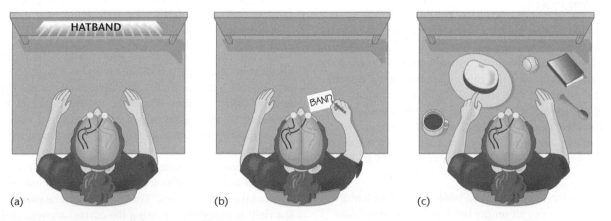

Figure 13.4 Effects of damage to the corpus callosum
(a) When the word *hatband* is flashed on a screen, **(b)** a woman with a split brain can report only what her left hemisphere saw, "band." **(c)** However, with her left hand, she can point to a hat, which is what the right hemisphere saw.

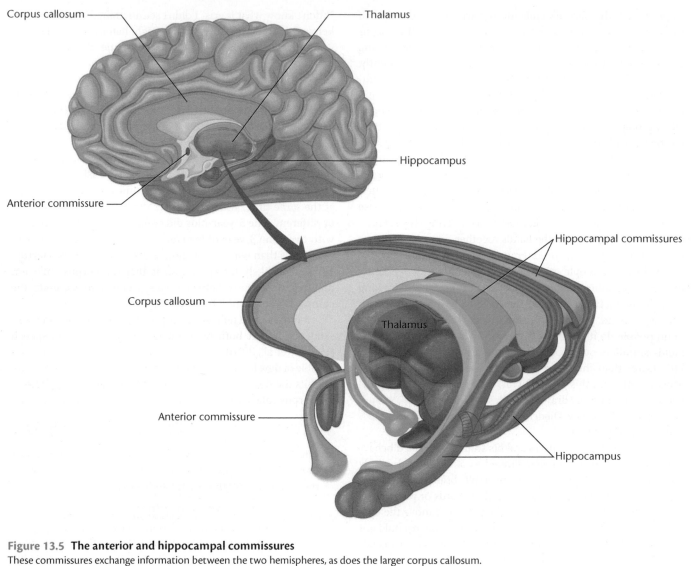

Figure 13.5 The anterior and hippocampal commissures
These commissures exchange information between the two hemispheres, as does the larger corpus callosum.
(*Source: Based on Nieuwenhuys, Voogd, & vanHuijzen, 1988, and others*)

Split Hemispheres: Competition and Cooperation

In the first weeks after split-brain surgery, the hemispheres act like separate people sharing one body. One split-brain person repeatedly took items from the grocery shelf with one hand and returned them with the other (Reuter-Lorenz & Miller, 1998). She explained, "I'd reach with my right for the thing I wanted, but the left would come in and they'd kind of fight." She had similar problems when she tried to get dressed, as each hand picked out different clothes and tried to put them on (Wolman, 2012). Another person—that is, his left hemisphere—described his experience as follows:

> If I'm reading, I can hold the book in my right hand; it's a lot easier to sit on my left hand, than to hold it with both hands. . . . You tell your hand—I'm going to turn so many pages in a book—turn three pages—then somehow the left hand will pick up two pages and you're at page 5, or whatever. It's better to let it go, pick it up with the right hand, and then turn to the right page. With your right hand, you correct what the left has done. (Dimond, 1979, p. 211)

Such conflicts become rare as time passes. The corpus callosum does not heal, but the brain learns to use the smaller connections between the left and right hemispheres (Myers & Sperry, 1985). In some situations, the hemispheres learn to cooperate. A split-brain person who was tested with the apparatus shown in Figure 13.4 used an interesting strategy to answer a yes–no question about what he saw in the left visual field. Suppose an experimenter flashes a picture in the left visual field and asks, "Was it green?" The left (speaking) hemisphere takes a guess: "Yes." That guess might be correct. If not, the right hemisphere, knowing the correct answer, makes the face frown. (Both hemispheres control facial muscles on both sides of the face.) The left hemisphere, feeling the frown, says, "Oh, I'm sorry, I meant 'no.'"

When the right hemisphere does something, the left hemisphere doesn't know why. So far as the left hemisphere is concerned, the true cause of the behavior was unconscious. How does it react? Rather than acting surprised, it invents an explanation. For example, if the right hemisphere sees something pleasant or unpleasant, the left hemisphere feels the change of mood and might say, "What a beautiful wall that is!" or "Right now you are making me sad." In one study, experimenters flashed different pictures to the two hemispheres and asked the person to point to pictures associated with what he or she saw. In one case, the left hemisphere saw a chicken claw and the right hemisphere saw a snow scene. The right hand then pointed to a picture of a chicken and the left hand pointed to a shovel. When asked to explain why he pointed at a shovel, he replied that you would need a shovel to clean out the chicken shed. From observations like these, Michael Gazzaniga (2000) proposed the concept of the **interpreter**, the tendency of the left hemisphere to invent and defend explanations for actions, even when the true causes are unconscious. This feature is not limited to split-brain people. We all think we know why we are doing something, when in fact we might be wrong.

The Right Hemisphere

After researchers discovered the importance of the left hemisphere for speech, they at first imagined the right hemisphere as something like a vice president, helping in a subordinate role but doing little unless the other hemisphere was damaged. Gradually observations showed that the right hemisphere has important functions of its own.

The right hemisphere is more adept than the left at comprehending spatial relationships. For example, one young woman with damage to her posterior right hemisphere had trouble finding her way around, even in familiar areas. To reach a destination, she needed directions with specific visual details, such as, "Walk to the corner where you see a building with a statue in front of it. Then turn left and go to the corner that has a flagpole and turn right. . . ." (Clarke, Assal, & deTribolet, 1993). Curiously, people who have right-hemisphere dominance for speech have left-hemisphere dominance for spatial relationships (Cai, Van der Haegen, & Brysbaert, 2013).

The right hemisphere is more responsive to emotional stimuli than the left, such as perceiving the emotions in people's gestures and tone of voice (Adolphs, Damasio, & Tranel, 2002). People with damage to the right hemisphere usually fail to understand humor and sarcasm (Beeman & Chiarello, 1998; H. J. Rosen et al., 2002).

In one fascinating study, people watched videotapes of 10 people. All 10 described themselves honestly during one speech and dishonestly during another. The task of the observers was to guess which of the two interviews was the honest one. The task is more difficult than you might guess, and most people are no more correct than chance. The group that performed best was people with left-hemisphere brain damage (Etcoff, Ekman, Magee, & Frank, 2000). They got only 60 percent correct—not great, but at least better than chance.

People with an intact left hemisphere relied on the left hemisphere's analysis of what people were saying. Those with left-hemisphere damage relied on the right hemisphere's more intuitive reactions to emotional expressions.

In another study, 11 patients went through a procedure in which one hemisphere at a time was anesthetized by drug injection into one of the carotid arteries, which provide blood to the head. (This procedure, called the Wada procedure, is sometimes used before certain kinds of brain surgery.) When they were tested with the right hemisphere inactivated, something fascinating happened: They could still describe any of the sad, frightening, or irritating events they had experienced in life, but they remembered only the facts, not the emotion. One patient remembered a car wreck, another remembered visiting his mother while she was dying, and another remembered a time his wife threatened to kill him. But they denied they had felt any significant fear, sadness, or anger. When they described the same events with both hemispheres active, they remembered strong emotions. So evidently, when the right hemisphere is inactive, people do not experience strong emotions and do not even remember feeling them (Ross, Homan, & Buck, 1994).

STOP & CHECK

5. Which hemisphere is dominant for the following in most people: speech, emotional inflection of speech, interpreting other people's emotional expressions, spatial relationships?

ANSWER 5. The left hemisphere is dominant for speech. The right hemisphere is dominant for the other items listed.

Avoiding Overstatements

The research on left-brain/right-brain differences is exciting, but has sometimes led to unscientific assertions. Occasionally, you may hear a person say something like, "I don't do well in science because it is a left-brain subject and I am a right-brain person." That kind of statement is based on two reasonable premises and a doubtful one. The scientific ideas are that (1) the hemispheres are specialized for different functions, and (2) certain tasks evoke greater activity in one hemisphere or the other. The doubtful premise is that any individual habitually relies mostly on one hemisphere.

What evidence do you suppose someone has for believing, "I am a right-brain person"? Did he or she undergo an MRI or PET scan to determine which hemisphere was larger or more active? Not likely. Generally, when people say, "I am right-brained," their only evidence is that they perform well on creative tasks or poorly on logical tasks. (Saying, "I am right-brained" sometimes implies that *because* I do poorly on logical tasks, *therefore,* I am creative. Unfortunately, illogical is not the same as creative.) In fact, most tasks, especially difficult ones, require cooperation by both hemispheres.

Evolution of Language

During your childhood, you heard, watched, and read many stories about animals—the three pigs, the three bears, various Disney and Warner Brothers cartoons, and others. In nearly all of them, the animals talked, right? In real life, *why don't they?*

Nonhuman animals do communicate through visual, auditory, tactile, or chemical displays, but those signals don't have much flexibility. A monkey might have one alarm call to indicate eagle in the air and another for snake on the ground, but it has no way to indicate eagle on the ground or snake in the tree (Cheney & Seyfarth, 2005). Human language stands out from other forms of communication because of its **productivity**, its ability to improvise new combinations of signals to represent new ideas.

We probably didn't evolve language out of nothing. Evolution almost always develops something by modifying a previous structure. Bat wings are modified arms, porcupine quills are modified hairs, and skunk stench is modified sweat gland secretion. If our language evolved from some ability our ancient apelike ancestors had, what was it?

Chimpanzees

Several early attempts to teach chimpanzees to talk failed. One reason is that humans vocalize while breathing out, whereas chimpanzees vocalize while breathing in. Go ahead, try to say something while inhaling. You'll probably want to try it in private so that other people don't laugh at you.

However, chimps in the wild do communicate with gestures, and investigators achieved better results by teaching them American Sign Language or other visual systems (Gardner & Gardner, 1975; Premack & Premack, 1972) (see Figure 13.6). In

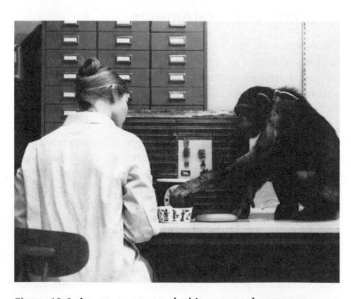

Figure 13.6 An attempt to teach chimpanzees language
One of the Premacks' chimps, Elizabeth, reacts to colored plastic chips that read "Not Elizabeth banana insert—Elizabeth apple wash."
(Source: Photo courtesy of Ann Premack)

one version, chimps learned to press keys bearing symbols to type messages on a computer (Rumbaugh, 1977), such as "Please machine give apple" or to another chimpanzee, "Please share your chocolate."

The chimpanzees' use of symbols differed from human language in several ways. They seldom used symbols in new, original combinations. That is, their symbol use was short on *productivity*. Also, they used symbols mainly to request, seldom to describe. However, they showed at least moderate understanding. For example, the chimp Washoe, trained in sign language, usually answered "Who" questions with names, "What" questions with objects, and "Where" questions with places, even when she used the wrong symbol for a name, object, or place (Van Cantfort, Gardner, & Gardner, 1989).

Bonobos

Amid skepticism about chimpanzee language, more promising results emerged from studies of a closely related species, *Pan paniscus,* known as the bonobo. Bonobos' social order resembles humans' in several regards. Males and females form strong, sometimes lasting, personal attachments. They often copulate face to face. The female is sexually responsive on almost any day and not just during her fertile period. The males contribute significantly to infant care. Adults often share food. They stand comfortably on their hind legs. In short, they resemble humans more than other primates do.

In the mid-1980s, Sue Savage-Rumbaugh, Duane Rumbaugh, and their associates tried to teach a female bonobo named Matata to press symbols that lit when touched. Each symbol represents a word (see Figure 13.7). Although Matata made little progress, her infant son Kanzi learned just by watching her. When given a chance to use the symbol board, he quickly excelled. Later, researchers noticed that Kanzi understood a fair amount of spoken language. For example, whenever anyone said the word *light,* Kanzi would flip the light switch. Kanzi and his younger sister, Mulika, developed language comprehension comparable to that of a typical 2- to 2½-year-old child:

- They understand more than they can produce.
- They follow unfamiliar, unlikely directions such as "Throw your ball in the river" or "Get the tomato in the microwave."
- They use symbols to name and describe objects even when they are not requesting them.
- They occasionally use the symbols to describe past events. Kanzi once pressed the symbols "Matata bite" to explain the cut that he had received on his hand an hour earlier.
- They frequently make original, creative requests, such as asking one person to chase another. (Hillix, Rumbaugh, & Savage-Rumbaugh, 2012; Savage-Rumbaugh, 1990; Savage-Rumbaugh, Sevcik, Brakke, & Rumbaugh, 1992; Savage-Rumbaugh et al., 1993)

Why have Kanzi and Mulika developed more impressive skills than other chimpanzees? Perhaps bonobos have more language potential than common chimpanzees. A second

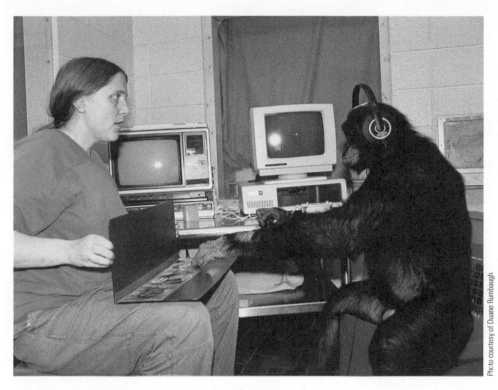

Figure 13.7 Language tests for Kanzi, a bonobo (*Pan paniscus*)
He listens to questions through earphones and points to answers on a board. The experimenter with him does not hear the questions.
(*Source: From Georgia State University's Language Research Center, operated with the Yerkes Primate Center of Emory.*)

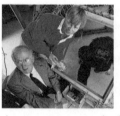

Duane Rumbaugh, Sue Savage-Rumbaugh, and chimpanzee Austin

Chimpanzees and bonobos are outstanding teachers of psychology. They never presume that we, as their students, know a damn thing about who they are. And they certainly aren't impressed with our degrees. Consequently, they are able to teach all manner of important things about what it means to be human and to be ape—that is, if we as students are quiet, listen carefully, and let them tell us as only they can.

explanation is that Kanzi and Mulika began language training when young. A third reason pertains to the method of training: Learning by observation and imitation (as humans do) promotes better language understanding than the formal training methods of previous studies (Savage-Rumbaugh et al., 1992).

✅ **STOP & CHECK** ▬▬▬▬▬

6. What are three likely explanations for why bonobos made more language progress than common chimpanzees?

ANSWER

6. Bonobos may be more predisposed to language than common chimpanzees. The bonobos started training at an earlier age. They learned by imitation instead of formal training techniques.

Nonprimates

What about nonprimate species? Spectacular results have been reported for Alex, an African gray parrot (see Figure 13.8). Parrots are, of course, famous for imitating sounds. Irene Pepperberg showed that parrots can use sounds meaningfully. She kept Alex in a stimulating environment and taught him by saying a word many times and offering rewards if Alex approximated the same sound. Gradually she moved on to more complex concepts (Pepperberg, 1981). Pepperberg generally used toys. For example, if Alex said "paper," "wood," or "key," she would give him what he asked for. In no case did she reward him with food for saying "paper" or "wood."

In one test, Alex viewed a tray of 12 objects and correctly answered 39 of 48 questions such as "What color is the key?" (answer: "green") and "What object is gray?" (answer: "circle"). He also answered questions of the form "How many blue keys?" in which he had to count the blue keys among objects of two shapes and two colors (Pepperberg, 1994).

It will not come as news to dog owners that dogs learn to respond to many human words. The extent of this possibility, however, goes beyond what most people, and certainly most scientists, expected. One border collie learned the names of over a thousand objects and remembered them over at least 32 months. She also learned categories such as "toy," which meant anything she had been allowed to play with. She also responded correctly to sentences requiring an understanding of simple grammar. For example, she responded correctly to the commands "to ball take Frisbee" and "to Frisbee take ball," even when other objects were present (Pilley, 2013). Another study found that part of dogs' left hemisphere responds to meaningful words, regardless of the tone of voice, whereas the right hemisphere responds to the intonation, which often indicates emotion (Andics et al., 2016). Those results match the pattern for human brains. If you do a YouTube search for "Chaser language," you can watch several videos.

What do we learn from studies of nonhuman language abilities? At a practical level, we gain insights into how best to teach language to those who do not learn it easily, such as people with brain damage or children with autism. At a more theoretical level, these studies indicate that human language evolved from precursors present in other species. These studies also point out the ambiguity of our concept: As psychologists have debated whether chimpanzees, parrots, or dogs are

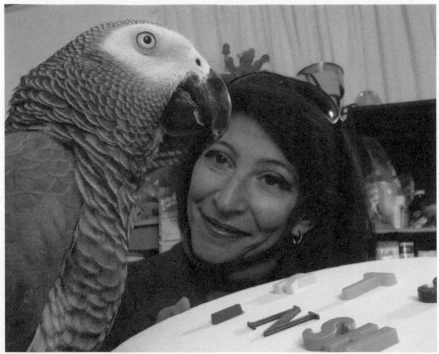

Figure 13.8 Language tests for Alex
Alex conversed about objects in simple English—for example, answering, "What color is the circle?" He received no food rewards.

showing language, they have been forced to think more carefully about how they define language.

How Did Humans Evolve Language?

Reconstructing the evolution of language is necessarily speculative, because no examination of fossils will help. One strong possibility is that language evolved from communication by gestures (Corballis, 2012a). All primates communicate by gestures, including humans. Children begin gesturing in the first year of life, and their use of gestures predicts how soon they will develop spoken language (Iverson & Goldin-Meadow, 2005). Most adults also accompany their speech with gestures, even when talking on a telephone, when the listener cannot see the gestures.

Mouth gestures may be particularly important. Monkeys use several mouth gestures to communicate, including a lip-smacking gesture, which has a rhythm similar to speech. Monkeys are known to watch one another's mouth movements, especially when another is vocalizing, and it is plausible that the combination of sound plus mouth gesture could have been a precursor to spoken language (Ghazanfar, 2013).

With regard to the brain, what changed to make language possible? Most theories fall into two categories: (1) We evolved it as a by-product of overall brain development, or (2) we evolved it as a specialization.

Is Language a By-Product of Intelligence?

One view is that humans evolved big brains for other reasons, and language developed as an accidental by-product. In its simplest form, this hypothesis faces several problems. First, if language is just a product of brain size, then anyone with a full-sized brain and normal overall intelligence should have normal language. However, not all do. In one family, 16 of 30 people over three generations show serious language deficits despite normal intelligence in other regards. Because of a particular dominant gene, the affected people have serious troubles in pronunciation and many other aspects of language (Fisher, Vargha-Khadem, Watkins, Monaco, & Pembrey, 1998; Gopnik & Crago, 1991; Lai, Fisher, Hurst, Vargha-Khadem, & Monaco, 2001). They have trouble with even simple grammatical rules, as shown in the following dialogue about making plurals:

Experimenter	Respondent
This is a wug; these are . . .	How should I know? *[Later]* These are wug.
This is a zat; these are . . .	These are zacko.
This is a sas; these are . . .	These are sasss. *[Not sasses]*

In another test, experimenters presented sentences and asked whether each sentence was correct and, if not, how to improve it. People in the affected family made many errors and odd corrections. For example:

Original Item	Attempted Correction
The boy eats three cookie.	The boys eat four cookie.

Despite the language difficulties, these people behave normally and intelligently in other regards. Evidently, language requires more than just a large brain and overall intelligence.

What about the reverse? Could someone with overall intellectual impairment have good language? Psychologists would have answered "no," until they discovered **Williams syndrome**,

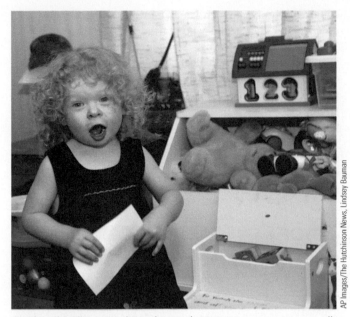

People with Williams syndrome have a characteristic appearance, as well as a special set of behavioral strengths and weaknesses.

a condition affecting about 1 person in 20,000, traceable to the loss of a gene that influences connections in the brain (Chailangkarn et al., 2016). Affected people are poor at tasks related to numbers, visuomotor skills (e.g., copying a drawing), and spatial perception (e.g., finding their way home). When asked to estimate the length of a bus, three people with Williams syndrome answered "30 inches," "3 inches or 100 inches maybe," and "2 inches, 10 feet" (Bellugi, Lichtenberger, Jones, Lai, & St. George, 2000). They show poor planning, frequent lapses of attention, and difficulty inhibiting inappropriate responses (Greer, Riby, Hamiliton, & Riby, 2013). They require supervision and have trouble with even simple jobs. Nevertheless, many of them speak grammatically and fluently. Many also show good ability to clap a complex rhythm and memorize songs (Levitin & Bellugi, 1998), and good ability to interpret facial expressions of emotion (Tager-Flusberg, Boshart, & Baron-Cohen, 1998).

In contrast to their impairments in other regards, many people with Williams syndrome develop remarkably good language. Figure 13.9 shows the result when a young woman was asked to draw an elephant and describe it. Contrast her almost poetic description to the unrecognizable drawing.

Let's not overstate the case. People with Williams syndrome do not handle language perfectly (Martens, Wilson, & Reutens, 2008; Meyer-Lindenberg, Mervis, & Berman, 2006). Their grammar is awkward, like that of someone who learned a second language late in life (Clahsen & Almazen, 1998; Karmiloff-Smith et al., 1998). They often use fancy words when a common word would work better, such as "I have to evacuate the glass" instead of "empty" or "pour out" the glass (Bellugi et al., 2000). Still, observations of Williams syndrome indicate that language is not simply a by-product of overall intelligence.

Language as a Specialization

If language is not just a by-product of overall intelligence, it must have evolved as a specialized brain mechanism. Noam Chomsky (1980) and Steven Pinker (1994) proposed that humans have a **language acquisition device**, a built-in mechanism for acquiring language. Most children develop language so quickly and easily that it seems they must have been biologically prepared for this learning. Deaf children quickly learn sign language, and if no one teaches them a sign language, they invent one and teach it to one another (Goldin-Meadow, McNeill, & Singleton, 1996; Goldin-Meadow & Mylander, 1998).

Researchers have begun to explore the genetic basis of this preparation for language. Remember that family whose members have such trouble with pronunciation and basic grammar? Their problem stems from a mutation in a gene designated *FOXP2*, which regulates a protein that promotes synapse formation in the cerebral cortex and the basal ganglia (Chen et al., 2016; Lai et al., 2001). Although both humans and chimpanzees have that gene, it differs in two places, resulting in proteins with different amino acids at two sites. The gene produces a multitude of effects, partly on brain development, but also on structures of the jaw and throat that are important for speech (Konopka et al., 2009). Another human specialization is that the part of our motor cortex that controls the vocal cords has much greater connections to the rest of the cortex than monkeys have (Kumar, Croxson, & Simonyan, 2016). The greater connections enable more complex and detailed control of sound production.

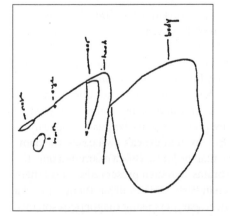

And what an elephant is, it is one of the animals. And what the elephant does, it lives in the jungle. It can also live in the zoo. And what it has, it has long gray ears, fan ears, ears that can blow in the wind. It has a long trunk that can pick up grass, or pick up hay . . . If they're in a bad mood it can be terrible . . . If the elephant gets mad it could stomp; it could charge, like a bull can charge. They have long big tusks. They can damage a car . . . it could be dangerous. When they're in a pinch, when they're in a bad mood it can be terrible. You don't want an elephant as a pet. You want a cat or a dog or a bird . . .

Figure 13.9 A young woman with Williams syndrome draws and describes an elephant
The investigator added the labels on the drawing based on what the woman said she was drawing.
(*Source: From "Williams syndrome: An unusual neuropsychological profile," by U. Bellugi, P. O. Wang, and T. L. Jernigan. In S. H. Broman and J. Grafman, Eds.,* Atypical Cognitive Deficits in Developmental Disorders. *Copyright © 1994 Lawrence Erlbaum. Reprinted by permission.*)

Why did humans evolve language and other species did not? One speculation is that language relates to the long period of dependency in childhood. Social interactions among people, including those between parents and children, favored the evolution of language. In that case, overall intelligence may be a by-product of language development more than language is a by-product of intelligence (Deacon, 1992, 1997).

STOP & CHECK

7. What evidence argues against the hypothesis that language evolution depended simply on the overall evolution of brain and intelligence?

8. List tasks that people with Williams syndrome do poorly and those that they do well.

ANSWERS

7. Some people have normal brain size but very poor language. Also, some people have intellectual disabilities but nevertheless develop nearly normal language. **8.** Poor: self-care skills, attention, planning, numbers, visual-motor skills, and spatial perception. Relatively good: language, interpretation of facial expressions, some aspects of music.

A Sensitive Period for Language Learning

If humans are specially adapted to learn language, perhaps we are adapted to learn best during a sensitive period early in life, just as sparrows learn their song best during an early period. The consistent result is that adults are better than children at memorizing the vocabulary of a second language, but children have a great advantage on mastering grammar and especially pronunciation (Huang, 2014; Saito, 2013). There is no sharp cutoff for learning a second language; starting at age 2 is better than 4, 4 is better than 6, and 13 is better than 16 (Hakuta, Bialystok, & Wiley, 2003; Harley & Wang, 1997; Weber-Fox & Neville, 1996). However, people who start learning a second language beyond age 12 or so almost never reach the level of a native speaker (Abrahamsson & Hyltenstam, 2009). Also, learning a second language from the start is different from learning one later. Many people guess that a bilingual person might rely on the left hemisphere for one language and the right hemisphere for the other. That guess is wrong. People who grow up in a bilingual home, speaking two languages from the start, show bilateral activity during speech for both languages, and stronger than average connections between the two hemispheres (Berken, Chai, Chen, Gracco, & Klein, 2016; Peng & Wang, 2011). People who learn a second language after about age 6 activate just the left hemisphere for both languages (Hull & Vaid, 2007; Peng & Wang, 2011).

Another way to test the sensitive-period idea is to study people who learned no language during early childhood. In some cases, hearing parents of deaf children concentrated unsuccessfully on teaching them spoken language and lip-reading, and eventually gave up and introduced sign language. Children who began sign language while still young learned much better than those who started later (Harley & Wang, 1997). A child who learns a spoken language early can learn sign language later, and a deaf child who learns sign language early can learn a spoken language later (except, of course, with poor pronunciation), but a child who learns no language while young is permanently impaired at learning any kind of language (Mayberry, Lock, & Kazmi, 2002). Even deaf children whose exposure to language is delayed for the first year of life show lasting deficits (Friedmann & Rusou, 2015). This observation strongly supports the importance of learning language in early childhood.

STOP & CHECK

9. What is the strongest evidence in favor of a sensitive period for language learning?

ANSWER

9. Deaf children who did not learn either spoken language or sign language while young do not become proficient at either type of language later.

Brain Damage and Language

Another way to study specializations for language is to examine the role of various brain areas. Much of our knowledge has come from studies of people with brain damage.

Broca's Aphasia (Nonfluent Aphasia)

In 1861, the French surgeon Paul Broca treated the gangrene of a patient who had been mute for 30 years. When the man died 5 days later, Broca did an autopsy and found a lesion in the left frontal cortex. Over the next few years, Broca examined the brains of additional patients with **aphasia** (language impairment), and nearly always found damage that included this same area, which is now known as **Broca's area** (see Figures 13.10 and 13.11). When brain damage impairs language production, we call it **Broca's aphasia**, or **nonfluent aphasia**, regardless of the exact location of damage. Broca published his results in 1865, slightly later than reports by other French physicians, Marc and Gustave Dax, who also pointed to the left hemisphere as the seat of language abilities (Finger & Roe, 1996). Broca received the credit, however, because his description was more detailed and more convincing. This discovery, the first demonstration of the function of a particular brain area, paved the way for modern neurology.

Modern methods have confirmed the importance of Broca's area for language production, but damage limited to that area produces only minor or brief language impairment (Long et al., 2016). In fact, even in Broca's own cases, the damage was more extensive than he knew. Broca examined only the external surface of the brains, and then preserved some of them at the Musée Dupuytren in Paris, which still has them. Almost a century and a half later, researchers using magnetic resonance

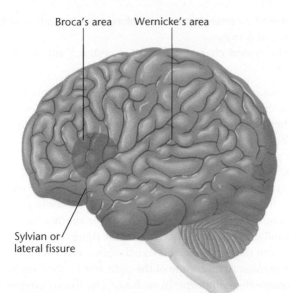

Broca's area Wernicke's area

Sylvian or
lateral fissure

Figure 13.10 Two areas important for language

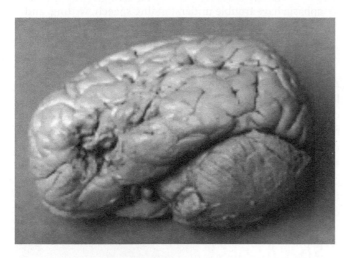

Figure 13.11 The brain of the first patient examined by Broca
Damage in the left frontal cortex is apparent. MRI has revealed that the
damage also extends deep into subcortical areas.

imaging showed that the original cases of Broca's aphasia had
damage extending deeper into the brain, including much of the
basal ganglia (Dronkers, Plaisant, Iba-Zizen, & Cabanis, 2007).
Today we recognize that Broca's aphasia relates to damage in
parts of the cortex, thalamus, and basal ganglia.

Impaired Language Production

People with Broca's aphasia are slow and awkward with all
forms of language communication, including speaking, writing, gesturing, and using sign language (Cicone, Wapner, Foldi,
Zurif, & Gardner, 1979; Neville et al., 1998; Petitto et al., 2000).
Broca's aphasia relates to language, not the vocal muscles. When
you read a word aloud, looking at the word activates your visual

system, which then exchanges information with Broca's area,
which then exchanges information with your motor cortex.
While you say the word, your motor cortex controls the output,
and Broca's area remains silent. That is, Broca's area helps to
organize speech, but it doesn't produce it (Flinker et al., 2015).

When people with Broca's aphasia speak, their speech is
meaningful but sparse. For example, they might say, "Weather
overcast" instead of "The weather is overcast." Although the
results vary among individuals, they generally omit pronouns,
prepositions, conjunctions, auxiliary (helping) verbs, quantifi-
ers, and tense and number endings. At least, that is the pattern
for people speaking English. German- or Italian-speaking people with aphasia use more word endings, because they are more
essential to the meaning than they are in English (Blackwell &
Bates, 1995). Prepositions, conjunctions, helping verbs, and so
forth are known as the *closed class* of grammatical forms because a language rarely adds new prepositions, conjunctions,
and the like. In contrast, new nouns and verbs (the *open class*)
enter a language frequently. People with Broca's aphasia seldom
use the closed-class words. They find it difficult or impossible
to repeat a phrase such as "No ifs, ands, or buts." However,
patients who cannot read aloud "To be or not to be" can read
"Two bee oar knot two bee" (Gardner & Zurif, 1975). The trouble pertains to the word meanings, not just pronunciation.

Why do people with Broca's aphasia omit the grammatical words and endings? Perhaps they have suffered damage to
a "grammar area" in the brain, but here is another possibility: When speaking is a struggle, people leave out the weakest
elements. Many people who are in pain speak as if they have
Broca's aphasia (Dick et al., 2001).

Problems in Comprehending Grammatical Words and Devices

People with Broca's aphasia understand most speech, except
when the meaning depends on prepositions, word endings,
or complex grammar—the same items that they omit when
speaking. If they hear a sentence with complex grammar, such
as "The girl that the boy is chasing is tall," they know that
someone is tall and someone is chasing, but they don't know
which is which (Zurif, 1980). Most English sentences are comprehensible even if we omit the prepositions and conjunctions.
You can demonstrate this for yourself by taking a paragraph
and deleting its prepositions, conjunctions, articles, helping
verbs, pronouns, and word endings to see how it might appear
to someone with Broca's aphasia. Here is an example, taken
from earlier in this section. Note how understandable it is despite the deletions:

> In 1861, the French surgeon Paul Broca treated
> the gangrene of a patient who had been mute for
> 30 years. When the man died 5 days later, Broca did
> an autopsy and found a lesion in the left frontal cor-
> tex. Over the next few years, Broca examined the
> brains of additional patients with aphasia (language
> impairment). In nearly all cases, he found damage
> (usually stroke-related) that included this same area,
> which is now known as Broca's area.

Still, people with Broca's aphasia have not totally lost their knowledge of grammar. For example, they generally recognize that something is wrong with the sentence "He written has songs," even if they cannot say how to improve it (Wulfeck & Bates, 1991). In many ways, their comprehension resembles that of intact people who are distracted. If you listen to someone speaking rapidly with a heavy accent in a noisy room, while you are trying to do something else at the same time, you catch bits and pieces of what the speaker says and try to guess the rest. Even when we hear a sentence clearly, we sometimes ignore the grammar. If you hear "The dog was bitten by the man," or "the ball kicked the girl," you might ignore the grammar and assume the dog bit the man and the girl kicked the ball (Ferreira, Bailey, & Ferraro, 2002). Patients with Broca's aphasia just rely on logical guesses more often than others do.

✓ STOP & CHECK

10. What kind of words are Broca's patients least likely to use?
11. What kind of words do Broca's patients have the most trouble understanding?

ANSWERS

10. They have the greatest trouble with "closed-class" words that are meaningful only in the context of a sentence, such as prepositions, conjunctions, and helping verbs. 11. They have the most trouble understanding the same kind of words they have trouble producing—the closed-class words.

Wernicke's Aphasia (Fluent Aphasia)

In 1874, Carl Wernicke (pronounced WER-nih-kee by most English speakers, although the German pronunciation is VAYR-nih-keh), a 26-year-old junior assistant in a German hospital, discovered that damage in part of the left temporal cortex produced a different kind of language impairment. Although patients could speak and write, their language comprehension was poor. Damage in and around **Wernicke's area** (see Figure 13.10), located near the auditory cortex, produces **Wernicke's aphasia,** characterized by poor language comprehension and impaired ability to remember the names of objects. It is also known as **fluent aphasia** because the person can still speak smoothly. As with Broca's aphasia, the symptoms and brain damage vary, and the damage generally extends beyond the cortex into the thalamus and basal ganglia. We use the term *Wernicke's aphasia,* or *fluent aphasia,*

to describe a certain pattern of behavior, independent of the location of damage.

The typical characteristics of Wernicke's aphasia are as follows:

1. *Articulate speech.* In contrast to people with Broca's aphasia, those with Wernicke's aphasia speak fluently, except when pausing to try to think of the name of something. They have no trouble with prepositions, conjunctions, or grammar.
2. *Difficulty finding the right word.* People with Wernicke's aphasia have **anomia** (ay-NOME-ee-uh), difficulty recalling the names of objects. They make up names (e.g., "thingamajig"), substitute one name for another, and use roundabout expressions such as "the thing that we used to do with the thing that was like the other one." When they do manage to find some of the right words, they might arrange them improperly, such as, "The Astros listened to the radio tonight" (instead of "I listened to the Astros on the radio tonight") (R. C. Martin & Blossom-Stach, 1986).
3. *Poor language comprehension.* People with Wernicke's aphasia have trouble understanding speech, writing, and sign language (Petitto et al., 2000). Impaired comprehension relates closely to difficulty remembering the names of objects.

Although Wernicke's area and surrounding areas are important, language comprehension also depends on the connections to other brain areas. For example, reading the word *lick* activates not only Wernicke's area but also the part of the motor cortex responsible for tongue movements. Reading *throw* activates the part of the premotor cortex controlling hand movements (Willems, Hagoort, & Casasanto, 2010). Apparently when you think about an action word, you imagine doing it. Table 13.1 contrasts Broca's aphasia and Wernicke's aphasia.

✓ STOP & CHECK

12. Describe the speech production of people with Wernicke's aphasia.
13. Describe the speech comprehension of people with Wernicke's aphasia.

ANSWERS

12. People with Wernicke's aphasia speak fluently and grammatically but omit most nouns and verbs and therefore make little sense. 13. People with Wernicke's aphasia have trouble understanding speech.

Table 13.1 | Broca's Aphasia and Wernicke's Aphasia

Type	Pronunciation	Content of Speech	Comprehension
Broca's aphasia	Poor	Mostly nouns and verbs; omits prepositions and other grammatical connectives	Okay unless the meaning depends on complex grammar
Wernicke's aphasia	Unimpaired	Grammatical but often nonsensical; has trouble finding the right word, especially names of objects	Seriously impaired

Dyslexia

Dyslexia is a specific impairment of reading in someone with adequate vision, motivation, cognitive skills, and educational opportunity. It is more common in boys than girls and linked to several identified genes (Field et al., 2013). Dyslexia is especially common in English, because it has so many words with odd spellings. (Consider *phlegm, bivouac, khaki, yacht, choir, physique,* and *gnat.*) However, dyslexia occurs in all languages and always pertains to a difficulty converting symbols into sounds (Ziegler & Goswami, 2005).

Many studies have reported abnormalities in the left hemisphere for people with dyslexia, and some of them appear very early in life, before children would be taught to read (Kraft et al., 2015; Raschle, Zuk, & Gaab, 2012; van Zuijen, Plakas, Maassen, Maurits, & van der Leij, 2013; Xia, Hoeft, Zhang, & Shu, 2016). One difference is that, unlike most normal readers, people with dyslexia have certain parts of the temporal cortex larger in the right hemisphere than in the left (Ma et al., 2015). You might wonder how anyone knew to test certain children before they were old enough to show symptoms of dyslexia. The researchers identified families that include several people with dyslexia, and then tested young children, expecting (correctly) that many of them would develop dyslexia later.

In the often confusing literature about dyslexia, one point that stands out is that different people have different kinds of reading problems, and no one explanation works for all. Most (but not all) have auditory problems, a smaller number have impaired control of eye movements, and some have both (Judge, Caravolas, & Knox, 2006). Some researchers distinguish between *dysphonetic dyslexia* and *dyseidetic dyslexia* (Flynn & Boder, 1991), although many people with dyslexia do not fit neatly into either category. People with dysphonetic dyslexia have trouble sounding out words, so they try to memorize each word as a whole, and when they don't recognize a word, they guess based on context. For example, they might read the word *laugh* as "funny." Readers with dyseidetic dyslexia sound out words well enough, but they fail to recognize a word as a whole. They read slowly and have trouble with irregularly spelled words.

Most but not all people with dyslexia have problems related to hearing, but not the kind of problem that could be corrected with hearing aids. People with dyslexia have no trouble carrying on a conversation, which would be difficult if their hearing were seriously impaired. In fact, even some good musicians have dyslexia. Tests found that they could easily detect small changes of pitch or tempo, but they had poor auditory memory. They had low accuracy at noting whether two sequences of tones, separated in time, were the same or different (Weiss, Granot, & Ahissar, 2014). That result suggests a problem with how the brain handles auditory information, not a problem with the auditory information itself. Other studies found that people with dyslexia have weaker than normal connections between the auditory cortex and Broca's area (Boets et al., 2013).

Many people with dyslexia have particular trouble detecting the temporal order of sounds, such as noticing the difference between beep-click-buzz and beep-buzz-click (Farmer & Klein, 1995; Kujala et al., 2000; Nagarajan et al., 1999). They also have difficulty making Spoonerisms—that is, trading the first consonants of two words, such as listening to "dear old queen" and saying "queer old dean" or hearing "way of life" and replying "lay of wife" (Paulesu et al., 1996). Doing so, of course, requires close attention to sounds and their order.

Many people with dyslexia also have abnormalities in their attention (Facoetti, Corradi, Ruffino, Gori, & Zorzi, 2010). Here is a demonstration. Fixate your eyes on the central dot in each display below and, without moving your eyes left or right, try to read the middle letter of each three-letter display:

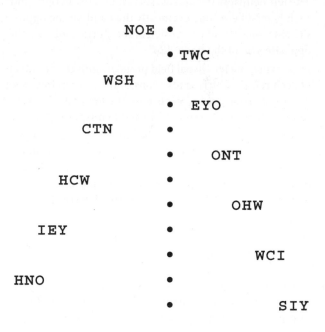

Most people find it easier to read the letters close to the fixation point, but some people with dyslexia are unusually adept at identifying letters well to the right of their fixation point. When they focus on a word, they are worse than average at reading it but better than average at perceiving letters 5 to 10 degrees to the right of it (Geiger, Lettvin, & Zegarra-Moran, 1992; Lorusso et al., 2004). That kind of attentional focus could certainly confuse attempts at reading (De Luca, Di Page, Judica, Spinelli, & Zoccolotti, 1999). In many cases, people with dyslexia also have difficulties when letters are too crowded together (Gori & Facoetti, 2015). In short, dyslexia can result from a variety of problems.

✓ STOP & CHECK

14. What evidence suggests that many of the brain abnormalities associated with dyslexia are a cause of the disorder rather than a result?

ANSWER

14. Certain abnormalities have been reported at an early age, before the start of language training.

Module 13.1 | In Closing

Language and the Brain

Many of the earliest home computers had no speech capacity, but users could plug in a device that would add speech, converting text output into sound. The evolution of human language was not like that. Our remote ancestors didn't just take a chimpanzee-type brain and add an independent module.

Language required widespread modifications throughout the brain and it made possible a great many additional changes in other functions. Trying to understand language is an important part of trying to understand what it means to be human.

Summary

1. The left hemisphere controls speech in most people, and each hemisphere controls mostly the hand on the opposite side, sees the opposite side of the world, and feels the opposite side of the body. **424**

2. In humans, the left visual field projects onto the right half of each retina, which sends axons to the right hemisphere. The right visual field projects onto the left half of each retina, which sends axons to the left hemisphere. **425**

3. After damage to the corpus callosum, each hemisphere can point or gesture to answer questions about the information that reaches it directly. However, because the left hemisphere controls speech in most people, only the left hemisphere of a split-brain person can give vocal answers about what it knows. **427**

4. Although the two hemispheres of a split-brain person are sometimes in conflict, they find ways to cooperate and cue each other. **428**

5. The right hemisphere is dominant for understanding and producing the emotional inflections of speech and for interpreting other people's emotional expressions. **429**

6. Bonobos have made significant progress in understanding language, and so have several other species to varying degrees. **430**

7. Evolution of language may have evolved from gestural communication in primates, and mouth gestures may have been especially important. **432**

8. The hypothesis that language emerged as a by-product of overall intelligence or brain size faces major problems: Some people have normal intelligence but impaired language, and many people with Williams syndrome have nearly normal language despite cognitive impairments. **432**

9. The best evidence for a sensitive period for language development is the observation that deaf children learn sign language much better if they start early than if their first opportunity comes later in life. Also, learning a second language in early childhood differs in many ways from learning it later. **434**

10. People with Broca's aphasia (nonfluent aphasia) have difficulty speaking and writing. They find prepositions, conjunctions, and other grammatical connectives especially difficult. They also fail to understand speech when its meaning depends on complex grammar. **434**

11. People with Wernicke's aphasia have trouble understanding speech and recalling the names of objects. **436**

12. Dyslexia (reading impairment) has many forms, resulting from diverse causes including impaired auditory memory and difficulties with visual attention. **437**

Key Terms

Terms are defined in the module on the page number indicated. They're also presented in alphabetical order with definitions in the book's Subject Index/Glossary, which begins on page 589. Interactive flash cards, audio reviews, and crossword puzzles are among the online resources available to help you learn these terms and the concepts they represent.

anomia **436**

aphasia **434**

Broca's aphasia (nonfluent aphasia) **434**

Broca's area **434**

corpus callosum **424**

dyslexia **437**

interpreter **429**

language acquisition device **433**

lateralization **424**

nonfluent aphasia **434**

optic chiasm **425**

planum temporale **425**

productivity **430**

split-brain people **427**

visual field **425**

Wernicke's aphasia (fluent aphasia) **436**

Wernicke's area **436**

Williams syndrome **432**

Thought Questions

1. Most people with Broca's aphasia suffer from partial paralysis on the right side of the body. Most people with Wernicke's aphasia do not. Why?
2. In a syndrome called *word blindness*, a person loses the ability to read (even single letters), although the person can still see and speak. What is a possible neurological explanation? That is, can you imagine a pattern of brain damage that might produce this result?

Module 13.1 | End of Module Quiz

1. In humans, what happens to visual information from the left visual field?

   A. It reaches the right half of each retina, which sends messages to the left hemisphere.

   B. It reaches the right half of each retina, which sends messages to the right hemisphere.

   C. It reaches the left half of each retina, which sends messages to the left hemisphere.

   D. It reaches the left half of each retina, which sends messages to the right hemisphere.

2. At the human optic chiasm, which axons cross to the opposite hemisphere?

   A. Those from the nasal (inside) half of each retina

   B. Those from the temporal (outside) half of each retina

   C. Those from the center of each retina

   D. All the axons from each retina

3. Under what condition can a split-brain person describe something he or she sees?

   A. After seeing it in the right visual field

   B. After seeing it in the left visual field

   C. After seeing it with the right eye

   D. After seeing it with the left eye

4. When the right hemisphere reacts to something it sees, causing a behavior that the left hemisphere can feel, how does the left hemisphere react?

   A. It expresses surprise.

   B. It pretends the action did not occur.

   C. It tries to stop the action or do the opposite.

   D. It invents a logical-sounding explanation.

5. Which of these does the right hemisphere control better than the left?

   A. Reactions to emotional stimuli

   B. Control of the right arm and hand

   C. Mathematical calculations

   D. Taste and smell

6. What is a likely explanation for bonobos' success at understanding speech?

   A. Bonobos' brains have larger neurons than most other primates.

   B. The experimenters combined both classical and operant conditioning.

   C. The bonobos spent much time with human children.

   D. The bonobos started young and learned by imitation.

7. If human language did not evolve from other primates' vocalizations, what else is a likely hypothesis?

   A. Language evolved from nothing at all.

   B. Language evolved from dancing.

   C. Language evolved from gestures including mouth gestures.

   D. Language evolved from the ability to perceive objects in three dimensions.

8. What is unusual about many people with Williams syndrome?

   A. Good language ability despite intellectual deficiencies

   B. Normal intelligence but poor language comprehension

   C. Good reading ability despite poor vision

   D. High intelligence during childhood but low during adulthood

9. The *FOXP* gene strongly affects what else, in addition to brain development?

   A. The stomach and intestines

   B. The pituitary and adrenal glands

   C. The jaw and throat

   D. Blood pressure and heart rate

10. If someone is bilingual from the start, how does the brain represent the two languages?

    A. One in the left hemisphere and the other in the right hemisphere

    B. Both in the left hemisphere

    C. Both in the right hemisphere

    D. Both in both hemispheres

11. People with Broca's aphasia are most impaired on producing and understanding which type of words?

    A. Common nouns

    B. Proper nouns

    C. Prepositions and conjunctions

    D. Adjectives and adverbs

12. Which of the following is characteristic of Wernicke's aphasia?

    A. Difficulty forming new long-term memories, especially episodic memories

    B. Inability to describe anything seen in the left visual field or felt with the left hand

    C. Poor pronunciation and difficulty using and understanding grammar

    D. Difficulty remembering names of objects

Answers: 1B, 2A, 3A, 4D, 5A, 6D, 7C, 8A, 9C, 10D, 11C, 12D.

Conscious and Unconscious Processes

[W]e know the meaning [of consciousness] so long as no one asks us to define it.

William James (1892/1961, p. 19)

The introduction to this book introduced the mind–body problem: In a universe composed of matter and energy, why is there such a thing as consciousness? And how does it relate to brain activity? Now armed with more understanding of the brain, it is time to return to those questions, even if the answers remain elusive.

The Mind–Brain Relationship

Suppose you say, "I became frightened because I saw a man with a gun." A neuroscientist says, "You became frightened because of increased electrochemical activity in the following areas of your brain. . . ." If both statements are right, what is the connection between them?

Biological explanations of behavior raise the **mind–body** or **mind–brain problem**: What is the relationship between the mind and the brain? Most nonscientists apparently assume **dualism**, the belief that mind and body exist separately. The French philosopher René Descartes defended dualism but recognized the vexing issue of how a mind that is not made of material could influence a physical brain. He proposed that mind and brain interact at a single point in space, which he suggested was the pineal gland, the smallest unpaired structure he could find in the brain (see Figure 13.12).

Although we credit Descartes with the first explicit defense of dualism, he hardly originated the idea. Our experiences seem so different from the physical actions of the brain that most people take it for granted that mind and brain must be different. Even outstanding psychologists sometimes lapse into dualistic thinking. One psychologist commented, "we know little about . . . whether neural events drive psychological events, or the converse" (G. A. Miller, 2010, p. 716). In other words, we don't know whether brain activity causes thoughts or whether thoughts cause brain activity. But if thoughts and brain activity are the same thing, the question doesn't make sense.

Nearly all current philosophers and neuroscientists reject dualism. A decisive objection is that dualism conflicts with one of the cornerstones of physics, known as the law of the conservation of matter and energy: Matter can transform into energy, and energy can transform into matter, but neither one emerges from nothing, disappears into nothing, or changes except because of influence from other matter or energy. Therefore, a mind that is not composed of matter or energy could not make anything happen, not even muscle movements. If you use a term like *mind* to mean a ghostlike something that is neither matter nor energy, don't underestimate the scientific and philosophical arguments that can be marshaled against you (Dennett, 1991).

The alternative to dualism is **monism**, the belief that the universe consists of only one kind of substance. Various forms of monism are possible in the following categories:

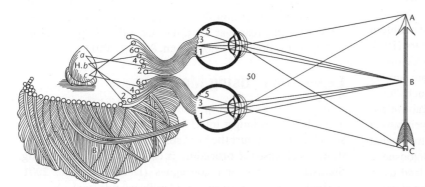

Figure 13.12 René Descartes's conception of brain and mind
Descartes understood how light from an object (the arrow) reached the retinas at the back of the eyes. The letters and numbers represent pathways that he imagined from the retinas to the pineal gland. (His guesses about those pathways were wrong.)
(Source: From Descartes's Treatise on Man)

- **materialism:** the view that everything that exists is material, or physical. According to one version of this view, "eliminative materialism," mental events don't exist at all, and any folk psychology that includes the concept of mind or mental activity is fundamentally mistaken. However, most of us find it difficult to believe that our minds are figments of our imagination. An alternative version of materialism is that researchers will eventually find a way to explain all psychological experiences in purely physical terms.
- **mentalism:** the view that only minds really exist and that the physical world could not exist unless some mind were aware of it. The philosopher George Berkeley was the primary defender of this position. It is not easy to test this idea. (Go ahead and try!)
- **identity position:** the view that mental processes and certain kinds of brain processes are the same thing, just described in different terms. By analogy, one could describe the *Mona Lisa* as an extraordinary painting, or one could list the exact color and brightness of each point on the painting. Although the two descriptions appear entirely different, they refer to the same item. The identity position says the mind is brain *activity*. Just as fire is not a "thing," but what happens to something, mental activity is what happens in the brain.

Can we be sure that monism is correct? No. However, researchers adopt it as the most reasonable working hypothesis, to see what progress they can make on that assumption. As you have seen throughout this text, experiences and brain activities appear inseparable. Stimulation of any brain area provokes an experience, and any experience evokes brain activity, and damage to any brain area leads to loss of some mental function. As far as we can tell, you cannot have mental activity without brain activity, and you cannot have certain types of brain activity without mental activity.

(Does a belief in monism mean that we are lowering our evaluation of minds? Maybe not. Maybe we are elevating our concept of the material world.)

David Chalmers (1995) distinguished between what he calls the easy problems and the hard problem of consciousness. The easy problems pertain to such questions as the difference between wakefulness and sleep and what brain activity occurs during consciousness. These issues are difficult scientifically but not philosophically. In contrast, the **hard problem** concerns why consciousness exists at all. As Chalmers (1995, p. 203) put it, "Why doesn't all this information-processing go on 'in the dark,' free of any inner feel?" Why does brain activity *feel* like anything at all? Many scientists (Crick & Koch, 2004) and philosophers (Chalmers, 2004) agree that we cannot answer that question, at least at present. We don't even have a clear hypothesis to test. The best we can do is determine what brain activity is necessary or sufficient for consciousness. Maybe research on such questions will some day lead us to an insight about the hard question, or maybe not. But starting with the "easy" questions seems the best strategy.

15. Why do nearly all scientists and philosophers reject the idea of dualism?

16. What is meant by the "hard problem"?

ANSWERS

15. Dualism contradicts the law of the conservation of matter and energy. According to that law, the only way to influence matter and energy, including that of your body, is to act on it with other matter and energy. **16.** The hard problem is why minds exist at all in a physical world. Why is there such a thing as consciousness?

Consciousness of a Stimulus

Although we don't have a good hypothesis about why consciousness exists at all, we might be able to answer some lesser questions about consciousness. The main research difficulty is that we cannot observe consciousness. Even defining it is difficult. For practical purposes, researchers use this operational definition: If a cooperative person reports awareness of one stimulus and not another, then he or she was **conscious** of the first and not the second. With individuals who cannot speak, including infants and nonhuman animals, this definition doesn't apply. Therefore, research on consciousness is limited to cooperative, healthy humans, ordinarily adults.

Using this definition, the next step is to present a given stimulus under two conditions, where we expect an observer to be conscious of it in one condition and not the other. Then researchers compare the brain responses in the two conditions. How could someone present a stimulus but prevent consciousness? Researchers have developed clever approaches based on interference. Suppose you clearly see a yellow dot. Then, although the dot remains on the screen, other dots around it flash on and off. While they are flashing, you do not see the stationary dot. This procedure is called **flash suppression** (Kreiman, Fried, & Koch, 2002). The strong response to the flashing stimulus decreases the response to the steady stimulus, as if it were a fainter light (Yuval-Greenberg & Heeger, 2013). Similarly, suppose you see a yellow dot, and then some blue dots all around it start moving rapidly. They grab your attention so strongly that you have trouble seeing the yellow dot. In fact, it seems to disappear for a few seconds, reappear for a few seconds, disappear again, and so forth (Bonneh, Cooperman, & Sagi, 2001).

Experiments Using Masking

Many studies use **masking**: A brief visual stimulus is preceded and followed by longer interfering stimuli. In many cases, researchers present just the brief stimulus and a longer one after it, in which case the procedure is called **backward masking**. Stanislas Dehaene and colleagues (Dehaene et al., 2001) flashed a word on a screen for 29 milliseconds (ms). On some trials, it was preceded and followed by a blank screen:

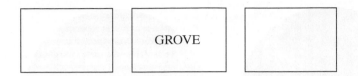

GROVE

In these cases, people identified the word almost 90 percent of the time. On other trials, the researchers flashed a word for the same 29 ms but preceded and followed it with masking patterns:

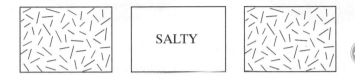

SALTY

In the masking condition, people almost never identified it. They usually said they saw no word at all. Using fMRI and evoked potentials, the researchers found that the stimulus initially activates the primary visual cortex in both the conscious and unconscious conditions but activates it more strongly in the conscious condition, because of less interference. Also, in the conscious condition, the activity spreads to additional brain areas, including the prefrontal cortex and parietal cortex, which amplify the signal and reflect it back to the visual cortex. For people with damage to the prefrontal cortex, a visual stimulus has to last longer before it becomes conscious, relative to other people (Del Cul, Dehaene, Reyes, Bravo, & Slachevsky, 2009).

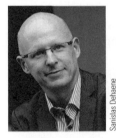

Stanislas Dehaene

Throughout the nineteenth and twentieth centuries, the question of consciousness lay outside the boundaries of normal science. . . . For many years, no serious researcher would touch the problem. . . . When I was a student in the late 1980s, I was surprised to discover that during lab meetings, we were not allowed to use the C-word. . . . And then in the late 1980s everything changed. Today the problem of consciousness is at the forefront of neuroscience research. (*Dehaene, 2014, pp. 7–8*)

A similar study found that the difference in response depending on whether a stimulus is or is not conscious becomes apparent 200 ms after onset of the stimulus, reaches maximum at 500 ms, and continues for the next 2 to 3 seconds. That study also found that consciousness of one stimulus inhibited responses to other stimuli at the same time (Q. Li, Hill, & He, 2014). That is, the stimuli present at any moment compete for your attention.

A conscious stimulus also synchronizes responses for neurons in various brain areas (Eckhorn et al., 1988; Gray, König, Engel, & Singer, 1989; Melloni et al., 2007; Womelsdorf et al., 2007). When you see something and recognize it, it evokes activity precisely synchronized in several brain areas, in the frequency of about 30 to 50 Hz (cycles per second), known as *gamma waves* (Doesburg, Green, McDonald, & Ward, 2009; Fisch et al., 2009). One consequence of synchronized action potentials is that their synaptic inputs arrive simultaneously at their target cells, producing maximal summation (Fell & Axmacher, 2011).

Overall, the data imply that consciousness of a stimulus depends on the amount and spread of brain activity. Becoming conscious of something means that its information takes over more of your brain's activity.

STOP & CHECK

17. In the experiment by Dehaene and colleagues, how were the conscious and unconscious stimuli similar? How were they different?
18. In this experiment, how did the brain's responses differ to the conscious and unconscious stimuli?

ANSWERS

17. The conscious and unconscious stimuli were physically the same (a word flashed on the screen for 29 ms). The difference was that a stimulus did not become conscious if it was preceded and followed by an interfering pattern. 18. A stimulus that reached consciousness activated the same brain areas as an unconscious stimulus but more strongly, and then the activity spread to additional areas. Also, brain responses became synchronized for a conscious pattern.

Experiments Using Binocular Rivalry

Here is another way to make a stimulus unconscious. Look at Figure 13.13, but hold it so close to your eyes that your nose touches the page, right between the two circles. Better yet, look at the two parts through a pair of tubes, such as the tubes inside rolls of paper towels or toilet paper, or roll up your hands like tubes. You should see red and black vertical stripes with your left eye, and green and black horizontal stripes with your right eye. (Close one eye and then the other to make sure your eyes see completely different patterns.) Seeing something requires perceiving *where* it is, and the red vertical stripes cannot be in the same place as the green horizontal stripes. Because your brain cannot perceive both patterns in the same location, your perception alternates between the two. For the average person, each perception lasts about 2 seconds before the other replaces it, although some people switch perceptions faster or slower. These shifts, demonstrating **binocular rivalry**, are gradual, sweeping from one side to another. You can voluntarily shift your attention to one or the other image, but only to a limited extent. Soon you see the other image anyway (Paffen & Alais, 2011). Instead of lines, the stimuli could be other images, such as a house versus a face.

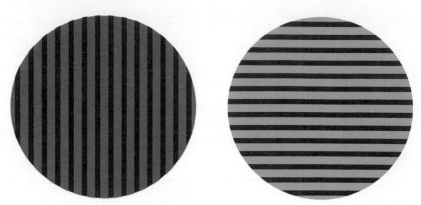

Figure 13.13 Binocular rivalry
If possible, look at the two circles through tubes, such as those from inside rolls of toilet paper or paper towels. Otherwise, touch your nose to the paper between the two parts so that your left eye sees one pattern while your right eye sees the other. The two views will compete for your consciousness, and your perception will alternate between them.

The two images do not necessarily divide your attention time equally. Some people see with one eye longer than the other. Also, an emotionally charged image, such as a face with an emotional expression, generally holds attention longer than a neutral image (Yoon, Hong, Joormann, & Kang, 2009). A happy face holds attention longer for someone in a happy mood, and a scowling face holds attention longer for someone in a sad mood (Anderson, Siegel, & Barrett, 2011; Anderson et al., 2013).

The stimulus seen by each eye evokes a brain response that researchers can measure. As the first perception fades and the stimulus seen by the other eye replaces it, the first pattern of brain activity fades also, and a different pattern replaces it. Both the red–black and green–black patterns you just experienced were stationary. To make the brain responses easier to distinguish, researchers presented to one eye a stationary stimulus and to the other eye a pattern that pulsated in size and brightness, as shown in Figure 13.14. Then they recorded brain activity in several areas. At times when people reported consciousness of the pulsating stimulus, pulsating activity at the same rhythm was prominent in much of

the brain, as shown in Figure 13.15. When people reported consciousness of the stationary stimulus, the pulsating activity was weak (Cosmelli et al., 2004). Again, the conclusion is that a conscious stimulus strongly activates much of the brain, virtually taking over brain activity. When the same stimulus is unconscious, it produces weaker and less widespread activity. A related study found that when someone switched between one perception and the other, the brain response changed first in the occipital cortex, and then spread to the other areas (de Jong et al., 2016).

The Fate of an Unattended Stimulus

Let's further consider binocular rivalry. While you are attending to, say, the green and black stripes, your brain does not completely discard information from the other eye. Certainly, if a bright stimulus suddenly flashed in that eye, it would capture your attention. More interestingly, suppose a word fades onto the screen slowly, and you are to report the time when your attention shifts to the previously unattended eye. The word captures your attention, causing you to shift your

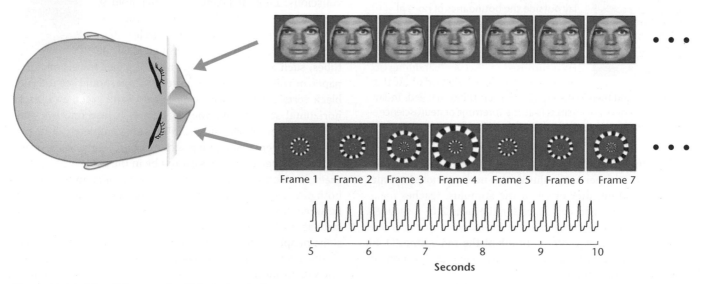

Figure 13.14 Stimuli for a study of binocular rivalry
The pattern in one eye was stationary. The one in the other eye pulsated a few times per second. Researchers could then examine brain activity to find cells that followed the rhythm of the pulsating stimulus.
(Source: Reprinted from "Waves of consciousness: Ongoing cortical patterns during binocular rivalry," by D. Cosmelli et al., 2004, NeuroImage, 23(1), pp. 128–140, with permission from Elsevier.)

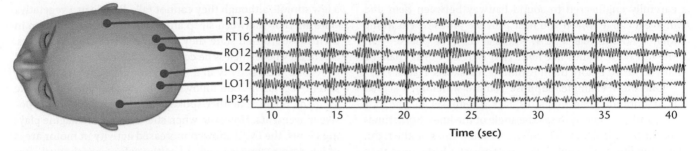

Figure 13.15 Brain activity during binocular rivalry
When the person reported seeing the pulsating stimulus, neurons throughout much of the brain responded vigorously at the same rhythm as the stimulus. When the person reported the stationary stimulus, the rhythmic activity subsided.
(Source: Reprinted from "Waves of consciousness: Ongoing cortical patterns during binocular rivalry," by D. Cosmelli et al., 2004, NeuroImage, 23(1), pp. 128–140, with permission from Elsevier.)

attention faster than you would have otherwise. Moreover, if it is a word from your own language, it captures your attention faster than a word from a language you do not understand (Jiang, Costello, & He, 2007). Other experiments with either binocular rivalry or flash suppression have shown that you more rapidly become aware of faces and other social stimuli than physically similar nonsocial stimuli, and more rapidly become aware of a signal previously associated with danger than one not paired with danger (Gayet et al., 2016; Su, van Boxtel, & Lu, 2016). If you have a strong interest in something—cars, for example—a picture of that kind of object gains your awareness more readily than it does for other people (Stein, Reeder, & Peelen, 2016). If you become aware of something highly meaningful faster than you do for something similar but less meaningful, evidently your brain decided the stimulus was meaningful *before* you became conscious of it! The conclusion is that much of brain activity is unconscious, and even unconscious activity can influence behavior.

✅ STOP & CHECK

19. How could someone use fMRI to determine which of two patterns in binocular rivalry is conscious at a given moment?
20. If someone is aware of the stimulus on the right in a case of binocular rivalry, what evidence indicates that the brain is also processing the stimulus on the left?

ANSWERS

19. Make one stimulus pulsate at a given rhythm and look for brain areas showing that rhythm of activity. The rhythm takes over widespread areas of the brain when that pattern is conscious. 20. If a stimulus gradually appears on the left side, attention shifts to the left faster if that stimulus is a meaningful word than if it is a word from an unfamiliar language.

Consciousness as a Threshold Phenomenon

Does consciousness come in degrees? That is, would it make sense to say you were "partly" conscious of some stimulus?

This is not an easy question to answer, but several studies suggest that consciousness is a yes–no phenomenon. Researchers flashed blurry words on a screen for brief fractions of a second and asked people to identify each word, if possible, and to rate *how* conscious they were of the word on a scale from 0 to 100. People almost always rated a word either 0 or 100. They almost never said they were partly conscious of something (Sergent & Dehaene, 2004). These results suggest that consciousness is a threshold phenomenon. When a stimulus activates enough neurons to a sufficient extent, the activity reverberates, magnifies, and extends over much of the brain. If a stimulus fails to reach that level, the pattern fades away. However, another study found that even when people report no consciousness of a stimulus, they could guess with 62 percent accuracy which of two possible stimuli it was (Q. Li et al., 2014). Again we see the point that stimuli can exert some effect even without conscious perception.

The Timing of Consciousness

Are you conscious of events instant by instant as they happen? It certainly seems that way, but if there were a delay between an event and your consciousness of it, how would you know? You wouldn't. Perhaps you sometimes construct a conscious experience after the event.

Consider the **phi phenomenon** that perceptual researchers noted long ago: If you see a dot in one position alternating with a similar dot nearby, it will appear that the dot is moving back and forth. Considering just the simplest case, imagine what happens if you see a dot in one position and then another: • ➡ •. You see a dot in one position, it appears to move, and you see it in the second position. Okay, but *when* did you see it move? When you saw it in the first position, you didn't know it was going to appear in the second position. You could not perceive it as moving until *after* it appeared in the second position. Evidently, you perceived it as moving from one position to the second after it appeared in the second position! In other words, the second position changed your perception of what occurred before it.

Another example: Suppose you hear a recorded word that is carefully engineered to sound halfway between *dent* and *tent*. We'll call it **ent*. If you hear it in the phrase "**ent in the fender*," it sounds like *dent*. If you hear it in the phrase "**ent in the forest*," it sounds like *tent*. That is, later words changed what you heard before them (Connine, Blasko, & Hall, 1991).

One more example: Suppose you are watching a screen that at unpredictable times displays a faint set of lines for 50 ms, and your task is to say the angle of the lines. Sometimes it appears on the left of the screen and sometimes on the right. The difficulty is adjusted so you are correct a little more than chance, and you often say you didn't see it at all. Now suppose that 400 ms *after* the stimulus, a cue flashes to tell you whether the stimulus was on the left or right of the screen. That stimulus increases the chance you will say you saw the stimulus, and increases your accuracy of identifying its angle (Sergent et al., 2013). So you are capable of becoming conscious of something after it is gone. Somehow your brain held it in reserve, capable of activating it after the fact.

STOP & CHECK

21. In what way does the phi phenomenon imply that a new stimulus sometimes changes consciousness of what went before it?

ANSWER

21. Someone who sees a dot on the left and then a dot on the right perceives the dot as moving from left to right. The perceived movement would have occurred before the dot appeared on the right, but the person had no reason to infer that movement until after the dot appeared on the right.

Conscious and Unconscious People

When we ask about the physiological basis for consciousness, we need to distinguish two questions. So far we have focused on what happens when a waking, alert, conscious person becomes conscious of a particular stimulus. The other question is what enables the person as a whole to be aware of anything at all. How do the brains of conscious people differ from those of people who are asleep, in a coma, or deeply anesthetized?

Two studies followed people as they lost consciousness under anesthesia and then regained it as the drug effects wore off. Loss of consciousness was marked by decreased overall activity and especially by decreased connectivity between the cerebral cortex and subcortical areas such as the thalamus, hypothalamus, and basal ganglia. Initial recovery of consciousness depended on increased connectivity between subcortical and cortical areas, and later increases in alertness depended on increased activity in the cortex (Långsjö et al., 2012; Schröter, 2012). A study with monkeys also found that a loss of synchrony and connectivity between cortical areas preceded a loss of consciousness (Ishizawa et al., 2016). Recall the earlier discussion that consciousness of a stimulus requires a spread of activity over much of the brain. With a loss of connectivity, no stimulus can spread its activity, and the person is conscious of nothing.

People in a minimally conscious state respond to at least a few stimuli, although they cannot talk. People in a vegetative state alternate between sleep and greater arousal, but even in their most aroused state they show no purposeful behaviors. Might they nevertheless be conscious? Researchers used fMRI to record brain activity in a young woman who was in a persistent vegetative state following a brain injury from a traffic accident. She had neither spoken nor made any other purposive movements. However, when she was told to imagine playing tennis, the fMRI showed increased activity in motor areas of her cortex, similar to what healthy volunteers showed after the same instruction. When she was told to imagine walking through her house, a different set of brain areas became active, again similar to the pattern for healthy volunteers (Owen et al., 2006). Follow-up studies found similar results in 4 of 53 patients in a vegetative state. One patient used brain activity—imagining tennis versus imagining walking through a house—to answer yes/no questions such as "Do you have a brother?" (Monti et al., 2010).

Another approach shows promise without requiring any response at all. Researchers used brief magnetic stimulation to activate a localized brain area, and then used EEG to observe the spread of activity. The activity spread only locally in anesthetized people, sleeping people, and most people in a vegetative state. It spread more widely for people in a minimally conscious state (Casali et al., 2013; Rosanova et al., 2012). This method offers a potentially quick way to probe for consciousness in an unresponsive person.

STOP & CHECK

22. As people lost consciousness under anesthesia and later regained it, what changed most strikingly in the brain?

ANSWER

22. Connectivity among brain areas increased as people regained consciousness.

Attention

Attention isn't synonymous with consciousness, but it is closely related. Of all the information that strikes your eyes, ears, and other receptors, you are conscious of only those few to which you direct your attention (Huang, Treisman, & Pashler, 2007). For example, consider **inattentional blindness** or *change blindness:* If something in a complex scene changes slowly, or changes while you blink your eyes, you probably will not notice it unless you are paying attention to the particular item that changes (Henderson & Hollingworth, 2003; Rensink, O'Regan, & Clark, 1997).

Brain Areas Controlling Attention

Psychologists distinguish bottom-up from top-down attention. A bottom-up process depends on the stimulus. If you are sitting on a park bench, gazing off into the distance, when suddenly a deer runs past you, it grabs your attention. A top-down process is intentional. You might be looking for someone you know in a crowd, and you check one face after another to find the one you want. Sometimes a top-down process overrules bottom-up processes. Suppose you are looking for a friend in a crowd, but it's a carnival crowd. Many people are dressed as clowns or wearing other gaudy attire, but your friend is wearing a plain shirt and blue jeans. You need to suppress the attention and activity that the unusual items would ordinarily attract (Mevorach, Hodsoll, Allen, Shalev, & Humphreys, 2010). Deliberate, top-down direction of attention depends on parts of the prefrontal cortex and parietal cortex (Buschman & Miller, 2007; Rossi, Bichot, Desimone, & Ungerleider, 2007). They direct attention by facilitating responsiveness in parts of the thalamus, which in turn increase the activation of appropriate areas of the sensory cortex (Engel et al., 2016; Wimmer et al., 2015).

You can control your attention (top-down) even without moving your eyes. To illustrate, keep your eyes fixated on the central *x* in the following display. Then attend to the *G* at the right and gradually shift your attention clockwise around the circle. Notice how you become aware of different parts of the circle without moving your eyes. As you deliberately shift your attention, you increase activity in one part after another of the visual cortex (Kamitani & Tong, 2005; Wegener, Freiwald, & Kreiter, 2004).

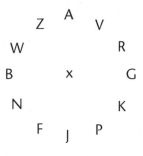

Another demonstration: What is the current sensation in your left foot? Chances are, before you read this question, you were not conscious of *any* sensation in your left foot. When you directed your attention to it, activity increased in the corresponding part of the somatosensory cortex (Lambie & Marcel, 2002).

One of psychologists' favorite ways to study attention is the **Stroop effect**, the difficulty of ignoring words and saying the color of ink. In the following display, say aloud the color of ink of each word, ignoring the words themselves:

RED BLUE GREEN **GREEN** BROWN **BLUE**
RED PURPLE GREEN RED

After all your years of learning to read words, it is hard to suppress that habit and respond to the color instead. However, when people successfully do so, they enhance the activity in

the color-vision areas of the cortex and decrease the activity in the areas responsible for identifying words (Polk, Drake, Jonides, Smith, & Smith, 2008).

Your ability to resist distraction fluctuates. Sometimes your "mind wanders," interfering with a task, especially a difficult one (Thomson, Besner, & Smilek, 2015). In one experiment, people's task was to find a circle within an array of squares. On some trials, one of the squares was red instead of green. Anything that is different attracts attention, and on the average, people responded a bit more slowly on trials with a red square present. However, the speed of responding varied from trial to trial. On trials when activity was enhanced in the middle frontal gyrus (part of the prefrontal cortex) at the *start* of the trial (before seeing the stimuli), people did best at ignoring the red square and thereby resisting distraction (Leber, 2010). This result confirms the importance of the prefrontal cortex in directing attention.

⊘ STOP & CHECK

23. What brain response was related to people's ability to resist distraction from an irrelevant red square among the green squares and circle?

ANSWER

23. Resistance to distraction related to the amount of activity in part of the prefrontal cortex before the presentation of stimuli.

Spatial Neglect

Brain damage can produce special types of attention problems. Many people with damage to the right hemisphere show **spatial neglect**—a tendency to ignore the left side of the body, the left side of objects, much of what they hear in the left ear, and much of what they feel in the left hand, especially in the presence of any competing sensation from the right side. Some people have been known to put clothes on only the right side of the body. These effects are most pronounced early after a stroke or other damage, and most people show at least partial recovery over the next 10 to 20 weeks (Nijboer, Kollen, & Kwakkel, 2013). (Damage in the left hemisphere seldom produces significant neglect of the right side.)

If asked to point straight ahead, most patients with neglect point to the right of center. If a patient with neglect is shown a long horizontal line and asked to divide it in half, generally he or she picks a spot to the right of center, as if part of the left side wasn't there (Richard, Honoré, Bernati, & Rousseaux, 2004).

Some patients with neglect also show deviations when estimating the midpoint of a numerical range. For example, what is halfway between 11 and 19? The correct answer is, of course, 15, but some people with neglect say "17." Evidently, they discount the lower numbers as if they were on the left side (Doricchi, Guariglia, Gasparini, & Tomaiuolo, 2005; Zorzi, Priftis, & Umiltà, 2002). At least in Western society, many people visualize the numbers as a line stretching to the right, as in the *x* axis of a graph. People also tend to imagine time as moving from left to right. Researchers presented some made-up statements about the past and the future, and then tested how well some people with spatial neglect remembered the statements. They forgot more statements about the past than about the future, again suggesting neglect of things imagined to be toward the left (Saj, Fuhrman, Vuilleumier, & Boroditsky, 2014).

Although some neglect patients have sensory losses, in many cases, the main problem is loss of attention rather than impaired sensation. One patient was shown a letter E, composed of small H's, as in Figure 13.16(a). She identified it as a big E composed of small H's, indicating that she saw the whole figure. However, when she was then asked to cross off all the H's, she crossed off only the ones on the right. When she was shown the figures in Figure 13.16(b), she identified them as an O composed of little O's and an X composed of little X's. Again, she could see both halves of both figures, but when she was asked to cross off all the elements, she crossed off only the ones on the right. The researchers summarized by saying she saw the forest but only half the trees (Marshall & Halligan, 1995).

Several procedures increase attention to the neglected side. Simply telling the person to pay attention to the left side helps briefly. So does having the person look left while at the same time feeling an object with the left hand (Vaishnavi, Calhoun, & Chatterjee, 2001) or hearing a sound from the left side of the world (Frassinetti, Pavani, & Làdavas, 2002).

Other manipulations also shift the attention. For example, some patients with neglect usually report feeling nothing

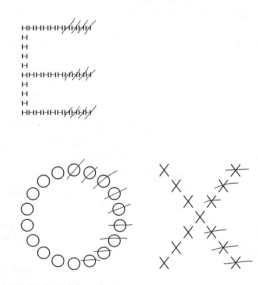

Figure 13.16 Spatial neglect
A patient with neglect identified the overall figures as E, O, and X, indicating that she saw the whole figures. However, when asked to cross off the elements that composed them, she crossed off only the parts on the right.
(Source: From "Seeing the forest but only half the trees?," by J. C. Marshall and P. W. Halligan, Nature, 373, pp. 521–523, Fig. 1 [parts C and E]. © 1995 Nature.)

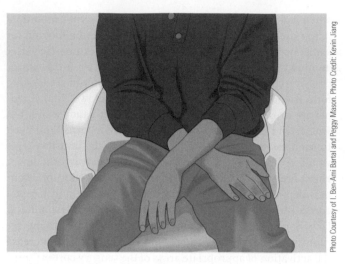

Figure 13.17 A way to reduce sensory neglect
Ordinarily, someone with right hemisphere damage neglects the left arm. However, if the left arm crosses over or under the right, attention to the left arm increases.

with the left hand, especially if the right hand feels something at the time. However, if you cross one hand over the other as shown in Figure 13.17, the person is more likely to report feeling the left hand, which is now on the right side of the body (Agliotti, Smania, & Peru, 1999). Also, the person ordinarily has trouble pointing to anything in the left visual field but has somewhat better success if the hand was so far to the left that he or she would have to move it to the right to point to the object (Mattingley, Husain, Rorden, Kennard, & Driver, 1998). Again, the conclusion is that neglect is not due to a loss of sensation but a difficulty in directing attention to the left side.

STOP & CHECK

24. What is the evidence that spatial neglect is a problem in attention, not just sensation?
25. What procedures increase attention to the left side in a person with spatial neglect?

ANSWERS

24. When a patient with neglect sees a large letter composed of small letters, he or she can identify the large letter but then neglects part of it when asked to cross off all the small letters. Also, someone who neglects the left hand pays attention to it when it is crossed over the right hand. 25. Simply telling the person to attend to something on the left helps temporarily. Having the person look to the left while feeling something on the left side increases attention to the felt object. Crossing the left hand over the right increases attention to the left hand. Moving a hand far to the left makes it easier for the person to point to something in the left visual field because the hand will move toward the right to point at the object.

Module 13.2 | In Closing

Attending to Attention and Being Conscious of Consciousness

Does research on the brain correlates of consciousness, like the studies described in this chapter, explain the relationship between brain activity and consciousness? Does it solve the mind–brain problem? No. Could it, if we improve our technology enough to explore brain activity in ever more complete detail? Some researchers believe it could, whereas others remain skeptical. One fundamental question is this: Suppose researchers establish exactly which neurons are responsible for a particular visual perception. The input to those neurons is just glutamate, GABA, and other neurotransmitters. How do those neurons "know" that the input of those transmitters came from visual stimuli? That is, why does activity of those particular neurons constitute a visual experience? Indeed, why does it constitute a conscious experience at all?

Perhaps someday someone—maybe you!—will propose a great insight into these difficult issues. In the meantime, researchers are learning much about what the brain has to do to produce conscious experiences, and we are moving toward using brain measurements to determine whether an unresponsive person is or is not conscious. Perhaps someday we can use similar strategies to infer consciousness or its absence in nonhuman animals, or to infer when consciousness emerges in early human development. Consciousness, which psychologists used to reject as a research topic, now has become an exciting one.

Summary

1. Dualism—the belief in a nonmaterial mind that exists separately from the body—conflicts with the conservation of matter and energy, one of the best-established principles of physics. Nearly all neuroscientists and philosophers accept some version of monism, the idea that mental activity is inseparable from brain activity. **441**

2. The hard problem is the question of why consciousness exists at all. Most scientists and philosophers agree that we cannot answer this question, at least at present. **442**

3. To identify the brain activities associated with consciousness, researchers present the same stimulus under conditions when an observer probably will or probably will not identify it consciously. **442**

4. When someone is conscious of a stimulus, the representation of that stimulus spreads over a large portion of the brain. **442**

5. A stimulus can influence our behavior without consciousness. Even before a stimulus becomes conscious, the brain processes the information enough to identify something as meaningful or meaningless. **444**

6. People almost never say they were partly conscious of something. It may be that consciousness is a threshold phenomenon: We become conscious of anything that exceeds a certain level of brain activity, and we are not conscious of other events. **445**

7. We are not always conscious of events instantaneously as they occur. Sometimes, a later event modifies our conscious perception of a stimulus that went before it. **445**

8. Researchers sometimes use brain recordings to infer whether someone is conscious. A few people diagnosed as being in a vegetative state have shown possible indications of consciousness. **446**

9. Attention to a stimulus requires increased brain responses to that stimulus and decreased responses to others. The prefrontal cortex is important for top-down control of attention. **446**

10. Damage to parts of the right hemisphere produce spatial neglect for the left side of the body or the left side of objects. **447**

11. Neglect results from a deficit in attention, not sensation. For example, someone with neglect can see an entire letter enough to say what it is, even though that same person ignores the left half when asked to cross out all the elements that compose it. **448**

Key Terms

Terms are defined in the module on the page number indicated. They're also presented in alphabetical order with definitions in the book's Subject Index/Glossary, which begins on page 589. Interactive flash cards, audio reviews, and crossword puzzles are among the online resources available to help you learn these terms and the concepts they represent.

backward masking **442**
binocular rivalry **443**
conscious **442**
dualism **441**
flash suppression **442**
hard problem **442**

identity position **442**
inattentional blindness **446**
masking **442**
materialism **442**
mentalism **442**
mind–brain problem **441**

monism **441**
phi phenomenon **445**
spatial neglect **447**
Stroop effect **447**

Thought Questions

1. Could a computer be conscious? What evidence, if any, would convince you that it was conscious?

2. How might one try to determine whether a nonhuman animal is conscious?

Module 13.2 | End of Module Quiz

1. Which of the following best states the identity position regarding mind and brain?
   A. The physical world cannot exist unless a mind is aware of it.
   B. Mental activity causes brain activity.
   C. Brain activity causes mental activity.
   D. Mental activity and brain activity are the same thing.

2. What do the following have in common: flash suppression, backward masking, and binocular rivalry?
   A. They prevent consciousness of a stimulus that someone would otherwise perceive.
   B. They measure the time required for a stimulus to reach consciousness.
   C. They increase the spread of information to widespread areas of the cortex.
   D. They improve someone's ability to maintain attention despite distraction.

3. What procedure is used in backward masking?
   A. participant views a stationary dot surrounded by bright flashing dots.
   B. Researchers present a brief visual stimulus followed by a second, longer stimulus.
   C. A participant views one scene in the left eye and an incompatible scene in the right eye.
   D. A participant views a dot in one position alternating with a similar dot nearby.

4. If your left eye views red vertical stripes and your right eye views green horizontal stripes, what do you perceive?
   A. Red and green stripes superimposed
   B. Yellow diagonal stripes
   C. A white field without stripes
   D. Alternation between seeing red stripes and seeing green stripes

5. What happens when you are conscious of a stimulus that does not happen when the same stimulus is present without your consciousness of it?
   A. Rhythms of activity in the brain become more variable.
   B. Activity increases in the pineal gland.
   C. The response in the right hemisphere is greater than in the left.
   D. The response to the stimulus spreads to much of the brain.

6. People are conscious of a prolonged stimulus, but not one with an extremely short presentation. What happens at an intermediate duration of presentation?
   A. People report being partly conscious of it.
   B. People are sometimes conscious of it and sometimes not, and the difference depends only on what happens at that moment.
   C. People are sometimes conscious of it and sometimes not, and stimuli after the event can influence the outcome.
   D. People report consciousness of a faint, blurry image.

7. What happens in the brain when people lose consciousness?
   A. Neurons stop producing action potentials.
   B. Synapses release only GABA and not glutamate.
   C. The eyes, ears, and other sensory receptors stop sending information to the brain.
   D. Activity in one brain area does not effectively spread to other areas.

8. Certain people in a vegetative state gave possible indication of consciousness by doing what?
   A. Laughing or crying in response to what someone said.
   B. Moving their eyes to the left or right to answer yes/no questions.
   C. Different brain activity after directions of what to imagine doing.
   D. Squeezing the hand of a loved one.

9. What happens in top-down attention?
   A. A strong sensory stimulus inhibits responses to other, simultaneous stimuli.
   B. The upper layers of the cerebral cortex inhibit the lower layers.
   C. Activity from upper layers of the cerebral cortex excites the lower layers.
   D. The prefrontal cortex facilitates activity in appropriate sensory areas.

10. Suppose someone who is trying to divide a horizontal line in half picks a spot far to the right of center. This result suggests probable damage or malfunction in which part of the brain?
    A. The left hemisphere
    B. The right hemisphere
    C. The prefrontal cortex
    D. The primary visual cortex

11. If someone has spatial neglect of the left side, which of these procedures, if any, would increase attention to a touch sensation on the left side?
    A. Ask the person to look to the left during the touch sensation.
    B. Ask the person to look to the right during the touch sensation.
    C. Ask the person to listen to music during the touch sensation.
    D. None of these procedures would have any noticeable effect.

Answers: 1D, 2A, 3B, 4D, 5D, 6C, 7D, 8C, 9D, 10B, 11A.

Making Decisions and Social Neuroscience

Life is full of decisions. Some are big ones: Where shall I go to college? What kind of job shall I seek? Should I marry this person or not? Some are small ones: Should I wear the green sweater or the blue one today? What kind of sandwich do I want for lunch? Shall I study a little longer tonight or go to sleep now? In each case, you consider the possible pluses and minuses.

Human life is also full of social interactions. Many couples spend their whole adult lifetime together, helping each other, their children, and their grandchildren. Many people devote great efforts to helping people they don't know, occasionally even risking their own lives. Economic cooperation makes possible enormous opportunities. Tonight you might drive a car made in Europe and powered by fuel from the Middle East so you can eat food grown by farmers in Asia, cooked according to a recipe from South America, at a restaurant built by people in a previous century. And you are protected from disease by the combined efforts of medical researchers from many countries and many centuries.

In this module we consider your brain activity during decision making and social behavior. These topics are not closely related, but we consider them together just because the treatment of each topic is short. Research on both topics began more recently than for the rest of neuroscience, and the conclusions are tentative.

Perceptual Decisions

One type of decision is factual: Should we expect rain today or not? Do these glasses improve my vision more than those do? Is the meal that I am cooking ready to come out of the oven, or not? To answer questions like these, you weigh the evidence.

The simplest way to imagine how the brain does this is to have one set of cells accumulate evidence in favor of one choice, another set accumulate evidence for the other choice, and a third set compare the two. Much evidence seems consistent with this idea (though not yet conclusive). In one study, a rat had to put its nose into a central port, listen to clicks, and then turn to the side with more clicks. Figure 13.18 shows the setup. Within the posterior parietal cortex, one set of cells responded in proportion to the number of clicks on the left, and another set responded in proportion to the number of clicks on the right. Within part of

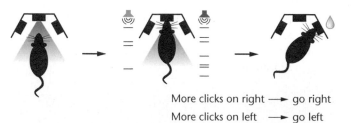

Figure 13.18 Design for a study of decision making in rats
If the rat heard more clicks on the left side, it can turn left for reward. If it heard more on the right side, it can turn right for reward.

the prefrontal cortex called the *frontal orienting fields*, adjacent to the motor cortex, one set of cells responded when the left side was ahead, and a different set responded when the right side was ahead. That is, responses in the posterior parietal cortex are graded, but responses in the frontal cortex produce an all-or-none outcome, like a scorekeeper who announces which team has won the game (Hanks et al., 2015). After damage to the frontal orienting fields, a rat is unable to keep track of the score, and it bases its decision on the last clicks it heard, instead of a running tally over even a brief period of time (Erlich, Brunton, Duan, Hanks, & Brody, 2015).

However, although these results seem to suggest that the cells in the posterior parietal cortex are counting the clicks, procedures that inactivate the posterior parietal cortex have little effect on the rat's behavior on this task (Brody & Hanks, 2016). Evidently the posterior parietal cortex is just echoing a process taking place somewhere else, and we do not yet know where that is.

In a similar type of study, a monkey gazes at a fixation point and responds with a left or right eye movement based on whether it sees dots moving left or right. The task is more difficult than it sounds, because only a few dots are moving, and a much larger number of dots are constantly appearing and then disappearing at random positions on the screen. The monkey watches for a while, and then has to wait a few seconds before responding. Within part of the parietal cortex, one set of cells is more active if the dots appeared to be moving left, and a different set responds if the dots were apparently moving right. During the delay before the monkey is allowed to respond, the relative response of the two types of cells shifts more and more strongly in one direction. For example, if the "look left" cells were a little ahead of the "look right" cells at the start of the delay, they become more and more ahead as time passes, as if the monkey is becoming more certain of the decision. However, as in the case of the click-counting study, inactivating this part of the parietal cortex has little effect on the decision, so these cells are echoing a decision process taking place somewhere else, not making the decision themselves (Katz, Yates, Pillow, & Huk, 2016; Latimer, Yates, Meister, Huk, & Pillow, 2015; Shadlen & Newsome, 1996).

Another type of research examines what happens when a rat in a difficult maze decides which direction to turn at a choice point. The rat stops and looks one way and then the other a few times before proceeding. By recording from place cells, as described in Chapter 12, researchers can "read a rat's mind" at that point. Recordings from the rat's hippocampus show that cells become active in the same order as if the rat were actually walking down one path or the other. That is, researchers watch the brain activity as the rat (apparently) imagines trying each route (Redish, 2016). Researchers get similar recordings from human brains while people imagine moving from one place to another (T. I. Brown et al., 2016; Jacobs et al., 2013; J. F. Miller et al., 2013). Many people have asserted that humans are the only species that can imagine the future. They are wrong about that. Even rats can imagine the future, at least the very near future.

⊘ STOP & CHECK

26. When a rat is deciding whether it hears more clicks on the left or right side, what happens in the frontal orienting fields?

27. What evidence says that rats can imagine the future?

ANSWERS

26. Depending on which ear is "ahead" at a given point, one set of cells or a different set of cells becomes active. 27. While pausing at a choice point in a maze, place cells in the hippocampus become active in the sequence that would occur as the rat traveled down one arm or the other in the maze.

Decisions Based on Values

Many decisions depend on preferences. You start by estimating what outcome each choice would bring, and then you decide which outcome seems better. In everyday life, you might consider many choices, but laboratory researchers simplify the situation by offering only two choices. For rats or mice, the choice might be to turn left or right for different types of reward or different probabilities of reward. For people, the choice might be to bet on one result or a different one. Suppose, as is realistic in everyday life, the payoff for one choice is usually better than the other, but not always. In that case, cells in the basal ganglia gradually learn which choice is better. Cells in the **ventromedial prefrontal cortex** also participate, apparently by modifying the responses of the basal ganglia.

For example, if choice A has usually been better than choice B, but something currently favors choice B, the rapid-learning prefrontal cortex can overrule the slower-learning basal ganglia (Brigman et al., 2013; Kovach et al., 2012). Suppose you have an opportunity to bet on "red" at a roulette wheel, but on some trials the wheel has mostly red slots and on other trials it has only a few red slots. You would, presumably, bet more heavily on red when you see more red slots. People with damage to the prefrontal cortex tend to bet about the same amount each time, based on their average expectation rather than what is true at the moment (Struder, Manes, Humphreys, Robbins, & Clark, 2015). Most, though not all, people with ventromedial prefrontal damage seem less sensitive than average to the possible rewards at the moment (Manohar & Husain, 2016).

An additional role of the ventromedial prefrontal cortex is to monitor confidence in one's decisions. People with damage to this area tend to be overconfident in many ways, such as gambling heavily or making impulsive decisions without carefully considering the likely consequences. People with Korsakoff's syndrome, discussed in Chapter 12, suffer damage to the ventromedial prefrontal cortex among other areas, and a common result is high confidence in the answers that they confabulate (Hebscher & Gilboa, 2016).

The ventromedial prefrontal cortex and other areas relay information to the nearby **orbitofrontal cortex** (see Figure 13.19), which responds based on how an expected reward compares to other possible choices. For example, getting a B+ on your term paper might be delightful or disappointing, depending on what grade you had been expecting (Frank & Claus, 2006). You might prefer a pizza at one time, but prefer cake at another time. The orbitofrontal cortex updates the expected value of one action or another, based on your current circumstances (Rudebeck & Murray, 2014). In one study

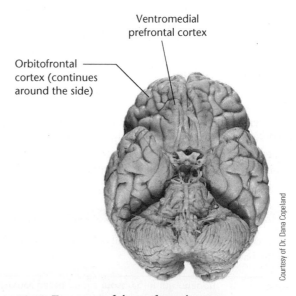

Ventromedial prefrontal cortex

Orbitofrontal cortex (continues around the side)

Courtesy of Dr. Dana Copeland

Figure 13.19 Two areas of the prefrontal cortex
The ventromedial prefrontal cortex and the orbitofrontal cortex are important contributors to decisions.

monkeys could choose (by moving their eyes left or right) between two juices. They had learned symbols representing different flavors of juice and different amounts of juice. So, on a given trial the choice might be between one drop of apple juice or two drops of cranberry juice, or between three drops of kiwi punch and one drop of peppermint tea. Many orbitofrontal cells responded to the preferred member of whatever pair was available. That is, a cell might respond to the sight of apple juice if it was preferred to cranberry, but respond to cherry on another trial if it was preferred to apple (Xie & Padoa-Schioppa, 2016). In a similar study, if a monkey had a choice between two rewards that were almost equal in value, its orbitofrontal neurons alternated many times between two patterns of activity, suggesting that the monkey was comparing two nearly equal values before deciding (Rich & Wallis, 2016).

Impairment or relative inactivity in the orbitofrontal cortex in humans is often associated with poor or impulsive decisions. Consider the Iowa Gambling Task: People can draw one card at a time from four piles. They always win $100 in play money from decks A and B, or $50 from C and D. However, some of the cards also have penalties:

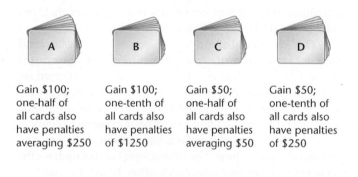

| Gain $100; one-half of all cards also have penalties averaging $250 | Gain $100; one-tenth of all cards also have penalties of $1250 | Gain $50; one-half of all cards also have penalties averaging $50 | Gain $50; one-tenth of all cards also have penalties of $250 |

When you examine all the payoffs, you can easily see that the best strategy is to pick cards from decks C and D. In the experiment, however, people have to discover the payoffs by trial and error. Ordinarily, as they sample from all four decks, they gradually start showing signs of tension whenever they draw a card from A or B, and they shift their preference toward C and D. People with orbitofrontal damage choose C and D also if their first few choices from A and B hit them with penalties. However, if they start with a streak of wins from A and B, they are very slow to switch to C and D (Stalnaker, Cooch, & Schoenbaum, 2015). Again, the point is that the prefrontal cortex, especially the orbitofrontal cortex, updates the relative advantage or disadvantage of each possible choice.

✅ **STOP & CHECK** ▰▰▰▰▰▰

28. How does the role of the prefrontal cortex differ from that of the basal ganglia?

ANSWER

28. The basal ganglia gradually learn a preference based on the usual result. The prefrontal cortex modifies that preference based on the most recent information.

The Biology of Love

Social neuroscience, the study of how genes, chemicals, and brain areas contribute to social behavior, is a relatively new area of study, but one that excites growing enthusiasm. We shall consider two topics, love and altruism.

Suppose you are passionately in love with someone. According to studies using fMRI, looking at pictures of the person you love strongly activates the brain areas associated with reward, in ways similar to the high that people report from addictive drugs (Burkett & Young, 2012). Viewing photos of your beloved also activates the hippocampus and other areas important for memory and cognition (Ortigue, Bianchi-Demicheli, Patel, Frum, & Lewis, 2010). (Thinking about someone you love evokes memories of what you have done together.) The point is that what we call love combines motivations, emotions, memories, and cognitions.

The role of **oxytocin** and the closely related hormone vasopressin has attracted much attention. Oxytocin stimulates contractions of the uterus during childbirth, stimulates breasts to produce milk, and tends to promote maternal behavior, social approach, and pair bonding in many mammalian species (Marlin, Mitre, D'amour, Chao, & Froemke, 2015; McCall & Singer, 2012; Sobota, Mihara, Forrest, Featherstone, & Siegel, 2015). Both men and women release it during sexual activity. It has been called the "love hormone," although a better term might be *love-enhancing* or *love-magnifying hormone*.

A convenient way to study oxytocin's effects is to give it to people as a nasal spray and compare its effects to a placebo. Oxytocin passes directly from the nasal cavity to the brain and exerts effects about half an hour later, although exactly how much reaches the brain is not certain. In one study, men who reported being passionately in love viewed photos of their female partner and other women, rating the attractiveness of each. They rated their partner higher when under the influence of oxytocin than that of a placebo. The oxytocin did not change their ratings of other women (Scheele et al., 2013). So oxytocin didn't increase attraction to everyone, but just to someone already loved.

In another study, heterosexual men received oxytocin or a placebo before meeting an attractive woman. The researchers simply measured how far away each man stood. Oxytocin did not influence single men's behavior, but it caused those in a monogamous relationship to stand *farther* away from the attractive woman (Scheele et al., 2012). That is, it apparently enhanced a man's fidelity to his partner, decreasing his willingness to face the temptation of another attractive woman.

Oxytocin helps people who have trouble recognizing faces, and people who can recognize faces but have trouble identifying their emotional expressions. In both cases, oxytocin has little or no effect on people who already recognize faces and expressions. It just helps those who were doing poorly (Bate et al., 2014; Guastella et al., 2010).

In many situations, oxytocin's effect on social relations depends on who the other people are. It increases conformity to the opinions of your in-group (people you perceive to be like yourself) but not to the opinions of an out-group (Stallen, De

Dreu, Shalvi, Smidts, & Sanfey, 2012). In certain economic games, you can protect your initial money or invest it in a cooperative venture with someone else, trusting that the other person won't cheat you. One study found that oxytocin increases trust toward your in-group members, but could increase, decrease, or have no effect on trust toward other people, depending on what you think of those people (van Ijzendoorn & Bakermans-Kranenburg, 2012). Unfortunately, the research on this topic has mostly presented small effects and we should be wary of drawing firm conclusions (Nave, Camerer, & McCullough, 2015).

The effects of oxytocin are not always pro-social. When people perceive themselves as being threatened, oxytocin increases their attention to possible dangers, increasing their anger, distress, and negative reactions to others, especially to strangers (Olff et al., 2013; Poulin, Holman, & Buffone, 2012). People who in general distrust others become even more distrustful under the influence of oxytocin (Bartz et al., 2011).

Definitely, we need more good research in this area. At this point, a tentative conclusion is that oxytocin increases attention to important social cues (Olff et al., 2013). The result is greater attention to facial expressions and stronger positive or negative responses to others, based on the information available. In any case, oxytocin does not appear to increase love, trust, or any other reaction on an absolute basis.

Empathy and Altruism

Civilized life depends on people helping one another. You might help explain something to a fellow student who is competing with you for a good grade in a course. You might contribute money to help victims of a natural disaster on the other side of the world. Helpfulness depends on **empathy**, the ability to identify with other people and feel their pain almost as if it were your own. Although empathy is not unique to humans, it is stronger in us than in other species. A monkey or chimpanzee

with a choice between rewarding just itself, or rewarding both itself and another monkey or chimpanzee seems almost indifferent to the other, unless the other is a relative or long-term associate (Chang, Gariépy, & Platt, 2013; Silk et al., 2005).

Moral and religious leaders teach us that we should extend kindness to everyone, but in fact most people tend to be more generous toward those they see as similar to themselves. For example, if you watch someone who is feeling socially rejected by others, you will "feel the pain" and your brain will react accordingly, but you will react more strongly if the person feeling rejected is one of your relatives or close friends (Beeney, Franklin, Levy, & Adams, 2011).

From an evolutionary standpoint, it makes sense to be altruistic toward your relatives, and someone who seems similar is more likely to be related to you than someone very different. However, some people show much stronger in-group biases than others do. Even rats show an in-group bias. Imagine a rat trapped in a plastic tube. A second rat outside the tube can open the door to let it escape. If they are from the same strain, such as two albino rats, the second rat opens the door. If they are from different strains, such as one albino rat and one hooded rat, the second rat ignores the trapped rat (see Figure 13.20). However, if an albino rat was reared throughout its life with other hooded rats, it helps a hooded rat but not another albino rat (Ben-Ami Bartal et al., 2014). Rats don't look at themselves in mirrors, and therefore a rat reared with hooded rats assumes it is one too!

Some people show much more empathy than others do. Much of that variation pertains to culture and family upbringing, but biological factors contribute also. The most profound effect occurs in a condition called **frontotemporal dementia** (or frontotemporal lobe degeneration), in which parts of the frontal and temporal lobes of the cerebral cortex gradually degenerate. The effects depend on the exact location of damage, but often the damage includes the ventromedial prefrontal cortex and

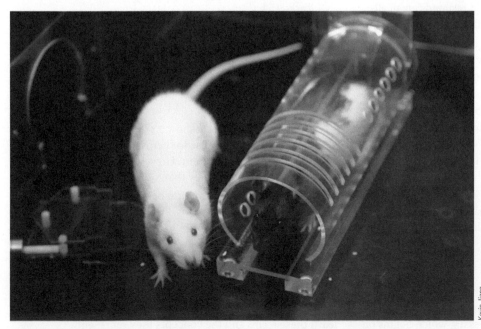

Figure 13.20 Out-group bias in rats
A rat will open the door to help a member of its own strain escape from a plastic tube, but it will not help a member of a different strain.
(Source: Photo Courtesy of I. Ben-Ami Bartal and Peggy Mason.)

Kevin Jiang

orbitofrontal cortex. These areas that are important for evaluating possible rewards are also important for interpreting and evaluating other people's emotional expressions (Delgado et al., 2016; Jenkins et al., 2014). Often, therefore, people with damage of this type do not recognize or respond to other's reactions, including reactions of distress, and therefore they show little empathy or concern (Oliver et al., 2015; Van den Stock et al., 2015). As mentioned in Chapter 11, people with damage in the ventromedial prefrontal cortex are more likely than others to calmly endorse a utilitarian moral position that it would be okay to kill one person to save five, under a variety of circumstances.

People with frontotemporal dementia also show little interest in how others perceive them. For example, they neglect their personal hygiene (Waldo, 2015). They also fail to show embarrassment. Suppose an experimenter asks you to sing, karaoke-style, in a room by yourself, but secretly videotapes your performance and then shows it to you while other people are watching. Unless you are a fine singer, you will presumably feel embarrassed. In contrast, people with frontotemporal dementia seem quite calm, even if their singing is dismally bad (Sturm, Ascher, Miller, & Levenson, 2008).

STOP & CHECK

29. Why is it misleading to call oxytocin the "love hormone"?
30. How is the role of the ventromedial prefrontal cortex and orbitofrontal cortex similar for value decisions and social behavior?

ANSWERS

29. Oxytocin apparently magnifies love that was already present, but it does not create love toward a stranger. 30. In both cases these brain areas are important for interpreting and evaluating information relevant to choices and actions.

Module 13.3 | In Closing

Biology of Decisions and Social Behavior

You may have noticed that this was a short module. Why do neuroscientists have so much more to say about vision, for example, than decisions or social behavior? The reason certainly has nothing to do with a lack of interest. The reason is that researchers prefer questions that they know how to answer. With vision or other senses, they can control the stimuli precisely and measure responses with reasonable accuracy. Decision making and social behavior are complicated. The effort to understand them biologically has just begun, but at least it has begun.

Summary

1. In a perceptual decision, cells (somewhere in the brain) respond in proportion to evidence favoring one choice or the other, but the frontal orienting field responds on an all-or-none basis to which choice the evidence favors so far. **452**
2. When a rat pauses at a choice point in a maze, hippocampal place cells respond in a sequence as if the rat is traveling down one arm of the maze or the other. **453**
3. For a decision of which outcome is preferable, the ventromedial prefrontal cortex responds to recent information by modifying the responses of the slower-learning basal ganglia. **453**
4. The ventromedial prefrontal cortex is also important for monitoring how confident one should be about a decision. **453**
5. The orbitofrontal cortex evaluates each possible choice relative to the value of other available choices. **453**
6. People with damage to the prefrontal cortex are slow to switch strategies in situations such as the Iowa Gambling Task. **454**
7. Passionate love excites the brain in ways that resemble those of addictive drugs. **454**
8. Based on current evidence, it appears that the role of the hormone oxytocin is to increase attention to social cues. The result could be either increased or decreased attraction and trust. **454**
9. Both humans and rats show a tendency to help those they perceive as similar to themselves, more than those they perceive as different. However, some show that tendency more strongly than others. **455**
10. People with frontotemporal dementia are poor at understanding others' emotions, and therefore unlikely to show empathy. **455**

Key Terms

Terms are defined in the module on the page number indicated. They're also presented in alphabetical order with definitions in the book's Subject Index/Glossary, which begins on page 589. Interactive flash cards, audio reviews, and crossword puzzles are among the online resources available to help you learn these terms and the concepts they represent.

Thought Questions

1. What effect would you predict that oxytocin would have on empathy?

2. What would you predict about the brain reactions of people with psychopathic traits?

Module 13.3 | End of Module Quiz

1. During a perceptual decision, what happens in the frontal orienting fields?

    A. Each cell responds in proportion to the evidence favoring one choice or the other.

    B. Cells compare inputs from elsewhere to determine which side is ahead.

    C. Cells send inhibitory messages to the muscles until the time for response arrives.

    D. Cells produce gamma waves to synchronize the visual areas with the auditory areas.

2. Can rats "think about the future"? And what is the evidence?

    A. No, they cannot, because they do not have a prefrontal cortex.

    B. Yes. Neuroscientists monitor rats' dreams that include possible activities.

    C. Yes. At a choice point, hippocampal place cells imagine possible routes.

    D. Yes. Their frontal orienting fields respond to choices before they are offered.

3. In a value decision, how do responses by the ventromedial prefrontal cortex differ from those of the basal ganglia?

    A. The ventromedial prefrontal cortex excites, whereas the basal ganglia inhibit.

    B. The ventromedial prefrontal cortex responds on an all-or-none basis.

    C. The ventromedial prefrontal cortex adjusts more rapidly to new information.

    D. The ventromedial prefrontal cortex is sensitive to rewards and punishments.

4. How would someone with prefrontal damage probably react on the Iowa Gambling Task?

    A. Normal decisions, but lack of confidence in those decisions

    B. Slow to switch from a poor strategy to a better strategy

    C. Extreme caution to avoid possible losses

    D. Random guessing

5. Which hypothesis best summarizes our current understanding about oxytocin?

    A. Oxytocin increases love and trust.

    B. Oxytocin helps people restrain their emotional responses.

    C. Oxytocin helps people overcome bad habits.

    D. Oxytocin increases attention toward social cues.

6. Which of the following helps explain why people with frontotemporal dementia fail to show empathy?

    A. They suffer a severe impairment of short-term memory.

    B. They are preoccupied with how they are regarded by others.

    C. They are impaired at understanding emotional expressions.

    D. They become more eager than average to compete.

Answers: 1B, 2C, 3C, 4B, 5D, 6C.

Suggestions for Further Reading

Dehaene, S. (2016). *Consciousness and the brain*. New York: Viking Press. Excellent review of research on how the brain's response differs between stimuli perceived consciously and those not perceived consciously.

Koch, C., Massimini, M., Boly, M., & Tononi, G. (2016). Neural correlates of consciousness: Progress and problems *Nature Reviews Neuroscience, 17*, 307–321. Detailed article reviewing research relating brain activity to conscious perception.

Kellogg, R. T. (2013). *The making of the mind: The neuroscience of human nature*. Amherst, NY: Prometheus. Theoretical view of what must have changed in our brains and behavior as humans evolved from primate ancestors.

Ornstein, R. (1997). *The right mind*. New York: Harcourt Brace. Very readable description of split-brain research and the differences between the left and right hemispheres.

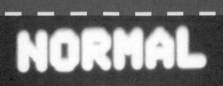

NORMAL

DEPRESSED

Psychological Disorders

Chapter 14

A physician who wants to treat your cough will start by diagnosing the cause. Did the cough come from the flu, a cold, allergy, lung cancer, tuberculosis, or something else? A lab test can identify the correct diagnosis with reasonable certainty, and a diagnosis informs the physician what treatment options are best.

Not many years ago, psychologists and psychiatrists were optimistic about using a similar approach for mental illness. The idea was to give each person a diagnosis such as depression or schizophrenia, and then find the cause and best treatment for each disorder. Research, however, has failed to support that approach. Most people who fit the diagnosis for one disorder fit the diagnosis for one or more other diagnoses also, and many people partly fit the diagnosis for several diagnoses without exactly fitting the diagnosis for any of them (Ahn, Flanagan, Marsh, & Sanislow, 2006; Caspi et al., 2014). The genes that predispose someone to schizophrenia largely overlap the genes that predispose to bipolar disorder, the genes that predispose to bipolar disorder overlap those that predispose to major depression, and those that predispose to major depression overlap those that predispose to attention deficit disorder (Cross-Disorder Group, 2013; Geschwind & Flint, 2015). The patterns of proteins, immune responses, and epigenetic changes also overlap for schizophrenia, bipolar disorder, and major depression (Network and Pathway Analysis Subgroup, 2015). In many cases a drug intended for the treatment of one diagnosis also helps many patients with other diagnoses.

In short, the categorical approach to mental illness is not quite right. This chapter is arranged around some traditional categories, mainly because most of the research has dealt with the causes and treatments of some category of problems, such as depression or schizophrenia. In defense of this organization, the categorical approach, though not quite right, is also not entirely wrong. Enough people have a primary difficulty of substance abuse, depression, or schizophrenia to justify research and tentative conclusions. Still, bear in mind that what pertains to one disorder also pertains to many people diagnosed with a different disorder.

> **Opposite:**
> PET scans show widespread areas of high activity (yellow) for someone in a normal mood, and decreased activity for someone in a depressed mood. (Photo Researchers, Inc./Alamy Stock Photo)

Learning Objectives

After studying this chapter, you should be able to:

1. Describe the role of the nucleus accumbens in reward.
2. Discuss cravings and their role in addiction.
3. Compare the role of genetics in substance abuse, depression, schizophrenia, and autism.
4. List important aspects of prenatal environment that may influence psychological disorders.
5. Describe medical and behavioral treatments for several psychological disorders.

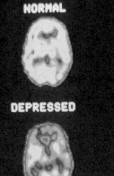

NORMAL

DEPRESSED

Substance Abuse

If you were doing something and you found that it did you more harm than good, you would stop doing it, right? That is why substance abuse (or *addiction* or *dependence*) is such a paradox. As an addiction progresses, the pleasures become weaker while the costs and risks increase. When we talk about addiction, we think mainly of alcohol and other drugs, but the same principles apply to gambling, overeating, excessive video game playing, and any other habit that dominates and harms someone's life.

Drug Mechanisms

Let's start with a brief description of how drugs work. Chapter 2 briefly mentioned the mechanisms of several drugs, but we now consider drugs from a different perspective. Most of the commonly abused drugs derive from plants. For example, nicotine comes from tobacco, caffeine from coffee and tea, opiates from poppies, and cocaine from coca. We might wonder why our brains respond to plant chemicals. An explanation is more apparent if we put it the other way: Why do plants produce chemicals that affect our brains? Nearly all neurotransmitters and hormones are the same in humans as in other species. So if a plant evolves a chemical to attract bees, repel caterpillars, or whatever, that chemical is likely to affect humans also.

Drugs either facilitate or inhibit transmission at synapses. A drug that blocks a neurotransmitter is an **antagonist**, whereas a drug that mimics or increases the effects is an **agonist.** (The term *agonist* is derived from a Greek word meaning "contestant." The term *agony* derives from the same root. An *antagonist* is an "anti-agonist," or member of the opposing team.) A *mixed agonist–antagonist* is an agonist for some effects and an antagonist for others, or an agonist at some doses and an antagonist at others.

Investigators say that a drug has an **affinity** for a receptor if it binds to it, like a key into a lock. Affinities vary from strong to weak. A drug's **efficacy** is its tendency to activate the receptor. A drug that binds to a receptor but fails to stimulate it has a high affinity but low efficacy.

The effectiveness and side effects of drugs vary from one person to another. Why? Most drugs affect several kinds of receptors. People vary in their abundance of each kind of

receptor. For example, one person might have a relatively large number of dopamine type D_4 receptors and relatively few D_1 or D_2 receptors, whereas someone else has the reverse (Cravchik & Goldman, 2000).

STOP & CHECK

1. Is a drug with high affinity and low efficacy an agonist or an antagonist?

ANSWER

1. It is an antagonist because, by occupying the receptor, it blocks out the neurotransmitter.

Predispositions

Most people drink alcohol in moderation, experiencing relaxation and decreased anxiety, whereas others develop a habit of alcohol abuse. With other substances also, some people try a drug a few times and then quit, whereas others develop an addiction. Evidently people differ in their predisposition to alcohol or drug abuse.

An important study examined brain and behavior in cases when someone with drug or alcohol abuse had a nonabusing brother or sister. Both siblings showed similar abnormalities of both gray matter and white matter, with certain brain areas larger than average and other areas smaller. Both also showed similar behavioral deficits on the stop signal task, in which the instruction is to respond quickly to a signal, but immediately inhibit the response if a second signal comes immediately after the first (Ersche et al., 2012). Evidently, certain aspects of brain and behavior are present from the start in people with a predisposition to addiction, regardless of their later substance use.

Genetic Influences

The probability of abusing alcohol or other drugs depends on both genetic and environmental influences. For example, parents' amount of alcohol use correlates with that of both biological and adopted children, although it correlates more strongly with that of the biological children (McGue, Malone, Keyes, & Iacono, 2014). Children who grow up in an unstable environment have an enhanced probability of substance use or abuse, and that probability is magnified if they also have a particular gene that affects serotonin synapses (Windle et al., 2016). Several other genes also affect the probability of substance use, but the effects vary from one environment to another (Guillot, Fanning, Liang, & Berman, 2015).

One gene with a well-confirmed influence on alcohol abuse controls the metabolism of alcohol. After anyone drinks ethyl alcohol, enzymes in the liver metabolize it to *acetaldehyde*, a toxic substance. The enzyme *acetaldehyde dehydrogenase* then converts acetaldehyde to *acetic acid*, a chemical that the body uses for energy:

$$\text{Ethyl alcohol} \xrightarrow{\quad} \underset{\text{dehydrogenase}}{\overset{\text{Acetaldehyde}}{\text{Acetaldehyde}}} \xrightarrow{\quad} \text{Acetic acid}$$

People with a gene for producing less acetaldehyde dehydrogenase metabolize acetaldehyde more slowly. If they drink much alcohol, they accumulate acetaldehyde, which produces flushing of the face, increased heart rate, nausea, headache, abdominal pain, impaired breathing, and tissue damage. Acetaldehyde is probably responsible for hangovers, although research on this topic is sparse. More than a third of the people in China and Japan have a gene that slows acetaldehyde metabolism. Probably for that reason, alcohol abuse has historically been uncommon in those countries (Luczak, Glatt, & Wall, 2006; Samochowiec, Samochowiec, Puls, Bienkowski, & Schott, 2014) (see Figure 14.1).

Environmental Influences

Prenatal environment also contributes to the risk for alcoholism. A mother who drinks alcohol during pregnancy increases the probability that her child will develop alcoholism

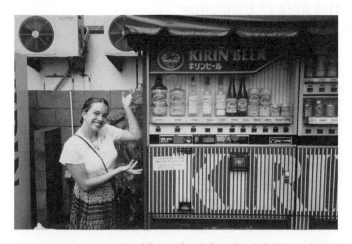

Figure 14.1 Robin Kalat (the author's daughter) finds an alcohol vending machine on a sidewalk in Tokyo in 1998
Restrictions against buying alcohol were traditionally weak in a country where most people cannot quickly metabolize acetaldehyde and therefore drink alcohol only in moderation. However, in 2000, Japan banned alcohol vending machines in public places.
(Source: James W. Kalat)

later, independently from the effect of how much she drinks as the child is growing up (Baer, Sampson, Barr, Connor, & Streissguth, 2003; Cornelius, De Genna, Goldschmidt, Larkby, & Day, 2016). Experiments with rats have also shown that prenatal exposure to alcohol increases alcohol consumption after birth (March, Abate, Spear, & Molina, 2009).

Childhood environment is critical also. Children who grow up in families with careful parental supervision are much less likely to develop impulse problems, even if they have genes linked to alcohol abuse or antisocial behavior (Dick et al., 2009). Adult environment is especially important for late-onset alcoholism. As a rule, people with early-onset alcoholism (before age 25) have a family history of alcoholism, a genetic predisposition, and a rapid onset of the problem. People with later onset are more likely to have reacted to life difficulties, less likely to have a family history of alcoholism, and more likely to respond well to treatment (Brown, Babor, Litt, & Kranzler, 1994).

STOP & CHECK

2. How does predisposition to alcohol abuse relate to how the liver metabolizes alcohol?

ANSWER

2. The liver metabolizes alcohol to acetaldehyde, which is toxic, and then to acetic acid. People whose enzymes are slow to metabolize acetaldehyde to acetic acid are less likely than others to abuse alcohol, because rapid or excessive drinking makes them ill.

Behavioral Predictors of Abuse

If genes, early environment, or anything else predisposes certain people to drug or alcohol abuse, presumably the predisposition alters behavioral reactions to the substance. If so, it should be possible to monitor behavior of young people and predict their risk for later problems. Doing so might be useful. By the time someone has developed a serious substance abuse problem, overcoming it is difficult. If we could identify people at risk before they develop a significant problem, could intervention be more successful? It is worth a try.

To identify people at risk, one strategy is to study huge numbers of people for years: Measure as many factors as possible for a group of children or adolescents, later determine which of them developed alcohol problems, and then see which early factors predicted the onset of alcoholism. Such studies find that alcoholism is more likely among those who were described in childhood as impulsive, risk taking, easily bored, sensation seeking, and outgoing (Dick, Johnson, Viken, & Rose, 2000; Legrand, Iacono, & McGue, 2005).

Other research follows this design: First, identify young men who are not yet problem drinkers. (Researchers focused first on men, because early-onset alcoholism is much more common in men than in women.) Compare men whose fathers had alcoholism to men who have no close relative with an alcohol problem. Because of the strong familial tendency

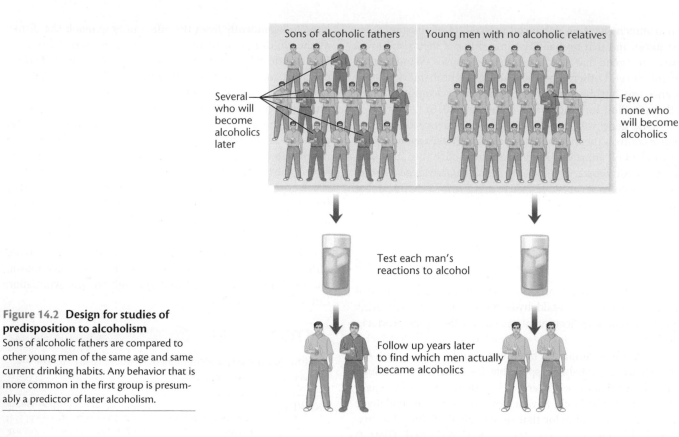

Figure 14.2 Design for studies of predisposition to alcoholism
Sons of alcoholic fathers are compared to other young men of the same age and same current drinking habits. Any behavior that is more common in the first group is presumably a predictor of later alcoholism.

toward alcoholism, researchers expect that many of the sons of alcoholics are future alcoholics themselves. The idea is that any behavior more common in the sons of alcoholics is probably a predictor of future alcoholism (see Figure 14.2).

The most robust finding is that sons of alcoholics show less than average intoxication after drinking a moderate amount of alcohol. They report feeling less drunk and show less body sway (Schuckit & Smith, 1996). Presumably, someone who starts feeling tipsy after a couple of drinks stops at that point. People who "hold their liquor well" continue drinking, perhaps enough to impair their judgment. Follow-up studies have found that men who report low intoxication after moderate drinking are more likely than others to abuse alcohol throughout their lives (Schuckit & Smith, 1997; Schuckit & Smith, 2013). Similar results have been reported for women (Eng, Schuckit, & Smith, 2005). A preliminary study with a modest number of college freshmen reported promising results based on simply explaining that if they "hold their liquor well," it is not something to brag about, but something to worry about. Students who learned that they were at increased risk tended to decrease their drinking (Schuckit et al., 2016).

✅ **STOP & CHECK** ▬▬▬▬▬▬▬

3. How do sons of alcoholics differ behaviorally, on average, from sons of nonalcoholics?

ANSWER 3. Sons of alcoholics show less intoxication, including less body sway, after drinking a moderate amount of alcohol.

Synaptic Mechanisms

Drugs affect synapses in different ways at different stages of someone's experiences. The effects while the drug is in the brain differ from effects that occur during withdrawal, and effects responsible for cravings. Efforts to alleviate drug abuse must consider a variety of mechanisms.

The Role of Dopamine

Attention to the role of dopamine in reinforcement began with a pair of young psychologists who were trying to answer an unrelated question. James Olds and Peter Milner (1954) wanted to test whether stimulation of a certain brain area might influence which direction a rat turns. When they implanted their electrode, they missed the intended target and instead hit an area called the septum. To their surprise, when the rat received the brain stimulation, it sat up, looked around, and sniffed, as if reacting to a favorable stimulus. Olds and Milner then gave rats the opportunity to press a lever to produce electrical **self-stimulation of the brain** (see Figure 14.3). With electrodes in the septum and certain other places, rats sometimes pressed as often as 2000 times per hour (Olds, 1958). Later researchers found that rats would work to stimulate many brain areas with axons that directly or indirectly increase the release of dopamine in the **nucleus accumbens**, as illustrated in Figure 14.4 (Wise, 1996).

The nucleus accumbens is important for many types of reinforcing experiences. Stimulant drugs such as cocaine and amphetamine increase or prolong the release of dopamine

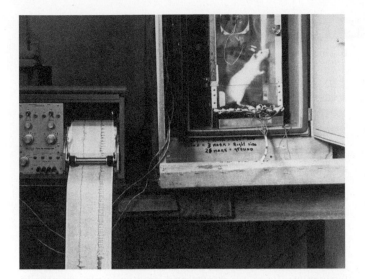

Figure 14.3 A rat pressing a lever for self-stimulation of its brain (*Source: Science Source*)

in the nucleus accumbens (Calipari & Ferris, 2013). Sexual excitement also releases dopamine there (Damsma, Pfaus, Wenkstern, Philips, & Fibiger, 1992; Lorrain, Riolo, Matuszewich, & Hull, 1999). So do music (Salimpoor et al., 2013), the taste of sugar (Roitman, Wheeler, Wightman, & Carelli, 2008), and simply imagining something pleasant (Costa, Lang, Sabatinelli, Versace, & Bradley, 2010). Gambling activates this area for habitual gamblers (Breiter, Aharon, Kahneman, Dale, & Shizgal, 2001), and video game playing activates it for habitual video game players (Ko et al., 2009; Koepp et al., 1998).

These results suggested that dopamine release might be essential for all addictions and all substance abuse. Besides

the stimulant drugs, most other abused drugs do increase dopamine release directly or indirectly. For example, nicotine stimulates neurons that release dopamine, and opiates inhibit neurons that inhibit dopamine release. However, growing evidence indicates that researchers have been overemphasizing the role of dopamine (Nutt, Lingford-Hughes, Erritzoe, & Stokes, 2015): First, although alcohol, marijuana, nicotine, and opiates do generally increase dopamine release, they do not increase it by much, and the amount of dopamine release does not correlate strongly with the pleasantness of the experience or the probability of addiction. Second, pharmaceutical companies have spent decades trying but failing to find drugs that would alleviate addictions via effects on dopamine. Drugs that block dopamine synapses do not reduce the reward properties of opiate drugs, and they do not decrease use. Although dopamine certainly contributes to reinforcement, it no longer appears to be as central as previously believed.

STOP & CHECK

4. What do drug use, sex, gambling, and video game playing have in common?
5. What evidence indicates that researchers have been overestimating the role of dopamine in addiction?

ANSWERS
4. They increase the release of dopamine in the nucleus accumbens. 5. Many drugs other than the stimulants can be highly addictive despite only small effects on dopamine synapses. Also, drugs that modify dopamine release have little effect on the use of opiates.

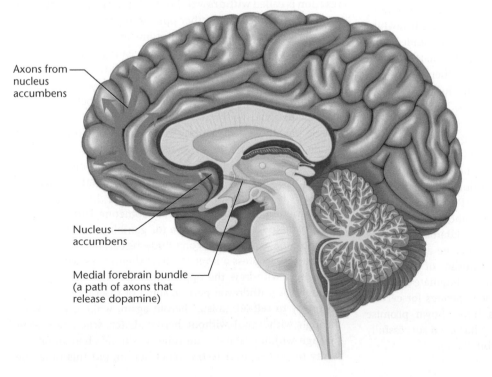

Axons from nucleus accumbens

Nucleus accumbens

Medial forebrain bundle (a path of axons that release dopamine)

Figure 14.4 The nucleus accumbens in the human brain
Many abused drugs and other reinforcing activities increase dopamine release in the nucleus accumbens.

Cravings

Addictions are persistent habits, and some evidence indicates that people with addictions have trouble breaking any habit, not just a drug habit. One study compared cocaine users to nonusers. First, all participants learned responses that would gain money or prevent electric shocks. Then the amount of money available decreased and the electric shock device was disconnected. At that point, nonusers quickly decreased their level of responding, but the cocaine users continued at close to their previous level (Ersche et al., 2016). The relevance for addiction is that a learned craving can persist long after the behavior has ceased to be rewarding. Recall from Chapter 13 a similar pattern for people with prefrontal cortex damage: After they have learned a response or a preference, they are slow to update it in response to new information.

A defining feature of addiction is **craving**, an insistent search for the substance. Even after a long period of abstinence, cues associated with the substance trigger a renewed craving. For example, seeing a lit cigarette triggers a craving in smokers (Hutchison, LaChance, Niaura, Bryan, & Smolen, 2002), a video of cocaine use triggers cravings in cocaine users (Volkow et al., 2006), and the sight of a video game triggers a craving in an excessive video game player (Thalemann, Wölfling, & Grüsser, 2007). The brain mechanism of craving differs from the response to the original activity.

Studies with laboratory rats show that exposure to addictive substances such as nicotine, cocaine, or alcohol alters neuronal structure and gene expression in several brain areas, especially if the exposure begins early in life (Korpi et al., 2015). Most of the research has used cocaine. One of the first effects of repeated cocaine use is that the nucleus accumbens, important for reward, becomes less sensitive to all types of reward, including cocaine. Thus, everyday pleasures become less intense, but users can still achieve a pleasurable state by increasing the dose or frequency of cocaine use. Meanwhile, responses to cues associated with the drug (reminders) become sensitized, attracting greater attention. That increased attention is magnified by the fact that other, competing rewards are less intense than before (Epping-Jordan, Watkins, Koob, & Markou, 1998; Volkow, Koob, & McLellan, 2016; Wolf, 2016).

Then, during a period of abstinence, the nucleus accumbens synapses responding to drug cues gradually become more and more sensitive, before later declining partly. These results match indications that craving increases during the early stage of abstinence, and slightly declines later (Parvaz, Moeller, & Goldstein, 2016; Scheyer et al., 2016). The increased response to drug cues has been traced to facilitated glutamate synapses in the nucleus accumbens, at least for cocaine and nicotine (Scofield et al., 2016; Wolf, 2016). The upshot of all this research is that a treatment that desensitizes glutamate synapses in the nucleus accumbens might reduce cravings for certain drugs. Although certain procedures have shown promise with laboratory rodents, so far nothing has been successfully applied to humans (Chesworth & Corbit, 2017).

STOP & CHECK

6. During a period of abstinence from cocaine, what happens in the nucleus accumbens?

ANSWER

6. Certain glutamate synapses in the nucleus accumbens become more responsive, causing increased excitation in response to cues associated with the substance. The result is craving, which increases for some time during abstinence.

Tolerance and Withdrawal

As an addiction develops, many of its effects, especially the enjoyable effects, decrease. That decrease is called **tolerance**. Because of tolerance, heroin users raise their amount and frequency of use to greater and greater levels, eventually taking amounts that could kill other people. Drug tolerance, a complex phenomenon, is to a large extent learned. For example, rats that consistently receive drugs in a distinctive location show more tolerance in that location than elsewhere (Cepeda-Benito, Davis, Reynoso, & Harraid, 2005; Siegel, 1983). That is, cues associated with receiving the drug activate learned mechanisms that counteract the effects of the drug. Because tolerance is learned, it can be weakened through extinction procedures. After many injections of morphine, a rat develops tolerance to it. If the rat then receives repeated injections of salt water without morphine, it weakens its learned connection between injection and morphine. The result is decreased tolerance the next time it receives a morphine injection (Siegel, 1977).

As the body comes to expect the drug under certain circumstances, it reacts strongly when the drug is absent. That reaction is called **withdrawal**. The withdrawal symptoms after someone quits heroin or other opiates include anxiety, sweating, vomiting, and diarrhea. Symptoms of alcohol withdrawal include irritability, fatigue, shaking, sweating, and nausea. In severe cases, alcohol withdrawal progresses to hallucinations, convulsions, fever, and cardiovascular problems.

One hypothesis has been that addictive behavior is an attempt to avoid withdrawal symptoms. However, that cannot be the whole explanation. Ex-smokers sometimes report strong cravings months or years after quitting. Cocaine is addictive even though the withdrawal symptoms are mild. Gambling can be a powerful addiction, even though no substance is withdrawn.

A modified explanation is that someone with an addiction learns to use the substance (or gambling habit or whatever) to cope with stress. In one study, researchers gave rats an opportunity to press a lever to inject themselves with heroin. Then they withdrew the opportunity for the drug. Midway through the withdrawal period, some of the rats had an opportunity to self-administer heroin again, while others went through withdrawal without heroin. Later, when rats went through withdrawal a second time, all the rats had an opportunity to press a lever to try to get heroin, but this time, the lever was inoperative. Although both groups of rats pressed the lever, those that had self-administered heroin during the previous withdrawal state pressed far more frequently (Hutcheson, Everitt, Robbins, & Dickinson, 2001). Evidently, receiving an addictive drug during a withdrawal period is a powerful experience. In effect, users—rat or human—learn that the drug relieves the distress caused by drug withdrawal. That learning can generalize to other situations, so that users crave the drug during other kinds of distress.

STOP & CHECK

7. Someone who is quitting an addictive substance for the first time is strongly counseled not to try it again. Why?

ANSWER

7. Taking an addictive drug during the withdrawal period is likely to lead to a habit of using the drug to relieve other kinds of distress.

Treatments

Some people who abuse alcohol or other substances manage to decrease their use without help. Those who discover that they cannot solve the problem on their own often try Alcoholics Anonymous, Narcotics Anonymous, or similar organizations, which are especially widespread in the United States. An alternative is to see a therapist, particularly a cognitive behavioral therapist. One version of therapy is *contingency management,* which includes rewards for remaining drug-free (Kaminer, 2000). Not many people turn to medications, but a few options are available.

Medications to Combat Alcohol Abuse

As mentioned, the liver metabolizes alcohol into acetaldehyde (a toxic substance) and then into acetic acid (harmless). The drug *disulfiram,* which goes by the trade name **Antabuse,** antagonizes the enzyme that metabolizes acetaldehyde. Consequently, anyone who takes Antabuse becomes nauseated after drinking alcohol. The effects of Antabuse were discovered by accident. The workers in one rubber-manufacturing plant found that when they got disulfiram on their skin, they developed a rash (Schwartz & Tulipan, 1933). If they inhaled it, they couldn't drink alcohol without getting sick. Soon therapists tried using disulfiram as a drug, hoping that those with alcoholism would associate alcohol with illness and stop drinking.

Most studies find that Antabuse is about equal to a placebo. Ordinarily, that result would indicate that a drug is ineffective, but Antabuse is a special case. When people take Antabuse, or a placebo that they think might be Antabuse, the threat of becoming ill strongly discourages any attempt to drink alcohol. As long as they do not try alcohol, of course, they do not know whether they were actually taking Antabuse. That is, Antabuse is about equal to placebo not because Antabuse is ineffective, but because thinking that a placebo might be Antabuse makes the placebo effective (Fuller & Roth, 1979; Skinner,

Lahmek, Pham, & Aubin, 2014). In either case, taking the daily pill reaffirms a pledge to avoid alcohol. Someone who takes an Antabuse pill and then drinks alcohol anyway becomes ill, and in most cases quits taking Antabuse instead of quitting alcohol.

A related idea is to have people drink alcohol and then immediately take a drug that produces nausea, thereby forming a learned aversion to the taste of the alcohol. That procedure usually produces quick and effective avoidance of alcohol, although its use has never been popular (Revusky, 2009).

Other medications are naloxone (trade name Revia) and naltrexone, which block opiate receptors and thereby decrease the pleasure from alcohol. Acamprosate is about equal to naltrexone in effectiveness, although its mechanism of effect remains uncertain (Jonas et al., 2014).

Medications to Combat Opiate Abuse

Heroin is an artificial substance invented in the 1800s as a supposedly safer alternative for people who were trying to quit morphine. Some physicians at the time recommended that people using alcohol switch to heroin (Siegel, 1987). They abandoned this idea when they discovered how addictive heroin is.

Still, the idea has persisted that people who cannot quit opiates might switch to a less harmful drug. **Methadone** (METH-uh-don), similar to heroin and morphine, activates the same brain receptors and produces the same effects. However, it has the advantage that it can be taken orally. (If heroin or morphine is taken orally, stomach acids break down most of it.) Methadone taken orally gradually enters the blood and then the brain, so its effects rise slowly, avoiding the "rush" experience that disrupts behavior. Because it is metabolized slowly and leaves the brain slowly, the withdrawal symptoms are also gradual. Furthermore, users avoid the risk of an injection with a possibly infected needle.

Buprenorphine and levomethadyl acetate (LAAM), similar to methadone, are also used to treat opiate addiction. LAAM has the advantage of producing a long-lasting effect so that the person visits a clinic three times a week instead of daily. People using any of these drugs live longer and healthier, on average, than heroin or morphine users, and they are far more likely to hold a job (Vocci, Acri, & Elkashef, 2005). However, these drugs do not end the addiction. They merely satisfy the craving in a less dangerous way.

STOP & CHECK

8. How does Antabuse work?
9. Methadone users who try taking heroin experience little effect from it. Why?

ANSWERS

8. Antabuse blocks the enzyme that converts acetaldehyde to acetic acid. It therefore makes people sick if they drink alcohol. Its effectiveness depends on the fact that someone knows or believes that drinking alcohol will cause illness. 9. Because methadone is already occupying the endorphin receptors, heroin cannot add much stimulation to them.

466 CHAPTER 14 | Psychological Disorders

Module 14.1 | In Closing

The Psychology and Biology of Substance Abuse

Many people say that alcoholism or other drug addiction is a disease. Is it? The medical profession has no firm definition of *disease.* Dis-ease is literally lack of ease, so in a sense anything that causes difficulty in life is a disease. However, the term is generally taken to imply that a disorder has a physiological basis and that medical intervention is the proper treatment.

As you have seen in this module, addiction does have a physiological basis, in part. Many genes increase the risk of

addiction. Addiction alters the brain's reaction to the drug, cues for the drug, and other events. However, none of the physiology provides a full explanation. Addiction also reflects a history of experiences. Although medical treatments sometimes help, behavioral interventions are still the most common treatments. Addiction is a complex problem that requires attention to both the physiology and the social environment.

Summary

1. A drug that increases activity at a synapse is an agonist; one that decreases activity is an antagonist. Drugs act in many ways, varying in their affinity (tendency to bind to a receptor) and efficacy (tendency to activate it). **460**

2. Predispositions to alcohol or drug abuse arise from genetics, prenatal environment, and later environment. Early-onset alcoholism reflects a stronger genetic predisposition than does later-onset alcoholism. **460**

3. People who drink alcohol with relatively little sign of intoxication are more likely than other people to develop alcohol abuse. **461**

4. Reinforcing brain stimulation, reinforcing experiences, and stimulant drugs increase the activity of axons that release dopamine in the nucleus accumbens. **462**

5. For abused drugs other than stimulants, the amount of dopamine release does not correlate well with pleasure or addiction, and blocking dopamine synapses

has little effect on opiate use. Evidently dopamine is not as essential to addiction as researchers previously believed. **463**

6. Repeated use of cocaine decreases the response of the nucleus accumbens to all pleasant experiences, but increases attention to cues reminding the individual of cocaine. **464**

7. During abstinence from cocaine, glutamate synapses in the nucleus accumbens become more responsive to cocaine-related cues. That increased sensitivity increases cue-induced cravings for cocaine. **464**

8. Repeated use of a drug leads to tolerance (decreased response) and withdrawal (unpleasant sensations during abstention). **464**

9. Several drugs including Antabuse and methadone help some people decrease their use of alcohol or opiates. **465**

Key Terms

Terms are defined in the module on the page number indicated. They're also presented in alphabetical order with definitions in the book's Subject Index/Glossary, which begins on

page 589. Interactive flash cards, audio reviews, and crossword puzzles are among the online resources available to help you learn these terms and the concepts they represent.

affinity **460**

agonist **460**

Antabuse **465**

antagonist **460**

craving **464**

efficacy **460**

methadone **465**

nucleus accumbens **462**

self-stimulation of the brain **462**

tolerance **464**

withdrawal **464**

Thought Question

The research on sensitization of the nucleus accumbens dealt with addictive drugs, mainly cocaine. Would you expect a gambling addiction to have similar effects? How could someone test this possibility?

Module 14.1 | End of Module Quiz

1. Which of the following types of drug would be a strong agonist?
   - **A.** One with high affinity and high efficacy
   - **B.** One with high affinity and low efficacy
   - **C.** One with low affinity and high efficacy
   - **D.** One with low affinity and low efficacy

2. The gene with the best-documented effect on predisposition to alcohol abuse exerts its effect in what way?
   - **A.** It alters the ratio of activity between the nucleus accumbens and the prefrontal cortex.
   - **B.** It alters how the liver metabolizes alcohol.
   - **C.** It alters the sensitivity of certain types of taste buds.
   - **D.** It alters the rate of secretion of stomach acid.

3. What evidence demonstrates predisposition toward drug or alcohol abuse?
   - **A.** Siblings of someone with drug addiction also show abnormalities of brain and behavior.
   - **B.** People with drug addiction remember having a positive experience in their first encounter with the drug.
   - **C.** Most young people can accurately predict whether they will eventually develop a drug addiction.
   - **D.** An fMRI study on newborns accurately predicted which ones would later develop drug addiction.

4. Genetic predisposition is most strongly evident for which type of alcohol abuser?
   - **A.** People with early-onset alcohol abuse
   - **B.** People with late-onset alcohol abuse
   - **C.** Women
   - **D.** Immigrants to a country

5. Of the following, which type of person is more likely than average to abuse alcohol?
   - **A.** Someone who shows little effect after moderate drinking
   - **B.** Someone who becomes intoxicated quickly after moderate drinking
   - **C.** Someone who was reared with strict rules in childhood
   - **D.** Someone with an introverted personality

6. What is the relationship between drug abuse and dopamine?
   - **A.** Probability of abusing a drug correlates strongly with how much dopamine it releases.
   - **B.** People seldom abuse the drugs that release dopamine.
   - **C.** Blocking dopamine synapses prevents any pleasure from a drug.
   - **D.** Most abused drugs release dopamine, but not in proportion to addictive potential.

7. What is the effect on the nucleus accumbens after repeated cocaine use?
   - **A.** The nucleus accumbens becomes less responsive to rewarding experiences.
   - **B.** The nucleus accumbens becomes more responsive to rewarding experiences.
   - **C.** The nucleus accumbens responds to events that were not previously rewarding.
   - **D.** The nucleus accumbens begins growing new neurons.

8. What accounts for increased cravings during cocaine abstinence?
   - **A.** Increased activity of certain enzymes in the liver.
   - **B.** Increased responsiveness of dopamine synapses to all types of reward.
   - **C.** Increased sensitivity of glutamate synapses to cues for cocaine.
   - **D.** Rapid fluctuations of heart beat.

9. What evidence indicates that tolerance is to a large extent learned?
   - **A.** Tolerance is greater in the location where one previously took the drug than elsewhere.
   - **B.** Tolerance is greater in highly educated people than in poorly educated people.
   - **C.** Tolerance is easily forgotten with the passage of time.
   - **D.** Telling people about the effects of a drug can produce tolerance.

10. In tests of Antabuse effectiveness, why are placebos so effective?
    - **A.** Antabuse has no physiological effects.
    - **B.** The chemicals used as placebos interact with liver enzymes.
    - **C.** Antabuse is effective mainly by the threat of illness after drinking.
    - **D.** Placebos tend to relieve pain.

11. What is the advantage of taking methadone instead of morphine or heroin?
    - **A.** Methadone is not addictive.
    - **B.** Someone can gradually taper off methadone and become drug-free.
    - **C.** Methadone is readily available without a prescription.
    - **D.** Methadone satisfies the craving without seriously disrupting behavior.

Answers: 1A, 2B, 3A, 4A, 5A, 6D, 7A, 8C, 9A, 10C, 11D.

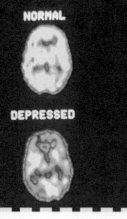
Module 14.2

Mood Disorders

Is it depressing to read about depression? It might be, but we shall spend much of this module considering how to relieve depression. People with depression look sad and act sad (see Figure 14.5), but most do recover.

Major Depressive Disorder

Everyone has times of feeling discouraged. Major depression is much more intense and prolonged. People with a **major depression** feel sad and helpless most of the day every day for weeks at a time. They can hardly even imagine enjoying anything. Their nucleus accumbens becomes less responsive to reward (Russo & Nestler, 2013). They feel worthless, contemplate suicide, and have trouble sleeping. They also have cognitive problems, including low motivation, attention problems, impaired memory, and impaired sense of smell. The cognitive limitations often persist even after successful treatment of the mood problems (Gonda et al., 2015; Siopi et al., 2016).

Absence of happiness is a more reliable symptom than increased sadness. In one study, people carried a beeper that sounded at unpredictable times to signal them to describe their emotional reactions at the moment. People with depression reported only an average number of unpleasant experiences but far below the average number of pleasant ones (Peters, Nicolson, Berkhof, Delespaul, & deVries, 2003). In other studies, people examined photographs or films as researchers recorded their reactions. People with depression reacted normally to sad or frightening depictions but seldom smiled at the comedies or pleasant pictures (Rottenberg, Kasch, Gross, & Gotlib, 2002; Sloan, Strauss, & Wisner, 2001).

Surveys have reported that about 5 to 6 percent of adults in the United States and Canada have a clinically significant depression (i.e., serious enough to warrant attention) within a given year, and more than 10 percent do at some point in life (Narrow, Rae, Robins, & Regier, 2002; Patten et al., 2015). Depression is more common in women than in men during the reproductive era, but about equal before puberty and after menopause (Mendle, Eisenlohr-Moul, & Kiesner, 2016). The reason for this trend is not known.

Although some people suffer from long-term depression, it is more common to have episodes of depression separated by periods of normal mood. Several studies reported that the

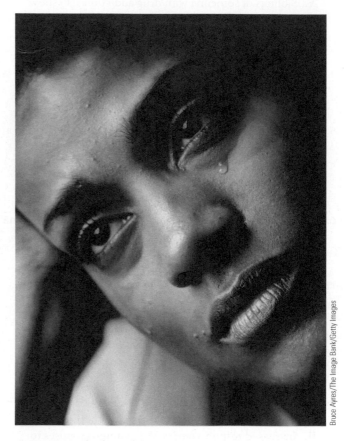

Bruce Ayres/The Image Bank/Getty Images

Figure 14.5 The face of depression
Depression shows in people's face, walk, voice, and mannerisms.

early episodes tend to be longer, whereas later episodes tend to be briefer but more frequent (e.g., Post, 1992). Although that idea seemed plausible, a later analysis showed that it reflected a statistical artifact: Suppose you measure the mean length of all first episodes. That will include anyone who ever became depressed, including some who had just one episode lasting many years. When you measure the mean length of all fifth episodes or all tenth episodes, you can study only people who had at least five or ten episodes. To have that many episodes, necessarily each of them had to be brief. So the comparison is invalid. If you compare the length of, say, first and fifth episodes but include only people who had at least five episodes, the mean length is about the same (Anderson, Monroe, Rohde, & Lewinsohn, 2016). The conclusion is simply that some people have shorter episodes, and possibly more of them, than other people do.

Genetics

Studies of twins and adopted children indicate a moderate degree of heritability for depression (Shih, Belmonte, & Zandi, 2004). Genetic factors are certainly not the only cause of depression. Several studies have found increased activity of the immune system, which can arise from injury, highly stressful experiences, poor diet, or other causes (Hodes, Kana, Menard, Merad, & Russo, 2015; Kaplan, Rucklidge, Romijn, & McLeod, 2015; Wohleb, Franklin, Iwata, & Duman, 2016).

Although many studies have identified one or more genes as being associated with depression, the results vary from one study to another (Cohen-Woods, Craig, & McGuffin, 2013). A likely explanation is that different genetic variations occur in different populations. A study of Chinese women with recurrent severe depression identified two genes with a strong effect. Those genes did not emerge in studies on Europeans, simply because those genes are rare in Europe (CONVERGE Consortium, 2015).

Another reason why it is hard to find a gene linked to depression is that when we talk about depression, we may be combining separate syndromes. People with early-onset depression (before age 30) have a high probability of having other relatives with depression (Bierut et al., 1999; Kendler, Gardner, & Prescott, 1999; Lyons et al., 1998), as well as relatives with anxiety disorders, neuroticism, attention deficit disorder, alcohol or marijuana abuse, obsessive-compulsive disorder, bulimia, migraine headaches, and irritable bowel syndrome (Fu et al., 2002; Gade, Kristoffersen, & Kessing, 2014; Hudson et al., 2003). Early-onset depression also tends to be more severe, more long-lasting, and more associated with suicidal tendencies (Park, Sohn, Seong, Suk, & Cho, 2015). People with late-onset depression (especially after age 45 to 50) have a high probability of relatives with circulatory problems (Kendler, Fiske, Gardner, & Gatz, 2009). Researchers have begun looking for genes that might be associated specifically with early-onset or late-onset depression (Power et al., 2012).

Another issue is that the effect of a gene varies with the environment. Much research concerns the gene that controls the serotonin transporter, a protein that regulates the ability of axons to reabsorb serotonin after its release. Investigators examined the serotonin transporter genes of 847 young adults, identifying two types: the *short* type and the *long* type. Each participant reported major stressful events over five years, such as financial setbacks, loss of job, and divorce. Figure 14.6 shows the results. For people with two short forms of the gene, increasing numbers of stressful experiences led to a major increase in the probability of depression. For those with two long forms, stressful events only slightly increased the risk of depression. Those with one short and one long gene were intermediate. In other words, the short form of the gene by itself

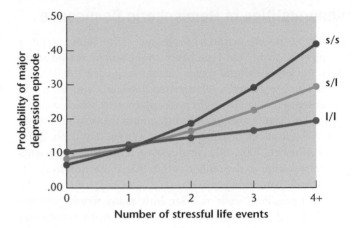

Figure 14.6 Genetics, stress, and depression
The effect of the serotonin transporter gene depended on the amount of stress.
(Source: From "Influence of life stress on depression: Moderation by a polymorphism in the 5-HTT gene," by A. Caspi et al., Science, 301, 2003, pp. 386–389. Reprinted with permission. © 2003 AAAS.)

did not lead to depression, but it magnified the reaction to stressful events (Caspi et al., 2003).

Although not all studies have replicated this result, an extensive review of the literature confirmed that the short form of the serotonin transporter gene increases the risk of a depressive reaction to major stressors, especially the stress of early childhood maltreatment (Karg, Burmeister, Shedden, & Sen, 2011). However, we should not think of the gene as a "risk for depression" gene. The same gene increases smiles, laughter, or anger depending on the event (Gyurak et al., 2013; Haase et al., 2015). That is, the short form of the serotonin transporter gene increases emotional reactivity of almost any type, good or bad.

Considering the high prevalence of depression and the links to genetics, evolutionary psychologists have raised the possibility that our ancestors evolved a tendency to become depressed under certain conditions. In particular, depression could be an adaptation to conserve energy after a defeat of some sort. It is possible that depression served a valid purpose for many of our ancestors after physical injuries, even if it is maladaptive today after more symbolic types of setback (Beck & Bredemeier, 2016).

✓ STOP & CHECK

10. What evidence suggests two types of depression are influenced by different genes?
11. What did Caspi and colleagues report to be the relationship between depression and genetics?

ANSWERS 10. Relatives of people with early-onset depression have a high risk of depression and many other psychological disorders. Relatives of people with late-onset depression have a high probability of circulatory problems. 11. People with the short form of the gene controlling the serotonin transporter are more likely than other people to react to stressful experiences by becoming depressed. However, in the absence of stressful experiences, their probability is not increased.

Abnormalities of Hemispheric Dominance

Studies of people without depression have found a fairly strong relationship between happy mood and increased activity in the left prefrontal cortex (Jacobs & Snyder, 1996). Most studies have reported a relationship between depression and increased activity in the right prefrontal cortex, which is stable over years despite changes in symptoms of depression (Davidson, 1984; Jesulola, Sharpley, Bitsika, Agnew, & Wilson, 2015; Pizzagalli et al., 2002; Vuga et al., 2006). It probably represents a predisposition to depression rather than a reaction to it.

Here's something you can try: Ask someone to solve a verbal problem, such as, "See how many words you can think of that start with *sa-*," or "see how many words you can think of that end with -us." Unobtrusively watch the person's eye movements. Most people gaze to the right during verbal tasks, suggesting left hemisphere dominance, but most individuals with depression gaze to the left (Lenhart & Katkin, 1986).

TRY IT YOURSELF

✅ **STOP & CHECK**

12. Some people offer to train you to use the right hemisphere of your brain more strongly, allegedly to increase creativity. If they were successful, can you see any disadvantage?

ANSWER

12. People with predominant right-hemisphere activity show an increased tendency toward depression.

Antidepressant Drugs

You might assume that investigators first determine the causes of a psychological disorder and then develop medications based on the causes. The opposite order has been more common: First investigators found drugs that seemed helpful, and then they tried to figure out how they work. Iproniazid, the first antidepressant drug, was originally marketed to treat tuberculosis, until physicians noticed that it relieved depression. Similarly, chlorpromazine was originally used for other purposes, until physicians noticed its ability to alleviate schizophrenia. For decades, researchers sought new drugs entirely by trial and error. Today, researchers evaluate new potential drugs in test tubes or tissue samples until they find one with a potential for strong or specific effects on neurotransmission. The result is the use of fewer laboratory animals.

Types of Antidepressants

Antidepressant drugs fall into several categories, including tricyclics, selective serotonin reuptake inhibitors, monoamine oxidase inhibitors, and atypical antidepressants. The **tricyclics** (e.g., imipramine, trade name Tofranil) operate by blocking the transporter proteins that reabsorb serotonin, dopamine, and norepinephrine into the presynaptic neuron

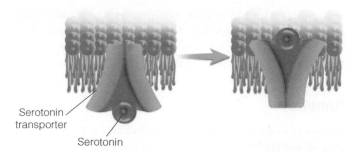

Serotonin transporter

Serotonin

Figure 14.7 Reuptake of serotonin into the presynaptic neuron The serotonin transporter protein is open to the outside of the neuron on the left. After it picks up a serotonin molecule, it flips position to deliver the serotonin to the inside of the presynaptic neuron. Tricyclic and SSRI antidepressants lock the transporter protein into the position shown at the left, preventing reuptake.

after their release. Figure 14.7 shows how the serotonin transporter protein picks up a serotonin molecule outside the membrane and then flips into position to deliver the molecule to the inside of the neuron. A tricyclic drug locks the transporter into the initial position, as shown on the left of the figure (Penmatsa, Wang, & Gouaux, 2013; H. Wang et al., 2013). The result is to prolong the presence of the neurotransmitters in the synaptic cleft, where they continue stimulating the postsynaptic cell. Tricyclics also block histamine receptors, acetylcholine receptors, and certain sodium channels (Horst & Preskorn, 1998). Blocking histamine produces drowsiness. Blocking acetylcholine leads to dry mouth and difficulty urinating. Blocking sodium channels causes heart irregularities, among other problems. People have to limit their use of tricyclic drugs to minimize these side effects.

The **selective serotonin reuptake inhibitors (SSRIs)** are similar to tricyclics but specific to the neurotransmitter serotonin. They attach to the center of the serotonin transporter protein and lock it into a shape that prevents serotonin from binding to it (Coleman, Green, & Gouaux, 2016). SSRIs produce milder side effects than the tricyclics, but their effectiveness is about the same. Common SSRIs include fluoxetine (trade name Prozac), sertraline (Zoloft), fluvoxamine (Luvox), citalopram (Celexa), and paroxetine (Paxil or Seroxat). As you might guess, **serotonin norepinephrine reuptake inhibitors (SNRIs)**, such as duloxetine (Cymbalta) and venlafaxine (Effexor), block reuptake of both serotonin and norepinephrine. Unlike other antidepressants, the SNRIs improve certain aspects of memory (Feltmann, Konradsson-Geuken, De Bundel, Lindskog, & Schilström, 2015). Many patients now take two or more drugs with different modes of action, although the effectiveness of this approach is uncertain (Millan, 2014).

The **monoamine oxidase inhibitors (MAOIs)** (e.g., phenelzine, trade name Nardil) block the enzyme monoamine oxidase (MAO), a presynaptic enzyme that metabolizes catecholamines and serotonin into inactive forms. When MAOIs block this enzyme, the presynaptic terminal has more of its transmitter available for release. The MAOIs were the earliest

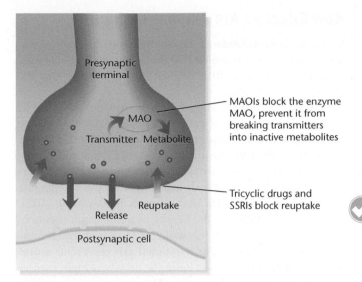

Figure 14.8 Routes of action of antidepressants
Tricyclics block the reuptake of dopamine, norepinephrine, and serotonin. SSRIs specifically block the reuptake of serotonin. SNRIs block reuptake of serotonin and norepinephrine. MAOIs block the enzyme MAO, which converts dopamine, norepinephrine, or serotonin into inactive chemicals.

antidepressants, but they are no longer the first choice for treatment. People taking MAOIs must avoid foods containing tyramine—including cheese, raisins, and many others—because a combination of tyramine and MAOIs increases blood pressure. Figure 14.8 summarizes the mechanisms of tricyclics, SSRIs, and MAOIs.

The **atypical antidepressants** include everything other than the types just discussed (Horst & Preskorn, 1998). One example is bupropion (Wellbutrin), which inhibits reuptake of dopamine and to some extent norepinephrine but not serotonin. Although antidepressants vary in which neurotransmitter(s) they target—serotonin, dopamine, norepinephrine, or some combination—all appear to be nearly equal in their effectiveness (Montgomery et al., 2007; Undurraga & Baldessarini, 2012).

Drug companies have not offered anything substantially new for depression in decades, but a couple of new possibilities are on the horizon. Ketamine, which antagonizes NMDA-type glutamate receptors but also increases formation of new synapses, produces rapid antidepressant effects in patients who don't respond to other medications. However, it also often produces hallucinations and delusions, and its benefits are not long-lasting (Bunney & Bunney, 2012; Duman & Aghajanian, 2012). Ketamine itself would not be a suitable antidepressant, but preliminary results suggest that one of ketamine's metabolites might be a potential candidate (Zanos et al., 2016).

Many people use St. John's wort, an herb, as an antidepressant. Because it is a nutritional supplement instead of a drug, the U.S. Food and Drug Administration does not regulate it, and its purity varies from one bottle to another. It has the advantage of being less expensive than antidepressant drugs. An advantage or disadvantage, depending on

your point of view, is that it is available without prescription. People can get it easily but often take inappropriate amounts. Its effectiveness appears to be comparable to that of standard antidepressant drugs (Sarris, Panossian, Schweitzer, Stough, & Scholey, 2011), but it has a worrisome side effect: St. John's wort increases the effectiveness of a liver enzyme that breaks down plant toxins, and also breaks down most medicines. Therefore, taking St. John's wort decreases the effectiveness of other drugs you might be taking—including other antidepressant drugs, cancer drugs, and AIDS drugs (He, Yang, Li, Du, & Zhou, 2010; Moore et al., 2000).

STOP & CHECK

13. What are the effects of tricyclic drugs?
14. What are the effects of SSRIs?
15. What are the effects of MAOIs?

ANSWERS

13. Tricyclic drugs block reuptake of serotonin and catecholamines. They also block histamine receptors, acetylcholine receptors, and certain sodium channels, thereby producing unpleasant side effects. 14. SSRIs selectively inhibit the reuptake of serotonin. 15. MAOIs block the enzyme MAO, which breaks down catecholamines and serotonin. The result is increased availability of these transmitters.

How Are Antidepressants Effective?

When researchers discovered that all the common antidepressants increase the availability of serotonin and other neurotransmitters, they at first assumed that the cause of depression was a deficiency of serotonin or other neurotransmitters. Gradually it became clear that this simple explanation cannot work. People with depression have approximately normal levels of neurotransmitters, and some studies have found *increased* serotonin release (Barton et al., 2008). Furthermore, it is possible to decrease serotonin levels suddenly by a diet with all the amino acids except tryptophan, the precursor to serotonin. For most people, this decrease in serotonin does not provoke any feelings of depression (Neumeister et al., 2004, 2006).

A major theoretical difficulty comes from the time course: Antidepressants produce their effects on neurotransmitters in the synapses within minutes to hours, depending on the drug, but people generally need to take the drugs for at least 2 weeks before they experience significant mood elevation (Stewart et al., 1998). Clearly, the current level of neurotransmitters does not explain depression or the benefits of the drugs.

How else might we explain the effects of antidepressant drugs? One hypothesis concerns neurotrophins. As discussed in Chapter 4, neurotrophins aid in the survival, growth, and connections of neurons. Most people with depression have lower than average levels of a neurotrophin called *brain-derived neurotrophic factor* (BDNF) that is important for synaptic plasticity, learning, and proliferation of new neurons in the hippocampus (Martinowich, Manji, & Lu, 2007; Sen, Duman, & Sanacora, 2008). As a result of low BDNF, most people with depression have a smaller than average hippocampus, impaired learning, and reduced production of new hippocampal neurons. Many studies suggest that antidepressant drugs increase BDNF levels, over the course of weeks (consistent with the time course for antidepressants to take effect), although the results have not been entirely consistent (Drzyzga, Marcinowska, & Obuchowicz, 2009; Matrisciano et al., 2008; Maya Vetencourt et al., 2008).

The proliferation of new neurons in the hippocampus, associated with new learning, does appear to be important for antidepressant effects. Procedures that block neuron production also block the behavioral benefits of antidepressant drugs (Airan et al., 2007). The importance of new learning may explain why antidepressants don't elevate the mood of people who are not depressed: Those people are not burdened with discouraging thoughts that they need to unlearn (Castrén & Rantamäki, 2010). However, the formation of new neurons is not the whole explanation for antidepressant drugs, as the drugs also exert essential effects on mature hippocampal neurons (Samuels et al., 2015).

✓ STOP & CHECK ▆▆▆▆▆

16. In what way does the time course of antidepressants conflict with the idea that they improve mood by increasing neurotransmitter levels?

17. As opposed to an interpretation in terms of neurotransmitter levels, what is an alternative explanation for the benefits of antidepressant drugs?

ANSWERS

16. Antidepressants produce their effects on serotonin and other neurotransmitters quickly, but their behavioral benefits develop gradually over 2 to 3 weeks. 17. Antidepressant drugs increase production of BDNF, which gradually promotes growth of new neurons in the hippocampus and new learning.

How Effective Are Antidepressants?

So far we have considered explanations of how antidepressants work. How sure are we that they *do* work? Not everyone is convinced (Kirsch, 2010), and we must at least say that the effectiveness is limited.

Most controlled studies find that antidepressants are at least moderately more effective than placebos, although the effect of placebos is strong and apparently increasing in recent years. Even when the advantage over placebos is statistically significant, it may be only slight in a clinical sense, and antidepressants have apparently little effect on the suicide rate (Bschor & Kilarski, 2016; Undurraga & Baldessarini, 2012). Figure 14.9 summarizes the results of many experiments in which people were randomly assigned to receive antidepressant drugs or placebos. The horizontal axis represents scores on the Hamilton Depression Rating Scale, where higher scores indicate more intense depression. The vertical axis represents amount of improvement. Triangles represent patients receiving the drug in a study, and circles represent patients receiving a placebo. The size of the triangle or circle is proportional to the number of patients in a group. Many people respond well on placebos, either because of spontaneous recovery over time or because of the expectation that comes from taking a pill. For patients with mild to moderate depression, the results for placebo groups overlap those for drug groups, and the differences between the groups appear too small to be meaningful. Only for people with severe depression did the drugs show a meaningful advantage (Kirsch et al., 2008).

For several reasons, it is possible that these data understate the effectiveness of the drugs. Some studies have used doses too low to get a reliable effect (Hieronymus, Nilsson, & Eriksson, 2016). Also, the Hamilton Depression Rating Scale is less reliable at lower levels of depression (Isaacson & Adler,

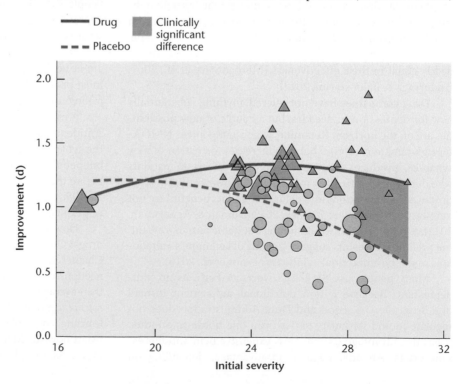

Figure 14.9 Mean improvement from depression by people taking antidepressants or placebos
Pink triangles represent people taking medications in a particular study. Gray circles represent people taking placebos. The size of the triangle or circle is proportional to the number of people in the study.
(Source: From Kirsch et al., 2008.)

2012). That is, it measures improvement for patients with severe depression more accurately than for patients with mild or moderate depression. Therefore, we should not necessarily conclude that the drugs are useful only in severe depression (Fountoulakis, Veroniki, Siamouli, & Moller, 2013). Nevertheless, the point remains that antidepressant drugs are only moderately helpful for most patients with depression, and in many cases not helpful at all.

When people take antidepressants, many fail to show any benefit from the first drug they try. After 6 weeks or so, the physician prescribes a different drug, and then if necessary another one, and so forth. It is not possible to predict which drug will work best for a given patient, so it is strictly a trial-and-error process. Switching to a different type of drug (SSRI versus tricyclic, for example) is no more likely to be helpful than switching to a drug of the same type. Most patients eventually show a favorable response to one of the drugs (Keers & Uher, 2012). However, at that point, how can we be sure the new drug was responsible for the improved mood? Depression occurs in episodes. That is, even without treatment, most people recover within a few months. When someone goes through a series of drugs before one of them finally seems to work, we don't know whether the patient would have recovered just as fast on the first drug, or without any drug at all. Unfortunately, many research studies have failed to include adequate control groups.

Alternatives to Antidepressant Drugs

Cognitive behavioral therapy and other forms of psychotherapy are often helpful. Reviews of the research literature find that antidepressant drugs and psychotherapy are about equally effective for treating all levels of depression, from mild to severe (Bortolotti, Menchetti, Bellini, Montaguti, & Berardi, 2008). Of course, considering that much of the response to antidepressant drugs is a placebo effect, the same must be true for psychotherapy. The effects of antidepressants and those of psychotherapy overlap more than we might have guessed. Brain scans show that antidepressants and psychotherapy increase metabolism in the same brain areas (Brody et al., 2001; S. D. Martin et al., 2001). That similarity should not be terribly surprising if we accept mind–body monism. If mental activity is the same thing as brain activity, then changing someone's thoughts should indeed change brain chemistry.

Psychotherapy has an advantage because its effects are more likely to last. That is, a relapse into depression is more likely after antidepressant drug treatment than after psychotherapy (Steinert, Hofmann, Kruse, & Leichsenring, 2014).

Would a combination of antidepressant drugs and psychotherapy work better than either one alone? On average, people receiving both treatments show more rapid improvement than people receiving either one alone, but the percentage of people showing improvement increases only slightly (de Maat et al., 2008; Hollon et al., 2014). If some people responded better to drugs and others to psychotherapy, we should expect the combination to help a much higher percentage of people, because everyone would be getting whichever one worked best.

Evidently, not many people respond to one treatment and not the other. Some people recover over time with no treatment or a placebo, another group improves equally well with either antidepressants or psychotherapy, a few respond better to one than to the other, and the remainder—one-third to one-half of all patients, by most estimates—do not respond well to either one (Friedman et al., 2009; Hollon, Thase, & Markowitz, 2002; Thase et al., 1997).

✓ STOP & CHECK

18. As depression becomes more severe, what happens to the percentage of patients showing improvement while taking antidepressant drugs or placebos?
19. What is an advantage of psychotherapy over antidepressant drugs?

ANSWERS 18. For more severe cases, the percentage of patients who improve remains about the same for patients taking antidepressant drugs, but fewer patients taking placebos show improvement. 19. People who respond well to psychotherapy have a lower risk of later relapse than people who respond to antidepressant drugs. Also, antidepressant drugs produce unpleasant side effects.

Electroconvulsive Therapy (ECT)

Another option, despite its stormy history, is treatment through an electrically induced seizure, known as **electroconvulsive therapy (ECT)**. ECT originated with the observation that for people with both epilepsy and schizophrenia, when symptoms of one disorder increase, symptoms of the other often decrease (Trimble & Thompson, 1986). In the 1930s, Ladislas Meduna and other physicians tried to relieve schizophrenia by inducing convulsions with a large dose of insulin. Insulin shock is a dreadful experience, however, and difficult to control. An Italian physician, Ugo Cerletti, after years of experimentation with animals, developed a method of inducing seizures with an electric shock through the head (Cerletti & Bini, 1938). Electroconvulsive therapy is quick, and most patients awaken calmly without remembering it.

Psychiatrists had only this shaky theoretical basis for expecting ECT to be helpful for schizophrenia. When it proved to be ineffective in most cases, you might guess that they would abandon it. Instead, they tried it for patients with other disorders, for whom they had no theoretical reason to expect it to work. Surprisingly, ECT did relieve depression in many cases. However, its misuse during the 1950s earned it a bad reputation, as some patients were given ECT hundreds of times without their consent and without any apparent benefit.

When antidepressant drugs became available in the late 1950s, the use of ECT declined abruptly. However, in the 1970s, psychiatrists brought back ECT for the patients who were not responding to the drugs. Today therapists use ECT mostly for patients with severe depression who have not responded to antidepressant drugs, and it is effective in most cases (Reisner, 2003). In most cases it is given

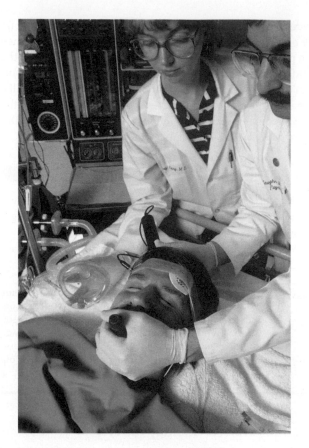

Figure 14.10 Electroconvulsive therapy (ECT)
In contrast to an earlier era, ECT today is administered with muscle
relaxants or anesthetics to minimize discomfort.
(Source: Will & Deni McIntyre / Science Source)

only with the patient's informed consent, although sometimes a court order requires it, such as for a patient at high
risk for suicide. Ordinarily it is applied every other day for
about 2 weeks. Patients are given muscle relaxants or anesthetics to minimize discomfort and the possibility of injury
(see Figure 14.10).

The most common side effect of ECT is memory impairment, but limiting the shock to the right hemisphere reduces
the memory loss. In any case, the memory impairment usually lasts only a few months, not forever (Reisner, 2003). The
main drawback to ECT is the high risk of relapse. Compared
to psychotherapy or antidepressant drugs, ECT generally
acts faster, but its benefits are less likely to persist. To prevent relapse, a patient periodically returns for additional ECT
treatments for at least several months, or follows ECT with
other treatments.

More than half a century after the introduction of ECT,
no one is yet sure how it relieves depression, but like antidepressant drugs, ECT increases the proliferation of new
neurons in the hippocampus (Perera et al., 2007). Most studies find that it increases BDNF levels, which antidepressant
drugs also increase, but this increase may or may not be related to the therapeutic benefits (Freire, Fleck, & da Rocha,
2016; Rocha et al., 2016).

Exercise and Diet

The simplest, least expensive antidepressant treatment is a
program of regular, moderate-intensity exercise (Leppämäki,
Partonen, & Lönnqvist, 2002). Controlled experiments have
confirmed modest antidepressant benefits, especially for
people over age 60 (Bridle, Spanjers, Patel, Atherton, &
Lamb, 2012). Even something so simple as walking improves
positive mood (Miller & Krizan, 2016). Exercise is best used
as a supplement to other treatments rather than as a therapy
by itself.

Several types of diet supplements are also worth considering. Research has suggested some value to omega-3
fatty acids, which are important for neuron membranes,
and vitamins B_6, B_9, and B_{12}. However, the research has not
been extensive or entirely conclusive (McGorry, Nelson, &
Markulev, 2017; Rechenberg, 2016).

Altered Sleep Patterns

Almost everyone with depression has sleep problems, and the
sleep problems generally precede the mood changes. Many
studies have reported that people who have trouble sleeping
are at high risk for later depression (Li, Wu, Gan, Qu, & Lu,
2016). The usual sleep pattern for someone with depression
resembles the sleep of healthy people who have traveled a couple of time zones west: They fall asleep when the clock says to
do so, but they enter REM sleep sooner than normal, and they
awaken early, as Figure 14.11 illustrates.

If you stay awake all night, how do you feel the next morning? Most people feel groggy and grouchy. Surprisingly, most
people with depression feel substantially improved (Benedetti
& Colombo, 2011). (Presumably someone discovered this
therapy by accident. It's hard to imagine any logical reason to
have tried it.) However, although the benefit from sleep deprivation is rapid, it is also brief, as depression usually returns
after the next night's sleep.

Another approach is to alter the sleep schedule, going to
bed hours earlier than usual. That is, if your circadian rhythm
is shifted, so why not sleep earlier, in phase with your rhythm?
The person then gets a normal amount of sleep with normal
timing of REM sleep. This procedure usually relieves depression quickly and its benefits last for a week or more (Riemann
et al., 1999). Eventually, however, the circadian rhythm shifts
again, as if the person had traveled a couple additional time
zones west without adjusting. So far, phase-advancing the
sleep schedule has not become a popular therapy, perhaps in
part because people have social reasons for wanting to stay
awake after early evening.

Still, the effectiveness of either sleep deprivation or a
change in sleep schedule implies that depression is related
to having a circadian rhythm out of phase with the environment. Supporting evidence comes from the phenomenon of **seasonal affective disorder (SAD)**—depression
that recurs during a particular season, such as winter. SAD
is most prevalent near the poles, where the winter nights
are long (Haggarty et al., 2002). In contrast to most other

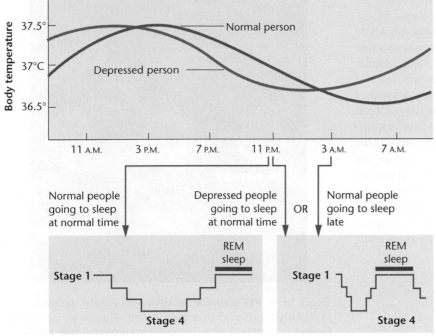

Figure 14.11 **Circadian rhythms and depression**
Most people with depression have their circadian rhythms advanced by several hours. They sleep as if they had gone to bed later than they actually did.
(*Source: Bottom graphs from Sleep, by J. Allan Hobson, ©1989, 1995 by J. Allan Hobson. Reprinted by permission of Henry Holt and Company, LLC.*)

patients with depression, who have phase-advanced circadian rhythms, people with seasonal affective disorder have phase-delayed rhythms (Teicher et al., 1997) (see Figure 14.12). Many people with SAD have a mutation in one of the genes responsible for regulating the circadian rhythm (Johansson et al., 2003).

It is possible to treat SAD with very bright lights—2500 lux for a couple of hours each morning, or even brighter lights for a shorter time (Dallaspezia, Suzuki, & Benedetti, 2015; Pail et al., 2011). Presumably this treatment works by resetting the circadian rhythm, although the research is not conclusive on that point. Regardless of the mechanisms, the benefits are substantial. Researchers have now tested bright-light therapy for nonseasonal depression, with results at least as good as those for antidepressant drugs, with quicker benefits (usually within one week), lower cost, and much less risk of side effects (Al-Karawi & Jubair, 2016; Dallaspezia et al., 2015).

✓ STOP & CHECK

20. What are the advantages and disadvantages of ECT?
21. What change in sleep habits sometimes relieves depression?
22. What are the advantages of bright-light treatment compared to antidepressant drugs?

ANSWERS 20. ECT helps many people who do not respond to antidepressant drugs or psychotherapy, and its benefits usually develop relatively quickly. However, the probability of a quick relapse is high. 21. Going to bed earlier sometimes relieves depression. 22. It is cheaper, has little risk of side effects, and produces its benefits more quickly.

Deep Brain Stimulation

Suppose you are getting desperate. You tried psychotherapy, you tried one antidepressant drug after another, you tried ECT, you exercised, and you changed your sleep schedule.

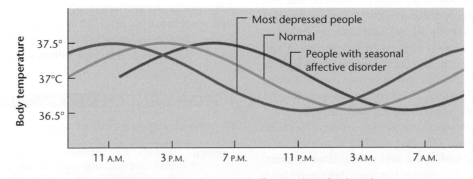

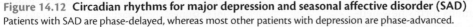

Figure 14.12 **Circadian rhythms for major depression and seasonal affective disorder (SAD)**
Patients with SAD are phase-delayed, whereas most other patients with depression are phase-advanced.

Nothing worked, and you are still miserably depressed. Do you have any other hope?

Another option is certainly not the first thing you would try: With **deep brain stimulation**, a physician implants a battery-powered device into the brain to deliver periodic stimulation to certain brain areas. Those areas are chosen because of studies showing that they increase their activity as a result of antidepressant drugs. Deep brain stimulation for depression is still in the experimental stage, but results have been encouraging. Most patients who failed to respond to all other treatments show gradual improvement over months, and about half get fully back to normal, as long as the stimulation continues (Riva-Posse, Holtzheimer, Garlow, & Mayberg, 2013). A possible refinement of this procedure is to use optogenetic stimulation, as described in Chapter 3. Optogenetic stimulation can control individual connections, rather than all the axons going from one area to another (Deisseroth, 2014).

Bipolar Disorder

Depression can be either unipolar or bipolar. People with unipolar depression vary between normality and depression. People with **bipolar disorder**, formerly known as *manic-depressive disorder*, alternate between two poles—depression and its opposite, mania. **Mania** is characterized by restless activity, excitement, laughter, excessive self-confidence, rambling speech, and loss of inhibitions. Some people with bipolar disorder have full-fledged manic episodes (known as *bipolar I disorder*), and some have mild or hypomanic episodes (*bipolar II disorder*). Bipolar disorder usually has its onset in the teenage years or early 20s. Although it is about equally common for men and women, men are more likely to have severe (bipolar I) cases, but women are more likely to get treatment (Merikangas & Pato, 2009).

Figure 14.13 shows the brain's increase in glucose use during mania and its decrease during depression (Baxter et al., 1985). Bipolar disorder has been linked to many genes, but apparently none of them are specific to bipolar disorder. The same genes also increase the risk of unipolar depression, schizophrenia, and other disorders (S.-H. Chang et al., 2013).

Treatments

The first successful treatment for bipolar disorder, and still the most common one, is **lithium** salts. Lithium's benefits were discovered accidentally by an Australian investigator, J. F. Cade, who believed uric acid might relieve mania and depression. Cade mixed uric acid (a component of urine) with a lithium salt to help it dissolve and then gave the solution to patients. It was indeed helpful, but investigators soon discovered that lithium was the effective agent, not uric acid.

Lithium stabilizes mood, preventing a relapse into either mania or depression. The dose must be regulated carefully, as a low dose is ineffective and a high dose is toxic. The mechanism of effect evidently has something to do with cells in the hippocampus. The hippocampus forms new neurons throughout life, and some of those that form in bipolar

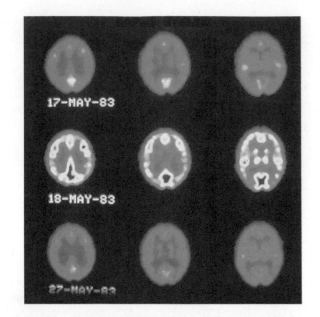

Figure 14.13 PET scans for a patient with bipolar disorder
Horizontal planes through three levels of the brain are shown for each day. On May 17 and May 27, when the patient was depressed, brain metabolic rates were low. On May 18, when the patient was in a cheerful, hypomanic mood, the brain metabolic rate was high. Red indicates the highest metabolic rate, followed by yellow, green, and blue.
(*Source: "Cerebral metabolic rates for glucose in mood disorders," by L. R. Baxter, M. E. Phelps, J. C. Mazziotta, J. M. Schwartz, R. H. Gerner, C. E. Selin, et al., 1985, Archives of General Psychiatry, 42, 441–447.*)

patients are hyperexcitable. Lithium relieves bipolar disorder only if it alleviates the hyperexcitability (Mertens et al., 2015).

Other drugs are the anticonvulsants valproate (trade names Depakene, Depakote, and others) and carbamazepine. If these drugs are not fully effective, physicians sometimes supplement them with antidepressant drugs or antipsychotic drugs—the ones also prescribed for schizophrenia. Antidepressant drugs are risky, as they sometimes provoke a switch from depression to mania. Antipsychotic drugs can be helpful, but they also produce unpleasant side effects.

Supplementary strategies include diet and sleep. As with major depression, omega-3 fatty acids, such as those in seafood, reduce the risk of bipolar disorder (Noaghiul & Hibbeln, 2003). Patients with bipolar disorder frequently have poor sleep quality during manic phases, depressed phases, and even when mood is normal (Altena et al., 2016). Getting consistent, adequate sleep helps stabilize mood and decrease the risk of a new episode (Harvey, Talbot, & Gershon, 2009).

STOP & CHECK

23. What are common treatments for bipolar disorder?

ANSWER 23. The common pharmaceutical treatments for bipolar disorder are lithium salts and certain anticonvulsant drugs—valproate and carbamazepine. A diet that includes omega-3 fatty acids also helps, as does a consistent sleep schedule.

Module 14.2 | In Closing

The Biology of Mood Swings

There is nothing abnormal about feeling sad if something unusually bad has just happened to you. For people with major depression or bipolar disorder, mood becomes largely independent of events. A bout of depression might persist for months or years, while even the best of news provides little cheer. A bipolar patient in a manic state has boundless energy and self-confidence that no contradiction can deter. Studying these states has great potential to inform us about the brain states that correspond to moods.

Summary

1. People with major depression find that almost nothing makes them happy. In most cases, depression occurs as a series of episodes. **468**

2. Depression has a genetic predisposition, but no one gene has a strong effect by itself. Stress can provoke depression by activating the immune system. **469**

3. Depression is associated with decreased activity in the left hemisphere of the cortex. **470**

4. Several kinds of antidepressant drugs are in wide use. Tricyclics block reuptake of serotonin and catecholamines. SSRIs block reuptake of serotonin. SNRIs block reuptake of both serotonin and norepinephrine. MAOIs block an enzyme that breaks down catecholamines and serotonin. **470**

5. Antidepressants probably do not produce their benefits simply by increasing synaptic levels of serotonin or any other transmitter. Ordinarily they affect synapses quickly but the mood benefits develop over weeks. **471**

6. One hypothesis is that antidepressants exert their effects by promoting development of new neurons in the hippocampus. New neurons facilitate new learning that competes with old, unpleasant thoughts. **471**

7. Most people do not respond quickly to antidepressant drugs, and part of the apparent benefit may be due to a placebo effect or the passage of time. **472**

8. Psychotherapy is about as effective as antidepressants. Psychotherapy is more likely than antidepressant drugs to produce long-lasting benefits. **473**

9. Other therapies for depression include exercise, electroconvulsive therapy, altered sleep patterns, and deep brain stimulation. **473**

10. Exposure to bright lights is an effective, inexpensive treatment not only for seasonal affective disorder, but also for other major depression. **475**

11. People with bipolar disorder alternate between depression and mania. Effective therapies include lithium salts and certain anticonvulsant drugs. A consistent sleep schedule is also recommended. **476**

Key Terms

Terms are defined in the module on the page number indicated. They're also presented in alphabetical order with definitions in the book's Subject Index/Glossary, which begins on page 589. Interactive flash cards, audio reviews, and crossword puzzles are among the online resources available to help you learn these terms and the concepts they represent.

atypical antidepressants **471**
bipolar disorder **476**
deep brain stimulation **476**
electroconvulsive therapy
    (ECT) **473**
lithium **476**

major depression **468**
mania **476**
monoamine oxidase inhibitors
    (MAOIs) **470**
seasonal affective disorder
    (SAD) **474**

selective serotonin reuptake
    inhibitors (SSRIs) **470**
serotonin norepinephrine reuptake
    inhibitors (SNRIs) **470**
tricyclics **470**

Thought Questions

1. Some people have suggested that ECT relieves depression by causing people to forget the events that caused it. What evidence opposes this hypothesis?

2. Suppose a person with depression rides a cruise ship that travels slowly around the world, one time zone east every day or two. What effect, if any, would you expect on the depression, and why?

Module 14.2 | End of Module Quiz

1. On average, how long does a first episode of depression last?

   A. Two months
   B. Longer than later episodes

   C. Shorter than later episodes
   D. About the same as later episodes

2. What is one reason why it may be hard to locate genes contributing to depression?

   A. The genes for depression in men differ from those in women.
   B. The genes for depression in one population may be rare in another.

   C. The genes for depression in adolescents differ from those in adults.
   D. The genes for depression in today's population differ from those in the past.

3. Relatives of people with late-onset depression have an increased probability of what type of disorder?

   A. Anxiety disorders
   B. Circulatory problems

   C. Alcohol abuse
   D. Migraine headaches

4. The short gene for the serotonin transporter relates to depression only in which people?

   A. People who have experienced severe stress
   B. People with dietary allergies

   C. People who have followed an irregular sleep schedule
   D. People who do not respond well to antidepressant drugs

5. How do SSRIs differ from tricyclic antidepressants?

   A. SSRIs act on just one type of synapse instead of several.
   B. SSRIs act on the hippocampus instead of the cerebral cortex.

   C. SSRIs enter the brain more rapidly and remain there longer.
   D. SSRIs are chemically similar to the brain's own neurotransmitters.

6. What is the disadvantage of using St. John's wort as an antidepressant?

   A. St. John's wort is more expensive than standard antidepressant drugs.
   B. St. John's wort is less effective and produces benefits more slowly.

   C. St. John's wort decreases the effectiveness of other drugs.
   D. St. John's wort is difficult to obtain legally.

7. If someone starts taking antidepressant drugs, when do behavioral benefits emerge?

   A. As soon as the drug reaches the brain
   B. As soon as the drug attaches to receptors on the synapses

   C. About one day after taking the first dose
   D. Two weeks or more after taking the first dose

8. Which of the following is important for relieving depression?

   A. Increasing the activity of the right hemisphere
   B. Forming new neurons in the hippocampus

   C. Blocking the production of BDNF
   D. Increasing the synthesis of GABA

9. If several patients who did not respond to drug A later improve after switching to drug B, what conclusion, if any, follows?

   A. Drug B is more effective than drug A.
   B. Some people respond to drug B but not to drug A.

   C. Any switch in drugs increases patients' motivation and therefore helps them recover.
   D. None of these conclusions follows.

10. Antidepressant effects resemble those of placebos except for which type of patient?

    A. Those with more severe depression
    B. Those with relatively mild depression

    C. Those with onset of depression late in life
    D. Those who are also receiving psychotherapy

11. Which treatment acts most rapidly, and which usually has the most lasting benefits?

    A. Antidepressants act most rapidly, and psychotherapy has the most lasting benefits.
    B. ECT acts most rapidly, and psychotherapy has the most lasting benefits.

    C. Psychotherapy acts most rapidly, and antidepressants have the most lasting benefits.
    D. ECT acts most rapidly, and antidepressants have the most lasting benefits.

12. Which of these often yields inexpensive relief from depression?
    A. Going to sleep hours later than usual
    B. Exposure to very bright lights in the morning
    C. Eating a fat-free diet
    D. Soothing music throughout the night

13. Which of these is a common treatment for bipolar disorder?
    A. Lithium salts
    B. Uric acid
    C. Vitamin C
    D. Avoidance of gluten

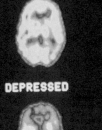

NORMAL

DEPRESSED

Module 14.3

Schizophrenia

Here is a conversation between two people diagnosed with schizophrenia:

A: Do you work at the air base?

B: You know what I think of work. I'm 33 in June, do you mind?

A: June?

B: 33 years old in June. This stuff goes out the window after I live this, uh—leave this hospital. So I can't get my vocal cords back. So I lay off cigarettes. I'm in a spatial condition, from outer space myself. . . .

A: I'm a real spaceship from across.

B: A lot of people talk that way, like crazy, but "Believe It or Not," by Ripley, take it or leave it—alone—it's in the Examiner, it's in the comic section, "Believe It or Not," by Ripley, Robert E. Ripley. Believe it or not, but we don't have to believe anything, unless I feel like it. Every little rosette—too much alone.

A: Yeah, it could be possible.

B: I'm a civilian seaman.

A: Could be possible. I take my bath in the ocean.

B: Bathing stinks. You know why? 'Cause you can't quit when you feel like it. You're in the service. (Haley, 1959, p. 321)

People with schizophrenia say and do things that other people (including other people with schizophrenia) find difficult to understand. Both biological and environmental factors contribute.

Diagnosis

Schizophrenia was originally called *dementia praecox,* Latin for "premature mental deterioration." In 1911, Eugen Bleuler introduced the term *schizophrenia.* Although the term is Greek for "split mind," it is *not* related to *dissociative identity disorder* (previously known as *multiple personality disorder*), in which someone alternates among personalities. What Bleuler meant by **schizophrenia** was a split between the emotional and intellectual aspects of experience: The person's emotional expression seems unconnected with current experiences. For example, someone might giggle or cry for no apparent reason, or fail to react to good or bad news. This detachment of emotion from intellect is no longer considered a central feature of schizophrenia, but the term lives on.

According to the *DSM-5* (American Psychiatric Association, 2013), to be diagnosed with schizophrenia, someone must have deteriorated in everyday functioning (work, interpersonal relations, self care, etc.) for at least 6 months for reasons not attributable to other disorders. The person must also have at least two symptoms from the following list, including at least one from the first three:

- **Delusions** (unjustifiable beliefs, such as "Beings from outer space are controlling my actions")
- **Hallucinations** (false sensory experiences, such as hearing voices when alone)
- Disorganized speech (rambling or incoherent)
- Grossly disorganized behavior
- Weak emotional expression, speech, and socialization

Diagnosis is sometimes a difficult judgment. An apparent delusion ("People are persecuting me") might be actually true, or at least a defensible belief. Many healthy people have occasionally heard a voice when they knew they were alone, most often when they were just waking up. The term "grossly disorganized behavior" encompasses a wide variety of possibilities. You could easily find several people diagnosed with schizophrenia who have almost nothing in common. As we shall see later in this module, the genetics vary among people diagnosed with schizophrenia, and so do the brain abnormalities. We are probably dealing with a family of related conditions, rather than a single disorder.

The first four items on the list—delusions, hallucinations, disorganized speech, and disorganized behavior—are called **positive symptoms**, meaning behaviors that are present that should be absent. Weak emotional expression, speech, and socialization are **negative symptoms**—behaviors that are absent that should be present. In most cases, negative symptoms are stable over time and difficult to treat.

480

It is also important to recognize *cognitive* symptoms. The cognitive symptoms are impairments of thought and reasoning that are common in people with schizophrenia, even in people of normal or above-normal intelligence (Woodward, 2016). People with schizophrenia typically have difficulty understanding and using abstract concepts. That is, they interpret sayings too literally. They also have trouble maintaining and focusing attention (Lakatos, Schroeder, Leitman, & Javitt, 2013). Memory impairments are also common, related to reduced connectivity between sensory areas of the cortex and the hippocampus (Haut et al., 2015).

One hypothesis is that impairments of attention and working memory are the central problem. One way to test this idea is to see whether we could make normal, healthy people talk or behave in incoherent ways if we overtaxed their working memory. Imagine yourself in the following study. A researcher shows a series of pictures for 30 seconds each, and you are supposed to tell a short story about each one. If you see a picture again, you should tell a new story about it, unlike your first one. You have an additional task to burden your working memory: While you are telling stories, letters appear on the screen, one at a time. You should pay attention to every second letter. Whenever it is the same as the last letter that you attended to, you should press a key. For example,

D L K F R F B L M T J T X H Q U B R B N

Attend to every second letter.

Press on these, because same as previous attended letter.

Do *not* press here. Same as previous *non*attended letter.

Most people's speech becomes less clear when they perform this memory task while trying to tell a story. If it is the second presentation of a picture, requiring them to avoid what they said the first time and tell a totally new story, the memory task causes even greater interference, and their speech becomes incoherent, much like schizophrenic speech (Kerns, 2007). The implication is that a limitation of working memory could explain several aspects of schizophrenia.

✓ STOP & CHECK

24. Why are hallucinations considered a positive symptom?

ANSWER

24. Hallucinations are considered a positive symptom because they are present when they should be absent. A "positive" symptom is not a "good" symptom.

Differential Diagnosis of Schizophrenia

In the description for diagnosing schizophrenia, did you notice the expression "not attributable to other disorders"? Even if someone's symptoms clearly match the description of schizophrenia, a therapist must make a **differential diagnosis**—that is, one that rules out other conditions. Here are a few conditions that sometimes resemble schizophrenia:

- *Substance abuse*: Abuse of amphetamine, methamphetamine, cocaine, LSD, or phencyclidine ("angel dust") can produce hallucinations or delusions. Substance abuse is more likely than schizophrenia to produce visual hallucinations.
- *Brain damage*: Damage or tumors in the temporal or prefrontal cortex can produce some of the symptoms of schizophrenia.
- *Undetected hearing deficits*: Sometimes, someone who is starting to have trouble hearing thinks that everyone else is whispering and starts to worry, "They're whispering about me!" Delusions of persecution can develop.
- *Huntington's disease*: The symptoms of Huntington's disease include hallucinations, delusions, and disordered thinking, as well as motor symptoms. An uncommon type of schizophrenia, *catatonic schizophrenia*, includes motor abnormalities. Therefore, a mixture of psychological and motor symptoms could represent either schizophrenia or Huntington's disease.
- *Nutritional problems*: Niacin deficiency can produce hallucinations and delusions (Hoffer, 1973), and so can a deficiency of vitamin C or an allergy to milk proteins (not the same as lactose intolerance). Some people who cannot tolerate wheat gluten or other proteins react with hallucinations and delusions (Reichelt, Seim, & Reichelt, 1996).

Demographic Data

According to one estimate, about half of one percent of people suffer from schizophrenia at some point in life (Brown, 2011). Some authorities cite higher or lower numbers, depending on how narrowly they define schizophrenia and how many mild cases they include. Because schizophrenia often produces long-term debilitation beginning in young adulthood, it is a major health problem in terms of the loss of productive, pleasant years of life.

Schizophrenia occurs in all ethnic groups and all parts of the world. However, it is more common in cities than in rural areas, especially for people who have lived in large cities since early childhood (Tost, Champagne, & Meyer-Lindenberg, 2015). Likely explanations include unstable social relationships, poverty, air pollution, exposure to toxic substances, and less exposure to the sun, resulting in less absorption of vitamin D.

Lifetime prevalence of schizophrenia is more common for men than women by a ratio of about 7:5. On average, it is also more severe in men and has an earlier onset—usually in the teens or early 20s for men, as compared to the mid- to late 20s for women (Aleman, Kahn, & Selten, 2003).

Researchers have documented several unexplained oddities about schizophrenia. The points that follow do not fit neatly into any currently prominent theory, illustrating how many mysteries remain:

- People with schizophrenia have a higher than average probability of autoimmune diseases such as Guillain-Barré syndrome or pernicious anemia (Benros et al., 2014).

- People with schizophrenia have an increased risk of colon cancer but a decreased risk of several other types of cancer, rheumatoid arthritis, and allergies (Goldman, 1999; Hippisley-Cox, Vinogradova, Coupland, & Parker, 2007; Roppel, 1978; Rubinstein, 1997; Tabarés-Seisdedos & Rubenstein, 2013).
- Women who have a schizophrenic breakdown during pregnancy usually give birth to daughters. However, those who have a breakdown shortly after giving birth usually gave birth to sons (Taylor, 1969).
- Many people with schizophrenia have a characteristic body odor, attributed to the chemical *trans*-3-methyl-2-hexenoic acid, and they also have decreased ability to smell that chemical (Brewer et al., 2007; Smith, Thompson, & Koster, 1969).
- Most people with schizophrenia and many of their unaffected relatives have deficits in pursuit eye movements—the ability to keep their eyes on a moving target (Keefe et al., 1997; Sereno & Holzman, 1993).

✅ STOP & CHECK

25. Someone with the symptoms of schizophrenia might not qualify for the diagnosis. Why not?

ANSWER

25. Other conditions such as drug abuse or brain damage can produce similar symptoms.

Genetics

Huntington's disease (Chapter 7) can be called a genetic disease: By examining part of chromosome 4, one can predict with almost perfect accuracy who will develop the disease and who will not. At one time, many researchers believed that schizophrenia might be a genetic disease in the same sense. However, accumulating evidence indicates it does not depend on any single gene.

Family Studies

The more closely you are biologically related to someone with schizophrenia, the greater your own probability of schizophrenia, as shown in Figure 14.14 (Gottesman, 1991). One of the most important points in Figure 14.14 is that monozygotic twins have a higher **concordance** (agreement) for schizophrenia than do dizygotic twins. Furthermore, twin pairs who are really monozygotic, but thought they weren't, are more concordant than twin pairs who thought they were, but really aren't (Kendler, 1983). That is, *being* monozygotic is more important than *being treated as* monozygotic.

The high concordance for monozygotic twins has long been taken as strong evidence for a genetic influence. However, note two limitations:

- Monozygotic twins have only about 50 percent concordance, not 100 percent.

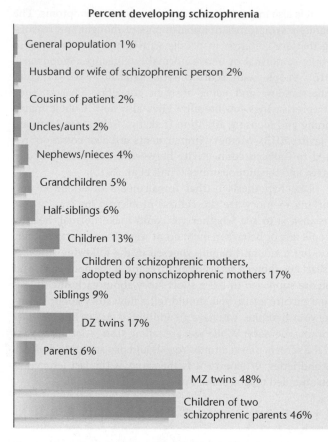

Percent developing schizophrenia

General population 1%
Husband or wife of schizophrenic person 2%
Cousins of patient 2%
Uncles/aunts 2%
Nephews/nieces 4%
Grandchildren 5%
Half-siblings 6%
Children 13%
Children of schizophrenic mothers, adopted by nonschizophrenic mothers 17%
Siblings 9%
DZ twins 17%
Parents 6%
MZ twins 48%
Children of two schizophrenic parents 46%

Figure 14.14 Probabilities of developing schizophrenia
People with a closer genetic relationship to someone with schizophrenia have a higher probability of developing it themselves.
(Source: Based on data from Gottesman, 1991)

- In Figure 14.14, note the greater similarity between dizygotic twins than between siblings. Dizygotic twins have the same genetic resemblance as siblings but greater environmental similarity, including prenatal environment.

Adopted Children Who Develop Schizophrenia

For adopted children who develop schizophrenia, the disorder is more common in their biological relatives than their adopting relatives. A Danish study found schizophrenia in 12.5 percent of the immediate biological relatives and none of the adopting relatives (Kety et al., 1994). Note in Figure 14.14 that children of a mother with schizophrenia have a moderately high probability of schizophrenia, even if adopted by mentally healthy parents.

These results suggest a genetic basis, but they are also consistent with a prenatal influence. A pregnant woman with schizophrenia passes her genes to her child, but she also provides the prenatal environment. Many women with schizophrenia abuse alcohol or other drugs, eat a poor diet, and have complications during pregnancy and delivery (Jablensky, Morgan, Zubrick, Bower, & Yellachich, 2005). If some of their

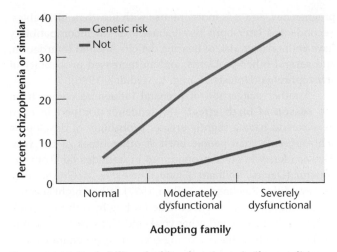

Figure 14.15 **Probability of schizophrenia or similar conditions in adopted children**
The probability was higher for children of a mother with schizophrenia, but growing up in a dysfunctional family magnified that risk.
(Source: Based on data from Wynne et al., 2006)

children develop schizophrenia, we cannot be sure that the reason is genetic.

Studies on adopted children also support a role for environmental influences. A study of adopted children in Finland found a high probability of schizophrenia or related conditions among children who had a biological mother with schizophrenia *and* a severely disordered adopting family. The genetic risk itself or the disordered family itself had less effect, as shown in Figure 14.15 (Wynne et al., 2006).

Efforts to Locate a Gene

Researchers working with various populations have identified more than a hundred genetic loci that differ on average between people with or without schizophrenia. Few of these genes actually change the structure of any protein. Mostly they control the amount of production of proteins that are important for brain function (Fromer et al., 2016; Schizophrenia Working Group, 2014). Many of these genes also increase the probability of other psychological disorders. The results vary from one study to another, partly because some genes are common in one ethnic group but not in another (Vieland et al., 2014).

No common gene produces more than a small increase in the probability of schizophrenia. Indeed, it would be difficult for any gene with a strong link to schizophrenia to become common, because people with schizophrenia have, on average, fewer than half as many children as other people do, and their brothers and sisters do not compensate by having more children than average (Bundy, Stahl, & MacCabe, 2011).

One individual gene worthy of mention, called *DISC1* *(disrupted in schizophrenia 1)*, controls differentiation and migration of neurons in brain development (Ishizuka et al., 2011; Steinecke, Gampe, Valkova, Kaether, & Bolz, 2012), production of dendritic spines (Hayashi-Takagi et al., 2010), the

generation of new neurons in the hippocampus (Duan et al., 2007), and learning (Greenhill et al., 2015). Certain variants in the *DISC1* gene are more common in people with schizophrenia than in the rest of the population (Moens et al., 2011).

Although no common gene has a strong effect, certain rare mutations do, especially mutations that alter the structure of proteins at synapses, or mutations that interfere with the major histocompatibility complex, which is part of the immune system (Dachtler et al., 2015; Fromer et al., 2014; Genovese et al., 2016; Purcell et al., 2014; Sekar et al., 2016). Although each of these mutations is rare, a great many mutations of this type are possible, potentially accounting for a significant number of cases. Another contributor is **microdeletion**, the deletion of a small part of a chromosome. Several studies have found that microdeletions are more common among people with schizophrenia than in other people (Buizer-Voskamp et al., 2011; Walsh et al., 2008). Thus, the hypothesis is that a new mutation or deletion of any of hundreds of genes disrupts brain development and increases the probability of schizophrenia. As fast as natural selection weeds out those mutations or deletions, new ones arise to replace them. Other cases may emerge from environmental factors, perhaps enhanced by some of the more common genetic variations that slightly increase vulnerability. The next section explores some of the known environmental influences.

STOP & CHECK

26. The fact that adopted children who develop schizophrenia usually have biological relatives with schizophrenia implies a probable genetic basis. What other interpretation is possible?
27. What is a microdeletion?

ANSWERS
26. A biological mother can influence her child's development through prenatal environment as well as genetics.
27. A microdeletion is an error in reproduction that deletes a small part of a chromosome.

The Neurodevelopmental Hypothesis

According to the **neurodevelopmental hypothesis**, prenatal or neonatal influences—genetic, environmental, or both—produce abnormalities in the developing brain. Even if these abnormalities by themselves do not cause schizophrenia, they leave the brain vulnerable to other disturbances at critical periods in childhood or adolescence. Those disturbances could include traumatic experiences, viral infections, dietary deficiencies or allergies, exposure to toxic chemicals, and other possible insults (Davis et al., 2016). The cumulative effect distorts brain function, and therefore behavior (Fatemi & Folsom, 2009; Weinberger, 1996).

The supporting evidence is that (1) several kinds of prenatal or early difficulties are linked to later schizophrenia; (2) people with schizophrenia have minor brain abnormalities that apparently originate early in life; and (3) it is plausible that abnormalities of early development could impair behavior in adulthood.

Prenatal and Neonatal Environment

E. F. Torrey and colleagues (2012) have argued that schizophrenia results from a combination of genetic and environmental influences. Among the environmental factors, they distinguished between intermediate risk factors and low risk factors. (Nothing was strong enough to count as a high risk factor.)

Intermediate Risk Factors

As already mentioned, living in a crowded city is a risk factor, presumably for environmental reasons. Another intermediate risk factor is prenatal or childhood infection with the parasite *Toxoplasma gondii*. This parasite, discussed in Chapter 11 in the context of anxiety and the amygdala, reproduces only in cats, but it can infect humans and other species also. People can be exposed to the parasite by handling infected cats, by playing in soil or sand where cats have defecated, or by eating chicken or pork after those animals fed in infected soil. If the parasite infects the brain of an infant or child, it impairs brain development. Antibodies against this parasite, indicating past exposure to it, are more common than average among people who have schizophrenia, major depression, bipolar disorder, or obsessive-compulsive disorder (Kramer & Bressan, 2015; Sutterland et al., 2015; Yolken, Dickerson, & Torrey, 2009). However, the parasite does not always enter the human brain, and it is possible to have antibodies against the parasite without developing psychological complications.

Low Risk Factors

The risk of schizophrenia is mildly elevated among people who had problems that could have affected their brain development, including poor nutrition of the mother during pregnancy, premature birth, low birth weight, and complications during delivery (Ballon, Dean, & Cadenhead, 2007). The risk is also elevated if the mother was exposed to extreme stress, such as the sudden death of a close relative, early in her pregnancy (Khashan et al., 2008) or if the mother had almost any prolonged illness during pregnancy (Brown, 2011). Illness triggers the immune system, which results in a fever, which interferes with brain development (Estes & McAllister, 2016). Schizophrenia has also been linked to head injuries in early childhood (AbdelMalik, Husted, Chow, & Bassett, 2003), although we do not know whether the head injuries led to schizophrenia or early symptoms of schizophrenia increased the risk of head injuries. Acute infections during adolescence are also common in people who later develop schizophrenia (Metcalf et al., 2017).

If a mother is Rh-negative and her baby is Rh-positive, the baby's Rh-positive blood factor may trigger an immunological rejection by the mother. The response is weak with the woman's first Rh-positive baby but stronger in later pregnancies, and it is more intense with boy than girl babies. Second- and later-born boy babies with Rh incompatibility have an increased risk of hearing deficits, mental retardation, and several other problems, and an increased probability of schizophrenia (Hollister, Laing, & Mednick, 1996).

Another suggestion of prenatal influences comes from the **season-of-birth effect**: the tendency for people born in winter to have a slightly greater probability of developing schizophrenia than people born at other times of the year. This tendency is more pronounced in latitudes far from the equator (Davies, Welham, Chant, Torrey, & McGrath, 2003; Torrey, Miller, Rawlings, & Yolken, 1997). What might account for the season-of-birth effect? The leading hypothesis is viral infection. Influenza and other viral epidemics are common in the fall. Therefore, the reasoning goes, many pregnant women become infected in the fall with a virus that impairs a crucial stage of brain development in a baby who will be born in the winter. Researchers retrieved blood samples that hospitals had taken from pregnant women and stored for decades. They found increased incidence of influenza virus among mothers whose children eventually developed schizophrenia (Brown et al., 2004; Buka et al., 2001). A virus that affects the mother might or might not cross the placenta into the fetus's brain, but the mother's cytokines (part of the immune system) do cross, and excessive cytokines can impair brain development (Zuckerman, Rehavi, Nachman, & Weiner, 2003). The mother's infection also causes a fever, which slows the division of fetal neurons. (Exercise during pregnancy does not overheat the abdomen and is not dangerous to the fetus. Hot baths and saunas pose a possible risk, however.) The overall conclusion is that a wide variety of genetic and environmental influences can lead to schizophrenia.

✓ STOP & CHECK

28. According to the neurodevelopmental hypothesis, when do the brain abnormalities associated with schizophrenia originate?

ANSWER
28. Initial problems begin before birth or soon after birth, but they combine with the effects of later difficulties.

Mild Brain Abnormalities

Many, but not all, people with schizophrenia show mild, variable abnormalities of brain anatomy, including less than average gray matter, especially in the hippocampus, amygdala, and thalamus (van Erp et al., 2016). White matter is reduced, and the ventricles (fluid-filled spaces within the brain) are enlarged (Kochunov & Hong, 2014; Meyer-Lindenberg, 2010; Wolkin et al., 1998; Wright et al., 2000) (see Figure 14.16). Minor abnormalities in subcortical areas are also common (Spoletini et al., 2011). Abnormalities visible in the blood vessels of the retina imply less than average blood flow to the brain (Meier et al., 2013). Still, the abnormalities are mild compared to those in people with Alzheimer's disease or

Ventricles

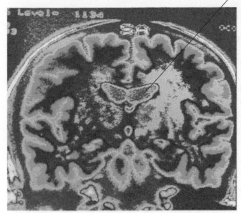 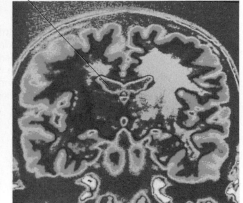

Figure 14.16 Coronal sections for identical twins
The twin on the left has schizophrenia; the twin on the right does not. The ventricles (near the center of each brain) are larger in the twin with schizophrenia.
(*Source: Photos courtesy of E. F. Torrey & M. F. Casanova/NIMH*)

many other disorders. On average, brain volume is only about 5 percent smaller than average, and many people show little or no anatomical abnormality (Woodward, 2016).

The brain areas with consistent signs of abnormality include some that mature slowly, such as the dorsolateral prefrontal cortex (Berman, Torrey, Daniel, & Weinberger, 1992; Fletcher et al., 1998; Gur et al., 2000). The abnormalities include weaker than average connections from the dorsolateral prefrontal cortex to other brain areas, and less than normal activity in this area during tasks requiring attention and memory (Lynall et al., 2010; van den Heuvel, Mandl, Stam, Kahn, & Pol, 2010; Weiss et al., 2009). As you might predict, people with schizophrenia perform poorly at tasks that depend on the prefrontal cortex (Goldberg, Weinberger, Berman, Pliskin, & Podd, 1987; Spindler, Sullivan, Menon, Lim, & Pfefferbaum, 1997). Most patients with schizophrenia show deficits of memory and attention similar to those of people with damage to the temporal or prefrontal cortex (Park, Holzman, & Goldman-Rakic, 1995).

An example of a task that tests for damage to the prefrontal cortex is the Wisconsin Card Sorting Test. Suppose someone hands you a shuffled deck of cards that differ in number, color, and shape of objects—for example, three red circles, five blue triangles, four green squares, and so forth. First you should sort the cards by color. Then the rule changes, and you are supposed to sort them by number, and later by shape. Shifting to a new rule requires suppressing the old one and activates the prefrontal cortex (Konishi et al., 1998). People with damage to the prefrontal cortex have no trouble following whichever rule comes first, but they have trouble shifting to a new rule. People with schizophrenia have the same difficulty.

Long-Term Course

Decades ago, psychiatrists regarded schizophrenia as a *progressive* disorder—that is, one that progresses to worse and worse outcome over time, analogous to Parkinson's disease or Alzheimer's disease. However, that conclusion was based largely on experience from the era when patients with

schizophrenia were confined to large, poorly staffed mental hospitals. It is understandable how someone who lived year after year in one of those grim places would deteriorate.

The more recent experience is that people diagnosed with schizophrenia vary in their outcome (Zipursky, Reilly, & Murray, 2013). Up to one-fourth show a serious disorder throughout life and possibly deteriorate, perhaps due to poverty, lack of social support, drug abuse, and poor care. Another group, perhaps 10 to 20 percent of all cases, recover from a first episode and do well from then on. The others—the majority—have one or more remissions and one or more relapses.

Much research has addressed the question of whether the brain abnormalities in schizophrenia become gradually worse as people age. Parkinson's disease and Alzheimer's disease are known as progressive disorders because the brain damage progresses to a worse and worse condition. In schizophrenia, some studies report that a few brain areas deteriorate over age slightly more than is typical for people of the same age (van Haren et al., 2016). However, most of the abnormality of both brain and behavior is present at the time of first diagnosis, with some further impairment in the next couple of years, but only slight deterioration after that in most patients (Andreasen et al., 2011; Chiapponi et al., 2013; Nesvag et al., 2012; Vita, De Peri, Deste, & Sacchetti, 2012; Woodward, 2016). Even when further deterioration does occur, it could be a result of drug use (common in people with schizophrenia) rather than a result of schizophrenia itself.

Early Development and Later Psychopathology

One question may have struck you. The neurodevelopmental hypothesis holds that schizophrenia results from factors that disrupt brain development before birth or during early childhood. Why, then, are most cases not diagnosed until age 20 or later? The time course may be less puzzling than it seems at first (Weinberger, 1996). Most of the people who receive a diagnosis of schizophrenia in adulthood had shown other

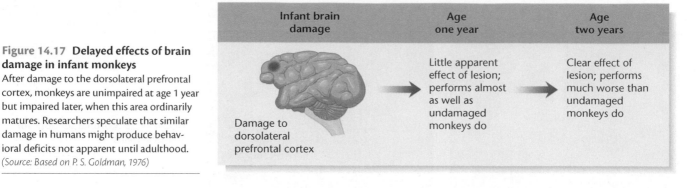

Figure 14.17 Delayed effects of brain damage in infant monkeys
After damage to the dorsolateral prefrontal cortex, monkeys are unimpaired at age 1 year but impaired later, when this area ordinarily matures. Researchers speculate that similar damage in humans might produce behavioral deficits not apparent until adulthood.
(Source: Based on P. S. Goldman, 1976)

problems since childhood, including deficits in attention, memory, and impulse control (Keshavan, Diwadkar, Montrose, Rajarethinam, & Sweeney, 2005). An analysis of home movies found that people who later developed schizophrenia showed movement abnormalities during infancy (Walker, Savoie, & Davis, 1994). These relatively minor problems developed into more serious problems later.

Furthermore, the dorsolateral prefrontal cortex, an area that shows consistent signs of deficit in schizophrenia, is one of the slowest brain areas to mature. Researchers damaged this area in infant monkeys and tested the monkeys later. At age 1 year, the monkeys' behavior was nearly normal, but by age 2 years, it had deteriorated markedly (Goldman, 1971, 1976). That is, the effects of the brain damage grew worse over age. Presumably, the effects of brain damage were minimal at age 1 year because the dorsolateral prefrontal cortex doesn't do much at that age anyway. Later, when it should begin assuming important functions, the damage begins to make a difference (see Figure 14.17).

✓ **STOP & CHECK** ▮▮▮▮▮▮▮▮▮▮

29. If brain abnormalities do not continue to grow worse over time, what is the implication for the possibility of recovery?

ANSWER

29. The prospects for recovery are more encouraging than they would seem if the brain were continuing to deteriorate over time. With any type of brain damage, some degree of recovery over time is likely.

Treatments

Before antipsychotic drugs became available in the mid-1950s, most people with schizophrenia were confined to mental hospitals with little hope of recovery. Today, mental hospitals are far less crowded because of drugs and outpatient treatment.

Antipsychotic Drugs and Dopamine

In the 1950s, psychiatrists discovered that **chlorpromazine** (trade name Thorazine) relieves the positive symptoms of

schizophrenia for most, though not all, patients. Researchers later discovered other **antipsychotic,** or **neuroleptic, drugs** (drugs that tend to relieve schizophrenia and similar conditions) in two chemical families: the **phenothiazines** (FEE-no-THI-uh-zeens), which include chlorpromazine, and the **butyrophenones** (BYOO-tir-oh-FEE-noans), which include haloperidol (trade name Haldol). Behavioral benefits of any of these drugs develop gradually over weeks. Symptoms may or may not return after cessation of treatment.

As Figure 14.18 illustrates, each of these drugs blocks dopamine synapses, specifically dopamine type D_2 synapses. For each drug, researchers determined the mean dose prescribed for patients with schizophrenia (displayed along the horizontal axis) and the amount needed to block dopamine receptors (displayed along the vertical axis). As the figure shows, the drugs that are most effective against schizophrenia (and therefore used in the smallest doses) are the most effective at blocking dopamine receptors (Seeman, Lee, Chau-Wong, & Wong, 1976).

That finding inspired the **dopamine hypothesis of schizophrenia,** which holds that schizophrenia results from excess activity at dopamine synapses in certain brain areas. Although the concentration of dopamine in the brain as a whole is no higher than normal, dopamine release is increased in the basal ganglia, especially in response to stressful events (Howes & Kapur, 2009; Simpson, Kellendonk, & Kandel, 2010). Further support for the dopamine hypothesis comes from the fact that extensive abuse of amphetamine, methamphetamine, or cocaine (which all increase dopamine at the synapses) induces **substance-induced psychotic disorder,** characterized by hallucinations and delusions. LSD, which also produces psychotic symptoms, is best known for its effects on serotonin synapses, but it also stimulates dopamine synapses.

In a clever study, researchers measured the number of dopamine receptors occupied at a given moment. They used a radioactively labeled drug, IBZM, that binds to type D_2 receptors. Because IBZM binds only to receptors that dopamine did not already bind, measuring the radioactivity counts the number of vacant dopamine receptors. Then the researchers used a second drug, AMPT, that blocks all synthesis of dopamine and again used IBZM to count the number of vacant D_2 receptors. Because AMPT had prevented production of

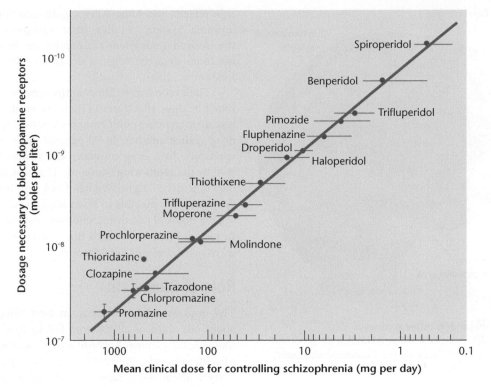

Figure 14.18 Dopamine-blocking effects of antipsychotic drugs
Drugs are arranged along the horizontal axis in terms of the average daily dose prescribed for patients with schizophrenia. (Horizontal lines indicate common ranges.) *Larger* doses are to the left, and *smaller* doses are to the right so that *more effective* drugs are to the right. Along the vertical axis is a measurement of the amount of each drug required to achieve a certain degree of blockage of postsynaptic dopamine receptors. *Larger* doses are toward the bottom, and *smaller* doses are toward the top so that the drugs on top are *more effective*.

(Source: From "Antipsychotic drug doses and neuroleptic/dopamine receptors," by P. Seeman, T. Lee, M. Chau-Wong, and K. Wong, 1976, Nature, 261, pp. 717–719. Copyright © 1976 Macmillan Magazines Limited. Reprinted by permission of Nature and Phillip Seeman.)

dopamine, *all* D_2 receptors should be vacant at this time, so the researchers got a count of the total. Then they subtracted the first count from the second count, yielding the number of D_2 receptors occupied by dopamine at the first count. The people with schizophrenia had about twice as many D_2 receptors occupied as normal:

- First count: IBZM binds to all D_2 receptors not already attached to dopamine.
- Second count: IBZM binds to all D_2 receptors (because AMPT eliminated production of dopamine).
- Second count minus first count equals the number of D_2 receptors bound to dopamine at the first count. (Abi-Dargham et al., 2000)

✓ STOP & CHECK

30. The ability of traditional antipsychotic drugs to relieve schizophrenia correlates strongly with what effect on neurotransmitters?

ANSWER

30. Their ability to relieve schizophrenia correlates strongly with how well they block activity at dopamine synapses.

Second-Generation Antipsychotic Drugs

The brain has several dopamine pathways with different functions. Drugs that block dopamine synapses produce their benefits by acting on neurons in the **mesolimbocortical system,** neurons that project from the midbrain to the limbic system and prefrontal cortex. However, these drugs also block dopamine neurons in the *mesostriatal system* that projects to the basal ganglia (see Figure 14.19). The effect on the basal ganglia produces **tardive dyskinesia** (TARD-eev dis-kih-NEE-zhee-uh), characterized by tremors and other involuntary movements that develop gradually and to varying degrees among patients (Kiriakakis, Bhatia, Quinn, & Marsden, 1998).

Once tardive dyskinesia emerges, it can last long after someone quits the drug (Kiriakakis et al., 1998). Consequently, the best strategy is to prevent it from starting. Certain drugs called **second-generation antipsychotics,** or *atypical antipsychotics,* reduce the risk of movement problems from 30 percent to 20 percent (Carbon, Hsieh, Kane, & Correll, 2017) (see Figure 14.20). The most common of these drugs are clozapine, amisulpride, risperidone, olanzapine, and aripiprazole. Compared to drugs like haloperidol, the second-generation antipsychotics have less effect on dopamine

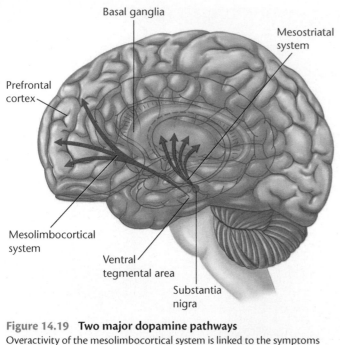

Figure 14.19 Two major dopamine pathways
Overactivity of the mesolimbocortical system is linked to the symptoms of schizophrenia. The path to the basal ganglia is associated with tardive dyskinesia, a movement disorder.
(Source: Adapted from Valzelli, 1980)

receptors but more strongly antagonize serotonin type 5-HT$_2$ receptors (Kapur et al., 2000; Meltzer, Matsubara, & Lee, 1989; Mrzljak et al., 1996; Roth, Willins, Kristiansen, & Kroeze, 1999). They also increase the release of glutamate (Melone et al., 2001). Unfortunately, they produce other

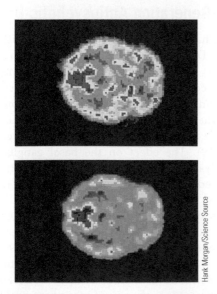
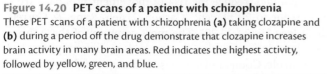

Figure 14.20 PET scans of a patient with schizophrenia
These PET scans of a patient with schizophrenia **(a)** taking clozapine and **(b)** during a period off the drug demonstrate that clozapine increases brain activity in many brain areas. Red indicates the highest activity, followed by yellow, green, and blue.

side effects, including weight gain and impairment of the immune system. Studies have disagreed about whether the second-generation antipsychotics improve quality of life more than the original drugs do (Grunder et al., 2016; Jones et al., 2006).

The second-generation antipsychotics do not differ by much in their effectiveness (Samara et al., 2016). Nevertheless, an interesting point emerges from studies comparing one drug against another: In 90 percent of the studies that were sponsored by a drug company, the results favored the drug sold by the sponsoring company (Heres et al., 2006). Interesting coincidence, right? We need not assume anything overtly dishonest. It is possible to bias a study in subtle ways, by altering the doses of two drugs, choosing patients who seem likely to respond to the sponsor's drug, or choosing one measurement instead of another to report.

Role of Glutamate

The dopamine hypothesis is, at best, incomplete, because about one-third of all patients fail to respond to the drugs that block dopamine. According to the **glutamate hypothesis of schizophrenia,** the problem relates in part to deficient activity at glutamate synapses in the prefrontal cortex. In many brain areas, dopamine inhibits glutamate release, or glutamate stimulates neurons that inhibit dopamine release. Therefore, increased dopamine could produce nearly the same effects as decreased glutamate.

Studies have consistently found decreased glutamate release in the prefrontal cortex for people with schizophrenia (Marsman et al., 2013). Further support for the glutamate hypothesis comes from the effects of **phencyclidine (PCP)** ("angel dust"), a drug that inhibits the NMDA glutamate receptors. At low doses, it produces intoxication and slurred speech. At larger doses, it produces both positive and negative symptoms of schizophrenia, including hallucinations, thought disorder, loss of emotions, and memory loss. PCP is an interesting model for schizophrenia in other regards also:

- PCP and the related drug *ketamine* produce little if any psychotic response in preadolescents. Just as the symptoms of schizophrenia usually begin to emerge well after puberty, so do the psychotic effects of PCP and ketamine.
- LSD, amphetamine, and cocaine produce temporary schizophrenic symptoms in almost anyone, and the effects are not much worse in people with a history of schizophrenia than in anyone else. However, PCP produces a relapse for someone who has recovered from schizophrenia. (Farber, Newcomer, & Olney, 1999; Hardingham & Do, 2016; Olney & Farber, 1995)

It might seem that the best test of the glutamate hypothesis would be to administer glutamate itself. However, glutamate is the brain's most widespread transmitter, and increasing it everywhere should cause confusion and possibly damage from overstimulation. The glutamate receptor has a second site that glycine activates to enhance the response to glutamate. Therefore, a possible approach would be to try to activate the glycine receptor. Unfortunately, so far all attempts to treat schizophrenia with drugs aimed at glutamate or glycine have produced only disappointing results (Beck, Javitt, & Howes, 2016; Iwata et al., 2015).

STOP & CHECK

31. What are the advantages of the second-generation antipsychotics?

ANSWER

31. Second-generation antipsychotics are less likely to cause tardive dyskinesia. Also, they alter synapses other than dopamine, in ways that may be helpful.

Module 14.3 | In Closing
Many Remaining Mysteries

Research is a little like reading a good mystery novel that presents a mixture of important clues and irrelevant information. In research on schizophrenia, we have an enormous amount of information, but also major gaps and occasional points that don't seem to fit. The final chapter of our mystery novel on schizophrenia is far from complete. However, although researchers have not yet solved the mystery, it should also be clear that they have made progress. It will be fascinating to see what develops in future research.

Summary

1. Positive symptoms of schizophrenia (behaviors that are not present in most other people) include hallucinations, delusions, inappropriate emotions, bizarre behaviors, and thought disorder. **480**

2. Negative symptoms (normal behaviors absent that should be present) include deficits of social interaction, emotional expression, and speech. **480**

3. Before diagnosing someone with schizophrenia, a therapist needs to rule out brain damage, drug abuse, and other conditions that could produce similar symptoms. **481**

4. Studies of twins and adopted children imply a genetic predisposition to schizophrenia. However, the adoption studies do not distinguish between the roles of genetics and prenatal environment. **482**

5. Researchers have identified many genes associated with schizophrenia, but no common gene increases the risk by much. A promising hypothesis is that schizophrenia results from new mutations or microdeletions of any of the hundreds of genes that are important for brain development. **483**

6. According to the neurodevelopmental hypothesis, either genes or difficulties early in life, often before birth, impair brain development in ways that increase vulnerability to later insults and predispose to behavioral abnormalities beginning in early adulthood. **483**

7. Many people with schizophrenia show mild abnormalities of brain development, especially in the temporal and frontal lobes. They also show cognitive deficits that make sense if their frontal and temporal lobes are less than fully functional. **484**

8. Contrary to what psychiatrists used to believe, most people with schizophrenia do not continue deteriorating throughout life. Some recover, some remain troubled throughout life, and some alternate between remission and relapse. Although the brain shows abnormalities during the first episode of schizophrenia, most people show little or no increase in those abnormalities as time passes. **485**

9. Parts of the prefrontal cortex are very slow to mature. It is plausible that early disruption of those areas might produce behavioral symptoms that manifest as schizophrenia in young adults. **485**

10. According to the dopamine hypothesis, schizophrenia is due to excess dopamine activity. Drugs that block dopamine synapses reduce the positive symptoms of schizophrenia, and drugs that increase dopamine activity induce the positive symptoms. **486**

11. Prolonged use of antipsychotic drugs may produce tardive dyskinesia, a movement disorder. Second-generation antipsychotic drugs reduce the risk of tardive dyskinesia. **487**

12. According to the glutamate hypothesis, part of the problem is deficient glutamate activity. Phencyclidine, which blocks NMDA glutamate synapses, produces both positive and negative symptoms of schizophrenia, especially in people predisposed to schizophrenia. **488**

Key Terms

Terms are defined in the module on the page number indicated. They're also presented in alphabetical order with definitions in the book's Subject Index/Glossary, which begins on page 589. Interactive flash cards, audio reviews, and crossword puzzles are among the online resources available to help you learn these terms and the concepts they represent.

antipsychotic (neuroleptic) drugs **486**

butyrophenones **486**

chlorpromazine **486**

concordance **482**

delusions **480**

differential diagnosis **481**

DISC1 **483**

dopamine hypothesis of schizophrenia **486**

glutamate hypothesis of schizophrenia **488**

hallucinations **480**

mesolimbocortical system **487**

microdeletion **483**

negative symptoms **480**

neurodevelopmental hypothesis **483**

phencyclidine (PCP) **488**

phenothiazines **486**

positive symptoms **480**

schizophrenia **480**

season-of-birth effect **484**

second-generation antipsychotics **487**

substance-induced psychotic disorder **486**

tardive dyskinesia **487**

Thought Question

On average, people who use much marijuana are more likely than others to develop schizophrenia. However, over the last several decades, the use of marijuana has increased while the prevalence of schizophrenia has not. What would be a reasonable hypothesis about the relationship between marijuana use and schizophrenia?

Module 14.3 | End of Module Quiz

1. Why is lack of emotional expression considered a "negative" symptom?

   A. It is disadvantageous to the patient.

   B. Only a small percentage of patients have this symptom.

   C. The symptom refers to the absence of something.

   D. It is caused by decreased activity in certain brain areas.

2. Schizophrenia is more common than average in which of the following types of people?

   A. People with allergies

   B. People who live in cities

   C. People who move from Europe to one of the Caribbean countries

   D. People who eat a diet rich in fish

3. Which of these is a likely conclusion about the role of genetics in schizophrenia?

   A. An aberrant form of the *DISC1* gene causes most cases of schizophrenia.

   B. Researchers believe one gene causes schizophrenia, but they have not found it yet.

   C. Rare mutations or microdeletions increase the probability of schizophrenia.

   D. Schizophrenia is not related to genetics.

4. According to the neurodevelopmental hypothesis, what starts schizophrenia?

   A. Disorders of brain development before or shortly after birth

   B. Tumors or other brain injuries between ages 8 and 12

   C. Difficult social experiences in adolescence

   D. Experiences shortly before the diagnosis

5. What is *Toxoplasma gondii?*

   A. A second-generation antipsychotic drug

   B. A parasite that can cause psychiatric disorders

   C. A chemical used for measuring dopamine concentrations

   D. A small nucleus of cells within the prefrontal cortex

6. Of these, which is the most likely explanation for the season-of-birth effect?

  A. Differences in the age of children when they start school

  B. Room temperature at the time of birth

  C. Availability of proteins in the diet

  D. Maternal illness during pregnancy

7. If schizophrenia is due to abnormal brain development in early life, how can we account for the fact that behavioral symptoms are not apparent until later in life?

  A. Schizophrenia impairs only social behavior, which is more important in adulthood.

  B. Other people do not notice the problems until the person is old enough to seek employment.

  C. A prime area of damage is the prefrontal cortex, which matures very slowly.

  D. Certain behavioral tests are inappropriate for use with children.

8. What is the time course of brain damage in schizophrenia?

  A. Most of the brain damage is present at diagnosis or soon after.

  B. The brain damage starts minimally and increases steadily throughout life.

  C. The brain damage occurs during adolescence and improves later.

  D. The brain damage is apparent only in patients who spent years in mental hospitals.

9. What is the effect of antipsychotic drugs on synapses?

  A. They stimulate oxytocin receptors.

  B. They interfere with reuptake of serotonin and other transmitters.

  C. They block certain dopamine synapses.

  D. They block certain glutamate synapses.

10. Of the following, which is an attempt to decrease tardive dyskinesia?

  A. Increased consumption of omega-3 fatty acids

  B. Exposure to bright lights in the morning

  C. Alternating between Thorazine and Haldol

  D. Use of second-generation antipsychotic drugs

Answers: 1C, 2B, 3C, 4A, 5B, 6D, 7C, 8A, 9C, 10D.

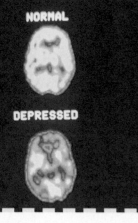

Autism Spectrum Disorders

Autism was once considered a rare condition. Today, estimates of its incidence vary substantially, with a median estimate of about one in 160 people worldwide (Elsabbagh et al., 2012). Part of the apparent increase is due to greater awareness and greater likelihood of using the label *autism* instead of something else. However, it is also possible that this condition has become more common than it used to be.

Symptoms and Characteristics

Therapists used to use the term *Asperger's syndrome* for people with a mild impairment similar to autism, but because Asperger's syndrome differs from autism only in degree, the new term **autism spectrum disorder** combines the two. In this module, for simplicity we use just the term *autism*, but you should understand that the term applies to the whole range of disorders.

Autism is about four times as common in boys as in girls. When it does occur in females, it tends to be more severe (Turner et al., 2015). Autism occurs throughout the world, and we have no convincing evidence that its prevalence varies by

geography, ethnic group, or socioeconomic status (Elsabbagh et al., 2012). The American Psychiatric Association (2013) identifies the following as important characteristics of autism spectrum disorder:

- Deficits in social and emotional exchange
- Deficits in gestures, facial expressions, and other nonverbal communication
- Stereotyped behaviors, such as repetitive movements (see Figure 14.21)
- Resistance to a change in routine
- Unusually weak or strong responses to stimuli, such as indifference to pain or a panicked reaction to a sound

Most people with autism have additional problems, such as epilepsy, anxiety, poor coordination, or deficits in attention or sleep (Bourgeron, 2015). Many have abnormalities in the cerebellum, resulting in clumsiness and impaired voluntary eye movements (Fatemi et al., 2012). Some have autistic symptoms secondary to brain tumors or other serious medical disorders (Sztainberg & Zoghbi, 2016). All of these symptoms vary substantially from one person to another. In the words of

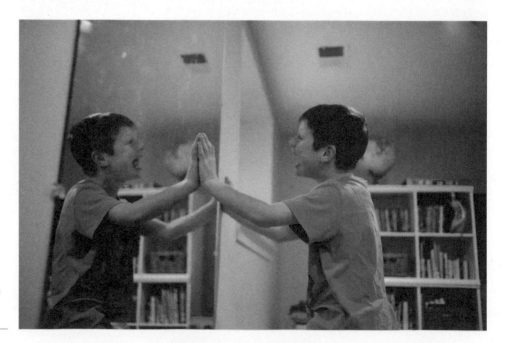

Figure 14.21 Stereotyped behaviors by an autistic child
Repetitive nonsocial behaviors are common in people with autism.
(Source: M. Scott Brauer/Alamy Stock Photo)

Steven Shore, "If you've met one child with autism, you've met one child with autism."

Parents of autistic children often notice a problem from the start, as an infant may not react comfortably to being held. Other problems increase over time. At age 2 months, children with autism make eye contact about as much as other children, but their eye contact gradually declines over the next two years (Jones & Klin, 2013). The problem is not an aversion to eye contact. Once they do make eye contact, they maintain it as long as other children, on average. The problem is that eyes and other social cues do not readily attract their attention (Moriuchi, Klin, & Jones, 2016).

In addition to the deficits characteristic of autism, certain strengths occur, too. Many develop narrow skills at which they excel. A surprising strength, not explained by any theory, is that children with autism tend to be substantially better than average at detecting visual motion (Foss-Feig, Tadin, Schauder, & Cascio, 2013).

Genetics and Other Causes

If you remember the information about genetics of drug abuse, depression, and schizophrenia, the genetic basis of autism will sound familiar: Many genes have been linked to autism, but no common gene exerts a large effect. Dozens of very rare genes can cause autism, but combined the identified genes account for only about 5 percent of cases (de la Torre-Ubieta, Won, Stein, & Geschwind, 2016). One identified mutation is to a gene in mitochondria (Aoki & Cortese, 2016). New mutations appear to be responsible for 10 percent or more of cases (Harris, 2016; Sanders et al., 2015; Tian et al., 2015). Although the number of possible mutations relevant to autism is large, their effects converge onto just a few chemical pathways that affect the early development of the brain (Krishnan et al., 2016). Exploring those pathways can help illuminate the basis of autism.

By examining the genes that surround a new mutation, and then comparing the results to the parents' chromosomes, researchers can infer whether a mutation came from the mother or the father, or whether it arose anew. Most of them occur on chromosomes inherited from the father, and the oldest fathers are slightly more likely to have children with autism than younger fathers are (Kong et al., 2012; O'Roak et al., 2012b). The same is true in schizophrenia. The explanation for the older-father effect is that women develop all their egg cells early in life, whereas men continue making new sperm throughout life, and mutations tend to accumulate (Lee & McGrath, 2015).

Prenatal environment can also contribute to autism. (Again note the parallel to schizophrenia.) The risk of autism increases if the mother is exposed during pregnancy to large amounts of pesticides, solvents, perfumes, or air pollutants (Mandy & Lai, 2016; Sealey et al., 2016).

A large-scale study found that after the birth of a child with autism, a brother or sister born less than 18 months later had a 14.4 percent chance of having autism also, whereas a brother or sister born 4 years later had only a 6.8 percent

chance (Risch et al., 2014). The genes were no more similar after a short delay than after a long delay, but the prenatal environments were more similar. For example, a mother who had an infection during the earlier pregnancy would be more likely to have the same infection after a shorter delay than after a longer one.

Some mothers of children with autism—about 12 percent—have antibodies that attack certain brain proteins. Few if any mothers of unaffected children have these antibodies. Identifying women with those antibodies might make it possible to intervene pharmacologically to prevent autism (Braunschweig et al., 2013). As further evidence for the relevance of those antibodies, researchers injected pregnant monkeys with antibodies from mothers of children with autism or mothers of unaffected children. Those injected with antibodies from children with autism—and not the others—had offspring that avoided social contacts with other monkeys (Bauman et al., 2013).

One more contributing factor: Nutritionists recommend that pregnant women and women planning to become pregnant get adequate amounts of **folic acid** (vitamin B_9), either from leafy green vegetables and orange juice, or from vitamin pills. Folic acid is important for development of the nervous system. Women who take folic acid pills during pregnancy have about half the probability of having a child with autism, compared to other women (Surén et al., 2013).

Children with autism have brain abnormalities that vary from one to another. A feature often noted is a large head. At age one year, the mean head size for autistic children is 10 percent greater than average. For the next several years, much of the cerebral cortex is larger than average. Some connections within the brain are stronger than average, whereas others are weaker than average. By young adulthood, the brain size is only about 1 percent greater than average (Hahamy, Behrmann, & Malach, 2015; Jumah, Ghannam, Jaber, Adeeb, & Tubbs, 2016; Schumann et al., 2010). Evidently brain development is progressing in an unusual way, but exactly how all this relates to the symptoms is not yet known.

STOP & CHECK

32. How can researchers determine whether a mutation or microdeletion has arisen anew?
33. Having a sibling with autism who is close to your age increases your own risk more than having a sibling with autism who is much older or younger. What conclusion does this observation imply?

ANSWERS **32.** They compare the child's chromosome to those of the parents. If neither parent has that mutation or microdeletion, then it arose anew. They can also examine surrounding genes to determine whether the chromosome came from the father or the mother. **33.** Genetics cannot be the whole explanation for autism. Factors in the prenatal environment may contribute. The prenatal environment would be more similar for siblings close in age.

Treatments

No medical treatment helps with the central problems of decreased social behavior and communication. Risperidone, a second-generation antipsychotic drug, sometimes reduces the stereotyped behaviors, but at the risk of serious side effects. In rare cases autism is due to mutation of a gene whose effects could be reversed chemically (Han et al., 2012; Novarino et al., 2012). At least, that is true theoretically. No attempts to apply this approach have been reported.

Behavioral treatments address the deficits in social behavior and communication. Parents, teachers, and therapists focus on eliciting the child's attention and reinforcing favorable behaviors. This procedure is successful with many children but not all. Treatments for stereotyped behaviors include reinforcing other behaviors or competing behaviors.

Not much solid research is available to evaluate the success of this approach (Reed, Hirst, & Hayman, 2012). Cognitive behavioral therapy provides moderate benefits according to therapists and parents, but not according to the people with autism themselves (Weston, Hodgekins, & Langdon, 2016).

Parents who grow understandably disappointed with these treatments are vulnerable to anyone who promises something better. A huge number of fad treatments have arisen, including special diets, chelation, music, and therapeutic touch. A treatment can become popular despite a lack of evidence to support it, or even the presence of evidence that it is useless or harmful. Many fad treatments make the parents feel good that they are trying something, but otherwise they are a waste of time and money (Matson, Adams, Williams, & Rieske, 2013).

Module 14.4 | In Closing

Development and Disorders

All the disorders discussed in this chapter—alcoholism and substance abuse, depression, schizophrenia, and autism—relate to many genes, not just one. Many of the genes that increase the risk of one disorder increase the risk of others, too. Many people have more than one disorder. Certainly many people have both depression and alcohol abuse, both

schizophrenia and alcohol or other substance abuse, or both autism and attention deficit disorder. In short, disorders that we discuss as if they were separate actually overlap. The early stages of brain development are complex and easily disrupted. Once the process goes off course, the risk increases for many undesirable outcomes.

Summary

1. Autism spectrum disorder is diagnosed more often now than in the past. The severity of symptoms varies greatly. **492**

2. Primary symptoms include a deficiency of social behavior and communication, including nonverbal communication. Many individuals also have repetitive stereotyped behaviors. **492**

3. No one gene is responsible for this condition. In some cases, it relates to new mutations or microdeletions, including one mutation to a mitochondrial gene. **493**

4. Difficulties in the prenatal environment also contribute. Some cases result because the mother during pregnancy produced certain antibodies that attack brain proteins. Consuming folic acid decreases the probability of having an autistic child. **493**

5. Behavioral treatments are the only effective approach to treating social and communicative deficits. Many parents try fad treatments of doubtful effectiveness. **494**

Key Terms

Terms are defined in the module on the page number indicated. They're also presented in alphabetical order with definitions in the book's Subject Index/Glossary, which begins on

page 589. Interactive flash cards, audio reviews, and crossword puzzles are among the online resources available to help you learn these terms and the concepts they represent.

autism spectrum disorder **492**
folic acid **493**

Thought Question

Some people have their chromosomes examined to check for predispositions to various illnesses, such as breast cancer. What would be the pros and cons of checking for genes associated with psychological disorders?

Module 14.4 | End of Module Quiz

1. In what way is the genetic basis of autism similar to that of schizophrenia?

   A. In both, most cases can be traced to a mutation in the *DISC1* gene.

   B. In both, many genes contribute.

   C. In both, a single dominant gene is responsible for the condition.

   D. In both, the genes exert their effects by altering serotonin reuptake.

2. Which of these is commonly observed for children with autism?

   A. If they see someone's eyes, they quickly look away.

   B. Eyes usually fail to capture their attention.

   C. When they see someone's eyes, they stare uninterrupted for an unusually long time.

   D. They move their eyes back and forth more rapidly than usual.

3. The probability of autism increases if which of these is true?

   A. The mother was significantly taller than the father.

   B. The mother was a vegetarian, but the father was not.

   C. The mother and father came from different ethnic groups.

   D. The father was much older than average.

4. Which of the following is common for children with autism, at age one year?

   A. The brain's norepinephrine concentration is 10 percent higher than average.

   B. The axons conduct impulses 10 percent faster than average.

   C. The head is 10 percent larger than average.

   D. The cerebral ventricles are 10 percent larger than average.

5. What dietary supplement during pregnancy decreases the probability of having a child with autism?

   A. Calcium

   B. Vitamin C

   C. Fish oil

   D. Folic acid

Answers: 1B, 2B, 3D, 4C, 5D.

Suggestions for Further Reading

Chahrour, M. et al. (2016). Current perspectives in autism spectrum disorder: From genes to therapy. *Journal of Neuroscience, vol. 36*, pp. 11402–11410. An excellent review of research on autism.

Kirsch, I. (2010). *The emperor's new drugs.* New York: Basic Books. A highly skeptical discussion of the effectiveness or ineffectiveness of antidepressant drugs.

Appendix A

Introduction

To understand certain aspects of biological psychology, particularly the action potential and the molecular mechanisms of synaptic transmission, you need to know a little about chemistry. If you have taken a high school or college course and remember the material reasonably well, you should have no trouble with the chemistry in this text. If your knowledge of chemistry is pretty hazy, this appendix will help. (If you plan to take other courses in biological psychology, you should study as much biology and chemistry as possible.)

Elements and Compounds

If you look around, you will see an enormous variety of materials—dirt, water, wood, plastic, metal, cloth, glass, your own body. Every object is composed of a small number of basic building blocks. If a piece of wood catches fire, it breaks down into ashes, gases, and water vapor. The same is true of your body. An investigator could take those ashes, gases, and water, and break them down by chemical and electrical means into carbon, oxygen, hydrogen, nitrogen, and a few other materials. Eventually, however, the investigator arrives at a set of materials that cannot be broken down further: Pure carbon or pure oxygen, for example, cannot be converted into anything simpler, at least not by ordinary chemical means. (High-power bombardment with subatomic particles is another story.) The matter we see is composed of **elements** (materials that cannot be broken down into other materials) and **compounds** (materials made up by combining elements).

Chemists have found 92 elements in nature, and they have constructed more in the laboratory. (Actually, one of the 92—technetium—is so rare as to be virtually unknown in nature.) Figure A.1, the periodic table, lists each of these

elements. Of these, only a few are important for life on Earth. Table A.1 shows the elements commonly found in the human body.

Note that each element has a one- or two-letter abbreviation, such as O for oxygen, H for hydrogen, and Ca for calcium. These are internationally accepted symbols that facilitate communication among chemists who speak different languages. For example, element number 19 is called potassium in English, potassio in Italian, kālijs in Latvian, and draslík in Czech. But chemists in all countries use the symbol K (from *kalium,* the Latin word for "potassium"). Similarly, the symbol for sodium is Na (from *natrium,* the Latin word for "sodium"), and the symbol for iron is Fe (from the Latin word *ferrum*).

A compound is represented by the symbols for the elements that compose it. For example, NaCl stands for sodium chloride (common table salt). H_2O, the symbol for water, indicates that water consists of two parts of hydrogen and one part of oxygen.

Table A.1	The Elements That Compose Almost All of the Human Body	
Element	Symbol	Percentage by Weight in Human Body
Oxygen	O	65
Carbon	C	18
Hydrogen	H	10
Nitrogen	N	3
Calcium	Ca	2
Phosphorus	P	1.1
Potassium	K	0.35
Sulfur	S	0.25
Sodium	Na	0.15
Chlorine	CI	0.15
Magnesium	Mg	0.05
Iron	Fe	Trace
Copper	Cu	Trace
Iodine	I	Trace
Fluorine	F	Trace
Manganese	Mn	Trace
Zinc	Zn	Trace
Selenium	Se	Trace
Molybdenum	Mo	Trace

Periodic Table of the Elements

Main group and transition elements (atomic number, symbol, name, atomic weight)

Group	1 IA	2 IIA	3 IIIB	4 IVB	5 VB	6 VIB	7 VIIB	8 VIIIB	9 VIIIB	10 VIIIB	11 IB	12 IIB	13 IIIA	14 IVA	15 VA	16 VIA	17 VIIA	18 VIIIA
Period 1	1 **H** hydrogen 1.008																	2 **He** helium 4.003
Period 2	3 **Li** lithium 6.941	4 **Be** beryllium 9.012											5 **B** boron 10.81	6 **C** carbon 12.011	7 **N** nitrogen 14.007	8 **O** oxygen 16.0	9 **F** fluorine 18.999	10 **Ne** neon 20.179
Period 3	11 **Na** sodium 22.99	12 **Mg** magnesium 24.305											13 **Al** aluminum 26.982	14 **Si** silicon 28.085	15 **P** phosphorous 30.974	16 **S** sulfur 32.060	17 **Cl** chlorine 35.453	18 **Ar** argon 39.948
Period 4	19 **K** potassium 39.098	20 **Ca** calcium 40.08	21 **Sc** scandium 44.955	22 **Ti** titanium 47.90	23 **V** vanadium 50.941	24 **Cr** chromium 51.996	25 **Mn** manganese 54.938	26 **Fe** iron 55.847	27 **Co** cobalt 58.933	28 **Ni** nickel 58.70	29 **Cu** copper 63.546	30 **Zn** zinc 65.38	31 **Ga** gallium 69.72	32 **Ge** germanium 72.59	33 **As** arsenic 74.922	34 **Se** selenium 78.96	35 **Br** bromine 79.904	36 **Kr** krypton 83.80
Period 5	37 **Rb** rubidium 85.468	38 **Sr** strontium 87.62	39 **Y** yttrium 88.906	40 **Zr** zirconium 91.22	41 **Nb** niobium 92.906	42 **Mo** molybdenum 95.940	43 **Tc** technetium (97)	44 **Ru** ruthenium 101.07	45 **Rh** rhodium 102.905	46 **Pd** palladium 106.40	47 **Ag** silver 107.868	48 **Cd** cadmium 112.41	49 **In** indium 114.82	50 **Sn** tin 118.69	51 **Sb** antimony 121.75	52 **Te** tellurium 127.60	53 **I** iodine 126.904	54 **Xe** xenon 131.30
Period 6	55 **Cs** cesium 132.905	56 **Ba** barium 137.33	57 **La** lanthanum 138.906 †	72 **Hf** hafnium 178.49	73 **Ta** tantalum 180.948	74 **W** tungsten 183.85	75 **Re** rhenium 186.207	76 **Os** osmium 190.20	77 **Ir** iridium 192.22	78 **Pt** platinum 195.09	79 **Au** gold 196.967	80 **Hg** mercury 200.59	81 **Tl** thallium 204.37	82 **Pb** lead 207.20	83 **Bi** bismuth 208.980	84 **Po** polonium (209)	85 **At** astatine (210)	86 **Rn** radon (222)
Period 7	87 **Fr** francium (223)	88 **Ra** radium 226.025	89 **Ac** actinium (227) ‡	104 **Rf** rutherfordium (261)	105 **Db** dubnium (262)	106 **Sg** seaborgium (266)	107 **Bh** bohrium (264)	108 **Hs** hassium (269)	109 **Mt** meitnerium (268)	110 **Ds** darmstadtium (271)	111 **Rg** roentgenium (272)	112 **Cn** copernicium (285)	113 **Nh** Nihonium (286)	114 **Uuq** ununquadium (289)	115 **Mc** Moscovium (289)	116 **Uuh** ununhexium (292)	117 **Ts** Tennessine (294)	118 **Og** Oganesson (294)

Inner Transition Elements

† Lanthanides 6:

58 **Ce** cerium 140.12	59 **Pr** praseodymium 140.908	60 **Nd** neodymium 144.24	61 **Pm** promethium (145)	62 **Sm** samarium 150.40	63 **Eu** europium 151.96	64 **Gd** gadolinium 157.25	65 **Tb** terbium 158.925	66 **Dy** dysprosium 162.50	67 **Ho** holmium 164.93	68 **Er** erbium 167.26	69 **Tm** thulium 168.934	70 **Yb** ytterbium 173.04	71 **Lu** lutetium 174.97

‡ Actinides 7:

90 **Th** thorium 232.038	91 **Pa** protactinium 231.036	92 **U** uranium 238.029	93 **Np** neptunium (237)	94 **Pu** plutonium (244)	95 **Am** americium (243)	96 **Cm** curium (247)	97 **Bk** berkelium (247)	98 **Cf** californium (251)	99 **Es** einsteinium (254)	100 **Fm** fermium (257)	101 **Md** mendelevium (258)	102 **No** nobelium (255)	103 **Lr** lawrencium (260)

Alkali Metals (Group IA) · Alkaline Earth Metals (Group IIA) · Transition Elements · Halogens (Group VIIA) · Noble Gases (Group VIIIA)

Key

atomic number — 1
symbol of element — **H**
element name — hydrogen
atomic weight — 1.008

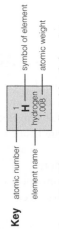

Figure A.1 The periodic table of chemistry
It is called "periodic" because certain properties show up at periodic intervals. For example, the column from lithium down consists of metals that readily form salts. The column at the far right consists of gases that do not readily form compounds. Elements 114 and 116 have only tentative names and symbols.

Atoms and Molecules

A block of iron can be chopped finer and finer until it is divided into tiny pieces that cannot be broken down any further. These pieces are called **atoms**. Every element is composed of atoms. A compound, such as water, can also be divided into tinier and tinier pieces. The smallest possible piece of a compound is called a **molecule**. A molecule of water can be further decomposed into two atoms of hydrogen and one atom of oxygen, but when that happens the compound is broken and is no longer water. A molecule is the smallest piece of a compound that retains the properties of the compound.

An atom is composed of subatomic particles, including protons, neutrons, and electrons. A proton has a positive electrical charge, a neutron has a neutral charge, and an electron has a negative charge. The nucleus of an atom—its center—contains one or more protons plus a number of neutrons. Electrons are found in the space around the nucleus. Because an atom has the same number of protons as electrons, the electrical charges balance out. (Ions, which we will soon consider, have an imbalance of positive and negative charges.)

The difference between one element and another is in the number of protons in the nucleus of the atom. Hydrogen has just one proton, for example, and oxygen has eight. The number of protons is the **atomic number** of the element; in the periodic table it is recorded at the top of the square for each element. The number at the bottom is the element's **atomic weight**, which indicates the weight of an atom relative to the weight of one proton. A proton has a weight of one unit, a neutron has a weight just trivially greater than one, and an electron has a weight just trivially greater than zero. The atomic weight of the element is the number of protons in the atom plus the average number of neutrons. For example, most hydrogen atoms have one proton and no neutrons; a few atoms per thousand have one or two neutrons, giving an average atomic weight of 1.008. Sodium ions have 11 protons; most also have 12 neutrons, and the atomic weight is slightly less than 23. (Can you figure out the number of neutrons in the average potassium atom? Refer to Figure A.1.)

Ions and Chemical Bonds

An atom that has gained or lost one or more electrons is called an **ion.** For example, if sodium and chloride come together, the sodium atoms readily lose one electron each and the chloride atoms gain one each. The result is a set of positively charged sodium ions (indicated Na^+) and negatively charged chloride ions (Cl^-). Potassium atoms, like sodium atoms, tend to lose an electron and to become positively charged ions (K^+); calcium ions tend to lose two electrons and gain a double positive charge (Ca^{++}).

Because positive charges attract negative charges, sodium ions attract chloride ions. When dry, sodium and chloride form a crystal structure, as Figure A.2 shows. (In water solution, the two kinds of ions move about haphazardly, occasionally attracting one another but then pulling apart.) The attraction of posi-

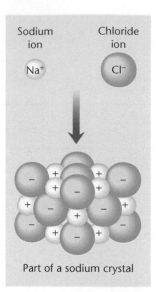

Figure A.2 **The crystal structure of sodium**
Each sodium ion is surrounded by chloride ions, and each chloride ion is surrounded by sodium ions; no ion is bound to any other single ion in particular.

tive ions for negative ions forms an **ionic bond.** In other cases, instead of transferring an electron from one atom to another, some pairs of atoms share electrons with each other, forming a **covalent bond.** For example, two hydrogen atoms bind, as shown in Figure A.3, and two hydrogen atoms bind with an oxygen atom, as shown in Figure A.4. Atoms that are attached by a covalent bond cannot move independently of one another.

Reactions of Carbon Atoms

Living organisms depend on the enormously versatile compounds of carbon. Because of the importance of these compounds for life, the chemistry of carbon is known as organic chemistry.

Carbon atoms form covalent bonds with hydrogen, oxygen, and a number of other elements. They also form covalent bonds with other carbon atoms. Two carbon atoms may share

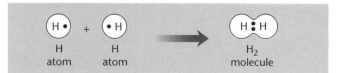

Figure A.3 **Structure of a hydrogen molecule**
A hydrogen atom has one electron; in the compound the two atoms share the two electrons equally.

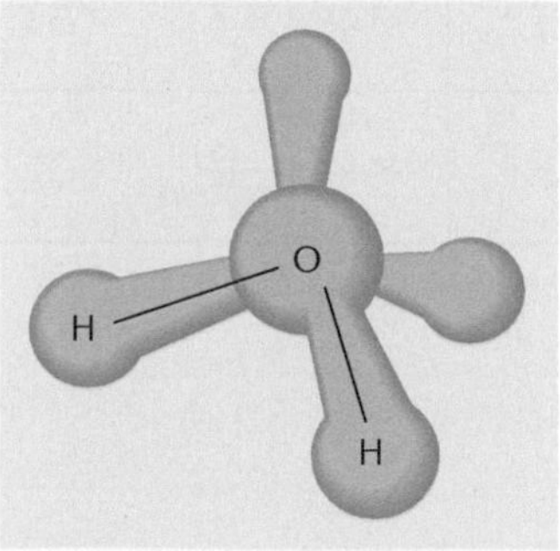

Figure A.4 **Structure of a water molecule**
The oxygen atom shares a pair of electrons with each hydrogen atom. Oxygen holds the electrons more tightly, making the oxygen part of the molecule more negatively charged than the hydrogen part of the molecule.

from one to three pairs of electrons. Such bonds can be indicated as follows:

C—C   Two atoms share one pair of electrons.
C=C   Two atoms share two pairs of electrons.
C≡C   Two atoms share three pairs of electrons.

Each carbon atom ordinarily forms four covalent bonds, either with other carbon atoms, with hydrogen atoms, or with other atoms. Many biologically important compounds include long chains of carbon compounds linked to one another, such as:

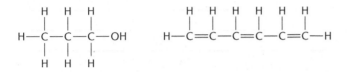

Note that each carbon atom has a total of four bonds, counting each double bond as two. In some molecules, the carbon chain loops around to form a ring:

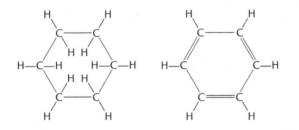

Ringed structures are common in organic chemistry. To simplify the diagrams, chemists often omit the hydrogen atoms. You can simply assume that each carbon atom in the diagram has four covalent bonds and that all the bonds not shown are with hydrogen atoms. To further simplify the diagrams, chemists often omit the carbon atoms themselves, showing only the carbon-to-carbon bonds. For example, the two molecules shown in the previous diagram might be rendered as follows:

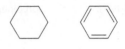

If a particular carbon atom has a bond with some atom other than hydrogen, the diagram shows the exception. For example, in each of the two molecules diagrammed below, one carbon has a bond with an oxygen atom, which in turn has a bond with a hydrogen atom. All the bonds that are not shown are carbon–hydrogen bonds.

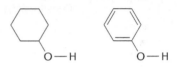

Figure A.5 illustrates some carbon compounds that are critical for animal life. Purines and pyrimidines form the central structure of DNA and RNA, the chemicals responsible for heredity. Proteins, fats, and carbohydrates are the primary types

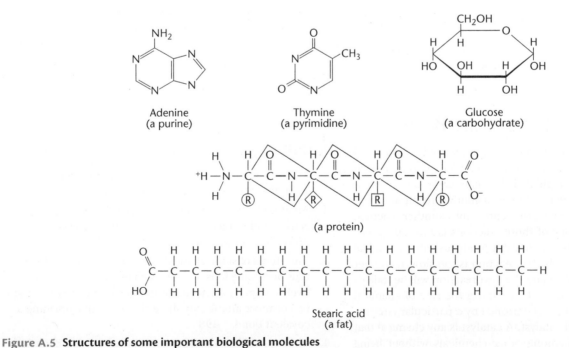

Adenine
(a purine)

Thymine
(a pyrimidine)

Glucose
(a carbohydrate)

(a protein)

Stearic acid
(a fat)

Figure A.5 Structures of some important biological molecules
The R in the protein represents a point of attachment for various chains that differ from one amino acid to another. Actual proteins are much longer than the chemical shown here.

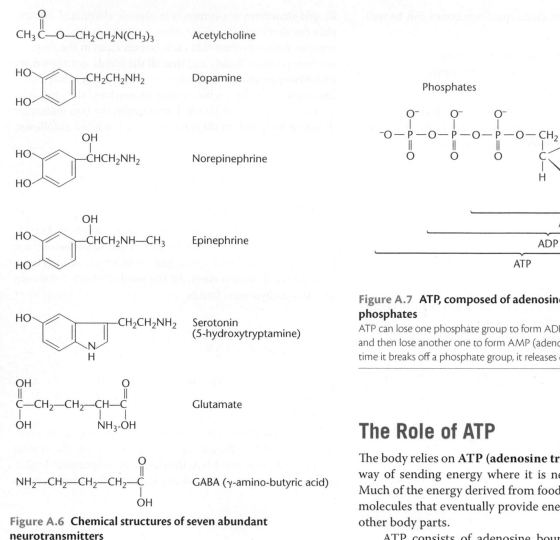

Figure A.6 Chemical structures of seven abundant neurotransmitters

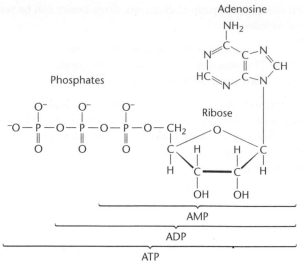

Figure A.7 ATP, composed of adenosine, ribose, and three phosphates
ATP can lose one phosphate group to form ADP (adenosine diphosphate) and then lose another one to form AMP (adenosine monophosphate). Each time it breaks off a phosphate group, it releases energy.

of fuel that the body uses. Figure A.6 displays the chemical structures of seven neurotransmitters that are extensively discussed in this text.

Chemical Reactions in the Body

A living organism is an immensely complicated, coordinated set of chemical reactions. Life requires that the rate of each reaction be carefully regulated. In many cases one reaction produces a chemical that enters into another reaction, which produces another chemical that enters into another reaction, and so forth. If any one of those reactions is too rapid compared to the others, the chemical it produces will accumulate to possibly harmful levels. If a reaction is too slow, it will not produce enough product and the next reaction will be stalled.

Enzymes are proteins that control the rate of chemical reactions. Each reaction is controlled by a particular enzyme. Enzymes are a type of catalyst. A catalyst is any chemical that facilitates a reaction among other chemicals without being altered itself in the process.

The Role of ATP

The body relies on **ATP (adenosine triphosphate)** as its main way of sending energy where it is needed (see Figure A.7). Much of the energy derived from food goes into forming ATP molecules that eventually provide energy for the muscles and other body parts.

ATP consists of adenosine bound to ribose and three phosphate groups (PO_3). Phosphates form high-energy covalent bonds. That is, a large amount of energy is required to form the bonds, and a large amount of energy is released when they break. ATP can break off one or two of its three phosphates to provide energy.

Summary

1. Matter is composed of 92 elements that combine to form an endless variety of compounds.   **496**

2. An atom is the smallest piece of an element. A molecule is the smallest piece of a compound that maintains the properties of the compound.   **498**

3. The atoms of some elements can gain or lose an electron, thus becoming ions. Positively charged ions attract negatively charged ions, forming an ionic bond. In some cases two or more atoms may share electrons, thus forming a covalent bond.   **498**

4. The principal carrier of energy in the body is a chemical called ATP.   **500**

Key Terms

atom **498**
atomic number **498**
atomic weight **498**
ATP (adenosine triphosphate) **500**
compound **496**

covalent bond **498**
element **496**
enzyme **500**
ion **498**
ionic bond **498**
molecule **498**

Introduction

The Society for Neuroscience, as a professional society for basic and clinical researchers in neuroscience, endorses and supports the appropriate and responsible use of animals as experimental subjects. Knowledge generated by neuroscience research on animals has led to important advances in the understanding of diseases and disorders that affect the nervous system and in the development of better treatments that reduce suffering in humans and animals. This knowledge also makes a critical contribution to our understanding of ourselves, the complexities of our brains and what makes us human. Continued progress in understanding how the brain works and further advances in treating and curing disorders of the nervous system require investigation of complex functions at all levels in the living nervous system. Because no adequate alternatives exist, much of this research must be done on animal subjects. The Society takes the position that neuroscientists have an obligation to contribute to this progress through responsible and humane research on animals.

Several functions of the Society are related to the use of animals in research. A number of these involve decisions about research conducted by members of the Society, including the scheduling of scientific presentations at the Annual Meeting, the review and publication of original research papers in *The Journal of Neuroscience* and the defense of members whose ethical use of animals in research is questioned by animal rights activists. The Society's support for the research of individual members defines a relationship between the Society and its members. The purpose of this document is to outline the policy that guides that relationship. Compliance with the following policy will be an important factor in determining the suitability of research for presentation at the Annual Meeting or for publication in *The Journal of Neuroscience* and in situations where the Society is asked to provide public and active support for a member whose use of animals in research has been questioned.

The responsibility for implementing the policy in each of these areas rests with the relevant administrative body (Program Committee, Publications Committee, Editorial Board and Committee on Animals in Research, respectively) in consultation with Council.

Policy on the Use of Animals in Neuroscience Research

Neuroscience research uses complicated, often invasive methods, each of which is associated with different problems, risks, and specific technical considerations. An experimental method that would be deemed inappropriate for one kind of research may be the method of choice for another kind of research. It is therefore impossible for the Society to define specific policies and procedures for the care and use of all research animals and for the design and conduct of every neuroscience experiment.

The U.S. Public Health Service Policy on Humane Care and Use of Laboratory Animals (PHS Policy) and the *Guide for the Care and Use of Laboratory Animals* (the Guide) describe general policies and procedures designed to ensure the humane and appropriate use of live vertebrate animals in all forms of biomedical research. The Society finds the policies and procedures set forth in the PHS Policy and the Guide to be both necessary and sufficient to ensure a high standard of animal care and use and adopts them as its official Policy on the Use of Animals in Neuroscience Research (Society Policy). All Society members are expected to conduct their animal research in compliance with this policy. Members are required to verify that they have done so when submitting abstracts for presentation at the Annual Meeting or manuscripts for publication in *The Journal of Neuroscience.* Adherence to the Society policy is also an important step toward receiving help from the Society in responding to questions about a member's use of animals in research. A complete description of what to do if your research is questioned is included in this handbook. Also, a complete description of SfN's policy and procedures for defending members whose research comes under attack can be obtained by contacting the Society's Central Office.

Local Committee Review

An important element of the Society Policy is the establishment of a local committee that is charged with reviewing and approving all proposed animal care and use procedures. In addition to scientists experienced in research involving animals and a veterinarian, the membership of this local committee should include a person who is not affiliated with the member's institution in any other way. In reviewing a proposed use of animals, the committee should evaluate the adequacy of institutional policies, animal husbandry, veterinary care, and the physical plant. The committee should pay specific attention to proposed procedures for animal procurement, quarantine and stabilization, separation by species, disease diagnosis and treatment, anesthesia and analgesia, surgery and postsurgical care, and euthanasia. The review committee also should ensure that procedures involving live vertebrate animals are designed and performed with due consideration of their relevance to human or animal health, the advancement of knowledge or the good of society. This review and approval of a member's use of live vertebrate animals in research by a local committee is an essential component of the Society Policy. For assistance in developing appropriate animal care and use procedures and establishing a local review committee, call the Society and consult the documents recommended at the end of this section.

Other Laws, Regulations, and Policies

In addition to complying with the policy described above, Society members who reside in North America must also adhere to all relevant national, state, or local laws and/or regulations that govern their use of animals in neuroscience research. Thus, U.S. members must observe the U.S. Animal Welfare Act (as amended in 1985) and its implementing regulations from the U.S. Department of Agriculture. Canadian members must abide by the January 1993 Guide to the Care and Use of Experimental Animals. Members in Mexico must comply with the "Seventh Title of the Regulations of the General Law of Health Regarding Health Research." In addition to complying with the laws and regulations of their home countries, foreign members of the Society should adhere to the official Society Policy outlined here.

Recommended References

Canadian Council on Animal Care. Guide to the Care and Use of Experimental Animals Vol. 1. 2d ed. Ontario, Canada: CCAC, 1993.

Foundation for Biomedical Research. The Biomedical Investigator's Handbook for Researchers Using Animal Models. Washington, D.C.: FBR, 1987.

Laws and Codes of Mexico. "Seventh Title of the Regulations of the General Law of Health Regarding Health Research." 12th updated ed. Porrua Collection, 430-31. Mexico: Porrua Publishers, 1995.

National Academy of Sciences. Guide for the Care and Use of Laboratory Animals, 7th ed. Washington, D.C.: National Research Council, Institute for Laboratory Animal Research, NAS, 1996.

National Institutes of Health. OPRR Public Health Service Policy on Humane Care and Use of Laboratory Animals. Rockville, MD: NIH/Office for Protection from Research Risks, 1996.

National Institutes of Health. Preparation and Maintenance of Higher Mammals During Neuroscience Experiments. Report of a National Institutes of Health Workshop. NIH Publication No. 94-3207. Bethesda, MD: NIH/National Eye Institute, 1994.

Society for Neuroscience. Handbook for the Use of Animals in Neuroscience Research. Washington, D.C.: SfN, 1991.

Visual Neuroscience. 1 (4): 421-6. "Anesthesia and Paralysis in Experimental Animals." Report of a Workshop held in Bethesda, Md., Oct. 27, 1984. Organized by the Division of Research Grants, National Institutes of Health. England: VN, 1984.

General Principles

The following principles, based largely on the PHS Policy on Humane Care and Use of Laboratory Animals, can be a useful guide to designing and implementing experimental procedures involving laboratory animals.

Animals selected for a procedure should be of an appropriate species and quality and the minimum number required to obtain valid results.

Proper use of animals, including the avoidance or minimization of discomfort, distress, and pain, is imperative.

Procedures with animals that may cause more than momentary or slight pain or distress should be performed with appropriate sedation, analgesia, or anesthesia. Surgical or other painful procedures should not be performed on unanesthetized animals paralyzed by chemical agents.

Postoperative care of animals should minimize discomfort and pain and, in any case, should be equivalent to accepted practices in schools of veterinary medicine.

Animals that would otherwise suffer severe or chronic pain or distress that cannot be relieved should be painlessly killed at the end of the procedure or, if appropriate, during the procedure. If the study requires the death of the animal, the animal must be killed in a humane manner.

Living conditions should be appropriate for the species and contribute to the animals' well-being. Normally, the housing, feeding, and care of all animals used for biomedical purposes must be directed by a veterinarian or other scientist trained and experienced in the proper care, handling, and use of the species being maintained or studied. In any case, appropriate veterinary care shall be provided.

Exceptions to these principles require careful consideration and should only be made by an appropriate review group such as an institutional animal care and use committee.

Policy on the Use of Human Subjects in Neuroscience Research

Experimental procedures involving human subjects must have been conducted in conformance with the policies and principles contained in the Federal Policy for the Protection of Human Subjects (U. S. Office of Science and Technology Policy) and in the Declaration of Helsinki. When publishing a paper in *The Journal of Neuroscience* or submitting an abstract for presentation at the Annual Meeting, authors must sign a statement of compliance with this policy.

Recommended References

"Declaration of Helsinki." Adopted by 18th World Medical Assembly, Helsinki, 1964; revised by 29th World Medical Assembly, Tokyo, 1975; Venice, 1983; and Hong Kong, 1989.

"Federal Policy for the Protection of Human Subjects; Notices and Rules." Federal Register (June 18, 1991) 56: 28002–32.

Varga, Andrew C., Ed. The Main Issue in Bioethics Revised Edition. New York: Paulist Press, 1984.

References

Numbers in parentheses following entries indicate the chapter in which a reference is cited.

Abbott, N. J., Rönnback, L., & Hansson, E. (2006). Astrocyte-endothelial interactions at the blood–brain barrier. *Nature Reviews Neuroscience, 7*, 41–53. (1)

Abbott, S. B. G., Machado, N. L. S., Geerling, J. C., & Saper, C. B. (2016). Reciprocal control of drinking behavior by median preoptic neurons in mice. *Journal of Neuroscience, 36*, 8228–8237. (9)

AbdelMalik, P., Husted, J, Chow, E. W. C., & Bassett, A. S. (2003). Childhood head injury and expression of schizophrenia in multiply affected families. *Archives of General Psychiatry, 60*, 231–236. (14)

Abi-Dargham, A., Rodenhiser, J., Printz, D., Zea-Ponce, Y., Gil, R., Kegeles, L. S., . . . Laruelle, M. (2000). Increased baseline occupancy of D2 receptors by dopamine in schizophrenia. *Proceedings of the National Academy of Sciences, USA, 97*, 8104–8109. (14)

Abrahamsson, N., & Hyltenstam, K. (2009). Age of onset and nativelikeness in a second language: Listener perception versus linguistic scrutiny. *Language Learning, 59*, 249–306. (13)

Ackman, J. B., Burbridge, T. J., & Crair, M. C. (2012). Retinal waves coordinate patterned activity throughout the developing visual system. *Nature, 490*, 219–225. (5)

Adamec, R. E., Stark-Adamec, C., & Livingston, K. E. (1980). The development of predatory aggression and defense in the domestic cat (*Felis catus*): 3. Effects on development of hunger between 180 and 365 days of age. *Behavioral and Neural Biology, 30*, 435–447. (11)

Adams, D. B., Gold, A. R., & Burt, A. D. (1978). Rise in female-initiated sexual activity at ovulation and its suppression by oral contraceptives. *New England Journal of Medicine, 299*, 1145–1150. (10)

Adams, R. B., Jr., Gordon, H. L., Baird, A. A., Ambady, N., & Kleck, R. E. (2003). Effects of gaze on amygdala sensitivity to anger and fear faces. *Science, 300*, 1536. (11)

Adams, R. B., Jr., & Kleck, R. E. (2005). Effects of direct and averted gaze on the perception of facially communicated emotion. *Emotion, 5*, 3–11. (11)

Addis, D. R., Wong, A. T., & Schacter, D. L. (2007). Remembering the past and imagining the future: Common and distinct neural substrates during event construction and elaboration. *Neuropsychologia, 45*, 1363–1377. (12)

Adkins, E. K., & Adler, N. T. (1972). Hormonal control of behavior in the Japanese quail. *Journal of Comparative and Physiological Psychology, 81*, 27–36. (10)

Admon, R., Lubin, G., Stern, O., Rosenberg, K., Sela, L., Ben-Ami, H., & Hendler, T. (2009). Human vulnerability to stress depends on amygdala's predisposition and hippocampal plasticity. *Proceedings of the National Academy of Sciences (U.S.A.), 106*, 14120–14125. (11)

Adolphs, R., Damasio, H., & Tranel, D. (2002). Neural systems for recognition of emotional prosody: A 3-D lesion study. *Emotion, 2*, 23–51. (13)

Adolphs, R., Tranel, D., & Buchanan, T. W. (2005). Amygdala damage impairs emotional memory for gist but not details of complex stimuli. *Nature Neuroscience, 8*, 512–518. (11)

Adolphs, R., Tranel, D., Damasio, H., & Damasio, A. (1995). Fear and the human amygdala. *Journal of Neuroscience, 15*, 5879–5891. (11)

Agarwal, N., Pacher, P., Tegeder, I., Amaya, F., Constantin, C. E., Brenner, G. J., . . . Kuner, R. (2007). Cannabinoids mediate analgesia largely via peripheral type 1 cannabinoid receptors in nociceptors. *Nature Neuroscience, 10*, 870–879. (6)

Aglioti, S., Smania, N., Atzei, A., & Berlucchi, G. (1997). Spatio-temporal properties of the pattern of evoked phantom sensations in a left index amputee patient. *Behavioral Neuroscience, 111*, 867–872. (4)

Aglioti, S., Smania, N., & Peru, A. (1999). Frames of reference for mapping tactile stimuli in brain-damaged patients. *Journal of Cognitive Neuroscience, 11*, 67–79. (13)

Agrati, D., Fernández-Guasti, A., Ferreño, M., & Ferreira, A. (2011). Coexpression of sexual behavior and maternal aggression: The ambivalence of sexually active mother rats toward male intruders. *Behavioral Neuroscience, 125*, 446–451. (10)

Ahlskog, J. E., & Hoebel, B. G. (1973). Overeating and obesity from damage to a noradrenergic system in the brain. *Science, 182*, 166–169. (9)

Ahlskog, J. E., Randall, P. K., & Hoebel, B. G. (1975). Hypothalamic hyperphagia: Dissociation from hyperphagia following destruction of noradrenergic neurons. *Science, 190*, 399–401. (9)

Ahmed, E. I., Zehr, J. L., Schulz, K. M., Lorenz, B. H., DonCarlos, L. L., & Sisk, C. L. (2008). Pubertal hormones modulate the addition of new cells to sexually dimorphic brain regions. *Nature Neuroscience, 11*, 995–997. (10)

Ahmed, I. I., Shryne, J. E., Gorski, R. A., Branch, B. J., & Taylor, A. N. (1991). Prenatal ethanol and the prepubertal sexually dimorphic nucleus of the preoptic area. *Physiology & Behavior, 49*, 427–432. (10)

Ahn, W., Flanagan, E. H., Marsh, J. K., & Sanislow, C. A. (2006). Beliefs about essences and the reality of mental disorders. *Psychological Science, 17*, 759–766. (14)

Airaksinen, M. S., & Saarma, M. (2002). The GDNF family: Signalling, biological functions and therapeutic value. *Nature Reviews Neuroscience, 3*, 383–394. (4)

Airan, R. D., Meltzer, L. A., Roy, M., Gong, Y., Chen, H., & Deisseroth, K. (2007). High-speed imaging reveals neurophysiological links to behavior in an animal model of depression. *Science, 317*, 819–823. (14)

Airavaara, M., Harvey, B. K., Voutilainen, M. H., Shen, H., Chou, J., Lindholm, P., . . . Wang, Y. (2012). CDNF protects the nigrostriatal dopamine system and promotes recovery after MPTP treatment in mice. *Cell Transplantation, 21*, 1213–1223. (7)

Ajina, S., Pestilli, F., Rokem, A., Kennard, C., & Bridge, H. (2015). Human blindsight is mediated by an intact geniculo-extrastriate pathway. *eLife, 4*, article 08935. (5)

Akers, K. G., Martinez-Canabal, A., Restivo, L., Yiu, A. P., De Cristofaro, A., Hsiang, H.-L., . . . Frankland, P. W. (2014). Hippocampal neurogenesis regulates forgetting during adulthood and infancy. *Science, 344*, 598–602. (12)

Alagiakrishnan, K., Gill, S. S., & Fagarasanu, A. (2012). Genetics and epigenetics of Alzheimer's disease. *Postgraduate Medical Journal, 88*, 522–529. (12)

Alanko, K., Santtila, P., Harlaar, N., Witting, K., Varjonen, M., Jern, P., . . . Sandnabba, N. K. (2010). Common genetic effects of gender atypical behavior in childhood and sexual orientation in adulthood: A study of Finnish twins. *Archives of Sexual Behavior, 39*, 81–92. (10)

Albouy, G., Sterpenich, V., Balteau, E., Vandewalle, G., Desseilles, M., Dang-Vu, T., . . . Maquet, P. (2008). Both the hippocampus and striatum are involved in consolidation of motor sequence memory. *Neuron, 58*, 261–272. (12)

Albuquerque, D., Stice, E., Rodríguez-Lopez, R., Manco, L., & Nóbrega, C. (2015). Current review of genetics of human obesity: From molecular mechanisms to an evolutionary perspective. *Molecular Genetics and Genomics, 290*, 1191–1221. (9)

Alcuter, S., Lin, W., Smith, J. K., Short, S. J., Goldman, B. D., Reznick, J. S., . . . Gao, W.

(2014). Development of thalamocortical connectivity during infancy and its cognitive correlations. *Journal of Neuroscience, 34*, 9067–9075. (4)

Aleman, A., Kahn, R. S., & Selten, J. P. (2003). Sex differences in the risk of schizophrenia. *Archives of General Psychiatry, 60*, 565–571. (14)

Alexander, G. M., & Hines, M. (2002). Sex differences in response to children's toys in nonhuman primates (*Cercopithecus aethiops sabaeus*). *Evolution and Human Behavior, 23*, 467–479. (10)

Alexander, G. M., Wilcox, T., & Woods, R. (2009). Sex differences in infants' visual interest in toys. *Archives of Sexual Behavior, 38*, 427–433. (10)

Al-Karawi, D., & Jubair, L. (2016). Bright light therapy for nonseasonal depression: Meta-analysis of clinical trials. *Journal of Affective Disorders, 198*, 64–71. (14)

Allen, H. L., Estrada, K., Lettre, G., Berndt, S. I., Weedon, M. N., Rivadeneira, F., . . . Hirschhorn, J. N. (2010). Hundreds of variants clustered in genomic loci and biological pathways affect human height. *Nature, 467*, 832–838. (4)

Allen, J. S., Damasio, H., Grabowski, T. J., Bruss, J., & Zhang, W. (2003). Sexual dimorphism and asymmetries in the gray-white composition of the human cerebrum. *NeuroImage, 18*, 880–894. (12)

Alleva, E., & Francia, N. (2009). Psychiatric vulnerability: Suggestions from animal models and role of neurotrophins. *Neuroscience and Biobehavioral Reviews, 33*, 525–536. (4)

Allison, T., & Cicchetti, D. V. (1976). Sleep in mammals: Ecological and constitutional correlates. *Science, 194*, 732–734. (8)

Almeida, J., He, D., Chen, Q., Mahon, B. Z., Zhang, F., Gonçalves, Ó. F., ... Bi, Y. (2015). Decoding visual location from neural patterns in the auditory cortex of the congenitally deaf. *Psychological Science, 26*, 1771–1782. (4)

Almli, C. R., Fisher, R. S., & Hill, D. L. (1979). Lateral hypothalamus destruction in infant rats produces consummatory deficits without sensory neglect or attenuated arousal. *Experimental Neurology, 66*, 146–157. (9)

Al-Rashid, R. A. (1971). Hypothalamic syndrome in acute childhood leukemia. *Clinical Pediatrics, 10*, 53–54. (9)

Altena, E., Micouland-Franchi, J.-A., Geoffroy, P.-A., Sanz-Arigita, E., Bioulac, S., & Philip, P. (2016). The bidirectional relation between emotional reactivity and sleep: From disruption to recovery. *Behavioral Neuroscience, 130*, 336–350. (8, 14)

Aman, J. E., Elangovan, N., Yeh, I-L., & Konczak, J. (2015). The effectiveness of proprioceptive training for improving motor function: A systematic review. *Frontiers in Human Neuroscience, 8*, Article 1075. (4)

Amateau, S. K., & McCarthy, M. M. (2004). Induction of PGE2 by estradiol mediates developmental masculinization of sex behavior. *Nature Neuroscience, 7*, 643–650. (10)

American Psychiatric Association. (2013). *Diagnostic and statistical manual of mental disorders*. Washington, DC: American Psychiatric Publishing. (14)

Amiry-Moghaddam, M., & Ottersen, O. P. (2003). The molecular basis of water transport in the brain. *Nature Reviews Neuroscience, 4*, 991–1001. (1)

Amting, J. M., Greening, S. G., & Mitchell, D. G. V. (2010). Multiple mechanisms of consciousness: The neural correlates of emotional awareness. *Journal of Neuroscience, 30*, 10039–10047. (11)

Anaclet, C., Ferrari, L., Arrigoni, E., Bass, C. E., Saper, C. B., Lu, J., & Fuller, P. M. (2014). GABAergic parafacial zone is a medullary slow wave sleep-promoting center. *Nature Neuroscience, 17*, 1217–1224. (8)

Anaclet, C., Parmentier, R., Ouk, K., Guidon, G., Buda, C., Sastre, J.-P., . . . Ohtsu, H. (2009). Orexin/hypocretin and histamine: Distinct roles in the control of wakefulness demonstrated using knock-out mouse models. *Journal of Neuroscience, 29*, 14423–14438. (8)

Anand, P., & Bley, K. (2011). Topical capsaicin for pain management: Therapeutic potential and mechanisms of action of the new high-concentration capsaicin 8% patch. *British Journal of Anaesthesia, 107*, 490–502. (6)

Andersen, J. L., Klitgaard, H., & Saltin, B. (1994). Myosin heavy chain isoforms in single fibres from m. vastus lateralis of sprinters: Influence of training. *Acta Physiologica Scandinavica, 151*, 135–142. (7)

Andersen, T. S., Tiippana, K., & Sams, M. (2004). Factors influencing audiovisual fission and fusion illusions. *Cognitive Brain Research, 21*, 301–308. (3)

Anderson, E., Dryman, M. T., Worthington, J., Hoge, E. A., Fischer, L. E., Pollack, M. H., . . . Simon, N. M. (2013). Smiles may go unseen in generalized social anxiety disorder: Evidence from binocular rivalry for reduced visual consciousness of positive facial expressions. *Journal of Anxiety Disorders, 27*, 619–626. (13)

Anderson, E., Siegel, E. H., & Barrett, L. F. (2011). What you feel influences what you see. The role of affective feelings in resolving binocular rivalry. *Journal of Experimental Social Psychology, 47*, 856–860. (13)

Anderson, M. A., Burda, J. E., Ren, Y., Ao, Y., O'Shea, T. M., Kawaguchi, R., . . . Sofroniew, M. V. (2016). Astrocyte scar formation aids central nervous system axon regeneration. *Nature, 532*, 195–200. (4)

Anderson, S. F., Monroe, S. M., Rohde, P., & Lewinsohn, P. M. (2016). Questioning kindling: An analysis of cycle acceleration in unipolar depression. *Clinical Psychological Science, 4*, 229–238. (14)

Anderson, S., Parbery-Clark, A., White-Schwoch, T., & Kraus, N. (2012). Aging affects neural precision of speech encoding. *Journal of Neuroscience, 32*, 14156–14164. (6)

Andics, A., Gábor, A., Gácsi, M., Faragó, T., Szabó, D., & Miklósi, Á. (2016). Neural mechanisms for lexical processing in dogs. *Science, 353*, 1030–1032. (13)

Andreasen, N. C. (1988). Brain imaging: Applications in psychiatry. *Science, 239*, 1381–1388. (3)

Andreasen, N. C., Nopoulos, P., Magnotta, V., Pierson, R., Ziebell, S., & Ho, B-C. (2011). Progressive brain change in schizophrenia: A prospective longitudinal study of first-episode schizophrenia. *Biological Psychiatry, 70*, 672–679. (14)

Andrew, D., & Craig, A. D. (2001). Spinothalamic lamina I neurons selectively sensitive to histamine: A central neural pathway for itch. *Nature Neuroscience, 4*, 72–77. (6)

Andrews, S. C., Enticott, P. G., Hoy, K. E., Thomson, R. H., & Fitzgerald, P. B. (2015). No evidence for mirror system dysfunction in schizophrenia from a multimodal TMS/EEG study. *Psychiatry Research, 228*, 431–440. (7)

Andrews, T. J., Halpern, S. D., & Purves, D. (1997). Correlated size variations in human visual cortex, lateral geniculate nucleus, and optic tract. *Journal of Neuroscience, 17*, 2859–2868. (5)

Andrillon, T., Poulsen, A. T., Hansen, L. K., Léger, D., & Kouider, S. (2016). Neural markers of responsiveness to the environment in human sleep. *Journal of Neuroscience, 36*, 6583–6596. (8)

Antanitus, D. S. (1998). A theory of cortical neuron-astrocyte interaction. *Neuroscientist, 4*, 154–159. (1)

Aoki, Y., & Cortese, S. (2016). Mitochondrial aspartate/glutamate carrier SLC25A12 and autism spectrum disorder: A meta-analysis. *Molecular Neurobiology, 53*, 1579–1588. (1, 14)

Apostolakis, E. M., Garai, J., Fox, C., Smith, C. L., Watson, S. J., Clark, J. H., & O'Malley, B. W. (1996). Dopaminergic regulation of progesterone receptors: Brain D5 dopamine receptors mediate induction of lordosis by D1-like agonists in rats. *Journal of Neuroscience, 16*, 4823–4834. (10)

Appleman, E. R., Albouy, G., Doyon, J., Cronin-Golomb, A., & King, B. R. (2016). Sleep quality influences subsequent motor skill acquisition. *Behavioral Neuroscience, 130*, 290–297. (8)

Araneda, R. C., Kini, A. D., & Firestein, S. (2000). The molecular receptive range of an odorant receptor. *Nature Neuroscience, 3*, 1248–1255. (6)

Archer, J. (2000). Sex differences in aggression between heterosexual partners: A meta-analytic review. *Psychological Bulletin, 126*, 651–680. (11)

Archer, J., Birring, S. S., & Wu, F. C. W. (1998). The association between testosterone and aggression in young men: Empirical findings and a meta-analysis. *Aggressive Behavior, 24,* 411–420. (11)

Archer, J., Graham-Kevan, N., & Davies, M. (2005). Testosterone and aggression: A reanalysis of Book, Starzyk, and Quinsey's (2001) study. *Aggression and Violent Behavior, 10,* 241–261. (11)

Arcurio, L. R., Gold, J. M., & James, T. W. (2012). The response of face-selective cortex with single face parts and part combinations. *Neuropsychologia, 50,* 2454–2459. (5)

Armstrong, J. B., & Schindler, D. E. (2011). Excess digestive capacity in predators reflects a life of feast and famine. *Nature, 476,* 84–87. (9)

Arnold, A. P. (2004). Sex chromosomes and brain gender. *Nature Reviews Neuroscience, 5,* 701–708. (10)

Arnold, A. P. (2009). The organizational-activational hypothesis as the foundation for a unified theory of sexual differentiation of all mammalian tissues. *Hormones and Behavior, 55,* 570–578. (10)

Arnold, A. P., & Breedlove, S. M. (1985). Organizational and activational effects of sex steroids on brain and behavior: A reanalysis. *Hormones and Behavior, 19,* 469–498. (10)

Arnsten, A. F. T. (2015). Stress weakens prefrontal networks: Molecular insults to higher cognition. *Nature Neuroscience, 18,* 1376–1385. (11)

Arvidson, K., & Friberg, U. (1980). Human taste: Response and taste bud number in fungiform papillae. *Science, 209,* 807–808. (6)

Asai, M., Ramachandrappa, S., Joachim, M., Shen, Y., Zhang, R., Nuthalapati, N., . . . Majzoub, J. A. (2013). Loss of function of the melanocortin 2 receptor accessory protein 2 is associated with mammalian obesity. *Science, 341,* 275–278. (9)

Ascoli, G. A. (2015). *Trees of the brain, roots of the mind.* Cambridge, MA: MIT Press. (1, 12)

Aserinsky, E., & Kleitman, N. (1955). Two types of ocular motility occurring in sleep. *Journal of Applied Physiology, 8,* 1–10. (8)

Ashmore, L. J., & Sehgal, A. (2003). A fly's eye view of circadian entrainment. *Journal of Biological Rhythms, 18,* 206–216. (8)

Aston-Jones, G., Chen, S., Zhu, Y., & Oshinsky, M. L. (2001). A neural circuit for circadian regulation of arousal. *Nature Neuroscience, 4,* 732–738. (8)

Athos, E. A., Levinson, B., Kistler, A., Zemansky, J., Bostrom, A., Freimer, N., & Gitschier, J. (2007). Dichotomy and perceptual distortions in absolute pitch ability. *Proceedings of the National Academy of Sciences, USA, 104,* 14795–14800. (6)

Attardo, A., Fitzgerald, J. E., & Schnitzer, M. J. (2015). Impermanence of dendritic spines in live adult CA1 hippocampus. *Nature, 523,* 592–596. (12)

Audero, E., Mlinar, B., Baccini, G., Skachokova, Z. K., Corradetti, R., & Gross, C. (2013). Suppression of serotonin neuron firing increases aggression in mice. *Journal of Neuroscience, 33,* 8678–8688. (11)

Avena, N. M., Rada, P., & Hoebel, B. G. (2008). Evidence for sugar addiction: Behavioral and neurochemical effects of intermittent, excessive sugar intake. *Neuroscience and Biobehavioral Reviews, 32,* 20–39. (9)

Aviezer, H., Trope, Y., & Todorov, A. (2012). Body cues, not facial expressions, discriminate between intense positive and negative emotions. *Science, 338,* 1225–1229. (11)

Avinun, R., Ebstein, R. P., & Knafo, A. (2012). Human maternal behaviour is associated with arginine vasopressin receptor 1A gene. *Biology Letters, 8,* 894–896. (10)

Avrabos, C., Sonikov, S. V., Dine, J., Markt, P. O., Holsboer, F., Landgraf, R., & Eder, M. (2013). Real-time imaging of amygdalar network dynamics *in vitro* reveals a neurophysiological link to behavior in a mouse model of extremes in trait anxiety. *Journal of Neuroscience, 33,* 16262–16267. (11)

Babich, F. R., Jacobson, A. L., Bubash, S., & Jacobson, A. (1965). Transfer of a response to naive rats by injection of ribonucleic acid extracted from trained rats. *Science, 149,* 656–657. (12)

Babikian, T., Merkley, T., Savage, R. C., Giza, C. C., & Levin, H. (2015). Chronic aspects of pediatric traumatic brain injury: Review of the literature. *Journal of Neurotrauma, 32,* 1849–1860. (4)

Backlund, E.-O., Granberg, P.-O., Hamberger, B., Sedvall, G., Seiger, A., & Olson, L. (1985). Transplantation of adrenal medullary tissue to striatum in Parkinsonism. In A. Björklund & U. Stenevi (Eds.), *Neural grafting in the mammalian CNS* (pp. 551–556). Amsterdam: Elsevier. (7)

Bäckman, J., & Alerstam, T. (2001). Confronting the winds: Orientation and flight behavior of roosting swifts, *Apus apus. Proceedings of the Royal Society of London. Series B—Biological Sciences, 268,* 1081–1087. (8)

Baddeley, A. D., & Hitch, G. J. (1994). Developments in the concept of working memory. *Neuropsychology, 8,* 485–493. (12)

Baer, J. S., Sampson, P. D., Barr, H. M., Connor, P. D., & Streissguth, A. P. (2003). A 21-year longitudinal analysis of the effects of prenatal alcohol exposure on young adult drinking. *Archives of General Psychiatry, 60,* 377–385. (14)

Bagemihl, B. (1999). *Biological exuberance.* New York: St. Martin's Press. (10)

Baghdoyan, H. A., Spotts, J. L., & Snyder, S. G. (1993). Simultaneous pontine and basal forebrain microinjections of carbachol suppress REM sleep. *Journal of Neuroscience, 13,* 229–242. (8)

Bailey, C. H., Giustetto, M., Huang, Y.-Y., Hawkins, R. D., & Kandel, E. R. (2000). Is heterosynaptic modulation essential for stabilizing Hebbian plasticity and memory? *Nature Reviews Neuroscience, 1,* 11–20. (12)

Bailey, J. M., & Pillard, R. C. (1991). A genetic study of male sexual orientation. *Archives of General Psychiatry, 48,* 1089–1096. (10)

Bailey, J. M., Pillard, R. C., Dawood, K., Miller, M. B., Farrer, L. A., Trivedi, S., & Murphy, R. L. (1999). A family history study of male sexual orientation using three independent samples. *Behavior Genetics, 29,* 79–86. (10)

Bailey, J. M., Pillard, R. C., Neale, M. C., & Agyei, Y. (1993). Heritable factors influence sexual orientation in women. *Archives of General Psychiatry, 50,* 217–223. (10)

Bailey, J. M., Vasey, P. L., Diamond, L. M., Breedlove, S. M., Vilain, E., & Epprecht, M. (2016). Sexual orientation, controversy, and science. *Psychological Science in the Public Interest, 17,* 45–101. (10)

Bailey, J. M., Willerman, L., & Parks, C. (1991). A test of the maternal stress theory of human male homosexuality. *Archives of Sexual Behavior, 20,* 277–293. (10)

Baillargeon, R. (1987). Object permanence in 3½- and 4½-month-old infants. *Developmental Psychology, 23,* 655–664. (5)

Bakken, T. E., Miller, J. A., Ding, S.-L., Sunkin, S. M., Smith, K. A., Ng, L., . . . Lein, E. S. (2016). A comprehensive transcriptional map of primate brain development. *Nature, 535,* 367–375. (12)

Bakken, T. E., Roddey, J. C., Djurovic, S., Akshoomoff, N., Amaral, D. G., Bloss, C. S., . . . Dale, A. M. (2012). Association of common genetic variants in GPCPD1 with scaling of visual cortical surface in humans. *Proceedings of the National Academy of Sciences (U.S.A.), 109,* 3985–3990. (5)

Bakker, J., De Mees, C., Douhard, Q., Balthazart, J., Gabant, P., Szpirer, J., & Szpirer, C. (2006). Alpha-fetoprotein protects the developing female mouse brain from masculinization and defeminization by estrogens. *Nature Neuroscience, 9,* 220–226. (10)

Bakker, J., Honda, S.-I., Harada, N., & Balthazart, J. (2002). The aromatase knockout mouse provides new evidence that estradiol is required during development in the female for the expression of sociosexual behaviors in adulthood. *Journal of Neuroscience, 22,* 9104–9112. (10)

Ballard, P. A., Tetrud, J. W., & Langston, J. W. (1985). Permanent human Parkinsonism due to 1-methyl-4-phenyl-1,2,3,6-tetrahydropyridine (MPTP). *Neurology, 35,* 949–956. (7)

Balleine, B. W., Delgado, M. R., & Hikosaka, O. (2007). The role of the dorsal striatum in reward and decision-making. *Journal of Neuroscience, 27,* 8161–8165. (12)

Ballon, J. S., Dean, K. A., & Cadenhead, K. S. (2007). Obstetrical complications in people at risk for developing schizophrenia. *Schizophrenia Research, 98,* 307–311. (14)

Banks, W. P., & Isham, E. A. (2009). We infer rather than perceive the moment we decided to act. *Psychological Science, 20,* 17–21. (7)

Barbour, D. L., & Wang, X. (2003). Contrast tuning in auditory cortex. *Science, 299,* 1073–1075. (6)

Bargary, G., Barnett, K. J., Mitchell, K. J., & Newell, F. N. (2009). Colored-speech synaesthesia is triggered by multisensory, not unisensory, perception. *Psychological Science, 20*, 529–533. (6)

Barger, L. K., Sullivan, J. P., Vincent, A. S., Fiedler, E. R., McKenna, L. M., Flynn-Evans, E. E., . . . Lockley, S. W. (2012). Learning to live on a Mars day: Fatigue countermeasures during the Phoenix Mars Lander Mission. *Sleep, 35*, 1423–1435. (8)

Barnea, G., O'Donnell, S., Mancia, F., Sun, X., Nemes, A., Mendelsohn, M., & Axel, R. (2004). Odorant receptors on axon termini in the brain. *Science, 304*, 1468. (6)

Barnes, B. M. (1996, September/October). Sang froid. *The Sciences, 36*(5), 13–14. (8)

Barnett, K. J., Finucane, C., Asher, J. E., Bargary, G., Corvin, A. P., Newell, F. N., & Mitchell, K. J. (2008). Familial patterns and the origins of individual differences in synaesthesia. *Cognition, 106*, 871–893. (6)

Barrett, L. F. (2012). Emotions are real. *Emotion, 12*, 413–429. (11)

Barrett, L. F., Bliss-Moreau, E., Duncan, S. L., Rauch, S. L., & Wright, C. I. (2007). The amygdala and the experience of affect. *Social Cognitive & Affective Neuroscience, 2*, 73–83. (11)

Barrett, L. F., & Simmons, W. K. (2015). Interoceptive predictions in the brain. *Nature Reviews Neuroscience, 16*, 419–429. (7)

Barretto, R. P. J., Gillis-Smith, S., Chandrashekar, J., Yarmolinsky, D. A., Schnitzer, M. J., Ryba, N. J. P., & Zuker, C. S. (2015). The neural representation of taste quality at the periphery. *Nature, 517*, 373–376. (6)

Barrientos, R. M., Frank, M. G., Crysdale, N. Y., Chapman, T. R., Ahrendsen, J. T., Day, H. E. W., . . . Maier, S. F. (2011). Little exercise, big effects: Reversing aging and infection-induced memory deficits, and underlying processes. *Journal of Neuroscience, 31*, 115778–11586. (4)

Barton, D. A., Esler, M. D., Dawood, T., Lambert, E. A., Haikerwal, D., Brenchley, C., . . . Lambert, G. W. (2008). Elevated brain serotonin turnover in patients with depression. *Archives of General Psychiatry, 65*, 38–46. (14)

Bartoshuk, L. M. (1991). Taste, smell, and pleasure. In R. C. Bolles (Ed.), *The hedonics of taste* (pp. 15–28). Hillsdale, NJ: Erlbaum. (6)

Bartoshuk, L. M., Gentile, R. L., Moskowitz, H. R., & Meiselman, H. L. (1974). Sweet taste induced by miracle fruit (*Synsephalum dulcificum*). *Physiology & Behavior, 12*, 449–456. (6)

Bartz, J. A., Simeon, D., Hamilton, H., Kim, S., Crystal, S., Braun, A., Vicens, V., & Hollander, E. (2011). Oxytocin can hinder trust and cooperation in borderline personality disorder. *Social, Cognitive, and Affective Neuroscience, 6*, 556–563. (13)

Barzilai, N., Alzmon, G., Derby, C. A., Bauman, J. M., & Lipton, R. B. (2006). A genotype of exceptional longevity is associated with preservation of cognitive function. *Neurology, 67*, 2170–2175. (4)

Bashford, J. A., Warren, R. M., & Lenz, P. W. (2013). Maintaining intelligibility at high speech intensities: Evidence of lateral inhibition in the lower auditory pathway. *Journal of the Acoustical Society of America, 134*, EL119–EL125. (5)

Basten, U., Hilger, K., & Fiebach, C. J. (2015). Where smart brains are different: A quantitative meta-analysis of functional and structural brain imaging studies on intelligence. *Intelligence, 51*, 10–27. (12)

Bate, S., Cook, S. J., Duchaine, B., Tree, J. J., Burns, E. J., & Hodgson, T. L. (2014). Intranasal inhalation of oxytocin improves face processing in developmental prosopagnosia. *Cortex, 50*, 55–63. (13)

Bates, T. C., Lewis, G. J., & Weiss, A. (2013). Childhood socioeconomic status amplifies genetic effects on adult intelligence. *Psychological Science, 24*, 2111–2116. (12)

Battersby, S. (1997). Plus c'est le même chews. *Nature, 385*, 679. (9)

Battleday, R. M., & Brem, A.-K. (2015). Modafinil for cognitive neuroenhancement in healthy non-sleep-deprived subjects: A systematic review. *European Neuropsychopharmacology, 25*, 1865–1881. (12)

Baum, A., Gatchel, R. J., & Schaeffer, M. A. (1983). Emotional, behavioral, and physiological effects of chronic stress at Three Mile Island. *Journal of Consulting and Clinical Psychology, 51*, 565–582. (11)

Bauman, M. D., Iosif, A.-M., Ashwood, P., Braunschweig, D., Lee, A., Schumann, C. M., . . . Amaral, D. G. (2013). Maternal antibodies from mothers of children with autism alter brain growth and social behavior development in the rhesus monkey. *Translational Psychiatry, 3*, e278. (14)

Baumann, O., Borra, R. J., Bower, J. M., Cullen, K. E., Habas, C., Ivry, R. B., . . . Sokolov, A. A. (2015). Consensus paper: The role of the cerebellum in perceptual processes. *Cerebellu, 14*, 197–220. (7)

Bautista, D. M., Sigal, Y. M., Milstein, A. D., Garrison, J. L., Zorn, J. A., Tsuruda, P. R., . . . Julius, D. (2008). Pungent agents from Szechuan peppers excite sensory neurons by inhibiting two-pore potassium channels. *Nature Neuroscience, 11*, 772–779. (6)

Baxter, L. R., Phelps, M. E., Mazziotta, J. C., Schwartz, J. M., Gerner, R. H., Selin, C. E., & Sumida, R. M. (1985). Cerebral metabolic rates for glucose in mood disorders. *Archives of General Psychiatry, 42*, 441–447. (14)

Bayley, P. J., Frascino, J. C., & Squire, L. R. (2005). Robust habit learning in the absence of awareness and independent of the medial temporal lobe. *Nature, 436*, 550–553. (12)

Bayley, P. J., Hopkins, R. O., & Squire, L. R. (2006). The fate of old memories after medial temporal lobe damage. *Journal of Neuroscience, 26*, 13311–13317. (12)

Baylis, G. C., & Driver, J. (2001). Shape-coding in IT cells generalizes over contrast and mirror reversal but not figure-ground reversal. *Nature Neuroscience, 4*, 937–942. (5)

Beall, A. T., & Tracy, J. L. (2013). Women are more likely to wear red or pink at peak fertility. *Psychological Science, 24*, 1837–1841. (10)

Beaton, E. A., Schmidt, L. A., Schulkin, J., Antony, M. M., Swinson, R. P., & Hall, G. B. (2008). Different neural responses to stranger and personally familiar faces in shy and bold adults. *Behavioral Neuroscience, 122*, 704–709. (11)

Beauchamp, M. S., & Ro, T. (2008). Neural substrates of sound-touch synesthesia after a thalamic lesion. *Journal of Neuroscience, 28*, 13696–13702. (6)

Beck, A. T., & Bredemeier, K. (2016). A unified model of depression: Integrating clinical, cognitive, biological, and evolutionary perspectives. *Clinical Psychological Science, 4*, 596–619. (14)

Beck, K., Javitt, D. C., & Howes, O. D. (2016). Targeting glutamate to treat schizophrenia: Lessons from recent clinical studies. *Psychopharmacology, 233*, 2425–2428. (14)

Beck, S., Richardson, S. P., Shamin, E. A., Dang, N., Schubert, M., & Hallett, M. (2008). Short intracortical and surround inhibition are selectively reduced during movement initiation in focal hand dystonia. *Journal of Neuroscience, 28*, 10363–10369. (4)

Becker, H. C. (1988). Effects of the imidazobenzodiazepine Ro15-4513 on the stimulant and depressant actions of ethanol on spontaneous locomotor activity. *Life Sciences, 43*, 643–650. (11)

Becker, H. G. T., Haarmeier, T., Tatagiba, M., & Gharabaghi, A. (2013). Electrical stimulation of the human homolog of the medial superior temporal area induces visual motion blindness. *Journal of Neuroscience, 33*, 18288–18297. (5)

Becks, L., & Agrawal, A. F. (2010). Higher rates of sex evolve in spatially heterogeneous environments. *Nature, 468*, 89–92. (10)

Bedny, M., Richardson, H., & Saxe, R. (2015). "Visual" cortex responds to spoken language in blind children. *Journal of Neuroscience, 35*, 11674–11681. (4)

Beebe, D. W., & Gozal, D. (2002). Obstructive sleep apnea and the prefrontal cortex: Towards a comprehensive model linking nocturnal upper airway obstruction to daytime cognitive and behavioral deficits. *Journal of Sleep Research, 11*, 1–16. (8)

Beeman, M. J., & Chiarello, C. (1998). Complementary right- and left-hemisphere language comprehension. *Current Directions in Psychological Science, 7*, 2–8. (13)

Beeney, J. E., Franklin, R. G. Jr., Levy, K. N., & Adams, R. B. Jr. (2011). I feel your pain: Emotional closeness modulates neural responses to empathically experienced rejection. *Social Neuroscience, 6*, 369–376. (13)

Bélanger, M., Allaman, I., & Magistretti, P. J. (2011). Brain energy metabolism: Focus on astrocyte-neuron metabolic cooperation. *Cell Metabolism, 14*, 724–738. (1)

Bellugi, U., Lichtenberger, L., Jones, W., Lai, Z., & St. George, M. (2000). I. The neurocognitive profile of Williams syndrome: A complex pattern of strengths and weaknesses. *Journal of Cognitive Neuroscience, 12*(Suppl.), 7–29. (13)

Belsky, D. W., Moffitt, T. E., Corcoran, D. L., Domingue, B., Harrington, H. L., Hogan, S., . . . Caspi, A. (2016). The genetics of success: How single-nucleotide polymorphisms associated with educational attainment relate to life-course development. *Psychological Science, 27,* 957–972. (12)

Ben Achour, S., & Pascual, O. (2012). Astrocyteneuron communication: Functional consequences. *Neurochemical Research, 37,* 2464–2473. (1)

Ben-Ami Bartal, I., Rodgers, D. A., Sarria, M. S. B., Decety, J., & Mason, P. (2014). Pro-social behavior in rats is modulated by social experience. *eLife, 3,* e01385. (13)

Benedetti, F., Arduino, C., & Amanzio, M. (1999). Somatotopic activation of opioid systems by target-directed expectations of analgesia. *Journal of Neuroscience, 19,* 3639–3648. (6)

Benedetti, F., & Colombo, C. (2011). Sleep deprivation in mood disorders. *Neuropsychobiology, 64,* 141–151. (14)

Benros, M. E., Pedersen, M. G., Rasmussen, H., Eaton, W. W., Nordentoft, M., & Mortensen, P. B. (2014). A nationwide study on the risk of autoimmune diseases in individuals with a personal or a family history of schizophrenia and related psychosis. *American Journal of Psychiatry, 171,* 218–226. (14)

Benschop, R. J., Godaert, G. L. R., Geenen, R., Brosschot, J. F., DeSmet, M. B. M., Olff, M., . . . Ballieux, R. E. (1995). Relationships between cardiovascular and immunologic changes in an experimental stress model. *Psychological Medicine, 25,* 323–327. (11)

Berdoy, M., Webster, J. P., & Macdonald, D. W. (2000). Fatal attraction in rats infected with *Toxoplasma gondii. Proceedings of the Royal Society of London, B, 267,* 1591–1594. (11)

Berenbaum, S. A. (1999). Effects of early androgens on sex-typed activities and interests in adolescents with congenital adrenal hyperplasia. *Hormones and Behavior, 35,* 102–110. (10)

Berenbaum, S. A., Bryk, K. L. K., & Beltz, A. M. (2012). Early androgen effects on spatial and mechanical abilities: Evidence from congenital adrenal hyperplasia. *Behavioral Neuroscience, 126,* 86–96. (10)

Berenbaum, S. A., Duck, S. C., & Bryk, K. (2000). Behavioral effects of prenatal versus postnatal androgen excess in children with 21-hydroxylase-deficient congenital adrenal hyperplasia. *Journal of Clinical Endocrinology & Metabolism, 85,* 727–733. (10)

Berger, R. J., & Phillips, N. H. (1995). Energy conservation and sleep. *Behavioural Brain Research, 69,* 65–73. (8)

Berger-Sweeney, J., & Hohmann, C. F. (1997). Behavioral consequences of abnormal cortical development: Insights into developmental disabilities. *Behavioural Brain Research, 86,* 121–142. (4)

Bergh, C., Callmar, M., Danemar, S., Hölcke, M., Isberg, S., Leon, M., . . . Södersten, P. (2013). Effective treatment of eating disorders: Results at multiple sites. *Behavioral Neuroscience, 127,* 878–889. (9)

Bergmann, O., Bhardwaj, R. D., Bernard, S., Zdunek, S., Barnabé-Heider, F., Walsh, S., . . . Druid, H. (2009). Evidence for cardiomyocyte renewal in humans. *Science, 324,* 98–102. (4)

Bergmann, O., Liebl, J., Bernard, S., Alkass, K., Yeung, M. S. Y., Steier, P., . . . Frisén, J. (2012). The age of olfactory bulb neurons in humans. *Neuron, 74,* 634–639. (4)

Berken, J. A., Chai, X., Chen, J.-K., Gracco, V. L., & Klein, D. (2016). Effects of early and late bilingualism on resting-state functional connectivity. *Journal of Neuroscience, 36,* 1165–1172. (13)

Berlucchi, G., Mangun, G. R., & Gazzaniga, M. S. (1997). Visuospatial attention and the split brain. *News in Physiological Sciences, 12,* 226–231. (13)

Berman, K. F., Torrey, E. F., Daniel, D. G., & Weinberger, D. R. (1992). Regional cerebral blood flow in monozygotic twins discordant and concordant for schizophrenia. *Archives of General Psychiatry, 49,* 927–934. (14)

Bernal, D., Donley, J. M., Shadwick, R. E., & Syme, D. A. (2005). Mammal-like muscles power swimming in a cold-water shark. *Nature, 437,* 1349–1352. (9)

Berntsen, D., & Rubin, D. C. (2015). Pretraumatic stress reactions in soldiers deployed to Afghanistan. *Clinical Psychological Science, 3,* 663–674.

Berntson, G. G., Bechara, A., Damasio, H., Tranel, D., & Cacioppo, J. T. (2007). Amygdala contribution to selective dimensions of emotion. *Social Cognitive & Affective Neuroscience, 2,* 123–129. (11)

Berryhill, M. E., Phuong, L., Picasso, L., Cabeza, R., & Olson, I. R. (2007). Parietal lobe and episodic memory: Bilateral damage causes impaired free recall of autobiographical memory. *Journal of Neuroscience, 27,* 14415–14423. (12)

Berson, D. M., Dunn, F. A., & Takao, M. (2002). Phototransduction by retinal ganglion cells that set the circadian clock. *Science, 295,* 1070–1073. (8)

Beuming, T., Kniazeff, J., Bergmann, M. L., Shi, L., Gracia, L., Raniszewska, K., . . . Loland, C. J. (2008). The binding sites for cocaine and dopamine in the dopamine transporter overlap. *Nature Neuroscience, 11,* 780–789. (2)

Bezzola, L., Mérillat, S., Gaser, C., & Jäncke, L. (2011). Training-induced neural plasticity in golf novices. *Journal of Neuroscience, 31,* 12444–12448. (4)

Bian, L., Hanson, R. L., Ossowski, V., Wiedrich, K., Mason, C. C., Traurig, M., . . . Bogardus, C. (2010). Variants in ASK1 are associated with skeletal muscle ASK1 expression, *in vivo* insulin resistance, and Type 2 diabetes in Pima Indians. *Diabetes, 59,* 1276–1282. (9)

Biben, M. (1979). Predation and predatory play behaviour of domestic cats. *Animal Behaviour, 27,* 81–94. (11)

Bickart, K. C., Wright, C. I., Dautoff, R. J., Dickerson, B. C., & Barrett, L. F. (2011). Amygdala volume and social network size in humans. *Nature Neuroscience, 14,* 163–164. (3)

Bidelman, G. M., & Alain, C. (2015). Musical training orchestrates coordinated neuroplasticity in auditory brainstem and cortex to counteract age-related declines in categorical vowel perception. *Journal of Neuroscience, 35,* 1240–1249. (4)

Bierut, L. J., Heath, A. C., Bucholz, K. K., Dinwiddie, S. H., Madden, P. A. F., Statham, D. J., . . . Martin, N. G. (1999). Major depressive disorder in a community-based twin sample. *Archives of General Psychiatry, 56,* 557–563. (14)

Bilalic, M., Langner, R., Ulrich, R., & Grodd, W. (2011). Many faces of expertise: Fusiform face area in chess experts and novices. *Journal of Neuroscience, 31,* 10206–10214. (5)

Billington, C. J., & Levine, A. S. (1992). Hypothalamic neuropeptide Y regulation of feeding and energy metabolism. *Current Opinion in Neurobiology, 2,* 847–851. (9)

Bimler, D., & Kirkland, J. (2009). Colour-space distortion in women who are heterozygous for colour deficiency. *Vision Research, 49,* 536–543. (5)

Bird, A. (2007). Perceptions of epigenetics. *Nature, 447,* 396–398. (4)

Bishop, E. G., Cherny, S. S., Corley, R., Plomin, R., DeFries, J. C., & Hewitt, J. K. (2003). Development genetic analysis of general cognitive ability from 1 to 12 years in a sample of adoptees, biological siblings, and twins. *Intelligence, 31,* 31–49. (12)

Biss, R. K., & Hasher, L. (2012). Happy as a lark: Morning-type younger and older people are higher in positive affect. *Emotion, 12,* 437–441. (8)

Bjork, J. M., & Pardini, D. A. (2015). Who are those "risk-taking adolescents"? Individual differences in developmental neuroimaging research. *Developmental Cognitive Neuroscience, 11,* 56–64. (4)

Bjorklund, A., & Kordower, J. H. (2013). Cell therapy for Parkinson's disease: What next? *Movement Disorders, 28,* 110–115. (7)

Björnsdotter, M., Löken, L., Olausson, H., Vallbo, Å., & Wessberg, J. (2009). Somatotopic organization of gentle touch processing in the posterior insular cortex. *Journal of Neuroscience, 29,* 9314–9320. (6)

Blackless, M., Charuvastra, A., Derryck, A., Fausto-Sterling, A., Lauzanne, K., & Lee, E. (2000). How sexually dimorphic are we? Review and synthesis. *American Journal of Human Biology, 12,* 151–166. (10)

Blackwell, A., & Bates, E. (1995). Inducing agrammatic profiles in normals: Evidence for the selective vulnerability of morphology under cognitive resource limitation. *Journal of Cognitive Neuroscience, 7,* 228–257. (13)

Blackwell, T., Yaffe, K., Laffan, A., Ancoli-Israel, S., Redline, S., Ensrud, K. E., . . . Stone, K. L. (2014). Associations of objectively and subjectively measured sleep quality with subsequent cognitive decline in older community-dwelling men: The MrOS sleep study. *Sleep, 37,* 655–663. (8)

Blake, R., & Hirsch, H. V. B. (1975). Deficits in binocular depth perception in cats after alternating monocular deprivation. *Science, 190,* 1114–1116. (5)

Blake, R., Palmeri, T. J., Marois, R., & Kim, C.-Y. (2005). On the perceptual reality of synesthetic color. In L. C. Robertson & N. Sagiv (Eds.), *Synesthesia* (pp. 47–73). Oxford, England: Oxford University Press. (6)

Blakemore, S.-J., Wolpert, D. M., & Frith, C. D. (1998). Central cancellation of self-produced tickle sensation. *Nature Neuroscience, 1,* 635–640. (6)

Blanchard, R. (2008). Review and theory of handedness, birth, order, and homosexuality in men. *Laterality, 13,* 51–70. (10)

Blanco, M. B., & Zehr, S. M. (2015). Striking longevity in a hibernating lemur. *Journal of Zoology, 296,* 177–188. (8)

Blanke, O. (2012). Multisensory brain mechanisms of bodily self-consciousness. *Nature Reviews Neuroscience, 13,* 556–571. (3)

Bliss, T. V., Collingridge, G. L., Kaang, B.-K., & Zhuo, M. (2016). Synaptic plasticity in the anterior cingulate in acute and chronic pain. *Nature Reviews Neuroscience, 17,* 485–496. (6)

Bliss, T. V. P., & Lømo, T. (1973). Long-lasting potentiation of synaptic transmission in the dentate area of the anaesthetized rabbit following stimulation of the perforant path. *Journal of Physiology (London), 232,* 331–356. (12)

Bloch, G., Barnes, B. M., Gerkema, M. P., & Helm, B. (2013). Animal activity around the clock with no overt circadian rhythms: patterns, mechanisms and adaptive value. *Proceedings of the Royal Society B, 280,* 20130019. (8)

Bloch, G. J., & Mills, R. (1995). Prepubertal testosterone treatment of neonatally gonadectomized male rats: Defeminization and masculinization of behavioral and endocrine function in adulthood. *Neuroscience and Biobehavioral Reviews, 59,* 187–200. (10)

Bloch, G. J., Mills, R., & Gale, S. (1995). Prepubertal testosterone treatment of female rats: Defeminization of behavioral and endocrine function in adulthood. *Neuroscience and Biobehavioral Reviews, 19,* 177–186. (10)

Bobrow, D., & Bailey, J. M. (2001). Is male homosexuality maintained via kin selection? *Evolution and Human Behavior, 22,* 361–368. (10)

Bock, A. S., Binda, P., Benson, N. C., Bridge, H., Watkins, K. E., & Fine, I. (2015). Resting-state retinotopic organization in the absence of retinal input and visual experience. *Journal of Neuroscience, 35,* 12366–12382. (5)

Boekel, W., Wagenmakers, E. J., Belay, L., Verhagen, J., Brown, S., & Forstmann, B. U. (2015). A purely confirmatory replication study of structural brain-behavior correlations. *Cortex, 66,* 115–133. (3)

Boets, B., Op de Beeck, H. P., Vandermosten, M., Scott, S. K., Gillebert, C. R., Mantini, D., . . . Ghesquière, P. (2013). Intact but less accessible phonetic representations in adults with dyslexia. *Science, 342,* 1251–1254. (13)

Bogaert, A. F. (2003a). The interaction of fraternal birth order and body size in male sexual orientation. *Behavioral Neuroscience, 117,* 381–384. (10)

Bogaert, A. F. (2003b). Number of older brothers and sexual orientation: New tests and the attraction/behavior distinction in two national probability samples. *Journal of Personality and Social Psychology, 84,* 644–652. (10)

Bogaert, A. F. (2006). Biological versus nonbiological older brothers and men's sexual orientation. *Proceedings of the National Academy of Sciences, USA, 103,* 10771–10774. (10)

Bogaert, A. F. (2010). Physical development and sexual orientation in men and women: An analysis of NATSAL-2000. *Archives of Sexual Behavior, 39,* 110–116. (10)

Boivin, D. B., Duffy, J. F., Kronauer, R. E., & Czeisler, C. A. (1996). Dose-response relationships for resetting of human circadian clock by light. *Nature, 379,* 540–542. (8)

Boksem, M. A. S., Mehta, P. H., Van den Bergh, B., van Son, V., Trautmann, S. T., Roelofs, K., . . . Sanfey, A. G. (2013). Testosterone inhibits trust but promotes reciprocity. *Psychological Science, 24,* 22306–22314. (11)

Boly, M., Perlbarg, V., Marrelec, G., Schabus, M., Laureys, S., Doyon, J., . . . Benali, H. (2012). Hierarchical clustering of brain activity during human nonrapid eye movement sleep. *Proceedings of the National Academy of Sciences (U.S.A.), 109,* 5856–5861. (8)

Bonath, B., Noesselt, T., Martinez, A., Mishra, J., Schwiecker, K., Heinze, H.-J., & Hillyard, S. A. (2007). Neural basis of the ventriloquist illusion. *Current Biology, 17,* 1697–1703. (3)

Bonini, F., Burle, B., Liégois-Chauvel, C., Régis, J., Chauvel, P., & Vidal, F. (2014). Action monitoring and medial frontal cortex: Leading role of supplementary motor area. *Science, 343,* 888–891. (7)

Bonneh, Y. S., Cooperman, A., & Sagi, D. (2001). Motion-induced blindness in normal observers. *Nature, 411,* 798–801. (13)

Bonner, M. F., & Grossman, M. (2012). Gray matter density of auditory association cortex relates to knowledge of sound concepts in primary progressive aphasia. *Journal of Neuroscience, 32,* 7986–7991. (6)

Booth, F. W., & Neufer, P. D. (2005, January/February). Exercise controls gene expression. *American Scientist, 93,* 28–35. (7)

Booth, W., Johnson, D. H., Moore, S., Schal, C., & Vargo, E. L. (2011). Evidence for viable, non-clonal but fatherless Boa constrictors. *Biology Letters, 7,* 253–256. (10)

Borisovska, M., Bensen, A. L., Chong, G., & Westbrook, G. L. (2013). Distinct modes of dopamine and GABA release in a dual transmitter neuron. *Journal of Neuroscience, 33,* 1790–1796. (2)

Born, S., Levit, A., Niv, M. Y., Meyerhof, W., & Belvens, M. (2013). The human bitter taste receptor TAS2R10 is tailored to accommodate numerous diverse ligands. *Journal of Neuroscience, 33,* 201–213. (6)

Borodinsky, L. N., Root, C. M., Cronin, J. A., Sann, S. B., Gu, X., & Spitzer, N. C. (2004). Activity-dependent homeostatic specification of transmitter expression in embryonic neurons. *Nature, 429,* 523–530. (2)

Borsutzky, S., Fujiwara, E., Brand, M., & Markowitsch, H. J. (2008). Confabulations in alcoholic Korsakoff patients. *Neuropsychologia, 46,* 3133–3143. (12)

Bortolotti, B., Menchetti, M., Bellini, F., Montaguti, M. B., & Berardi, D. (2008). Psychological interventions for major depression in primary care: A meta-analytic review of randomized controlled trials. *General Hospital Psychiatry, 30,* 293–302. (14)

Bouchard, T. J., Jr., & McGue, M. (1981). Familial studies of intelligence: A review. *Science, 212,* 1055–1059. (12)

Boucsein, K., Weniger, G., Mursch, K., Steinhoff, B. J., & Irle, E. (2001). Amygdala lesion in temporal lobe epilepsy subjects impairs associative learning of emotional facial expressions. *Neuropsychologia, 39,* 231–236. (11)

Bourane, S., Duan, B., Koch, S. C., Dalet, A., Britz, O., Garcia Campmany, L., Kim, E., . . . Goulding, M. (2015). Gate control of mechanical itch by a subpopulation of spinal cord interneurons. *Science, 350,* 550–554. (6)

Bourgeron, T. (2015). From the genetic architecture to synaptic plasticity in autism spectrum disorder. *Nature Reviews Neuroscience, 16,* 551–563. (14)

Bourque, C. W. (2008). Central mechanisms of osmosensation and systemic osmoregulation. *Nature Reviews Neuroscience, 9,* 519–531. (9)

Bouton, C. E., Shaikhouni, A., Annetta, N. V., Bockbrader, M. A., Friedenberg, D. A., Nielson, D. M., . . . Rezai, A. R. (2016). Restoring cortical control of functional movement in a human with quadriplegia. *Nature, 533,* 247–250. (7)

Boutrel, B., Franc, B., Hen, R., Hamon, M., & Adrien, J. (1999). Key role of 5-HT1B receptors in the regulation of paradoxical sleep as evidenced in 5-HT1B knock-out mice. *Journal of Neuroscience, 19,* 3204–3212. (8)

Bowles, S. (2006). Group competition, reproductive leveling, and the evolution of human altruism. *Science, 314,* 1569–1572. (4)

Bowles, S., & Posel, B. (2005). Genetic relatedness predicts South African migrant workers' remittances to their families. *Nature, 434,* 380–383. (1)

Bowmaker, J. K. (1998). Visual pigments and molecular genetics of color blindness. *News in Physiological Sciences, 13,* 63–69. (5)

Bowmaker, J. K. (2008). Evolution of vertebrate visual pigments. *Vision Research, 48,* 2022–2041. (5)

Bowmaker, J. K., & Dartnall, H. J. A. (1980). Visual pigments of rods and cones in a human retina. *Journal of Physiology (London), 298,* 501–511. (5)

Boyce, R., Glasgow, S. D., Williams, S., & Adamantidis, A. (2016). Causal evidence for the role of REM sleep theta rhythm in contextual memory consolidation. *Science, 352,* 812–816. (8)

Bozkurt, A., Bozkurt, O. H., & Sonmez, I. (2015). Birth order and sibling sex ratio in a population with high fertility: Are Turkish male-to-female transsexuals different? *Archives of Sexual Behavior, 44,* 1331–1337. (10)

Braams, B. R., van Duijvenvoorde, A. C. K., Peper, J. S., & Crone, E. A. (2015). Longitudinal changes in adolescent risk-taking: A comprehensive study of neural responses to rewards, pubertal development, and risk-taking behavior. *Journal of Neuroscience, 35,* 7226–7238. (4)

Branco, T., Clark, B. A., & Häusser, M. (2010). Dendritic discrimination of temporal input sequences in cortical neurons. *Science, 329,* 1671–1675. (2)

Brandt, T. (1991). Man in motion: Historical and clinical aspects of vestibular function. *Brain, 114,* 2159–2174. (6)

Brans, R. G. H., Kahn, R. S., Schnack, H. G., van Baal, G. C. M., Posthuma, D., van Haren, N. E. M., . . . Pol, H. E. H. (2010). Brain plasticity and intellectual ability are influenced by shared genes. *Journal of Neuroscience, 30,* 5519–5524. (4)

Braun, A. R., Balkin, T. J., Wesensten, N. J., Guadry, F., Carson, R. E., Varga, M., . . . Herscovitch, P. (1998). Dissociated pattern of activity in visual cortices and their projections during human rapid eye movement sleep. *Science, 279,* 91–95. (7, 8)

Braunschweig, D., Krakowiak, P., Duncanson, P., Boyce, R., Hansen, R. L., Ashwood, P., . . . Van de Water, J. (2013). Autism-specific maternal autoantibodies recognize critical proteins in developing brain. *Translational Psychiatry, 3,* e277. (14)

Braus, H. (1960). Anatomie des Menschen, 3. Band: Periphere Leistungsbahnen II. Centrales Nervensystem, Sinnesorgane. 2. Auflage [Human anatomy: Vol. 3. Peripheral pathways II. Central nervous system, sensory organs (2nd ed.)]. Berlin: Springer-Verlag. (3)

Bray, G. A., Nielsen, S. J., & Popkin, B. M. (2004). Consumption of high-fructose corn syrup in beverages may play a role in the epidemic of obesity. *American Journal of Clinical Nutrition, 79,* 537–543. (9)

Breiter, H. C., Aharon, I., Kahneman, D., Dale, A., & Shizgal, P. (2001). Functional imaging of neural responses to expectancy and experience of monetary gains and losses. *Neuron, 30,* 619–639. (14)

Bremmer, F., Kubischik, M., Hoffmann, K.-P., & Krekelberg, B. (2009). Neural dynamics of saccadic suppression. *Journal of Neuroscience, 29,* 12374–12383. (5)

Brewer, W. J., Wood, S. J., Pantelis, C., Berger, G. E., Copolov, D. L., & McGorry, P. D. (2007). Olfactory sensitivity through the course of psychosis: Relationships to olfactory identification, symptomatology and the schizophrenia odour. *Psychiatry Research, 149,* 97–104. (14)

Brickman, A. M., Khan, U. A., Provenzano, F. A., Yeung, L.-K., Suzuki, W., Schroeter, H., . . . Small, S. A. (2014). Enhancing dentate gyrus function with dietary flavanols improves cognition in older adults. *Nature Neuroscience, 17,* 1798–1803. (12)

Bridge, H., Thomas, O. M., Minini, L., Cavina-Pratesi, C., Milner, A. D., & Parker, A. J. (2013). Structural and functional changes across the visual cortex of a patient with visual form agnosia. *Journal of Neuroscience, 33,* 12779–12791. (5)

Bridgeman, B., & Staggs, D. (1982). Plasticity in human blindsight. *Vision Research, 22,* 1199–1203. (5)

Bridle, C., Spanjers, K., Patel, S., Atherton, N. M., & Lamb, S. E. (2012). Effect of exercise on depression severity in older people: Systematic review and meta-analysis of randomised controlled trials. *British Journal of Psychiatry, 201,* 180–185. (14)

Briggs, R., Brooks, N., Tate, R., & Lah, S. (2015). Duration of post-traumatic amnesia as a predictor of functional outcome in school-age children: A systematic review. *Developmental Medicine & Child Neurology, 57,* 618–627. (4)

Brigman, J. L., Daut, R. A., Wright, T., Gunduz-Cinar, O., Graybeal, C., Davis, M. I., . . . Holmes, A. (2013). GluN2B in corticostriatal circuits governs choice learning and choice shifting. *Nature Neuroscience, 16,* 1101–1110. (12)

Brock, O., Baum, M. J., & Bakker, J. (2011). The development of female sexual behavior requires prepubertal estradiol. *Journal of Neuroscience, 31,* 5574–5578. (10)

Brodin, T., Fick, J., Jonsson, M., & Klaminder, J. (2013). Dilute concentrations of a psychiatric drug alter behavior of fish from natural populations. *Science, 339,* 814–815. (11)

Brody, A. L., Saxena, S., Stoessel, P., Gillies, L. A., Fairbanks, L. A., Alborzian, S., .. Baxter, L. R. (2001). Regional brain metabolic changes in patients with major depression treated with either paroxetine or interpersonal therapy. *Archives of General Psychiatry, 58,* 631–640. (14)

Brody, C. D., & Hanks, T. D. (2016). Neural underpinnings of the evidence accumulator. *Current Opinion in Neurobiology, 37,* 149–157. (13)

Brooks, P. L., & Peever, J. H. (2011). Impaired GABA and glycine transmission triggers cardinal features of rapid eye movement sleep behavior disorder in mice. *Journal of Neuroscience, 31,* 7111–7121. (8)

Brooks, P. L., & Peever, J. H. (2012). Identification of the transmitter and receptor mechanisms responsible for REM sleep paralysis. *Journal of Neuroscience, 32,* 9785–9795. (8)

Brooks, D. C., & Bizzi, E. (1963). Brain stem electrical activity during deep sleep. *Archives Italiennes de Biologie, 101,* 648–665. (8)

Brown, A., & Weaver, L. C. (2012). The dark side of neuroplasticity. *Experimental Neurology, 235,* 133–141. (4)

Brown, A. S. (2011). The environment and susceptibility to schizophrenia. *Progress in Neurobiology, 93,* 23–58. (14)

Brown, A. S., Begg, M. D., Gravenstein, S., Schaefer, C. A., Wyatt, R. J., Bresnahan, M., . . . Susser, E. S. (2004). Serologic evidence of prenatal influenza in the etiology of schizophrenia. *Archives of General Psychiatry, 61,* 774–780. (14)

Brown, C. E., Li, P., Boyd, J. D., Delaney, K. R., & Murphy, T. H. (2007). Extensive turnover of dendritic spines and vascular remodeling in cortical tissues recovering from stroke. *Journal of Neuroscience, 27,* 4101–4109. (4)

Brown, G. C., & Neher, J. J. (2014). Microglial phagocytosis of live neurons. *Nature Reviews Neuroscience, 15,* 209–216. (1)

Brown, G. L., Ebert, M. H., Goyer, P. F., Jimerson, D. C., Klein, W. J., Bunney, W. E., & Goodwin, F. K. (1982). Aggression, suicide, and serotonin: Relationships of CSF amine metabolites. *American Journal of Psychiatry, 139,* 741–746. (11)

Brown, J., Babor, T. F., Litt, M. D., & Kranzler, H. R. (1994). The type A/type B distinction. *Annals of the New York Academy of Sciences, 708,* 23–33. (14)

Brown, J. R., Ye, H., Bronson, R. T., Dikkes, P., & Greenberg, M. E. (1996). A defect in nurturing in mice lacking the immediate early gene *fos B. Cell, 86,* 297–309. (10)

Brown, K. L., & Freeman, J. H. (2016). Retention of eyeblink conditioning in periweanling and adult rats. *Developmental Psychobiology, 58,* 1055–1065. (12)

Brown, T. I., Carr, V. A., La Rocque, K. F., Favila, S. E., Gordon, A. M., Bowles, B., . . . Wagner, A. D. (2016). Prospective representation of navigational goals in the human hippocampus. *Science, 352,* 1323–1326. (12, 13)

Bruck, M., Cavanagh, P., & Ceci, S. J. (1991). Fortysomething: Recognizing faces at one's 25th reunion. *Memory & Cognition, 19,* 221–228. (5)

Brumpton, B., Langhammer, A., Romundstad, P., Chen, Y., & Mai, X. M. (2013). The associations of anxiety and depression symptoms with weight change and incident obesity: The HUNT study. *International Journal of Obesity, 37,* 1268–1274. (9)

Bruns, P., Liebnau, R., & Röder, B. (2011). Cross-modal training induces changes in spatial representations early in the auditory processing pathway. *Psychological Science, 22,* 1120–1126. (3)

Bschor, T., & Kilarski, L. L. (2016). Are antidepressants effective? A debate on their efficacy for the treatment of major depression in adults. *Expert Review of Neurotherapeutics, 16*, 367–374. (14)

Bucci, M. P., & Seessau, M. (2012). Saccadic eye movements in children: A developmental study *Experimental Brain Research, 222*, 21–30. (7)

Buck, L., & Axel, R. (1991). A novel multigene family may encode odorant receptors: A molecular basis for odor recognition. *Cell, 65*, 175–187. (6)

Buell, S. J., & Coleman, P. D. (1981). Quantitative evidence for selective dendritic growth in normal human aging but not in senile dementia. *Brain Research, 214*, 23–41. (4)

Buhle, J. T., Stevens, B. L., Friedman, J. J., & Wager, T. D. (2012). Distraction and placebo: Two separate routes to pain control. *Psychological Science, 23*, 246–253. (6)

Bühren, K., Schwarte, R., Fluck, F., Timmesfeld, N., Krei, M., Egberts, K., . . . Herpertz-Dahlmann, B. (2014). Comorbid psychiatric disorders in female adolescents with first-onset anorexia nervosa. *European Eating Disorders Review, 22*, 39–44. (9)

Buizer-Voskamp, J. E., Muntjewerff, J. W., Strengman, E., Sabatti, C., Stefansson, H., Vorstman, J. A. S., & Ophoff, R. A. (2011). Genome-wide analysis shows increased frequency of copy number variations deletions in Dutch schizophrenia patients. *Biological Psychiatry, 70*, 655–662. (14)

Buka, S. L., Tsuang, M. T., Torrey, E. F., Klebanoff, M. A., Bernstein, D., & Yolken, R. H. (2001). Maternal infections and subsequent psychosis among offspring. *Archives of General Psychiatry, 58*, 1032–1037. (14)

Bulbena, A., Gago, J., Martin-Santos, R., Porta, M., Dasquens, J., & Berrios, G. E. (2004). Anxiety disorder & joint laxity: A definitive link. *Neurology, Psychiatry and Brain Research, 11*, 137–140. (11)

Bulbena, A., Gago, J., Sperry, L., & Bergé, D. (2006). The relationship between frequency and intensity of fears and a collagen condition. *Depression and Anxiety, 23*, 412–417. (11)

Bundgaard, M. (1986). Pathways across the vertebrate blood–brain barrier: Morphological viewpoints. *Annals of the New York Academy of Sciences, 481*, 7–19. (1)

Bundy, H., Stahl, B. H., & MacCabe, J. H. (2011). A systematic review and meta-analysis of the fertility of patients with schizophrenia and their unaffected relatives. *Acta Psychiatrica Scandinavica, 123*, 98–106. (14)

Bunney, B. G., & Bunney, W. E. (2012). Rapid-acting antidepressant strategies: Mechanisms of action. *International Journal of Neuropsychopharmacology, 15*, 695–713. (14)

Burgaleta, M., Head, K., Álvarez-Linera, J., Martinez, K., Escorial, S., Haier, R., & Colom, R. (2012). Sex differences in brain volume are related to specific skills, not general intelligence. *Intelligence, 40*, 60–68. (3)

Burke, T. M., Markwald, R. R., McHill, A. M., Chinoy, E. D., Snider, J. A., Bessman, S. C., . . . Wright, K. P. Jr. (2015). Effects of caffeine on the human circadian clock *in vivo* and *in vitro*. *Science Translational Medicine, 7*, 305ra146. (8)

Burkett, J. P., & Young, L. J. (2012). The behavioral, anatomical, and pharmacological parallels between social attachment, love, and addiction. *Psychopharmacology, 224*, 1–26. (13)

Burman, D. D., Lie-Nemeth, T., Brandfonbrener, A. G., Parisi, T., & Meyer, J. R. (2009). Altered finger representations in sensorimotor cortex of musicians with focal dystonia: Precentral cortex. *Brain Imaging and Behavior, 3*, 10–23. (4)

Burr, D. C., Morrone, M. C., & Ross, J. (1994). Selective suppression of the magnocellular visual pathway during saccadic eye movements. *Nature, 371*, 511–513. (5)

Burra, N., Hervais-Adelman, A., Kerzel, D., Tamietto, M., de Gelder, B., & Pegna, A. J. (2013). Amygdala activation for eye contact despite complete cortical blindness. *Journal of Neuroscience, 33*, 10483–10489. (11)

Burrell, B. (2004). *Postcards from the brain museum.* New York: Broadway Books. (3, 12)

Burri, A., Cherkas, L., Spector, T., & Rahman, Q. (2011). Genetic and environmental influences on female sexual orientation, childhood gender typicality and adult gender identity. *PLoS One, 6*, e21982. (10)

Burt, S. A. (2009). Rethinking environmental contributions to child and adolescent psychopathology: A meta-analysis of shared environmental influences. *Psychological Bulletin, 135*, 608–637. (4)

Burt, S. A., Klump, K. L., Gorman-Smith, D., & Neiderhiser, J. M. (2016). Neighborhood disadvantage alters the origins of children's nonaggressive conduct problems. *Clinical Psychological Science, 4*, 511–526. (11)

Burton, H., Snyder, A. Z., Conturo, T. E., Akbudak, E., Ollinger, J. M., & Raichle, M. E. (2002). Adaptive changes in early and late blind: A fMRI study of Braille reading. *Journal of Neurophysiology, 87*, 589–607. (4)

Burton, R. F. (1994). *Physiology by numbers.* Cambridge, England: Cambridge University Press. (9)

Buschman, T. J., & Miller, E. K. (2007). Top-down versus bottom-up control of attention in the prefrontal and posterior parietal cortices. *Science, 315*, 1860–1862. (13)

Bushdid, C., Magnasco, M. O., Vosshall, L. B., & Keller, A. (2014). Humans can discriminate more than 1 trillion olfactory stimuli. *Science, 343*, 1370–1372. (6)

Buss, D. M. (1994). The strategies of human mating. *American Scientist, 82*, 238–249. (4)

Buss, D. M. (2000). Desires in human mating. *Annals of the New York Academy of Sciences, 907*, 39–49. (10)

Buss, D. M. (2001). Cognitive biases and emotional wisdom in the evolution of conflict

between the sexes. *Current Directions in Psychological Science, 10*, 219–223. (10)

Byars, J. A., Beglinger, L. J., Moser, D. J., Gonzalez-Alegre, P., & Nopoulos, P. (2012). Substance abuse may be a risk factor for earlier onset of Huntington's disease. *Journal of Neurology, 259*, 1824–1831. (7)

Byl, N. N., McKenzie, A., & Nagarajan, S. S. (2000). Differences in somatosensory hand organization in a healthy flutist and a flutist with focal hand dystonia: A case report. *Journal of Hand Therapy, 13*, 302–309. (4)

Byne, W., Tobet, S., Mattiace, L. A., Lasco, M. S., Kemether, E., Edgar, M. A., . . . Jones, L. B. (2001). The interstitial nuclei of the human anterior hypothalamus: An investigation of variation with sex, sexual orientation, and HIV status. *Hormones and Behavior, 40*, 86–92. (10)

Cabeza, R., & Moscovitch, M. (2013). Memory systems, processing modes, and components: Functional neuroimaging evidence. *Perspectives on Psychological Science, 8*, 49–55. (3)

Cahill, L. (2006). Why sex matters for neuroscience. *Nature Reviews Neuroscience, 7*, 477–484. (10)

Cahill, L., & McGaugh, J. L. (1998). Mechanisms of emotional arousal and lasting declarative memory. *Trends in Neurosciences, 21*, 294–299. (12)

Cai, D. J., Mednick, S. A., Harrison, E. M., Kanady, J. C., & Mednick, S. C. (2009). REM, not incubation, improves creativity by priming associative networks. *Proceedings of the National Academy of Sciences (U.S.A.), 106*, 10130–10134. (8)

Cai, H., Haubensak, W., Anthony, T. E., & Anderson, D. J. (2014). Central amygdala PKC-δ⁺neurons mediate the influence of multiple anorexigenic signals. *Nature Neuroscience, 17*, 1240–1248. (9)

Cai, Q., Van der Haegen, L., & Brysbaert, M. (2013). Complementary hemispheric specialization for language production and visuospatial attention. *Proceedings of the National Academy of Sciences (U.S.A.), 110*, E322–E330. (13)

Cajal, S. R. (1937). Recollections of my life. *Memoirs of the American Philosophical Society, 8.* (Original work published 1901–1917) (1)

Calabresi, P., Picconi, B., Tozzi, A., Ghiglieri, V., & Di Filippo, M. (2014). Direct and indirect pathways of basal ganglia: A critical reappraisal. *Nature Neuroscience, 17*, 1022–1030. (7)

Caldara, R., & Seghier, M. L. (2009). The fusiform face area responds automatically to statistical regularities optimal for face categorization. *Human Brain Mapping, 30*, 1615–1625. (5)

Calipari, E. S., & Ferris, M. J. (2013). Amphetamine mechanisms and actions at the dopamine terminal revisited. *Journal of Neuroscience, 33*, 8923–8925. (14)

Cameron, N. M., Champagne, F. A., Parent, C., Fish, E. W., Ozaki-Kuroda, K., & Meaney, M. J. (2005). The programming of individual differences in defensive responses and reproductive strategies in the rat through variations in maternal care. *Neuroscience and Biobehavioral Reviews, 29,* 843–865. (4)

Campbell, S. S., & Tobler, I. (1984). Animal sleep: A review of sleep duration across phylogeny. *Neuroscience and Biobehavioral Reviews, 8,* 269–300. (8)

Camperio-Ciani, A., Corna, F., & Capiluppi, C. (2004). Evidence for maternally inherited factors favouring male homosexuality and promoting female fecundity. *Proceedings of the Royal Society of London, B, 271,* 2217–2221. (10)

Campfield, L. A., Smith, F. J., Guisez, Y., Devos, R., & Burn, P. (1995). Recombinant mouse OB protein: Evidence for a peripheral signal linking adiposity and central neural networks. *Science, 269,* 546–552. (9)

Campi, K. L., Collins, C. E., Todd, W. D., Kaas, J., & Krubitzer, L. (2011). Comparison of area 17 cellular composition in laboratory and wild-caught rats including diurnal and nocturnal species. *Brain Behavior and Evolution, 77,* 116–130. (4)

Canal, C. E., & Gold, P. E. (2007). Different temporal profiles of amnesia after intra-hippocampus and intra-amygdala infusions of anisomycin. *Behavioral Neuroscience, 121,* 732–741. (12)

Canepari, M., Rossi, R., Pellegrino, M. A., Orell, R. W., Cobbold, M., Harridge, S., & Bottinelli, R. (2005). Effects of resistance training on myosin function studies by the in vitro motility assay in young and older men. *Journal of Applied Physiology, 98,* 2390–2395. (7)

Cannon, J. R., & Greenamyre, J. T. (2013). Gene-environment interactions in Parkinson's disease: Specific evidence in humans and mammalian models. *Neurobiology of Disease, 57,* 38–46. (7)

Cannon, W. B. (1927). The James-Lange theory of emotions: Critical examinations and an alternative theory. *American Journal of Psychology, 39,* 106–124. (11)

Cannon, W. B. (1929). Organization for physiological homeostasis. *Physiological Reviews, 9,* 399–431. (9)

Cannon, W. B. (1945). *The way of an investigator.* New York: Norton. (11)

Canter, R. G., Penney, J., & Tsai, L.-H. (2016). The road to restoring neural circuits for the treatment of Alzheimer's disease. *Nature, 539,* 187–196. (12)

Cantú, S. M., Simpson, J. A., Griskevicius, V., Weisberg, Y. J., Durante, K. M., & Beal, D. J. (2014). Fertile and selectively flirty: Women's behavior toward men changes across the ovulatory cycle. *Psychological Science, 25,* 431–438. (10)

Cao, M., & Guilleminault, C. (2010). Families with sleepwalking. *Sleep Medicine, 11,* 726–734. (8)

Cappelletti, M., & Wallen, K. (2016). Increasing women's sexual desire: The comparative effectiveness of estrogens and androgens. *Hormones and Behavior, 78,* 178–193. (10)

Carbon, M., Hsieh, C. H., Kane, J. M., & Correll, C. U. (2017). Tardive dyskinesia prevalence in the period of second-generation antipsychotic use: A meta-analysis. *Journal of Clinical Psychology,* in press. (14)

Cardoso, F. L. (2009). Recalled sex-typed behavior in childhood and sports' preferences in adulthood of heterosexual, bisexual, and homosexual men from Brazil, Turkey, and Thailand. *Archives of Sexual Behavior, 38,* 726–736. (10)

Carey, I. M., Shah, S. M., DeWilde, S., Harris, T., Victor, C. R., & Cook, D. G. (2014). Increased risk of acute cardiovascular events after partner bereavement. *JAMA Internal Medicine, 174,* 598–605. (11)

Carhart-Harris, R. L., Muthukumaraswamy, S., Roseman, L., Kaelen, M., Droog, W., Murphy, K., . . . Nutt, D. J. (2016). Neural correlates of the LSD experience revealed by multimodal neuroimaging. *Proceedings of the National Academy of Sciences (U.S.A.), 113,* 4853–4858. (2)

Carlsson, A. (2001). A paradigm shift in brain research. *Science, 294,* 1021–1024. (2)

Carpenter, C. J. (2012). Meta-analyses of sex differences in responses to sexual versus emotional infidelity: Men and women are more similar than different. *Psychology of Women Quarterly, 36,* 25–37. (10)

Carpenter, G. A., & Grossberg, S. (1984). A neural theory of circadian rhythms: Aschoff's rule in diurnal and nocturnal mammals. *American Journal of Physiology, 247,* R1067–R1082. (8)

Carré, J. M., Iselin, A.-M. R., Welker, K. M., Hariri, A. R., & Dodge, K. A. (2014). Testosterone reactivity to provocation mediates the effect of early intervention on aggressive behavior. *Psychological Science, 25,* 1140–1146. (11)

Carrera, O., Adan, R. A. H., Gutiérrez, E., Danner, U. N., Hoek, H. W., van Elburg, A. A., & Kas, M. J. H. (2012). Hyperactivity in anorexia nervosa: Warming up not just burning-off calories. *PLoS One, 7,* e41851. (9)

Carruth, L. L., Reisert, I., & Arnold, A. P. (2002). Sex chromosome genes directly affect brain sexual differentiation. *Nature Neuroscience, 5,* 933–934. (10)

Carter, M. E., Soden, M. E., Zweifel, L. S., & Palmiter, R. D. (2013). Genetic identification of a neural circuit that suppresses appetite. *Nature, 503,* 111–114. (9)

Carver, C. S., Johnson, S. L., Joormann, J., Kim, Y., & Nam, J. Y. (2011). Serotonin transporter polymorphism interacts with childhood adversity to predict aspects of impulsivity. *Psychological Science, 22,* 589–595. (11)

Casali, A. G., Gosseries, O., Rosanova, M., Boly, M., Sarasso, S., Casali, K. R., . . . Massimini, M. (2013). A theoretically based index of consciousness independent of sensory processes and behavior. *Science Translational Medicine, 5,* 198ra105. (13)

Case, L. K., Laubacher, C. M., Olausson, H., Wang, B., Spagnolo, P. A., & Bushnell, M. C. (2016). Encoding of touch intensity but not pleasantness in human primary somatosensory cortex. *Journal of Neuroscience, 36,* 5850–5860. (6)

Casey, B. J., & Caudle, K. (2013). The teenage brain: Self control. *Current Directions in Psychological Science, 22,* 82–87. (4)

Cash, S. S., Halgren, E., Dehghani, N., Rosssetti, A. O., Thesen, T., Wang, C. M., . . . Ulbert, I. (2009). The human K-complex represents an isolated cortical down-state. *Science, 324,* 1084–1087. (8)

Caspi, A., Houts, R. M., Belsky, D. W., Goldman-Mellor, S. J., Harrington, H. L., Israel, S., . . . Moffitt, T. E. (2014). The *p* factor: One general psychopathology factor in the structure of psychiatric disorders? *Clinical Psychological Science, 2,* 119–137. (14)

Caspi, A., McClay, J., Moffitt, T. E., Mill, J., Martin, J., Craig, I. W., . . . Poulton, R. (2002). Role of genotype in the cycle of violence in maltreated children. *Science, 297,* 851–854. (11)

Caspi, A., Sugden, K., Moffitt, T. E., Taylor, A., Craig, I. W., Harrington, H., . . . Poulton, R. (2003). Influence of life stress on depression: Moderation by a polymorphism in the 5-HTT gene. *Science, 301,* 386–389. (14)

Cassia, V. M., Turati, C., & Simion, F. (2004). Can a nonspecific bias toward top-heavy patterns explain newborns' face preference? *Psychological Science, 15,* 379–383. (5)

Castellucci, V. F., Pinsker, H., Kupfermann, I., & Kandel, E. (1970). Neuronal mechanisms of habituation and dishabituation of the gill-withdrawal reflex in *Aplysia. Science, 167,* 1745–1748. (12)

Castrén, E., & Rantamäki, T. (2010). The role of BDNF and its receptors in depression and antidepressant drug action: Reactivation of developmental plasticity. *Developmental Neurobiology, 70,* 289–296. (14)

Castro-Alvarez, J. F., Gutierrez-Vargas, J., Darnaudéry, M., & Cardona-Gómez, G. P. (2011). ROCK inhibition prevents tau hyperphosphorylation and p25/CDK5 increase after global cerebral ischemia. *Behavioral Neuroscience, 125,* 465–472. (4)

Catalano, S. M., & Shatz, C. J. (1998). Activity-dependent cortical target selection by thalamic axons. *Science, 281,* 559–562. (4)

Catania, K. C. (2006). Underwater "sniffing" by semi-aquatic mammals. *Nature, 444,* 1024–1025. (6)

Catchpole, C. K., & Slater, P. J. B. (1995). *Bird song: Biological themes and variations.* Cambridge, England: Cambridge University Press. (0)

Catmur, C., Walsh, V., & Heyes, C. (2007). Sensorimotor learning configures the human mirror system. *Current Biology, 17,* 1527–1531. (7)

Catterall, W. A. (1984). The molecular basis of neuronal excitability. *Science, 223,* 653–661. (1)

Cavina-Pratesi, C., Connolly, J. D., & Milner, A. D. (2013). Optic ataxia as a model to investigate the role of the posterior parietal cortex in visually guided action: Evidence from studies of patient M. H. *Frontiers in Human Neuroscience, 7*, article 336. (5)

Cepeda-Benito, A., Davis, K. W., Reynoso, J. T., & Harraid, J. H. (2005). Associative and behavioral tolerance to the analgesic effects of nicotine in rats: Tail-flick and paw-lick assays. *Psychopharmacology, 180*, 224–233. (14)

Cerletti, U., & Bini, L. (1938). L'Elettroshock. *Archivio Generale di Neurologia e Psichiatria e Psicoanalisi, 19*, 266–268. (14)

Cerrato, M., Carrera, O., Vazquez, R., Echevarria, E., & Gutiérrez, E. (2012). Heat makes a difference in activity-based anorexia: A translational approach to treatment development in anorexia nervosa. *International Journal of Eating Disorders, 45*, 26–35. (9)

Chafee, M. V., & Goldman-Rakic, P. S. (1998). Matching patterns of activity in primate prefrontal area 8a and parietal area 7ip neurons during a spatial working memory task. *Journal of Neurophysiology, 79*, 2919–2940. (12)

Chailangkarn, T., Trujillo, C. A., Freitas, B., Hrvoy-Mihic, B., Herai, R. H., Yu, D. X., . . . Moutri, A. R. (2016). A human neurodevelopmental model for Williams syndrome. *Nature, 536*, 338–343. (13)

Chalmers, D. J. (1995). Facing up to the problem of consciousness. *Journal of Consciousness Studies, 2*, 200–219. (13)

Chalmers, D. L. (2004). How can we construct a science of consciousness? In M. S. Gazzaniga (Ed.), *The cognitive neurosciences* (3rd ed.) (pp. 1111–1119). Cambridge, MA: MIT Press. (13)

Chalmers, D. (2007). Naturalistic dualism. In M. Velmans & S. Schneider (Eds.), *The Blackwell companion to consciousness* (pp. 359–368). Malden, MA: Blackwell. (0)

Chang, E. F., & Merzenich, M. M. (2003). Environmental noise retards auditory cortical development. *Science, 300*, 498–502. (6)

Chang, G.-Q., Gaysinskaya, V., Karatayev, O., & Leibowitz, S. F. (2008). Maternal high-fat diet and fetal programming: Increased proliferation of hypothalamic peptide-producing neurons that increase risk for overeating and obesity. *Journal of Neuroscience, 28*, 12107–12119. (9)

Chang, S.-H., Gao, L., Li, Z., Zhang, W.-N., Du, Y., & Wang, J. (2013). BDgene: A genetic database for bipolar disorder and its overlap with schizophrenia and major depressive disorder. *Biological Psychiatry, 74*, 727–733. (14)

Chang, S. W. C., Gariépy, J.-F., & Platt, M. L. (2013). Neuronal reference frames for social decisions in primate frontal cortex. *Nature Neuroscience, 16*, 243–250. (13)

Chao, M. V. (2010). A conversation with Rita Levi-Montalcini. *Annual Review of Physiology, 72*, 1–13. (4)

Chapman, S. B., Aslan, S., Spence, J. S., DeFina, L. F., Keebler, M. W., Didehbani, N., & Lu, H. (2013). Shorter term aerobic exercise improves brain, cognition, and cardiovascular fitness in aging. *Frontiers in Aging Neuroscience, 5*, Article 75. (12)

Chatterjee, R. (2015). Out of the darkness. *Science, 350*, 372–375. (5)

Chaudhari, N., Landin, A. M., & Roper, S. D. (2000). A metabotropic glutamate receptor variant functions as a taste receptor. *Nature Neuroscience, 3*, 113–119. (6)

Chee, M. J. S., Myers, M. G. Jr., Price, C. J., & Colmers, W. F. (2010). Neuropeptide Y suppresses anorexigenic output from the ventromedial nucleus of the hypothalamus. *Journal of Neuroscience, 30*, 3380–3390. (9)

Chen, L. M., Friedman, R. M., & Roe, A. W. (2003). Optical imaging of a tactile illusion in area 3b of the primary somatosensory cortex. *Science, 302*, 881–885. (6)

Chen, Y.-C., Kuo, H.-Y., Bornschein, U., Takahashi, H., Chen, S.-Y., Lu, K.-M., . . . Liu, F.-C. (2016). *Foxp2* controls synaptic wiring of corticostriatal circuits and vocal communication by opposing Mef2c. *Nature Neuroscience, 19*, 1513–1522. (13)

Cheney, D. L. (2011). Cooperation in nonhuman primates. In R. Menzel & J. Fischer (Eds.), *Animal thinking* (pp. 239–252). Cambridge, MA: MIT Press. (4)

Cheney, D. L., & Seyfarth, R. M. (2005). Constraints and adaptations in the earliest stages of language evolution. *Linguistic Review, 22*, 135–159. (13)

Chesworth, R., & Corbit, L. H. (2017). Recent developments in the behavioural and pharmacological enhancement of extinction of drug seeking. *Addiction Biology, 22*, 2–43. (14)

Cheyne, J. A., & Pennycook, G. (2013). Sleep paralysis postepisode distress: Modeling potential effects of episode characteristics, general psychological distress, beliefs, and cognitive style. *Clinical Psychological Science, 1*, 135–148. (8)

Chiapponi, C., Piras, F., Fagioli, S., Piras, F., Caltagirone, C., & Spalletta, G. (2013). Age-related brain trajectories in schizophrenia: A systematic review of structural MRI studies. *Psychiatry Research—Neuroimaging, 214*, 83–93. (14)

Chiang, M.-C., Barysheva, M., Shattuck, D. W., Lee, A. D., Madsen, S. K., Avedissian, C., . . . Thompson, P. M. (2009). Genetics of brain fiber architecture and intellectual performance. *Journal of Neuroscience, 29*, 2212–2224. (12)

Cho, K. (2001). Chronic "jet lag" produces temporal lobe atrophy and spatial cognitive deficits. *Nature Neuroscience, 4*, 567–568. (8)

Chomsky, N. (1980). *Rules and representations.* New York: Columbia University Press. (13)

Chong, S. Y. C., Ptácek, L. J., & Fu, Y. H. (2012). Genetic insights on sleep schedules: This time it's PERsonal. *Trends in Genetics, 28*, 598–605. (8)

Chong, S. C., Jo, S., Park, K. M., Joo, E. Y., Lee, M.-J., Hong, S. C., & Hong, S. B. (2013). Interaction between the electrical stimulation of a face-selective area and the perception of face stimuli. *NeuroImage, 77*, 70–76. (5)

Chou, E. Y., Parmar, B. L., & Galinsky, A. D. (2016). Economic insecurity increases physical pain. *Psychological Science, 27*, 443–454. (6)

Christensen, C. B., Christensen-Dalsgaard, J., & Madsen, P. T. (2015). Hearing of the African lungfish (*Protopterus annectens*) suggests underwater pressure detection and rudimentary aerial hearing in early tetrapods. *Journal of Experimental Biology, 218*, 381–387. (6)

Chuang, H., Prescott, E. D., Kong, H., Shields, S., Jordt, S.-E., Basbaum, A. I., . . . Julius, D. (2001). Bradykinin and nerve growth factor release the capsaicin receptor from Ptdlns(4, 5)P2-mediated inhibition. *Nature, 411*, 957–962. (6)

Chung, W. C. J., de Vries, G. J., & Swaab, D. F. (2002). Sexual differentiation of the bed nucleus of the stria terminalis in humans may extend into adulthood. *Journal of Neuroscience, 22*, 1027–1033. (10)

Churchland, P. S. (1986). *Neurophilosophy.* Cambridge, Massachusetts: MIT Press. (0)

Ciaramelli, E., Muccioli, M., Làdavas, E., & di Pellegrino, G. (2007). Selective deficit in personal moral judgment following damage to ventromedial prefrontal cortex. *Social Cognitive and Affective Neuroscience, 2*, 84–92. (11)

Cichon, J., & Gan, W.-B. (2015). Branch-specific dendritic Ca^{2+} spikes cause persistent synaptic plasticity. *Nature, 520*, 180–185. (12)

Cicone, N., Wapner, W., Foldi, N. S., Zurif, E., & Gardner, H. (1979). The relation between gesture and language in aphasic communication. *Brain and Language, 8*, 342–349. (13)

Clahsen, H., & Almazen, M. (1998). Syntax and morphology in Williams syndrome. *Cognition, 68*, 167–198. (13)

Clark, D. A., Mitra, P. P., & Wang, S. S.-H. (2001). Scalable architecture in mammalian brains. *Nature, 411*, 189–193. (3)

Clark, R. E., & Lavond, D. G. (1993). Reversible lesions of the red nucleus during acquisition and retention of a classically conditioned behavior in rabbits. *Behavioral Neuroscience, 107*, 264–270. (12)

Clark, W. S. (2004). Is the zone-tailed hawk a mimic? *Birding, 36*, 494–498. (0)

Clarke, S., Assal, G., & deTribolet, N. (1993). Left hemisphere strategies in visual recognition, topographical orientation and time planning. *Neuropsychologia, 31*, 99–113. (13)

Cleary, L. J., Hammer, M., & Byrne, J. H. (1989). Insights into the cellular mechanisms of short-term sensitization in *Aplysia*. In T. J. Carew & D. B. Kelley (Eds.), *Perspectives in neural systems and behavior* (pp. 105–119). New York: Liss. (12)

Clelland, C. D., Choi, M., Romberg, C., Clemenson, G. D. Jr., Fragniere, A., Tyers, P., . . . Bussey, T. J. (2009). A functional role for adult hippocampal neurogenesis in spatial pattern separation. *Science, 325*, 210–213. (4)

Clemenson, G. D., & Stark, C. E. L. (2015). Virtual environmental enrichment through video games improves hippocampal-associated memory. *Journal of Neuroscience, 35,* 16116–16125. (4)

Clements, K. M., Smith, L. M., Reynolds, J. N. J., Overton, P. G., Thomas, J. D., & Napper, R. M. (2012). Early postnatal ethanol exposure: Glutamatergic excitotoxic cell death during acute withdrawal. *Neurophysiology, 44,* 376–386. (4)

Clutton-Brock, T. H., O'Riain, M. J., Brotherton, P. N. M., Gaynor, D., Kansky, R., Griffin, A. S., & Manser, M. (1999). Selfish sentinels in cooperative mammals. *Science, 284,* 1640–1644. (4)

Coan, J. A., Schaefer, H. S., & Davidson, R. J. (2006). Lending a hand: Social regulation of the neural response to threat. *Psychological Science, 17,* 1032–1039. (11)

Cobos, P., Sánchez, M., Pérez, N., & Vila, J. (2004). Effects of spinal cord injuries on the subjective component of emotions. *Cognition and Emotion, 18,* 281–287. (11)

Coderre, T. J., Katz, J., Vaccarino, A. L., & Melzack, R. (1993). Contribution of central neuroplasticity to pathological pain: Review of clinical and experimental evidence. *Pain, 52,* 259–285. (6)

Coenen, A. M. L. (1995). Neuronal activities underlying the electroencephalogram and evoked potentials of sleeping and waking: Implications for information-processing. *Neuroscience and Biobehavioral Reviews, 19,* 447–463. (8)

Cohen, D., & Nicolelis, M. A. L. (2004). Reduction of single-neuron firing uncertainty by cortical ensembles during motor skill learning. *Journal of Neuroscience, 24,* 3574–3582. (7)

Cohen, L. G., Celnik, P., Pascual-Leone, A., Corwell, B., Faiz, L., Dambrosia, J., . . . Hallett, M. (1997). Functional relevance of cross-modal plasticity in blind humans. *Nature, 389,* 180–183. (4)

Cohen, S., Frank, E., Doyle, W. J., Skoner, D. P., Rabin, B. S., & Swaltney, J. M., Jr. (1998). Types of stressors that increase susceptibility to the common cold in healthy adults. *Health Psychology, 17,* 214–223. (11)

Cohen, S., Janicki-Deverts, D., Turner, R. B., & Doyle, W. J. (2015). Does hugging provide stress-buffering social support? A study of susceptibility to upper respiratory infection and illness. *Psychological Science, 26,* 135–147. (11)

Cohen-Kettenis, P. T. (2005). Gender change in 46, XY persons with 5a-reductase-2 deficiency and 17b-hydroxysteroid dehydrogenase-3 deficiency. *Archives of Sexual Behavior, 34,* 399–410. (10)

Cohen-Tannoudji, M., Babinet, C., & Wassef, M. (1994). Early determination of a mouse somatosensory cortex marker. *Nature, 368,* 460–463. (4)

Cohen-Woods, S., Craig, I. W., & McGuffin, P. (2013). The current state of play on the molecular genetics of depression. *Psychological Medicine, 43,* 673–687. (14)

Colantuoni, C., Rada, P., McCarthy, J., Patten, C., Avena, N. M., Chadeayne, A., & Hoebel, B. G. (2002). Evidence that intermittent, excessive sugar intake causes endogenous opioid dependence. *Obesity Research, 10,* 478–488. (9)

Colantuoni, C., Schwenker, J., McCarthy, J., Rada, P., Ladenheim, B., Cadet, J.-L., . . . Hoebel, B. G. (2001). Excessive sugar intake alters binding to dopamine and mu-opioid receptors in the brain. *NeuroReport, 12,* 3549–3552. (9)

Colapinto, J. (1997, December 11). The true story of John/Joan. *Rolling Stone,* pp. 54–97. (10)

Coleman, J. A., Green, E. M., & Gouaux, E. (2016). X-ray structures and mechanism of the human serotonin transporter. *Nature, 532,* 334–339. (14)

Collingridge, G. L., Peineau, S., Howland, J. G., & Wang, Y. T. (2010). Long-term depression in the CNS. *Nature Reviews Neuroscience, 11,* 459–473. (12)

Collins, C. E. (2011). Variability in neuron densities across the cortical sheet in primates. *Brain, Behavior and Evolution, 78,* 37–50. (3)

Colom, R., Burgaleta, M., Román, F. J., Karama, S., Alvarez-Linera, J., Abad, F. J., . . . Haier, R. J. (2013). Neuroanatomic overlap between intelligence and cognitive factors: Morphometry methods provide support for the key role of the frontal lobes. *NeuroImage, 72,* 143–152. (12)

Colom, R., Quiroga, M. A., Solana, A. B., Burgaleta, M., Román, F. J., Privado, J., . . . Karama, S. (2012). Structural changes after videogame practice related to a brain network associated with intelligence. *Intelligence, 40,* 479–489. (4)

Coltheart, M. (2013). How can functional neuroimaging inform cognitive theories? *Perspectives on Psychological Science, 8,* 98–103. (3)

Conn, P. M., & Parker, J. V. (2008). Winners and losers in the animal-research war. *American Scientist, 96,* 184–186. (0)

Connine, C. M., Blasko, D. G., & Hall, M. (1991). Effects of subsequent sentence context in auditory word recognition: Temporal and linguistic constraints. *Journal of Memory and Language, 30,* 234–250. (13)

Considine, R. V., Sinha, M. K., Heiman, M. L., Kriauciunas, A., Stephens, T. W., Nyce, M. R., . . . Caro, J. F. (1996). Serum immunoreactive-leptin concentrations in normal-weight and obese humans. *New England Journal of Medicine, 334,* 292–295. (9)

Constantinidis, C., & Klingberg, T. (2016). The neuroscience of working memory capacity and training. *Nature Reviews Neuroscience, 17,* 438–449. (12)

Conti, V., Marini, C., Gana, S., Sudi, J., Dobyns, W. B., & Guerrini, R. (2011). Corpus callosum agenesis, severe mental retardation, epilepsy, and dyskinetic quadriparesis due to a novel mutation in the homeodomain of ARX. *American Journal of Medical Genetics Part A, 155A,* 892–897. (4)

CONVERGE Consortium. (2015). Sparse whole-genome sequencing identifies two loci for major depression. *Nature, 523,* 588–591. (14)

Cooke, B. M., Tabibnia, G., & Breedlove, S. M. (1999). A brain sexual dimorphism controlled by adult circulating androgens. *Proceedings of the National Academy of Sciences, USA, 96,* 7538–7540. (10)

Coppola, D. M., Purves, H. R., McCoy, A. N., & Purves, D. (1998). The distribution of oriented contours in the real world. *Proceedings of the National Academy of Sciences, USA, 95,* 4002–4006. (5)

Corballis, M. C. (2012a). How language evolved from manual gestures. *Gesture, 12,* 200–226. (13)

Corballis, M. C. (May–June, 2012b). Mind wandering. *American Scientist, 100(3),* 210–217. (3)

Corcoran, A. J., Barber, J. R., & Conner, W. E. (2009). Tiger moth jams bat sonar. *Science, 325,* 325–327. (6)

Corkin, S. (1984). Lasting consequences of bilateral medial temporal lobectomy: Clinical course and experimental findings in H. M. *Seminars in Neurology, 4,* 249–259. (12)

Corkin, S. (2002). What's new with the amnesic patient H. M.? *Nature Reviews Neuroscience, 3,* 153–159. (12)

Corkin, S. (2013). *Permanent present tense.* New York: Basic books. (12)

Corkin, S., Rosen, T. J., Sullivan, E. V., & Clegg, R. A. (1989). Penetrating head injury in young adulthood exacerbates cognitive decline in later years. *Journal of Neuroscience, 9,* 3876–3883. (4)

Cornelius, M. D., De Genna, N. M., Goldschmidt, L., Larkby, C., & Day, N. L. (2016). Prenatal alcohol and other early childhood adverse exposures: Direct and indirect pathways to adolescent drinking. *Neurotoxicology and Teratology, 55,* 8–15. (14)

Corradi-Dell'Acqua, C., Hofstetter, C., & Vuilleumier, P. (2011). Felt and seen pain evoke the same local patterns of cortical activity in insular and cingulate cortex. *Journal of Neuroscience, 31,* 17996–18006. (6)

Cosmelli, D., David, O., Lachaux, J.-P., Martinerie, J., Garnero, L., Renault, B., & Varela, F. (2004). Waves of consciousness: Ongoing cortical patterns during binocular rivalry. *NeuroImage, 23,* 128–140. (13)

Coss, R. G., Brandon, J. G., & Globus, A. (1980). Changes in morphology of dendritic spines on honeybee calycal interneurons associated with cumulative nursing and foraging experiences. *Brain Research, 192,* 49–59. (4)

Costa, R. P., Froemke, R. C., Sjöström, P. J., & van Rossum, M. C. W. (2015). Unified pre-and postsynaptic long-term plasticity enables reliable and flexible learning. *eLife, 4,* e09457. (12)

Costa, V. D., Lang, P. J., Sabatinelli, D., Versace, F., & Bradley, M. M. (2010). Emotional imagery: Assessing pleasure and arousal in the brain's reward circuitry. *Human Brain Mapping, 31,* 1446–1457. (14)

Courchesne, E., Townsend, J., Akshoomoff, N. A., Saitoh, O., Yeung-Courchesne, R., Lincoln, A. J., . . . Lau, L. (1994). Impairment in shifting attention in autistic and cerebellar patients. *Behavioral Neuroscience, 108,* 848–865. (3)

Cowart, B. J. (2005, Spring). Taste, our body's gustatory gatekeeper. *Cerebrum, 7*(2), 7–22. (6)

Cox, J. J., Reimann, F., Nicholas, A. K., Thornton, G., Roberts, E., Springell, K., . . . Woods, C. G. (2006). An *SCN9A* channelopathy causes congenital inability to experience pain. *Nature, 304,* 115–117. (6)

Craig, A. M., & Boudin, H. (2001). Molecular heterogeneity of central synapses: Afferent and target regulation. *Nature Neuroscience, 4,* 569–578. (2)

Crair, M. C., Gillespie, D. C., & Stryker, M. P. (1998). The role of visual experience in the development of columns in cat visual cortex. *Science, 279,* 566–570. (5)

Cravchik, A., & Goldman, D. (2000). Neurochemical individuality. *Archives of General Psychiatry, 57,* 1105–1114. (14)

Cressey, D. (2016). Q&A: Fabulous fact fisher. *Nature, 534,* 325. (10)

Crick, F. C., & Koch, C. (2004). A framework for consciousness. In M. S. Gazzaniga (Ed.), *The cognitive neurosciences* (3rd ed., pp. 1133–1143). Cambridge, MA: MIT Press. (13)

Crick, F., & Mitchison, G. (1983). The function of dream sleep. *Nature, 304,* 111–114. (8)

Critchley, H. D., Mathias, C. J., & Dolan, R. J. (2001). Neuroanatomical basis for first- and second-order representations of bodily states. *Nature Neuroscience, 4,* 207–212. (11)

Critchley, H. D., & Rolls, E. T. (1996). Hunger and satiety modify the responses of olfactory and visual neurons in the primate orbitofrontal cortex. *Journal of Neurophysiology, 75,* 1673–1686. (9)

Crivelli, C., Jarillo, S., Russell, J. A., & Fernández-Dols, J. M. (2016). Reading emotions from faces in two indigenous societies. *Journal of Experimental Psychology: General, 145,* 830–843. (11)

Crone, E. A., & Dahl, R. E. (2012). Understanding adolescence as a period of social-affective engagement and goal flexibility. *Nature Reviews Neuroscience, 13,* 636–650. (4)

Cross-Disorder Group of the Psychiatric Genomic Consortium. (2013). Identification of risk loci with shared effects on five major psychiatric disorders: A genome-wide analysis. *Lancet, 381,* 1371–1379. (14)

Crossin, K. L., & Krushel, L. A. (2000). Cellular signaling by neural cell adhesion molecules of the immunoglobulin family. *Developmental Dynamics, 218,* 260–279. (4)

Crowley, S. J., & Eastman, C. I. (2013). Melatonin in the afternoons of a gradually advancing sleep schedule enhances the circadian phase advance. *Psychopharmacology, 225,* 825–837. (8)

Cryan, J. F., & Dinan, T. G. (2012). Mind-altering microorganisms: The impact of the gut microbiota on brain and behavior. *Nature Reviews Neuroscience, 13,* 701–712. (9)

Cui, G., Jun, S. B., Jin, X., Pham, M. D., Vogel, S. S., Lovinger, D. M., & Costa, R. M. (2013). Concurrent activation of striatal direct and indirect pathways during action initiation. *Nature, 494,* 238–242. (7)

Cummings, D. E., Clement, K., Purnell, J. Q., Vaisse, C., Foster, K. E., Frayo, R. S., . . . Weigle, D. S. (2002). Elevated plasma ghrelin levels in Prader-Willi syndrome. *Nature Medicine, 8,* 643–644. (9)

Cummings, D. E., & Overduin, J. (2007). Gastrointestinal regulation of food intake. *Journal of Clinical Investigation, 117,* 13–23. (9)

Curry, A. (2013). The milk revolution. *Nature, 500,* 20–22. (9)

Cushman, F., Gray, K., Gaffey, A., & Mendes, M. B. (2012). Simulating murder: The aversion to harmful action. *Emotion, 12,* 2–7. (11)

Cutler, W. B., Preti, G., Krieger, A., Huggins, G. R., Garcia, C. R., & Lawley, H. J. (1986). Human axillary secretions influence women's menstrual cycles: The role of donor extract from men. *Hormones and Behavior, 20,* 463–473. (6)

Cvijanovic, N., Feinle-Bisset, C., Young, R. L., & Little, T. J. (2015). Oral and intestinal sweet and fat tasting: Impact of receptor polymorphisms and dietary modulation for metabolic disease. *Nutrition Reviews, 73,* 318–334. (9)

Czeisler, C. (2013). Casting light on sleep deficiency. *Nature, 497,* S13. (8)

Czeisler, C. A., Johnson, M. P., Duffy, J. F., Brown, E. N., Ronda, J. M., & Kronauer, R. E. (1990). Exposure to bright light and darkness to treat physiologic maladaptation to night work. *New England Journal of Medicine, 322,* 1253–1259. (8)

Czeisler, C. A., Weitzman, E. D., Moore-Ede, M. C., Zimmerman, J. C., & Knauer, R. S. (1980). Human sleep: Its duration and organization depend on its circadian phase. *Science, 210,* 1264–1267. (8)

Dachtler, J., Ivorra, J. L., Rowland, T. E., Lever, C., Rodgers, R. J., & Clapcote, S. J. (2015). Heterozygous deletion of alpha-neurexin I or alpha-neurexin II results in behaviors relevant to autism and schizophrenia. *Behavioral Neuroscience, 129,* 765–776. (14)

Dabbs, J. M., Jr., Carr, T. S., Frady, R. L., & Riad, J. K. (1995). Testosterone, crime, and misbehavior among 692 male prison inmates. *Personality and Individual Differences, 18,* 627–633. (11)

Dale, N., Schacher, S., & Kandel, E. R. (1988). Long-term facilitation in *Aplysia* involves increase in transmitter release. *Science, 239,* 282–285. (12)

Dale, P. S., Harlaar, N., Haworth, C. M. A., & Plomin, R. (2010). Two by two: A twin study of second-language acquisition. *Psychological Science, 21,* 635–640. (4)

Dallaspezia, S., Suzuki, M., & Benedetti, F. (2015). Chronobiology for mood disorders. *Current Psychiatry Reports, 17,* article 95. (14)

Dalterio, S., & Bartke, A. (1979). Perinatal exposure to cannabinoids alters male reproductive function in mice. *Science, 205,* 1420–1422. (10)

Dalton, K. (1968). Ante-natal progesterone and intelligence. *British Journal of Psychiatry, 114,* 1377–1382. (10)

Dalton, P., Doolittle, N., & Breslin, P. A. (2002). Gender-specific induction of enhanced sensitivity to odors. *Nature Neuroscience, 5,* 199–200. (6)

Damasio, A. (1999). *The feeling of what happens.* New York: Harcourt Brace. (11)

Damasio, A. R. (1994). *Descartes' error.* New York: Putnam's Sons. (11)

Damsma, G., Pfaus, J. G., Wenkstern, D., Phillips, A. G., & Fibiger, H. C. (1992). Sexual behavior increases dopamine transmission in the nucleus accumbens and striatum of male rats: A comparison with novelty and locomotion. *Behavioral Neuroscience, 106,* 181–191. (14)

Darweesh, S. K. L., Verlinden, V. J. A., Adams, H. H. H., Uitterlinden, A. G., Hofman, A., Stricker, B. H., . . . Ikram, M. A. (2016). Genetic risk of Parkinson's disease in the general population. *Parkinsonism & Related Disorders, 29,* 54–59. (7)

Darwin, C. (1859). *The origin of species.* New York: D. Appleton. (4)

Das, A., Tadin, D., & Huxlin, K. R. (2014). Beyond blindsight: Properties of visual relearning in cortically blind fields. *Journal of Neuroscience, 34,* 11652–11664. (5)

Daum, I., Schugens, M. M., Ackermann, H., Lutzenberger, W., Dichgans, J., & Birbaumer, N. (1993). Classical conditioning after cerebellar lesions in humans. *Behavioral Neuroscience, 107,* 748–756. (12)

Davidson, R. J. (1984). Affect, cognition, and hemispheric specialization. In C. E. Izard, J. Kagan, & R. B. Zajonc (Eds.), *Emotions, cognition, & behavior* (pp. 320–365). Cambridge, England: Cambridge University Press. (14)

Davidson, R. J., & Fox, N. A. (1982). Asymmetrical brain activity discriminates between positive and negative affective stimuli in human infants. *Science, 218,* 1235–1237. (11)

Davidson, R. J., & Henriques, J. (2000). Regional brain function in sadness and depression. In J. C. Borod (Ed.), *The neuropsychology of emotion* (pp. 269–297). London: Oxford University Press. (11)

Davidson, S., Zhang, X., Khasabov, S. G., Simone, D. A., & Giesler, G. J. Jr. (2009). Relief of itch by scratching: State-dependent inhibition of primate spinothalamic tract neurons. *Nature Neuroscience, 12,* 544–546. (6)

Davies, G., Armstrong, N., Bis, J. C., Bressler, J., Chouraki, V., Giddaluru, S., . . . Deary, I. J. (2015). Genetic contributions to variation in general cognitive function: A meta-analysis of genome-wide association studies in the CHARGE consortium (N = 53 949). *Molecular Psychiatry, 20,* 183–192. (12)

Davies, G., Welham, J., Chant, D., Torrey, E. F., & McGrath, J. (2003). A systematic review and meta-analysis of Northern hemisphere season of birth effects in schizophrenia. *Schizophrenia Bulletin, 29,* 587–593. (14)

Davies, P. (2006). *The Goldilocks enigma.* Boston, MA: Houghton Mifflin. (0)

Davis, E. C., Shryne, J. E., & Gorski, R. A. (1995). A revised critical period for the sexual differentiation of the sexually dimorphic nucleus of the preoptic area in the rat. *Neuroendocrinology, 62,* 579–585. (10)

Davis, J., Eyre, H., Jacka, F. N., Dodd, S., Dean, O., McEwen, S., & Berk, M. (2016). A review of vulnerability and risks for schizophrenia: Beyond the two hit hypothesis. *Neuroscience and Biobehavioral Reviews, 65,* 185–194. (14)

Davis, J. I., Senghas, A., Brandt, F., & Ochsner, K. N. (2010). The effects of BOTOX injections on emotional experience. *Emotion, 10,* 433–440. (11)

Davis, K. D., Kiss, Z. H. T., Luo, L., Tasker, R. R., Lozano, A. M., & Dostrovsky, J. O. (1998). Phantom sensations generated by thalamic microstimulation. *Nature, 391,* 385–387. (4)

Dawkins, R. (1989). *The selfish gene* (new ed.). Oxford, England: Oxford University Press. (4)

Dawson, T. M., Gonzalez-Zulueta, M., Kusel, J., & Dawson, V. L. (1998). Nitric oxide: Diverse actions in the central and peripheral nervous system. *The Neuroscientist, 4,* 96–112. (2)

Day, S. (2005). Some demographic and sociocultural aspects of synesthesia. In L. C. Robertson & N. Sagiv (Eds.), *Synesthesis* (pp. 11–33). Oxford, England: Oxford University Press. (6)

Dayan, E., Censor, N., Buch, E. R., Sandrini, M., & Cohen, L. G. (2013). Noninvasive brain stimulation: From physiology to network dynamics and back. *Nature Neuroscience, 16,* 838–844. (3)

de Bruin, J. P. C., Swinkels, W. A. M., & de Brabander, J. M. (1997). Response learning of rats in a Morris water maze: Involvement of the medial prefrontal cortex. *Behavioral Brain Research, 85,* 47–55. (12)

de Castro, J. M. (2000). Eating behavior: Lessons from the real world of humans. *Nutrition, 16,* 800–813. (9)

de Jong, M. C., Hendriks, R. J. M., Vansteensel, M. J., Raemaekers, M., Verstraten, F. A. J., Ramsey, N. F., . . . van Ee, R. (2016). Intracranial recordings of occipital cortex responses to illusory visual events. *Journal of Neuroscience, 36,* 6297–6311. (13)

de Jong, W. W., Hendriks, W., Sanyal, S., & Nevo, E. (1990). The eye of the blind mole rat (*Spalax ehrenbergi*): Regressive evolution at the molecular level. In E. Nevo & O. A. Reig (Eds.), *Evolution of subterranean mammals at the organismal and molecular levels* (pp. 383–395). New York: Liss. (8)

De Luca, M., Di Page, E., Judica, A., Spinelli, D., & Zoccolotti, P. (1999). Eye movement patterns in linguistic and non-linguistic tasks in developmental surface dyslexia. *Neuropsychologia, 37,* 1407–1420. (13)

de Maat, S., Dekker, J., Schoevers, R., van Aalst, G., Gijsbers-van Wijk, C., Hendriksen, M., . . . de Jonghe, F. (2008). Short psychodynamic supportive psychotherapy, antidepressants, and their combination in the treatment of major depression: A mega-analysis based on three randomized clinical trials. *Depression and Anxiety, 25,* 565–574. (14)

De Pitta, M., Brunel, N., & Volterra, A. (2016). Astrocytes: Orchestrating synaptic plasticity? *Neuroscience, 323,* 43–61. (1)

De Wall, C. N., Mac Donald, G., Webster, G. D., Masten, C. L., Baumeister, R. F., Powell, C., . . . Eisenberger, N. I. (2010). Acetaminophen reduces social pain: Behavioral and neural evidence. *Psychological Science, 21,* 931–937. (6)

Deacon, T. W. (1990). Problems of ontogeny and phylogeny in brain-size evolution. *International Journal of Primatology, 11,* 237–282. (3)

Deacon, T. W. (1992). Brain-language coevolution. In J. A. Hawkins & M. Gell-Mann (Eds.), *The evolution of human languages* (pp. 49–83). Reading, MA: Addison-Wesley. (13)

Deacon, T. W. (1997). *The symbolic species.* New York: Norton. (3, 13)

Deady, D. K., North, N. T., Allan, D., Smith, M. J. L., & O'Carroll, R. E. (2010). Examining the effect of spinal cord injury on emotional awareness, expressivity and memory for emotional material. *Psychology, Health and Medicine, 15,* 406–419. (11)

DeArmond, S. J., Fusco, M. M., & Dewey, M. M. (1974). *Structure of the human brain.* New York: Oxford University Press. (9)

DeCoursey, P. (1960). Phase control of activity in a rodent. *Cold Spring Harbor Symposia on Quantitative Biology, 25,* 49–55. (8)

Deeb, S. S. (2005). The molecular basis of variation in human color vision. *Clinical Genetics, 67,* 369–377. (5)

Dees, E. W., & Baraas, R. C. (2014). Performance of normal females and carriers of color-vision deficiencies on standard color-vision tests. *Journal of the Optical Society of America A, 31,* A401–A409. (5)

de Groot, J. H. B., Smeets, M. A. M., Kaldewaij, A., Duijndam, M. J. A., & Semin, G. R. (2012). Chemosignals communicate human emotions. *Psychological Science, 23,* 1417–1424. (6)

Dehaene, S. (2014). *Consciousness and the brain.* New York: Viking. (13)

Dehaene-Lambertz, G., Montavont, A., Jobert, A., Allirol, L., Dubois, J., Hertz-Pannier, L., & Dehaene, S. (2010). Language or music, mother or Mozart? Structural and environmental influences on infants' language networks. *Brain & Language, 114,* 53–65. (13)

Dehaene, S., Naccache, L., Cohen, L., LeBihan, D., Mangin, J.-F., Poline, J.-B., & Riviere, D. (2001). Cerebral mechanisms of word masking and unconscious repetition priming. *Nature Neuroscience, 4,* 752–758. (13)

Dehaene, S., Pegado, F., Braga, L. W., Ventura, P., Filho, G. N., Jobert, A., . . . Cohen, L. (2010). How learning to read changes the cortical networks for vision and language. *Science, 330,* 1359–1364. (5, 13)

de Hemptinne, C., Swann, N. C., Ostrem, J. L., Ryapolova-Webb, E. S., San Luciano, M., Galifianakis, N. B., & Starr, P. A. (2015). Therapeutic deep brain stimulation reduces cortical phase-amplitude coupling in Parkinson's disease. *Nature Neuroscience, 18,* 779–786. (7)

Deisseroth, K. (2014). Circuit dynamics of adaptive and maladaptive behaviour. *Nature, 505,* 309–317. (14)

Deisseroth, K. (2015). Optogenetics: 10 years of microbial opsins in neuroscience. *Nature Neuroscience, 18,* 1213–1225. (3)

De Jager, P. L., Srivastava, G., Lunnon, K., Burgess, J., Schalkwyk, L. C., Yu, L., . . . Bennett, D. A. (2014). Alzheimer's disease: Early alterations in brain DNA methylation at *ANK1, BIN1, RHBDF2,* and other loci. *Nature Neuroscience, 17,* 1156–1163. (12)

de la Iglesia, H. O., Fernández-Duque, E., Golombek, D. A., Lanza, N., Duffy, J. F., Czeisler, C. A., & Valeggia, C. R. (2015). Access to electric light is associated with shorter sleep duration in a traditionally hunter-gatherer community. *Journal of Biological Rhythms, 30,* 342–350. (8)

de la Torre-Ubieta, L., Won, H., Stein, J. L., & Geschwind, D. H. (2016). Advancing the understanding of autism disease mechanisms through genetics. *Nature Medicine, 22,* 345–361. (14)

de la Vega, A., Chang, L. J., Banich, M. T., Wager, T. D., & Yarkoni, T. (2016). Large-scale meta-analysis of human medial frontal cortex reveals tripartite functional organization. *Journal of Neuroscience, 36,* 6553–6562. (3)

Del Cul, A., Dehaene, S., Reyes, P., Bravo, E., & Slachevsky, A. (2009). Causal role of prefrontal cortex in the threshold for access to consciousness. *Brain, 132,* 2531–2540. (13)

Delgado, M. R., Beer, J. S., Fellows, L. K., Huettel, S. A., Platt, M. L., Quirk, G. J., & Schiller, D. (2016). Viewpoints: Dialogues on the functional role of the ventromedial prefrontal cortex. *Nature Neuroscience, 19,* 1545–1552. (13)

Deliagina, T. G., Orlovsky, G. N., & Pavlova, G. A. (1983). The capacity for generation of rhythmic oscillations is distributed in the lumbosacral spinal cord of the cat. *Experimental Brain Research, 53,* 81–90. (7)

Dement, W. (1972). *Some must watch while some must sleep.* San Francisco: Freeman. (8)

Dement, W., & Kleitman, N. (1957a). Cyclic variations in EEG during sleep and their relation to eye movements, body motility, and dreaming. *Electroencephalography and Clinical Neurophysiology, 9*, 673–690. (8)

Dement, W., & Kleitman, N. (1957b). The relation of eye movements during sleep to dream activity: An objective method for the study of dreaming. *Journal of Experimental Psychology, 53*, 339–346. (8)

Dement, W. C. (1990). A personal history of sleep disorders medicine. *Journal of Clinical Neurophysiology, 7*, 17–47. (8)

Dennett, D. C. (1991). *Consciousness explained.* Boston, MA: Little, Brown. (0, 13)

Derégnaucourt, S., Mitra, P. P., Fehér, O., Pytte, C., & Tchernichovski, O. (2005). How sleep affects the developmental learning of bird song. *Nature, 433*, 710–716. (8)

DeSimone, J. A., Heck, G. L., & Bartoshuk, L. M. (1980). Surface active taste modifiers: A comparison of the physical and psychophysical properties of gymnemic acid and sodium lauryl sulfate. *Chemical Senses, 5*, 317–330. (6)

DeSimone, J. A., Heck, G. L., Mierson, S., & DeSimone, S. K. (1984). The active ion transport properties of canine lingual epithelia in vitro. *Journal of General Physiology, 83*, 633–656. (6)

Desmurget, M., Reilly, K. T., Richard, N., Szathmari, A., Mottolese, C., & Sirigu, A. (2009). Movement intention after parietal cortex stimulation in humans. *Science, 324*, 811–813. (7)

Detre, J. A., & Floyd, T. F. (2001). Functional MRI and its applications to the clinical neurosciences. *Neuroscientist, 7*, 64–79. (3)

Deutsch, D., Henthorn, T., Marvin, E., & Xu, H. S. (2006). Absolute pitch among American and Chinese conservatory students: Prevalence differences, and evidence for a speech-related critical period. *Journal of the Acoustical Society of America, 119*, 719–722. (6)

Deutsch, J. A., Young, W. G., & Kalogeris, T. J. (1978). The stomach signals satiety. *Science, 201*, 165–167. (9)

DeValois, R. L., Albrecht, D. G., & Thorell, L. G. (1982). Spatial frequency selectivity of cells in macaque visual cortex. *Vision Research, 22*, 545–559. (5)

Devor, M. (1996). Pain mechanisms. *The Neuroscientist, 2*, 233–244. (6)

de Vries, G. J., & Södersten, P. (2009). Sex differences in the brain: The relation between structure and function. *Hormones and Behavior, 55*, 589–596. (10)

De Young, C. G., Hirsch, J. B., Shane, M. S., Papademetris, X., Rajeevan, N., & Gray, J. R. (2010). Testing predictions from personality neuroscience: Brain structure and the big five. *Psychological Science, 21*, 820–828. (3)

Dhingra, R., Sullivan, L., Jacques, P. F., Wang, T. J., Fox, C. S., Meigs, J. B., . . . Vasan, R. S. (2007). Soft drink consumption and risk of developing cardiometabolic risk factors and the metabolic syndrome in middle-aged adults in the community. *Circulation, 116*, 480–488. (9)

Di Lorenzo, P. M., Chen, J.-Y., & Victor, J. D. (2009). Quality time: Representation of a multidimensional sensory domain through temporal coding. *Journal of Neuroscience, 29*, 9227–9238. (6)

Di Lorenzo, P. M., Leshchinskiy, S., Moroney, D. N., & Ozdoba, J. M. (2009). Making time count: Functional evidence for temporal coding of taste sensation. *Behavioral Neuroscience, 123*, 14–25. (1)

Diamond, L. M. (2007). A dynamical systems approach to the development and expression of female same-sex sexuality. *Perspectives on Psychological Science, 2*, 142–161. (10)

Diamond, M., & Sigmundson, H. K. (1997). Management of intersexuality: Guidelines for dealing with persons with ambiguous genitalia. *Archives of Pediatrics and Adolescent Medicine, 151*, 1046–1050. (10)

Dias, B. G., & Ressler, K. J. (2014). Parental olfactory experience influences behavior and neural structure in subsequent generations. *Nature Neuroscience, 17*, 89–96. (4)

Dibb-Hajj, S. D., Black, J. A., & Waxman, S. G. (2015). $Na_v1.9$: A sodium channel linked to human pain. *Nature Reviews Neuroscience, 16*, 511–519. (6)

Dichgans, J. (1984). Clinical symptoms of cerebellar dysfunction and their topodiagnostic significance. *Human Neurobiology, 2*, 269–279. (7)

Dick, D. M., Agrawal, A., Keller, M. C., Adkins, A., Aliev, F., Monroe, S., . . . Sher, K. J. (2015). Candidate gene-environment interaction research: Reflections and recommendations. *Perspectives on Psychological Science, 10*, 37–59. (4)

Dick, D. M., Johnson, J. K., Viken, R. J., & Rose, R. J. (2000). Testing between-family associations in within-family comparisons. *Psychological Science, 11*, 409–413. (14)

Dick, D. M., Latendresse, S. J., Lansford, J. E., Budde, J. P., Goate, A., Dodge, K. A., . . . Bates, J. E. (2009). Role of *GABRA2* in trajectories of externalizing behavior across development and evidence of moderation by parental monitoring. *Archives of General Psychiatry, 66*, 649–657. (14)

Dick, F., Bates, E., Wulfeck, B., Utman, J. A., Dronkers, N., & Gernsbacher, M. A. (2001). Language deficits, localization, and grammar: Evidence for a distributive model of language breakdown in aphasic patients and neurologically intact individuals. *Psychological Review, 108*, 759–788. (13)

Dicke, U., & Roth, G. (2016). Neuronal factors determining high intelligence. *Philosophical Transactions of the Royal Society B, 371*, 20150180. (12)

Diéguez, C., Vazquez, M. J., Romero, A., López, M., & Nogueiras, R. (2011). Hypothalamic control of lipid metabolism: Focus on leptin, ghrelin and melanocortins. *Neuroendocrinology, 94*, 1–11. (9)

Dierks, T., Linden, D. E. J., Jandl, M., Formisano, E., Goebel, R., & Lanfermann, H. (1999). Activation of Heschl's gyrus during auditory hallucinations. *Neuron, 22*, 615–621. (3)

Dijk, D.-J., & Archer, S. N. (2010). *PERIOD3*, circadian phenotypes, and sleep homeostasis. *Sleep Medicine Reviews, 14*, 151–160. (8)

Dijk, D.-J., Neri, D. F., Wyatt, J. K., Ronda, J. M., Riel, E., Ritz-deCecco, A., . . . Czeisler, C. A. (2001). Sleep, performance, circadian rhythms, and light-dark cycles during two space shuttle flights. *American Journal of Physiology: Regulatory, Integrative, and Comparative Physiology, 281*, R1647–R1664. (8)

Diller, L., Packer, O. S., Verweij, J., McMahon, M. J., Williams, D. R., & Dacey, D. M. (2004). L and M cone contributions to the midget and parasol ganglion cell receptive fields of macaque monkey retina. *Journal of Neuroscience, 24*, 1079–1088. (5)

Dimitriou, M. (2014). Human spindle sensitivity reflects the balance of activity between antagonistic muscles. *Journal of Neuroscience, 34*, 13644–13655. (1)

Dimond, S. J. (1979). Symmetry and asymmetry in the vertebrate brain. In D. A. Oakley & H. C. Plotkin (Eds.), *Brain, behaviour, and evolution* (pp. 189–218). London: Methuen. (13)

Di Napoli, M., Zha, A. M., Godoy, D. A., Masotti, L., Schreuder, F. H. B. M., Popa-Wagner, A., & Behrouz, R. (2016). Prior cannabis use is associated with outcome after intracerebral hemorrhage. *Cerebrovascular Diseases, 41*, 248–255. (4)

Ding, F., O'Donnell, J., Xu, Q., Kang, N., Goldman, N., & Nedergaard, M. (2016). Changes in the composition of brain interstitial ions control the sleep-wake cycle. *Science, 352*, 550–555. (8)

Dinstein, I., Hasson, U., Rubin, N., & Heeger, D. J. (2007). Brain areas selective for both observed and executed movements. *Journal of Neurophysiology, 98*, 1415–1427. (7)

Dinstein, I., Thomas, C., Humphreys, K., Minshew, N., Behrmann, M., & Heeger, D. J. (2010). Normal movement selectivity in autism. *Neuron, 66*, 461–469. (7)

Di Paola, M., Caltagirone, C., & Petrosini, L. (2013). Prolonged rock climbing activity induces structural changes in cerebellum and parietal lobe. *Human Brain Mapping, 34*, 2707–2714. (7)

Disner, S. G., Beevers, C. G., Lee, H.-J., Ferrell, R. E., Hariri, A. R., & Telch, M. J. (2013). War zone stress interacts with the 5-HTTLPR polymorphism to predict the development of sustained attention for negative emotion stimuli in soldiers returning from Iraq. *Clinical Psychological Science, 1*, 413–425. (11)

Doesburg, S. M., Green, J. J., McDonald, J. J., & Ward, L. M. (2009). Rhythms of consciousness: Binocular rivalry reveals large-scale oscillatory network dynamics mediating visual perception. *PLoS One, 4*, e6142. (13)

Doremus-Fitzwater, T. L., Barretto, M., & Spear, L. P. (2012). Age-related differences in impulsivity among adolescent and adult Sprague-Dawley rats. *Behavioral Neuroscience, 126*, 735–741. (4)

Doricchi, F., Guariglia, P., Gasparini, M., & Tomaiuolo, F. (2005). Dissociation between physical and mental number line bisection in right hemisphere brain damage. *Nature Neuroscience, 8*, 1663–1665. (13)

Dormal, G., Lepore, F., & Collignon, O. (2012). Plasticity of the dorsal "spatial" stream in visually deprived individuals. *Neural Plasticity*, Article 687659. (5)

Doty, R. L., Applebaum, S., Zusho, H., & Settle, R. G. (1985). Sex differences in odor identification ability: A cross-cultural analysis. *Neuropsychologia, 23*, 667–672. (6)

Doty, R. L., & Kamath, V. (2014). The influences of age on olfaction: A review. *Frontiers in Psychology, 5*, PMC 3916729. (6)

Douaud, G., Groves, A. R., Tamnes, C. K., Westlye, L. T., Duff, E. P., Engvig, A., . . . Johansen-Berg, H. (2014). A common brain network links development, aging, and vulnerability to disease. *Proceedings of the National Academy of Sciences (U.S.A.), 111*, 17648–17653. (4)

Dowling, J. E. (1987). *The retina.* Cambridge, MA: Harvard University Press. (5)

Dowling, J. E., & Boycott, B. B. (1966). Organization of the primate retina. *Proceedings of the Royal Society of London, B, 166*, 80–111. (5)

Downing, P. E., Chan, A. W.-Y., Peelen, M. V., Dodds, C. M., & Kanwisher, N. (2005). Domain specificity in visual cortex. *Cerebral Cortex, 16*, 1453–1461. (5)

Draganski, B., Gaser, C., Busch, V., Schuierer, G., Bogdahn, U., & May, A. (2004). Changes in grey matter induced by training. *Nature, 427*, 311–312. (4)

Dreger, A. D. (1998). *Hermaphrodites and the medical invention of sex.* Cambridge, MA: Harvard University Press. (10)

Dreher, J. C., Dunne, S., Pazderska, A., Frodl, T., Nolan, J. J., & O'Doherty, J. P. (2016). Testosterone causes both prosocial and antisocial status-enhancing behaviors in human males. *Proceedings of the National Academy of Sciences (U.S.A.), 113*, 11633–11638. (11)

Dresler, M., Koch, S. P., Wehrle, R., Spoormaker, V. I., Hosboer, F., Steiger, A., . . . Czisch, M. (2011). Dreamed movement elicits activation in the sensorimotor cortex. *Current Biology, 21*, 1833–1837. (8)

Dronkers, N. F., Plaisant, O., Iba-Zizen, M. T., & Cabanis, E. A. (2007). Paul Broca's historic cases: high resolution MR imaging of the brains of Leborgne and Lelong. *Brain, 130*, 1432–1441. (13)

Drzyzga, L. R., Marcinowska, A., & Obuchowicz, E. (2009). Antiapoptotic and neurotrophic effects of antidepressants: A review of clinical and experimental studies. *Brain Research Bulletin, 79*, 248–257. (14)

Duan, X., Chang, J. H., Ge, S., Faulkner, R. L., Kim, J. Y., Kitabatake, Y., . . . Song, H. (2007). Disrupted-in-schizophrenia 1 regulated integration of newly generated neurons in the adult brain. *Cell, 130*, 1146–1158. (14)

Duboué, E. R., & Keene, A. C. (2016). Chapter 15–Investigating the evolution of sleep in the Mexican cavefish. In A. C. Keene, M. Yoshizawa, & S. E. McGaugh (Eds.), *Biology and Evolution of the Mexican cavefish* (pp. 291–308). Amsterdam: Elsevier. (8)

Deboué, E. R., Keene, A. C., & Borowsky, R. L. (2011). Evolutionary convergence on sleep loss in cavefish populations. *Current Biology, 21*, 671–676. (8)

Ducommun, C. Y., Michel, C. M., Clarke, S., Adriani, M., Seeck, M., Landis, T., & Blanke, O. (2004). Cortical motion deafness. *Neuron, 43*, 765–777. (6)

Duff, M. C., Hengst, J., Tranel, D., & Cohen, N. J. (2006). Development of shared information in communication despite hippocampal amnesia. *Nature Neuroscience, 9*, 140–146. (12)

Duke, A. A., Bègue, L., Bell, R., & Eisenlohr-Moul, T. (2013). Revisiting the serotonin-aggression relation in humans: A meta-analysis. *Psychological Bulletin, 139*, 1148–1172. (11)

Duman, R. S., & Aghajanian, G. K. (2012). Synaptic dysfunction in depression: Potential therapeutic targets. *Science, 338*, 68–72. (14)

Dunn, B. D., Galton, H. C., Morgan, R., Evans, D., Olliver, C., Meyer, M., . . . Dalgeish, T. (2010). Listening to your heart: How interoception shapes emotion experience and intuitive decision making. *Psychological Science, 21*, 1835–1844. (11)

Dunsmoor, J. E., Murty, V. P., Davachi, L., & Phelps, E. A. (2015). Emotional learning selectively and retroactively strengthens memories for related events. *Nature, 520*, 345–348. (12)

Durante, K. M., & Li, N. P. (2009). Oestradiol level and opportunistic mating in women. *Biology Letters, 5*, 179–182. (10)

Durso, G. R. O., Luttrell, A., & Way, B. M. (2015). Over-the-counter relief from pains and pleasures alike: Acetaminophen blunts evaluation sensitivity to both negative and positive stimuli. *Psychological Science, 26*, 750–758. (6)

Duvarci, S., Bauer, E. P., & Paré, D. (2009). The bed nucleus of the stria terminalis mediates inter-individual variations in anxiety and fear. *Journal of Neuroscience, 29*, 10357–10361. (11)

Dyal, J. A. (1971). Transfer of behavioral bias: Reality and specificity. In E. J. Fjerdingstad (Ed.), *Chemical transfer of learned information* (pp. 219–263). New York: American Elsevier. (12)

Earnest, D. J., Liang, F.-Q., Ratcliff, M., & Cassone, V. M. (1999). Immortal time: Circadian clock properties of rat suprachiasmatic cell lines. *Science, 283*, 693–695. (8)

Eastman, C. I., Hoese, E. K., Youngstedt, S. D., & Liu, L. (1995). Phase-shifting human circadian rhythms with exercise during the night shift. *Physiology & Behavior, 58*, 1287–1291. (8)

Eaves, L. J., Martin, N. G., & Heath, A. C. (1990). Religious affiliation in twins and their parents: Testing a model of cultural inheritance. *Behavior Genetics, 20*, 1–22. (4)

Eccles, J. C. (1964). *The physiology of synapses.* Berlin: Springer-Verlag. (2)

Eckhorn, R., Bauer, R., Jordan, W., Brosch, M., Kruse, W., Munk, M., & Reitboeck, H. J. (1988). Coherent oscillations: A mechanism of feature linking in the visual cortex? *Biological Cybernetics, 60*, 121–130. (13)

Eckstrand, K. L., Ding, Z. H., Dodge, N. C., Cowan, R. L., Jacobson, J. L., Jacobson, S. W., & Avison, M. J. (2012). Persistent dose-dependent changes in brain structure in young adults with low-to-moderate alcohol exposure *in utero. Alcoholism—Clinical & Experimental Research, 36*, 1892–1902. (4)

Edelman, G. M. (1987). *Neural Darwinism.* New York: Basic Books. (4)

Edelstein, R. S., Wardecker, B. M., Chopik, W. J., Moors, A. C., Shipman, E. L., & Lin, N. J. (2015). Prenatal hormones in first-time expectant parents: Longitudinal changes and within-couple correlations. *American Journal of Human Biology, 27*, 317–325. (10)

Eden, A. S., Schreiber, J., Anwander, A., Keuper, K., Laeger, I., Zwanzger, P., . . . Dobel, C. (2015). Emotion regulation and trait anxiety are predicted by the microstructure of fibers between amygdala and prefrontal cortex. *Journal of Neuroscience, 35*, 6020–6027. (11)

Edman, G., Åsberg, M., Levander, S., & Schalling, D. (1986). Skin conductance habituation and cerebrospinal fluid 5-hydroxy-indoleacic acid in suicidal patients. *Archives of General Psychiatry, 43*, 586–592. (11)

Ehrhardt, A. A., & Money, J. (1967). Progestin-induced hermaphroditism: IQ and psychosexual identity in a study of ten girls. *Journal of Sex Research, 3*, 83–100. (10)

Ehrlich, P. R., Dobkin, D. S., & Wheye, D. (1988). *The birder's handbook.* New York: Simon & Schuster. (9)

Eichenbaum, H. (2000). A cortical-hippocampal system for declarative memory. *Nature Reviews Neuroscience, 1*, 41–50. (12)

Eichenbaum, H. (2002). *The cognitive neuroscience of memory.* New York: Oxford University Press. (12)

Eichenbaum, H. (2016). Still searching for the engram. *Learning & Behavior, 44*, 209–222. (12)

Eidelberg, E., & Stein, D. G. (1974). Functional recovery after lesions of the nervous system. *Neurosciences Research Program Bulletin, 12*, 191–303. (4)

Eippert, F., Finsterbusch, J., Binget, U., & Büchel, C. (2009). Direct evidence for spinal cord involvement in placebo analgesia. *Science, 326*, 404. (6)

Eisenberger, N. I., Lieberman, M. D., & Williams, K. D. (2003). Does rejection hurt?

An fMRI study of social exclusion. *Science, 302,* 290–292. (6)

Eisenbruch, A. B., Simmons, Z. L., & Roney, J. R. (2015). Lady in red: Hormonal predictors of women's clothing choices. *Psychological Science, 26,* 1332–1338. (10)

Eisenstein, E. M., & Cohen, M. J. (1965). Learning in an isolated prothoracic insect ganglion. *Animal Behaviour, 13,* 104–108. (12)

Ejaz, N., Hamada, M., & Diedrichsen, J. (2015). Hand use predicts the structure of representations in sensorimotor cortex. *Nature Neuroscience, 18,* 1034–1040. (3)

Ek, M., Engblom, D., Saha, S., Blomqvist, A., Jakobsson, P.-J., & Ericsson-Dahlstrand, A. (2001). Pathway across the blood–brain barrier. *Nature, 410,* 430–431. (9)

Ekman, P., & Friesen, W. V. (1984). *Unmasking the face* (2nd ed.). Palo Alto, CA: Consulting Psychologists Press. (11)

Elbert, T., Candia, V., Altenmüller, E., Rau, H., Sterr, A., Rockstroh, B., . . . Taub, E. (1998). Alteration of digital representations in somatosensory cortex in focal hand dystonia. *Neuroreport, 9,* 3571–3575. (4)

Elbert, T., Pantev, C., Wienbruch, C., Rockstroh, B., & Taub, E. (1995). Increased cortical representation of the fingers of the left hand in string players. *Science, 270,* 305–307. (4)

Eldar, E., Cohen, J. D., & Niv, Y. (2013). The effects of neural gain on attention and learning. *Nature Neuroscience, 16,* 1146–1153. (8)

Eldridge, L. L., Engel, S. A., Zeineh, M. M., Bookheimer, S. Y., & Knowlton, B. J. (2005). A dissociation of encoding and retrieval processes in the human hippocampus. *Journal of Neuroscience, 25,* 3280–3286. (12)

Elias, C. F., Lee, C., Kelly, J., Aschkenazi, C., Ahima, R. S., Couceyro, P. R., . . . Elmquist, J. K. (1998). Leptin activates hypothalamic CART neurons projecting to the spinal cord. *Neuron, 21,* 1375–1385. (9)

Ellacott, K. L. J., & Cone, R. D. (2004). The central melanocortin system and the integration of short- and long-term regulators of energy homeostasis. *Recent Progress in Hormone Research, 59,* 395–408. (9)

Ellemberg, D., Lewis, T. L., Maurer, D., Brar, S., & Brent, H. P. (2002). Better perception of global motion after monocular than after binocular deprivation. *Vision Research, 42,* 169–179. (5)

Elliott, T. R. (1905). The action of adrenalin. *Journal of Physiology (London), 32,* 401–467. (2)

Ellis, L., & Ames, M. A. (1987). Neurohormonal functioning and sexual orientation: A theory of homosexuality–heterosexuality. *Psychological Bulletin, 101,* 233–258. (10)

Ellis, L., Ames, M. A., Peckham, W., & Burke, D. (1988). Sexual orientation of human offspring may be altered by severe maternal stress during pregnancy. *Journal of Sex Research, 25,* 152–157. (10)

Ellis, L., & Cole-Harding, S. (2001). The effects of prenatal stress, and of prenatal alcohol and nicotine exposure, on human sexual orientation. *Physiology & Behavior, 74,* 213–226. (10)

Ells, L. J., Hillier, F. C., Shucksmith, J., Crawley, H., Harbige, L., Shield, J., . . . Summerbell, C. D. (2008). A systematic review of the effect of dietary exposure that could be achieved through normal dietary intake on learning and performance of school-aged children of relevance to UK schools. *British Journal of Nutrition, 100,* 927–936. (9)

Elgoyhen, A. B., Langguth, B., De Ridder, D., & Vanneste, S. (2015). Tinnitus: Perspectives from human neuroimaging. *Nature Reviews Neuroscience, 16,* 632–642. (6)

Elsabbagh, M., Divan, G., Koh, Y. J., Kim, Y. S., Kauchali, S., Marcin, C., . . . Fombonne, E. (2012). Global prevalence of autism and other pervasive developmental disorders. *Autism Research, 5,* 160–179. (14)

Eng, M. Y., Schuckit, M. A., & Smith, T. L. (2005). The level of response to alcohol in daughters of alcoholics and controls. *Drug and Alcohol Dependence, 79,* 83–93. (14)

Engel, T. A., Steinmetz, N. A., Gieselmann, M. A., Thiele, A., Moore, T., & Boahen, K. (2016). Selective modulation of cortical state during spatial attention. *Science, 354,* 1140–1144. (13)

Epp, J. R., Mera, R. S., Kohler, S., Josselyn, S. A., & Frankland, P. W. (2016). Neurogenesis-mediated forgetting minimizes proactive interference. *Nature Communications, 7,* article 10838. (12)

Epping-Jordan, M. P., Watkins, S. S., Koob, G. F., & Markou, A. (1998). Dramatic decreases in brain reward function during nicotine withdrawal. *Nature, 393,* 76–79. (14)

Erickson, C., & Lehrman, D. (1964). Effect of castration of male ring doves upon ovarian activity of females. *Journal of Comparative and Physiological Psychology, 58,* 164–166. (10)

Erickson, K. I., Prakash, R. S., Voss, M. W., Chaddock, L., Heo, S., McLaren, M., . . . Kramer, A. F. (2010). Brain-derived neurotrophic factor is associated with age-related decline in hippocampal volume. *Journal of Neuroscience, 30,* 5368–5375. (4)

Erlich, J. C., Brunton, B. W., Duan, C. A., Hanks, T. D., & Brody, C. D. (2015). Distinct effects of prefrontal and parietal cortex inactivations on an accumulation of evidence task in the rat. *eLife, 4,* e05457. (13)

Ernst, A., Alkass, K., Bernard, S., Salehpour, M., Perl, S., Tisdale, J., . . . Frisén, J. (2014). Neurogenesis in the striatum of the adult human brain. *Cell, 156,* 1072–1083. (4)

Ersche, K. D., Gillan, C. M., Jones, P. S., Williams, G. B., Ward, L. H. E., Luijten, M., . . . Robbins, T. W. (2016). Carrots and sticks fail to change behavior in cocaine addiction. *Science, 352,* 1468–1471. (14)

Ersche, K. D., Jones, P. S., Williams, G. B., Turton, A. J., Robbins, T. W., & Bullmore, E. T. (2012). Abnormal brain structure implicated in stimulant drug addiction. *Science, 335,* 601–604. (14)

Eschenko, O., Mölle, M., Born, J., & Sara, S. J. (2006). Elevated sleep spindle density after learning or after retrieval in rats. *Journal of Neurophysiology, 26,* 12914–12920. (8)

Esser, S. K., Hill, S., & Tononi, G. (2009). Breakdown of effective connectivity during slow wave sleep: Investigating the mechanism underlying a cortical gate using large-scale modeling. *Journal of Neurophysiology, 102,* 2096–2111. (8)

Estes, M. L., & McAllister, A. K. (2016). Maternal immune activation: Implications for neuropsychiatric disorders. *Science, 353,* 772–777. (14)

Etcoff, N. L., Ekman, P., Magee, J. J., & Frank, M. G. (2000). Lie detection and language comprehension. *Nature, 405,* 139. (13)

Etgen, A. M., Chu, H.-P., Fiber, J. M., Karkanias, G. B., & Morales, J. M. (1999). Hormonal integration of neurochemical and sensory signals governing female reproductive behavior. *Behavioural Brain Research, 105,* 93–103. (10)

Euston, D. R., Tatsuno, M., & McNaughton, B. L. (2007). Fast-forward playback of recent memory sequences in prefrontal cortex during sleep. *Science, 318,* 1147–1150. (8)

Evans, D. A., Funkenstein, H. H., Albert, M. S., Scherr, P. A., Cook, N. R., Chown, M. J., . . . Taylor, J. O. (1989). Prevalence of Alzheimer's disease in a community population of older persons. *Journal of the American Medical Association, 262,* 2551–2556. (12)

Evarts, E. V. (1979). Brain mechanisms of movement. *Scientific American, 241*(3), 164–179. (7)

Facoetti, A., Corradi, N., Ruffino, M., Gori, S., & Zorzi, M. (2010). Visual spatial attention and speech segmentation are both impaired in preschoolers at familial risk for developmental dyslexia. *Dyslexia, 16,* 22–239. (13)

Falk, D., Lepore, F. E., & Noe, A. (2013). The cerebral cortex of Albert Einstein: A description and preliminary analysis of unpublished photographs. *Brain, 136,* 1304–1327. (3)

Falkner, A. L., Grosenick, L., Davidson, T. J., Deisseroth, K., & Lin, D. (2016). Hypothalamic control of male aggression-seeking behavior. *Nature Neuroscience, 19,* 596–604. (11)

Falleti, M. G., Maruff, P., Collie, A., Darby, D. G., & McStephen, M. (2003). Qualitative similarities in cognitive impairment associated with 24 h of sustained wakefulness and a blood alcohol concentration of 0.05%. *Journal of Sleep Research, 12,* 265–274. (8)

Fan, W., Ellacott, K. L. J., Halatchev, I. G., Takahashi, K., Yu, P., & Cone, R. D. (2004). Cholecystokinin-mediated suppression of feeding involves the brainstem melanocortin system. *Nature Neuroscience, 7,* 335–336. (9)

Fantz, R. L. (1963). Pattern vision in newborn infants. *Science, 140,* 296–297. (5)

Farah, M. J., Wilson, K. D., Drain, M., & Tanaka, J. N. (1998). What is "special" about face perception? *Psychological Review, 105,* 482–498. (5)

Farber, N. B., Newcomer, J. W., & Olney, J. W. (1999). Glycine agonists: What can they teach us about schizophrenia? *Archives of General Psychiatry, 56,* 13–17. (14)

Farber, S. L. (1981). *Identical twins reared apart: A reanalysis.* New York: Basic Books. (12)

Farivar, R. (2009). Dorsal-ventral integration in object recognition. *Brain Research Reviews, 61,* 144–153. (5)

Farmer, M. E., & Klein, R. M. (1995). The evidence for a temporal processing deficit linked to dyslexia: A review. *Psychonomic Bulletin & Review, 2,* 460–493. (13)

Fatemi, S. H., Aldinger, K. A., Ashwood, P., Bauman, M. L., Blaha, C. D., Blatt, G. J., . . . Welsh, J. P. (2012). Consensus paper: Pathological role of the cerebellum in autism. *Cerebellum, 11,* 777–807. (14)

Fatemi, S. H., & Folsom, T. D. (2009). The neurodevelopmental hypothesis of schizophrenia, revisited. *Schizophrenia Bulletin, 35,* 528–548. (14)

Fedrigo, O., Pfefferle, A. D., Babbitt, C. C., Haygood, R., Wall, C. E., & Wray, G. A. (2011). A potential role for glucose transporters in the evolution of human brain size. *Brain, Behavior and Evolution, 78,* 315–326. (4)

Feeney, D. M., & Sutton, R. L. (1988). Catecholamines and recovery of function after brain damage. In D. G. Stein & B. A. Sabel (Eds.), *Pharmacological approaches to the treatment of brain and spinal cord injury* (pp. 121–142). New York: Plenum Press. (4)

Feeney, D. M., Sutton, R. L., Boyeson, M. G., Hovda, D. A., & Dail, W. G. (1985). The locus coeruleus and cerebral metabolism: Recovery of function after cerebral injury. *Physiological Psychology, 13,* 197–203. (4)

Feinstein, J. S., Adolphs, R., Damasio, A., & Tranel, D. (2011). The human amygdala and the induction and experience of fear. *Current Biology, 21,* 34–38. (11)

Feinstein, J. S., Buzza, C., Hurlemann, R., Follmer, R. L., Dahdaleh, N. S., Coryell, W. H., . . . Wemmie, J. A. (2013). Fear and panic in humans with bilateral amygdala damage. *Nature Neuroscience, 16,* 270–272. (11)

Fell, J., & Axmacher, N. (2011). The role of phase synchronization in memory processes. *Nature Reviews Neuroscience, 12,* 105–118. (13)

Feller, G. (2010). Protein stability and enzyme activity at extreme biological temperatures. *Journal of Physics—Condensed Matter, 22,* article 323101. (9)

Feltmann, K., Konradsson-Geuken, Å., De Bundel, D., Lindskog, M., & Schilström, B. (2015). Antidepressant drugs specifically inhibiting norepinephrine reuptake enhance recognition memory in rats. *Behavioral Neuroscience, 129,* 701–708. (14)

Fendrich, R., Wessinger, C. M., & Gazzaniga, M. S. (1992). Residual vision in a scotoma: Implications for blindsight. *Science, 258,* 1489–1491. (5)

Feng, J., Fouse, S., & Fan, G. (2007). Epigenetic regulation of neural gene expression and neuronal function. *Pediatric Research, 61 (5), Part 2,* 58R–63R. (4)

Feng, J., Spence, I., & Pratt, J. (2007). Playing an action video game reduces gender differences in spatial cognition. *Psychological Science, 18,* 850–855. (10)

Fenselau, H., Campbell, J. N., Verstegen, A. M. J., Madara, J. C., Xu, J., Shah, B. P., . . . Lowell, B. B. (2017). A rapidly acting glutamatergic ARC → PVH satiety circuit postsynaptically regulated by alpha-MSH. *Nature Neuroscience, 20,* 42–51. (9)

Fentress, J. C. (1973). Development of grooming in mice with amputated forelimbs. *Science, 179,* 704–705. (7)

Ferando, I., Faas, G. C., & Mody. I. (2016). Diminished KCC2 confounds synapse specificity of LTP during senescence. *Nature Neuroscience, 19,* 1197–1200. (12)

Ferbinteanu, J. (2016). Contributions of hippocampus and striatum to memory-guided behavior depend on past experience. *Journal of Neuroscience, 36,* 6459–6470. (12)

Fergusson, D. M., Boden, J. M., Horwood, L. J., Miller, A., & Kennedy, M. A. (2012). Moderating role of the *MAOA* genotype in antisocial behavior. *British Journal of Psychiatry, 200,* 116–123. (11)

Fernández-Ruiz, J., Moro, M. A., & Martiínez-Orgado, J. (2015). Cannabinoids in neurodegenerative disorders and stroke/brain trauma: From preclinical models to clinical applications. *Neurotherapeutics, 12,* 793–806. (4)

Ferreira, F., Bailey, K. G. D., & Ferraro, V. (2002). Good-enough representations in language comprehension. *Current Directions in Psychological Science, 11,* 11–15. (13)

Field, L. L., Shumansky, K., Ryan, J., Truong, D, Swiergala, E., & Kaplan, B. J. (2013). Dense-map genome scan for dyslexia supports loci at 4q13, 16p12, 17q22; suggests novel locus at 7q36. *Genes, Brain and Behavior, 12,* 56–69. (13)

Fields, R. D. (2015). A new mechanism of nervous system plasticity: Activity-dependent myelination. *Nature Reviews Neuroscience, 16,* 756–766. (4)

Filosa, J. A., Bonev, A. D., Straub, S. V., Meredith, A. L., Wilkerson, M. K., Aldrich, R. W., & Nelson, M. T. (2006). Local potassium signaling couples neuronal activity to vasodilation in the brain. *Nature Neuroscience, 9,* 1397–1403. (1)

Fine, I. Wade, A. R., Brewer, A. A., May, M. G., Goodman, D. F., Boynton, G. M., . . . McLeod, D. I. A. (2003). Long-term deprivation affects visual perception and cortex. *Nature Neuroscience, 6,* 915–916. (5)

Finger, S., & Roe, D. (1996). Gustave Dax and the early history of cerebral dominance. *Archives of Neurology, 53,* 806–813. (13)

Fink, B., Hugill, N., & Lange, B. P. (2012). Women's body movements are a potential cue to ovulation. *Personality and Individual Differences, 53,* 759–763. (10)

Finn, E. S., Shen, X., Scheinost, D., Rosenberg, M. D., Huang, J., Chun, M. M., . . . Constable, R. T. (2015). Functional connectome fingerprinting: identifying individuals using patterns of brain connectivity. *Nature Neuroscience, 18,* 1664–1671. (3)

Fisch, L., Privman, E., Ramot, M., Harel, M., Nir, Y., Kipervasser, S., . . . Malach, R. (2009). Neural "ignition": Enhanced activation linked to perceptual awareness in human ventral stream visual cortex. *Neuron, 64,* 562–574. (13)

Fisher, S. E., Vargha-Khadem, F., Watkins, K. E., Monaco, A. P., & Pembrey, M. E. (1998). Localisation of a gene implicated in a severe speech and language disorder. *Nature Genetics, 18,* 168–170. (13)

Fitts, D. A., Starbuck, E. M., & Ruhf, A. (2000). Circumventricular organs and ANGII-induced salt appetite: Blood pressure and connectivity. *American Journal of Physiology, 279,* R2277–R2286. (9)

Fjell, A. M., Walhovd, K. B., Fennema-Notestine, C., McEvoy, L. K., Hagler, D. J., Holland, D., . . . Dale, A. M. (2009). One-year brain atrophy evident in healthy aging. *Journal of Neuroscience, 29,* 15223–15231. (4)

Fjell, A. M., Westlye, L. T., Amlien, I., Tamnes, C. K., Grydeland, H., Engvig, A., . . . Walhovd, K. B. (2015). High-expanding cortical regions in human development and evolution are related to higher intellectual abilities. *Cerebral Cortex, 25,* 26–34. (12)

Fjerdingstad, E. J. (1973). Transfer of learning in rodents and fish. In W. B. Essman & S. Nakajima (Eds.), *Current biochemical approaches to learning and memory* (pp. 73–98). Flushing, NY: Spectrum. (12)

Flatz, G. (1987). Genetics of lactose digestion in humans. *Advances in Human Genetics, 16,* 1–77. (9)

Fleet, W. S., & Heilman, K. M. (1986). The fatigue effect in hemispatial neglect. *Neurology, 36*(Suppl. 1), 258. (4)

Fletcher, M. A., Low, K. A., Boyd, R., Zimmerman, B., Gordon, B. A., Tan, C. H., . . . Fabiani, M. (2016). Comparing aging and fitness effects on brain anatomy. *Frontiers in Human Neuroscience, 10,* Article 286. (4)

Fletcher, G. J. O., Simpson, J. A., Campbell, L., & Overall, N. C. (2015). Pair-bonding, romantic love, and evolution: The curious case of *Homo sapiens. Perspectives on Psychological Science, 10,* 20–36. (12)

Fletcher, P. C., McKenna, P. J., Frith, C. D., Grasby, P. M., Friston, K. J., & Dolan, R. J. (1998). Brain activations in schizophrenia during a graded memory task studied with functional neuroimaging. *Archives of General Psychiatry, 55,* 1001–1008. (14)

Fletcher, R., & Voke, J. (1985). *Defective colour vision.* Bristol, England: Hilger. (5)

Flinker, A., Korzeniewska, A., Shestyuk, A. Y., Franaszcuk, P. J., Dronkers, N. F., Knight, R. T., & Crone, N. E. (2015). Redefining the role of Broca's area in speech. *Proceedings of the National Academy of Sciences (U.S.A.), 112,* 2871–2875. (13)

Flor, H., Elbert, T., Knecht, S., Wienbruch, C., Pantev, C., Birbaumer, N., . . . Taub, E. (1995). Phantom-limb pain as a perceptual correlate of cortical reorganization following arm amputation. *Nature, 375,* 482–484. (4)

Florence, S. L., & Kaas, J. H. (1995). Large-scale reorganization at multiple levels of the somatosensory pathway follows therapeutic amputation of the hand in monkeys. *Journal of Neuroscience, 15,* 8083–8095. (4)

Flowers, K. A., & Hudson, J. M. (2013). Motor laterality as an indicator of speech laterality. *Neuropsychology, 27,* 256–265. (13)

Flynn, J. M., & Boder, E. (1991). Clinical and electrophysiological correlates of dysphonetic and dyseidetic dyslexia. In J. F. Stein (Ed.), *Vision and visual dyslexia* (pp. 121–131). Vol. 13 of J. R. Cronly-Dillon (Ed.), *Vision and visual dysfunction.* Boca Raton, FL: CRC Press. (13)

Foerde, K., Knowlton, B. J., & Poldrack, R. A. (2006). Modulation of competing memory systems by distraction. *Proceedings of the National Academy of Sciences, USA, 103,* 11778–11783. (12)

Foerde, K., Race, E., Verfaellie, M., & Shohamy, D. (2013). A role for the medial temporal lobe in feedback-driven learning: Evidence from amnesia. *Journal of Neuroscience, 33,* 5698–5704. (12)

Foerde, K., & Shohamy, D. (2011). Feedback timing modulates brain systems for learning in humans. *Journal of Neuroscience, 31,* 13157–13167. (12)

Foerde, K., Steinglass, J. E., Shohamy, D., & Walsh, B. T. (2015). Neural mechanisms supporting maladaptive food choices in anorexia nervosa. *Nature Neuroscience, 18,* 1571–1573. (9)

Fogel, S. M., Nader, R., Cote, K. A., & Smith, C. T. (2007). Sleep spindles and learning potential. *Behavioral Neuroscience, 121,* 1–10. (8)

Foltz, E. I., & White, L. E. Jr. (1962). Pain "relief" by frontal cingulumotomy. *Journal of Neurosurgery, 19,* 89–100. (6)

Foo, H., & Mason, P. (2009). Analgesia accompanying food consumption requires ingestion of hedonic foods. *Journal of Neuroscience, 29,* 13053–13062. (6)

Forger, N. G., & Breedlove, S. M. (1987). Motoneuronal death during human fetal development. *Journal of Comparative Neurology, 234,* 118–122. (4)

Foroni, F., & Semin, G. R. (2009). Language that puts you in touch with your bodily feelings. *Psychological Science, 20,* 974–980. (7)

Forster, B., & Corballis, M. C. (2000). Interhemispheric transfer of colour and shape information in the presence and absence of the corpus callosum. *Neuropsychologia, 38,* 32–45. (13)

Fortin, N. J., Agster, K. L., & Eichenbaum, H. B. (2002). Critical role of the hippocampus in memory for sequences of events. *Nature Neuroscience, 5,* 458–462. (12)

Foss-Feig, J. H., McGugin, R. W., Gauthier, I., Mash, L. E., Ventola, P., & Cascio, C. J. (2016). A functional neuroimaging study of fusiform response to restricted interests in children and adolescents with autism spectrum disorder. *Journal of Neurodevelopmental Disorders, 8,* article 15. (5)

Foss-Feig, J. H., Tadin, D., Schauder, K. B., & Cascio, C. J. (2013). A substantial and unexpected enhancement of motion perception in autism. *Journal of Neuroscience, 33,* 8243–8249. (14)

Fotopoulou, A., Solms, M., & Turnbull, O. (2004). Wishful reality distortions in confabulation: A case report. *Neuropsychologia, 47,* 727–744. (12)

Foulkes, D., & Domhoff, G. W. (2014). Bottom-up or top-down in dream neuroscience? A top-down critique of two bottom-up studies. *Consciousness and Cognition, 27,* 168–171. (8)

Fountoulakis, K. N., Veroniki, A. A., Siamouli, M., & Moller, H. J. (2013). No role for initial severity on the efficacy of antidepressants: Results of a multi-meta-analysis. *Archives of General Psychiatry, 12,* Article 26. (14)

Frank, M. J., & Claus, E. D. (2006). Anatomy of a decision: Striato-orbitofrontal interactions in reinforcement learning, decision making, and reversal. *Psychological Review, 113,* 300–326. (12)

Frank, R. A., Mize, S. J. S., Kennedy, L. M., de los Santos, H. C., & Green, S. J. (1992). The effect of *Gymnema sylvestre* extracts on the sweetness of eight sweeteners. *Chemical Senses, 17,* 461–479. (6)

Franz, E. A., Waldie, K. E., & Smith, M. J. (2000). The effect of callosotomy on novel versus familiar bimanual actions: A neural dissociation between controlled and automatic processes? *Psychological Science, 11,* 82–85. (13)

Frassinetti, F., Pavani, F., & Làdavas, E. (2002). Acoustical vision of neglected stimuli: Interaction among spatially converging audiovisual inputs in neglect patients. *Journal of Cognitive Neuroscience, 14,* 62–69. (13)

Frayling, T. M., Timpson, N. J., Weedon, M. N., Zeggini, E., Freathy, R. M., Lindgren, C. M., . . . McCarthy, M. I. (2007). A common variant in the *FTO* gene is associated with body mass index and predisposes to childhood and adult obesity. *Science, 316,* 889–894. (9)

Freed, C. R., Greene, P. E., Breeze, R. E., Tsai, W.-Y., DuMouchel, W., Kao, R., . . . Fahn, S. (2001). Transplantation of embryonic dopamine neurons for severe Parkinson's disease. *New England Journal of Medicine, 344,* 710–719. (7)

Freedman, M. S., Lucas, R. J., Soni, B., von Schantz, M., Muñoz, M., David-Gray, Z., &

Foster, R. (1999). Regulation of mammalian circadian behavior by non-rod, non-cone, ocular photoreceptors. *Science, 284,* 502–504. (8)

Freeman, J., Ziemba, C. M., Heeger, D. J., Simoncelli, E. P., & Movshon, J. A. (2013). A functional and perceptual signature of the second visual area in primates. *Nature Neuroscience, 16,* 974–981. (5)

Freeman, J. H. (2015). Cerebellar learning mechanisms. *Brain Research, 1621,* 260–269. (12)

Freire, C., & Koifman, S. (2012). Pesticide exposure and Parkinson's disease: Epidemiological evidence of association. *Neurotoxicology, 33,* 947–971. (7)

Freire, T. F. V., Fleck, M. P. D., & da Rocha, N. S. (2016). Remission of depression following electroconvulsive therapy (ECT) is associated with higher levels of brain-derived neurotrophic factor (BDNF). *Brain Research Bulletin, 121,* 263–269. (14)

Frese, M., & Harwich, C. (1984). Shiftwork and the length and quality of sleep. *Journal of Occupational Medicine, 26,* 561–566. (8)

Frey, S. H., Bogdanov, S., Smith, J. C., Watrous, S., & Breidenbach, W. C. (2008). Chronically deafferented sensory cortex recovers a grossly typical organization after allogenic hand transplantation. *Current Biology, 18,* 1530–1534. (4)

Friedman, E. S., Thase, M. E., Wisniewski, S. R., Trivedi, M. H., Biggs, M. M., Fava, M., . . . Rush, A. J. (2009). Cognitive therapy augmentation versus CT switch treatment: A STAR*D report. *International Journal of Cognitive Therapy, 2,* 66–87. (14)

Friedman, M. I., & Stricker, E. M. (1976). The physiological psychology of hunger: A physiological perspective. *Psychological Review, 83,* 409–431. (9)

Friedmann, N., & Rusou, D. (2015). Critical period for first language: the crucial role of language input during the first year of life. *Current Opinion in Neurobiology, 35,* 27–34. (13)

Frisén, L., Nordenström, A., Falhammar, H., Filipsson, H., Holmdahl, G., Janson, P. O., . . . Nordenskjold, A. (2009). Gender role behavior, sexuality, and psychosocial adaptation in women with congenital adrenal hyperplasia due to CYP21A2 deficiency. *Journal of Clinical Endocrinology & Metabolism, 94,* 3432–3439. (10)

Fritsch, G., & Hitzig, E. (1870). Über die elektrische Erregbarkeit des Grosshirns [Concerning the electrical stimulability of the cerebrum]. *Archiv für Anatomie Physiologie und Wissenschaftliche Medicin,* 300–332. (7)

Fromer, M., Pocklington, A. J., Kavanagh, D. H., Williams, H. J., Dwyer, S., Gormley, P., . . . O'Donovan, M. C. (2014). *De novo* mutations in schizophrenia implicate synaptic networks. *Nature, 506,* 179–184. (14)

Fromer, M., Roussos, P., Sieberts, S. K., Johnson, J. S., Kavanagh, D. H., Perumal,

T. M., . . . Sklar, P. (2016). Gene expression elucidates functional impact of polygenic risk for schizophrenia. *Nature Neuroscience, 19*, 1442–1453. (14)

Frost, S., Kanagasingam, Y., Sohrabi, H., Bourgeat, P., Villemagne, V., Rowe, C. C., . . . Martins, R. N. (2013). Pupil response biomarkers for early detection and monitoring of Alzheimer's disease. *Current Alzheimer Research, 10*, 931–939. (12)

Fu, L.-Y., Acuna-Goycolea, C., & van den Pol, A. N. (2004). Neuropeptide Y inhibits hypocretin/orexin neurons by multiple presynaptic and postsynaptic mechanisms: Tonic depression of the hypothalamic arousal system. *Journal of Neuroscience, 24*, 8741–8751. (9)

Fu, Q. A., Heath, A. C., Bucholz, K. K., Nelson, E., Goldberg, J., Lyons, M. J., . . . Eisen, S. A. (2002). Shared genetic risk of major depression, alcohol dependence, and marijuana dependence. *Archives of General Psychiatry, 59*, 1125–1132. (14)

Fu, W., Sugai, T., Yoshimura, H., & Onoda, N. (2004). Convergence of olfactory and gustatory connections onto the endopiriform nucleus in the rat. *Neuroscience, 126*, 1033–1041. (6)

Fuchs, T., Haney, A., Jechura, T. J., Moore, F. R., & Bingman, V. P. (2006). Daytime naps in night-migrating birds: Behavioural adaptation to seasonal sleep deprivation in the Swainson's thrush, *Catharus ustulatus*. *Animal Behaviour, 72*, 951–958. (8)

Fuller, R. K., & Roth, H. P. (1979). Disulfiram for the treatment of alcoholism: An evaluation in 128 men. *Annals of Internal Medicine, 90*, 901–904. (14)

Funato, H., Miyoshi, C., Fujiyama, T., Kanda, T., Sato, M., Wang, Z., . . . Yanagisawa, M. (2016). Forward-genetics analysis of sleep in randomly mutagenized mice. *Nature, 539*, 378–383. (8)

Furuya, S., & Hanakawa, T. (2016). The curse of motor expertise: Use-dependent focal dystonia as a manifestation of maladaptive changes in body representation. *Neuroscience Research, 104*, 112–119. (4)

Fuster, J. M. (1989). *The prefrontal cortex* (2nd ed.). New York: Raven Press. (3)

Gabrieli, J. D. E., Corkin, S., Mickel, S. F., & Growdon, J. H. (1993). Intact acquisition of mirror-tracing skill in Alzheimer's disease and in global amnesia. *Behavioral Neuroscience, 107*, 899–910. (12)

Gade, A., Kristoffersen, M., & Kessing, L. V. (2015). Neuroticism in remitted major depression: Elevated with early onset but not late onset of depression. *Psychopathology, 48*, 400–407. (14)

Gage, F. H. (2000). Mammalian neural stem cells. *Science, 287*, 1433–1438. (4)

Gais, S., Plihal, W., Wagner, U., & Born, J. (2000). Early sleep triggers memory for early visual discrimination skills. *Nature Neuroscience, 3*, 1335–1339. (8)

Galin, D., Johnstone, J., Nakell, L., & Herron, J. (1979). Development of the capacity for tactile information transfer between hemispheres in normal children. *Science, 204*, 1330–1332. (13)

Gallardo-Pujol, D., Andrés-Pueyo, A., Maydeu-Olivares, A. (2013). *MAOA* genotype, social exclusion and aggression: An experimental test of a gene-enviornmental interaction. *Genes, Brain and Behavior, 12*, 140–145. (11)

Gallese, V., Fadiga, L., Fogassi, L., & Rizzolatti, G. (1996). Action recognition in the premotor cortex. *Brain, 119*, 593–609. (7)

Gamaldo, A. A., An, Y., Allaire, J. C., Kitner-Triolo, M. H., & Zonderman, A. B. (2012). Variability in performance: Identifying early signs of future cognitive impairment. *Neuropsychology, 26*, 534–540. (12)

Gamer, M., & Büchel, C. (2009). Amygdala activation predicts gaze toward fearful eyes. *Journal of Neuroscience, 29*, 9123–9126. (11)

Gandhi, T. K., Ganesh, S., & Sinha, P. (2014). Improvement in spatial imagery following sight onset late in childhood. *Psychological Science, 25*, 693–701. (5)

Gangestad, S. W., & Simpson, J. A. (2000). The evolution of human mating: Trade-offs and strategic pluralism. *Behavioral and Brain Sciences, 23*, 573–644. (10)

Ganguly, K., Kiss, L., & Poo, M. (2000). Enhancement of presynaptic neuronal excitability by correlated presynaptic and postsynaptic spiking. *Nature Neuroscience, 3*, 1018–1026. (12)

Ganis, G., Keenan, J. P., Kosslyn, S. M., & Pascual-Leone, A. (2000). Transcranial magnetic stimulation of primary motor cortex affects mental rotation. *Cerebral Cortex, 10*, 175–180. (3)

Ganna, A., Genovese, G., Howrigan, D. P., Byrnes, A., Kurki, M. I., Zekavat, S. M., . . . Neale, B. M. (2016). Ultra-rare disruptive and damaging mutations influence educational attainment in the general population. *Nature Neuroscience, 19*, 1563–1565. (12)

Gao, J.-H., Parsons, L. M., Bower, J. M., Xiong, J., Li, J., & Fox, P. T. (1996). Cerebellum implicated in sensory acquisition and discrimination rather than motor control. *Science, 272*, 545–547. (7)

Garcia-Falgueras, A., & Swaab, D. F. (2008). A sex difference in the hypothalamic uncinate nucleus: Relationship to gender identity. *Brain, 131*, 3132–3146. (10)

Gardner, B. T., & Gardner, R. A. (1975). Evidence for sentence constituents in the early utterances of child and chimpanzee. *Journal of Experimental Psychology: General, 104*, 244–267. (13)

Gardner, H., & Zurif, E. B. (1975). Bee but not be: Oral reading of single words in aphasia and alexia. *Neuropsychologia, 13*, 181–190. (13)

Gaser, C., & Schlaug, G. (2003). Brain structures differ between musicians and non-musicians. *Journal of Neuroscience, 23*, 9240–9245. (4)

Gates, G. J. (2011). *How many people are lesbian, gay, bisexual, and transgender?* Los Angeles: The Williams Institute. (10)

Gayet, S., Paffen, C. L. E., Belopolsky, A. V., Theeuwes, J., & Van der Stigchel, S., (2016). Visual input signaling threat gains preferential access to awareness in a breaking continuous flash suppression paradigm. *Cognition, 149*, 77–83. (13)

Gazzaniga, M. S. (2000). Cerebral specialization and interhemispheric communication: Does the corpus callosum enable the human condition? *Brain, 123*, 1293–1326. (13)

Ge, S., Yang, C.-H., Hsu, K.-S., Ming, G.-L., & Song, H. (2007). A critical period for enhanced synaptic plasticity in newly generated neurons of the adult brain. *Neuron, 54*, 559–566. (4)

Geerling, J. C., & Loewy, A. D. (2008). Central regulation of sodium appetite. *Experimental Physiology, 93*, 177–209. (9)

Geier, C. F., Terwilliger, R., Teslovich, T., Velanova, K., & Luna, B. (2010). Immaturities in reward processing and its influence on inhibitory control in adolescence. *Cerebral Cortex, 20*, 1613–1629. (4)

Geiger, B. M., Haburcak, M., Avena, N. M., Moyer, M. C., Hoebel, B. G., & Pothos, E. N. (2009). Deficits of mesolimbic dopamine neurotransmission in rat dietary obesity. *Neuroscience, 159*, 1193–1199. (9)

Geiger, G., Lettvin, J. Y., & Zegarra-Moran, O. (1992). Task-determined strategies of visual process. *Cognitive Brain Research, 1*, 39–52. (13)

Gendron, M., Roberson, D., van der Vyver, J. M., & Barrett, L. F. (2014). Perceptions of emotion from facial expressions are not culturally universal: Evidence from a remote culture. *Emotion, 14*, 251–262. (11)

Genovese, G., Fromer, M., Stahl, E. A., Ruderfer, D. M., Chambert, K., Landén, M., . . . McCarroll, S. A. (2016). Increased burden of ultra-rare protein-altering variants among 7,877 individuals with schizophrenia. *Nature Neuroscience, 19*, 1433–1441. (14)

Gerber, P., Schlaffke, L., Heba, S., Greenlee, M. W., Schultz, T., & Schmidt-Wilcke, T. (2014). Juggling revisited—A voxel-based morphometry study with expert jugglers. *NeuroImage, 95*, 320–325. (4)

Gerwig, M., Hajjar, K., Dimitrova, A., Maschke, M., Kolb, F. P., Frings, M., . . . Timmann, D. (2005). Timing of conditioned eyeblink responses is impaired in cerebellar patients. *Journal of Neuroscience, 25*, 3919–3931. (12)

Geschwind, D. H., & Flint, J. (2015). Genetics and genomics of psychiatric disease. *Science, 349*, 1489–1494. (14)

Geschwind, N., & Levitsky, W. (1968). Human brain: Left–right asymmetries in temporal speech region. *Science, 161*, 186–187. (13)

Geuter, S., & Büchel, C. (2013). Facilitation of pain in the human spinal cord by nocebo treatment. *Journal of Neuroscience, 33*, 13784–13790. (6)

Ghazanfar, A. A. (2013). Multisensory vocal communication in primates and the evolution of rhythmic speech. *Behavioral Ecology and Sociobiology, 67*, 1441–1448. (13)

Ghosh, S., & Chattarji, S. (2015). Neuronal encoding of the switch from specific to generalized fear. *Nature Neuroscience, 18,* 112–120. (11)

Gibbs, F. P. (1983). Temperature dependence of the hamster circadian pacemaker. *American Journal of Physiology, 244,* R607–R610. (8)

Gibbs, J., Young, R. C., & Smith, G. P. (1973). Cholecystokinin decreases food intake in rats. *Journal of Comparative and Physiological Psychology, 84,* 488–495. (9)

Giber, K., Diana, M. A., Plattner, V. M., Dugué, G. P., Bokor, H., Rousseau, C. V., . . . Acsády, L. (2015). A subcortical inhibitory signal for behavioral arrest in the thalamus. *Nature Neuroscience, 18,* 562–568. (8)

Gilaie-Dotan, S., Tymula, A., Cooper, N., Kable, J. W., Gllimcher, P. W., & Levy, I. (2014). Neuroanatomy predicts individual risk attitudes. *Journal of Neuroscience, 34,* 12394–12401. (4)

Gilbertson, M. W., Shenton, M. E., Ciszewski, A., Kasai, K., Lasko, N. B., Orr, S. P., & Pitman, R. K. (2002). Smaller hippocampal volume predicts pathological vulnerability to psychological trauma. *Nature Neuroscience, 5,* 1242–1247. (11)

Gilissen, C., Hehir-Kwa, J. Y., Thung, D. T., van de Vorst, M., van Bon, B. W. M., Willemsen, M. H., . . . Veltman, J. A. (2014). Genome sequencing identifies major causes of severe intellectual disability. *Nature, 511,* 344–347. (12)

Gilmore, J. H., Lin, W., Prastawa, M. W., Looney, C. B., Vetsa, Y. S. K., Knickmeyer, R. C., . . . Gerig, G. (2007). Regional gray matter growth, sexual dimorphism, and cerebral asymmetry in the neonatal brain. *Journal of Neuroscience, 27,* 1255–1260. (12)

Giuliani, D., & Ferrari, F. (1996). Differential behavioral response to dopamine D2 agonists by sexually naive, sexually active, and sexually inactive male rats. *Behavioral Neuroscience, 110,* 802–808. (10)

Giummarra, M. J., Georgiou-Karistianis, N., Nicholls, M. E. R., Gibson, S. J., Chou, M., & Bradshaw, J. L. (2010). Corporeal awareness and proprioceptive sense of the phantom. *British Journal of Psychology, 101,* 791–808. (4)

Gizowki, C., Zaelzer, C., & Bourque, C. W. (2016). Clock-driven vasopressin neurotransmission mediates anticipatory thirst prior to sleep. *Nature, 536,* 685–688. (9)

Glendenning, K. K., Baker, B. N., Hutson, K. A., & Masterton, R. B. (1992). Acoustic chiasm V: Inhibition and excitation in the ipsilateral and contralateral projections of LSO. *Journal of Comparative Neurology, 319,* 100–122. (6)

Glykys, J., Peng, Z., Chandra, D., Homanics, G. E., Houser, C. R., & Mody, I. (2007). A new naturally occurring GABAA receptor subunit partnership with high sensitivity to ethanol. *Nature Neuroscience, 10,* 40–48. (11)

Goate, A., Chartier-Harlin, M. C., Mullan, M., Brown, J., Crawford, F., Fidani, L., . . . Owen, M. (1991). Segregation of a missense mutation in the amyloid precursor protein gene with familial Alzheimer's disease. *Nature, 349,* 704–706. (12)

Godfrey, K. M., Lillycrop, K. A., Burdge, G. C., Gluckman, P. D., & Hanson, M. A. (2007). Epigenetic mechanisms and the mismatch concept of the developmental origins of health and disease. *Pediatric Research, 61 (5), Part 2,* 5R–10R. (4)

Gogos, J. A., Osborne, J., Nemes, A., Mendelsohn, M., & Axel, R. (2000). Genetic ablation and restoration of the olfactory topographic map. *Cell, 103,* 609–620. (4)

Gold, R. M. (1973). Hypothalamic obesity: The myth of the ventromedial hypothalamus. *Science, 182,* 488–490. (9)

Goldberg, T. E., Weinberger, D. R., Berman, K. F., Pliskin, N. H., & Podd, M. H. (1987). Further evidence for dementia of the prefrontal type in schizophrenia? *Archives of General Psychiatry, 44,* 1008–1014. (14)

Goldin-Meadow, S., McNeill, D., & Singleton, J. (1996). Silence is liberating: Removing the handcuffs on grammatical expression in the manual modality. *Psychological Review, 103,* 34–55. (13)

Goldin-Meadow, S., & Mylander, C. (1998). Spontaneous sign systems created by deaf children in two cultures. *Nature, 391,* 279–281. (13)

Goldman, L. S. (1999). Medical illness in patients with schizophrenia. *Journal of Clinical Psychiatry, 60*(Suppl 21), 10–15. (14)

Goldman, P. S. (1971). Functional development of the prefrontal cortex in early life and the problem of neuronal plasticity. *Experimental Neurology, 32,* 366–387. (14)

Goldman, P. S. (1976). The role of experience in recovery of function following orbital prefrontal lesions in infant monkeys. *Neuropsychologia, 14,* 401–412. (14)

Goldstein, A. (1980). Thrills in response to music and other stimuli. *Physiological Psychology, 8,* 126–129. (6)

Golestani, N., Molko, N., Dehaene, S., LeBihan, D., & Pallier, C. (2007). Brain structure predicts the learning of foreign speech sounds. *Cerebral Cortex, 17,* 575–582. (4)

Golestani, N., Price, C. J., & Scott, S. K. (2011). Born with an ear for dialects? Structural plasticity in the expert phonetician brain. *Journal of Neuroscience, 31,* 4213–4220. (4)

Goller, A. I., Richards, K., Novak, S., & Ward, J. (2013). Mirror-touch synaesthesia in the phantom limbs of amputees. *Cortex, 49,* 243–251. (4)

Golombok, S., Rust, J., Zervoulis, K., Golding, J., & Hines, M. (2012). Continuity in sex-typed behavior from preschool to adolescence: A longitudinal population study of boys and girls aged 3–13 year. *Archives of Sexual Behavior, 41,* 591–597. (10)

Golumbic, E. Z., Cogan, G. B., Schroeder, C. E., & Poeppel, D. (2013). Visual input enhances selective speech envelope tracking in auditory cortex at a "cocktail party." *Journal of Neuroscience, 33,* 1417–1426. (6)

Gomez, A., Rodriguez-Exposito, B., Duran, E., Martín-Monzón, I., Broglio, C., Salas, C., & Rodríguez, F. (2016). Relational and procedural memory systems in the goldfish brain revealed by trace and delay eyeblink-like conditioning. *Physiology & Behavior, 167,* 332–340. (12)

Gonda, X., Pompili, M., Serafini, G., Carvalho, A. F., Rihmer, R., & Dome, P. (2015). The role of cognitive dysfunction in the symptoms and remission from depression. *Annals of General Psychiatry, 14,* article 27. (14)

Gong, G., He, Y., & Evans, A. C. (2011). Brain connectivity: Gender makes a difference. *Neuroscientist, 17,* 575–591. (3)

Gonzalez Andino, S. L., de Peralta Menendez, R. G., Khateb, A., Landis, T., & Pegna, A. J. (2009). Electrophysiological correlates of affective blindsight. *NeuroImage, 44,* 581–589. (5)

Goodale, M. A. (1996). Visuomotor modules in the vertebrate brain. *Canadian Journal of Physiology and Pharmacology, 74,* 390–400. (7)

Goodale, M. A., Milner, A. D., Jakobson, L. S., & Carey, D. P. (1991). A neurological dissociation between perceiving objects and grasping them. *Nature, 349,* 154–156. (7)

Gooley, J. J., Rajaratnam, S. M. W., Brainard, G. C., Kronauer, R. E., Czeisler, C. A., & Lockley, S. W. (2010). Spectral responses of the human circadian system depend on the irradiance and duration of exposure to light. *Science Translational Medicine, 2,* 31ra33. (8)

Gopnik, M., & Crago, M. B. (1991). Familial aggregation of a developmental language disorder. *Cognition, 39,* 1–50. (13)

Gordon, I., Zagoory-Sharon, O., Leckman, J. F., & Feldman, R. (2010). Prolactin, oxytocin, and the development of paternal behavior across the first six months of fatherhood. *Hormones and Behavior, 58,* 513–518. (10)

Gori, S., & Facoetti, A. (2015). How the visual aspects can be crucial in reading acquisition: The intriguing case of crowding and developmental dyslexia. *Journal of Vision, 15,* article 8. (13)

Gorski, R. A. (1980). Sexual differentiation of the brain. In D. T. Krieger & J. C. Hughes (Eds.), *Neuroendocrinology* (pp. 215–222). Sunderland, MA: Sinauer. (10)

Gorski, R. A. (1985). The 13th J. A. F. Stevenson memorial lecture. Sexual differentiation of the brain: Possible mechanisms and implications. *Canadian Journal of Physiology and Pharmacology, 63,* 577–594. (10)

Gorski, R. A., & Allen, L. S. (1992). Sexual orientation and the size of the anterior commissure in the human brain. *Proceedings of the National Academy of Sciences, USA, 89,* 7199–7202. (10)

Gottesman, I. I. (1991). *Schizophrenia genesis.* New York: Freeman. (14)

Gougoux, F., Belin, P., Voss, P., Lepore, F., Lassonde, M., & Zatorre, R. J. (2009). Voice perception in blind persons: A functional magnetic resonance imaging study. *Neuropsychologia, 47,* 2967–2974. (4)

Grabowska, A. (2017). Sex on the brain: Are gender-dependent structural and functional differences associated with behavior? *Journal of Neuroscience Research, 95,* 200–212. (12)

Grace, P. M., Strand, K. A., Galer, E. L., Urban, D. J., Wang, X., Baratta, M. V., . . . Watkins, L. R. (2016). Morphine paradoxically prolongs neuropathic pain in rats by amplifying spinal NLRP3 inflammasome activation. *Proceedings of the National Academy of Sciences, 113,* 113, E3441–E3450. (6)

Gradisar, M., Gardner, G., & Dohnt, H. (2011). Recent worldwide sleep patterns and problems during adolescence: A review and meta-analysis of age, region, and sleep. *Sleep Medicine, 12,* 110–118. (8)

Gray, C. M., König, P., Engel, A. K., & Singer, W. (1989). Oscillatory responses in cat visual cortex exhibit inter-columnar synchronization which reflects global stimulus properties. *Nature, 338,* 334–337. (13)

Gray, J. A. (1970). The psychophysiological basis of introversion–extraversion. *Behavioural Research Therapy, 8,* 249–266. (11)

Gray, S. M., Meijer, R. I., & Barrett, E. J. (2014). Insulin regulates brain function, but how does it get there? *Diabetes, 63,* 3992–3997. (1)

Graziadei, P. P. C., & deHan, R. S. (1973). Neuronal regeneration in frog olfactory system. *Journal of Cell Biology, 59,* 525–530. (4)

Graziano, M. S. A., Taylor, C. S. R., & Moore, T. (2002). Complex movements evoked by microstimulation of precentral cortex. *Neuron, 34,* 841–851. (3, 7)

Grazioplene, R. G., Ryman, S., Gray, J. R., Rustichini, A., Jung, R. E., & De Young, C. G. (2015). Subcortical intelligence: Caudate volume predicts IQ in healthy twins. *Human Brain Mapping, 36,* 1407–1416. (12)

Graziottin, A., Koochaki, P. E., Rodenberg, C. A., & Dennerstein, L. (2009). The prevalence of hypoactive sexual desire disorder in surgically menopausal women: An epidemiological study of women in four European countries. *Journal of Sexual Medicine, 6,* 2143–2153. (10)

Greene, J. D., Sommerville, R. B., Nystrom, L. E., Darley, J. M., & Cohen, J. D. (2001). An fMRI investigation of emotional engagement in moral judgment. *Science, 293,* 2105–2108. (11)

Greenhill, S. D., Juczewski, K., de Haan, A. M., Seaton, G., Fox, K., & Hardingham, N. R. (2015). Adult cortical plasticity depends on an early postnatal critical period. *Science, 349,* 424–427. (14)

Greenough, W. T. (1975). Experiential modification of the developing brain. *American Scientist, 63,* 37–46. (4)

Greer, J., Riby, D. M., Hamiliton, C., & Riby, L. M. (2013). Attentional lapse and inhibition control in adults with Williams syndrome. *Research in Developmental Disabilities, 34,* 4170–4177. (13)

Gregerson, P. K., Kowalsky, E., Lee, A., Baron-Cohen, S., Fisher, S. E., Asher, J. E., . . . Li, W. T. (2013). Absolute pitch exhibits phenotypic and genetic overlap with synesthesia. *Human Molecular Genetics, 22,* 2097–2104. (6)

Gregory, M. D., Kippenhan, J. S., Dickinson, D., Carrasco, J., Mattay, V. S., Weinberger, D. R., & Berman, K. F. (2016). Regional variations in brain gyrification are associated with general cognitive ability in humans. *Current Biology, 26,* 1301–1305. (12)

Griffin, D. R., Webster, F. A., & Michael, C. R. (1960). The echolocation of flying insects by bats. *Animal Behaviour, 8,* 141–154. (6)

Griffiths, T. D., Uppenkamp, S., Johnsrude, I., Josephs, O., & Patterson, R. D. (2001). Encoding of the temporal regularity of sound in the human brainstem. *Nature Neuroscience, 4,* 633–637. (6)

Grillon, C., Morgan, C. A., III, Davis, M., & Southwick, S. M. (1998). Effect of darkness on acoustic startle in Vietnam veterans with PTSD. *American Journal of Psychiatry, 155,* 812–817. (11)

Gritton, H. J., Sutton, B. C., Martinez, V., Sarter, M., & Lee, T. M. (2009). Interactions between cognition and circadian rhythms: Attentional demands modify circadian entrainment. *Behavioral Neuroscience, 123,* 937–948. (8)

Groeger, J. A., Lo, J. C. Y., Burns, C. G., & Dijk, D.-J. (2011). Effects of sleep inertia after daytime naps vary with executive load and time of day. *Behavioral Neuroscience, 125,* 252–260. (8)

Gross, C. G. (1999). The fire that comes from the eye. *The Neuroscientist, 5,* 58–64. (5)

Gross, C. T., & Canteras, N. S. (2012). The many paths to fear. *Nature Reviews Neuroscience, 13,* 651–658. (11)

Grossman, S. P., Dacey, D., Halaris, A. E., Collier, T., & Routtenberg, A. (1978). Aphagia and adipsia after preferential destruction of nerve cell bodies in hypothalamus. *Science, 202,* 537–539. (9)

Grueter, M., Grueter, T., Bell, V., Horst, J., Laskowki, W., Sperling, K., & Kennerknecht, I. (2007). Hereditary prosopagnosia: The first case series. *Cortex, 43,* 734–749. (5)

Grunder, G., Heinze, M., Cordes, J., Muhlbauer, B., Juckel, G., Schulz, C., . . . Timm, J. (2016). Effects of first-generation antipsychotics versus second-generation antipsychotics on quality of life in schizophrenia: A double-blind, randomized study. *Lancet Psychiatry, 3,* 717–729. (14)

Guastella, A. J., Einfeld, S. L., Gray, K. M., Rinehart, N. J., Tonge, B. J., Lambert, T. J., & Hickie, I. B. (2010). Intranasal oxytocin improves emotion recognition for youth with autism spectrum disorders. *Biological Psychology, 67,* 692–694. (13)

Gubernick, D. J., & Alberts, J. R. (1983). Maternal licking of young: Resource exchange and proximate controls. *Physiology & Behavior, 31,* 593–601. (10)

Guéguen, N. (2012). Gait and menstrual cycle: Ovulating women use sexier gaits and walk slowly ahead of men. *Gait & Posture, 35,* 621–624. (10)

Guggisberg, A. G., & Mottaz, A. (2013). Timing and awareness of movement decisions: Does consciousness really come too late? *Frontiers in Human Neuroscience, 7,* article 385. (7)

Guidotti, A., Ferrero, P., Fujimoto, M., Santi, R. M., & Costa, E. (1986). Studies on endogenous ligands (endocoids) for the benzodiazepine/beta carboline binding sites. *Advances in Biochemical Pharmacology, 41,* 137–148. (11)

Guillot, C. R., Fanning, J. R., Liang, T., & Berman, M. E. (2015). COMT associations with disordered gambling and drinking measures. *Journal of Gambling Studies, 31,* 513–524. (14)

Güler, A. D., Ecker, J. L., Lall, G. S., Haq, S., Altimus, C. M., Liao, H.-W., . . . Hattar, S. (2008). Melanopsin cells are the principal conduits for rod-cone input to non-image-forming vision. *Nature, 453,* 102–105. (8)

Gunia, B. C., Barnes, C. M., & Sah, S. (2014). The morality of larks and owls: Unethical behavior depends on chronotype as well as time of day. *Psychological Science, 25,* 2272–2274. (8)

Gunn, S. R., & Gunn, W. S. (2007). Are we in the dark about sleepwalking's dangers? In C. A. Read (Ed.), *Cerebrum 2007: Emerging ideas in brain science* (pp. 71–84). New York: Dana Press. (8)

Guo, J., Xue, L.-J., Huang, Z.-Y., Wang, Y.-S., Zhang, L., Zhou, G.-H., & Yuan, L.-X. (2016). Effect of CPAP therapy on cardiovascular events and mortality in patients with obstructive sleep apnea: A meta-analysis. *Sleep and Breathing, 20,* 965–974. (8)

Guo, S.-W., & Reed, D. R. (2001). The genetics of phenylthiocarbamide perception. *Annals of Human Biology, 28,* 111–142. (6)

Gur, R. E., Cowell, P. E., Latshaw, A., Turetsky, B. I., Grossman, R. I., Arnold, S. E., . . . Gur, R. C. (2000). Reduced dorsal and orbital prefrontal gray matter volumes in schizophrenia. *Archives of General Psychiatry, 57,* 761–768. (14)

Gusella, J. F., & MacDonald, M. E. (2000). Molecular genetics: Unmasking polyglutamine triggers in neurodegenerative disease. *Nature Reviews Neuroscience, 1,* 109–115. (7)

Gustafsson, B., & Wigström, H. (1990). Basic features of long-term potentiation in the hippocampus. *Seminars in the Neurosciences, 2,* 321–333. (12)

Guterstam, A., Petkova, V. I., & Ehrsson, H. H. (2011). The illusion of owning a third arm. *PLoS One, 6,* e17208. (3)

Gvilia, I., Turner, A., McGinty, D., & Szymusiak, R. (2006). Preoptic area neurons and the homeostatic regulation of rapid eye movement sleep. *Journal of Neuroscience, 26,* 3037–3044. (8)

Gwinner, E. (1986). Circannual rhythms in the control of avian rhythms. *Advances in the Study of Behavior, 16,* 191–228. (8)

Gyurak, A., Haase, C. M., Sze, J., Goodkind, M. S., Coppola, G., Lane, J., Miller, B. L., & Levenson, R. W. (2013). The effect of the serotonin transporter polymorphism (5-HTTLPR) on empathic and self-conscious emotional reactivity. *Emotion, 13,* 25–35. (14)

Haase, C. M., Beermann, U., Saslow, L. R., Shiota, M. N., Saturn, S. R., Lwi, S. J., . . . Levenson, R. W. (2015). Short alleles, bigger smiles: The effect of 5-HTTLPR on positive emotional expressions. *Emotion, 15,* 438–448. (14)

Hagenauer, M. H., & Lee, T. M. (2012). The neuroendocrine control of the circadian system: Adolescent chronotype. *Frontiers in Neuroendocrinology, 33,* 211–229. (8)

Hagenbuch, B., Gao, B., & Meier, P. J. (2002). Transport of xenobiotics across the blood–brain barrier. *News in Physiological Sciences, 17,* 231–234. (1)

Haggarty, J. M., Cernovsky, Z., Husni, M., Minor, K., Kermean, P., & Merskey, H. (2002). Seasonal affective disorder in an Arctic community. *Acta Psychiatrica Scandinavica, 105,* 378–384. (14)

Hägglund, M., Dougherty, K. J., Borgius, L., Itohara, S., Iwasato, T., & Kiehn, O. (2013). Optogenetic dissection reveals multiple rhythmogenic modules underlying locomotion. *Proceedings of the National Academy of Sciences, 110,* 11589–11594. (7)

Hahamy, A., Behrmann, M., & Malach, R. (2015). The idiosyncratic brain: Distortion of spontaneous connectivity patterns in autism spectrum disorder. *Nature Neuroscience, 18,* 302–309. (14)

Haimov, I., & Arendt, J. (1999). The prevention and treatment of jet lag. *Sleep Medicine Reviews, 3,* 229–240. (8)

Haimov, I., & Lavie, P. (1996). Melatonin—A soporific hormone. *Current Directions in Psychological Science, 5,* 106–111. (8)

Haist, F., Adamo, M., Wazny, J. H., Lee, K., & Stiles, J. (2013). The functional architecture for face-processing expertise: fMRI evidence of the developmental trajectory of the core and the extended face systems. *Neuropsychologia, 51,* 2893–2908. (5)

Hakuta, K., Bialystok, E., & Wiley, E. (2003). Critical evidence: A test of the critical-period hypothesis for second-language acquisition. *Psychological Science, 14,* 31–38. (13)

Halaas, J. L, Gajiwala, K. S., Maffei, M., Cohen, S. L., Chait, B. T., Rabinowitz, D., . . . Friedman, J. M. (1995). Weight-reducing effects of the plasma protein encoded by the obese gene. *Science, 269,* 543–546. (9)

Halaschek-Wiener, J., Amirabbasi-Beik, M., Monfared, N., Pieczyk, M., Sailer, C., Kollar, A., . . . Brooks-Wilson, A. R. (2009). Genetic variation in healthy oldest-old. *PLoS ONE, 4,* e6641. (4)

Halder, R., Hennion, M., Vidal, R. O., Shomroni, O., Rahman, R.-U., Rajput, A., . . . Bonn, S. (2016). DNA methylation changes in plasticity genes accompany the formation and maintenance of memory. *Nature Neuroscience, 19,* 102–110. (12)

Haley, J. (1959). An interactional description of schizophrenia. *Psychiatry, 22,* 321–332. (14)

Hallmayer, J., Faraco, J., Lin, L., Hesselson, S., Winkelmann, J., Kawashima, M., . . . Mignot, E. (2009). Narcolepsy is strongly associated with the T-cell receptor alpha locus. *Nature Genetics, 41,* 708–711. (8)

Halpern, S. D., Andrews, T. J., & Purves, D. (1999). Interindividual variation in human visual performance. *Journal of Cognitive Neuroscience, 11,* 521–534. (5)

Hamann, K., Warneken, F., Greenberg, J. R., & Tomasello, M. (2011). Collaboration encourages equal sharing in children but not in chimpanzees. *Nature, 476,* 328–331. (4)

Hamann, S. B., & Squire, L. R. (1995). On the acquisition of new declarative knowledge in amnesia. *Behavioral Neuroscience, 109,* 1027–1044. (12)

Hamer, D. H., Hu, S., Magnuson, V. L., Hu, N., & Pattatucci, A. M. L. (1993). A linkage between DNA markers on the X chromosome and male sexual orientation. *Science, 261,* 321–327. (10)

Hamilton, W. D. (1964). The genetical evolution of social behavior (I and II). *Journal of Theoretical Biology, 7,* 1–16, 17–52. (4)

Hampson, E., & Rovet, J. F. (2015). Spatial function in adolescents and young adults with congenital adrenal hyperplasia: Clinical phenotype and implications for the androgen hypothesis. *Psychoneuroendocrinology, 54,* 60–70. (10)

Han, J.-H., Kushner, S. A., Yiu, A. P., Cole, C. J., Matynia, A., Brown, R. A., . . . Josselyn, S. A. (2007). Neuronal competition and selection during memory formation. *Science, 316,* 457–460. (12)

Han, S., Tai, C., Westenbroek, R. E., Yu, F. H., Cheah, C. S., Potter, G. B., . . . Catterall, W. A. (2012). Autistic-like behaviour in *Scn1a+/-* mice and rescue by enhanced GABA-mediated neurotransmission. *Nature, 489,* 385–390. (14)

Hanada, R., Leibbrandt, A., Hanada, T., Kitaoka, S., Furuyashiki, T., Fujihara, H., . . . Penninger, J. M. (2009). Central control of fever and female body temperature by RANKL/RANK. *Nature, 462,* 505–509. (9)

Hanaway, J., Woolsey, T. A., Gado, M. H., & Roberts, M. P., Jr. (1998). *The brain atlas.* Bethesda, MD: Fitzgerald Science Press. (11)

Hanchate, N. K., Kondoh, K., Lu, Z., Kuang, D., Ye, X., Qiu, X., . . . Buck, L. B. (2015). Single-cell transcriptomics reveals receptor transformations during olfactory neurogenesis. *Science, 350,* 1251–1255. (6)

Hanks, T. D., Kopec, C. D., Brunton, B. W., Duan, C. A., Erlich, J. C., & Brody, C. D. (2015). Distinct relationships of parietal and prefrontal cortices to evidence accumulation. *Nature, 520,* 220–223. (13)

Hannibal, J., Hindersson, P., Knudsen, S. M., Georg, B., & Fahrenkrug, J. (2001). The photopigment melanopsin is exclusively present in pituitary adenylate cyclase-activating polypeptide-containing retinal ganglion cells of the retinohypothalamic tract. *Journal of Neuroscience, 21,* RC191: 1–7. (8)

Hannon, E., Spiers, H., Viana, J., Pidsley, R., Burrage, J., Murphy, T. M., . . . Mill, J. (2016). Methylation QTLs in the developing brain and their enrichment in schizophrenia risk loci. *Nature Neuroscience, 19,* 48–54. (4)

Haqq, C. M., & Donahoe, P. K. (1998). Regulation of sexual dimorphism in mammals. *Physiological Reviews, 78,* 1–33. (10)

Hara, J., Beuckmann, C. T., Nambu, T., Willie, J. T., Chemelli, R. M., Sinton, C. M., . . . Sakurai, T. (2001). Genetic ablation of orexin neurons in mice results in narcolepsy, hypophagia, and obesity. *Neuron, 30,* 345–354. (8)

Hardingham, G. E., & Do, K. Q. (2016). Linking early-life NMDAR hypofunction and oxidative stress in schizophrenia pathogenesis. *Nature Reviews Neuroscience, 17,* 126–134. (14)

Hargreaves, R. (2007). New migraine and pain research. *Headache, 47* (Suppl. 1), S26–S43. (3)

Hari, R. (1994). Human cortical functions revealed by magnetoencephalography. *Progress in Brain Research, 100,* 163–168. (3)

Harley, B., & Wang, W. (1997). The critical period hypothesis: Where are we now? In A. M. B. deGroot & J. F. Knoll (Eds.), *Tutorials in bilingualism* (pp. 19–51). Mahwah, NJ: Erlbaum. (13)

Harmon-Jones, E., & Gable, P. A. (2009). Neural activity underlying the effect of approach-motivated positive affect on narrowed attention. *Psychological Science, 20,* 406-409. (9)

Harmon-Jones, E., & Peterson, C. K. (2009). Supine body position reduces neural response to anger evocation. *Psychological Science, 20,* 1209–1210. (11)

Harris, C. R. (1999, July/August). The mystery of ticklish laughter. *American Scientist, 87*(4), 344–351. (6)

Harris, K. D., & Shepherd, G. M. G. (2015). The neocortical circuit: Themes and variations. *Nature Neuroscience, 18,* 170–181. (3, 12)

Harris, J. C. (2016). The origin and natural history of autism spectrum disorders. *Nature Neuroscience, 11,* 1390–1391. (14)

Harris, K. M., & Stevens, J. K. (1989). Dendritic spines of CA1 pyramidal cells in the rat hippocampus: Serial electron microscopy with reference to their biophysical characteristics. *Journal of Neuroscience, 9,* 2982–2997. (1)

Harrison, G. H. (2008, January). How chickadees weather winter. *National Wildlife, 46*(1), 14–15. (9)

Harrison, Y. (2013). Individual response to the end of Daylight Saving Time is largely dependent on habitual sleep duration. *Biological Rhythm Research, 44,* 391–401. (8)

Hart, B. L. (Ed.). (1976). *Experimental psychobiology.* San Francisco: Freeman. (9)

Hartline, H. K. (1949). Inhibition of activity of visual receptors by illuminating nearby retinal areas in the limulus eye. *Federation Proceedings, 8,* 69. (5)

Harvey, A. G., & Bryant, R. A. (2002). Acute stress disorder: A synthesis and critique. *Psychological Bulletin, 128,* 886–902. (11)

Harvey, A. G., Talbot, L. S., & Gershon, A. (2009). Sleep disturbance in bipolar disorder across the lifespan. *Clinical Psychology: Science & Practice, 16,* 256–277. (14)

Harvie, D. S., Broecker, M., Smith, R. T., Meuldeers, A., Madden, V. J., & Moseley, G. L. (2015). Bogus visual feedback alters onset of movement-evoked pain in people with neck pain. *Psychological Science, 26,* 385–392. (6)

Hasler, B. P., & Clark, D. B. (2013). Circadian misalignment, reward-related brain function, and adolescent alcohol involvement. *Alcoholism: Clinical and Experimental Research, 37,* 558–565. (8)

Hassabis, D., Kumaran, D., Vann, S. D., & Maguire, E. A. (2007). Patients with hippocampal amnesia cannot imagine new experiences. *Proceedings of the National Academy of Sciences, USA, 104,* 1726–1731. (12)

Hassan, B., & Rahman, Q. (2007). Selective sexual orientation-related differences in object location memory. *Behavioral Neuroscience, 121,* 625–633. (10)

Hassett, J. M., Siebert, E. R., & Wallen, K. (2008). Sex differences in rhesus monkey toy preferences parallel those of children. *Hormones and Behavior, 54,* 359–364. (10)

Haueisen, J., & Knösche, T. R. (2001). Involuntary motor activity in pianists evoked by music perception. *Journal of Cognitive Neuroscience, 13,* 786–792. (7)

Haut, K. M., van Erp, T. G. M., Knowlton, B., Bearden, C. E., Subotnik, K., Ventura, J., . . . Cannon, T. D. (2015). Contributions of feature binding during encoding and functional connectivity of the medial temporal lobe structures to episodic memory deficits across the prodromal and first-episode phases of schizophrenia. *Clinical Psychological Science, 3,* 159–174. (14)

Havlicek, J., & Roberts, S. C. (2009). MHC-correlated mate choice in humans: A review. *Psychoneuroendocrinology, 34,* 497–512. (6)

Haworth, C. M. A., Wright, M. J., Luciano, M., Martin, N. G., de Geus, E. J. C., van Beijsterveldt, C. E. M., . . . Plomin, R. (2010). The heritability of general cognitive ability increases linearly from childhood to young adulthood. *Molecular Psychiatry, 15,* 1112–1120. (12)

Hayashi-Takagi, A., Takaki, M., Graziane, N., Seshadri, S., Murdoch, H., Dunlop, A. J., . . . Sawa, A. (2010). Disrupted-in-schizophrenia 1(*DISC-1*) regulates spines of the glutamate synapse via Rac1. *Nature Neuroscience, 13,* 327–332. (14)

Hayes, J. E., Bartoshuk, L. M., Kidd, J. R., & Duffy, V. B. (2008). Supertasting and PROP bitterness depends on more than the *TAS2R38* gene. *Chemical Senses, 33,* 255–265. (6)

Hayes, S. M., Hayes, J. P., Cadden, M., & Verfaellie, M. (2013). A review of cardio-respiratory fitness-related neuroplasticity in the aging brain. *Frontiers in Aging Neuroscience, 5,* Article 31. (4)

He, S. M., Yang, A. K., Li, X. T., Du, Y. M., & Zhou, S. F. (2010). Effects of herbal products on the metabolism and transport of anticancer agents. *Expert Opinion on Drug Metabolism & Toxicity, 6,* 1195–1213. (14)

Hebb, D. O. (1949). *Organization of behavior.* New York: Wiley. (12)

Heuer, E., & Bachevalier, J. (2011). Neonatal hippocampal lesions in rhesus macaques alter the monitoring, but not maintenance, of information in working memory. *Behavioral Neuroscience, 125,* 859–870. (12)

Heims, H. C., Critchley, H. D., Dolan, R., Mathias, C. J., & Cipolotti, L. (2004). Social and motivational functioning is not critically dependent on feedback of autonomic responses: Neuropsychological evidence from patients with pure autonomic failure. *Neuropsychologia, 42,* 1979–1988. (11)

Held, R., Ostrovsky, Y., deGelder, B., Gandhi, T., Ganesh, S., Mathur, U., & Sinha, P. (2011). The newly sighted fail to match seen with felt. *Nature Neuroscience, 14,* 551–553. (5)

Helder, E. J., Mulder, E., & Gunnoe, M. L. (2016). A longitudinal investigation of children internationally adopted at school age. *Child Neuropsychology, 22,* 39–64. (4)

Heller, A. S., van Reekum, C. M., Schaefer, S. M., Lapate, R. C., Radler, B. T., Ryff, C. D., & Davidson, R. J. (2013). Sustained striatal activity predicts eudaimonic well-being and cortisol output. *Psychological Science, 24,* 2191–2200. (11)

Henderson, J. M., & Hollingworth, A. (2003). Global transsaccadic change blindness during scene perception. *Psychological Science, 14,* 493–497. (13)

Hendry, S. H. C., & Reid, R. C. (2000). The koniocellular pathway in primate vision. *Annual Review of Neuroscience, 23,* 127–153. (5)

Henley, C. L., Nunez, A. A., & Clemens, L. G. (2011). Hormones of choice: The neuroendocrinology of partner preference in animals. *Frontiers in Neuroendocrinology, 32,* 146–154. (10)

Hennies, N., Ralph, M. A. L., Kempkes, M., Cousins, J. N., & Lewis, P. A. (2016). Sleep spindle density predicts the effect of prior knowledge on memory consolidation. *Journal of Neuroscience, 36,* 3799–3810. (8)

Hennig, R., & Lømo, T. (1985). Firing patterns of motor units in normal rats. *Nature, 314,* 164–166. (7)

Herculano-Houzel, S. (2011a). Brains matter, bodies maybe not: The case for examining neuron numbers irrespective of body size. *Annals of the New York Academy of Sciences, 1225,* 191–199. (12)

Herculano-Houzel, S. (2011b). Not all brains are made the same: New views on brain scaling in evolution. *Brain, Behavior and Evolution, 78,* 22–36. (3)

Herculano-Houzel, S. (2012). The remarkable, yet not extraordinary, human brain as a scaled-up primate brain and its associated cost. *Proceedings of the National Academy of Sciences (U.S.A.), 109,* 10661–10668. (12)

Herculano-Houzel, S., Catania, K., Manger, P. R., & Kaas, J. H. (2015). Mammalian brains are made of these: A data set of the numbers and densities of neuronal and non-neural cells in the brain of glires, primates, scandentia, eulipotyphians, afrotherians, and artiodactyls, and their relationship with body mass. *Brain Behavior and Evolution, 86,* 145–163. (1, 3)

Herdener, M., Esposito, F., di Salle, F., Boller, C., Hilti, C. C., Habermeyer, B., . . . Cattapan-Ludewig, K. (2010). Musical training induces functional plasticity in human hippocampus. *Journal of Neuroscience, 30,* 1377–1384. (4)

Heres, S., Davis, J., Maino, K., Jetzinger, E., Kissling, W., & Leucht, S. (2006). Why olanzapine beats risperidone, risperidone beats quetiapine, and quetiapine beats olanzapine: an exploratory analysis of head-to-head comparison studies of second-generation antipsychotics. *American Journal of Psychiatry, 163,* 185–194. (14)

Herman, A. M., Ortiz-Guzman, J., Kochukov, M., Herman, I., Quast, K. B., Patel, J. M., . . . Arenkiel, B. R. (2016). A cholinergic basal forebrain feeding circuit modulates appetite suppression. *Nature, 538,* 253–256. (9)

Herrero, S. (1985). *Bear attacks: Their causes and avoidance.* Piscataway, NJ: Winchester. (6)

Herrup, K. (2015). The case for rejecting the amyloid cascade hypothesis. *Nature Neuroscience, 18,* 794–799. (12)

Herry, C., & Johansen, J. P. (2014). Encoding of fear learning and memory in distributed neuronal circuits. *Nature Neuroscience, 17,* 1644–1654. (11)

Hervé, P. Y., Zago, L., Petit, L., Mazoyer, B., & Tzourio-Mazoyer, N. (2013). Revisiting human hemispheric specialization with neuroimaging. *Trends in Cognitive Sciences, 17,* 69–80. (13)

Herz, R. S., McCall, C., & Cahill, L. (1999). Hemispheric lateralization in the processing of odor pleasantness versus odor names. *Chemical Senses, 24,* 691–695. (13)

Hess, B. J. M. (2001). Vestibular signals in self-orientation and eye movement control. *News in Physiological Sciences, 16,* 234–238. (6)

Hesse, M. D., Thiel, C. M., Stephan, K. E., & Fink, G. R. (2006). The left parietal cortex and motor intention: An event-related functional magnetic resonance imaging study. *Neuroscience, 140,* 1209–1221. (7)

Hesselmann, G., Hebart, M., & Malach, R. (2011). Differential BOLD activity associated with subjective and objective reports during "blindsight" in normal observers. *Journal of Neuroscience, 31,* 12936–12944. (5)

Heyes, C. (2010). Where do mirror neurons come from? *Neuroscience and Biobehavioral Reviews, 34,* 575–583. (7)

Hebscher, M., & Gilboa, A. (2016). A boost of confidence: The role of the ventromedial prefrontal cortex in memory, decision-making, and schemas. *Neuropsychologia, 90,* 46–58. (13)

Hieronymus, F., Nilsson, S., & Eriksson, E. (2016). A mega-analysis of fixed-dose trials reveals dose-dependency and a rapid onset of action for the antidepressant effect of three selective serotonin reuptake inhibitors. *Translational Psychiatry, 6,* article e834. (14)

Higgs, S., Williamson, A. C., Rotshtein, P., & Humphreys, G. W. (2008). Sensory-specific satiety is intake in amnesics who eat multiple meals. *Psychological Science, 19,* 623–628. (12)

Hillix, W. A., Rumbaugh, D. M., & Savage-Rumbaugh, E. S. (2012). The emergence of reason, intelligence, and language in humans and animals. In L. L'Abate (Ed.), *Paradigms in theory construction* (pp. 397–420). New York: Springer. (13)

Hines, M., Golombok, S., Rust, J., Johnston, K. J., Golding, J., & the Avon Longitudinal Study of Parents and Children Study Team. (2002). Testosterone during pregnancy and gender role behavior of preschool children: A longitudinal, population study. *Child Development, 73,* 1678–1687. (10)

Hines, M., Pasterski, V., Spencer, D., Neufeld, S., Patalay, P., Hindmarsh, P. C., . . . Acerini, C. L. (2016). Prenatal androgen exposure alters girls' responses to information indicating gender-appropriate behaviour. *Philosophical Transactions of the Royal Society B, 371,* article 20150125. (10)

Hinkley, L. B. N., Marco, E. J., Brown, E. G., Bukshpun, P., Gold, J., Hill, S., . . . Nagarajan, S. S. (2016). The contribution of the corpus callosum to language lateralization. *Journal of Neuroscience, 36,* 4522–4533. (13)

Hippisley-Cox, J., Vinogradova, Y., Coupland, C., & Parker, C. (2007). Risk of malignancy in patients with schizophrenia or bipolar disorder. *Archives of General Psychiatry, 64,* 1368–1376. (14)

Hitchcock, J. M., & Davis, M. (1991). Efferent pathway of the amygdala involved in conditioned fear as measured with the fear-potentiated startle paradigm. *Behavioral Neuroscience, 105,* 826–842. (11)

Hiyama, T. Y., Watanabe, E., Okado, H., & Noda, M. (2004). The subfornical organ is the primary locus of sodium-level sensing by Nax sodium channels for the control of salt-intake behavior. *Journal of Neuroscience, 24,* 9276–9281. (9)

Hobson, J. A. (1989). *Sleep.* New York: Scientific American Library. (14)

Hobson, J. A. (2009). REM sleep and dreaming: Towards a theory of protoconsciousness. *Nature Reviews Neuroscience, 10,* 803–813. (8)

Hobson, J. A., & McCarley, R. W. (1977). The brain as a dream state generator: An activation-synthesis hypothesis of the dream process. *American Journal of Psychiatry, 134,* 1335–1348. (8)

Hobson, J. A., Pace-Schott, E. F., & Stickgold, R. (2000). Dreaming and the brain: Toward a cognitive neuroscience of conscious states. *Behavioral and Brain Sciences, 23,* 793–1121. (8)

Hochberg, L. R., Bacher, D., Jarosiewicz, B., Masse, N. Y., Simeral, J. D., Vogel, J., . . . Donoghue, J. P. (2012). Reach and grasp by people with tetraplegia using a neurally controlled robotic arm. *Nature, 485,* 372–375. (7)

Hodes, G. E., Kana, V., Menard, C., Merad, M., & Russo, S. J. (2015). Neuroimmune mechanisms of depression. *Nature Neuroscience, 18,* 1386–1393. (14)

Hoebel, B. G., & Hernandez, L. (1993). Basic neural mechanisms of feeding and weight regulation. In A. J. Stunkard & T. A. Wadden (Eds.), *Obesity: Theory and therapy* (2nd ed., pp. 43–62). New York: Raven Press. (9)

Hoebel, B. G., Rada, P. V., Mark, G. P., & Pothos, E. (1999). Neural systems for reinforcement and inhibition of behavior: Relevance to eating, addiction, and depression. In D. Kahneman, E. Diener, & N. Schwartz (Eds.), *Well-being: Foundations of hedonic psychology* (pp. 560–574). New York: Russell Sage Foundation. (9)

Hoffer, A. (1973). Mechanism of action of nicotinic acid and nicotinamide in the treatment of schizophrenia. In D. Hawkins & L. Pauling (Eds.), *Orthomolecular psychiatry* (pp. 202–262). San Francisco: Freeman. (14)

Hoffman, P. L., Tabakoff, B., Szabó, G., Suzdak, P. D., & Paul, S. M. (1987). Effect of an imidazobenzodiazepine, Ro15-4513, on the incoordination and hypothermia produced by ethanol and pento-barbital. *Life Sciences, 41,* 611–619. (11)

Hoffmann, F., & Curio, G. (2003). REM-Schlaf und rezidivierende Erosio corneae—eine Hypothese. [REM sleep and recurrent corneal erosion—A hypothesis.] *Klinische Monatsblatter für Augenheilkunde, 220,* 51–53. (8)

Holcombe, A. O., & Cavanagh, P. (2001). Early binding of feature pairs for visual perception. *Nature Neuroscience, 4,* 127–128. (3)

Hollis, E. R. II, Ishiko, N., Yu, T., Lu, C.-C., Haimovich, A., Tolentino, K., . . . Zou, Y. (2016). Ryk controls remapping of motor cortex during functional recovery after spinal cord injury. *Nature Neuroscience, 19,* 697–705. (4)

Hollister, J. M., Laing, P., & Mednick, S. A. (1996). Rhesus incompatibility as a risk factor for schizophrenia in male adults. *Archives of General Psychiatry, 53,* 19–24. (14)

Hollon, S. D., DeRubeis, R. J., Fawcett, J., Amsterdam, J. D., Shelton, R. C., Zajecka, J., . . . Gallop, R. (2014). Effect of cognitive therapy with antidepressant medications versus antidepressants alone on the rate of recovery in major depressive disorder. A randomized clinical trial. *JAMA Psychiatry, 71,* 1157–1164. (14)

Hollon, S. D., Thase, M. E., & Markowitz, J. C. (2002). Treatment and prevention of depression. *Psychological Science in the Public Interest, 3,* 39–77. (14)

Holy, T. E., Dulac, C., & Meister, M. (2000). Responses of vomeronasal neurons to natural stimuli. *Science, 289,* 1569–1572. (6)

Homewood, J., & Stevenson, R. J. (2001). Differences in naming accuracy of odors presented to the left and right nostrils. *Biological Psychology, 58,* 65–73. (13)

Hopkins, W. D. (2006). Comparative and familial analysis of handedness in great apes. *Psychological Bulletin, 132,* 538–559. (13)

Hopkins, W. D., Misiura, M., Pope, S. M., & Latash, E. M. (2015). Behavioral and brain asymmetries in primates: A preliminary evaluation of two evolutionary hypotheses. *Annals of the New York Academy of Sciences, 1359,* 65–83. (13)

Horikawa, T., Tamaki, M., Miyawaki, Y., & Kamitani, Y. (2013). Neural decoding of visual imagery during sleep. *Science, 340,* 639–642. (3)

Horn, S. R., Charney, D. S., & Feder, A. (2016). Understanding resilience: New approaches for preventing and treating PTSD. *Experimental Neurology, 284,* 119–132. (11)

Horne, J. A. (1992). Sleep and its disorders in children. *Journal of Child Psychology & Psychiatry & Allied Disciplines, 33,* 473–487. (8)

Horne, J. A., & Minard, A. (1985). Sleep and sleepiness following a behaviourally "active" day. *Ergonomics, 28,* 567–575. (8)

Horowitz, L. F., Saraiva, L. R., Kuang, D., Yoon, K.-h., & Buck, L. B. (2014). Olfactory receptor patterning in a higher primate. *Journal of Neuroscience, 34,* 12241–12252. (6)

Horridge, G. A. (1962). Learning of leg position by the ventral nerve cord in headless insects. *Proceedings of the Royal Society of London, B, 157,* 33–52. (12)

Horst, W. D., & Preskorn, S. H. (1998). Mechanisms of action and clinical characteristics of three atypical antidepressants: Venlafaxine, nefazodone, bupropion. *Journal of Affective Disorders, 51,* 237–254. (14)

Horvath, T. L. (2005). The hardship of obesity: A soft-wired hypothalamus. *Nature Neuroscience, 8,* 561–565. (9)

Hoshi, E., & Tanji, J. (2000). Integration of target and body-part information in the premotor cortex when planning action. *Nature, 408,* 466–470. (7)

Hötting, K., & Röder, B. (2013). Beneficial effects of physical exercise on neuroplasticity and cognition. *Neuroscience and Biobehavioral Reviews, 37,* 2243–2257. (4)

Houk, C. P., & Lee, P. A. (2010). Approach to assigning gender in 46,XX congenital adrenal hyperplasia with male external genitalia: Replacing dogmatism with pragmatism. *Journal of Clinical Endocrinology & Metabolism, 95,* 4501–4508. (10)

Hourai, A., & Miyata, S. (2013). Neurogenesis in the circumventricular organs of adult mouse brains. *Journal of Neuroscience Research, 91,* 757–770. (9)

Hovda, D. A., & Feeney, D. M. (1989). Amphetamine-induced recovery of visual cliff performance after bilateral visual cortex ablation in cats: Measurements of depth perception thresholds. *Behavioral Neuroscience, 103,* 574–584. (4)

Howard, J. D., Plailly, J., Grueschow, M., Haynes, J.-D., & Gottfried, J. A. (2009). Odor quality coding and categorization in human posterior piriform cortex. *Nature Neuroscience, 12,* 932–938. (6)

Howes, O. D., & Kapur, S. (2009). The dopamine hypothesis of schizophrenia: Version III—the final common pathway. *Schizophrenia Bulletin, 35,* 549–562. (14)

Hrdy, S. B. (2000). The optimal number of fathers. *Annals of the New York Academy of Sciences, 907,* 75–96. (10)

Hróbjartsson, A., & Gøtzsche, P. C. (2001). Is the placebo powerless? *New England Journal of Medicine, 344,* 1594–1602. (6)

Hsieh, P.-J., Vul, E., & Kanwisher, N. (2010). Recognition alters the spatial pattern of fMRI activation in early retinotopic cortex. *Journal of Neurophysiology, 103,* 1501–1507. (5)

Hu, P., Stylos-Allan, M., & Walker, M. P. (2006). Sleep facilitates consolidation of emotional declarative memory. *Psychological Science, 17,* 891–898. (8)

Hua, J. Y., & Smith, S. J. (2004). Neural activity and the dynamics of central nervous system development. *Nature Neuroscience, 7,* 327–332. (4)

Huang, A. L., Chen, X., Hoon, M. A., Chandrashekar, J., Guo, W., Tränker, D., . . . Zuker, C. S. (2006). The cells and logic for mammalian sour taste detection. *Nature, 442,* 934–938. (6)

Huang, B. H. (2014). The effects of age on second language grammar and speech production. *Journal of Psycholinguistic Research, 43,* 397–420. (13)

Huang, L., Treisman, A., & Pashler, H. (2007). Characterizing the limits of human visual awareness. *Science, 317,* 823–825. (13)

Huang, Y.-J., Maruyama, Y., Lu, K.-S., Pereira, E., Plonsky, I., Baur, J. E., . . . Roper, S. D. (2005). Mouse taste buds use serotonin as a neurotransmitter. *Journal of Neuroscience, 25,* 843–847. (2)

Hubbard, E. M., Piazza, M., Pinel, P., & Dehaene, S. (2005). Interactions between number and space in parietal cortex. *Nature Reviews Neuroscience, 6,* 435–448. (3)

Hubel, D. H. (1963, November). The visual cortex of the brain. *Scientific American, 209*(5), 54–62. (5)

Hubel, D. H., & Wiesel, T. N. (1959). Receptive fields of single neurons in the cat's striate cortex. *Journal of Physiology, 148,* 574–591. (5)

Hubel, D. H., & Wiesel, T. N. (1965). Binocular interaction in striate cortex of kittens reared with artificial squint. *Journal of Neurophysiology, 28,* 1041–1059. (5)

Hubel, D. H., & Wiesel, T. N. (1977). Functional architecture of macaque monkey visual

cortex. *Proceedings of the Royal Society of London, B, 198,* 1–59. (5)

Hubel, D. H., & Wiesel, T. N. (1998). Early exploration of the visual cortex. *Neuron, 20,* 401–412. (5)

Huber, E., Webster, J. M., Brewer, A. A., MacLeod, D. I. A., Wandell, B. A., Boynton, G. M., . . . Fine, I. (2015). A lack of experience-dependent plasticity after more than a decade of recovered sight. *Psychological Science, 26,* 393–401. (5)

Huber, R., Ghilardi, M. F., Massimini, M., & Tononi, G. (2004). Local sleep and learning. *Nature, 430,* 78–81. (8)

Hudson, J. I., Hiripi, E., Pope, H. G., Jr., & Kessler, R. C. (2007). The prevalence and correlates of eating disorders in the National Comorbidity Survey Replication. *Biological Psychiatry, 61,* 348–358. (9)

Hudson, J. I., Mangweth, B., Pope, H. G., Jr., De Col, C., Hausmann, A., Gutweniger, S., . . . Tsuang, M. T. (2003). Family study of affective spectrum disorder. *Archives of General Psychiatry, 60,* 170–177. (14)

Hudspeth, A. J. (2014). Integrating the active process of hair cells with cochlear function. *Nature Reviews Neuroscience, 15,* 600–614. (6)

Hugdahl, K. (1996). Brain laterality—Beyond the basics. *European Psychologist, 1,* 206–220. (13)

Hull, E. M., Du, J., Lorrain, D. S., & Matuszewich, L. (1997). Testosterone, preoptic dopamine, and copulation in male rats. *Brain Research Bulletin, 44,* 327–333. (10)

Hull, E. M., Eaton, R. C., Markowski, V. P., Moses, J., Lumley, L. A., & Loucks, J. A. (1992). Opposite influence of medial preoptic D_1 and D_2 receptors on genital reflexes: Implications for copulation. *Life Sciences, 51,* 1705–1713. (10)

Hull, E. M., Lorrain, D. S., Du, J., Matuszewich, L., Lumley, L. A., Putnam, S. K., & Moses, J. (1999). Hormone-neurotransmitter interactions in the control of sexual behavior. *Behavioural Brain Research, 105,* 105–116. (10)

Hull, E. M., Nishita, J. K., Bitran, D., & Dalterio, S. (1984). Perinatal dopamine-related drugs demasculinize rats. *Science, 224,* 1011–1013. (10)

Hull, R., & Vaid, J. (2007). Bilingual language lateralization: A meta-analytic tale of two hemispheres. *Neuropsychologia, 45,* 1987–2008. (13)

Hunt, L. T., Kolling, N., Soltani, A., Woolrich, M. W., Rushworth, M. F. S., & Behrens, T. E. J. (2012). Mechanisms underlying cortical activity during value-guided choice. *Nature Neuroscience, 15,* 470–476. (3)

Hunt, S. P., & Mantyh, P. W. (2001). The molecular dynamics of pain control. *Nature Reviews Neuroscience, 2,* 83–91. (6)

Huntington's Disease Collaborative Research Group. (1993). A novel gene containing a trinucleotide repeat that is expanded and unstable on Huntington's disease chromosomes. *Cell, 72,* 971–983. (7)

Hurovitz, C. S., Dunn, S., Domhoff, G. W., & Fiss, H. (1999). The dreams of blind men and women: A replication and extension of previous findings. *Dreaming, 9,* 183–193. (5)

Hurvich, L. M., & Jameson, D. (1957). An opponent-process theory of color vision. *Psychological Review, 64,* 384–404. (5)

Huszar, D., Lynch, C. A., Fairchild-Huntress, V., Dunmore, J. H., Fang, Q., Berkemeier, L. R., . . . Lee, F. (1997). Targeted disruption of the melanocortin-4 receptor results in obesity in mice. *Cell, 88,* 131–141. (9)

Hutcherson, C. A., Montaser-Kouhsari, L., Woodward, J., & Rangel, A. (2015). Emotional and utilitarian appraisals of moral dilemmas are encoded in separate areas and integrated in ventromedial prefrontal cortex. *Journal of Neuroscience, 35,* 12593–12605. (11)

Hutcheson, D. M., Everitt, B. J., Robbins, T. W., & Dickinson, A. (2001). The role of withdrawal in heroin addiction: Enhances reward or promotes avoidance? *Nature Neuroscience, 4,* 943–947. (14)

Hutchison, K. E., LaChance, H., Niaura, R., Bryan, A., & Smolen, A. (2002). The DRD4 VNTR polymorphism influences reactivity to smoking cues. *Journal of Abnormal Psychology, 111,* 134–143. (14)

Huth, A. G., de Heer, W. A., Griffiths, T. L., Theunissen, F. E., & Gallant, J. L. (2016). Natural speech reveals the semantic maps that tile human cerebral cortex. *Nature, 532,* 453–458. (13)

Huttner, H. B., Bergmann, O., Salehpour, M., Rácz, A., Tatarishvili, J., Lindgren, E., . . . Frisén, J. (2014). The age and genomic integrity of neurons after cortical stroke in humans. *Nature Neuroscience, 17,* 801–803. (4)

Hyde, J. S., Lindberg, S. M., Linn, M. C., Ellis, A. B., & Williams, C. C. (2008). Gender similarities characterize math performance. *Science, 321,* 494–495. (12)

Hyde, K. L., Lerch, J., Norton, A., Forgeard, M., Winner, E., Evans, A. C., & Schlaug, G. (2009a). Musical training shapes structural brain development. *Journal of Neuroscience, 29,* 3019–3025. (4)

Hyde, K. L., Lerch, J., Norton, A., Forgeard, M., Winner, E., Evans, A. C., . . . Schlaug, G. (2009b). The effects of musical training on structural brain development: A longitudinal study. *Annals of the New York Academy of Sciences, 1169,*182–186. (4)

Hyde, K. L., Lerch, J. P., Zatorre, R. J., Griffiths, T. D., Evans, A. C., & Peretz, I. (2007). Cortical thickness in congenital amusia: When less is better than more. *Journal of Neuroscience, 27,* 13028–13032. (6)

Hyde, K. L., & Peretz, I. (2004). Brains that are out of tune but in time. *Psychological Science, 15,* 356–360. (6)

Iggo, A., & Andres, K. H. (1982). Morphology of cutaneous receptors. *Annual Review of Neuroscience, 5,* 1–31. (6)

Ikemoto, S., Yang, C., & Tan, A. (2015). Basal ganglia circuit loops, dopamine and motivation: A review and enquiry. *Behavioural Brain Research, 290*, 17–31. (7)

Ikonomidou, C., Bittigau, P. Ishimaru, M. J., Wozniak, D. F., Koch, C., Genz, K., . . . Olney, J. W. (2000). Ethanol-induced apoptotic neurodegeneration and fetal alcohol syndrome. *Science, 287*, 1056–1060. (4)

Ilieva, I. P., Hook, C. J., & Farah, M. J. (2015). Prescription stimulants' effects on healthy inhibitory control, working memory, and episodic memory: A meta-analysis. *Journal of Cognitive Neuroscience, 27*, 1069–1089. (12)

Imamura, K., Mataga, N., & Mori, K. (1992). Coding of odor molecules by mitral/tufted cells in rabbit olfactory bulb: I. Aliphatic compounds. *Journal of Neurophysiology, 68*, 1986–2002. (6)

Immordino-Yang, M. H., Christodoulou, J. A., & Singh, V. (2012). Rest is not idleness: Implications of the brain's default mode for human development and education. *Perspectives on Psychological Science, 7*, 352–364. (3)

Imperato-McGinley, J., Guerrero, L., Gautier, T., & Peterson, R. E. (1974). Steroid 5 alpha-reductase deficiency in man: An inherited form of male pseudohermaphroditism. *Science, 186*, 1213–1215. (10)

Ingram, C. J. E., Mulcare, C. A., Itan, Y., Thomas, M. G., & Swallow, D. M. (2009). Lactose digestion and the evolutionary genetics of lactase persistence. *Human Genetics, 124*, 579–591. (9)

Innocenti, G. M. (1980). The primary visual pathway through the corpus callosum: Morphological and functional aspects in the cat. *Archives Italiennes de Biologie, 118*, 124–188. (13)

Inouye, S. T., & Kawamura, H. (1979). Persistence of circadian rhythmicity in a mammalian hypothalamic "island" containing the suprachiasmatic nucleus. *Proceedings of the National Academy of Sciences, USA, 76*, 5962–5966. (8)

Isaacson, G., & Adler, M. (2012). Randomized clinical trials underestimate the efficacy of antidepressants in less severe depression. *Acta Psychiatrica Scandinavica, 125*, 453–459. (14)

Ishizawa, Y., Ahmed, O. J., Patel, S. R., Gale, J. T., Sierra-Mercado, D., Brown, E. N., & Eskandar, E. N. (2016). Dynamics of propofol-induced loss of consciousness across primate neocortex. *Journal of Neuroscience, 36*, 7718–7726. (13)

Ishizuka, K., Kamiya, A., Oh, E. C., Kanki, H., Seshadri, S., Robinson, J. F., . . . Sawa, A. (2011). DISC-1-dependent switch from progenitor proliferation to migration in the developing cortex. *Nature, 473*, 92–96. (14)

Isler, K., & van Schaik, C. P. (2009). The expensive brain: A framework for explaining evolutionary changes in brain size. *Journal of Human Evolution, 57*, 392–400. (12)

Isoda, M., & Hikosaka, O. (2007). Switching from automatic to controlled action by monkey medial frontal cortex. *Nature Neuroscience, 10*, 240–248. (7)

Iuculano, T., & Kadosh, R. C. (2013). The mental cost of cognitive enhancement. *Journal of Neuroscience, 33*, 4482–4486. (12)

Iverson, J. M., & Goldin-Meadow, S. (2005). Gesture paves the way for language development. *Psychological Science, 16*, 367–371. (13)

Ivry, R. B., & Diener, H. C. (1991). Impaired velocity perception in patients with lesions of the cerebellum. *Journal of Cognitive Neuroscience, 3*, 355–366. (7)

Iwata, Y., Nakajima, S., Suzuki, T., Keefe, R. S. E., Plitman, E., Chung, J. K., . . . Uchida, H. (2015). Effects of glutamate positive modulators on cognitive deficits in schizophrenia: A systematic review and meta-analysis of double-blind randomized controlled trials. *Molecular Psychiatry, 20*, 1151–1160. (14)

Iwema, C. L., Fang, H., Kurtz, D. B., Youngentob, S. L., & Schwob, J. E. (2004). Odorant receptor expression patterns are restored in lesion-recovered rat olfactory epithelium. *Journal of Neuroscience, 24*, 356–369. (6)

Jablensky, A. V., Morgan, V., Zubrick, S. R., Bower, C., & Yellachich, L.-A. (2005). Pregnancy, delivery, and neonatal complications in a population cohort of women with schizophrenia and major affective disorders. *American Journal of Psychiatry, 162*, 79–91. (14)

Jacobs, B., & Scheibel, A. B. (1993). A quantitative dendritic analysis of Wernicke's area in humans: I. Lifespan changes. *Journal of Comparative Neurology, 327*, 83–96. (4)

Jacobs, G. D., & Snyder, D. (1996). Frontal brain asymmetry predicts affective style in men. *Behavioral Neuroscience, 110*, 3–6. (14)

Jacobs, G. H. (2014). The discovery of spectral opponency in visual systems and its impact on understanding the neurobiology of color vision. *Journal of the History of the Neurosciences, 23*, 287–314. (5)

Jacobs, J., Weidemann, C. T., Miller, J. F., Solway, A., Burke, J. F., Wei, X.-X., . . . Kahana, M. J. (2013). Direct recordings of grid-like neuronal activity in human spatial navigation. *Nature Neuroscience, 16*, 1188–1190. (13)

Jaffe, A. E., Gao, Y., Deep-Soboslay, A., Tao, R., Hyde, T. M., Weinberger, D. R., & Kleinman, J. E. (2016). Mapping DNA methylation across development, genotype and schizophrenia in the human frontal cortex. *Nature Neuroscience, 19*, 40–47. (4)

Jahanshahi, M., Obeso, I., Rothwell, J. C., & Obeso, J. A. (2015). A fronto-striato-subthalamic-pallidal network for goal-directed and habitual inhibition. *Nature Reviews Neuroscience, 16*, 719–732. (7)

James, R. S. (2013). A review of the thermal sensitivity of the mechanics of vertebrate skeletal muscle. *Journal of Comparative Physiology B: Biochemical, Systemic, and Environmental Physiology, 183*, 723–733. (9)

James, T. W., & James, K. H. (2013). Expert individuation of objects increases activation in the fusiform face area of children. *NeuroImage, 67*, 182–192. (5)

James, W. (1884). What is an emotion? *Mind, 9*, 188–205. (11)

James, W. (1894). The physical basis of emotion. *Psychological Review, 1*, 516–529. (11)

James, W. (1961). *Psychology: The briefer course.* New York: Harper. (Original work published 1892) (13)

Jameson, K. A., Highnote, S. M., & Wasserman, L. M. (2001). Richer color experience in observers with multiple photopigment opsin genes. *Psychonomic Bulletin and Review, 8*, 244–261. (5)

Jäncke, L., Beeli, G., Eulig, C., & Hänggi, J. (2009). The neuroanatomy of grapheme-color synesthesia. *European Journal of Neuroscience, 29*, 1287–1293. (6)

Janak, P. H., & Tye, K. M. (2015). From circuits to behaviour in the amygdala. *Nature, 517*, 284–292. (11)

Jarrard, L. E., Okaichi, H., Steward, O., & Goldschmidt, R. B. (1984). On the role of hippocampal connections in the performance of place and cue tasks: Comparisons with damage to hippocampus. *Behavioral Neuroscience, 98*, 946–954. (12)

Jenkins, L. M., Andrewes, D. G., Nicholas, C. L., Drummond, K. L., Moffat, B. A., Phal, P., . . . Kessels, R. P. C. (2014). Social cognition in patients following surgery to the prefrontal cortex. *Psychiatry Research: Neuroimaging, 224*, 192–203. (13)

Jennings, J. H., Rizzi, G., Stamatakis, A. M., Ung, R. L., & Stuber, G. D. (2013). The inhibitory circuit architecture of the lateral hypothalamus orchestrates feeding. *Science, 341*, 1517–1521. (9)

Jerison, H. J. (1985). Animal intelligence as encephalization. *Philosophical Transactions of the Royal Society of London, B, 308*, 21–35. (3)

Jesulola, E., Sharpley, C. F., Bitsika, V., Agnew, L. L., & Wilson, P. (2015). Frontal alpha asymmetry as a pathway to behavioural withdrawal in depression: Research findings and issues. *Behavioural Brain Research, 292*, 56–67. (14)

Ji, D., & Wilson, M. A. (2007). Coordinated memory replay in the visual cortex and hippocampus during sleep. *Nature Neuroscience, 10*, 100–107. (8)

Jiang, P., Josue, J., Li, X., Glaser, D., Li, W., Brand, J. G., . . . Beauchamp, G. K. (2012). Major taste loss in carnivorous mammals. *Proceedings of the National Academy of Sciences (U.S.A.), 109*, 4956–4961. (6)

Jiang, Y., Costello, P., & He, S. (2007). Processing of invisible stimuli. *Psychological Science, 18*, 349–355. (13)

Jirout, J. J., & Newcombe, N. S. (2015). Building blocks for developing spatial skills: Evidence from a large, representative U.S. sample. *Psychological Science, 26*, 302–310. (12)

Joel, D., Berman, Z., Tavor, I., Wexler, N., Gaber, O., Stein, Y., . . . Assaf, Y. (2015). *Proceedings of the National Academy of Sciences (U.S.A.), 50*, 15468–15473. (10)

Johanek, L. M., Meyer, R. A., Hartke, T., Hobelmann, J. G., Maine, D. N., LaMotte, R.

H., & Ringkamp, M. (2007). Psychophysical and physiological evidence for parallel afferent pathways mediating the sensation of itch. *Journal of Neuroscience, 27*, 7490–7497. (6)

Johansson, C., Willeit, M., Smedh, C., Ekholm, J., Paunio, T., Kieseppä, T., . . . Partonen, T. (2003). Circadian clock-related polymorphisms in seasonal affective disorder and their relevance to diurnal preference. *Neuropsychopharmacology, 28*, 734–739. (14)

Johnsen, E. L., Tranel, D., Lutgendorf, S., & Adolphs, R. (2009). A neuroanatomical dissociation for emotion induced by music. *International Journal of Psychophysiology, 72*, 24–33. (11)

Johnson, M. R., Shkura, K., Langley, S. R., Delahaye-Duriez, A., Srivastava, P., Hill, W. D., . . . Petretto, E. (2016). Systems genetics identifies a convergent gene network for cognition and neurodevelopmental disease. *Nature Neuroscience, 19*, 223–232. (12)

Johnson, P. L., Federici, L. M., Fitz, S. D., Renger, J. J., Shireman, B., Winrow, C. J., . . . Shekhar, A. (2015). Orexin 1 and 2 receptor involvement in CO_2-induced panic-associated behavior and autonomic responses. *Depression and Anxiety, 32*, 671–683. (11)

Johnsrude, I. S., Mackey, A., Hakyemez, H., Alexander, E., Trang, H. P., & Carlyon, R. P. (2013). Swinging at a cocktail party: Voice familiarity aids speech perception in the presence of a competing voice. *Psychological Science, 24*, 1995–2004. (6)

Jonas, D. E., Amick, H. R., Feltner, C., Bobashev, G., Thomas, K., Wines, R., . . . Garbutt, J. C. (2014). Pharmacology for adults with alcohol use disorders in outpatient settings: A systematic review and meta-analysis. *Journal of the American Medical Association, 311*, 1889–1900. (14)

Jones, A. R., & Shusta, E. V. (2007). Blood–brain barrier transport of therapeutics via receptor-mediation. *Pharmaceutical Research, 24*, 1759–1771. (1)

Jones, C. R., Campbell, S. S., Zone, S. E., Cooper, F., DeSano, A., Murphy, P. J., . . . Ptacek, L. J. (1999). Familial advanced sleep-phase syndrome: A short-period circadian rhythm variant in humans. *Nature Medicine, 5*, 1062–1065. (8)

Jones, C. R., Huang, A. L., Ptácek, L. J., & Fu, Y.-H. (2013). Genetic basis of human circadian rhythm disorders. *Experimental Neurology, 243*, 28–33. (8)

Jones, E. G., & Pons, T. P. (1998). Thalamic and brainstem contributions to large-scale plasticity of primate somatosensory cortex. *Science, 282*, 1121–1125. (4)

Jones, H. S., & Oswald, I. (1968). Two cases of healthy insomnia. *Electroencephalography and Clinical Neurophysiology, 24*, 378–380. (8)

Jones, P. B., Barnes, T. R. E., Davies, L., Dunn, G., Lloyd, H., Hayhurst, K. P., . . . Lewis, S. W. (2006). Randomized controlled trial of the effect on quality of life of second- vs. first-generation antipsychotic drugs in schizophrenia. *Archives of General Psychiatry, 63*, 1079–1087. (14)

Jones, W., & Klin, A. (2013). Attention to eyes is present but in decline in 2-6-month-old infants later diagnosed with autism. *Nature, 504*, 427–431. (14)

Jordan, H. A. (1969). Voluntary intragastric feeding. *Journal of Comparative and Physiological Psychology, 62*, 237–244. (9)

Jouvet, M. (1960). Telencephalic and rhombencephalic sleep in the cat. In G. E. W. Wolstenholme & M. O'Connor (Eds.), *CIBA Foundation symposium on the nature of sleep* (pp. 188–208). Boston: Little, Brown. (8)

Juda, M., Vetter, C., & Roenneberg, T. (2013). Chronotype modulates sleep duration, sleep quality, and social jet lag in shift-workers. *Journal of Biological Rhythms, 28*, 141–151. (8)

Judge, J., Caravolas, M., & Knox, P. C. (2006). Smooth pursuit eye movements and phonological processing in adults with dyslexia. *Cognitive Neuropsychology, 23*, 1174–1189. (13)

Jueptner, M., & Weiller, C. (1998). A review of differences between basal ganglia and cerebellar control of movements as revealed by functional imaging studies. *Brain, 121*, 1437–1449. (7)

Julvez, J., Méndez, M., Fernandez-Barres, S., Romaguera, D., Vioque, J., Llop, S., . . . Sunyer, J. (2016). Maternal consumption of seafood in pregnancy and child neuropsychological development: A longitudinal study based on a population with high consumption levels. *American Journal of Epidemiology, 183*, 169–182. (9)

Jumah, F., Ghannam, M., Jaber, M., Adeeb, N., & Tubbs, R. S. (2016). Neuroanatomical variation in autism spectrum disorder: A comprehensive review. *Clinical Anatomy, 29*, 454–465. (14)

Jürgensen, M., Kleinemeier, E., Lux, A., Steensma, T. D., Cohen-Kettenis, P. T., Hiort, O., . . . DSD Network Working Group. (2013). Psychosexual development in adolescents and adults with disorders of sexual development—Results from the German Clinical Evaluation Study. *Journal of Sexual Medicine, 10*, 2703–2714. (10)

Kaas, J. H. (1983). What, if anything, is SI? Organization of first somatosensory area of cortex. *Physiological Reviews, 63*, 206–231. (6)

Kaas, J. H., Merzenich, M. M., & Killackey, H. P. (1983). The reorganization of somatosensory cortex following peripheral nerve damage in adult and developing mammals. *Annual Review of Neuroscience, 6*, 325–356. (4)

Kaas, J. H., Nelson, R. J., Sur, M., Lin, C.-S., & Merzenich, M. M. (1979). Multiple representations of the body within the primary somatosensory cortex of primates. *Science, 204*, 521–523. (3)

Kaas, J. H., & Stepniewska, I. (2016). Evolution of posterior parietal cortex and parietal-frontal networks for specific actions in primates. *Journal of Comparative Neurology, 524*, 595–608. (7)

Kagan, J. (2016). An overly pessimistic extension. *Perspectives on Psychological Science, 11*, 442–450. (11)

Kaiser, A., Haller, S., Schmitz, S., & Nitsch, C. (2009). On sex/gender related similarities and differences in fMRI language research. *Brain Research Reviews, 61*, 49–59. (10)

Kales, A., Scharf, M. B., & Kales, J. D. (1978). Rebound insomnia: A new clinical syndrome. *Science, 201*, 1039–1041. (8)

Kalin, N. H., Shelton, S. E., Davidson, R. J., & Kelley, A. E. (2001). The primate amygdala mediates acute fear but not the behavioral and physiological components of anxious temperament. *Journal of Neuroscience, 21*, 2067–2074. (11)

Kaminer, Y. (2000). Contingency management reinforcement procedures for adolescent substance abuse. *Journal of the American Academy of Child and Adolescent Psychiatry, 39*, 1324–1326. (14)

Kamitani, Y., & Tong, F. (2005). Decoding the visual and subjective contents of the human brain. *Nature Neuroscience, 8*, 679–685. (13)

Kandel, E. R., & Schwartz, J. H. (1982). Molecular biology of learning: Modulation of transmitter release. *Science, 218*, 433–443. (12)

Kántor, O., Mezey, S., Adeghate, J., Naumann, A., Nitschke, R., Énzsöly, A., . . . Völgyi, B. (2016). Calcium buffer proteins are specific markers of human retinal neurons. *Cell and Tissue Research, 365*, 29–50. (5)

Kanwisher, N. (2010). Functional specificity in the human brain: A window into the functional architecture of the mind. *Proceedings of the National Academy of Sciences, 107*, 11163–11170. (5)

Kanwisher, N., & Yovel, G. (2006). The fusiform face area: A cortical region specialized for the perception of faces. *Philosophical Transactions of the Royal Society, B, 361*, 2109–2128. (5)

Kaplan, B. J., Rucklidge, J. J., Romijn, A., & McLeod, K. (2015). The emerging field of nutritional mental health: Inflammation, the microbiome, oxidative stress, and mitochondrial function. *Clinical Psychological Science, 3*, 964–980. (14)

Kapur, S., Zipusky, R., Jones, C., Shammi, C. S., Remington, G., & Seeman, P. (2000). A positron emission tomography study of quetiapine in schizophrenia. *Archives of General Psychiatry, 57*, 553–559. (14)

Karg, K., Burmeister, M., Shedden, K., & Sen, S. (2011). The serotonin transporter promoter variant (5-HTTLPR), stress, and depression meta-analysis revisited. *Archives of General Psychiatry, 68*, 444–454. (14)

Kargo, W. J., & Nitz, D. A. (2004). Improvements in the signal-to-noise ratio of motor cortex cells distinguish early versus late phases of motor skill learning. *Journal of Neuroscience, 24*, 5560–5569. (7)

Karlsson, M., & Frank, L. M. (2009). Awake replay of remote experiences in the hippocampus. *Nature Neuroscience, 12*, 913–918. (8)

Karmiloff-Smith, A., Tyler, L. K., Voice, K., Sims, K., Udwin, O., Howlin, P., & Davises,

M. (1998). Linguistic dissociations in Williams syndrome: Evaluating receptive syntax in on-line and off-line tasks. *Neuropsychologia, 36,* 343–351. (13)

Karnath, H. O., Rüter, J., Mandler, A., & Himmelbach, M. (2009). The anatomy of object recognition: Visual form agnosia caused by medial occipitotemporal stroke. *Journal of Neuroscience, 29,* 5854–5862. (5)

Karns, C. M., Dow, M. W., & Neville, H. J. (2012). Altered cross-modal processing in the primary auditory cortex of congenitally deaf adults: A visual-somatosensory fMRI study with a double-flash illusion. *Journal of Neuroscience, 32,* 9626–638. (4)

Karra, E., O'Daly, O. G., Choudhury, A. I., Yousseif, A., Millership, S., Neary, M. T., . . . Batterham, R. L. (2013). A link between FTO, ghrelin, and impaired brain food-cue responsivity. *Journal of Clinical Investigation, 123,* 3539–3551. (9)

Karrer, T., & Bartoshuk, L. (1991). Capsaicin desensitization and recovery on the human tongue. *Physiology & Behavior, 49,* 757–764. (6)

Kas, M. J. H., Tiesjema, B., van Dijk, G., Garner, K. M., Barsh, G. S., Ter Brake, O., . . . Adan, R. A. H. (2004). Induction of brain region-specific forms of obesity by agouti. *Journal of Neuroscience, 24,* 10176–10181. (9)

Katz, L. N., Yates, J. L., Pillow, J. W., & Huk, A. C. (2016). Dissociated functional significance of decision-related activity in the primate dorsal stream. *Nature, 535,* 285–288. (13)

Kavanau, J. L. (1998). Vertebrates that never sleep: Implications for sleep's basic function. *Brain Research Bulletin, 46,* 269–279. (8)

Kay, C., Collins, J. A., Miedzybrodzka, Z., Madore, S. J., Gordon, E. S., Gerry, N., . . . Hayden, M. R. (2016). Huntington disease reduced penetrance alleles occur at high frequency in the general population. *Neurology, 87,* 282–288. (7)

Kayyal, M. H., & Russell, J. A. (2013). Americans and Palestinians judge spontaneous facial expressions of emotion. *Emotion, 13,* 891–904. (11)

Kazama, A. M., Heurer, E., Davis, M., & Bachevalier, J. (2012). Effects of neonatal amygdala lesions on fear learning, conditioned inhibition, and extinction in adult macaques. *Behavioral Neuroscience, 126,* 392–403. (11)

Kazén, M., Kuenne, T., Frankenberg, H., & Quirin, M. (2012). Inverse relation between cortisol and anger and their relation to performance and explicit memory. *Biological Psychology, 91,* 28–35. (11)

Keefe, R. S. E., Silverman, J. M., Mohs, R. C., Siever, L. J., Harvey, P. D., Friedman, L., . . . Davis, K. L. (1997). Eye tracking, attention, and schizotypal symptoms in nonpsychotic relatives of patients with schizophrenia. *Archives of General Psychiatry, 54,* 169–176. (14)

Keele, S. W., & Ivry, R. (1990). Does the cerebellum provide a common computation for diverse tasks? *Annals of the New York Academy of Sciences, 608,* 179–207. (7)

Keers, R., & Uher, R. (2012). Gene-environment interaction in major depression and antidepressant treatment response. *Current Psychiatry Reports, 14,* 129–137. (14)

Keiser, M. S., Kordasiewicz, H. B., & McBride, J. L. (2016). Gene suppression strategies for dominantly inherited neurodegenerative diseases: Lessons from Huntington's disease and spinocerebellar ataxia. *Human Molecular Genetics, 25,* R53–R64. (7)

Kelly, T. L., Neri, D. F., Grill, J. T., Ryman, D., Hunt, P. D., Dijk, D.-J., . . . Czeisler, C. A. (1999). Nonentrained circadian rhythms of melatonin in submariners scheduled to an 18-hour day. *Journal of Biological Rhythms, 14,* 190–196. (8)

Kendler, K. S. (1983). Overview: A current perspective on twin studies of schizophrenia. *American Journal of Psychiatry, 140,* 1413–1425. (14)

Kendler, K. S., Fiske, A., Gardner, C. O., & Gatz, M. (2009). Delineation of two genetic pathways to major depression. *Biological Psychiatry, 65,* 808–811. (14)

Kendler, K. S., Gardner, C. O., & Prescott, C. A. (1999). Clinical characteristics of major depression that predict risk of depression in relatives. *Archives of General Psychiatry, 56,* 322–327. (14)

Kendler, K. S., Turkheimer, E., Ohlsson, H., Sundquist, J., & Sundquist, K. (2015). Family environment and the malleability of cognitive ability: A Swedish national home-reared and adopted-away cosibling control study. *Proceedings of the National Academy of Sciences (U.S.A.), 112,* 4612–4617. (12)

Kennard, C., Lawden, M., Morland, A. B., & Ruddock, K. H. (1995). Colour identification and colour constancy are impaired in a patient with incomplete achromatopsia associated with prestriate cortical lesions. *Proceedings of the Royal Society of London, B, 260,* 169–175. (5)

Kennaway, D. J., & Van Dorp, C. F. (1991). Free-running rhythms of melatonin, cortisol, electrolytes, and sleep in humans in Antarctica. *American Journal of Physiology, 260,* R1137–R1144. (8)

Kennedy, D. P., & Adolphs, R. (2010). Impaired fixation to eyes following amygdala damage arises from abnormal bottom-up attention. *Neuropsychologia, 48,* 3392–3398. (11)

Kennedy, D. P., Gläscher, J., Tyszka, J. M., & Adolphs, R. (2009). Personal space regulation by the human amygdala. *Nature Neuroscience, 12,* 1226–1227. (11)

Kennerley, S. W., Diedrichsen, J., Hazeltine, E., Semjen, A., & Ivry, R. B. (2002). Callosotomy patients exhibit temporal uncoupling during continuous bimanual movements. *Nature Neuroscience, 5,* 376–381. (13)

Kerchner, G. A., & Nicoll, R. A. (2008). Silent synapses and the emergence of a postsynaptic mechanism for LTP. *Nature Reviews Neuroscience, 9,* 813–825. (12)

Kerns, J. G. (2007). Experimental manipulation of cognitive control processes causes an increase in communication disturbances in healthy volunteers. *Psychological Medicine, 37,* 995–1004. (14)

Keshavan, M. S., Diwadkar, V. A., Montrose, D. M., Rajarethinam, R., & Sweeney, J. A. (2005). Premorbid indicators and risk for schizophrenia: A selective review and update. *Schizophrenia Research, 79,* 45–57. (14)

Kesner, R. P., Gilbert, P. E., & Barua, L. A. (2002). The role of the hippocampus in meaning for the temporal order of a sequence of odors. *Behavioral Neuroscience, 116,* 286–290. (12)

Kety, S. S., Wender, P. H., Jacobson, B., Ingraham, L. J., Jansson, L., Faber, B., & Kinney, D. K. (1994). Mental illness in the biological and adoptive relatives of schizophrenic adoptees. *Archives of General Psychiatry, 51,* 442–455. (14)

Keverne, E. B. (1999). The vomeronasal organ. *Science, 286,* 716–720. (6)

Khakh, B. J., & Sofroniew, M. V. (2015). Diversity of astrocyte functions and phenotypes in neural circuits. *Nature Reviews Neuroscience, 18,* 942–952. (1)

Khashan, A. S., Abel, K. M., McNamee, R., Pedersen, M. G., Webb, R. T., Baker, P. N., . . . Mortensen, P. B. (2008). Higher risk of offspring schizophrenia following antenatal maternal exposure to severe adverse life events. *Archives of General Psychiatry, 65,* 146–152. (14)

Kiesner, J., Mendle, J., Eisenlohr-Moul, T. A., & Pastore, M. (2016). Clinical symptom change across the menstrual cycle: Attributional, affective, and physical symptoms. *Clinical Psychological Science, 4,* 882–894. (10)

Kilgour, A. R., de Gelder, B., & Lederman, S. J. (2004). Haptic face recognition and prosopagnosia. *Neuropsychologia, 42,* 707–712. (5)

Killeffer, F. A., & Stern, W. E. (1970). Chronic effects of hypothalamic injury. *Archives of Neurology, 22,* 419–429. (9)

Kilner, J. M., Neal, A., Weiskopf, N., Friston, K. J., & Frith, C. D. (2009). Evidence of mirror neurons in human inferior frontal gyrus. *Journal of Neuroscience, 29,* 10153–10159. (7)

Kim, E. J., Pellman, B., & Kim, J. J. (2015). Stress effects on the hippocampus: A critical review. *Learning & Memory, 22,* 411–416. (11)

Kim, J. G., Suyama, S., Koch, M., Jin, S., Argente-Arizon, P., . . . Horvath, T. L. (2014). Leptin signaling in astrocytes regulates hypothalamic neuronal circuits and feeding. *Nature Neuroscience, 17,* 908–910. (1)

Kim, P., Strathearn, L., & Swain, J. E. (2016). The maternal brain and its plasticity in humans. *Hormones and Behavior, 77,* 113–123. (10)

Kim, S.-Y., Adhikari, A., Lee, S. Y., Marshel, J. H., Kim, C. K., Mallory, C. S., . . . Deisseroth, K. (2013). Diverging neural pathways assemble a behavioural state from separable features in anxiety. *Nature, 496,* 219–223. (11)

Kim, U., Jorgenson, E., Coon, H., Leppert, M., Risch, N., & Drayna, D. (2003). Positional cloning of the human quantitative trait locus underlying taste sensitivity to phenylthiocarbamide. *Science, 299,* 1221–1225. (6)

Kim-Han, J. S., Antenor-Dorsey, J. A., & O'Malley, K. L. (2011). The Parkinsonian mimetic, MPP+, specifically impairs mitochondrial transport in dopamine axons. *Journal of Neuroscience, 31,* 7212–7221. (7)

King, B. M., Smith, R. L., & Frohman, L. A. (1984). Hyperinsulinemia in rats with ventromedial hypothalamic lesions: Role of hyperphagia. *Behavioral Neuroscience, 98,* 152–155. (9)

Kinnamon, J. C. (1987). Organization and innervation of taste buds. In T. E. Finger & W. L. Silver (Eds.), *Neurobiology of taste and smell* (pp. 277–297). New York: Wiley. (6)

Kinoshita, M., Matsui, R., Kato, S., Hasegawa, T., Kasahara, H., . . . Isa, T. (2012). Genetic dissection of the circuit for hand dexterity in primates. *Nature, 487,* 235–238. (7)

Kinsey, A. C., Pomeroy, W. B., & Martin, C. E. (1948). *Sexual behavior in the human male.* Philadelphia: Saunders. (10)

Kinsey, A. C., Pomeroy, W. B., Martin, C. E., & Gebhard, P. H. (1953). *Sexual behavior in the human female.* Philadelphia: Saunders. (10)

Kiriakakis, V., Bhatia, K. P., Quinn, N. P., & Marsden, C. D. (1998). The natural history of tardive dyskinesia: A long-term follow-up study of 107 cases. *Brain, 121,* 2053–2066. (14)

Kirkpatrick, P. J., Smielewski, P., Czosnyka, M., Menon, D. K., & Pickard, J. D. (1995). Near-infrared spectroscopy in patients with head injury. *Journal of Neurosurgery, 83,* 963–970. (4)

Kirsch, I. (2010). *The Emperor's New Drugs.* New York: Basic Books. (14)

Kirsch, I., Deacon, B. J., Huedo-Medina, T. B., Scoboria, A., Moore, T. J., & Johnson, B. T. (2008). Initial severity and antidepressant benefits: A meta-analysis of data submitted to the Food and Drug Administration. *PLoS Medicine, 5,* e45. (14)

Klawans, H. L. (1988). *Toscanini's fumble and other tales of clinical neurology.* Chicago: Contemporary Books. (3)

Kleen, J. K., Sitomer, M. T., Killeen, P. R., & Conrad, C. D. (2006). Chronic stress impairs spatial memory and motivation for reward without disrupting motor ability and motivation to explore. *Behavioral Neuroscience, 120,* 842–851. (11)

Kleiber, M. L., Mantha, K., Stringer, R. L., & Singh, S. M. (2013). Neurodevelopmental alcohol exposure elicits long-term changes to gene expression that alter distinct molecular pathways dependent on timing of exposure. *Journal of Neurodevelopmental Disorders, 5,* article 6. (4)

Klein, D. F. (1993). False suffocation alarms, spontaneous panics, and related conditions. *Archives of General Psychiatry, 50,* 306–317. (11)

Kleitman, N. (1963). *Sleep and wakefulness* (Rev. ed.). Chicago: University of Chicago Press. (8)

Klengel, T., Mehta, D., Anacker, C., Rex-Haffner, M., Pruessner, J. C., Pariante, C. M., . . . Binder, E. B. (2013). Allele-specific *FKBP5* DNA demethylation mediates gene-childhood trauma interactions. *Nature Neuroscience, 16,* 33–41. (4)

Kluger, M. J. (1991). Fever: Role of pyrogens and cryogens. *Physiological Reviews, 71,* 93–127. (9)

Klüver, H., & Bucy, P. C. (1939). Preliminary analysis of functions of the temporal lobes in monkeys. *Archives of Neurology and Psychiatry, 42,* 979–1000. (3)

Knyazev, G. G., Slobodskaya, H. R., & Wilson, G. D. (2002). Psychophysiological correlates of behavioural inhibition and activation. *Personality and Individual Differences, 33,* 647–660. (11)

Ko, C.-H., Liu, G.-C., Hsiao, S., Yen, J.-Y., Yang, M.-J., Lin, W.-C., . . . Chen, C. S. (2009). Brain activities associated with gaming urge of online gaming addiction. *Journal of Psychiatric Research, 43,* 739–747. (14)

Koban, L., & Wager, T. D. (2016). Beyond conformity: Social influences on pain reports and physiology. *Emotion, 16,* 24–32. (6)

Kobayakawa, K., Kobayakawa, R., Matsumoto, H., Oka, Y., Imai, T., Ikawa, M., . . . Sakano, H. (2007). Innate versus learned odour processing in the mouse olfactory bulb. *Nature, 450,* 503–508. (6)

Kobelt, P., Paulitsch, S., Goebel, M., Stengel, A., Schmidtmann, M., van der Voort, I. R., . . . Monnikes, H. (2006). Peripheral injection of CCK-8S induces Fos expression in the dorsomedial hypothalamic nucleus in rats. *Brain Research, 1117,* 109–117. (9)

Kochunov, P., & Hong, L. E. (2014). Neurodevelopmental and neurodegenerative models of schizophrenia: White matter at the center stage. *Schizophrenia Bulletin, 40,* 721–728. (14)

Koenigs, M., Huey, E. D., Raymont, V., Cheon, B., Solomon, J., Wassermann, E. M., & Grafman, J. (2008). Focal brain damage protects against post-traumatic stress disorder in combat veterans. *Nature Neuroscience, 11,* 232–237. (11)

Koenigs, M., Young, L., Adolphs, R., Tranel, D., Cushman, F., Hauser, M., & Damasio, A. (2007). Damage to the prefrontal cortex increases utilitarian moral judgments. *Nature, 446,* 908–911. (11)

Koepp, M. J., Gunn, R. N., Lawrence, A. D., Cunningham, V. J., Dagher, A., Jones, T., . . . Grasby, P. M. (1998). Evidence for striatal dopamine release during a video game. *Nature, 393,* 266–268. (14)

Kogan, A., Oveis, C., Carr, E. W., Gruber, J., Mauss, I. B., Shallcross, A., . . . Keltner, D. (2014). Vagal activity is quadratically related to prosocial traits, prosocial emotions, and observer perceptions of prosociality. *Journal of Personality and Social Psychology, 107,* 1051–1063. (11)

Kohler, E., Keysers, C., Umiltà, M. A., Fogassi, L., Gallese, V., & Rizzolatti, G. (2002). Hearing sounds, understanding actions: Action representation in mirror neurons. *Science, 297,* 846–848. (7)

Kohn, M. (2008). The needs of the many. *Nature, 456,* 296–299. (4)

Koleske, A. J. (2013). Molecular mechanisms of dendrite stability. *Nature Reviews Neuroscience, 14,* 536–550. (4)

Komisaruk, B. R., Adler, N. T., & Hutchison, J. (1972). Genital sensory field: Enlargement by estrogen treatment in female rats. *Science, 178,* 1295–1298. (10)

Komorowski, R. W., Manns, J. R., & Eichenbaum, H. (2009). Robust conjunctive item-lace coding by hippocampal neurons parallels learning what happens where. *Journal of Neuroscience, 29,* 9918–9929. (12)

Komura, Y., Tamura, R., Uwano, T., Nishijo, H., Kaga, K., & Ono, T. (2001). Retrospective and prospective coding for predicted reward in the sensory thalamus. *Nature, 412,* 546–549. (3)

Konadhode, R. R., Pelluru, D., & Shiromani, P. J. (2015). Neurons containing orexin or melanin concentrating hormone reciprocally regulate wake and sleep. *Frontiers in Systems Neuroscience, 8,* article UNSP244. (8)

Kondoh, K. Lu, Z., Ye, X., Olson, D. P., Lowell, B. B., & Buck, L. B. (2016). A specific area of olfactory cortex involved in stress hormone responses to predator odours. *Nature, 532,* 103–106. (6)

Kong, A., Frigge, M. L., Masson, G., Besenbacher, S., Sulem, P., Magnusson, G., . . . Stefansson, K. (2012). Rate of *de novo* mutations and the importance of father's age to disease risk. *Nature, 488,* 471–475. (14)

Konishi, S., Nakajima, K., Uchida, I., Kameyama, M., Nakahara, K., Sekihara, K., & Miyashita, Y. (1998). Transient activation of inferior prefrontal cortex during cognitive set shifting. *Nature Neuroscience, 1,* 80–84. (14)

Konopka, G., Bomar, J. M., Winden, K., Coppola, G., Jonsson, Z. O., Gao, F., . . . Geschwind, D. H. (2009). Human specific transcriptional regulation of CNS development genes by *FOXP2. Nature, 462,* 213–217. (4, 13)

Koralek, A. C., Jin, X., Long, J. D. II, Costa, R. M., & Carmena, J. M. (2012). Corticostriatal plasticity is necessary for learning intentional neuroprosthetic skills. *Nature, 483,* 331–335. (12)

Korman, M., Doyon, J., Doljansky, J., Carrier, J., Dagan, Y., & Karni, A. (2007). Daytime sleep condenses the time course of motor memory consolidation. *Nature Neuroscience, 10,* 1206–1213. (8)

Kornhuber, H. H. (1974). Cerebral cortex, cerebellum, and basal ganglia: An introduction to their motor functions. In F. O. Schmitt & F. G. Worden (Eds.), *The neurosciences: Third study program* (pp. 267–280). Cambridge, MA: MIT Press. (7)

Korpi, E. R., den Hollander, B., Farooq, U., Vashchinkina, E., Rajkumar, R., Nutt, D. J., . . . Dawe, G. S. (2015). Mechanisms of action and persistent neuroplasticity by drugs of abuse. *Pharmacological Reviews, 67*, 872–1004. (14)

Kosslyn, S. M., Ganis, G., & Thompson, W. L. (2001). Neural foundations of imagery. *Nature Reviews Neuroscience, 2*, 635–642. (5)

Kosslyn, S. M., & Thompson, W. L. (2003). When is early visual cortex activated during visual mental imagery? *Psychological Bulletin, 129*, 723–746. (5)

Kostrzewa, R. M., Kostrzewa, J. P., Brown, R. W., Nowak, P., & Brus, R. (2008). Dopamine receptor supersensitivity: Development, mechanisms, presentation, and clinical applicability. *Neurotoxicity Research, 14*, 121–128. (4)

Kotowicz, Z. (2007). The strange case of Phineas Gage. *History of the Human Sciences, 20*, 115–131. (11)

Kotrschal, A., Rogell, B., Bundsen, A., Svensson, B., Zajitschek, S., Brännström, I., . . . Kolm, N. (2013). Artificial selection on relative brain size in the guppy reveals costs and benefits of evolving a larger brain. *Current Biology, 23*, 168–171. (4)

Kourtzi, Z., & Kanwisher, N. (2000). Activation in human MT/MST by static images with implied motion. *Journal of Cognitive Neuroscience, 12*, 48–55. (5)

Kovach, C. K., Daw, N. D., Rudrauf, D., Tranel, D., & O'Doherty, J. P. (2012). Anterior prefrontal cortex contributes to action selection through tracking of recent reward trends. *Journal of Neuroscience, 32*, 8434–8442. (12)

Kraemer, D. J. M., Macrae, C. N., Green, A. E., & Kelley, W. M. (2005). Sound of silence activates auditory cortex. *Nature, 434*, 158. (6)

Kraft, I., Cafiero, R., Schaadt, G., Brauer, J., Neef, N. E., Müller, B., . . . Skeide, M. A. (2015). Cortical differences in preliterate children at familiar risk of dyslexia are similar to those observed in dyslexic readers. *Brain, 138*, e378. (13)

Krajbich, I., Adolphs, R., Tranel, D., Denburg, N. L., & Camerer, C. F. (2009). Economic games quantify diminished sense of guilt in patients with damage to the prefrontal cortex. *Journal of Neuroscience, 29*, 2188–2192. (11)

Krakauer, A. H. (2005). Kin selection and cooperative courtship in wild turkeys. *Nature, 434*, 69–72. (4)

Kramer, P., & Bressan, P. (2015). Humans as superorganisms: How microbes, viruses, imprinted genes, and other selfish entities shape our behavior. *Perspectives on Psychological Science, 10*, 464–481. (14)

Krashes, M. J., Lowell, B. B., & Garfield, A. S. (2016). Melanocortin-4 receptor-regulated energy homeostasis. *Nature Neuroscience, 19*, 206–219. (9)

Krause, E. G., & Sakal, R. R. (2007). Richter and sodium appetite: From adrenalectomy to molecular biology. *Appetite, 49*, 353–367. (9)

Kravitz, A. V., Tye, L. D., & Kreitzer, A. C. (2012). Distinct roles for direct and indirect pathway striatal neurons in reinforcement. *Nature Neuroscience, 15*, 816–818. (7)

Kreiman, G., Fried, I., & Koch, C. (2002). Single-neuron correlates of subjective vision in the human medial temporal lobe. *Proceedings of the National Academy of Sciences (U.S.A.), 99*, 8378–8383. (13)

Krishnan, A., Zhang, R., Yao, V., Theesfeld, C. L., Wong, A. K., Tadych, A., . . . Troyanskaya, O. G. (2016). Genome-wide prediction and functional characterization of the genetic basis of autism spectrum disorder. *Nature Neuroscience, 19*, 1454–1462. (14)

Kristensson, K. (2011). Microbes' roadmap to neurons. *Nature Reviews Neuroscience, 12*, 345–357. (1)

Kropff, E., Carmichael, J. E., Moser, M.-B., & Moser, E. I. (2015). Speed cells in the medial entorhinal cortex. *Nature, 523*, 419–424. (12)

Kross, E., Berman, M. G., Mischel, W., Smith, E. E., & Wager, T. D. (2011). Social rejection shares somatosensory representations with physical pain. *Proceedings of the National Academy of Sciences (U.S.A.), 108*, 6270–6275. (6)

Krueger, J. M., Rector, D. M., Roy, S., Van Dongen, H. P. A., Belenky, G., & Panksepp, J. (2008). Sleep as a fundamental property of neuronal assemblies. *Nature Reviews Neuroscience, 9*, 910–919. (8)

Krupa, D. J., Thompson, J. K., & Thompson, R. F. (1993). Localization of a memory trace in the mammalian brain. *Science, 260*, 989–991. (12)

Kuba, H., Ishii, T. M., & Ohmori, H. (2006). Axonal site of spike initiation enhances auditory coincidence detection. *Nature, 444*, 1069–1072. (1)

Kubista, H., & Boehm, S. (2006). Molecular mechanisms underlying the modulation of exocytotic noradrenaline release via presynaptic receptors. *Pharmacology & Therapeutics, 112*, 213–242. (2)

Kuczewski, N., Porcer, C., Ferrand, N., Fiorentino, H., Pellegrino, C., Kolarow, R., . . . Gaiarsa, J. L. (2008). Backpropagating action potentials trigger dendritic release of BDNF during spontaneous network activity. *Journal of Neuroscience, 28*, 7013–7023. (12)

Kujala, T., Myllyviita, K., Tervaniemi, M., Alho, K., Kallio, J., & Näätänen, R. (2000). Basic auditory dysfunction in dyslexia as demonstrated by brain activity measurements. *Psychophysiology, 37*, 262–266. (13)

Kujawa, S. G., & Liberman, M. C. (2009). Adding insult to injury: Cochlear nerve degeneration after "temporary" noise-induced hearing loss. *Journal of Neuroscience, 29*, 14077–14085. (6)

Kukkonen, J. P. (2013). Physiology of the orexinergic/hypocretinergic system: A revisit in 2012. *American Journal of Physiology, 304*, C2–C32. (8)

Kullmann, D. M., & Lamsa, K. P. (2007). Long-term synaptic plasticity in hippocampal interneurons. *Nature Reviews Neuroscience, 8*, 687–699. (2)

Kumar, V., Croxson, P. L., & Simonyan, K. (2016). Structural organization of the laryngeal motor cortical network and its implication for evolution of speech production. *Journal of Neuroscience, 36*, 4170–4181. (13)

Kumpik, D. P., Kacelnik, O., & King, A. J. (2010). Adaptive reweighting of auditory localization cues in response to chronic unilateral earplugging in humans. *Journal of Neuroscience, 30*, 4883–4894. (6)

Kupfermann, I., Castellucci, V., Pinsker, H., & Kandel, E. (1970). Neuronal correlates of habituation and dishabituation of the gill withdrawal reflex in *Aplysia*. *Science, 167*, 1743–1745. (12)

Kurth, F., Jancke, L., & Luders, E. (2017). Sexual dimorphism of Broca's area: More gray matter in female brains in Brodmann areas 44 and 45. *Journal of Neuroscience Research, 95*, 626–632. (12)

Kuypers, H. G. J. M. (1989). Motor system organization. In G. Adelman (Ed.), *Neuroscience year* (pp. 107–110). Boston: Birkhäuser. (7)

Labouèbe, G., Boutrel, B., Tarussio, D., & Thorens, B. (2016). Glucose-responsive neurons of the paraventricular thalamus control sucrose-seeking behavior. *Nature Neuroscience, 19*, 999–1002. (9)

Laburn, H. P. (1996). How does the fetus cope with thermal challenges? *News in Physiological Sciences, 11*, 96–100. (4, 14)

La Delfa, N. J., Garcia, D. B. L., Cappelletto, J. A. M., McDonald, A. C., Lyons, J. L., & Lee, T. D. (2013). The gunslinger effect: Why are movements made faster when responding to versus initiating an action? *Journal of Motor Behavior, 45*, 85–90. (7)

Laeng, B., & Caviness, V. S. (2001). Prosopagnosia as a deficit in encoding curved surfaces. *Journal of Cognitive Neuroscience, 13*, 556–576. (5)

Laeng, B., Svartdal, F., & Oelmann, H. (2004). Does color synesthesia pose a paradox for early-selection theories of attention? *Psychological Science, 15*, 277–281. (6)

Lahti, T. A., Leppämäki, S., Ojanen, S.-M., Haukka, J., Tuulio-Henriksson, A., Lönnqvist, J., & Partonen, T. (2006). Transition into daylight saving time influences the fragmentation of the rest–activity cycle. *Journal of Circadian Rhythms, 4*, 1. (8)

Lai, C. S. L., Fisher, S. E., Hurst, J. A., Vargha-Khadem, F., & Monaco, A. P. (2001). A forkhead-domain gene is mutated in a severe speech and language disorder. *Nature, 413*, 519–523. (13)

Lake, R. I. E., Eaves, L. J., Maes, H. H. M., Heath, A. C., & Martin, N. G. (2000). Further evidence against the environmental transmission of individual differences in neuroticism from a collaborative study of 45,850 twins and relatives on two continents. *Behavior Genetics, 30*, 223–233. (4)

Lakatos, P., Schroeder, C. E., Leitman, D. I., & Javitt, D. C. (2013). Predictive suppression of cortical excitability and its deficit in schizophrenia. *Journal of Neuroscience, 33*, 11692–11702. (14)

Lambie, J. A., & Marcel, A. J. (2002). Consciousness and the varieties of emotion experience: A theoretical framework. *Psychological Review, 109,* 219–259. (13)

Lamminmäki, A., Hines, M., Kuiri-Hänninen, T., Kilpeläinen, L., Dunkel, L., & Sankilampi, U. (2012). Testosterone measured in infancy predicts subsequent sex-typed behavior in boys and girls. *Hormones and Behavior, 61,* 611–616. (10)

Land, E. H., Hubel, D. H., Livingstone, M. S., Perry, S. H., & Burns, M. M. (1983). Colour-generating interactions across the corpus callosum. *Nature, 303,* 616–618. (5)

Landis, D. M. D. (1987). Initial junctions between developing parallel fibers and Purkinje cells are different from mature synaptic junctions. *Journal of Comparative Neurology, 260,* 513–525. (2)

Lang, P. J. (2014). Emotion's response patterns: The brain and the autonomic nervous system. *Emotion Review, 6,* 93–99. (11)

Långsjö, J. W., Alkire, M. T., Kaskinoro, K., Hayama, H., Maksimow, A., Kaisti, K. K., . . . Scheinin, H. (2012). Returning from oblivion: Imagining the neural core of consciousness. *Journal of Neuroscience, 32,* 4935–4943. (13)

Långström, N., Rahman, Q., Carlström, E., & Lichtenstein, P. (2010). Genetic and environmental effects on same-sex sexual behavior: A population study of twins in Sweden. *Archives of Sexual Behavior, 39,* 75–80. (10)

Larsen, B., & Luna, B. (2015). In vivo evidence of neurophysiological maturation of the human adolescent striatum. *Developmental Cognitive Neuroscience, 12,* 74–85. (4)

Lashley, K. S. (1929). *Brain mechanisms and intelligence.* Chicago: University of Chicago Press. (12)

Lashley, K. S. (1930). Basic neural mechanisms in behavior. *Psychological Review, 37,* 1–24. (12)

Lashley, K. S. (1950). In search of the engram. *Symposia of the Society for Experimental Biology, 4,* 454–482. (12)

Latimer, K. W., Yates, J. L., Meister, M. L. R., Huk, A. C., & Pillow, J. W. (2015). Single-trial spike trains in parietal cortex reveal discrete steps during decision-making. *Science, 349,* 184–187. (13)

Lau, H. C., Rogers, R. D., Haggard, P., & Passingham, R. E. (2004). Attention to intention. *Science, 303,* 1208–1210. (7)

Laurent, J.-P., Cespuglio, R., & Jouvet, M. (1974). Dèlimitation des voies ascendantes de l'activité ponto-génículo-occipitale chez le chat [Demarcation of the ascending paths of ponto-geniculo-occipital activity in the cat]. *Brain Research, 65,* 29–52. (8)

Lauterborn, J. C., Palmer, L. C., Jia, Y., Pham, D. T., Hou, B., Wang, W., . . . Lynch, G. (2016). Chronic ampakine treatments stimulate dendritic growth and promote learning in middle-aged rats. *Journal of Neuroscience, 36,* 1636–1646. (12)

Lavidor, M., & Walsh, V. (2004). The nature of foveal representation. *Nature Reviews Neuroscience, 5,* 729–735. (13)

Lavzin, M., Rapoport, S., Polsky, A., Garion, L., & Schiller, J. (2012). Nonlinear dendritic processing determines angular tuning of barrel cortex neurons in vivo. *Nature, 490,* 397–401. (2)

Leaver, A. M., & Rauschecker, J. P. (2016). Functional topography of human auditory cortex. *Journal of Neuroscience, 36,* 1416–1428. (6)

Leber, A. B. (2010). Neural predictors of within-subject fluctuations in attentional control. *Journal of Neuroscience, 30,* 11458–11465. (13)

LeDoux, J. (1996). *The emotional brain.* New York: Simon & Schuster. (11)

Lee, B. K., & McGrath, J. J. (2015). Advancing parental age and autism: multifactorial pathways. *Trends in Molecular Medicine, 21,* 118–125. (14)

Lee, P.-C., Bordelon, Y., Bronstein, J., & Ritz, B. (2012). Traumatic brain injury, paraquat exposure, and their relationship to Parkinson disease. *Neurology, 79,* 2061–2066. (7)

Lee, H. L., Devlin, J. T., Shakeshaft, C., Stewart, L. H., Brennan, A., Glensman, J., . . . Price, C. J. (2007). Anatomical traces of vocabulary acquisition in the adolescent brain. *Journal of Neuroscience, 27,* 1184–1189. (3)

Lee, K. M., Skoe, E., Kraus, N., & Ashley, R. (2009). Selective subcortical enhancement of musical intervals in musicians. *Journal of Neuroscience, 29,* 5832–5840. (4)

Lee, M. G., Hassani, O. K., & Jones, B. E. (2005). Discharge of identified orexin/hypocretin neurons across the sleep-waking cycle. *Journal of Neuroscience, 25,* 6716–6720. (8)

Lee, Y., Morrison, B. M., Li, Y., Lengacher, S., Farah, M. H., . . . Rothstein, J. D. (2012). Oligodendroglia metabolically support axons and contribute to neurodegeneration. *Nature, 487,* 443–448. (1)

Lee, Y.-J., Lee, S., Chang, M., & Kwak, H.-W. (2015). Saccadic movement deficiencies in adults with ADHD tendencies. *ADHD Attention Deficit and Hyperactivity Disorders, 7,* 271–280. (7)

Legrand, L. N., Iacono, W. G., & McGue, M. (2005, March/April). Predicting addiction. *American Scientist, 93,* 140–147. (14)

Lehky, S. R. (2000). Deficits in visual feature binding under isoluminant conditions. *Journal of Cognitive Neuroscience, 12,* 383–392. (3)

Lehrman, D. S. (1964). The reproductive behavior of ring doves. *Scientific American, 211*(5), 48–54. (10)

Lehrer, J. (2009). Small, furry . . . and smart. *Nature, 461,* 862–864. (12)

Leibniz, G. (1989). *The Principles of Nature and Grace, Based on Reason.* Dordrecht, Netherlands: Kluwer Publishers. (Original work published 1714) (0)

Leibowitz, S. F., & Alexander, J. T. (1991). Analysis of neuropeptide Y-induced feeding: Dissociation of Y_1 and Y_2 receptor effects on natural meal patterns. *Peptides, 12,* 1251–1260. (9)

Leibowitz, S. F., & Hoebel, B. G. (1998). Behavioral neuroscience of obesity. In G. A. Bray, C. Bouchard, & P. T. James (Eds.), *Handbook of obesity* (pp. 313–358). New York: Dekker. (9)

Lein, E. S., & Shatz, C. J. (2001). Neurotrophins and refinement of visual circuitry. In W. M. Cowan, T. C. Südhof, & C. F. Stevens (Eds.), *Synapses* (pp. 613–649). Baltimore: Johns Hopkins University Press. (5)

Leinders-Zufall, T., Lane, A. P., Puche, A. C., Ma, W., Novotny, M. V., Shipley, M. T., & Zufall, F. (2000). Ultrasensitive pheromone detection by mammalian vomeronasal neurons. *Nature, 405,* 792–796. (6)

Lelieveld, S. H., Reijnders, M. R. F., Pfundt, R., Yntema, H. G., Kamsteeg, E.-J., de Vries, P., . . . Gilissen, C. (2016). Meta-analysis of 2,104 trios provides support for 10 new genes for intellectual disability. *Nature Neuroscience, 19,* 1194–1196. (12)

Lemos, B., Araripe, L. O., & Hartl, D. L. (2008). Polymorphic Y chromosomes harbor cryptic variation with manifold functional consequences. *Science, 319,* 91–93. (10)

Lenggenhager, B., Tadi, T., Metzinger, T., & Blanke, O. (2007). Video ergo sum: Manipulating bodily self-consciousness. *Science, 317,* 1096–1099. (3)

Lenhart, R. E., & Katkin, E. S. (1986). Psychophysiological evidence for cerebral laterality effects in a high-risk sample of students with subsyndromal bipolar depressive disorder. *American Journal of Psychiatry, 143,* 602–607. (14)

Lenz, F. A., & Byl, N. N. (1999). Reorganization in the cutaneous core of the human thalamic principal somatic sensory nucleus (ventral caudal) in patients with dystonia. *Journal of Neurophysiology, 82,* 3204–3212. (4)

Lenz, K. M., Nugent, B. M., Haliyur, R., & McCarthy, M. M. (2013). Microglia are essential to masculinization of brain and behavior. *Journal of Neuroscience, 33,* 2761–2772. (10)

Leon, L. R. (2002). Invited review: Cytokine regulation of fever: Studies using gene knockout mice. *Journal of Applied Physiology, 92,* 2648–2655. (9)

Leppämäki, S., Partonen, T., & Lönnqvist, J. (2002). Bright-light exposure combined with physical exercise elevates mood. *Journal of Affective Disorders, 72,* 572–575. (14)

Lesku, J. A., Rattenborg, N. C., Valcu, M., Vyssotski, A. L., Kuhn, S., Kuemmeth, F., . . . Kempenaers, B. (2012). Adaptive sleep loss in polygynous pectoral sandpipers. *Science, 337,* 1654–1658. (8)

LeVay, S. (1991). A difference in hypothalamic structure between heterosexual and homosexual men. *Science, 253,* 1034–1037. (10)

LeVay, S. (1993). *The sexual brain.* Cambridge, MA: MIT Press. (10)

Levi-Montalcini, R. (1987). The nerve growth factor 35 years later. *Science, 237,* 1154–1162. (4)

Levi-Montalcini, R. (1988). *In praise of imperfection.* New York: Basic Books. (4)

Levin, E. D., & Rose, J. E. (1995). Acute and chronic nicotine interactions with dopamine systems and working memory performance. *Annals of the New York Academy of Sciences, 757,* 245–252. (2)

Levine, J. D., Fields, H. L., & Basbaum, A. I. (1993). Peptides and the primary afferent nociceptor. *Journal of Neuroscience, 13,* 2273–2286. (2)

Levitin, D. J., & Bellugi, U. (1998). Musical abilities in individuals with Williams syndrome. *Music Perception, 15,* 357–389. (13)

Lévy, F., Keller, M., & Poindron, P. (2004). Olfactory regulation of maternal behavior in mammals. *Hormones and Behavior, 46,* 284–302. (10)

Lewis, T. L., & Maurer, D. (2005). Multiple sensitive periods in human visual development: Evidence from visually deprived children. *Developmental Psychobiology, 46,* 163–183. (5)

Lewis, V. G., Money, J., & Epstein, R. (1968). Concordance of verbal and nonverbal ability in the adrenogenital syndrome. *Johns Hopkins Medical Journal, 122,* 192–195. (10)

Li, G., Wang, L., Shi, F., Lyall, A. E., Lin, W., Gilmore, J. H., & Shen, D. (2014). Mapping longitudinal development of local cortical gyrification in infants from birth to 2 years of age. *Journal of Neuroscience, 34,* 4228–4238. (4)

Li, J., Chen, C., Wu, K., Zhang, M., Zhu, B., Chen, C., . . . Dong, Q. (2015). Genetic veriations in the serotonergic system contribute to amygdala volume in humans. *Frontiers in Neuroanatomy, 9,* article 129. (11)

Li, L., Wu, C., Gan, Y., Qu, X. G., & Lu, Z. X. (2016). Insomnia and the risk of depression: A meta-analysis of prospective cohort studies. *BMC Psychiatry, 16,* article 375. (14)

Li, Q., Hill, Z., & He, B. J. (2014). Spatiotemporal dissociation of brain activity underlying subjective awareness, objective performance and confidence. *Journal of Neuroscience, 34,* 4382–4395. (13)

Li, S. L., Jost, R. M., Morale, S. E., Stager, D. R., Dao, L., Stager, D., & Birch, E. E. (2014). A binocular iPad treatment for amblyopic children. *Eye, 28,* 1246–1253. (5)

Li, S., Nie, E. H., Yin, Y., Benowitz, L. I., Tung, S., Vinters, H. V., . . . Carmichael, S. T. (2015). GDF10 is a signal for axonal sprouting and functional recovery after a stroke. *Nature Neuroscience, 18,* 1737–1745. (4)

Li, W., Englund, E., Widner, H., Mattsson, B., van Westen, D., Lätt, J., . . . Li, J.-Y. (2016). Extensive graft-derived dopaminergic innervation is maintained 24 years after transplantation in the degenerating parkinsonian brain. *Proceedings of the National Academy of Sciences (U.S.A.), 113,* 6544–6549. (7)

Li, X., Li, W., Liu, G., Shen, X., & Tang, Y. (2015). Association between cigarette smoking and Parkinson's disease: A meta-analysis. *Archives of Gerontology and Geriatrics, 61,* 510–516. (7)

Liberles, S. D., & Buck, L. B. (2006). A second class of chemosensory receptors in the olfactory epithelium. *Nature, 442,* 645–650. (6)

Libet, B., Gleason, C. A., Wright, E. W., & Pearl, D. K. (1983). Time of conscious intention to act in relation to onset of cerebral activities (readiness potential): The unconscious initiation of a freely voluntary act. *Brain, 106,* 623–642. (7)

Liebman, M., Pelican, S., Moore, S. A., Holmes, B., Wardlaw, M. K., Melcher, L. M., . . . Haynes, G. W. (2006). Dietary intake-, eating behavior-, and physical activity-related determinants of high body mass index in the 2003 Wellness IN the Rockies cross-sectional study. *Nutrition Research, 26,* 111–117. (9)

Lim, A. S. P., Ellison, B. A., Wang, J. L., Yu, L., Schneider, J. A., Buchman, A. S., . . . Saper, C. B. (2014). Sleep is related to neuron numbers in the ventrolateral preoptic/intermediate nucleus in older adults with and without Alzheimer's disease. *Brain, 137,* 2847–2861. (8)

Lim, B. K., Huang, K. W., Grueter, B. A., Rothwell, P. E., & Malenka, R. C. (2012). Anhedonia requires MC4R-mediated synaptic adaptations in nucleus accumbens. *Nature, 487,* 183–189. (11)

Lim, J.-H. A., Stafford, B. K., Nguyen, P. L., Lien, B. V., Wang, C., Zukor, K., . . . Huberman, A. D. (2016). Neural activity promotes long-distance, target-specific regeneration of adult retinal axons. *Nature Neuroscience, 19,* 1073–1084. (4)

Lim, M. M., Wang, Z., Olazábal, D. E., Ren, X., Terwilliger, E. F., & Young, L. J. (2004). Enhanced partner preference in a promiscuous species by manipulating the expression of a single gene. *Nature, 429,* 754–757. (10)

Lin, D. Y., Shea, S. D., & Katz, L. C. (2006). Representation of natural stimuli in the rodent main olfactory bulb. *Neuron, 50,* 937–949. (6)

Lin, J.-S., Hou, Y., Sakai, K., & Jouvet, M. (1996). Histaminergic descending inputs to the mesopontine tegmentum and their role in the control of cortical activation and wakefulness in the cat. *Journal of Neuroscience, 16,* 1523–1537. (8)

Lin, L., Faraco, J., Li, R., Kadotani, H., Rogers, W., Lin, X., . . . Mignot, E. (1999). The sleep disorder canine narcolepsy is caused by a mutation in the hypocretin (orexin) receptor 2 gene. *Cell, 98,* 365–376. (8)

Lindberg, N. O., Coburn, C., & Stricker, E. M. (1984). Increased feeding by rats after subdiabetogenic streptozotocin treatment: A role for insulin in satiety. *Behavioral Neuroscience, 98,* 138–145. (9)

Lindgren, L., Bergdahl, J., & Nyberg, L. (2016). Longitudinal evidence for smaller hippocampus volume as a vulnerability factor for perceived stress. *Cerebral Cortex, 26,* 3527–3533. (11)

Lindner, A., Iyer, A., Kagan, I., & Andersen, R. A. (2010). Human posterior parietal cortex plans where to reach and what to avoid. *Journal of Neuroscience, 30,* 11715–11725. (7)

Lindquist, K. A., Wager, T. D., Kober, H., Bliss-Moreau, E., & Barrett, L. F. (2012). The brain basis of emotion: A meta-analytic review. *Behavioral and Brain Sciences, 35,* 121–202. (11)

Lindsay, P. H., & Norman, D. A. (1972). *Human information processing.* New York: Academic Press. (6)

Ling, S., Pratte, M. S., & Tong, F. (2015). Attention alters orientation processing in the human lateral geniculate nucleus. *Nature Neuroscience, 18,* 496–498. (5)

Liou, Y.-C., Tocilj, A., Davies, P. L., & Jia, Z. (2000). Mimicry of ice structure by surface hydroxyls and water of a beta-helix antifreeze protein. *Nature, 406,* 322–324. (9)

Lisman, J., Schulman, H., & Cline, H. (2002). The molecular basis of CaMKII function in synaptic and behavioural memory. *Nature Reviews Neuroscience, 3,* 175–190. (12)

Lisman, J., Yasuda, R., & Raghavachari, S. (2012). Mechanisms of CaMKII action in long-term potentiation. *Nature Reviews Neuroscience, 13,* 169–182. (12)

Lisman, J. E., Raghavachari, S., & Tsien, R. W. (2007). The sequence of events that underlie quantal transmission at central glutamatergic synapses. *Nature Reviews Neuroscience, 8,* 597–609. (2)

Liu, F., Wollstein, A., Hysi, P. G., Ankra-Badu, G. A., Spector, T. D., Park, D, . . . Kayser, M. (2010). Digital quantification of human eye color highlights genetic association of three new loci. *PLoS Genetics, 6,* e1000934. (4)

Liu, G., & Tsien, R. W. (1995). Properties of synaptic transmission at single hippocampal synaptic boutons. *Nature, 375,* 404–408. (2)

Liu, L., She, L., Chen, M., Liu, T., Lu, H. D., Dan, Y., & Poo, M. (2016). Spatial structure of neuronal receptive field in awake monkey secondary visual cortex (V2). *Proceedings of the National Academy of Sciences (U.S.A.), 113,* 1913–1918. (5)

Liu, P., & Bilkey, D. K. (2001). The effect of excitotoxic lesions centered on the hippocampus or perirhinal cortex in object recognition and spatial memory tasks. *Behavioral Neuroscience, 115,* 94–111. (12)

Liu, S., Globa, A. K., Mills, F., Naef, L., Qiao, M., Bamji, S. X., & Borgland, S. L. (2016). Consumption of palatable food primes food approach behavior by rapidly increasing synaptic density in the VTA. *Proceedings of the National Academy of Sciences (U.S.A.), 113,* 2520–2525. (9)

Liu, X., Zwiebel, L. J., Hinton, D., Benzer, S., Hall, J. C., & Rosbash, M. (1992). The period gene encodes a predominantly nuclear protein in adult Drosophila. *Journal of Neuroscience, 12,* 2735–2744. (8)

Liu, Y., Samad, O. A., Zhang, L., Duan, B., Tong, Q., Lopes, C., . . . Ma, Q. (2010). VGLUT2-dependent glutamate release from nociceptors is required to sense pain and suppress itch. *Neuron, 68,* 543–556. (6)

Liu, Z.-W., Faraguna, U., Cirelli, C., Tononi, G., & Gao, X.-B. (2010). Direct evidence for wake-related increases and sleep-related decreases in synaptic strength in rodent cortex. *Journal of Neuroscience, 30,* 8671–8675. (8)

Livingstone, M. S. (1988, January). Art, illusion and the visual system. *Scientific American, 258*(1), 78–85. (5)

Livingstone, M. S., & Hubel, D. (1988). Segregation of form, color, movement, and depth: Anatomy, physiology, and perception. *Science, 240,* 740–749. (5)

Loe, I. M., Feldman, H. M., Yasui, E., & Luna, B. (2009). Oculomotor performance identifies underlying cognitive deficits in attention-deficit/hyperactivity disorder. *Journal of the American Academy of Child and Adolescent Psychiatry, 48,* 431–440. (7)

Loehlin, J. C., Horn, J. M., & Willerman, L. (1989). Modeling IQ change: Evidence from the Texas adoption project. *Child Development, 60,* 993–1004. (12)

Loewenstein, W. R. (1960, August). Biological transducers. *Scientific American, 203*(2), 98–108. (6)

Loewi, O. (1960). An autobiographic sketch. *Perspectives in Biology, 4,* 3–25. (2)

Lohse, M., Garrido, L., Driver, J., Dolan, R. J., Duchaine, B. C., & Furl, N. (2016). Effective connectivity from early visual cortex to posterior occipitotemporal face areas supports face selectivity and predicts developmental prosopagnosia. *Journal of Neuroscience, 36,* 3821–3828. (5)

Loman, M. M., Johnson, A. E., Westerlund, A., Pollak, S. D., Nelson, C. A., & Gunnar, M. R. (2013). The effect of early deprivation on executive attention in middle childhood. *Journal of Child Psychology and Psychiatry, 54,* 37–45. (4)

Lomber, S. G., & Malhotra, S. (2008). Double dissociation of "what" and "where" processing in auditory cortex. *Nature Neuroscience, 11,* 609–617. (6)

Lomniczi, A., Loche, A., Castellano, J. M., Ronnekleiv, O. K., Bosch, M., Kaidar, G., . . . Ojeda, S. R. (2013). Epigenetic control of female puberty. *Nature Neuroscience, 16,* 281–289. (4)

Long, M. A., Jutras, M. J., Connors, B. W., & Burwell, R. D. (2005). Electrical synapses coordinate activity in the suprachiasmatic nucleus. *Nature Neuroscience, 8,* 61–66. (8)

Long, M. A., Katlowitz, K. A., Svirsky, M. A., Clary, R. C., Byun, T. M., Majaj, N., . . . Greenlee, J. D. W. (2016). Functional segregation of cortical regions underlying speech timing and articulation. *Neuron, 89,* 1187–1193. (13)

Lorincz, A., & Nusser, Z. (2010). Molecular identity of dendritic voltage-gated sodium channels. *Science, 328,* 906–909. (1)

Lorrain, D. S., Riolo, J. V., Matuszewich, L., & Hull, E. M. (1999). Lateral hypothalamic serotonin inhibits nucleus accumbens dopamine: Implications for sexual refractoriness. *Journal of Neuroscience, 19,* 7648–7652. (14)

Lorusso, M. L., Facoetti, A., Pesenti, S., Cattaneo, C., Molteni, M., & Geiger, G. (2004). Wider recognition in peripheral vision common to different subtypes of dyslexia. *Vision Research, 44,* 2413–2424. (13)

Lott, I. T. (1982). Down's syndrome, aging, and Alzheimer's disease: A clinical review. *Annals of the New York Academy of Sciences, 396,* 15–27. (12)

Lotto, R. B., & Purves, D. (2002). The empirical basis of color perception. *Consciousness and Cognition, 11,* 609–629. (5)

Lotze, M., Grodd, W., Birbaumer, N., Erb, M., Huse, E., & Flor, H. (1999). Does use of a myoelectric prosthesis prevent cortical reorganization and phantom limb pain? *Nature Neuroscience, 2,* 501–502. (4)

Loui, P., Alsop, D., & Schlaug, G. (2009). Tone deafness: A new disconnection syndrome? *Journal of Neuroscience, 29,* 10215–10220. (6)

Löw, A., Weymar, M., & Hamm, A. O. (2015). When threat is near, get out of here: Dynamics of defensive behavior during freezing and active avoidance. *Psychological Science, 26,* 1706–1716. (11)

Lucas, R. J., Douglas, R. H., & Foster, R. G. (2001). Characterization of an ocular photopigment capable of driving pupillary constriction in mice. *Nature Neuroscience, 4,* 621–626. (8)

Lucas, R. J., Freedman, M. S., Muñoz, M., Garcia-Fernández, J.-M., & Foster, R. G. (1999). Regulation of the mammalian pineal by non-rod, non-cone ocular photoreceptors. *Science, 284,* 505–507. (8)

Luczak, S. E., Glatt, S. J., & Wall, T. L. (2006). Meta-analysis of *ALDHx* and *ADHIB* with alcohol dependence in Asians. *Psychological Bulletin, 132,* 607–621. (14)

Luczak, A., McNaughton, B. L., & Harris, K. D. (2015). Packet-based communication in the cortex. *Nature Reviews Neuroscience, 16,* 745–755. (3)

Luders, E., Gaser, C., Narr, K. L., & Toga, A. W. (2009). Why sex matters: Brain size independent differences in gray matter distributions between men and women. *Journal of Neuroscience, 29,* 14265–14270. (10)

Luders, E., Narr, K. I., Thompson, P. M., Rex, D. E., Jancke, L., Steinmetz, H., & Toga, A. W. (2004). Gender differences in cortical complexity. *Nature Neuroscience, 7,* 799–800. (12)

Ludwig, M., & Leng, G. (2006). Dendritic peptides release and peptide-dependent behaviours. *Nature Reviews Neuroscience, 7,* 126–136. (2)

Lumley, A. J., Michalczyk, L., Kitson, J. J. N., Spurgin, L. G., Morrison, C. A., Godwin, J. L., . . . Gage, M. J. G. (2015). Sexual selection protects against extinction. *Nature, 522,* 470–473. (10)

Luna, B., Padmanabhan, A., & O'Hearn, K. (2010). What has fMRI told us about the development of cognitive control through adolescence? *Brain and Cognition, 72,* 101–113. (4)

Lund, R. D., Lund, J. S., & Wise, R. P. (1974). The organization of the retinal projection to the dorsal lateral geniculate nucleus in pigmented and albino rats. *Journal of Comparative Neurology, 158,* 383–404. (5)

Lundqvist, M., Rose, J., Herman, P., Brincat, S. L., Buschman, T. J., & Miller, E. K. (2016). Gamma and beta bursts underlie working memory. *Neuron, 90,* 152–164. (12)

Lunnon, K., Smith, R., Hannon, E., De Jager, P. L., Srivastava, G., Volta, M., Troakes, C., . . . Mill, J. (2014). Methylomic profiling implicates cortical deregulation of *ANK1* in Alzheimer's disease. *Nature Neuroscience, 17,* 1164–1170. (12)

Lutz, B., Marsicano, G., Maldonado, R., & Hillard, C. J. (2015). The endocannabinoid system in guarding against fear, anxiety and stress. *Nature Reviews Neuroscience, 16,* 705–718. (2)

Lyamin, O. I., Kosenko, P. O., Lapierre, J. L., Mukhametov, L. M., & Siegel, J. (2008). Fur seals display a strong drive for bilateral slow-wave sleep while on land. *Journal of Neuroscience, 28,* 12614–12621. (8)

Lyamin, O., Pryaslova, J., Lance, V., & Siegel, J. (2005). Continuous activity in cetaceans after birth. *Nature, 435,* 1177. (8)

Lyman, C. P., O'Brien, R. C., Greene, G. C., & Papafrangos, E. D. (1981). Hibernation and longevity in the Turkish hamster *Mesocricetus brandti. Science, 212,* 668–670. (8)

Lynall, M.-E., Bassett, D. S., Kerwin, R., McKenna, P. J., Kitzbichler, M., Muller, U., & Bullmore, E. (2010). Functional connectivity and brain networks in schizophrenia. *Journal of Neuroscience, 30,* 9477–9487. (14)

Lyons, M. J., Eisen, S. A., Goldberg, J., True, W., Lin, N., Meyer, J. M., . . . Tsuang, M. T. (1998). A registry-based twin study of depression in men. *Archives of General Psychiatry, 55,* 468–472. (14)

Lyons, M. J., York, T. P., Franz, C. E., Grant, M. D., Eaves, L. J., Jacobson, K. C., . . . Kremen, W. S. (2009). Genes determine stability and the environment determines change in cognitive ability during 35 years of adulthood. *Psychological Science, 20,* 1146–1152. (12)

Ma, Y., Koyama, M. S., Milham, M. P., Castellanos, F. X., Quinn, B. T., Pardoe, H., . . . Blackmon, K. (2015). Cortical thickness abnormalities associated with dyslexia, independent of remediation status. *NeuroImage: Clinical, 7,* 177–186. (13)

Macdonald, R. L., Weddle, M. G., & Gross, R. A. (1986). Benzodiazepine, beta-carboline, and barbiturate actions on GABA responses. *Advances in Biochemical Psychopharmacology, 41,* 67–78. (11)

Macey, P. M., Henderson, L. A., Macey, K. E., Alger, J. R., Frysinger, R. C., Woo, M. A., . . . Harper, R. M. (2002). Brain morphology associated with obstructive sleep apnea.

American Journal of Respiratory & Critical Care Medicine, 166, 1382–1387. (8)

MacFarlane, J. G., Cleghorn, J. M., & Brown, G. M. (1985a, September). *Circadian rhythms in chronic insomnia.* Paper presented at the World Congress of Biological Psychiatry, Philadelphia. (8)

MacFarlane, J. G., Cleghorn, J. M., & Brown, G. M. (1985b). Melatonin and core temperature rhythms in chronic insomnia. In G. M. Brown & S. D. Wainwright (Eds.), *The pineal gland: Endocrine aspects* (pp. 301–306). New York: Pergamon Press. (8)

MacFarquhar, L. (2009, July 27). The kindest cut. *The New Yorker, 85*(22), 38–51. (4)

MacLean, P. D. (1949). Psychosomatic disease and the "visceral brain": Recent developments bearing on the Papez theory of emotion. *Psychosomatic Medicine, 11,* 338–353. (11)

MacLusky, N. J., & Naftolin, F. (1981). Sexual differentiation of the central nervous system. *Science, 211,* 1294–1303. (10)

Macphail, E. M. (1985). Vertebrate intelligence: The null hypothesis. *Philosophical Transactions of the Royal Society of London, B, 308,* 37–51. (3)

Madsen, H. B., & Kim, J. H. (2016). Ontogeny of memory: An update on 40 years of work with infantile amnesia. *Behavioural Brain Research, 298,* 4–14. (12)

Maffei, A., Nataraj, K., Nelson, S. B., & Turrigiano, G. G. (2006). Potentiation of cortical inhibition by visual deprivation. *Nature, 443,* 81–84. (5)

Maguire, E. A., Gadian, D. G., Johnsrude, I. S., Good, C. D., Ashburner, J., Frackowiak, R. S. J., & Frith, C. D. (2000). Navigation-related structural change in the hippocampi of taxi drivers. *Proceedings of the National Academy of Sciences, USA, 97,* 4398–4403. (12)

Mahler, S. V., Moorman, D. E., Smith, R. J., James, M. H., & Aston-Jones, G. (2014). Motivational activation: A unifying hypothesis of orexin/hypocretin function. *Nature Neuroscience, 17,* 1298–1303. (9)

Manohar, S. G., & Husain, M. (2016). Human ventromedial prefrontal lesions alter incentivisation by reward. *Cortex, 76,* 104–120. (13)

Maier, S. F., & Watkins, L. R. (1998). Cytokines for psychologists: Implications of bidirectional immune-to-brain communication for understanding behavior, mood, and cognition. *Psychological Review, 105,* 83–107. (11)

Mainland, J. D., Keller, A., Li, Y. R., Zhou, T., Trimmer, C., Snyder, L. L., . . . Matsunami, H. (2014). The missense of smell: Functional variability in the human odorant receptor repertoire. *Nature Neuroscience, 17,* 114–120. (6)

Malik, S., Vinukonda, G., Vose, L. R., Diamond, D., Bhimavarapu, B. B. R., Hu, F., . . . Ballabh, P. (2013). Neurogenesis continues in the third trimester of pregnancy and is suppressed by premature birth. *Journal of Neuroscience, 33,* 411–423. (4)

Mallis, M. M., & DeRoshia, C. W. (2005). Circadian rhythms, sleep, and performance in space. *Aviation, Space, and Environmental Medicine, 76*(Suppl. 6), B94–B107. (8)

Malmberg, A. B., Chen, C., Tonegawa, S., & Basbaum, A. I. (1997). Preserved acute pain and reduced neuropathic pain in mice lacking PKCg. *Science, 278,* 279–283. (6)

Man, K., Kaplan, J. T., Damasio, A., & Meyer, K. (2012). Sight and sound converge to form modality-invariant representations in temporoparietal cortex. *Journal of Neuroscience, 32,* 16629–16636. (3)

Mancuso, K., Hauswirth, W. W., Li, Q., Connor, T. B., Kuchenbecker, J. A., Mauck, M. C., . . . Neitz, M. (2009). Gene therapy for red-green colour blindness. *Nature, 461,* 784–787. (5)

Mander, B. A., Marks, S. M., Vogel, J. W., Rao, V., Lu, B., Saletin, J. M., . . . Walker, M. P. (2015). β-amyloid disrupts human NREM slow waves and related hippocampus-dependent memory consolidation. *Nature Neuroscience, 18,* 1051–1057. (8)

Mandy, W., & Lai, M.-C. (2016). Annual research review: The role of the environment in the developmental psychopathology of autism spectrum condition. *Journal of Child Psychology and Psychiatry, 57,* 271–292. (14)

Mangan, M. A. (2004). A phenomenology of problematic sexual behavior. *Archives of Sexual Behavior, 33,* 287–293. (8)

Mangiapane, M. L., & Simpson, J. B. (1980). Subfornical organ: Forebrain site of pressor and dipsogenic action of angiotensin II. *American Journal of Physiology, 239,* R382–R389. (9)

Mann, J. J., Arango, V., & Underwood, M. D. (1990). Serotonin and suicidal behavior. *Annals of the New York Academy of Sciences, 600,* 476–485. (11)

Mann, T., Tomiyama, J., & Ward, A. (2015). Promoting public health in the context of the "obesity epidemic": False starts and promising new directions. *Perspectives on Psychological Science, 10,* 706–710. (9)

Maquet, P., Laureys, S., Peigneux, P., Fuchs, S., Petiau, C., Phillips, C., . . . Cleermans, A. (2000). Experience-dependent changes in cerebral activation during human REM sleep. *Nature Neuroscience, 3,* 831–836. (8)

Maquet, P., Peters, J.-M., Aerts, J., Delfiore, G., Degueldre, C., Luxen, A., & Franck, G. (1996). Functional neuroanatomy of human rapid-eye-movement sleep and dreaming. *Nature, 383,* 163–166. (7, 8)

Marcar, V. L., Zihl, J., & Cowey, A. (1997). Comparing the visual deficits of a motion blind patient with the visual deficits of monkeys with area MT removed. *Neuropsychologia, 35,* 1459–1465. (5)

March, S. M., Abate, P., Spear, N. E., & Molina, J. C. (2009). Fetal exposure to moderate ethanol doses: Heightened operant responsiveness elicited by ethanol-related reinforcers. *Alcoholism: Clinical and Experimental Research, 33,* 1981–1993. (14)

Marek, R., Strobel, C., Bredy, T. W., & Sah, P. (2013). Partners in the fear circuit. *Journal of Physiology, 591,* 2381–2391. (11)

Maret, S., Faraguna, U., Nelson, A. B., Cirelli, C., & Tononi, G. (2011). Sleep and waking modulate spine turnover in the adolescent mouse cortex. *Nature Neuroscience, 14,* 1418–1420. (8)

Mariño, G., Fernández, A. F., Cabrera, S., Lundberg, Y. W., Cabanillas, R., Rodríguez, F., & Lopez-Otin, C. (2010). Autophagy is essential for mouse sense of balance. *Journal of Clinical Investigation, 120,* 2331–2344. (6)

Mark, A. L. (2013). Selective leptin resistance revisited. *American Journal of Physiology: Regulatory, Integrative, and Comparative Physiology, 305,* R566–R581. (9)

Marlatt, M. W., Potter, M. C., Lucassen, P. J., & van Praag, H. (2012). Running throughout middle-age improves memory function, hippocampal neurogenesis, and BDNF levels in female C57B1/6J mice. *Developmental Neurobiology, 72*(S1), 943–952. (4)

Marlin, B. J., Mitre, M., D'amour, J. A., Chao, M. V., & Froemke, R. C. (2015). Oxytocin enables maternal behaviour by balancing cortical inhibition. *Nature, 520,* 499–504. (13)

Marquié, J.-C., Tucker, P., Folkard, S., Gentil, C., & Ansiau, D. (2015). Chronic effects of shift work on cognition: Findings from the VISAT longitudinal study. *Occupational and Environmental Medicine, 72,* 258–264. (8)

Marris, E. (2006). Grey matters. *Nature, 444,* 808–810. (0)

Marshall, J. C., & Halligan, P. W. (1995). Seeing the forest but only half the trees? *Nature, 373,* 521–523. (13)

Marshall, J. F. (1985). Neural plasticity and recovery of function after brain injury. *International Review of Neurobiology, 26,* 201–247. (4)

Marsman, A., van den Heuvel, M. P., Klomp, D. W. J., Kahn, R. S., Luijten, P. R., & Pol, H. E. H. (2013). Glutamate in schizophrenia: A focused review and meta-analysis of H-1-MRS studies. *Schizophrenia Bulletin, 39,* 120–129. (14)

Martens, M. A., Wilson, S. J., & Reutens, D. C. (2008). Research review: Williams syndrome: A critical review of the cognitive, behavioral, and neuroanatomical phenotype. *Journal of Child Psychology and Psychiatry, 49,* 576–608. (13)

Martin, A., & Olson, K. R. (2015). Beyond good and evil: What motivations underlie children's prosocial behavior? *Perspectives on Psychological Science, 10,* 159–175. (4)

Martin, G., Rojas, L. M., Ramírez, Y., & McNeil, R. (2004). The eyes of oilbirds (*Steatornis caripensis*): Pushing at the limits of sensitivity. *Naturwissenschaften, 91,* 26–29. (5)

Martin, P. R., Lee, B. B., White, A. J. R., Solomon, S. G., & Rütiger, L. (2001). Chromatic sensitivity of ganglion cells in the peripheral primate retina. *Nature, 410,* 933–936. (5)

Martín, R., Bajo-Grañeras, R., Moratalla, R., Perea, G., & Araque, A. (2015).

Circuit-specific signaling in astrocyte-neuron networks in basal ganglia pathways. *Science, 349*, 730–734. (1)

Martin, R. C., & Blossom-Stach, C. (1986). Evidence of syntactic deficits in a fluent aphasic. *Brain and Language, 28*, 196–234. (13)

Martin, S. D., Martin, E., Rai, S. S., Richardson, M. A., Royall, R., & Eng, C. (2001). Brain blood flow changes in depressed patients treated with interpersonal psychotherapy or venlafaxine hydrochloride. *Archives of General Psychiatry, 58*, 641–648. (14)

Martindale, C. (2001). Oscillations and analogies: Thomas Young, MD, FRS, genius. *American Psychologist, 56*, 342–345. (5)

Martínez-Horta, S., Perez-Perez, J., van Duijn, E., Fernandez-Bobadilla, R., Carceller, M., Pagonabarrage, J., . . . Kulisevsky, J. (2016). Neuropsychiatric symptoms are very common in premanifest and early stage Huntington's disease. *Parkinsonism & Related Disorders, 25*, 58–64. (7)

Martínez-Horta, S., Riba, J., de Bobadilla, R. F., Pagonabarraga, J., Pascual-Sedano, B., Antonijoan, R. M., . . . Kulisevsky, J. (2014). Apathy in Parkinson's disease: Neurophysiological evidence of impaired incentive processing. *Journal of Neuroscience, 34*, 5918–5926. (7)

Martinez-Vargas, M. C., & Erickson, C. J. (1973). Some social and hormonal determinants of nest-building behaviour in the ring dove (*Streptopelia risoria*). *Behaviour, 45*, 12–37. (10)

Martinowich, K., Manji, H., & Lu, B. (2007). New insights into BDNF function in depression and anxiety. *Nature Neuroscience, 10*, 1089–1093. (14)

Masal, E., Randler, C., Besoluk, S., Önder, I., Horzum, M. B., & Vollmer, C. (2015). Effects of longitude, latitude and social factors on chronotype in Turkish students. *Personality and Individual Differences, 86*, 73–81. (8)

Mascaro, J. S., Hackett, P. D., & Rilling, J. K. (2013). Testicular volume is inversely correlated with nurturing-related brain activity in human fathers. *Proceedings of the National Academy of Sciences, 110*, 15746–15751. (10)

Masland, R. H. (2012). The tasks of amacrine cells. *Visual Neuroscience, 29*, 3–9. (5)

Masland, R. H. (2001). The fundamental plan of the retina. *Nature Neuroscience, 4*, 877–886. (5)

Maslen, H., Douglas, T., Cohen Kadosh, R., Levy, N., & Savulescu, J. (2014). The regulation of cognitive enhancement devices: Extending the medical model. *Journal of Law and the Biosciences, 1*, 68–93. (12)

Mason, M. F., Norton, M. I., Van Horn, J. D., Wegner, D. M., Grafton, S. T., & Macrae, C. N. (2007). Wandering minds: The default network and stimulus-independent thought. *Science, 315*, 393–395. (3)

Massimini, M., Ferrarelli, F., Huber, R., Esser, S. K., Singh, H., & Tononi, G. (2005). Breakdown of cortical effective connectivity during sleep. *Science, 309*, 2228–2232. (8)

Mathews, G. A., Fane, B. A., Conway, G. S., Brook, C. G. D., & Hines, M. (2009). Personality and congenital adrenal androgen exposure. *Hormones and Behavior, 55*, 285–291. (10)

Matrisciano, F., Bonaccorso, S., Ricciardi, A., Scaccianoce, S., Panaccione, I., Wang, L., . . . Shelton, R. C. (2008). Changes in BDNF serum levels in patients with major depression disorder (MDD) after 6 months treatment with sertraline, escitalopram, or venlafaxine. *Journal of Psychiatric Research, 43*, 247–254. (14)

Matson, J. L., Adams, H. L., Williams, L. W., & Rieske, R. D. (2013). Why are there so many unsubstantiated treatments in autism? *Research in Autism Spectrum Disorders, 7*, 466–474. (14)

Matsumoto, Y., Mishima, K., Satoh, K., Tozawa, T., Mishima, Y., Shimizu, T., & Hishikawa, Y. (2001). Total sleep deprivation induces an acute and transient increase in NK cell activity in healthy young volunteers. *Sleep, 24*, 804–809. (8)

Matsunami, H., Montmayeur, J.-P., & Buck, L. B. (2000). A family of candidate taste receptors in human and mouse. *Nature, 404*, 601–604. (6)

Mattavelli, G., Sormaz, M., Flack, T., Asghar, A. V. R., Fan, S., Frey, J., . . . Andrews, T. J. (2014). Neural responses to facial expressions support the role of the amygdala in processing threat. *Social Cognitive and Affective Neuroscience, 9*, 1684–1689. (11)

Mattingley, J. B., Husain, M., Rorden, C., Kennard, C., & Driver, J. (1998). Motor role of human inferior parietal lobe revealed in unilateral neglect patients. *Nature, 392*, 179–182. (13)

Matuszewich, L., Lorrain, D. S., & Hull, E. M. (2000). Dopamine release in the medial preoptic area of female rats in response to hormonal manipulation and sexual activity. *Behavioral Neuroscience, 114*, 772–782. (10)

Maurice, D. M. (1998). The Von Sallmann lecture of 1996: An ophthalmological explanation of REM sleep. *Experimental Eye Research, 66*, 139–145. (8)

May, P. R. A., Fuster, J. M., Haber, J., & Hirschman, A. (1979). Woodpecker drilling behavior: An endorsement of the rotational theory of impact brain injury. *Archives of Neurology, 36*, 370–373. (4)

Maya Vetencourt, J. F., Sale, A., Viegi, A., Baroncelli, L., DePasquale, R., O'Leary, O. F., . . . Maffei, L. (2008). The antidepressant fluoxetine restores plasticity in the adult visual cortex. *Science, 320*, 385–388. (14)

Mayberry, R. I., Lock, E., & Kazmi, H. (2002). Linguistic ability and early language exposure. *Nature, 417*, 38. (13)

Mayer, A. D., & Rosenblatt, J. S. (1979). Hormonal influences during the ontogeny of maternal behavior in female rats. *Journal of Comparative and Physiological Psychology, 93*, 879–898. (10)

Mazur, A., & Michalek, J. (1998). Marriage, divorce, and male testosterone. *Social Forces, 77*, 315–330. (10)

Mazza, S., Gerber, E., Gustin, M.-P., Kasikci, Z., Koenig, O., Toppino, T. C., & Magnin, M. (2016). Relearn faster and retain longer: Along with practice, sleep makes perfect. *Psychological Science, 27*, 1321–1330. (8)

McBride, C. S., Baier, F., Omondi, A. B., Spitzer, S. A., Lutomiah, J., Sang, R., . . . Vosshall, L. B. (2014). Evolution of mosquito preference for humans linked to an odorant receptor. *Nature, 515*, 222–227. (6)

McBurney, D. H., & Bartoshuk, L. M. (1973). Interactions between stimuli with different taste qualities. *Physiology & Behavior, 10*, 1101–1106. (6)

McCall, C., & Singer, T. (2012). The animal and human neuroendocrinology of social cognition, motivation and behavior. *Nature Neuroscience, 15*, 681–688. (13)

McCarley, R. W., & Hoffman, E. (1981). REM sleep, dreams, and the activation-synthesis hypothesis. *American Journal of Psychiatry, 138*, 904–912. (8)

McCarthy, M. M. (2010). How it's made: Organizational effects of hormones on the developing brain. *Journal of Neuroendocrinology, 22*, 736–742. (10)

McCarthy, M. M. (2016). Multifaceted origins of sex differences in the brain. *Philosophical Transactions of the Royal Society B, 371*, article number 20150106. (10)

McCarthy, M. M., & Arnold, A. P. (2011). Reframing sexual differentiation of the brain. *Nature Neuroscience, 14*, 677–683. (10)

McClintock, M. K. (1971). Menstrual synchrony and suppression. *Nature, 229*, 244–245. (6)

McConnell, J. V. (1962). Memory transfer through cannibalism in planarians. *Journal of Neuropsychiatry, 3*(Suppl. 1), 42–48. (12)

McConnell, S. K. (1992). The genesis of neuronal diversity during development of cerebral cortex. *Seminars in the Neurosciences, 4*, 347–356. (4)

McDermott, R., Dawes, C., Prom-Wormley, E., Eaves, L., & Hatemi, P. K. (2013). MAOS and aggression: A gene-environment interaction in two populations. *Journal of Conflict Resolution, 57*, 1043–1064. (11)

McDonald, M. J., Rice, D. P., & Desai, M. M. (2016). Sex speeds adaptation by altering the dynamics of molecular evolution. *Nature, 531*, 233–236. (10)

McEwen, B. S. (2000). The neurobiology of stress: From serendipity to clinical relevance. *Brain Research, 886*, 172–189. (9, 11)

McGorry, P. D., Nelson, B., & Markulev, C. (2017). Effect of omega-3 polysaturated fatty acids in young people at ultrahigh risk for psychotic disorders. *JAMA Psychiatry, 74*, 19–27. (14)

McGue, M., & Bouchard, T. J., Jr. (1998). Genetic and environmental influences on human behavioral differences. *Annual Review of Neuroscience, 21*, 1–24. (12)

McGue, M., Malone, S., Keyes, M., & Iacono, W. G. (2014). Parent-offspring similarity for drinking: A longitudinal adoption study. *Behavior Genetics, 44,* 620–628. (14)

McGuire, S., & Clifford, J. (2000). Genetic and environmental contributions to loneliness in children. *Psychological Science, 11,* 487–491. (4)

McHugh, P. R., & Moran, T. H. (1985). The stomach: A conception of its dynamic role in satiety. *Progress in Psychobiology and Physiological Psychology, 11,* 197–232. (9)

McIntyre, M., Gangestad, S. W., Gray, P. B., Chapman, J. F., Burnham, T. C., O'Rourke, M. T., & Thornhill, R. (2006). Romantic involvement often reduces men's testosterone levels—but not always: The moderating effect of extrapair sexual interest. *Journal of Personality and Social Psychology, 91,* 642–651. (10)

McIntyre, R. S., Konarski, J. Z., Wilkins, K., Soczynska, J. K., & Kennedy, S. H. (2006). Obesity in bipolar disorder and major depressive disorder: Results from a National Community Health Survey on Mental Health and Well-Being. *Canadian Journal of Psychiatry, 51,* 274–280. (9)

McKeever, W. F., Seitz, K. S., Krutsch, A. J., & Van Eys, P. L. (1995). On language laterality in normal dextrals and sinistrals: Results from the bilateral object naming latency task. *Neuropsychologia, 33,* 1627–1635. (13)

McKemy, D. D., Neuhausser, W. M., & Julius, D. (2002). Identification of a cold receptor reveals a general role for TRP channels in thermosensation. *Nature, 416,* 52–58. (6)

McKenzie, I. A., Ohayon, D., Li, H., Paes de Faria, J., Emery, B., Tohyama, K., & Richardson, W. D. (2014). Motor skill learning requires active central myelination. *Science, 346,* 318–322. (4)

McKinnon, W., Weisse, C. S., Reynolds, C. P., Bowles, C. A., & Baum, A. (1989). Chronic stress, leukocyte-subpopulations, and humoral response to latent viruses. *Health Psychology, 8,* 839–402. (11)

McMillan, K. A., Asmundson, G. J. G., Zvolensky, M. J., & Carleton, R. N. (2012). Startle response and anxiety sensitivity: Subcortical indices of physiologic arousal and fear responding. *Emotion, 12,* 1264–1272. (11)

McNay, E. (2014). Your brain on insulin: From heresy to dogma. *Perspectives on Psychological Science, 9,* 88–90. (1)

Meddis, R., Pearson, A. J. D., & Langford, G. (1973). An extreme case of healthy insomnia. *EEG and Clinical Neurophysiology, 35,* 213–214. (8)

Mednick, S. C., McDevitt, E. A., Walsh, J. K., Wamsley, E., Paulus, M., Kanady, J. C., & Drummond, S. P. A. (2013). The critical role of sleep spindles in hippocampal-dependent memory: A pharmacological study. *Journal of Neuroscience, 13,* 4494–4504. (8)

Mehta, P. H., Welker, K. M., Zilioli, S., & Carré, J. M. (2015). Testosterone and cortisol jointly modulate risk-taking. *Psychoneuroendocrinology, 56,* 88–99. (11)

Meier, M. H., Shaler, I., Moffitt, T. E., Kapur, S., Keefe, R. S. E., Wong, T. Y., . . . Poulton, R. (2013). Microvascular abnormality in schizophrenia as shown by retinal imaging. *American Journal of Psychiatry, 170,* 1451–1459. (14)

Meister, M., Wong, R. O. L., Baylor, D. A., & Shatz, C. J. (1991). Synchronous bursts of action potentials in ganglion cells of the developing mammalian retina. *Science, 252,* 939–943. (4)

Melby-Lervåg, M., Redick, T. S., & Hulme, C. (2016). Working memory training does not improve performance on measures of intelligence or other measures of "far transfer": Evidence from a meta-analytic review. *Perspectives on Psychological Science, 11,* 512–534. (4)

Melis, A. P., Grocke, P., Kalbitz, J., & Tomasello, M. (2016). One for you, one for me: Humans' unique turn-taking skills. *Psychological Science, 27,* 987–996. (12)

Melloni, L., Molina, C., Pena, M., Torres, D., Singer, W., & Rodriguez, E. (2007). Synchronization of neural activity across cortical areas correlates with conscious perception. *Journal of Neuroscience, 27,* 2858–2865. (13)

Melone, M., Vitellaro-Zuccarello, L., Vallejo-Illarramendi, A., Pérez-Samartin, A., Matute, C., Cozzi, A., . . . Conti, F. (2001). The expression of glutamate transporter GLT-1 in the rat cerebral cortex is down-regulated by the antipsychotic drug clozapine. *Molecular Psychiatry, 6,* 380–386. (14)

Meltzer, H. Y., Matsubara, S., & Lee, J.-C. (1989). Classification of typical and atypical antipsychotic drugs on the basis of dopamine D-1, D-2 and serotonin2 pKi values. *Journal of Pharmacology and Experimental Therapeutics, 251,* 238–246. (14)

Meltzoff, A. N., & Moore, M. K. (1977). Imitation of facial and manual gestures by human neonates. *Science, 198,* 75–78. (7)

Melzack, R., & Wall, P. D. (1965). Pain mechanisms: A new theory. *Science, 150,* 971–979. (6)

Méndez-Bértolo, C., Moratti, S., Toledano, R., Lopez-Sosa, F., Martínez-Alvarez, R., Mah, Y. H., . . . Strange, B. A. (2016). A fast pathway for fear in human amygdala. *Nature Neuroscience, 19,* 1041–1049. (11)

Mendieta-Zéron, H., López, M., & Diéguez, C. (2008). Gastrointestinal peptides controlling body weight homeostasis. *General and Comparative Endocrinology, 155,* 481–495. (9)

Mendle, J., Eisenlohr-Moul, T., & Kiesner, J. (2016). From menarche to menopause: Women's reproductive milestones and risk for psychopathology—An introduction to the special series. *Clinical Psychological Science, 4,* 859–866. (14)

Mergen, M., Mergen, H., Ozata, M., Oner, R., & Oner, C. (2001). A novel melanocortin 4 receptor (MC4R) gene mutation associated with morbid obesity. *Journal of Clinical Endocrinology & Metabolism, 86,* 3448–3451. (9)

Merikangas, K. R., & Pato, M. (2009). Recent developments in the epidemiology of bipolar disorder in adults and children: Magnitude, correlates, and future directions. *Clinical Psychology: Science and Practice, 16,* 121–133. (14)

Mertens, J., Wang, Q.-W., Kim, Y., Yu, D. X., Pham, S., Yang, B., . . . Yao, J. (2015). Differential responses to lithium in hyperexcitable neurons from patients with bipolar disorder. *Nature, 527,* 95–99. (14)

Merzenich, M. M., Nelson, R. J., Stryker, M. P., Cynader, M. S., Schoppman, A., & Zook, J. M. (1984). Somatosensory cortical map changes following digit amputation in adult monkeys. *Journal of Comparative Neurology, 224,* 591–605. (4)

Mesgarani, N., & Chang, E. F. (2013). Selective cortical representation of attended speaker in multi-talker speech perception. *Nature, 485,* 233–236. (6)

Meshi, D., Drew, M. R., Saxe, M., Ansorge, M. S., David, D., Santarelli, L., . . . Hen, R. (2006). Hippocampal neurogenesis is not required for behavioral effects of environmental enrichment. *Nature Neuroscience, 9,* 729–731. (4)

Mesgarani, N., Cheung, C., Johnson, K., & Chang, E. F. (2014). Phonetic feature encoding in human superior temporal gyrus. *Science, 343,* 1006–1010. (6)

Metcalf, S. A., Jones, P. B., Nordstrom, T., Timonen, M., Maki, P., Miettunen, J., . . . Khandaker, G. M. (2017). Serum C-reactive protein in adolescence and risk of schizophrenia in adulthood: A prospective birth cohort study. *Brain, Behavior, and Immunity, 59,* 253–259. (14)

Mevorach, C., Hodsoll, J., Allen, H., Shalev, L., & Humphreys, G. (2010). Ignoring the elephant in the room: A neural circuit to downregulate salience. *Journal of Neuroscience, 30,* 6072–6079. (13)

Meyer, B., Yuen, K. S. L., Ertl, M., Polomac, N., Mulert, C., Büchel, C., & Kalish, R. (2015). Neural mechanisms of placebo anxiolysis. *Journal of Neuroscience, 35,* 7365–7373. (6)

Meyer, K., Kaplan, J. T., Essex, R., Webber, C., Damasio, H., & Damasio, A. (2010). Predicting visual stimuli on the basis of activity in auditory cortices. *Nature Neuroscience, 13,* 667–671. (6)

Meyer-Bahlburg, H. F. L., Dalke, K. B., Berenbaum, S. A., Cohen-Kettenis, P. T., Hines, M., & Schober, J. M. (2016). Gender assignment, reassignment and outcome in disorders of sex development: Update of the 2005 Consensus Conference. *Hormone Research in Paediatrics, 85,* 112–118. (10)

Meyer-Bahlburg, H. F. L., Dolezal, C., Baker, S. W., & New, M. I. (2008). Sexual orientation in women with classical or non-classical congenital adrenal hyperplasia as a function of degree of prenatal androgen excess. *Archives of Sexual Behavior, 37,* 85–99. (10)

Meyer-Lindenberg, A. (2010). From maps to mechanisms through neuroimaging of schizophrenia. *Nature, 468,* 194–202. (14)

Meyer-Lindenberg, A., Mervis, C. B., & Berman, K. F. (2006). Neural mechanisms in Williams syndrome: A unique window to genetic influences on cognition and behaviour. *Nature Reviews Neuroscience, 7,* 380–393. (13)

Mezzanotte, W. S., Tangel, D. J., & White, D. P. (1992). Waking genioglossal electromyogram in sleep apnea patients versus normal controls (a neuromuscular compensatory mechanism). *Journal of Clinical Investigation, 89,* 1571–1579. (8)

Mihalcescu, I., Hsing, W., & Leibler, S. (2004). Resilient circadian oscillator revealed in individual cyanobacteria. *Nature, 430,* 81–85. (8)

Mika, A., Mazur, G. J., Hoffman, A. N., Talboom, J. S., Bimonte-Nelson, H. A., Sanabria, F., & Conrad, C. D. (2012). Chronic stress impairs prefrontal cortex-dependent response inhibition and spatial working memory. *Behavioral Neuroscience, 126,* 605–619. (11)

Milich, R., & Pelham, W. E. (1986). Effects of sugar ingestion on the classroom and playgroup behavior of attention deficit disordered boys. *Journal of Consulting and Clinical Psychology, 54,* 714–718. (9)

Millan, M. J. (2014). On "polypharmacy" and multi-target agents, complementary strategies for improving the treatment of depression: A comparative appraisal. *International Journal of Neuropsychopharmacology, 17,* 1009–1037. (14)

Miller, C. A., Gavin, C. F., White, J. A., Parrish, R. R., Honasoge, A., Yancey, C. R., . . . Sweatt, J. D. (2010). Cortical DNA methylation maintains remote memory. *Nature Neuroscience, 13,* 664–666. (12)

Miller, G. (2007a). Animal extremists get personal. *Science, 318,* 1856–1585. (0)

Miller, G. A. (2010). Mistreating psychology in the decades of the brain. *Perspectives on Psychological Science, 5,* 716–743. (0, 13)

Miller, G., Tybur, J. M., & Jordan, B. D. (2007). Ovulatory cycle effects on tip earnings by lap dancers: Economic evidence for human estrus? *Evolution and Human Behavior, 28,* 375–381. (10)

Miller, I. N., Neargarder, S., Risi, M. M., & Cronin-Golomb, A. (2013). Frontal and posterior subtypes of neuropsychological deficit in Parkinson's disease. *Behavioral Neuroscience, 127,* 175–183. (7)

Miller, J. C., & Krizan, Z. (2016). Walking facilitates positive affect (even when expecting the opposite). *Emotion, 16,* 775–785. (14)

Miller, J. F., Neufang, M., Solway, A., Brandt, A., Trippel, M., Mader, I., . . . Schulze-Bonhage, A. (2013). Neural activity in human hippocampal formation reveals the spatial context of retrieved memories. *Science, 342,* 1111–1114. (13)

Miller, S. L., & Maner, J. K. (2010). Scent of a woman: Men's testosterone responses to olfactory ovulation cues. *Psychological Science, 21,* 276–283. (6)

Milner, B. (1959). The memory defect in bilateral hippocampal lesions. *Psychiatric Research Reports, 11,* 43–58. (12)

Milner, A. D. (2012). Is visual processing in the dorsal stream accessible to consciousness? *Proceedings of the Royal Society, B, 279,* 2289–2298. (5)

Min, J., Chiu, D. T., & Wang, Y. (2013). Variation in the heritability of body mass index based on diverse twin studies: A systematic review. *Obesity Reviews, 14,* 871–882. (9)

Mineur, Y. S., Abizaid, A., Rao, Y., Salas, R., DiLeone, R. J., Gündisch, D., . . . Picciotto, M. R. (2011). Nicotine decreases food intake through activation of POMC neurons. *Science, 332,* 1330–1332. (9)

Minichiello, L. (2009). TrkB signaling pathways in LTP and learning. *Nature Reviews Neuroscience, 10,* 850–860. (12)

Minkel, J. D., Banks, S., Htaik, O., Moreta, M. C., Jones, C. W., McGlinchey, E. L., . . . Dinges, D. F. (2012). Sleep deprivation and stressors: Evidence for elevated negative affect in response to mild stressors when sleep deprived. *Emotion, 12,* 1015–1020. (8)

Minokoshi, Y., Alquier, T., Furukawa, N., Kim, Y.-B., Lee, A., Xue, B., . . . Kahn, B. B. (2004). AMP-kinase regulates food intake by responding to hormonal and nutrient signals in the hypothalamus. *Nature, 428,* 569–574. (9)

Minto, C. L., Liao, L.-M., Woodhouse, C. R. J., Ransley, P. G., & Creighton, S. M. (2003). The effect of clitoral surgery in individuals who have intersex conditions with ambiguous genitalia: A cross-sectional study. *Lancet, 361,* 1252–1257. (10)

Misrahi, M., Meduri, G., Pissard, S., Bouvattier, C., Beau, I., Loosfelt, H., . . . Bougneres, P. (1997). Comparison of immunocytochemical and molecular features with the phenotype in a case of incomplete male pseudohermaphroditism associated with a mutation of the luteinizing hormone receptor. *Journal of Clinical Endocrinology & Metabolism, 82,* 2159–2165. (10)

Mistlberger, R. E., & Skene, D. J. (2004). Social influences on mammalian circadian rhythms: Animal and human studies. *Biological Rhythms, 79,* 533–556. (8)

Mitchell, D. E. (1980). The influence of early visual experience on visual perception. In C. S. Harris (Ed.), *Visual coding and adaptability* (pp. 1–50). Hillsdale, NJ: Erlbaum. (5)

Miu, A. C., Vulturar, R., Chis, A., Ungureanu, L., & Gross, J. J. (2013). Reappraisal as a mediator in the link between 5-HTTLPR and social anxiety symptoms. *Emotion, 13,* 1012–1022. (11)

Miyazawa, A., Fujiyoshi, Y., & Unwin, N. (2003). Structure and gating mechanism of the acetylcholine receptor pore. *Nature, 423,* 949–955. (2)

Mochizuki, T., Crocker, A., McCormack, S., Yanagisawa, M., Sakurai, T., & Scammell, T. E. (2004). Behavioral state instability in orexin knock-out mice. *Journal of Neuroscience, 24,* 6291–6300. (8)

Moens, L. N., De Rijk, P., Reumers, J., Van den Bossche, M. J. A., Glassee, W., De Zutter, S., . . . Del-Favero, J. (2011). Sequencing of *DISC1* pathway genes reveals increased burden of rare missense variants in schizophrenia patients from a northern Swedish population. *PLoS One, 6,* e23450. (14)

Mokalled, M. H., Patra, C., Dickson, A. L., Endo, T., Stainer, D. Y. R., & Poss, K. D. (2016). Injury-induced *ctgfa* directs glial bridging and spinal cord regeneration in zebrafish. *Science, 354,* 630–634. (4)

Molloy, K., Griffiths, T. D., Chait, M., & Lavie, N. (2015). Inattentional deafness: Visual load leads to time-specific suppression of auditory evoked responses. *Journal of Neuroscience, 35,* 16046–16054. (6)

Money, J., & Ehrhardt, A. A. (1972). *Man & woman, boy & girl.* Baltimore: Johns Hopkins University Press. (10)

Money, J., & Lewis, V. (1966). IQ, genetics and accelerated growth: Adrenogenital syndrome. *Bulletin of the Johns Hopkins Hospital, 118,* 365–373. (10)

Money, J., & Schwartz, M. (1978). Biosocial determinants of gender identity differentiation and development. In J. B. Hutchison (Ed.), *Biological determinants of sexual behaviour* (pp. 765–784). Chichester, England: Wiley. (10)

"Monkeying around." (2016). *Nature, 532,* 281. (0)

Monk, T. H., & Aplin, L. C. (1980). Spring and autumn daylight time changes: Studies of adjustment in sleep timings, mood, and efficiency. *Ergonomics, 23,* 167–178. (8)

Monteleone, P., Serritella, C., Scognamiglio, P., & Maj, M. (2010). Enhanced ghrelin secretion in the cephalic phase of food ingestion in women with bulimia nervosa. *Psychoneuroendocrinology, 35,* 284–288. (9)

Montgomery, K. J., Seeherman, K. R., & Haxby, J. V. (2009). The well-tempered social brain. *Psychological Science, 20,* 1211–1213. (7)

Montgomery, S. A., Baldwin, D. S., Blier, P., Fineberg, N. A., Kasper, S., Lader, M., . . . Thase, M. E. (2007). Which antidepressants have demonstrated superior efficacy? A review of the evidence. *International Clinical Psychopharmacology, 22,* 323–329. (14)

Monti, M. M., Vanhaudenhuyse, A., Coleman, M. R., Boly, M., Pickard, J. D., Tshibanda, L., . . . Laureys, S. (2010). Willful modulation of brain activity in disorders of consciousness. *New England Journal of Medicine, 362,* 579–589. (13)

Monti-Bloch, L., Jennings-White, C., Dolberg, D. S., & Berliner, D. L. (1994). The human vomeronasal system. *Psychoneuroendocrinology, 19,* 673–686. (6)

Montoya, E. R., Terburg, D., Bos, P. A., & van Honk, J. (2012). Testosterone, cortisol, and serotonin as key regulators of social aggression: A review. *Motivation & Emotion, 36*, 65–73. (11)

Moody, T. D., Chang, G. Y., Vanek, Z. F., & Knowlton, B. J. (2010). Concurrent discrimination learning in Parkinson's disease. *Behavioral Neuroscience, 124*, 1–8. (12)

Moore, L. B., Goodwin, B., Jones, S. A., Wisely, G. B., Serabjit-Singh, C. J., Willson, T. M., . . . Kliewer, S. A. (2000). St. John's wort induces hepatic drug metabolism through activation of the pregnane X receptor. *Proceedings of the National Academy of Sciences, USA, 97*, 7500–7502. (14)

Moore, T. L., Schetter, S. P., Killiany, R. J., Rosene, D. L., & Moss, M. B. (2012). Impairment in delayed nonmatching to sample following lesions of dorsal prefrontal cortex. *Behavioral Neuroscience, 126*, 772–780. (12)

Moore-Ede, M. C., Czeisler, C. A., & Richardson, G. S. (1983). Circadian timekeeping in health and disease. *New England Journal of Medicine, 309*, 469–476. (8)

Moors, A. (2009). Theories of emotion causation: A review. *Cognition & Emotion, 23*, 625–662. (11)

Moretti, A., Ferrari, F., & Villa, R. F. (2015). Neuroprotection for ischaemic stroke: Current status and challenges. *Pharmacology & Therapeutics, 146*, 23–34. (4)

Morfini, G. A., You, Y-M., Pollema, S. L., Kaminska, A., Liu, K., Yoshioka, K., . . . Brady, S. T. (2009). Pathogenic huntingtin inhibits fast axonal transport by activating JNK3 and phosphorylating kinesin. *Nature Neuroscience, 12*, 864–871. (7)

Mori, K., Mataga, N., & Imamura, K. (1992). Differential specificities of single mitral cells in rabbit olfactory bulb for a homologous series of fatty acid odor molecules. *Journal of Neurophysiology, 67*, 786–789. (6)

Moriuchi, J. M., Klin, A., & Jones, W. (2016). Mechanisms of diminished attention to eyes in autism. *American Journal of Psychiatry, 174*, 26–35. (14)

Morley, J. E., Levine, A. S., Grace, M., & Kneip, J. (1985). Peptide YY (PYY), a potent orexigenic agent. *Brain Research, 341*, 200–203. (9)

Moroz, L. L., Kocot, K. M., Citarella, M. R., Dosung, S., Norekian, T. P., Povolotskaya, I. S., . . . Kohn, A. B. (2014). The ctenophore genome and the evolutionary origin of nervous systems. *Nature, 510*, 109–114. (2)

Morquette, P., Verdier, D., Kodala, A., Féthière, J., Philippe, A. G., Robitaille, R., & Kolta, A. (2015). An astrocyte-dependent mechanism for neuronal rhythmogenesis. *Nature Neuroscience, 18*, 844–854. (1)

Morran, L. T., Schmidt, O. G., Gelarden, I. A., Parrish, R. C. II, & Lively, C. M. (2011). Running with the red queen: Host-parasite coevolution selects for biparental sex. *Science, 333*, 216–218. (10)

Morris, J. S., deBonis, M., & Dolan, R. J. (2002). Human amygdala responses to fearful eyes. *NeuroImage, 17*, 214–222. (11)

Morris, M., Lack, L., & Dawson, D. (1990). Sleep-onset insomniacs have delayed temperature rhythms. *Sleep, 13*, 1–14. (8)

Morrison, A. R., Sanford, L. D., Ball, W. A., Mann, G. L., & Ross, R. J. (1995). Stimulus-elicited behavior in rapid eye movement sleep without atonia. *Behavioral Neuroscience, 109*, 972–979. (8)

Morrison, J. H., & Baxter, M. G. (2012). The ageing cortical synapse: Hallmarks and implications for cognitive decline. *Nature Reviews Neuroscience, 13*, 240–250. (4)

Morrison, S. F. (2016). Central neural control of thermoregulation and brown adipose tissue. *Autonomic Neuroscience, 196*, 14–24. (9)

Morton, A. J., Wood, N. I., Hastings, M. H., Hurelbrink, C., Barker, R. A., & Maywood, E. S. (2005). Disintegration of the sleep–wake cycle and circadian timing in Huntington's disease. *Journal of Neuroscience, 25*, 157–163. (8)

Morton, G. J., Cummings, D. E., Baskin, D. G., Barsh, G. S., & Schwartz, M. W. (2006). Central nervous system control of food intake and body weight. *Nature, 443*, 289–295. (9)

Moruzzi, G., & Magoun, H. W. (1949). Brain stem reticular formation and activation of the EEG. *Electroencephalography and Clinical Neurophysiology, 1*, 455–473. (8)

Moscarello, J. M., & LeDoux, J. E. (2013). Active avoidance learning requires prefrontal suppression of amygdala-mediated defensive reactions. *Journal of Neuroscience, 33*, 3815–3823. (11)

Moser, H. R., & Giesler, G. J. Jr. (2013). Itch and analgesia resulting from intrathecal application of morphine: Contrasting effects on different populations of trigeminothalamic tract neurons. *Journal of Neuroscience, 33*, 6093–6101. (6)

Moser, M.-B., & Moser, E. I. (2016, January). Where am I? Where am I going? *Scientific American, 314*(1), 26–33. (12)

Moss, C. F., & Simmons, A. M. (1986). Frequency selectivity of hearing in the green treefrog, *Hyla cinerea*. *Journal of Comparative Physiology, A, 159*, 257–266. (6)

Moss, S. J., & Smart, T. G. (2001). Constructing inhibitory synapses. *Nature Reviews Neuroscience, 2*, 240–250. (2)

Mrzljak, L., Bergson, C., Pappy, M., Huff, R., Levenson, R., & Goldman-Rakic, P. S. (1996). Localization of dopamine D4 receptors in GABAergic neurons of the primate brain. *Nature, 381*, 245–248. (14)

Mueller, K., Fritz, T., Mildner, T., Richter, M., Schulze, K., Lepsien, J., . . . Möller, H. E. (2015). Investigating the dynamics of the brain response to music: A central role of the ventral striatum/nucleus accumbens. *NeuroImage, 116*, 68–79. (11)

Muller, Y. L., Hanson, R. L., Bian, L., Mack, J., Shi, X. L., Pakyz, R., . . . Baier, L. J. (2010). Functional variants in MBL2 are associated with type 2 diabetes and pre-diabetes traits in Pima Indians and the Old Order Amish. *Diabetes, 59*, 2080–2085. (9)

Munoz, D. P., & Everling, S. (2004). Look away: The anti-saccade task and the voluntary control of eye movement. *Nature Reviews Neuroscience, 5*, 218–228. (7)

Muraskin, J., Sherwin, J., & Sajda, P. (2015). Knowing when not to swing: EEG evidence that enhanced perception-action coupling underlies baseball batter expertise. *NeuroImage, 123*, 1–10. (5)

Murata, Y., Higo, N., Hayashi, T., Nishimura, Y., Sugiyama, Y., Oishi, T., . . . Onoe, H. (2015). Temporal plasticity involved in recovery from manual dexterity deficit after motor cortex lesion in macaque monkeys. *Journal of Neuroscience, 35*, 84–95. (4)

Murphy, F. C., Nimmo-Smith, I., & Lawrence, A. D. (2003). Functional neuroanatomy of emotions: A meta-analysis. *Cognitive, Affective, & Behavioral Neuroscience, 3*, 207–233. (11)

Murphy, M. L. M., Slavich, G. M., Chen, E., & Miller, G. E. (2015). Targeted rejection predicts decreased symptom severity in youth with asthma. *Psychological Science, 26*, 111–121. (11)

Murphy, M. R., Checkley, S. A., Seckl, J. R., & Lightman, S. L. (1990). Naloxone inhibits oxytocin release at orgasm in man. *Journal of Clinical Endocrinology & Metabolism, 71*, 1056–1058. (10)

Murray, G., Carrington, M. J., Nicholas, C. L., Kleiman, J., Dwyer, R., Allen, N. B., & Trinder, J. (2009). Nature's clocks and human mood: The circadian system modulates reward motivation. *Emotion, 9*, 705–716. (8)

Murrell, J., Farlow, M., Ghetti, B., & Benson, M. D. (1991). A mutation in the amyloid precursor protein associated with hereditary Alzheimer's disease. *Science, 254*, 97–99. (12)

Murty, N. A. R., & Arun, S. P. (2015). Dynamics of 3D view invariance in monkey inferotemporal cortex. *Journal of Neurophysiology, 113*, 2180–2194. (5)

Murty, V. P., LaBar, K. S., & Adcock, R. A. (2012). Threat of punishment motivates memory encoding via amygdala, not midbrain, interactions with the medial temporal lobe. *Journal of Neuroscience, 32*, 8969–8976. (12)

Musacchia, G., Sams, M., Skoe, E., & Kraus, N. (2007). Musicians have enhanced subcortical auditory and audiovisual processing of speech and music. *Proceedings of the National Academy of Sciences, USA, 104*, 15894–15898. (4)

Musiek, E. S., & Holtzman, D. M. (2015). Three dimensions of the amyloid hypothesis: Time, space, and "wingmen." *Nature Neuroscience, 18*, 800–806. (12)

Muto, V., Jaspar, M., Meyer, C., Kussé, C., Chellappa, S. L., Degueldre, C., . . . Maquet,

P. (2016). Local modulation of human brain responses by circadian rhythmicity and sleep debt. *Science, 353*, 687–690. (8)

Myers, C. A., Vandermosten, M., Farris, E. A., Hancock, R., Gimenez, P., Black, J. M., . . . Hoeft, F. (2014). White matter morphometric changes uniquely predict children's reading acquisition. *Psychological Science, 25*, 1870–1883. (12)

Myers, J. J., & Sperry, R. W. (1985). Interhemispheric communication after section of the forebrain commissures. *Cortex, 21*, 249–260. (13)

Nadal, A., Díaz, M., & Valverde, M. A. (2001). The estrogen trinity: Membrane, cytosolic, and nuclear effects. *News in Physiological Sciences, 16*, 251–255. (10)

Nagarajan, S., Mahncke, H., Salz, T., Tallal, P., Roberts, T., & Merzenich, M. M. (1999). Cortical auditory signal processing in poor readers. *Proceedings of the National Academy of Sciences, USA, 96*, 6483–6488. (13)

Nagy, E. (2011). Sharing the moment: The duration of embraces in humans. *Journal of Ethology, 29*, 389–393. (7)

Nahum, L., Bouzerda-Wahlen, A., Guggisberg, A., Ptak, R., & Schnider, A. (2012). Forms of confabulation: Dissociations and associations. *Neuropsychologia, 50*, 2224–2234. (12)

Najt, P., Bayer, U., & Hausmann, M. (2013). Models of hemispheric specialization in facial emotion perception—A reevaluation. *Emotion, 13*, 159–167. (11)

Nakamura, K. (2011). Central circuitries for body temperature regulation and fever. *American Journal of Physiology—Regulatory, Integrative, and Comparative Physiology, 301*, R1207–R1228. (9)

Nakata, H., Yoshie, M., Miura, A., & Kudo, K. (2010). Characteristics of the athletes' brain: Evidence from neurophysiology and neuroimaging. *Brain Research Reviews, 62*, 197–211. (5)

Nalls, M. A., Pankratz, N., Lill, C. M., Do, C. B., Hernandez, D. G., Saad, M., . . . Singleton, A. B. (2014). Large-scale meta-analysis of genome-wide association data identifies six new risk loci for Parkinson's disease. *Nature Genetics, 46*, 989–993. (7)

Narr, K. L., Woods, R. P., Thompson, P. M., Szeszko, P., Robinson, D., Dimtcheva, T., . . . Bilder, R. M. (2007). Relationships between IQ and regional cortical gray matter thickness in healthy adults. *Cerebral Cortex, 17*, 2163–2171. (12)

Narrow, W. E., Rae, D. S., Robins, L. N., & Regier, D. A. (2002). Revised prevalence estimates of mental disorders in the United States. *Archives of General Psychiatry, 59*, 115–123. (14)

Nasr, S., Polimeni, J. R., & Tootell, R. B. H. (2016). Interdigitated color- and disparity-selective columns within human visual cortical areas V2 and V3. *Journal of Neuroscience, 36*, 1841–1857. (5)

Nassi, J. J., & Callaway, E. M. (2006). Multiple circuits relaying primate parallel visual pathways to the middle temporal cortex. *Journal of Neuroscience, 26*, 12789–12798. (5)

Nassi, J. J., & Callaway, E. M. (2009). Parallel processing strategies of the primate visual system. *Nature Reviews Neuroscience, 10*, 360–372. (5)

Nathans, J., Davenport, C. M., Maumenee, I. H., Lewis, R. A., Hejtmancik, J. F., Litt, M., . . . Fishman, G. (1989). Molecular genetics of human blue cone monochromacy. *Science, 245*, 831–838. (5)

Naumer, M. J., & van den Bosch, J. J. F. (2009). Touching sounds: Thalamocortical plasticity and the neural basis of multisensory integration. *Journal of Neurophysiology, 102*, 7–8. (6)

Navarrete, C. D., McDonald, M. M., Mott, M. L., & Asher, B. (2012). Virtual morality: Emotion and action in a simulated three-dimensional "trolley problem." *Emotion, 12*, 364–370. (11)

Nave, G., Camerer, C., & McCullough, M. (2015). Does oxytocin increase trust in humans? A critical review of the literature. *Perspectives on Psychological Science, 10*, 772–789. (13)

Nebes, R. D. (1974). Hemispheric specialization in commissurotomized man. *Psychological Bulletin, 81*, 1–14. (13)

Nedergaard, M., & Verkhatsky, A. (2012). Artifact versus reality: How astrocytes contribute to synaptic events. *Glia, 60*, 1013–1023. (1)

Nef, P. (1998). How we smell: The molecular and cellular bases of olfaction. *News in Physiological Sciences, 13*, 1–5. (6)

Nelson, D. L., Orr, H. T., & Warren, S. T. (2013). The unstable repeats—three evolving faces of neurological disease. *Neuron, 77*, 825–843. (7)

Nelson, C. A., Wewerka, S., Thomas, K. M., Tribby-Walbridge, S., deRegnier, R., & Georgieff, M. (2000). Neurocognitive sequelae of infants of diabetic mothers. *Behavioral Neuroscience, 114*, 950–956. (4)

Nesvag, R., Bergmann, O., Rimol, L. M., Lange, E. H., Haukvik, U. K., Hartberg, C. B., . . . Agartz, I. (2012). A 5-year follow-up study of brain cortical and subcortical abnormalities in a schizophrenia cohort. *Schizophrenia Research, 142*, 209–216. (14)

Netter, F. H. (1983). *CIBA collection of medical illustrations: Vol. 1. Nervous system.* New York: CIBA. (10)

Nettersheim, A., Hallschmid, M., Born, J., & Diekelmann, S. (2015). The role of sleep in motor sequence consolidation: Stabilization rather than enhancement. *Journal of Neuroscience, 35*, 6696–6702. (8)

Network and Pathway Analysis Subgroup of the Psychiatric Genomics Consortium. (2015). Psychiatric genome-wide association study analyses implicate neuronal, immune and histone pathways. *Nature Neuroscience, 18*, 199–209. (14)

Neumeister, A., Hu, X.-Z., Luckenbaugh, D. A., Schwarz, M., Nugent, A. C., Bonne, O., . . . Charney, D. S. (2006). Differential effects of *5-HTTLPR* genotypes on the behavioral and neural responses to tryptophan depletion in patients with major depression and controls. *Archives of General Psychiatry, 63*, 978–986. (14)

Neumeister, A., Nugent, A. C., Waldeck, T., Geraci, M., Schwarz, M., Bonne, O., . . . Drevets, W. C. (2004). Neural and behavioral responses to tryptophan depletion in unmedicated patients with remitted major depressive disorder and controls. *Archives of General Psychiatry, 61*, 765–773. (14)

Neville, H. J., Bavelier, D., Corina, D., Rauschecker, J., Karni, A., Lalwani, A., . . . Turner, R. (1998). Cerebral organization for language in deaf and hearing subjects: Biological constraints and effects of experience. *Proceedings of the National Academy of Sciences, USA, 95*, 922–929. (13)

Nevin, R. (2007). Understanding international crime trends: The legacy of preschool lead exposure. *Environmental Research, 104*, 315–336. (11)

Nicklas, W. J., Saporito, M., Basma, A., Geller, H. M., & Heikkila, R. E. (1992). Mitochondrial mechanisms of neurotoxicity. *Annals of the New York Academy of Sciences, 648*, 28–36. (7)

Nicolelis, M. A. L., Ghazanfar, A. A., Stambaugh, C. R., Oliveira, L. M. O., Laubach, M., Chapin, J. K., . . . Kaas, J. H. (1998). Simultaneous encoding of tactile information by three primate cortical areas. *Nature Neuroscience, 1*, 621–630. (3)

Nielsen, J., Hedeholm, R. B., Heinemeier, J., Bushnell, P. G., Christiansen, J. S., Olsen, J., . . . Steffensen, J. F. (2016). Eye lens radiocarbon reveals centuries of longevity in the Greenland shark (*Somniosus microcephaus*). *Science, 353*, 702–707. (4)

Nieuwenhuys, R., Voogd, J., & vanHuijzen, C. (1988). *The human central nervous system* (3rd rev. ed.). Berlin: Springer-Verlag. (3, 9, 11, 13)

Nijboer, T. C. W., Kollen, B. J., & Kwakkel, G. (2013). Time course of visuospatial neglect early after stroke: A longitudinal cohort study. *Cortex, 59*, 2021–2027. (13)

Nikolova, Y. S., Koenen, K. C., Galea, S., Wang, C.-M., Seney, M. L., Sibille, E., . . . Hariri, A. R. (2014). Serotonin transporter epigenetic modification predicts human brain function. *Nature Neuroscience, 17*, 1153–1155. (12)

Nilsson, G. E. (1999, December). The cost of a brain. *Natural History, 108*, 66–73. (3)

Nir, Y., & Tononi, G. (2010). Dreaming and the brain: From phenomenology to neurophysiology. *Trends in Cognitive Sciences, 14*, 88–100. (8)

Nishimaru, H., Restrepo, C. E., Ryge, J., Yanagawa, Y., & Kiehn, O. (2005). Mammalian motor neurons corelease glutamate and acetylcholine at central synapses. *Proceedings of the National Academy of Sciences, USA, 102,* 5245–5249. (2)

Nishimura, Y., Onoe, H., Morichika, Y., Perfiliev, S., Tsukada, H., & Isa, T. (2007). Time-dependent central compensatory mechanisms of finger dexterity after spinal cord injury. *Science, 318,* 1150–1155. (4)

Nishizawa, K., Fukabori, R., Okada, K., Kai, N., Uchigashima, M., Watanabe, M., . . . Kobayashi, K. (2012). Striatal indirect pathway contributes to selection accuracy of learned motor actions. *Journal of Neuroscience, 32,* 13421–13432. (7)

Nitabach, M. N., & Taghert, P. H. (2008). Organization of the *Drosophila* circadian control circuit. *Current Biology, 18,* R84–R93. (8)

Noaghiul, S., & Hibbeln, J. R. (2003). Cross-national comparisons of seafood consumption and rates of bipolar disorders. *American Journal of Psychiatry, 160,* 2222–2227. (14)

Nørby, S., (2015). Why forget? On the adaptive value of memory loss. *Perspectives on Psychological Science, 10,* 551–578. (12)

Nordenström, A., Frisén, L., Falhammar, H., Filipsson, H., Holmdahl, G., Janson, P. O., . . . Nordenskjold, A. (2010). Sexual function and surgical outcome in women with congenital adrenal hyperplasia due to CYP21A2 deficiency: Clinical perspective and the patients' perception. *Journal of Clinical Endocrinology & Metabolism, 95,* 3633–3640. (10)

Nordenström, A., Servin, A., Bohlin, G., Larsson, A., & Wedell, A. (2002). Sex-typed toy play behavior correlates with the degree of prenatal androgen exposure assessed by *CYP21* genotype in girls with congenital adrenal hyperplasia. *Journal of Clinical Endocrinology & Metabolism, 87,* 5119–5124. (10)

Norman-Haignere, S. V., Albouy, P., Caclin, A., McDermott, J. H., Kanwisher, N. G., & Tillman, B. (2016). Pitch-responsive cortical regions in congenital amusia. *Journal of Neuroscience, 36,* 2986–2994. (6)

Norris, A. L., Marcus, D. K., & Green, B. A. (2015). Homosexuality as a discrete class. *Psychological Science, 26,* 1843–1853. (10)

North, R. A. (1989). Neurotransmitters and their receptors: From the clone to the clinic. *Seminars in the Neurosciences, 1,* 81–90. (2)

Nosenko, N. D., & Reznikov, A. G. (2001). Prenatal stress and sexual differentiation of monoaminergic brain systems. *Neurophysiology, 33,* 197–206. (10)

Nottebohm, F. (2002). Why are some neurons replaced in adult brain? *Journal of Neuroscience, 22,* 624–628. (4)

Novarino, G., El-Fishawy, P., Kayserili, H., Meguid, N. A., Scott, E. M., Schroth, J., . . . Gleeson, J. G. (2012). Mutations in *BCKD-kinase* lead to a potentially treatable form of autism with epilepsy. *Science, 338,* 394–397. (14)

Nugent, B. M., Wright, C. L., Shetty, A. C., Hodes, G. E., Lenz, K. M., Mahurkar, A., . . . McCarthy, M. M. (2015). Brain feminization requires active repression of masculinization via DNA methylation. *Nature Neuroscience, 18,* 690–697. (10)

Nugent, F. S., Penick, S. C., & Kauer, J. A. (2007). Opioids block long-term potentiation of inhibitory synapses. *Nature, 446,* 1086–1090. (12)

Numan, M., & Woodside, B. (2010). Maternity: Neural mechanisms, motivational processes, and physiological adaptations. *Behavioral Neuroscience, 124,* 715–741. (10, 11)

Nutt, D. J., Lingford-Hughes, A., Erritzoe, D., & Stokes, P. R. A. (2015). The dopamine theory of addiction: 40 years of highs and lows. *Nature Reviews Neuroscience, 16,* 305–312. (14)

Obeso, J. A., Marin, C., Rodriguez-Oroz, C., Blesa, J., Benitez-Temiño, B., Mena-Segovia, J., . . . Olanow, C. W. (2008). The basal ganglia in Parkinson's disease: Current concepts and unexplained observations. *Annals of Neurology, 64*(Suppl.), S30–S46. (7)

O'Connor, E. C., Kremer, Y., Lefort, S., Harada, M., Pascoli, V., Rohner, C., & Lüscher, C. (2015). Accumbal D1R neurons projecting to lateral hypothalamus authorize feeding. *Neuron, 88,* 553–564. (9)

Offidani, E., Guidi, J., Tomba, E., & Fava, G. A. (2013). Efficacy and tolerability of benzodiazepines versus antidepressants in anxiety disorders: A systematic review and meta-analysis. *Psychotherapy and Psychosomatics, 82,* 355–362. (11)

Oka, Y., Ye, M., & Zuker, C. S. (2015). Thirst driving and suppressing signals encoded by distinct neural populations in the brain. *Nature, 520,* 349–352. (9)

O'Kane, G., Kensinger, E. A., & Corkin, S. (2004). Evidence for semantic learning in profound amnesia: An investigation with patient H. M. *Hippocampus, 14,* 417–425. (12)

Okbay, A., Beauchamp, J. P., Fontana, M. A., Lee, J. J., Pers, T. H., Rietveld, C. A., . . . Benjamin, D. J. (2016). Genome-wide association study identifies 74 loci associated with educational attainments. *Nature, 533,* 539–542. (12)

O'Keefe, J., & Burgess, N. (1996). Geometric determinants of the place fields of hippocampal neurons. *Nature, 381,* 425–434. (12)

O'Keefe, J., & Dostrovsky, J. (1971). The hippocampus as a spatial map. Preliminary evidence from unit activity in the freely-moving rat. *Brain Research, 34,* 171–175. (12)

Okhovat, M., Berrio, A., Wallace, G., Ophir, A. G., & Phelps, S. M. (2015). Sexual fidelity trade-offs promote regulatory variation in the prairie vole brain. *Science, 350,* 1371–1374. (10)

Olanow, C. W., Goetz, C. G., Kordower, J. H., Stoessl, A. J., Sossi, V., Brin, M. F., . . . Freeman, T. B. (2003). A double-blind controlled trial of bilateral fetal nigral transplantation in Parkinson's disease. *Annals of Neurology, 54,* 403–414. (7)

Olds, J. (1958). Satiation effects in self-stimulation of the brain. *Journal of Comparative and Physiological Psychology, 51,* 675–678. (14)

Olds, J., & Milner, P. (1954). Positive reinforcement produced by electrical stimulation of the septal area and other regions of the rat brain. *Journal of Comparative and Physiological Psychology, 47,* 419–428. (14)

Oliver, L. D., Mitchell, D. G. V., Dziobek, I., MacKinley, J., Coleman, K., Rankin, K. P., & Finger, E. C. (2015). Parsing cognitive and emotional empathy deficits for negative and positive stimuli in frontotemporal dementia. *Neuropsychologia, 67,* 14–26. (13)

Olkowicz, S., Kocourek, M., Lucan, R. K., Portes, M., Fitch, T., Herculano-Houzel, S., & Nemec, P. (2016). Birds have primate-like numbers of neurons in the forebrain. *Proceedings of the National Academy of Sciences, 113,* 7255–7260. (12)

Oler, J. A., Fox, A. S., Shelton, S. E., Rogers, J., Dyer, T. D., Davidson, R. J., . . . Kalin, N. H. (2010). Amygdalar and hippocampal substrates of anxious temperament differ in their heritability. *Nature, 466,* 864–868. (11)

Olff, M., Frijling, J. L., Kubzansky, L. D., Bradley, B., Ellenbogen, M. A., Cardoso, C., . . . van Zuiden, M. (2013). The role of oxytocin in social bonding, stress regulation and mental health: An update on the moderating effects of context and individual differences. *Psychoneuroendocrinology, 38,* 1883–1894. (13)

Olney, J. W., & Farber, N. B. (1995). Glutamate receptor dysfunction and schizophrenia. *Archives of General Psychiatry, 52,* 998–1007. (14)

Olson, E. J., Boeve, B. F., & Silber, M. H. (2000). Rapid eye movement sleep behaviour disorder: Demographic, clinical and laboratory findings in 93 cases. *Brain, 123,* 331–339. (8)

Olsson, A., Kopsida, E., Sorjonen, K., & Savic, I. (2016). Testosterone and estrogen impact social evaluations and vicarious emotions: A double-blind placebo-controlled study. *Emotion, 16,* 515–523. (10)

Olsson, M. J., Lundström, J. N., Kimball, B. A., Gordon, A. R., Karshikoff, B., Hosseini, N., . . . Lekander, M. (2014). The scent of disease: Human body odor contains an early chemosensory cue of sickness. *Psychological Science, 25,* 817–823. (6)

Olton, D. S., & Papas, B. C. (1979). Spatial memory and hippocampal function. *Neuropsychologia, 17,* 669–682. (12)

Olton, D. S., Walker, J. A., & Gage, F. H. (1978). Hippocampal connections and spatial discrimination. *Brain Research, 139,* 295–308. (12)

Ono, M., Igarashi, T., Ohno, E., & Sasaki, M. (1995). Unusual thermal defence by a honeybee against mass attack by hornets. *Nature, 377,* 334–336. (9)

Oostenbroek, J., Suddendorf, T., Nielsen, M., Redshaw, J., Kennedy-Costantini, S., Davis, J., . . . Slaughter, V. (2016). Comprehensive longitudinal study challenges the existence of neonatal imitation in humans. *Current Biology, 26*, 1334–1338. (7)

O'Roak, B. J., Vives, L., Girirajan, S., Karakoc, E., Krumm, N., . . . Eichler, E. E. (2012). Sporadic autism exomes reveal a highly interconnected protein network of *de novo* mutations. *Nature, 485*, 246–250. (14)

O'Rourke, N. A., Weiler, N. C., Micheva, K. D., & Smith, S. J. (2012). Deep molecular diversity of mammalian synapses: Why it matters and how to measure it. *Nature Reviews Neuroscience, 13*, 365–379. (2)

Ortigue, S., Bianchi-Demicheli, F., Patel, N., Frum, C., & Lewis, J. W. (2010). Neuroimaging of love: fMRI meta-analysis evidence towards new perspectives in sexual medicine. *Journal of Sexual Medicine, 7*, 3541–3552. (13)

Otmakhov, N., Tao-Cheng, J.-H., Carpenter, S., Asrican, B., Dosemici, A., & Reese, T. S. (2004). Persistent accumulation of calcium/calmodulin-dependent protein kinase II in dendritic spines after induction of NMDA receptor-dependent chemical long-term potentiation. *Journal of Neuroscience, 25*, 9324–9331. (12)

Ousman, S. S., & Kubes, P. (2012). Immune surveillance in the central nervous system. *Nature Neuroscience, 15*, 1096–1101. (1)

Owen, A. M., Coleman, M. R., Boly, M., Davis, M. H., Laureys, S., & Pickard, J. D. (2006). Detecting awareness in the vegetative state. *Science, 313*, 1402. (13)

Oxley, D. R., Smith, K. B., Alford, J. R., Hibbing, M. V., Miller, J. L., Scalora, M., . . . Hibbing, J. R. (2008). Political attitudes vary with physiological traits. *Science, 321*, 1667–1670. (11)

Packer, A. M., Roska, B., & Häusser, M. (2013). Targeting neurons and photons for optogenetics. *Nature Neuroscience, 16*, 805–815. (3)

Padilla, S. L., Qiu, J., Soden, M. E., Sanz, E., Nestor, C. C., Barker, F. D., . . . Palmiter, R. D. (2016). Agouti-related peptide neural circuits mediate adaptive behaviors in the starved state. *Nature Neuroscience, 19*, 734–741. (9)

Paffen, C. L. E., & Alais, D. (2011). Attentional modulation of binocular rivalry. *Frontiers in Human Neuroscience, 5*, Article 105. (13)

Pail, G., Huf, W., Pjrek, E., Winkler, D., Willeit, M., Praschak-Rider, N., & Kasper, S. (2011). Bright-light therapy in the treatment of mood disorders. *Neuropsychobiology, 64*, 152–162. (14)

Palop, J. J., Chin, J., & Mucke, L. (2006). A network dysfunction perspective on neurodegenerative diseases. *Nature, 443*, 768–773. (12)

Palva, S., Linkenkaer-Hansen, K., Näätänen, R., & Palva, J. M. (2005). Early neural correlates of conscious somatosensory perception. *Journal of Neuroscience, 25*, 5248–5258. (6)

Pandey, G. N., Pandey, S. C., Dwivedi, Y., Sharma, R. P., Janicak, P. G., & Davis, J. M. (1995). Platelet serotonin-2A receptors: A potential biological marker for suicidal behavior. *American Journal of Psychiatry, 152*, 850–855. (11)

Panov, A. V., Gutekunst, C.-A., Leavitt, B. R., Hayden, M. R, Burke, J. R., Strittmatter, W. J., & Greenamyre, J. T. (2002). Early mitochondrial calcium defects in Huntington's disease are a direct effect of polyglutamines. *Nature Neuroscience, 5*, 731–736. (7)

Panula, P., & Nuutinen, S. (2013). The histaminergic network in the brain: Basic organization and role in disease. *Nature Reviews Neuroscience, 14*, 472–487. (8)

Pardal, R., & López-Barneo, J. (2002). Low glucose-sensing cells in the carotid body. *Nature Neuroscience, 5*, 197–198. (9)

Paredes, M. F., James, D., Gil-Perotin, S., Kim, H., Cotter, J. A., Ng, C., . . . Alvarez-Buylla, A. (2016). Extensive migration of young neurons into the infant human frontal lobe. *Science, 354*, 81. (4)

Parent, M. B., Habib, M. K., & Baker, G. B. (1999). Task-dependent effects of the antidepressant/antipanic drug phenelzine on memory. *Psychopharmacology, 142*, 280–288. (8)

Parise, E., & Csibra, G. (2012). Electrophysiological evidence for the understanding of maternal speech by 9-month-old infants. *Psychological Science, 23*, 728–733. (3)

Park, D. C., & McDonough, I. M. (2013). The dynamic aging mind: Revelations from functional neuroimaging research. *Perspectives on Psychological Science, 8*, 62–67. (4)

Park, I. S., Lee, K. J., Han, J. W., Lee, N. J., Lee, W. T., Park, K. A., & Rhyu, I. J. (2009). Experience-dependent plasticity of cerebellar vermis in basketball players. *Cerebellum, 8*, 334–339. (7)

Park, I. S., Lee, N. J., Kim, T.-Y., Park, J.-H., Won, Y.-M., Jung, Y.-J., . . . Rhyu, I. J. (2012). Volumetric analysis of cerebellum in short-track speed skating players. *Cerebellum, 11*, 925–930. (7)

Park, J. E., Sohn, J. H., Seong, S. J., Suk, H. W., & Cho, M. J. (2015). General similarities but consistent differences between early- and late-onset depression among Korean adults aged 40 and older. *Journal of Nervous and Mental Disease, 203*, 617–625. (14)

Park, S., Holzman, P. S., & Goldman-Rakic, P. S. (1995). Spatial working memory deficits in the relatives of schizophrenic patients. *Archives of General Psychiatry, 52*, 821–828. (14)

Parker, G. H. (1922). *Smell, taste, and allied senses in the vertebrates.* Philadelphia: Lippincott. (6)

Parton, L. E., Ye, C. P., Coppari, R., Enriori, P. J., Choi, B., Zhang, C.-Y., . . . Lowell, B. B. (2007). Glucose sensing by POMC neurons regulates glucose homeostasis and is impaired in obesity. *Nature, 449*, 228–232. (9)

Parvaz, M. A., Moeller, S. J., & Goldstein, R. Z. (2016). Incubation of cue-induced craving in adults addicted to cocaine measured by electroencephalography. *JAMA Psychiatry, 73*, 1127–1134. (14)

Parvizi, J., Jacques, C., Foster, B. L., Withoft, N., Rangarajan, V., Weiner, K. S., & Grill-Spector, K. (2012). Electrical stimulation of human fusiform face-selective regions distorts face perception. *Journal of Neuroscience, 32*, 14915–14920. (5)

Pascual, A., Hidalgo-Figueroa, M., Piruat, J. I., Pintado, C. O., Gómez-Díaz, R., & López-Barneo, J. (2008). Absolute requirement of GDNF for adult catecholaminergic neuron survival. *Nature Neuroscience, 11*, 755–761. (4)

Pasterski, V. L., Geffner, M. E., Brain, C., Hindmarsh, P., Brook, C., & Hines, M. (2005). Prenatal hormones and postnatal socialization by parents as determinants of male-typical toy play in girls with congenital adrenal hyperplasia. *Child Development, 76*, 264–278. (10)

Pasterski, V., Geffner, M. E., Brain, C., Hindmarsh, P., Brook, C., & Hines, M. (2011). Prenatal hormones and childhood sexual selection: Playmate and play style preferences in girls with congenital adrenal hyperplasia. *Hormones and Behavior, 59*, 549–555. (10)

Patten, S. B., Williams, J. V. A., Lavorato, D. H., Fiest, K. M., Bulloch, A. G. M., & Wang, J. L. (2015). The prevalence of major depression is not changing. *Canadian Journal of Psychiatry, 60*, 31–34. (14)

Patterson, K., Nestor, P. J., & Rogers, T. T. (2007). Where do you know what you know? The representation of semantic knowledge in the human brain. *Nature Reviews Neuroscience, 8*, 976–987. (12)

Paulesu, E., Frith, U., Snowling, M., Gallagher, A., Morton, J., Frackowiak, R. S. J., & Frith, C. D. (1996). Is developmental dyslexia a disconnection syndrome? *Brain, 119*, 143–157. (13)

Paus, T., Marrett, S., Worsley, K. J., & Evans, A. C. (1995). Extraretinal modulation of cerebral blood flow in the human visual cortex: Implications for saccadic suppression. *Journal of Neurophysiology, 74*, 2179–2183. (5)

Pavlov, I. P. (1927). *Conditioned reflexes.* Oxford, England: Oxford University Press. (12)

Payne, J. D., Kensinger, E. A., Wamsley, E. J., Spreng, R. N., Alger, S. E., Gibler, K., . . . Stickgold, R. (2015). Napping and the selective consolidation of negative aspects of scenes. *Emotion, 15*, 176–186. (8)

Pearson, H. (2006). Freaks of nature? *Nature, 444*, 1000–1001. (7)

Peck, C. J., Lau, B., & Salzman, C. D. (2013). The primate amygdala combines information about space and value. *Nature Neuroscience, 16*, 340–348. (11)

Peelle, J. E., Troiani, V., Grossman, M., & Wingfield, A. (2011). Hearing loss in older adults affects neural systems supporting speech comprehension. *Journal of Neuroscience, 31*, 12638–12643. (6)

Peeters, R., Simone, L., Nelissen, K., Fabbri-Desstro, M., Vanduffel, W., Rizzolatti, G., & Orban, G. A. (2009). The representation of tool use in humans and monkeys: Common and uniquely human features. *Journal of Neuroscience, 29,* 11523–11539. (0)

Peigneux, P., Laureys, S., Fuchs, S., Collette, F., Perrin, F., Reggers, J., . . . Maquet, P. (2004). Are spatial memories strengthened in the human hippocampus during slow wave sleep? *Neuron, 44,* 535–545. (8)

Peleg, G., Katzir, G., Peleg, O., Kamara, M., Brodsky, L., Hel-Or, H., . . . Nevo, E. (2006). Hereditary family signature of facial expression. *Proceedings of the National Academy of Sciences, USA, 103,* 15921–15926. (4)

Pelli, D. G., & Tillman, K. A. (2008). The uncrowded window of object recognition. *Nature Neuroscience, 11,* 1129–1135. (5)

Pellis, S. M., O'Brien, D. P., Pellis, V. C., Teitelbaum, P., Wolgin, D. L., & Kennedy, S. (1988). Escalation of feline predation along a gradient from avoidance through "play" to killing. *Behavioral Neuroscience, 102,* 760–777. (11)

Pelleymounter, M. A., Cullen, M. J., Baker, M. B., Hecht, R., Winters, D., Boone, T., & Collins, F. (1995). Effects of the obese gene product on body weight regulation in *ob/ob* mice. *Science, 269,* 540–543. (9)

Pembrey, M. E., Bygren, L. O., Kaati, G., Edvinsson, S., Northstone, K., Sjöstrom, M., . . . The ALSPAC Study Team. (2006). Sex-specific male-line transgenerational responses in humans. *European Journal of Human Genetics, 14,* 159–166. (4)

Penagos, H., Melcher, J. R., & Oxenham, A. J. (2004). A neural representation of pitch salience in nonprimary human auditory cortex revealed with functional magnetic resonance imaging. *Journal of Neuroscience, 24,* 6810–6815. (6)

Penfield, W. (1955). The permanent record of the stream of consciousness. *Acta Psychologica, 11,* 47–69. (12)

Penfield, W., & Milner, B. (1958). Memory deficit produced by bilateral lesions in the hippocampal zone. *Archives of Neurology and Psychiatry, 79,* 475–497. (12)

Penfield, W., & Perot, P. (1963). The brain's record of auditory and visual experience. *Brain, 86,* 595–696. (12)

Penfield, W., & Rasmussen, T. (1950). *The cerebral cortex of man.* New York: Macmillan. (3, 7)

Peng, G., & Wang, W. S.-Y. (2011). Hemisphere lateralization is influenced by bilingual status and composition of words. *Neuropsychologia, 49,* 1981–1986. (13)

Peng, Y., Gillis-Smith, S., Jin, H., Tränker, D., Ryba, N. J. P., & Zuker, C. S. (2015). Sweet and bitter taste in the brain of awake behaving animals. *Nature, 527,* 512–515. (6)

Penmatsa, A., Wang, K. H., & Gouaux, E. (2013). X-ray structure of dopamine transporter elucidates antidepressant mechanism. *Nature, 503,* 85–90. (14)

Pennisi, E. (2015). Of mice and men. *Nature, 349,* 21–22. (12)

Penzo, M. A., Robert, V., Tucciarone, J., De Bundel, D., Wang, M., Van Aelst, L., . . . Li, B. (2015). The paraventricular thalamus controls a central amygdala fear circuit. *Nature, 519,* 455–459. (11)

Pepperberg, I. M. (1981). Functional vocalizations by an African grey parrot. *Zeitschrift für Tierpsychologie, 55,* 139–160. (13)

Pepperberg, I. M. (1994). Numerical competence in an African gray parrot (*Psittacus erithacus*). *Journal of Comparative Psychology, 108,* 36–44. (13)

Pereda, A. E. (2014). Electrical synapses and their functional interactions with chemical synapses. *Nature Reviews Neuroscience, 15,* 250–263. (2)

Pereira, M., & Ferreira, A. (2016). Neuroanatomical and neurochemical basis of parenting: Dynamic coordination of motivational, affective and cognitive processes. *Hormones and Behavior, 77,* 72–85. (10)

Perera, T. D., Coplan, J. D., Lisanby, S. H., Lipira, C. M., Arif, M., Carpio, C., . . . Dwork, A. J. (2007). Antidepressant-induced neurogenesis in the hippocampus of adult nonhuman primates. *Journal of Neuroscience, 27,* 4894–4901. (14)

Perlow, M. J., Freed, W. J., Hoffer, B. J., Seiger, A., Olson, L., & Wyatt, R. J. (1979). Brain grafts reduce motor abnormalities produced by destruction of nigrostriatal dopamine system. *Science, 204,* 643–647. (7)

Perrone, J. A., & Thiele, A. (2001). Speed skills: Measuring the visual speed analyzing properties of primate MT neurons. *Nature Neuroscience, 4,* 526–532. (5)

Peretti, D., Bastide, A., Radford, H., Verity, N., Molloy, C., Martin, M. G., . . . Mallucci, G. R. (2015). RBM3 mediates structural plasticity and protective effects of cooling in neurodegeneration. *Nature, 518,* 236–239. (8)

Pert, C. B., & Snyder, S. H. (1973). The opiate receptor: Demonstration in nervous tissue. *Science, 179,* 1011–1014. (2, 6)

Pesold, C., & Treit, D. (1995). The central and basolateral amygdala differentially mediate the anxiolytic effect of benzodiazepines. *Brain Research, 671,* 213–221. (11)

Peters, F., Nicolson, N. A., Berkhof, J., Delespaul, P., & deVries, M. (2003). Effects of daily events on mood states in major depressive disorder. *Journal of Abnormal Psychology, 112,* 203–211. (14)

Peters, R. M., Hackeman, E., & Goldreich, D. (2009). Diminutive digits discern delicate details: Fingertip size and the sex difference in tactile spatial acuity. *Journal of Neuroscience, 29,* 15756–15761. (6)

Peterson, C., Warren, K. L., & Short, M. M. (2011). Infantile amnesia across the years: A 2-year follow-up of children's earliest memories. *Child Development, 82,* 1092–1105. (12)

Peterson, C. K., & Harmon-Jones, E. (2012). Anger and testosterone: Evidence that situationally-induced anger relates to situationally-induced testosterone. *Emotion, 12,* 899–902. (11)

Peterson, L. R., & Peterson, M. J. (1959). Short-term retention of individual verbal items. *Journal of Experimental Psychology, 58,* 193–198. (12)

Petitto, L. A., Zatorre, R. J., Gauna, K., Nikelski, E. J., Dostie, D., & Evans, A. C. (2000). Speech-like cerebral activity in profoundly deaf people processing signed languages: Implications for the neural basis of human language. *Proceedings of the National Academy of Sciences, USA, 97,* 13961–13966. (13)

Petrovic, P., Kalso, E., Petersson, K. M., & Ingvar, M. (2002). Placebo and opioid analgesia—Imaging a shared neuronal network. *Science, 295,* 1737–1740. (6)

Pezzoli, G., & Cereda, E. (2013). Exposure to pesticides or solvents and risk of Parkinson's disease. *Neurology, 80,* 2035–2041. (7)

Phan, K. L., Wager, T., Taylor, S. F., & Liberzon, I. (2002). Functional neuroanatomy of emotion: A meta-analysis of emotion activation studies in PET and fMRI. *NeuroImage, 16,* 331–348. (11)

Phelps, M. E., & Mazziotta, J. C. (1985). Positron emission tomography: Human brain function and biochemistry. *Science, 228,* 799–809. (3)

Pietropaolo, S., Feldon, J., Alleva, E., Cirulli, F., & Yee, B. K. (2006). The role of voluntary exercise in enriched rearing: A behavioral analysis. *Behavioral Neuroscience, 120,* 787–803. (4)

Pietschnig, J., Penke, L., Wicherts, J. M., Zeiler, M., & Voracek, M. (2015). Meta-analysis of associations between human brain volume and intelligence differences: How strong are they and what do they mean? *Neuroscience and Biobehavioral Reviews, 57,* 411–432. (12)

Pilley, J. W. (2013). Border collie comprehends sentences containing a prepositional object, verb, and direct object. *Learning and Motivation, 44,* 229–240. (13)

Pinker, S. (1994). *The language instinct.* New York: HarperCollins. (13)

Pinkston, J. W., & Lamb, R. J. (2011). Delay discounting in C57BL/6J and DBA/2J mice: Adolescent-limited and life-persistent patterns of impulsivity. *Behavioral Neuroscience, 125,* 194–201. (4)

Pinto, L., & Götz, M. (2007). Radial glial cell heterogeneity: The source of diverse progeny in the CNS. *Progress in Neurobiology, 83,* 2–23. (1)

Pishnamazi, M., Tafakhori, A., Loloee, S., Modabbernia, A., Aghamollaii, V., Bahrami, B., & Winston, J. S. (2016). Attentional bias towards and away from fearful faces is modulated by developmental amygdala damage. *Cortex, 81,* 24–34. (11)

Pizzagalli, D. A., Nitschke, J. B., Oakes, T. R., Hendrick, A. M., Horras, K. A., Larson, C.

L., . . . Davidson, R. J. (2002). Brain electrical tomography in depression: The importance of symptom severity, anxiety, and melancholic features. *Biological Psychiatry, 52,* 73–85. (14)

Plant, G. T., James-Galton, M., & Wilkinson, D. (2015). Progressive cortical visual failure associated with occipital calcification and coeliac disease with relative preservation of the dorsal "action" pathway. *Cortex, 71,* 160–170. (5)

Platje, E., Popma, A., Vermeiren, R. R. J. M., Doreleijers, T. A. H., Meeus, W. H. J., van Lier, P. A. C., . . . Jansen, L. M. C. (2015). Testosterone and cortisol in relation to aggression in a non-clinical sample of boys and girls. *Aggressive Behavior, 41,* 478–487. (11)

Plihal, W., & Born, J. (1997). Effects of early and late nocturnal sleep on declarative and procedural memory. *Journal of Cognitive Neuroscience, 9,* 534–547. (8)

Plomin, R., Corley, R., DeFries, J. C., & Fulker, D. (1990). Individual differences in television viewing in early childhood: Nature as well as nurture. *Psychological Science, 1,* 371–377. (4)

Plomin, R., DeFries, J. C., Knopik, V. S., & Neiderhiser, J. M. (2016). Top 10 replicated findings from behavioral genetics. *Perspectives on Psychological Science, 11,* 3–23. (4)

Plomin, R., Fulker, D. W., Corley, R., & DeFries, J. C. (1997). Nature, nurture, and cognitive development from 1 to 16 years: A parent-offspring adoption study. *Psychological Science, 8,* 442–447. (12)

Plomin, R., Haworth, C. M. A., Meaburn, E. L., Price, T. S., Wellcome Trust Case Control Consortium 2, & Davis, O. S. P. (2013). Common DNA markers can account for more than half of the genetic influence on cognitive abilities. *Psychological Science, 24,* 562–568. (4, 12)

Plutchik, R. (1982). A psychoevolutionary theory of emotions. *Social Science Information, 21,* 529–553. (11)

Pochedly, J. T., Widen, S. C., & Russell, J. A. (2012). What emotion does the "facial expression of disgust" express? *Emotion, 12,* 1315–1319. (11)

Poduslo, S. E., Huang, R., & Spiro, A. III (2009). A genome screen of successful aging without cognitive decline identifies LRP1B by haplotype analysis. *American Journal of Medical Genetics, B, 153B,* 114–119. (4)

Poldrack, R. A. (2006). Can cognitive processes be inferred from neuroimaging data? *Trends in Cognitive Sciences, 10,* 59–63. (3)

Poldrack, R. A., Sabb, F. W., Foerde, K., Tom, S. M., Asarnow, R. F., Bookheimer, S. Y., & Knowlton, B. J. (2005). The neural correlates of motor skill automaticity. *Journal of Neuroscience, 25,* 5356–5364. (7)

Polk, T. A., Drake, R. M., Jonides, J. J., Smith, M. R., & Smith, E. E. (2008). Attention enhances the neural processing of relevant features and suppresses the processing of irrelevant features in humans: A functional magnetic resonance imaging study of the Stroop task. *Journal of Neuroscience, 28,* 13786–13792. (13)

Pons, T. P., Garraghty, P. E., Ommaya, A. K., Kaas, J. H., Taub, E., & Mishkin, M. (1991). Massive cortical reorganization after sensory deafferentation in adult macaques. *Science, 252,* 1857–1860. (4)

Pontieri, F. E., Tanda, G., Orzi, F., & DiChiara, G. (1996). Effects of nicotine on the nucleus accumbens and similarity to those of addictive drugs. *Nature, 382,* 255–257. (3)

Pontzer, H., Brown, M. H., Raichlen, D. A., Dunsworth, H., Hare, B., Walker, K., . . . Ross, S. R. (2016). Metabolic acceleration and the evolution of human brain size and life history. *Nature, 533,* 390–392. (12)

Poremba, A., Saunders, R. C., Crane, A. M., Cook, M., Sokoloff, L., & Mishkin, M. (2003). Functional mapping of the primate auditory system. *Science, 299,* 568–572. (6)

Porter, J., Craven, B., Khan, R. M., Chang, S.-J., Kang, I., Judkewicz, B., . . . Sobel, N. (2007). Mechanisms of scent-tracking in humans. *Nature Neuroscience, 10,* 27–29. (6)

Posner, S. F., Baker, L., Heath, A., & Martin, N. G. (1996). Social contact, social attitudes, and twin similarity. *Behavior Genetics, 26,* 123–133. (4)

Post, R. M. (1992). Transduction of psychological stress into the neurobiology of recurrent affective disorder. *American Journal of Psychiatry, 149,* 999–1010. (14)

Posthuma, D., De Geus, E. J. C., Baaré, W. F. C., Pol, H. E. H., Kahn, R. S., & Boomsma, D. I. (2002). The association between brain volume and intelligence is of genetic origin. *Nature Neuroscience, 5,* 83–84. (12)

Potegal, M. (1994). Aggressive arousal: The amygdala connection. In M. Potegal & J. F. Knutson (Eds.), *The dynamics of aggression* (pp. 73–111). Hillsdale, NJ: Erlbaum. (11)

Potegal, M., Ferris, C., Hebert, M., Meyerhoff, J. M., & Skaredoff, L. (1996). Attack priming in female Syrian golden hamsters is associated with a *c-fos* coupled process within the corticomedial amygdala. *Neuroscience, 75,* 869–880. (11)

Potegal, M., Hebert, M., DeCoster, M., & Meyerhoff, J. L. (1996). Brief, high-frequency stimulation of the corticomedial amygdala induces a delayed and prolonged increase of aggressiveness in male Syrian golden hamsters. *Behavioral Neuroscience, 110,* 401–412. (11)

Potegal, M., Robison, S., Anderson, F., Jordan, C., & Shapiro, E. (2007). Sequence and priming in 15 month-olds' reactions to brief arm restraint: Evidence for a hierarchy of anger responses. *Aggressive Behavior, 33,* 508–518. (11)

Pouchelon, G., Gambino, F., Bellone, C., Telley, L., Vitali, I., Lüscher, C., . . . Jabaudon, D. (2014). Modality-specific thalamocortical inputs instruct the identity of postsynaptic L4 neurons. *Nature, 511,* 471–477. (4)

Poulos, A. M., & Thompson, R. F. (2015). Localization and characterization of an essential associative memory trace in the mammalian brain. *Brain Research, 1621,* 252–259. (12)

Poulin, M. J., Holman, E. A., & Buffone, A. (2012). The neruogenetics of nice: Oxytocin and vasopressin receptor genes and prosocial behavior. *Psychological Science, 23,* 446–452. (13)

Power, R. A., Keers, R., Ng, M. Y., Butler, A. W., Uher, R., Cohen-Woods, S., . . . Lewis, C. M. (2012). Dissecting the genetic heterogeneity of depression through age at onset. *American Journal of Medical Genetics, 159B,* 859–868. (14)

Preckel, F., Lipnevich, A. A., Anastasiya, A., Schneider, S., & Roberts, R. D. (2011). Chrono-type, cognitive abilities, and academic achievement: A meta-analytic investigation. *Learning and Individual Differences, 21,* 483–492. (8)

Preckel, F., Lipnevich, A. A., Boehme, K., Brandner, L., Georgi, K., Könen, T., . . . Roberts, R. D. (2013). Morningness-eveningness and educational outcomes: The lark has an advantage over the owl at high school. *British Journal of Educational Psychology, 83,* 114–134. (8)

Premack, A. J., & Premack, D. (1972). Teaching language to an ape. *Scientific American, 227*(4), 92–99. (13)

Preti, G., Cutler, W. B., Garcia, C. R., Huggins, G. R., & Lawley, H. J. (1986). Human axillary secretions influence women's menstrual cycles: The role of donor extract of females. *Hormones and Behavior, 20,* 474–482. (6)

Pritchard, T. C., Hamilton, R. B., Morse, J. R., & Norgren, R. (1986). Projections of thalamic gustatory and lingual areas in the monkey, *Macaca fascicularis. Journal of Comparative Neurology, 244,* 213–228. (6)

Provine, R. R. (1979). "Wing-flapping" develops in wingless chicks. *Behavioral and Neural Biology, 27,* 233–237. (7)

Provine, R. R. (1981). Wing-flapping develops in chickens made flightless by feather mutations. *Developmental Psychobiology, 14,* 48 B 1–486. (7)

Provine, R. R. (1984). Wing-flapping during development and evolution. *American Scientist, 72,* 448–455. (7)

Provine, R. R. (1986). Yawning as a stereotyped action pattern and releasing stimulus. *Ethology, 72,* 109–122. (7)

Provine, R. R. (1972). Ontogeny of bioelectric activity in the spinal cord of the chick embryo and its behavioral implications. *Brain Research, 41,* 365–378. (4)

Prutkin, J., Duffy, V. B., Etter, L., Fast, K., Gardner, E., Lucchina, L. A., . . . Bartoshuk, L. M. (2000). Genetic variation and inferences about perceived taste intensity in mice and men. *Physiology & Behavior, 69,* 161–173. (6)

Puca, A. A., Daly, M. J., Brewster, S. J., Matise, T. C., Barrett, J., Shea-Drinkwater,

M., . . . Perls, T. (2001). A genome-wide scan for linkage to human exceptional longevity identifies a locus on chromosome 4. *Proceedings of the National Academy of Sciences (U.S.A.), 98*, 10505–10508. (4)

Pudas, S., Persson, J., Josefsson, M., de Luna, X., Nilsson, L.-G., & Nyberg, L. (2013). Brain characteristics of individuals resisting age-related cognitive decline over two decades. *Journal of Neuroscience, 33,* 8668–8677. (4)

Puneeth, N. C., & Arun, S. P. (2016). A neural substrate for object permanence in monkey inferotemporal cortex. *Scientific Reports, 6,* Article 30808. (5)

Purcell, D. W., Blanchard, R., & Zucker, K. J. (2000). Birth order in a contemporary sample of gay men. *Archives of Sexual Behavior, 29*, 349–356. (10)

Purcell, S. M., Moran, J. L., Fromer, M., Ruderfer, D., Solovieff, N., Roussos, P., . . . Sklar, P. (2014). A polygenic burden of rare disruptive mutations in schizophrenia. *Nature, 506*, 185–190. (14)

Purves, D., & Hadley, R. D. (1985). Changes in the dendritic branching of adult mammalian neurones revealed by repeated imaging *in situ. Nature, 315*, 404–406. (4)

Purves, D., & Lotto, R. B. (2003). *Why we see what we do: An empirical theory of vision.* Sunderland, MA: Sinauer Associates. (5)

Purves, D., Shimpi, A., & Lotto, R. B. (1999). An empirical explanation of the Cornsweet effect. *Journal of Neuroscience, 19,* 8542–8551. (5)

Putnam, S. K., Du, J., Sato, S., & Hull, E. M. (2001). Testosterone restoration of copulatory behavior correlates with medial preoptic dopamine release in castrated male rats. *Hormones and Behavior, 39*, 216–224. (10)

Puzziferri, N., Roshek, T. B. III, Mayo, H. G., Gallagher, R., Belle, S. H., & Livingston, E. H. (2014). Long-term follow-up after bariatric surgery: A systematic review. *Journal of the American Medical Association, 312,* 934–942. (9)

Queen, T. L., & Hess, T. M. (2010). Age differences in the effects of conscious and unconscious thought in decision making. *Psychology and Aging, 25*, 251–261. (4)

Race, E., Keane, M. M., & Verfaellie, M. (2011). Medial temporal lobe damage causes deficits in episodic memory and episodic future thinking not attributable to deficits in narrative construction. *Journal of Neuroscience, 31*, 10262–10269. (12)

Radoeva, P. D., Prasad, S., Brainard, D. H., & Aguirre, G. K. (2008). Neural activity within area V1 reflects unconscious visual performance in a case of blindsight. *Journal of Cognitive Neuroscience, 20*, 1927–1939. (5)

Rahman, Q., & Wilson, G. D. (2003). Born gay? The psychobiology of human sexual orientation. *Personality and Individual Differences, 34,* 1337–1382. (10)

Rainville, P., Duncan, G. H., Price, D. D., Carrier, B., & Bushnell, M. C. (1997). Pain affect encoded in human anterior cingulate but not somatosensory cortex. *Science, 277,* 968–971. (6)

Rakic, P. (1998). Cortical development and evolution. In M. S. Gazzaniga & J. S. Altman (Eds.), *Brain and mind: Evolutionary perspectives* (pp. 34–40). Strasbourg, France: Human Frontier Science Program. (4)

Ralph, M. R., Foster, R. G., Davis, F. C., & Menaker, M. (1990). Transplanted suprachiasmatic nucleus determines circadian period. *Science, 247*, 975–978. (8)

Ralph, M. R., & Menaker, M. (1988). A mutation of the circadian system in golden hamsters. *Science, 241*, 1225–1227. (8)

Ramachandran, V. S. (2003, May). Hearing colors, tasting shapes. *Scientific American, 288*(5), 52–59. (6)

Ramachandran, V. S., & Blakeslee, S. (1998). *Phantoms in the brain.* New York: Morrow. (4)

Ramachandran, V. S., & Hirstein, W. (1998). The perception of phantom limbs: The D. O. Hebb lecture. *Brain, 121*, 1603–1630. (4)

Ramirez, J. J. (2001). The role of axonal sprouting in functional reorganization after CNS injury: Lessons from the hippocampal formation. *Restorative Neurology and Neuroscience, 19*, 237–262. (4)

Ramirez, J. J., Bulsara, K. R., Moore, S. C., Ruch, K., & Abrams, W. (1999). Progressive unilateral damage of the entorhinal cortex enhances synaptic efficacy of the crossed entorhinal afferent to dentate granule cells. *Journal of Neuroscience, 19*: RC42, 1–6. (4)

Ramirez, J. J., Campbell, D., Poulton, W., Barton, C., Swails, J., Geghman, K., . . . Courchesne, S. L. (2007). Bilateral entorhinal cortex lesions impair acquisition of delayed spatial alternation in rats. *Neurobiology of Learning and Memory, 87*, 264–268. (4)

Ramirez, J. J., McQuilkin, M., Carrigan, T., MacDonald, K., & Kelley, M. S. (1996). Progressive entorhinal cortex lesions accelerate hippocampal sprouting and spare spatial memory in rats. *Proceedings of the National Academy of Sciences, USA, 93*, 15512–15517. (4)

Ramón y Cajal, S. *see* Cajal, S. R.

Randler, C., Ebenhöh, N., Fischer, A., Höchel, S., Schroff, C., Stoll, J. C., & Vollmer, C. (2012). Chronotype but not sleep length is related to salivary testosterone in young men. *Psychoneuroendocrinology, 37,* 1740–1744. (8)

Ran, C., Hoon, M. A., & Chen, X. (2016). The coding of cutaneous temperature in the spinal cord. *Nature Neuroscience, 19,* 1201–1209. (6)

Ranson, S. W., & Clark, S. L. (1959). *The anatomy of the nervous system: Its development and function* (10th ed.). Philadelphia: Saunders. (3)

Rapoport, S. I., & Robinson, P. J. (1986). Tight-junctional modification as the basis of osmotic opening of the blood–brain barrier. *Annals of the New York Academy of Sciences, 481*, 250–267. (1)

Rasch, B., Pommer, J., Diekelmann, & Born, J. (2009). Pharmacological REM sleep suppression paradoxically improves rather than impairs skill memory. *Nature Neuroscience, 12*, 396–397. (8)

Raschle, N. M., Zuk, J., & Gaab, N. (2012). Functional characteristics of developmental dyslexia in left-hemispheric posterior brain regions predate reading onset. *Proceedings of the National Academy of Sciences (U.S.A.), 109*, 2156–2161. (13)

Rattenborg, N. C., Amlaner, C. J., & Lima, S. L. (2000). Behavioral, neurophysiological and evolutionary perspectives on unihemispheric sleep. *Neuroscience and Biobehavioral Reviews, 24*, 817–842. (8)

Rattenborg, N. C., Mandt, B. H., Obermeyer, W. H., Winsauer, P. J., Huber, R., Wikelski, M., & Benca, R. M. (2004). Migratory sleeplessness in the white-crowned sparrow (*Zonotrichia leucophrys gambelii*). *PLoS Biology, 2*, 924–936. (8)

Rattenborg, N. C., Voirin, B., Cruz, S. M., Tisdale, R., Dell'Omo, G., Llipp, H.-P., . . . Vyssotski, A. L. (2016). Evidence that birds sleep in mid-flight. *Nature Communications, 7*, article 12468. (8)

Raum, W. J., McGivern, R. F., Peterson, M. A., Shryne, J. H., & Gorski, R. A. (1990). Prenatal inhibition of hypothalamic sex steroid uptake by cocaine: Effects on neurobehavioral sexual differentiation in male rats. *Developmental Brain Research, 53*, 230–236. (10)

Rauschecker, A. M., Dastjerdi, M., Weiner, K. S., Witthoft, N., Chen, J., Selimbeyoglu, A., & Parvizi, J. (2011). Illusions of visual motion elicited by electrical stimulation of human MT complex. *PLoS One, 6*, e21798. (5)

Rauskolb, S., Zagrebelsky, M., Dreznjak, A., Deogracias, R., Matsumoto, T., Wiese, S., . . . Barde, Y. A. (2010). Global deprivation of brain-derived neurotrophic factor in the CNS reveals an area-specific requirement for dendritic growth. *Journal of Neuroscience, 30*, 1739–1749. (4)

Ravussin, Y., Leibel, R. L., & Ferrante, A. W. Jr. (2014). A missing link in body weight homeostasis: The catabolic signal of the overfed state. *Cell Metabolism, 20*, 565–572. (9)

Rawlins, M. D., Wexler, N. S., Wexler, A. R., Tabrizi, S. J., Douglas, I., Evans, S. J. W., & Smeeth, L. (2016). The prevalence of Huntington's disease. *Neuroepidemiology, 46*, 144–153. (7)

Rechenberg, K. (2016). Nutritional interventions in clinical depression. *Clinical Psychological Science, 4*, 144–162. (14)

Redish, A. D. (2016). Vicarious trial and error. *Nature Reviews Neuroscience, 17*, 147–159. (12, 13)

Redmond, D. E., Jr., Bjugstad, K. B., Teng, Y. D., Ourednik, V., Ourednik, J., Wakeman, D. R., . . . Snyder, E. Y. (2007). Behavioral improvement in a primate Parkinson's model is associated with multiple homeostatic effects of human neural stem cells. *Proceedings of the National Academy of Sciences, USA, 104,* 12175–12180. (7)

Redondo, R. L., & Morris, R. G. M. (2011). Making memories last: The synaptic tagging and capture hypothesis. *Nature Reviews Neuroscience, 12,* 17–30. (12)

Reed, F. D. D., Hirst, J. M., & Hayman, S. R. (2012). Assessment and treatment of stereotypic behavior in children with autism and other developmental disabilities: A thirty year review. *Research in Autism Spectrum Disorders, 6,* 422–430. (14)

Reeves, A. G., & Plum, F. (1969). Hyperphagia, rage, and dementia accompanying a ventromedial hypothalamic neoplasm. *Archives of Neurology, 20,* 616–624. (9)

Refinetti, R. (2000). *Circadian physiology.* Boca Raton, FL: CRC Press. (8)

Refinetti, R., & Carlisle, H. J. (1986). Complementary nature of heat production and heat intake during behavioral thermoregulation in the rat. *Behavioral and Neural Biology, 46,* 64–70. (9)

Refinetti, R., & Menaker, M. (1992). The circadian rhythm of body temperature. *Physiology & Behavior, 51,* 613–637. (8)

Regan, T. (1986). The rights of humans and other animals. *Acta Physiologica Scandinavica, 128*(Suppl. 554), 33–40. (0)

Reichelt, K. L., Seim, A. R., & Reichelt, W. H. (1996). Could schizophrenia be reasonably explained by Dohan's hypothesis on genetic interaction with a dietary peptide overload? *Progress in Neuro-Psychopharmacology & Biological Psychiatry, 20,* 1083–1114. (14)

Reick, M., Garcia, J. A., Dudley, C., & McKnight, S. L. (2001). NPAS2: An analog of clock operative in the mammalian forebrain. *Science, 293,* 506–509. (8)

Reid, C. A., Dixon, D. B., Takahashi, M., Bliss, T. V. P., & Fine, A. (2004). Optical quantal analysis indicates that long-term potentiation at single hippocampal mossy fiber synapses is expressed through increased release probability, recruitment of new release sites, and activation of silent synapses. *Journal of Neuroscience, 24,* 3618–3626. (12)

Reiner, W. G., & Gearhart, J. P. (2004). Discordant sexual identity in some genetic males with cloacal exstrophy assigned to female sex at birth. *New England Journal of Medicine, 350,* 333–341. (10)

Reinius, B., Saetre, P., Leonard, J. A., Blekhman, R., Merino-Martinez, R., Gilad, Y., & Jazin, E. (2008). An evolutionarily conserved sexual signature in the primate brain. *PLoS Genetics,* e1000100. (10)

Reisner, A. D. (2003). The electroconvulsive therapy controversy: Evidence and ethics. *Neuropsychology Review, 13,* 199–219. (14)

Rennaker, R. L., Chen, C.-F. F., Ruyle, A. M., Sloan, A. M., & Wilson, D. A. (2007). Spatial and temporal distribution of odorant-evoked activity in the piriform cortex. *Journal of Neuroscience, 27,* 1534–1542. (6)

Rensch, B. (1964). Memory and concepts of higher animals. *Proceedings of the Zoological Society of Calcutta, 17,* 207–221. (12)

Rensch, B. (1977). Panpsychic identism and its meaning for a universal evolutionary picture. *Scientia, 112,* 337–349. (0)

Rensink, R. A., O'Regan, J. K., & Clark, J. J. (1997). To see or not to see: The need for attention to perceive changes in scenes. *Psychological Science, 8,* 368–373. (13)

Renzel, R., Baumann, C. R., & Poryazova, R. (2016). EEG after sleep deprivation is a sensitive tool in the first diagnosis of idiopathic generalized but not focal epilepsy. *Clinical Neurophysiology, 127,* 209–213. (3)

Reuter-Lorenz, P., & Davidson, R. J. (1981). Differential contributions of the two cerebral hemispheres to the perception of happy and sad faces. *Neuropsychologia, 19,* 609–613. (11)

Reuter-Lorenz, P. A., & Miller, A. C. (1998). The cognitive neuroscience of human laterality: Lessons from the bisected brain. *Current Directions in Psychological Science, 7,* 15–20. (13)

Revusky, S. (2009). Chemical aversion treatment of alcoholism. In S. Reilly & T. R. Schachtman (Eds.), *Conditioned taste aversion* (pp. 445–472). New York: Oxford University Press. (14)

Rhees, R. W., Shryne, J. E., & Gorski, R. A. (1990). Onset of the hormone-sensitive perinatal period for sexual differentiation of the sexually dimorphic nucleus of the preoptic area in female rats. *Journal of Neurobiology, 21,* 781–786. (10)

Rhodes, J. S., van Praag, H., Jeffrey, S., Girard, I., Mitchell, G. S., Garland, T., Jr., & Gage, F. H. (2003). Exercise increases hippocampal neurogenesis to high levels but does not improve spatial learning in mice bred for increased voluntary wheel running. *Behavioral Neuroscience, 117,* 1006–1016. (4)

Ricciardi, E., Bonino, D., Sani, L., Vecchi, T., Guazzelli, M., Haxby, J. V., . . . Pietrini, P. (2009). Do we really need vision? How blind people "see" the actions of others. *Journal of Neuroscience, 29,* 9719–9724. (7)

Rice, G., Anderson, C., Risch, N., & Ebers, G. (1999). Male homosexuality: Absence of linkage to microsatellite markers at Xq28. *Science, 284,* 665–667. (10)

Rice, W. R., Friberg, U., & Gavrilets, S. (2012). Homosexuality as a consequence of epigenetically canalized sexual development. *Quarterly Review of Biology, 87,* 343–368. (10)

Rich, E. L., & Wallis, J. D. (2016). Decoding subjective decisions from orbitofrontal cortex. *Nature Neuroscience, 19,* 973–980. (13)

Richard, C., Honoré, J., Bernati, T., & Rousseaux, M. (2004). Straight-ahead pointing correlates with long-line bisection in neglect patients. *Cortex, 40,* 75–83. (13)

Richter, C. P. (1922). A behavioristic study of the activity of the rat. *Comparative Psychology Monographs, 1,* 1–55. (8)

Richter, C. P. (1936). Increased salt appetite in adrenalectomized rats. *American Journal of Physiology, 115,* 155–161. (9)

Richter, C. P. (1950). Taste and solubility of toxic compounds in poisoning of rats and humans. *Journal of Comparative and Physiological Psychology, 43,* 358–374. (6)

Richter, C. P. (1967). Psychopathology of periodic behavior in animals and man. In J. Zubin & H. F. Hunt (Eds.), *Comparative psychopathology* (pp. 205–227). New York: Grune & Stratton. (8)

Richter, C. P. (1975). Deep hypothermia and its effect on the 24-hour clock of rats and hamsters. *Johns Hopkins Medical Journal, 136,* 1–10. (8)

Ridaura, V. K., Faith, J. J., Rey, F. E., Cheng, J., Duncan, A. E., Kau, A. L., . . . Gordon, J. I. (2013). Gut microbiota from twins discordant for obesity modulate metabolism in mice. *Science, 341,* 1079. (9)

Rieger, G., Chivers, M. L., & Bailey, J. M. (2005). Sexual arousal patterns of bisexual men. *Psychological Science, 16,* 579–584. (10)

Riek, R., & Eisenberg, D. S. (2016). The activities of amyloids from a structural perspective. *Nature, 539,* 227–235. (12)

Riemann, D., König, A., Hohagen, F., Kiemen, A., Voderholzer, U., Backhaus, J., . . . Berger, M. (1999). How to preserve the antidepressive effect of sleep deprivation: A comparison of sleep phase advance and sleep phase delay. *European Archives of Psychiatry and Clinical Neuroscience, 249,* 231–237. (14)

Rietveld, C. A., Medland, S. E., Derringer, J., Yang, J., Esko, T., Martin, N. W., . . . Koellinger, P. D. (2013). GWAS of 126,559 individuals identifies genetic variants associated with educational attainment. *Science, 340,* 1467–1471. (4)

Rigoni, D., Brass, M., & Sartori, G. (2010). Postaction determinants of the reported time of conscious intentions. *Frontiers in Human Neuroscience, 4,* article 38. (7)

Rilling, J. K., & Young, L. J. (2014). The biology of mammalian parenting and its effect on offspring social development. *Science, 345,* 771–776. (10)

Rinn, W. E. (1984). The neuropsychology of facial expression: A review of the neurological and psychological mechanisms for producing facial expressions. *Psychological Bulletin, 95,* 52–77. (7)

Risch, N., Hoffmann, T. J., Anderson, M., Croen, L. A., Grether, J. K., & Windham, G. C. (2014). Familial recurrence of autism spectrum disorder: Evaluating genetic and environmental contributions. *American Journal of Psychiatry, 171,* 1206–1213. (14)

Ritchie, S. J., Bastin, M. E., Tucker-Drob, E. M., Maniega, S. M., Englehardt, L. E., Cox, S. R., . . . Deary, I. J. (2015). Coupled changes in brain white matter microstructure and fluid intelligence in later life. *Journal of Neuroscience, 35,* 8672–8682. (12)

Rittenhouse, C. D., Shouval, H. Z., Paradiso, M. A., & Bear, M. F. (1999). Monocular deprivation induces homosynaptic long-term depression in visual cortex. *Nature, 397,* 347–350. (5)

Ritz, B., Ascherio, A., Checkoway, H., Marder, K. S., Nelson, L. M., Rocca, W. A., . . . Gorell, J. (2007). Pooled analysis of tobacco use and risk of Parkinson's disease. *Archives of Neurology, 64,* 990–997. (7)

Riva-Posse, P., Holtzheimer, P. E., Garlow, S. J., & Mayberg, H. S. (2013). Practical considerations in the development and refinement of subcallosal cingulate white matter deep brain stimulation for treatment-resistant depression. *World Neurosurgery, 80,* S27. E25–S27.E34. (14)

Rizzolatti, G., & Sinigaglia, C. (2010). The functional role of the parieto-frontal mirror circuit: Interpretations and misinterpretations. *Nature Reviews Neuroscience, 11,* 264–274. (7)

Roberson, D. P., Gudes, S., Sprague, J. M., Patoski, H. A. W., Robson, V. K., Blasl, F., . . . Woolf, C. J. (2013). Activity-dependent silencing reveals functionally distinct itch-generating sensory neurons. *Nature Neuroscience, 16,* 910–918. (6)

Roberts, S. C., Gosling, L. M., Carter, V., & Petrie, M. (2008). MHC-correlated odour preferences in humans and the use of oral contraceptives. *Proceedings of the Royal Society B, 275,* 2715–2722. (6)

Robertson, I. H. (2005, Winter). The deceptive world of subjective awareness. *Cerebrum, 7*(1), 74–83. (3)

Robinson, A. M., Buttolph, T., Green, J. T., & Bucci, D. J. (2015). Physical exercise affects attentional orienting behavior through noradrenergic mechanisms. *Behavioral Neuroscience, 129,* 361–367. (4)

Robinson, M. J. F., & Berridge, K. C. (2013). Instant transformation of learned repulsion into motivational "wanting." *Current Biology, 23,* 282–289. (9)

Rocha, R. B., Dondossola, E. R., Grande, A. J., Colonetti, T., Ceretta, L. B., Passos, I. C., . . . da Rosa, M. I. (2016). Increased BDNF levels after electroconvulsive therapy in patients with major depressive disorder: A meta-analysis study. *Journal of Psychiatric Research, 83,* 47–53. (14)

Rodgers, A. B., Morgan, C. P., Leu, A. N., & Bale, T. L. (2015). Transgenerational epigenetic programming via sperm micro RNA recapitulates effects of paternal stress. *Proceedings of the National Academy of Sciences (U.S.A.), 112,* 13699–13704. (4)

Rodriguez, I., Greer, C. A., Mok, M. Y., & Mombaerts, P. A. (2000). A putative pheromone receptor gene expressed in human olfactory mucosa. *Nature Genetics, 26,* 18–19. (6)

Roenneberg, T., Allebrandt, K. V., Merrow, M., & Vetter, C. (2012). Social jetlag and obesity. *Current Biology, 22,* 939–943. (8)

Roenneberg, T., Kuehnle, T., Pramstaller, P. P., Ricken, J., Havel, M., Guth, A., & Merrow, M. (2004). A marker for the end of adolescence. *Current Biology, 14,* R1038–R1039. (8)

Roenneberg, T., Kumar, C. J., & Merrow, M. (2007). The human circadian clock entrains to sun time. *Current Biology, 17,* R44–R45. (8)

Roffwarg, H. P., Muzio, J. N., & Dement, W. C. (1966). Ontogenetic development of human sleep-dream cycle. *Science, 152,* 604–609. (8)

Roitman, M. F., Wheeler, R. A., Wightman, R. M., & Carelli, R. M. (2008). Real-time chemical responses in the nucleus accumbens differentiate rewarding and aversive stimuli. *Nature Neuroscience, 11,* 1376–1377. (14)

Rokers, B., Cormack, L. K., & Huk, A. C. (2009). Disparity- and velocity-based signals for three-dimensional motion perception in human MT1. *Nature Neuroscience, 12,* 1050–1055. (5)

Rolls, E. T. (1995). Central taste anatomy and neurophysiology. In R. L. Doty (Ed.), *Handbook of olfaction and gustation* (pp. 549–573). New York: Dekker. (6)

Rome, L. C., Loughna, P. T., & Goldspink, G. (1984). Muscle fiber activity in carp as a function of swimming speed and muscle temperature. *American Journal of Psychiatry, 247,* R272–R279. (7)

Romer, A. S. (1962). *The vertebrate body.* Philadelphia: Saunders. (4)

Romero, E., Cha, G.-H., Verstreken, P., Ly, C. V., Hughes, R. E., Bellen, H. J., & Botas, J. (2007). Suppression of neurodegeneration and increased neurotransmission caused by expanded full-length huntingtin accumulating in the cytoplasm. *Neuron, 57,* 27–40. (7)

Rommel, S. A., Pabst, D. A., & McLellan, W. A. (1998). Reproductive thermoregulation in marine mammals. *American Scientist, 86,* 440–448. (9)

Roney, J. R., & Simmons, Z. L. (2013). Hormonal predictors of sexual motivation in natural menstrual cycles. *Hormones and Behavior, 63,* 636–645. (10)

Roorda, A., & Williams, D. R. (1999). The arrangement of the three cone classes in the living human eye. *Nature, 397,* 520–522. (5)

Roppel, R. M. (1978). Cancer and mental illness. *Science, 201,* 398. (14)

Rosanova, M., Gosseries, O., Casarotto, S., Boly, M., Casali, A. G., Bruno, M.-A., . . . Massimini, M. (2012). Recovery of cortical effective connectivity and recovery of consciousness in vegetative patients. *Brain, 135,* 1308–1320. (13)

Rose, J. E., Brugge, J. F., Anderson, D. J., & Hind, J. E. (1967). Phase-locked response to low-frequency tones in single auditory nerve fibers of the squirrel monkey. *Journal of Neurophysiology, 30,* 769–793. (6)

Rose, T., Jaepel, J., Hübener, M., & Bonhoeffer, T. (2016). Cell-specific restoration of stimulus preference after monocular deprivation in the visual cortex. *Science, 352,* 1319–1322. (5)

Roselli, C. E., Larkin, K., Resko, J. A., Stellflug, J. N., & Stormshak, F. (2004). The volume of a sexually dimorphic nucleus in the ovine medial preoptic area/anterior hypothalamus varies with sexual partner preference. *Endocrinology, 145,* 478–483. (10)

Roselli, C. E., Stadelman, H., Reeve, R., Bishop, C. V., & Stormshak, F. (2007). The ovine sexually dimorphic nucleus of the medial preoptic area is organized prenatally by testosterone. *Endocrinology, 148,* 4450–4457. (10)

Rosen, H. J., Perry, R. J., Murphy, J., Kramer, J. H., Mychack, P., Schuff, N., . . . Miller, B. L. (2002). Emotion comprehension in the temporal variant of frontotemporal dementia. *Brain, 125,* 2286–2295. (13)

Rosenbaum, R. S., Köhler, S., Schacter, D. L., Moscovitch, M., Westmacott, R., Black, S. E., . . . Tulving, E. (2005). The case of K. C.: Contributions of a memory-impaired person to memory theory. *Neuropsychologia, 43,* 989–1021. (12)

Rosenblatt, J. S. (1967). Nonhormonal basis of maternal behavior in the rat. *Science, 156,* 1512–1514. (10)

Rosenblatt, J. S. (1970). Views on the onset and maintenance of maternal behavior in the rat. In L. R. Aronson, E. Tobach, D. S. Lehrman, & J. S. Rosenblatt (Eds.), *Development and evolution of behavior* (pp. 489–515). San Francisco: Freeman. (10)

Rosenblatt, J. S., Olufowobi, A., & Siegel, H. I. (1998). Effects of pregnancy hormones on maternal responsiveness, responsiveness to estrogen stimulation of maternal behavior, and the lordosis response to estrogen stimulation. *Hormones and Behavior, 33,* 104–114. (10)

Rosenkranz, K., Butler, K., Williamson, A., & Rothwell, J. C. (2009). Regaining motor control in musician's dystonia by restoring sensorimotor organization. *Journal of Neuroscience, 29,* 14627–14636. (4)

Rosenzweig, E. (2016). With eyes wide open: How and why awareness of the psychological immune is compatible with its efficacy. *Perspectives on Psychological Science, 11,* 222–238. (6)

Rosenzweig, M. R., & Bennett, E. L. (1996). Psychobiology of plasticity: Effects of training and experience on brain and behavior. *Behavioural Brain Research, 78,* 57–65. (4)

Ross, E. D., Homan, R. W., & Buck, R. (1994). Differential hemispheric lateralization of primary and social emotions. *Neuropsychiatry, Neuropsychology, and Behavioral Neurology, 7,* 1–19. (13)

Rossi, A. F., Bichot, N. P., Desimone, R., & Ungerleider, L. G. (2007). Top-down attentional deficits in macaques with lesions of lateral prefrontal cortex. *Journal of Neuroscience, 27,* 11306–11314. (13)

Rossi, D. J., Oshima, T., & Attwell, D. (2000). Glutamate release in severe brain ischaemia is mainly by reversed uptake. *Nature, 403,* 316–321. (4)

Rossi, E. A., & Roorda, A. (2010). The relationship between visual resolution and cone spacing in the human fovea. *Nature Neuroscience, 13,* 156–157. (5)

Roth, B. L., Willins, D. L., Kristiansen, K., & Kroeze, W. K. (1999). Activation is hallucinogenic and antagonism is therapeutic:

Role of 5-HT2A receptors in atypical antipsychotic drug actions. *Neuroscientist, 5,* 254–262. (14)

Roth, M. M., Dahmen, J. C., Muir, D. R., Imhof, F., Martini, F. J., & Hofer, S. B. (2016). Thalamic nuclei convey diverse contextual information to layer 1 of visual cortex. *Nature Neuroscience, 19,* 299–307. (5)

Rottenberg, J., Kasch, K. L., Gross, J. J., & Gotlib, I. H. (2002). Sadness and amusement reactivity differentially predict concurrent and prospective functioning in major depressive disorder. *Emotion, 2,* 135–146. (14)

Routtenberg, A., Cantallops, I., Zaffuto, S., Serrano, P., & Namgung, U. (2000). Enhanced learning after genetic overexpression of a brain growth protein. *Proceedings of the National Academy of Sciences, USA, 97,* 7657–7662. (12)

Rouw, R., & Scholte, H. S. (2007). Increased structural connectivity in grapheme-color synesthesia. *Nature Neuroscience, 10,* 792–797. (6)

Roy, A., DeJong, J., & Linnoila, M. (1989). Cerebrospinal fluid monoamine metabolites and suicidal behavior in depressed patients. *Archives of General Psychiatry, 46,* 609–612. (11)

Royer, S., & Paré, D. (2003). Conservation of total synaptic weight through balanced synaptic depression and potentiation. *Nature, 422,* 518–522. (12)

Rozin, P., Dow, S., Moscovitch, M., & Rajaram, S. (1998). What causes humans to begin and end a meal? A role for memory for what has been eaten, as evidenced by a study of multiple meal eating in amnesic patients. *Psychological Science, 9,* 392–396. (12)

Rozin, P., & Kalat, J. W. (1971). Specific hungers and poison avoidance as adaptive specializations of learning. *Psychological Review, 78,* 459–486. (9, 12)

Rozin, P., & Pelchat, M. L. (1988). Memories of mammaries: Adaptations to weaning from milk. *Progress in Psychobiology and Physiological Psychology, 13,* 1–29. (9)

Rozin, P., & Schull, J. (1988). The adaptive-evolutionary point of view in experimental psychology. In R. C. Atkinson, R. J. Herrnstein, G. Lindzey, & R. D. Luce (Eds.), *Stevens' handbook of experimental psychology* (2nd ed.): Vol. 1. *Perception and motivation* (pp. 503–546). New York: Wiley. (12)

Rubens, A. B., & Benson, D. F. (1971). Associative visual agnosia. *Archives of Neurology, 24,* 305–316. (5)

Rubin, B. D., & Katz, L. C. (2001). Spatial coding of enantiomers in the rat olfactory bulb. *Nature Neuroscience, 4,* 355–356. (6)

Rubin, M., Shvil, E., Papini, S., Chhetry, B. T., Helpman, L., Markowitz, J. C., . . . Neria, Y. (2016). Greater hippocampal volume is associated with PTSD treatment response. *Psychiatry Research—Neuroimaging, 252,* 36–39. (11)

Rubinow, M. J., Arseneau, L. M., Beverly, J. L., & Juraska, J. M. (2004). Effect of the estrous cycle on water maze acquisition depends on the temperature of the water. *Behavioral Neuroscience, 118,* 863–868. (9)

Rubinstein, G. (1997). Schizophrenia, rheumatoid arthritis and natural resistance genes. *Schizophrenia Research, 25,* 177–181. (14)

Rudebeck, P. H., & Murray, E. A. (2014). The orbitofrontal oracle: cortical mechanisms for the prediction and evaluation of specific behavioral outcomes. *Neuron, 84,* 1143–1156. (13)

Rugg, M. D., & Thompson-Schill, S. L. (2013). Moving forward with fMRI data. *Perspectives on Psychological Science, 8,* 84–87. (3)

Rumbaugh, D. M. (Ed.). (1977). *Language learning by a chimpanzee: The Lana Project.* New York: Academic Press. (13)

Running, C. A., Craig, B. A., & Mattes, R. D. (2015). Oleogustus: The unique taste of fat. *Chemical Senses, 40,* 507–516. (6)

Rupprecht, R., di Michele, F., Hermann, B., Ströhle, A., Lancel, M., Romeo, E., & Holsboer, F. (2001). Neuroactive steroids: Molecular mechanisms of action and implications for neuropsychopharmacology. *Brain Research Reviews, 37,* 59–67. (10)

Rusak, B., & Zucker, I. (1979). Neural regulation of circadian rhythms. *Physiological Reviews, 59,* 449–526. (8)

Ruschel, J., Hellal, F., Flynn, K. C., Dupraz, S., Elliott, D. A., Tedeschi, A., . . . Bradke, F. (2015). Systemic administration of epothilone B promotes axon regeneration after spinal cord injury. *Science, 348,* 347–352. (4)

Russell, M. J., Switz, G. M., & Thompson, K. (1980). Olfactory influences on the human menstrual cycle. *Pharmacology, Biochemistry, and Behavior, 13,* 737–738. (6)

Russo, S. J., & Nestler, E. J. (2013). The brain reward circuitry in mood disorders. *Nature Reviews Neuroscience, 14,* 609–625. (14)

Rütgen, M., Seidel, E.-M., Riecansky, I., & Lamm, C. (2015). Reduction of empathy for pain by placebo analgesia suggests functional equivalence of empathy and first-hand emotion experience. *Journal of Neuroscience, 35,* 8938–8947. (6)

Saad, W. A., Luiz, A. C., Camargo, L. A. A., Renzi, A., & Manani, J. V. (1996). The lateral preoptic area plays a dual role in the regulation of thirst in the rat. *Brain Research Bulletin, 39,* 171–176. (9)

Sääksjärvi, K., Knekt, P., Rissanen, H., Laaksonen, M. A., Reunanen, A., & Männistö, S. (2008). Prospective study of coffee consumption and risk of Parkinson's disease. *European Journal of Clinical Nutrition, 62,* 908–915. (7)

Sabelström, H., Stenudd, M., Réu, P., Dias, D. O., Elfineh, M., Zdunek, S., . . . Frisén, J. (2013). Resident neural stem cells restrict tissue damage and neuronal loss after spinal cord injury in mice. *Science, 342,* 637–640. (4)

Sabo, K. T., & Kirtley, D. D. (1982). Objects and activities in the dreams of the blind. *International Journal of Rehabilitation Research, 5,* 241–242. (3)

Sack, R. L., & Lewy, A. J. (2001). Circadian rhythm sleep disorders: Lessons from the blind. *Sleep Medicine Reviews, 5,* 189–206. (8)

Sacks, O. (2010, August 30). Face-blind. *The New Yorker, 86(31),* 36–43. (5)

Sadato, N., Pascual-Leone, A., Grafman, J., Deiber, M.-P., Ibañez, V., & Hallett, M. (1998). Neural networks for Braille reading by the blind. *Brain, 121,* 1213–1229. (4)

Sadato, N., Pascual-Leone, A., Grafman, J., Ibañez, V., Deiber, M.-P., Dold, G., & Hallett, M. (1996). Activation of the primary visual cortex by Braille reading in blind subjects. *Nature, 380,* 526–528. (4)

Sadri-Vakili, G., Kumaresan, V., Schmidt, H. D., Famous, K. R., Chawla, P., Vassoler, F. M., . . . Cha, J. H. J. (2010). Cocaine-induced chromatin remodeling increases brain-derived neurotrophic factor transcription in the rat medial prefrontal cortex, which alters the reinforcing efficacy of cocaine. *Journal of Neuroscience, 30,* 11735–11744. (4)

Sagarin, B. J., Martin, A. L., Coutinho, S. A., Edlund, J. E., Patel, L., Skowronski, J. J., & Zengel, B. (2012). Sex differences in jealousy: A meta-analytic examination. *Evolution and Human Behavior, 33,* 595–614. (10)

Saito, K. (2013). Age effects on late bilingualism: The production development of /r/ by high-proficiency Japanese learners of English. *Journal of Memory and Language, 69,* 546–562. (13)

Saj, A., Fuhrman, O., Vuilleumier, P., & Boroditsky, L. (2014). Patients with left spatial neglect also neglect the "left side" of time. *Psychological Science, 25,* 207–214. (13)

Sakurai, T. (2007). The neural circuit of orexin (hypocretin): Maintaining sleep and wakefulness. *Nature Reviews Neuroscience, 8,* 171–181. (8)

Salimpoor, V. N., van den Bosch, I., Kovacevic, N., McIntosh, A. R., Dagher, A., & Zatorre, R. J. (2013). Interactions between the nucleus accumbens and auditory cortices predict music reward value. *Science, 340,* 216–219. (14)

Salinsky, M., Kanter, R., & Dasheiff, R. M. (1987). Effectiveness of multiple EEGs in supporting the diagnosis of epilepsy: An operational curve. *Epilepsia, 28,* 331–334. (3)

Salmelin, R., Hari, R., Lounasmaa, O. V., & Sams, M. (1994). Dynamics of brain activation during picture naming. *Nature, 368,* 463–465. (3)

Salthouse, T. A. (2006). Mental exercise and mental aging. *Perspectives on Psychological Science, 1,* 68–87. (4)

Salz, D. M., Tiganj, Z., Khasnabish, S., Kohley, A., Sheehan, D., Howard, M. W., & Eichenbaum, H. (2016). Time cells in hippocampal area CA3. *Journal of Neuroscience, 36,* 7476–7484. (12)

Samara, M. T., Dold, M., Gianatsi, M., Nikolakopoulou, A., Helfer, B., Salanti, G., . . . Leucht, S. (2016). Efficacy, acceptability, and tolerability of antipsychotics in treatment-resistant schizophrenia: A network meta-analysis. *JAMA Psychiatry, 73,* 199–210. (14)

Sami, M. B., & Faruqui, R. (2015). The effectiveness of dopamine agonists for treatment of neuropsychiatric symptoms post brain injury and stroke. *Acta Neuropsychiatrica, 27,* 317–326. (4)

Samochowiec, J., Samochowiec, A., Puls, I., Bienkowski, P., & Schott, B. H. (2014). Genetics of alcohol dependence: A review of clinical studies. *Neuropsychobiology, 70,* 77–94. (14)

Samuels, B. A., Anacker, C., Hu, A., Levinstein, M. R., Pickenhagen, A., Tsetsenis, T., . . . Hen, R. (2015). 5-HT1A receptors on mature dentate gyrus granule cells are critical for the antidepressant response. *Nature Neuroscience, 18,* 1606–1616. (14)

Sanai, N., Nguyen, T., Ihrie, R. A., Mirzadeh, Z., Tsai, H.-H., Wong, M., . . . Alvarez-Buylla, A., (2011). Corridors of migrating neurons in the human brain and their decline during infancy. *Nature, 478,* 382–386. (4)

Sánchez-Navarro, J. P., Driscoll, D., Anderson, S. W., Tranel, D., Bechara, A., & Buchanan, T. W. (2014). Alterations of attention and emotional processing following childhood-onset damage to the prefrontal cortex. *Behavioral Neuroscience, 128,* 1–11. (11)

Sanders, A. R., Martin, E. R., Beecham, G. W., Guo, S., Dawood, K., Rieger, G., . . . Bailey, J. M. (2015). Genome-wide scan demonstrates significant linkage for male sexual orientation. *Psychological Medicine, 45,* 1379–1388. (10)

Sanders, C. E., Tattersall, G. J., Reichert, M., Andrade, D. V., Abe, A. S., & Milsom, W. K. (2015). Daily and annual cycles in thermoregulatory behaviour and cardio-respiratory physiology of black and white tegu lizards. *Journal of Comparative Physiology B, 185,* 905–915. (8)

Sanders, S. J., Xin, H., Willsey, A. J., Ercan-Sencicek, A. G., Samocha, K. E., Cicek, A. E., . . . State, M. W. (2015). Insights into autism spectrum disorder genomic architecture and biology from 71 risk loci. *Neuron, 87,* 1215–1233. (14)

Sanders, S. K., & Shekhar, A. (1995). Anxiolytic effects of chlordiazepoxide blocked by injection of GABA$_A$ and benzodiazepine receptor antagonists in the region of the anterior basolateral amygdala of rats. *Biological Psychiatry, 37,* 473–476. (11)

Sanes, J. N., Donoghue, J. P., Thangaraj, V., Edelman, R. R., & Warach, S. (1995). Shared neural substrates controlling hand movements in human motor cortex. *Science, 268,* 1775–1777. (7)

Sanes, J. R. (1993). Topographic maps and molecular gradients. *Current Opinion in Neurobiology, 3,* 67–74. (4)

Sanger, T. D., Pascual-Leone, A., Tarsy, D., & Schlaug, G. (2001). Nonlinear sensory cortex response to simultaneous tactile stimuli in writer's cramp. *Movement Disorders, 17,* 105–111. (4)

Sanger, T. D., Tarsy, D., & Pascual-Leone, A. (2001). Abnormalities of spatial and temporal sensory discrimination in writer's cramp. *Movement Disorders, 16,* 94–99. (4)

Santarnecchi, E., Galli, G., Polizzotto, N. R., Rossi, A., & Rossi, S. (2014). Efficiency of weak brain connections support general cognitive functioning. *Human Brain Mapping, 35,* 4566–4582. (12)

Saper, C. B., Romanovsky, A. A., & Scammell, T. E. (2012). Neural circuitry engaged by prostaglandins during the sickness syndrome. *Nature Neuroscience, 15,* 1088–1095. (11)

Sapolsky, R. M. (1992). *Stress, the aging brain, and the mechanisms of neuron death.* Cambridge, MA: MIT Press. (11)

Sapolsky, R. M. (1998). *Why zebras don't get ulcers.* New York: Freeman. (11)

Sapolsky, R. M. (2015). Stress and the brain: Individual variability and the inverted-U. *Nature Neuroscience, 18,* 1344–1346. (11)

Sargolini, F., Fyhn, M., Hafting, T., McNaughton, B. L., Witter, M. P., Moser, M.-B., & Moser, E. I. (2006). Conjunctive representation of position, direction, and velocity in entorhinal cortex. *Science, 312,* 758–762. (12)

Sarris, J., Panossian, A., Schweitzer, I., Stough, C., & Scholey, A. (2011). Herbal medicine for depression, anxiety and insomnia: A review of psychopharmacology and clinical evidence. *European Neuropsychopharmacology, 21,* 841–860. (14)

Satinoff, E. (1991). Developmental aspects of behavioral and reflexive thermoregulation. In H. N. Shanir, G. A. Barr, & M. A. Hofer (Eds.), *Developmental psychobiology: New methods and changing concepts* (pp. 169–188). New York: Oxford University Press. (9)

Satinoff, E., McEwen, G. N., Jr., & Williams, B. A. (1976). Behavioral fever in newborn rabbits. *Science, 193,* 1139–1140. (9)

Satinoff, E., & Rutstein, J. (1970). Behavioral thermoregulation in rats with anterior hypothalamic lesions. *Journal of Comparative and Physiological Psychology, 71,* 77–82. (9)

Sato, M., & Stryker, M. P. (2008). Distinctive features of adult ocular dominance plasticity. *Journal of Neuroscience, 28,* 10278–10286. (5)

Saunders, A., Oldenburg, I. A., Berezovskii, V. K., Johnson, C. A., Kingery, N. D., Elliott, H. L., . . . Satatini, B. L. (2015). A direct GABAergic output from the basal ganglia to the frontal cortex. *Nature, 521,* 85–89. (7)

Savage-Rumbaugh, E. S. (1990). Language acquisition in a nonhuman species: Implications for the innateness debate. *Developmental Psychobiology, 23,* 599–620. (13)

Savage-Rumbaugh, E. S., Murphy, J., Sevcik, R. A., Brakke, K. E., Williams, S. L., & Rumbaugh, D. M. (1993). Language comprehension in ape and child. *Monographs of the Society for Research in Child Development, 58* (Serial no. 233). (13)

Savage-Rumbaugh, E. S., Sevcik, R. A., Brakke, K. E., & Rumbaugh, D. M. (1992). Symbols: Their communicative use, communication, and combination by bonobos (*Pan paniscus*). In L. P. Lipsitt & C. Rovee-Collier (Eds.), *Advances in infancy research* (Vol. 7, pp. 221–278). Norwood, NJ: Ablex. (13)

Savic, I., & Arver, S. (2014). Sex differences in cortical thickness and their possible genetic and sex hormonal underpinnings. *Cerebral Cortex, 24,* 3246–3257. (12)

Savic, I., Berglund, H., & Lindström, P. (2005). Brain response to putative pheromones in homosexual men. *Proceedings of the National Academy of Sciences (U.S.A.), 102,* 7356–7361. (6)

Savic, I., & Lindström, P. (2008). PET and MRI show differences in cerebral asymmetry and functional connectivity between homo- and heterosexual subjects. *Proceedings of the National Academy of Sciences, USA, 105,* 9403–9408. (10)

Savin-Williams, R. C. (2016). Sexual orientation: Categories or continuum? Commentary on Bailey et al. (2016). *Psychological Science in the Public Interest, 17,* 37–44. (10)

Saxton, T. K., Nováková, L. M., Jash, R., Sandová, A., Plotená, D., & Havlícek, J. (2014). Sex differences in olfactory behavior in Namibian and Czech children. *Chemical Perception, 7,* 117–125. (6)

Schaal, N. K., Pfeifer, J., Krause, V., & Pollok, B. (2015). From amusic to musical? Improving pitch memory in congenital amusia with transcranial alternating current stimulation. *Behavioural Brain Research, 294,* 141–148. (6)

Schacter, D. L. (1983). Amnesia observed: Remembering and forgetting in a natural environment. *Journal of Abnormal Psychology, 92,* 236–242. (12)

Scheele, D., Striepens, N., Güntürkün, O., Deutschländer, S., Maier, W., Kendrick, K. M., & Hurlemann, R. (2012). Oxytocin modulates social distance between males and females. *Journal of Neuroscience, 32,* 16074–16079. (13)

Scheele, D., Wille, A., Kendrick, K. M., Stoffel-Wagner, B., Becker, B., Güntürkün, O., . . . Hurlemann, R. (2013). Oxytocin enhances brain reward system responses in men viewing the face of their female partner. *Proceedings of the National Academy of Sciences (U.S.A.), 110,* 20308–20313. (13)

Scheibel, A. B. (1983). Dendritic changes. In B. Reisberg (Ed.), *Alzheimer's Disease* (pp. 69–73). New York: Free Press. (12)

Schellenberg, E. G., & Trehub, S. E. (2003). Good pitch memory is widespread. *Psychological Science, 14,* 262–266. (6)

Schenk, T. (2006). An allocentric rather than perceptual deficit in patient D. F. *Nature Neuroscience, 9,* 1369–1370. (5)

Schenck, C. H. (2015). Update on sexsomnia, sleep related sexual seizures, and forensic implications. *NeuroQuantology, 13,* 518–541. (8)

Schenk, T., Mai, N., Ditterich, J., & Zihl, J. (2000). Can a motion-blind patient reach for moving objects? *European Journal of Neuroscience, 12,* 3351–3360. (5)

Scherrer, G., Imamachi, N., Cao, Y.-Q., Contet, C., Mennicken, F., O'Donnell, D., . . . Basbaum, A. I. (2009). Dissociation of the opioid receptor mechanisms that control mechanical and heat pain. *Cell, 137*, 1148–1159. (6)

Scheyer, A. F., Loweth, J. A., Christian, D. T., Uejima, J., Rabei, R., Le, T., . . . Wolf, M. E. (2016). AMPA receptor plasticity in accumbens core contributes to incubation of methamphetamine craving. *Biological Psychiatry, 80*, 661–670. (14)

Schiffman, S. S. (1983). Taste and smell in disease. *New England Journal of Medicine, 308*, 1275–1279, 1337–1343. (6)

Schiffman, S. S., & Erickson, R. P. (1971). A psychophysical model for gustatory quality. *Physiology & Behavior, 7*, 617–633. (6)

Schiffman, S. S., & Erickson, R. P. (1980). The issue of primary tastes versus a taste continuum. *Neuroscience and Biobehavioral Reviews, 4*, 109–117. (6)

Schiffman, S. S., Lockhead, E., & Maes, F. W. (1983). Amiloride reduces the taste intensity of Na$^+$ and Li$^+$ salts and sweeteners. *Proceedings of the National Academy of Sciences, USA, 80*, 6136–6140. (6)

Schiffman, S. S., McElroy, A. E., & Erickson, R. P. (1980). The range of taste quality of sodium salts. *Physiology & Behavior, 24*, 217–224. (6)

Schizophrenia Working Group of the Psychiatric Genomics Consortium. (2014). Biological insights from 108 schizophrenia-associated genetic loci. *Nature, 511*, 421–427. (14)

Schlack, A., Krekelberg, B., & Albright, T. D. (2007). Recent history of stimulus speeds affects the speed tuning of neurons in area MT. *Journal of Neuroscience, 27*, 11009–11018. (5)

Schlerf, J., Ivry, R. B., & Diedrichsen, J. (2012). Encoding of sensory prediction errors in the human cerebellum. *Journal of Neuroscience, 32*, 4913–4922. (7)

Schlinger, H. D., Jr. (1996). How the human got its spots. *Skeptic, 4*, 68–76. (4)

Schmid, A., Koch, M., & Schnitzler, H.-U. (1995). Conditioned pleasure attenuates the startle response in rats. *Neurobiology of Learning and Memory, 64*, 1–3. (11)

Schmid, M. C., Schmiedt, J. T., Peters, A. J., Saunders, R. C., Maier, A., & Leopold, D. A. (2013). Motion-sensitive responses in visual area V4 in the absence of primary visual cortex. *Journal of Neuroscience, 33*, 18740–18745. (5)

Schmidt, L. A. (1999). Frontal brain electrical activity in shyness and sociability. *Psychological Science, 10*, 316–320. (11)

Schmidt, R., Leventhal, D. K., Mallet, N., Chen, F., & Berke, J. D. (2013). Canceling actions involves a race between basal ganglia pathways. *Nature Neuroscience, 16*, 1118–1124. (7)

Schmidt-Hieber, C, Jonas, P., & Bischofberger, J. (2004). Enhanced synaptic plasticity in newly generated granule cells of the adult hippocampus. *Nature, 429*, 184–187. (4)

Schmitt, K. C., & Reith, M. E. A. (2010). Regulation of the dopamine transporter. *Annals of the New York Academy of Sciences, 1187*, 316–340. (2)

Schneider, B. A., Trehub, S. E., Morrongiello, B. A., & Thorpe, L. A. (1986). Auditory sensitivity in preschool children. *Journal of the Acoustical Society of America, 79*, 447–452. (6)

Schneider, P., Scherg, M., Dosch, G., Specht, H. J., Gutschalk, A., & Rupp, A. (2002). Morphology of Heschl's gyrus reflects enhanced activation in the auditory cortex of musicians. *Nature Neuroscience, 5*, 688–694. (4)

Schnider, A. (2003). Spontaneous confabulation and the adaptation of thought to ongoing reality. *Nature Reviews Neuroscience, 4*, 662–671. (12)

Schomacher, M., Müller, H. D., Sommer, C., Schwab, S., & Schäbitz, W.-R. (2008). Endocannabinoids mediate neuroprotection after transient focal cerebral ischemia. *Brain Research, 1240*, 213–220. (4)

Schroeder, J. A., & Flannery-Schroeder, E. (2005). Use of herb *Gymnema sylvestre* to illustrate the principles of gustatory sensation: An undergraduate neuroscience laboratory exercise. *Journal of Undergraduate Neuroscience Education, 3*, A59–A62. (6)

Schröter, M. S., Spoormaker, V. I., Schorer, A., Wohlschläger, A., Czisch, M., Kochs, E. F., . . . Ilg, R. (2012). Spatiotemporal reconfiguration of large-scale brain functional networks during propofol-induced loss of consciousness. *Journal of Neuroscience, 32*, 12832–12840. (13)

Schuckit, M. A., & Smith, T. L. (1996). An 8-year follow-up of 450 sons of alcoholic and control subjects. *Archives of General Psychiatry, 53*, 202–210. (14)

Schuckit, M. A., & Smith, T. L. (1997). Assessing the risk for alcoholism among sons of alcoholics. *Journal of Studies on Alcohol, 58*, 141–145. (14)

Schuckit, M. A., & Smith, T. L. (2013). Stability of scores and correlations with drinking behaviors over 15 years for the self-report of the effects of alcohol questionnaire. *Drug and Alcohol Dependence, 128*, 194–199. (14)

Schuckit, M. A., Smith, T. L., Clausen, P., Fromme, K., Skidmore, J., Shafir, A., & Kalmijn, J. (2016). The low level of response to alcohol-based heavy drinking prevention program: One-year follow-up. *Journal of Studies on Alcohol and Drugs, 77*, 25–37. (14)

Schulkin, J. (1991). *Sodium hunger: The search for a salty taste*. Cambridge, England: Cambridge University Press. (9)

Schulz, K. M., Molenda-Figueira, H. A., & Sisk, C. L. (2009). Back to the future: The organizational-activational hypothesis adapted to puberty and adolescence. *Hormones and Behavior, 55*, 597–604. (10)

Schumann, C. M., Bloss, C. S., Barnes, C. C., Wideman, G. M., Carper, R. A., Akshoomoff, N., . . . Courchesne, E. (2010). Longitudinal magnetic resonance imaging study of cortical development through early childhood in autism. *Journal of Neuroscience, 30*, 4419–4427. (14)

Schwartz, C. E., Wright, C. I., Shin, L. M., Kagan, J., & Rauch, S. L. (2003). Inhibited and uninhibited infants "grown up": Adult amygdalar response to novelty. *Science, 300*, 1952–1953. (11)

Schwartz, G., Kim, R. M., Kolundzija, A. B., Rieger, G., & Sanders, A. R. (2010). Biodemographic and physical correlates of sexual orientation in men. *Archives of Sexual Behavior, 39*, 93–109. (10)

Schwartz, G. J. (2000). The role of gastrointestinal vagal afferents in the control of food intake: Current prospects. *Nutrition, 16*, 866–873. (9)

Schwartz, J. A. (2015). Socioeconomic status as a moderator of the genetic and shared environmental influence on verbal IQ: A multilevel behavioral genetic approach. *Intelligence, 52*, 80–89. (12)

Schwartz, L., & Tulipan, L. (1933). An outbreak of dermatitis among workers in a rubber manufacturing plant. *Public Health Reports, 48*, 809–814. (14)

Schwartz, M. F. (1995). Re-examining the role of executive functions in routine action production. *Annals of the New York Academy of Sciences, 769*, 321–335. (7)

Schwartz, N., Temkin, P., Jurado, S., Lim, B. K., Heifets, B. D., . . . Malenka, R. C. (2014). Decreased motivation during chronic pain requires long-term depression in the nucleus accumbens. *Science, 345*, 535–542. (6)

Schwartz, W. J., & Gainer, H. (1977). Suprachiasmatic nucleus: Use of ^{14}C-labeled deoxyglucose uptake as a functional marker. *Science, 197*, 1089–1091. (8)

Schwarz, J. M., Liang, S.-L., Thompson, S. M., & McCarthy, M. M. (2008). Estradiol induces hypothalamic dendritic spines by enhancing glutamate release: A mechanism for organizational sex differences. *Neuron, 58*, 584–598. (10)

Schweinhardt, P., Seminowicz, D. A., Jaeger, E., Duncan, G. H., & Bushnell, M. C. (2009). The anatomy of the mesolimbic reward system: A link between personality and the placebo analgesic response. *Journal of Neuroscience, 29*, 4882–4887. (6)

Scofield, M. D., Heinsbroek, J. A., Gipson, C. D., Kupchik, Y. M., Spencer, S., Smith, A. C. W., . . . Kalivas, P. W. (2016). The nucleus accumbens: Mechanisms of addiction across drug classes reflect the importance of glutamate homeostasis. *Pharmacological Reviews, 68*, 816–871. (14)

Scott, S. H. (2004). Optimal feedback control and the neural basis of volitional motor control. *Nature Reviews Neuroscience, 5*, 532–544. (7)

Scoville, W. B., & Milner, B. (1957). Loss of recent memory after bilateral hippocampal lesions. *Journal of Neurology, Neurosurgery, and Psychiatry, 20*, 11–21. (12)

Scullin, M. K., & Bliwise, D. L. (2015). Sleep, cognition, and normal aging: Integrating a half century of multidisciplinary research. *Perspectives on Psychological Science, 10,* 97–137. (8)

Sealey, L. A., Hughes, B. W., Sriskanda, A. N., Guest, J. R., Gibson, A. D., Johnson-Williams, L., . . . Bagasra, O. (2016). Environmental factors in the development of autism spectrum disorders. *Environment International, 88,* 288–298. (14)

Seeley, R. J., Kaplan, J. M., & Grill, H. J. (1995). Effect of occluding the pylorus on intraoral intake: A test of the gastric hypothesis of meal termination. *Physiology & Behavior, 58,* 245–249. (9)

Seeman, P., Lee, T., Chau-Wong, M., & Wong, K. (1976). Antipsychotic drug doses and neuroleptic/dopamine receptors. *Nature, 261,* 717–719. (14)

Seery, M. D., Leo, R. J., Lupien, S. P., Kondrak, C. L., & Almonte, J. L. (2013). An upside to adversity? Moderate cumulative lifetime adversity is associated with resilient responses in the face of controlled stressors. *Psychological Science, 24,* 1181–1189. (11)

Segal, N. L. (2000). Virtual twins: New findings on within-family environmental influences on intelligence. *Journal of Educational Psychology, 92,* 442–448. (4)

Segal, N. L., McGuire, S. A., & Stohs, J. H. (2012). What virtual twins reveal about general intelligence and other behaviors. *Personality and Individual Differences, 53,* 405–410. (12)

Segerstrom, S. C., & Miller, G. E. (2004). Psychological stress and the human immune system: A meta-analytic study of 30 years of inquiry. *Psychological Bulletin, 130,* 601–630. (11)

Sehgal, A., Ousley, A., Yang, Z., Chen, Y., & Schotland, P. (1999). What makes the circadian clock tick: Genes that keep time? *Recent Progress in Hormone Research, 54,* 61–85. (8)

Seid, M. A., Castillo, A, & Wcislo, W. T. (2011). The allometry of brain miniaturization in ants. *Brain, Behavior and Evolution, 77,* 5–13. (3)

Sekar, A., Bialas, A. R., de Rivera, H., Davis, A., Hammond, T. R., Kamitaki, N., . . . McCarroll, S. A. (2016). Schizophrenia risk from complex variation of complement component 4. *Nature, 530,* 177–183. (14)

Selkoe, D. J. (2000). Toward a comprehensive theory for Alzheimer's disease. *Annals of the New York Academy of Sciences, 924,* 17–25. (12)

Selye, H. (1979). Stress, cancer, and the mind. In J. Taché, H. Selye, & S. B. Day (Eds.), *Cancer, stress, and death* (pp. 11–27). New York: Plenum Press. (11)

Semendeferi, K., Lu, A., Schenker, N., & Damasio, H. (2002). Humans and great apes share a large frontal cortex. *Nature Neuroscience, 5,* 272–276. (3)

Semenya, S. W., & Vasey, P. L. (2016). The relationship between adult occupational preferences and childhood gender nonconformity among Samoan women, men, and *Fa'afafine. Human Nature, 27,* 283–295. (10)

Sen, S., Duman, R., & Sanacora, G. (2008). Serum brain-derived neurotrophic factor, depression, and antidepressant medications: Meta-analyses and implications. *Biological Psychiatry, 64,* 527–532. (14)

Sens, E., Teschner, U., Meissner, W., Preul, C., Huonker, R., Witte, O. W., . . . Weiss, T. (2012). Effects of temporary functional deafferentation on the brain, sensation, and behavior of stroke patients. *Journal of Neuroscience, 32,* 11773–11779. (4)

Seow, Y.-X., Ong, P. K. C., & Huang, D. (2016). Odor-specific loss of smell sensitivity with age as revealed by the specific sensitivity test. *Chemical Senses, 41,* 487–495. (6)

Sereno, A. B., & Holzman, P. S. (1993). Express saccades and smooth pursuit eye movement function in schizophrenic, affective disorder, and normal subjects. *Journal of Cognitive Neuroscience, 5,* 303–316. (14)

Sergent, C., & Dehaene, S. (2004). Is consciousness a gradual phenomenon? *Psychological Science, 15,* 720–728. (13)

Sergent, C., Wyart, V., Babo-Rebelo, M., Cohen, L., Naccache, L., & Tallon-Baudry, C. (2013). Cueing attention after the stimulus is gone can retrospectively trigger conscious perception. *Current Biology, 23,* 150–155. (13)

Serino, A., Pizzoferrato, F., & Làdavas, E. (2008). Viewing a face (especially one's own face) being touched enhances tactile perception on the face. *Psychological Science, 19,* 434–438. (6)

Severens, M., Farquhar, J., Desain, P., Duysens, J., & Gielen, C. (2010). Transient and steady-state responses to mechanical stimulation of different fingers reveal interactions based on lateral inhibition. *Clinical Neurophysiology, 121,* 2090–2096. (5)

Shackman, A. J., McMenamin, B. W., Maxwell, J. S., Greischar, L. L., & Davidson, R. J. (2009). Right dorsolateral prefrontal cortical activity and behavioral inhibition. *Psychological Science, 20,* 1500–1506. (11)

Shadlen, M. N., & Newsome, W. T. (1996). Motion perception: Seeing and deciding. *Proceedings of the National Academy of Sciences (U.S.A.), 93,* 628–633. (13)

Shah, B., Shine, R., Hudson, S., & Kearney, M. (2003). Sociality in lizards: Why do thick-tailed geckos (*Nephrurus milii*) aggregate? *Behaviour, 140,* 1039–1052. (9)

Shah, N. M., Pisapia, D. J., Maniatis, S., Mendelsohn, M. M., Nemes, A., & Axel, R. (2004). Visualizing sexual dimorphism in the brain. *Neuron, 43,* 313–319. (10)

Shalev, A. Y., Peri, T., Brandes, D., Freedman, S., Orr, S. P., & Pitman, R. K. (2000). Auditory startle response in trauma survivors with posttraumatic stress disorder: A prospective study. *American Journal of Psychiatry, 157,* 255–261. (11)

Shapiro, C. M., Bortz, R., Mitchell, D., Bartel, P., & Jooste, P. (1981). Slow-wave sleep: A recovery period after exercise. *Science, 214,* 1253–1254. (8)

Sharbaugh, S. M. (2001). Seasonal acclimatization to extreme climatic conditions by black-capped chickadees (*Poecile atricapilla*) in interior Alaska (64° N). *Physiological and Biochemical Zoology, 74,* 568–575. (9)

Sharma, J., Angelucci, A., & Sur, M. (2000). Induction of visual orientation modules in auditory cortex. *Nature, 404,* 841–847. (4)

Shatz, C. J. (1992, September). The developing brain. *Scientific American, 267*(9), 60–67. (4)

Shatz, C. J. (1996). Emergence of order in visual-system development. *Proceedings of the National Academy of Sciences, USA, 93,* 602–608. (5)

Shaw, D. J., & Czekóová, K. (2013). Exploring the development of the mirror neuron system: Finding the right paradigm. *Developmental Neuropsychology, 38,* 256–271. (7)

Shawa, N., & Roden, L. C. (2016). Chronotype of South African adults is affected by solar entrainment. *Chronobiology International, 33,* 315–323. (8)

Shema, R., Haramati, S., Ron, S., Hazvi, S., Chen, A., Sacktor, T. C., . . . Dudai, Y. (2011). Enhancement of consolidated long-term memory by overexpression of protein kinase Mζ in the neocortex. *Science, 331,* 1207–1210. (12)

Shema, R., Sacktor, T. C., & Dudai, Y. (2007). Rapid erasure of long-term memory associations in the cortex by an inhibitor of PKMζ. *Science, 317,* 951–953. (12)

Shen, H., Gong, Q. H., Aoki, C., Yuan, M., Ruderman, Y., Dattilo, M., . . . Smith, S. S. (2007). Reversal of neurosteroid effects at alpha 4 beta 2 delta GABA$_A$ receptors triggers anxiety at puberty. *Nature Neuroscience, 10,* 469–477. (11)

Shenhav, A., & Greene, J. D. (2014). Integrative moral judgment: Dissociating the roles of the amygdala and ventromedial prefrontal cortex. *Journal of Neuroscience, 34,* 4741–4749. (11)

Sher, L., Carballo, J. J., Grunebaum, M. F., Burke, A. K., Zalsman, G., Huang, Y.-Y., . . . Oquendo, M. A. (2006). A prospective study of the association of cerebrospinal fluid monoamine metabolite levels with lethality of suicide attempts in patients with bipolar disorder. *Bipolar Disorders, 8,* 543–550. (11)

Sherrington, C. S. (1906). *The integrative action of the nervous system* (2nd ed.). New York: Scribner's. New Haven, CT: Yale University Press, 1947. (2)

Sherrington, C. S. (1941). *Man on his nature.* New York: Macmillan. (2)

Shih, R. A., Belmonte, P. L., & Zandi, P. P. (2004). A review of the evidence from family, twin and adoption studies for a genetic contribution to adult psychiatric disorders. *International Review of Psychiatry, 16,* 260–283. (14)

Shima, K., Isoda, M., Mushiake, H., & Tanji, J. (2007). Categorization of behavioural sequences in the prefrontal cortex. *Nature, 445*, 315–318. (7)

Shimada-Sugimoto, M., Otowa, T., & Hettema, J. M. (2015). Genetics of anxiety disorders: Genetic epidemiological and molecular studies in humans. *Psychiatry and Clinical Sciences, 69*, 388–401. (11)

Shimojo, S., Kamitani, Y., & Nishida, S. (2001). Afterimage of perceptually filled-in surface. *Science, 293*, 1677–1680. (5)

Shine, R., Phillips, B., Waye, H., LeMaster, M., & Mason, R. T. (2001). Benefits of female mimicry in snakes. *Nature, 414*, 267. (9)

Shiv, B., Loewenstein, G., Bechara, A., Damasio, H., & Damasio, A. R. (2005). Investment behavior and the negative side of emotion. *Psychological Science, 16*, 435–439. (11)

Shohamy, D. (2011). Learning and motivation in the human striatum. *Current Opinion in Neurobiology, 21*, 408–414. (12)

Shohamy, D., Myers, C. E., Kalanithi, J., & Gluck, M. A. (2008). Basal ganglia and dopamine contributions to probabilistic category learning. *Neuroscience and Biobehavioral Reviews, 32*, 219–236. (12)

Shoulson, I. (1990). Huntington's disease: Cognitive and psychiatric features. *Neuropsychiatry, Neuropsychology, and Behavioral Neurology, 3*, 15–22. (7)

Shrager, Y., Levy, D. A., Hopkins, R. O., & Squire, L. R. (2008). Working memory and the organization of brain systems. *Journal of Neuroscience, 28*, 4818–4822. (12)

Shulman, E. P. (2014). Deciding in the dark: Differences in intuitive risk judgment. *Developmental Psychology, 50*, 167–177. (4)

Shutts, D. (1982). *Lobotomy: Resort to the knife.* New York: Van Nostrand Reinhold. (3)

Siegel, C. S., Fink, K. L., Strittmatter, S. M., & Cafferty, W. B. J. (2015). Plasticity of intact rebral projections mediates spontaneous recovery of function after corticospinal tract injury. *Journal of Neuroscience, 35*, 1443–1457. (4)

Siegel, J. M. (1995). Phylogeny and the function of REM sleep. *Behavioural Brain Research, 69*, 29–34. (8)

Siegel, J. M. (2009). Sleep viewed as a state of adaptive inactivity. *Nature Reviews Neuroscience, 10*, 747–753. (8)

Siegel, J. M. (2012). Suppression of sleep for mating. *Science, 337*, 1610–1611. (8)

Siegel, S. (1977). Morphine tolerance as an associative process. *Journal of Experimental Psychology: Animal Behavior Processes, 3*, 1–13. (14)

Siegel, S. (1983). Classical conditioning, drug tolerance, and drug dependence. *Research Advances in Alcohol and Drug Problems, 9*, 279–314. (14)

Siegel, S. (1987). Alcohol and opiate dependence: Reevaluation of the Victorian perspective. *Research Advances in Alcohol and Drug Problems, 9*, 279–314. (14)

Silber, B. Y., & Schmitt, J. A. J. (2010). Effects of tryptophan loading on human cognition, mood, and sleep. *Neuroscience and Biobehavioral Reviews, 34*, 387–407. (9)

Silbersweig, D. A., Stern, E., Frith, C., Cahill, C., Holmes, A., Grootoonk, S., . . . Frackowiak, R. S. J. (1995). A functional neuroanatomy of hallucinations in schizophrenia. *Nature, 378*, 176–179. (14)

Silk, J. B., Brosnan, S. F., Vonk, J., Henrich, J., Povinelli, D. J., Richardson, A. S., . . . Schapiro, S. J. (2005). Chimpanzees are indifferent to the welfare of unrelated group members. *Nature, 437*, 1357–1359. (1, 13)

Silva, A. J., Zhou, Y., Rogerson, T., Shobe, J., & Balaji, J. (2009). Molecular and cellular approaches to memory allocation in neural circuits. *Science, 326*, 391–395. (12)

Silva, B. A., Mattucci, C., Krzywkowski, P., Cuozzo, R., Carbonari, L., & Gross, C. T. (2016). The ventromedial hypothalamus mediates predator fear memory. *European Journal of Neuroscience, 43*, 1431–1439. (9)

Silventoinen, K., Jelenkovic, A., Sund, R., Hur, Y.-M., Yokoyama, Y., Honda, C., . . . Kaprio, J. (2016). Genetic and environmental effects on body mass index from infancy to the onset of adulthood: An individual-based pooled analysis of 45 twin cohorts participating in the COllaborative project of Development of Anthropometrical measures in Twins (CODATwins) study. *American Journal of Clinical Nutrition, 104*, 371–379 (9)

Silver, R. A. (2010). Neuronal arithmetic. *Nature Reviews Neuroscience, 11*, 474–489. (2)

Silvers, J. A., Lumian, D. S., Gabard-Durnam, L., Gee, D. G., Goff, B., Fareri, D. S., . . . Tottenham, N. (2016). Previous institutionalization is followed by broader amygdala-hippocampal-PFC network connectivity during aversive learning in human development. *Journal of Neuroscience, 36*, 6420–6430. (11)

Simner, J., & Ward, J. (2006). The taste of words on the tip of the tongue. *Nature, 444*, 438. (6)

Simon, B., Fletcher, J. A., & Doebeli, M. (2013). Towards a general theory of group selection. *Evolution, 67*, 1561–1572. (4)

Simons, D. J., Boot, W. R., Charness, N., Gathercole, S. E., Chabris, C. F., Hambrick, D. Z., & Stine-Morrow, E. A. L. (2016). Do "brain-training" programs work? *Psychological Science in the Public Interest, 17*, 103–186. (4)

Simpson, E. H., Kellendonk, C., & Kandel, E. (2010). A possible role for the striatum in the pathogenesis of the cognitive symptoms of schizophrenia. *Neuron, 65*, 585–596. (14)

Sincich, L. C., Park, K. F., Wohlgemuth, M. J., & Horton, J. C. (2004). Bypassing V1: A direct geniculate input to area MT. *Nature Neuroscience, 7*, 1123–1128. (5)

Singer, T., Seymour, B., O'Doherty, J., Kaube, H., Dolan, R. J., & Frith, C. D. (2004). Empathy for pain involves the affective but not sensory components of pain. *Science, 303*, 1157–1162. (6)

Singh, S., & Mallick, B. N. (1996). Mild electrical stimulation of pontine tegmentum around locus coeruleus reduces rapid eye movement sleep in rats. *Neuroscience Research, 24*, 227–235. (8)

Siopi, E., Denizet, M., Gabellec, M.-M., deChaumont, F., Olivo-Marin, J.-C., Guilloux, J.-P., . . . Lazarini, F. (2016). Anxiety- and depression-like states lead to pronounced olfactory deficits and impaired adult neurogenesis in mice. *Journal of Neuroscience, 36*, 518–531. (14)

Sirigu, A., Grafman, J., Bressler, K., & Sunderland, T. (1991). Multiple representations contribute to body knowledge processing. Evidence from a case of autopagnosia. *Brain, 114*, 629–642. (6)

Sirotin, Y. B., Hillman, E. M. C., Bordier, C., & Das, A. (2009). Spatiotemporal precision and hemodynamic mechanism of optical point spreads in alert primates. *Proceedings of the National Academy of Sciences, 106*, 18390–18395. (3)

Sjöström, M., Friden, J., & Ekblom, B. (1987). Endurance, what is it? Muscle morphology after an extremely long distance run. *Acta Physiologica Scandinavica, 130*, 513–520. (7)

Skinner, M. D., Lahmek, P., Pham, H., & Aubin, H. J. (2014). Disulfiram efficacy in the treatment of alcohol dependence: A meta-analysis. *PLoS One*, e87366. (14)

Skitzki, J. J., Chen, Q., Wang, W. C., & Evans, S. S. (2007). Primary immune surveillance: Some like it hot. *Journal of Molecular Medicine, 85*, 1361–1367. (9)

Skoe, E., & Kraus, N. (2012). A little goes a long way: How the adult brain is shaped by musical training in childhood. *Journal of Neuroscience, 32*, 11507–11510. (4)

Skorska, M. N., Geniole, S. N., Vrysen, B. M., McCormick, C. M., & Bogaert, A. F. (2015). Facial structure predicts sexual orientation in both men and women. *Archives of Sexual Behavior, 44*, 1377–1394. (10)

Slavich, G. M., & Cole, S. W. (2013). The emerging field of human social genomics. *Clinical Psychological Science, 1*, 331–348. (4)

Sloan, D. M., Strauss, M. E., & Wisner, K. L. (2001). Diminished response to pleasant stimuli by depressed women. *Journal of Abnormal Psychology, 110*, 488–493. (14)

Smith, G. B., Sederberg, A., Elyada, Y. M., Van Hooser, S. D., Kaschube, M., & Fitzpatrick, D. (2015). The development of cortical circuits for motion discrimination. *Nature Neuroscience, 18*, 252–261. (5)

Smith, G. P. (1998). Pregastric and gastric satiety. In G. P. Smith (Ed.), *Satiation: From gut to brain* (pp. 10–39). New York: Oxford University Press. (9)

Smith, G. P., & Gibbs, J. (1998). The satiating effects of cholecystokinin and bombesin-like peptides. In G. P. Smith (Ed.), *Satiation:*

From gut to brain (pp. 97–125). New York: Oxford University Press. (9)

Smith, K., Thompson, G. F., & Koster, H. D. (1969). Sweat in schizophrenic patients: Identification of the odorous substance. *Science, 166,* 398–399. (14)

Smith, K. S., Bucci, D. J., Luikart, B. W., & Mahler, S. V. (2016). DREADDs: Use and application in behavioral neuroscience. *Behavioral Neuroscience, 130,* 137–155. (3)

Smith, L. T. (1975). The interanimal transfer phenomenon: A review. *Psychological Bulletin, 81,* 1078–1095. (12)

Smith, M. A., Brandt, J., & Shadmehr, R. (2000). Motor disorder in Huntington's disease begins as a dysfunction in error feedback control. *Nature, 403,* 544–549. (7)

Smith, M. E., & Farah, M. J. (2011). Are prescription stimulants "smart pills"? The epidemiology and cognitive neuroscience of prescription stimulant use by normal healthy individuals. *Psychological Science, 137,* 717–741. (12)

Smolker, H. R., Depue, B. E., Reineberg, A. E., Orr, J. M., & Banich, M. T. (2015). Individual differences in regional prefrontal gray matter morphometry and fractional anisotropy are associated with different constructs of executive function. *Brain Structure & Function, 220,* 1291–1306. (3)

Smulders, T. V., Shiflett, M. W., Sperling, A. J., & DeVoogd, T. J. (2000). Seasonal changes in neuron numbers in the hippocampal formation of a food-hoarding bird: The black-capped chickadee. *Journal of Neurobiology, 44,* 414–422. (4)

Snyder, L. H., Grieve, K. L., Brotchie, P., & Andersen, R. A. (1998). Separate body- and world-referenced representations of visual space in parietal cortex. *Nature, 394,* 887–891. (7)

Sobota, R., Mihara, T., Forrest, A., Featherstone, R. E., & Siegel, S. J. (2015). Oxytocin reduces amygdala activity, increases social interactions, and reduces anxiety-like behavior irrespective of NMDAR antagonism. *Behavioral Neuroscience, 129,* 389–398. (13)

Sodersten, P., Bergh, C., Leon, M., & Zandian, M. (2016). Dopamine and anorexia nervosa. *Neuroscience and Biobehavioral Reviews, 60,* 26–30. (9)

Solms, M. (1997). *The neuropsychology of dreams.* Mahwah, NJ: Erlbaum. (8)

Solms, M. (2000). Dreaming and REM sleep are controlled by different brain mechanisms. *Behavioral and Brain Sciences, 23,* 843–850. (8)

Solomon, S. G., & Lennie, P. (2007). The machinery of colour vision. *Nature Reviews Neuroscience, 8,* 276–286. (5)

Solter, A. (2008). A 2-year-old child's memory of hospitalization during early infancy. *Infant and Child Development, 17,* 593–605. (12)

Song, H., Stevens, C. F., & Gage, F. H. (2002). Neural stem cells from adult hippocampus develop essential properties of functional CNS neurons. *Nature Neuroscience, 5,* 438–445. (4)

Song, K., Wang, H., Kamm, G. B., Pohle, J., de Castro Reis, F., Heppenstall, P., Wende, H., & Siemens, J. (2016). The TRPM2 channel is a hypothalamic heat sensor that limits fever and can drive hypothermia. *Science, 353,* 1393–1398. (9)

Song, Y., Zhu, Q., Li, J., Wang, X., & Liu, J. (2015). Typical and atypical development of functional connectivity in the face network. *Journal of Neuroscience, 35,* 14624–14635. (5)

Soon, C. S., Brass, M., Heinze, H.-J., & Haynes, J.-D. (2008). Unconscious determinants of free decisions in the human brain. *Nature Neuroscience, 11,* 543–545. (7)

Sorger, B., Reithler, J., Dahmen, B., & Goebel, R. (2012). A real-time fMRI-based spelling device immediately enabling robust motor-independent communication. *Current Biology, 22,* 1333–1338. (3)

Southwell, D. G., Froemke, R. C., Alvarez-Buylla, A., Stryker, M. P., & Gandhi, S. P. (2010). Cortical plasticity induced by inhibitory neuron transplantation. *Science, 327,* 1145–1148. (5)

Southwell, D. G., Paaredes, M. F., Galvao, R. P., Jones, D. L., Froemke, R. C., Sebe, J. Y., . . . Alvarez-Buylla, A. A. (2012). Intrinsically determined cell death of developing cortical interneurons. *Nature, 491,* 109–113. (4)

Spalding, K. L., Bergmann, O., Alkass, K., Bernard, S., Salehpour, M., Huttner, H. B., . . . Frisén, J. (2013). Dynamics of hippocampal neurogenesis in adult humans. *Cell, 153,* 1219–1227. (4)

Spalding, K. L., Bhardwaj, R. D., Buchholz, B. A., Druid, H., & Frisén, J. (2005). Retrospective birth dating of cells in humans. *Cell, 122,* 133–143. (4)

Spangler, R., Wittkowski, K. M., Goddard, N. L., Avena, N. M., Hoebel, B. G., & Leibowitz, S. F. (2004). Opiate-like effects of sugar on gene expression in reward areas of the rat brain. *Molecular Brain Research, 124,* 134–142. (9)

Spearman, C. (1904). "General intelligence," objectively determined and measured. *American Journal of Psychology, 15,* 201–293. (12)

Speer, N. K., Reynolds, J. R., Swallow, K. M., & Zacks, J. M. (2009). Reading stories activates neural representations of visual and motor experiences. *Psychological Science, 20,* 989–999. (7)

Spelke, E. S. (2005). Sex differences in intrinsic aptitude for mathematics and science? *American Psychologist, 60,* 950–958. (12)

Spencer, R. M. C., Zelaznik, H. N., Diedrichsen, J., & Ivry, R. B. (2003). Disrupted timing of discontinuous but not continuous movements by cerebellar lesions. *Science, 300,* 1437–1439. (7)

Sperandie, I., Chouinard, P. A., & Goodale, M. A. (2012). Retinotopic activity in V1 reflects the perceived and not the retinal size of an afterimage. *Nature Neuroscience, 15,* 540–542. (5)

Sperry, R. W. (1943). Visuomotor coordination in the newt (*Triturus viridescens*) after regeneration of the optic nerve. *Journal of Comparative Neurology, 79,* 33–55. (4)

Sperry, R. W. (1975). In search of psyche. In F. G. Worden, J. P. Swazey, & G. Adelman (Eds.), *The neurosciences: Paths of discovery* (pp. 425–434). Cambridge, MA: MIT Press. (4)

Spezio, M. L., Huang, P.-Y. S., Castelli, F., & Adolphs, R. (2007). Amygdala damage impairs eye contact during conversations with real people. *Journal of Neuroscience, 27,* 3994–3997. (11)

Spiegel, T. A. (1973). Caloric regulation of food intake in man. *Journal of Comparative and Physiological Psychology, 84,* 24–37. (9)

Spindler, K. A., Sullivan, E. V., Menon, V., Lim, K. O., & Pfefferbaum, A. (1997). Deficits in multiple systems of working memory in schizophrenia. *Schizophrenia Research, 27,* 1–10. (14)

Spitzer, N. C. (2015). Neurotransmitter switching? No surprise. *Neuron, 86,* 1131–1144. (2)

Spoletini, I., Cherubini, A., Banfi, G., Rubino, I. A., Peran, P., Caltagirone, C., & Spalletta, G. (2011). Hippocampi, thalami, and accumbens microstructural damage in schizophrenia: A volumetry, diffusivity, and neuropsychological study. *Schizophrenia Bulletin, 37,* 118–130. (14)

Spreux-Varoquaux, O., Alvarez, J.-C., Berlin, I., Batista, G., Despierre, P.-G., Gilton, A., & Cremniter, D. (2001). Differential abnormalities in plasma 5-HIAA and platelet serotonin concentrations in violent suicide attempters. *Life Sciences, 69,* 647–657. (11)

Spurzheim, J. G. (1908). *Phrenology* (rev. ed.) Philadelphia: Lippincott. (3)

Squire, L. R. (1992). Memory and the hippocampus: A synthesis from findings with rats, monkeys, and humans. *Psychological Review, 99,* 195–231. (12)

Squires, T. M. (2004). Optimizing the vertebrate vestibular semicircular canal: Could we balance any better? *Physical Review Letters, 93,* 198106. (6)

Stallen, M., De Dreu, C. K. W., Shalvi, S., Smidts, A., & Sanfey, A. G. (2012). The herding hormone: Oxytocin stimulates in-group conformity. *Psychological Science, 23,* 1288–1292. (13)

Stalnaker, T. A., Cooch, N. K., & Schoenbaum, G. (2015). What the orbitofrontal cortex does not do. *Nature Neuroscience, 18,* 620–625. (13)

Stanford, L. R. (1987). Conduction velocity variations minimize conduction time differences among retinal ganglion cell axons. *Science, 238,* 358–360. (1)

Starr, C., & Taggart, R. (1989). *Biology: The unity and diversity of life.* Pacific Grove, CA: Brooks/Cole. (2, 3, 7, 10)

Steele, C. J., Bailey, J. A., Zatorre, R. J., & Penhune, V. B. (2013). Early musical training and white-matter plasticity in the corpus callosum: Evidence for a sensitive period. *Journal of Neuroscience, 33,* 1282–1290. (4)

Steffens, B. (2007). *Ibn al-Haytham: First Scientist.* Greensboro, NC: Morgan Reynolds Publishing. (5)

Stein, B. E., Stanford, T. R., & Rowland, B. A. (2014). Development of multisensory integration from the perspective of the individual neuron. *Nature Reviews Neuroscience, 15*, 520–535. (3)

Stein, M. B., Hanna, C., Koverola, C., Torchia, M., & McClarty, B. (1997). Structural brain changes in PTSD. *Annals of the New York Academy of Sciences, 821*, 76–82. (11)

Stein, T., Reeder, R. R., & Peelen, M. V. (2016). Privileged access to awareness for faces and objects of expertise. *Journal of Experimental Psychology—Human Perception and Performance, 42*, 788–798. (13)

Steinberg, L. (2013). The influence of neuroscience on U.S. Supreme Court decisions about adolescents' criminal culpability. *Nature Reviews Neuroscience, 14*, 513–518. (4)

Steinberg, L., Graham, S., O'Brien, L., Woolard, J., Cauffman, E., & Banich, M. (2009). Age differences in future orientation and delay discounting. *Child Development, 80*, 28–44. (4)

Steinecke, A., Gampe, C., Valkova, C., Kaether, C., & Bolz, J. (2012). Disrupted-in-schizophrenia 1 (DISC1) is necessary for the correct migration of cortical interneurons. *Journal of Neuroscience, 32*, 738–745. (14)

Steinert, C., Hofmann, M., Kruse, J., & Leichsenring, F. (2014). Relapse rates after psychotherapy for depression—stable long term effects? *Journal of Affective Disorders, 168*, 107–118. (14)

Stellar, J. E., Cohen, A., Oveis, C., & Keltner, D. (2015). Affective and physiological responses to the suffering of others: Compassion and vagal activity. *Journal of Personality and Social Psychology, 108*, 572–585. (11)

Stensola, H., Stensola, T., Solstad, T., Frøland, K., Moser, M.-B., & Moser, E. I. (2012). The entorhinal grid map is discretized. *Nature, 492*, 72–78. (12)

Stephens, T. W., Basinski, M., Bristow, P. K., Bue-Valleskey, J. M., Burgett, S. G., Craft, L., . . . Heiman, M. (1995). The role of neuropeptide Y in the antiobesity action of the obese gene product. *Nature, 377*, 530–532. (9)

Sterling, P. (2012). Allostasis: A model of predictive regulation. *Physiology & Behavior, 106*, 5–15. (9)

Sterpenich, V., D'Argembeau, A., Desseiles, M., Balteau, E., Albouy, G., Vandewalle, G., . . . Maquet, P. (2006). The locus ceruleus is involved in the successful retrieval of emotional memories in humans. *Journal of Neuroscience, 26*, 7416–7423. (8)

Stevens, C. F. (2001). An evolutionary scaling law for the primate visual system and its basis in cortical function. *Nature, 411*, 193–195. (5)

Stevens, M., & Cuthill, I. C. (2007). Hidden messages: Are ultraviolet signals a special channel in avian communication? *Bioscience, 57*, 501–507. (5)

Stevenson, R. J., Hodgson, D., Oaten, M. J., Moussavi, M., Langberg, R., Case, T. I., &
Barouei, J. (2012). Disgust elevates core body temperature and up-regulates certain oral immune markers. *Brain Behavior and Immunity, 26*, 1160–1168. (11)

Stevenson, R. J. (2014). Flavor binding: Its nature and cause. *Psychological Bulletin, 140*, 487–510. (3)

Stevenson, R. J., Miller, L. A., & McGrillen, K. (2013). The lateralization of gustatory function and the flow of information from tongue to cortex. *Neuropsychologia, 51*, 1408–1416. (6, 13)

Stewart, J. W., Quitkin, F. M., McGrath, P. J., Amsterdam, J., Fava, M., Fawcett, J., . . . Roback, P. (1998). Use of pattern analysis to predict differential relapse of remitted patients with major depression during 1 year of treatment with fluoxetine or placebo. *Archives of General Psychiatry, 55*, 334–343. (14)

Stice, E., & Yokum, S. (2016). Gain in body fat is associated with increased striatal response to palatable food cues, whereas body fat stability is associated with decreased striatal response. *Journal of Neuroscience, 36*, 6949–6956. (9)

Stickgold, R., Malia, A., Maguire, D., Roddenberry, D., & O'Connor, M. (2000). Replaying the game: Hypnagogic images in normals and amnesics. *Science, 290*, 350–353. (12)

Stillman, P., Van Bavel, J., & Cunningham, W. (2015). Valence asymmetries in the human amygdala: Task relevance modulates amygdala responses to positive more than negative affective cues. *Journal of Cognitive Neuroscience, 27*, 842–851. (11)

Stokes, M., Thompson, R., Cusack, R., & Duncan, J. (2009). Top-down activation of shape-specific population codes in visual cortex during mental imagery. *Journal of Neuroscience, 29*, 1565–1572. (5)

Stolzenberg, D. S., & Champagne, F. A. (2016). Hormonal and non-hormonal bases of maternal behavior: The role of experience and epigenetic mechanisms. *Hormones and Behavior, 77*, 204–210. (10)

Storey, A. E., & Ziegler, T. E. (2016). Primate paternal care: Interactions between biology and social experience. *Hormones and Behavior, 77*, 260–271. (10)

Storey, K. B., & Storey, J. M. (1999, May/June). Lifestyles of the cold and frozen. *The Sciences, 39*(3), 33–37. (9)

Stough, C., & Pase, M. P. (2015). Improving cognition in the elderly with nutritional supplements. *Current Directions in Psychological Science, 24*, 177–183. (12)

Stricker, E. M. (1969). Osmoregulation and volume regulation in rats: Inhibition of hypovolemic thirst by water. *American Journal of Physiology, 217*, 98–105. (9)

Stricker, E. M., Swerdloff, A. F., & Zigmond, M. J. (1978). Intrahypothalamic injections of kainic acid produce feeding and drinking deficits in rats. *Brain Research, 158*, 470–473. (9)
Striemer, C. L., Chapman, C. S., & Goodale, M. A. (2009). "Real-time" obstacle avoidance in the absence of primary visual cortex. *Proceedings of the National Academy of Sciences (U.S.A.), 106*, 15996–16001. (5)

Stroebele, N., de Castro, J. M., Stuht, J., Catenacci, V., Wyatt, H. R., & Hill, J. O. (2008). A small-changes approach reduces energy intake in free-living humans. *Journal of the American College of Nutrition, 28*, 63–68. (9)

Strotmann, J., Levai, O., Fleischer, J., Schwarzenbacher, K., & Breer, H. (2004). Olfactory receptor proteins in axonal processes of chemosensory neurons. *Journal of Neuroscience, 224*, 7754–7761. (6)

Struder, B., Manes, F., Humphreys, G., Robbins, T. W., & Clark, L. (2015). Risk-sensitive decision-making in patients with posterior parietal and ventromedial prefrontal cortex injury. *Cerebral Cortex, 25*, 1–9. (13)

Stryker, M. P., & Sherk, H. (1975). Modification of cortical orientation selectivity in the cat by restricted visual experience: A reexamination. *Science, 190*, 904–906. (5)

Stryker, M. P., Sherk, H., Leventhal, A. G., & Hirsch, H. V. B. (1978). Physiological consequences for the cat's visual cortex of effectively restricting early visual experience with oriented contours. *Journal of Neurophysiology, 41*, 896–909. (5)

Stuber, G. D., & Wise, R. A. (2016). Lateral hypothalamic circuits for feeding and reward. *Nature Neuroscience, 19*, 198–205. (9)

Sturm, V. E., Ascher, E. A., Miller, B. L., & Levenson, R. W. (2008). Diminished self-conscious emotional responding in frontotemporal lobar degeneration patients. *Emotion, 8*, 861–869. (13)

Stuss, D. T., & Benson, D. F. (1984). Neuropsychological studies of the frontal lobes. *Psychological Bulletin, 95*, 3–28. (3)

Su, J., van Boxtel, J. J. A., & Lu, H. (2016). Social interactions receive priority to conscious perception. *PLoS One, 11*, article e0160468. (13)

Suez, J., Korem, T., Zeevi, D., Zilberman-Schapira, G., Thais, C. A., Maza, O., . . . Elinav, E. (2014). Artificial sweeteners induce glucose intolerance by altering the gut microbiota. *Nature, 514*, 181–186. (9)

Sugamura, G., & Higuchi, R. (2015). Do we feel afraid because we tremble?: The effect of physical coldness on feelings of fear. Poster at the International Convention of Psychological Science, Amsterdam, March 13, 2015. (11)

Sun, Y.-G., Zhao, Z.-Q., Meng, X.-L., Yin, J., Liu, X.-Y., & Chen, Z. F. (2009). Cellular basis of itch sensation. *Science, 325*, 1531–1534. (6)

Sur, M., & Leamey, C. A. (2001). Development and plasticity of cortical areas and networks. *Nature Reviews Neuroscience, 2*, 251–262. (5)

Surén, P., Roth, C., Bresnahan, M., Haugen, M., Hornig, M., Hirtz, D., . . . Stoltenberg, C., (2013). Association between maternal use of folic acid supplements and risk of autism spectrum disorders in children. *Journal of the American Medical Association, 309,* 570–577. (14)

Sutterland, A. L., Fond, G., Kuin, A., Koeter, M. W. J., Lutter, R., van Gool, T., . . . de Haan, L. (2015). Beyond the association. *Toxoplasma gondii* in schizophrenia, bipolar disorder, and addiction: Systematic review and meta-analysis. *Psychiatrica Scandinavica, 132,* 161–179. (14)

Sutton, A. K., Pei, H., Burnett, K. H., Myers, M. G. Jr., Rhodes, C. J., & Olson, D. P. (2014). Control of food intake and energy expenditure by Nos1 neurons of the paraventricular hypothalamus. *Journal of Neuroscience, 34,* 15306–15318. (9)

Sutton, L. C., Lea, E., Will, M. J., Schwartz, B. A., Hartley, C. E., Poole, J. C., . . . Maier, S. F. (1997). Inescapable shock-induced potentiation of morphine analgesia. *Behavioral Neuroscience, 111,* 1105–1113. (6)

Sutton, R. L., Hovda, D. A., & Feeney, D. M. (1989). Amphetamine accelerates recovery of locomotor function following bilateral frontal cortex ablation in rats. *Behavioral Neuroscience, 103,* 837–841. (4)

Suzdak, P. D., Glowa, J. R., Crawley, J. N., Schwartz, R. D., Skolnick, P., & Paul, S. M. (1986). A selective imidazobenzodiazepine antagonist of ethanol in the rat. *Science, 234,* 1243–1247. (11)

Swaab, D. F., & Hofman, M. A. (1990). An enlarged suprachiasmatic nucleus in homosexual men. *Brain Research, 537,* 141–148. (10)

Swan, S. H., Liu, F., Hines, M., Kruse, R. L., Wang, C., Redmon, J. B., . . . Weiss, B. (2010). Prenatal phthalate exposure and reduced masculine play in boys. *International Journal of Andrology, 33,* 259–269. (10)

Sweeney, J. A., Rosano, C., Berman, R. A., & Luna, B. (2001). Inhibitory control of attention declines more than working memory during normal aging. *Neurobiology of Aging, 22,* 39–47. (7)

Swoboda, H., Amering, M., Windhaber, J., & Katschnig, H. (2003). The long-term course of panic disorder—An 11 year follow-up. *Journal of Anxiety Disorders, 17,* 223–232. (11)

Sztainberg, Y., & Zoghbi, H. Y. (2016). Lessons learned from studying syndromic autism spectrum disorders. *Nature Neuroscience, 19,* 1408–1417. (14)

Tabarean, I. V., Sanchez-Alavez, M., & Sethi, J. (2012). Mechanisms of H-2 histamine receptor dependent modulation of body temperature and neuronal activity in the medial preoptic nucleus. *Neuropharmacology, 63,* 171–180. (9)

Tabarés-Seisdedos, R., & Rubenstein, J. L. (2013). Inverse cancer comorbidity: A serendipitous opportunity to gain insight into CNS disorders. *Nature Reviews Neuroscience, 14,* 293–304. (14)

Taber-Thomas, B. C., Asp, E. W., Koenigs, M., Sutterer, M., Anderson, S. W., & Tranel, D. (2014). Arrested development: Early prefrontal lesions impair the maturation of moral judgment. *Brain, 137,* 1254–1261. (11)

Tabrizi, S. J., Cleeter, M. W. J., Xuereb, J., Taanman, J.-W., Cooper, J. M., & Schapira, A. H. V. (1999). Biochemical abnormalities and excitotoxicity in Huntington's disease brain. *Annals of Neurology, 45,* 25–32. (7)

Taddese, A., Nah, S. Y., & McCleskey, E. W. (1995). Selective opioid inhibition of small nociceptive neurons. *Science, 270,* 1366–1369. (6)

Tagawa, Y., Kanold, P. O., Majdan, M., & Shatz, C. J. (2005). Multiple periods of functional ocular dominance plasticity in mouse visual cortex. *Nature Neuroscience, 8,* 380–388. (5)

Tager-Flusberg, H., Boshart, J., & Baron-Cohen, S. (1998). Reading the windows to the soul: Evidence of domain-specific sparing in Williams syndrome. *Journal of Cognitive Neuroscience, 10,* 631–639. (13)

Tagliazucchi, E., Roseman, L., Kaelen, M., Orban, C., Muthukumaraswamy, S. D., Murphy, K., Laufs, H., . . . Carhart-Harris, R. (2016). Increased global functional connectivity correlates with LSD-induced ego dissolution. *Current Biology, 26,* 1043–1050. (2)

Tai, L.-H., Lee, A. M., Benavidez, N., Bonci, A., & Wilbrecht, L. (2012). Transient stimulation of distinct subpopulations of striatal neurons mimics changes in action value. *Nature Neuroscience, 15,* 1281–1289. (7)

Taillard, J., Philip, P., Coste, O., Sagaspe, P., & Bioulac, B. (2003). The circadian and homeostatic modulation of sleep pressure during wakefulness differs between morning and evening chronotypes. *Journal of Sleep Research, 12,* 275–282. (8)

Takano, T., Tian, G.-F., Peng, W., Lou, N., Libionka, W., Han, X., & Nedergaard, M. (2006). Astrocyte-mediated control of cerebral blood flow. *Nature Neuroscience, 9,* 260–267. (1)

Takehara-Nishiuchi, K., & McNaughton, B. L. (2008). Spontaneous changes of neocortical code for associative memory during consolidation. *Science, 322,* 960–963. (12)

Takemura, H., Ashida, H., Amano, K., Kitaoka, A., & Murakami, I. (2012). Neural correlates of induced motion perception in the human brain. *Journal of Neuroscience, 32,* 14344–14354. (5)

Takeuchi, T., Duszkiewicz, A. J., Sonneborn, A., Spooner, P. A., Yamasaki, M., Watanabe, M., . . . Morris, R. G. M. (2016). Locus coeruleus and dopaminergic consolidation of everyday memory. *Nature, 537,* 357–362. (12)

Tamietto, M., Castelli, L., Vighetti, S., Perozzo, P., Geminiani, G., Weiskrantz, L., & de Gelder, B. (2009). Unseen facial and bodily expressions trigger fast emotional reactions. *Proceedings of the National Academy of Sciences (U.S.A.), 106,* 17661–17666. (5)

Tanaka, J., Hayashi, Y., Nomura, S., Miyakubo, H., Okumura, T., & Sakamaki, K. (2001). Angiotensinergic and noradrenergic mechanisms in the hypothalamic paraventricular nucleus participate in the drinking response induced by activation of the subfornical organ in rats. *Behavioural Brain Research, 118,* 117–122. (9)

Tanaka, J., Hori, K., & Nomura, M. (2001). Dipsogenic response induced by angiotensinergic pathways from the lateral hypothalamic area to the subfornical organ in rats. *Behavioural Brain Research, 118,* 111–116. (9)

Tanaka, M., Nakahara, T., Muranaga, T., Kojima, S., Yasuhara, D., Ueno, H., . . . Inui, A. (2006). Ghrelin concentrations and cardiac vagal tone are decreased after pharmacologic and cognitive-behavioral treatment in patients with bulimia nervosa. *Hormones and Behavior, 50,* 261–265. (9)

Tanaka, Y., Kamo, T., Yoshida, M., & Yamadori, A. (1991). "So-called" cortical deafness. *Brain, 114,* 2385–2401. (6)

Tandon, S., Simon, S. A., & Nicolelis, M. A. L. (2012). Appetitive changes during salt deprivation are paralleled by widespread neuronal adaptations in nucleus accumbens, lateral hypothalamus, and central amygdala. *Journal of Neurophysiology, 108,* 1089–1105. (9)

Tanji, J., & Shima, K. (1994). Role for supplementary motor area cells in planning several movements ahead. *Nature, 371,* 413–416. (7)

Tanner, C. M., Kamel, F., Ross, G. W., Hoppin, J. A., Goldman, S. M., Korell, M., . . . Langston, J. W. (2011). Rotenone, paraquat, and Parkinson's disease. *Environmental Health Perspectives, 119,* 866–872. (7)

Tappy, L., & Lê, K.-A. (2010). Metabolic effects of fructose and the worldwide increase in obesity. *Physiological Reviews, 90,* 23–46. (9)

Tarampi, M. R., Heydari, N., & Hegarty, M. (2016). A tale of two types of perspective taking: Sex differences in spatial ability. *Psychological Science, 27,* 1507–1516. (10)

Taravosh-Lahn, K., Bastida, C., & Delville, Y. (2006). Differential responsiveness to fluoxetine during puberty. *Behavioral Neuroscience, 120,* 1084–1092. (11)

Tattersall, G. J., Andrade, D. V., & Abe, A. S. (2009). Heat exchange from the toucan bill reveals a controllable vascular thermal radiator. *Science, 325,* 468–470. (9)

Tattersall, G. J., Leite, C. A. C., Sanders, C. E., Cadena, V., Andrade, D. V., Abe, A. S., & Milsom, W. K. (2016). Seasonal reproductive endothermy in tegu lizards. *Science Advances, 2,* e1500951. (9)

Taub, E., & Berman, A. J. (1968). Movement and learning in the absence of sensory feedback. In S. J. Freedman (Ed.), *The neuropsychology of spatially oriented behavior* (pp. 173–192). Homewood, IL: Dorsey. (4)

Taylor, J. P., Hardy, J., & Fischbeck, K. H. (2002). Toxic proteins in neurodegenerative disease. *Science, 296,* 1991–1995. (12)

Taylor, M. A. (1969). Sex ratios of newborns: Associated with prepartum and postpartum schizophrenia. *Science, 164,* 723–721. (14)

Teff, K. L., Elliott, S. S., Tschöp, M., Kieffer, T. J., Rader, D., Heiman, M., . . . Havel, P. J. (2004). Dietary fructose reduces circulating insulin and leptin, attenuates postprandial suppression of ghrelin, and increases triglycerides in women. *Journal of Clinical Endocrinology & Metabolism, 89,* 2963–2972. (9)

Teicher, M. H., Glod, C. A., Magnus, E., Harper, D., Benson, G., Krueger, K., & McGreenery, C. E. (1997). Circadian rest–activity disturbances in seasonal affective disorder. *Archives of General Psychiatry, 54,* 124–130. (14)

Teitelbaum, P. (1961). Disturbances in feeding and drinking behavior after hypothalamic lesions. In M. R. Jones (Ed.), *Nebraska Symposia on Motivation 1961* (pp. 39–69). Lincoln: University of Nebraska Press. (9)

Teitelbaum, P., & Epstein, A. N. (1962). The lateral hypothalamic syndrome. *Psychological Review, 69,* 74–90. (9)

Teitelbaum, P., Pellis, V. C., & Pellis, S. M. (1991). Can allied reflexes promote the integration of a robot's behavior? In J. A. Meyer & S. W. Wilson (Eds.), *From animals to animats: Simulation of animal behavior* (pp. 97–104). Cambridge, MA: MIT Press/ Bradford Books. (7)

Terburg, D., Aarts, H., & van Honk, J. (2012). Testosterone affects gaze aversion from angry faces outside of conscious awareness. *Psychological Science, 23,* 459–463. (11)

Terzaghi, M., Sartori, I., Tassi, L., Rustioni, V., Proserpio, P., Lorusso, G., . . . Nobili, L. (2012). Dissociated local arousal states underlying essential features of non-rapid eye movement arousal parasomnia: An intracerebral stereo-electroencephalographic study. *Journal of Sleep Research, 21,* 502–506. (8)

Tesoriero, C., Codita, A., Zhang, M.-D., Cherninsky, A., Karlsson, H., Grassi-Zucconi, G., . . . Kristensson, K. (2016). H1N1 influenza virus induces narcolepsy-like sleep disruption and targets sleep-wake regulatory neurons in mice. *Proceedings of the National Academy of Sciences (U.S.A.), 113,* E368–E377. (8)

Tetrud, J. W., Langston, J. W., Garbe, P. L., & Ruttenber, A. J. (1989). Mild Parkinsonism in persons exposed to 1-methyl-4-phenyl-1,2,3,6-tetrahydropyridine (MPTP). *Neurology, 39,* 1483–1487. (7)

Thalemann, R., Wölfling, K., & Grüsser, S. M. (2007). Specific cue reactivity on computer game-related cues in excessive gamers. *Behavioral Neuroscience, 121,* 614–618. (14)

Thannickal, T. C., Moore, R. Y., Nienhuis, R., Ramanathan, L., Gulyani, S., Aldrich, M., . . . Siegel, J. M. (2000). Reduced number of hypocretin neurons in human narcolepsy. *Neuron, 27,* 469–474. (8)

Thase, M. E., Greenhouse, J. B., Frank, E., Reynolds, C. F., III, Pilkonis, P. A., Hurley, K., . . . Kupfer, D. J. (1997). Treatment of major depression with psychotherapy or psychotherapy-psychopharmacology combinations. *Archives of General Psychiatry, 54,* 1009–1015. (14)

Theunissen, F. E., & Elie, J. E. (2014). Neural processing of natural sounds. *Nature Reviews Neuroscience, 15,* 355–366. (6)

Theusch, E., Basu, A., & Gitschier, J. (2009). Genome-wide study of families with absolute pitch reveals linkage to 8q24.21 and locus heterogeneity. *American Journal of Human Genetics, 85,* 112–119. (6)

Thier, P., Dicke, P. W., Haas, R., & Barash, S. (2000). Encoding of movement time by populations of cerebellar Purkinje cells. *Nature, 405,* 72–76. (7)

Thomas, B. C., Croft, K. E., & Tranel, D. (2011). Harming kin to save strangers: Further evidence for abnormally utilitarian moral judgments after ventromedial prefrontal damage. *Journal of Cognitive Neuroscience, 23,* 2186–2196. (11)

Thomas, C., Avidan, G., Humphreys, K., Jung, K., Gao, F., & Behrmann, M. (2009). Reduced structural connectivity in ventral visual cortex in congenital prosopagnosia. *Nature Neuroscience, 12,* 29–31. (5)

Thomas, C., & Baker, C. I. (2013). Teaching an adult brain new tricks: A critical review of evidence for training-dependent structural plasticity in humans. *NeuroImage, 73,* 225–236. (4)

Thomson, D. R., Besner, D., & Smilek, D. (2015). A resource-control account of sustained attention: Evidence from mind-wandering and vigilance paradigms. *Perspectives on Psychological Science, 10,* 82–96. (13)

Thompson, R. F. (1986). The neurobiology of learning and memory. *Science, 233,* 941–947. (12)

Thompson, W. F., Marin, M. M., & Stewart, L. (2012). Reduced sensitivity to emotional prosody in congenital amusia rekindles the musical protolanguage hypothesis. *Proceedings of the National Academy of Sciences (U.S.A.), 109,* 19027–19032. (6)

Thurman, D. J. (2016). The epidemiology of traumatic brain injury in children and youths: A review of research since 1990. *Journal of Child Neurology, 31,* 20–27. (4)

Tian, D., Stoppel, J. L., Heynen, A. J., Lindemann, L., Jaeschke, G., Mills, A. A., . . . Bear, M. F. (2015). Contribution of mGluR5 to pathophysiology in a mouse model of human chromosome 16p11.2 microdeletion. *Nature Neuroscience, 18,* 182–184. (14)

Ticku, M. K., & Kulkarni, S. K. (1988). Molecular interactions of ethanol with GABAergic system and potential of Ro15-4513 as an ethanol antagonist. *Pharmacology Biochemistry and Behavior, 30,* 501–510. (11)

Tillman, B., Leveque, Y., Fornoni, L., Abouy, P., & Caclin, A. (2016). Impaired short-term memory for pitch in congenital amusia. *Brain Research, 1640,* 251–263. (6)

Timms, B. G., Howdeshell, K. L., Barton, L., Richter, C. A., & vom Saal, F. S. (2005). Estrogenic chemicals in plastic and oral contraceptives disrupt development of the fetal mouse prostate and urethra. *Proceedings of the National Academy of Sciences, USA, 102,* 7014–7019. (10)

Tinbergen, N. (1951). *The study of instinct.* Oxford, England: Oxford University Press. (0)

Tinbergen, N. (1973). The search for animal roots of human behavior. In N. Tinbergen (Ed.), *The animal in its world* (Vol. 2, pp. 161–174). Cambridge, MA: Harvard University Press. (0)

Tingate, T. R., Lugg, D. J., Muller, H. K., Stowe, R. P., & Pierson, D. L. (1997). Antarctic isolation: Immune and viral studies. *Immunology and Cell Biology, 75,* 275–283. (11)

Tiruneh, M. A., Huang, B. S., & Leenen, F. H. H. (2013). Role of angiotensin II type 1 receptors in the pressor responses to central sodium in rats. *Brain Research, 1527,* 79–86. (9)

Tishkoff, S. A., Reed, F. A., Ranciaro, A., Voight, B. F., Babbitt, C. C., Silverman, J. S., Deloukas, P. (2007). Convergent adaptation of human lactase persistence in Africa and Europe. *Nature Genetics, 39,* 31–40. (9)

Tizzano, M., Gulbransen, B. D., Vandenbeuch, A., Clapp, T. R., Herman, J. P., Sibhatu, H. M., . . . Finger, T. E. (2010). Nasal chemosensory cells use bitter taste signaling to detect irritants and bacterial signals. *Proceedings of the National Academy of Sciences (U.S.A.), 107,* 3210–3215. (6)

Tobin, V. A., Hashimoto, H., Wacker, D. W., Takayanagi, Y., Langnaese, K., Caquíneau, C., . . . Ludwig, M. (2010). An intrinsic vasopressin system in the olfactory bulb is involved in social recognition. *Nature, 464,* 413–417. (10)

Tøien, Ø., Blake, J., Edgar, D. M., Grahn, D. A., Heller, H. C., & Barnes, B. M. (2011). Hibernation in black bears: Independence of metabolic suppression from body temperature. *Science, 331,* 906–909. (8)

Tokizawa, K., Yasuhara, S., Nakamura, M., Uchida, Y., Crawshaw, L. I., & Nagashma, K. (2010). Mild hypohydration induced by exercise in the heat attenuates autonomic thermoregulatory responses to the heat, but not thermal pleasantness in humans. *Physiology & Behavior, 100,* 340–345. (9)

Tolman, E. C. (1949). There is more than one kind of learning. *Psychological Review, 56,* 144–155. (12)

Tominaga, M., Caterina, M. J., Malmberg, A. B., Rosen, T. A., Gilbert, H., Skinner, K., . . . Julius, D. (1998). The cloned capsaicin receptor integrates multiple pain-producing stimuli. *Neuron, 21,* 531–543. (6)

Tomasino, B., & Gremese, M. (2016). The cognitive side of M1. *Frontiers in Human Neuroscience, 10,* article 298. (7)

Tomson, S. N., Narayan, M., Allen, G. I., & Eagleman, D. M. (2013). Neural networks of colored sequence synesthesia. *Journal of Neuroscience, 33,* 14098–14106. (6)

Tong, Q., Ye, C.-P., Jones, J. E., Elmquist, J. K., & Lowell, B. B. (2008). Synaptic release of GABA by AgRP neurons is required for normal regulation of energy balance. *Nature Neuroscience, 11,* 998–1000. (9)

Tong, X., Ao, Y., Faas, G. C., Nwaobi, S. E., Xu, J., Haustein, M. D., . . . Khakh, B. S. (2014). Astrocyte Kir4.1 ion channel deficits contribute to neuronal dysfunction in

Huntington's disease model mice. *Nature Neuroscience, 17,* 694–703. (7)

Torrey, E. F., Bartko, J. J., & Yolken, R. H. (2012). *Toxoplasma gondii* and other risk factors for schizophrenia: An update. *Schizophrenia Bulletin, 38,* 642–647. (14)

Torrey, E. F., Miller, J., Rawlings, R., & Yolken, R. H. (1997). Seasonality of births in schizophrenia and bipolar disorder: A review of the literature. *Schizophrenia Research, 28,* 1–38. (14)

Tosches, M. A., Bucher, D., Vopalensky, P., & Arendt, D. (2014). Melatonin signaling controls circadian swimming behavior in marine zooplankton. *Cell, 159,* 46–57. (8)

Tost, H., Champagne, F. A., & Meyer-Lindenberg, A. (2015). Environmental influence in the brain, human welfare and mental health. *Nature Neuroscience, 18,* 1421–1431. (14)

Toufexis, D. (2007). Region- and sex-specific modulation of anxiety behaviours in the rat. *Journal of Neuroendocrinology, 19,* 461–473. (11)

Tovote, P., Esposito, M. S., Botta, P., Chaudun, F., Fadok, J. P., Markovic, M., . . . Lüthi, A. (2016). Midbrain circuits for defensive behaviour. *Nature, 534,* 206–212. (11)

Townsend, J., Courchesne, E., Covington, J., Westerfield, M., Harris, N. S., Lyden, P., . . . Press, G. A. (1999). Spatial attention deficits in patients with acquired or developmental cerebellar abnormality. *Journal of Neuroscience, 19,* 5632–5643. (7)

Tran, P. B., & Miller, R. J. (2003). Chemokine receptors: Signposts to brain development and disease. *Nature Reviews Neuroscience, 4,* 444–455. (4)

Tranel, D., & Damasio, A. (1993). The covert learning of affective valence does not require structures in hippocampal system or amygdala. *Journal of Cognitive Neuroscience, 5,* 79–88. (12)

Travaglia, A., Bisaz, R., Sweet, E. S., Blitzer, R. D., & Alberini, C. M. (2016). Infantile amnesia reflects a developmental period for hippocampal learning. *Nature Neuroscience, 19,* 1225–1233. (12)

Travers, S. P., Pfaffmann, C., & Norgren, R. (1986). Convergence of lingual and palatal gustatory neural activity in the nucleus of the solitary tract. *Brain Research, 365,* 305–320. (6)

Trevena, J. A., & Miller, J. (2002). Cortical movement preparation before and after a conscious decision to move. *Consciousness and Cognition, 11,* 162–190. (7)

Trimble, M. R., & Thompson, P. J. (1986). Neuropsychological and behavioral sequelae of spontaneous seizures. *Annals of the New York Academy of Sciences, 462,* 284–292. (14)

Tritsch, N. X., Ding, J. B., & Sabatini, B. L. (2012). Dopaminergic neurons inhibit striatal output through non-canonical release of GABA. *Nature, 490,* 262–266. (2, 7)

Trivers, R. L. (1985). *Social evolution.* Menlo Park, CA: Benjamin/Cummings. (4)

Trudel, E., & Bourque, C. W. (2010). Central clock excites vasopressin neurons by waking osmosensory afferents during late sleep. *Nature Neuroscience, 13,* 467–474. (9)

Tsankova, N., Renthal, W., Kumar, A., & Nestler, E. J. (2007). Epigenetic regulation in psychiatric disorders. *Nature Reviews Neuroscience, 8,* 355–367. (4)

Tsui, W. K., Yang, Y., Cheung, L. K., & Leung, Y. Y. (2016). Distraction osteogenesis as a treatment of obstructive sleep apnea syndrome. *Medicine, 95,* e4674. (8)

Tsunematsu, T., Kilduff, T. S., Boyden, E. S., Takahashi, S., & Yamanaka, A. (2011). Acute optogenetic silencing of orexin/hypocretin neurons induces slow-wave sleep in mice. *Journal of Neuroscience, 31,* 10529–10539. (8)

Tucker, D. M., Luu, P., & Pribram, K. H. (1995). Social and emotional self-regulation. *Annals of the New York Academy of Sciences, 769,* 213–239. (7)

Tucker-Drob, E. M., & Bates, T. C. (2016). Large cross-national differences in gene x socioeconomic status interaction on intelligence. *Psychological Science, 27,* 138–149. (12)

Tunc, B., Solmaz, B., Parker, D., Satterthwaite, T. D., Elliott, M. A., Calkins, M. E., . . . Verma, R. (2016). Establishing a link between sex-related differences in the structural connectome and behaviour. *Philosophical Transactions of the Royal Society B, 371,* article 20150111. (12)

Turkheimer, E. (2016). Weak genetic explanation 20 years later: Reply to Plomin et al. (2016). *Perspectives on Psychological Science, 11,* 24–28. (4)

Turner, R. S., & Anderson, M. E. (2005). Context-dependent modulation of movement-related discharge in the primate globus pallidus. *Journal of Neuroscience, 25,* 2965–2976. (7)

Turner, R. S., & Desmurget, M. (2010). Basal ganglia contributions to motor control: A vigorous tutor. *Current Opinion in Neurobiology, 20,* 704–716. (7)

Turner, T. N., Sharma, K., Oh, E. C., Liu, Y. P., Collins, R. L., . . . Sosa, M. X., . . . Chakravarti, A. (2015). Loss of delta-catenin function in severe autism. *Nature, 520,* 51–56. (14)

Udry, J. R., & Chantala, K. (2006). Masculinity–femininity predicts sexual orientation in men but not in women. *Journal of Biosocial Science, 38,* 797–809. (10)

Udry, J. R., & Morris, N. M. (1968). Distribution of coitus in the menstrual cycle. *Nature, 220,* 593–596. (10)

Uekita, T., & Okaichi, H. (2005). NMDA antagonist MK-801 does not interfere with the use of spatial representation in a familiar environment. *Behavioral Neuroscience, 119,* 548–556. (12)

Undurraga, J., & Baldessarini, R. J. (2012). Randomized, placebo-controlled trials of antidepressants for acute major depression: Thirty-year meta-analytic review. *Neuropsychopharmacology, 37,* 851–864. (14)

Unterberg, A. W., Stover, J., Kress, B., & Kiening, K. L. (2004). Edema and brain trauma. *Neuroscience, 129,* 1021–1029. (4)

Urry, H. L., Nitschke, J. B., Dolski, I., Jackson, D. C., Dalton, K. M., Mueller, C. J., . . . Davidson, R. J. (2004). Making a life worth living: Neural correlates of well-being. *Psychological Science, 15,* 367–372. (11)

Ursano, R. J., Kessler, R. C., Stein, M. B., Naifeh, J. A., Aliaga, P. A., Fullerton, C. S., . . . Heeringa, S. G. (2016). Risk factors, methods, and timing of suicide attempts among U.S. Army soldiers. *JAMA Psychiatry, 73,* 741–749. (11)

Uslaner, J. M., Tye, S. J., Eddins, D. M., Wang, X. H., Fox, S. V., Savitz, A. T., . . . Renger, J. J. (2013). Orexin receptor anatgonists differ from standard sleep drugs by promoting sleep at doses that do not disrupt cognition. *Science Translational Medicine, 5,* 179ra44. (8)

U.S.–Venezuela Collaborative Research Project. (2004). Venezuelan kindreds reveal that genetic and environmental factors modulate Huntington's disease age of onset. *Proceedings of the National Academy of Sciences, USA, 101,* 3498–3503. (7)

Vaishnavi, S., Calhoun, J., & Chatterjee, A. (2001). Binding personal and peripersonal space: Evidence from tactile extinction. *Journal of Cognitive Neuroscience, 13,* 181–189. (13)

Vallines, I., & Greenlee, M. W. (2006). Saccadic suppression of retinotopically localized blood oxygen level-dependent responses in human primary visual area V1. *Journal of Neuroscience, 26,* 5965–5969. (5)

Valzelli, L. (1973). The "isolation syndrome" in mice. *Psychopharmacologia, 31,* 305–320. (11)

Valzelli, L. (1980). *An approach to neuroanatomical and neurochemical psychophysiology.* Torino, Italy: C. G. Edizioni Medico Scientifiche. (14)

Valzelli, L., & Bernasconi, S. (1979). Aggressiveness by isolation and brain serotonin turnover changes in different strains of mice. *Neuropsychobiology, 5,* 129–135. (11)

van Anders, S. M., & Goldey, K. L. (2010). Testosterone and parnering are linked via relationship status for women and "relationship orientation" for men. *Hormones and Behavior, 58,* 820–826. (10)

van Anders, S. M., Hamilton, L. D., & Watson, N. V. (2007). Multiple partners are associated with higher testosterone in North American men and women. *Hormones and Behavior, 51,* 454–459. (10)

van Anders, S. M., & Watson, N. V. (2006). Relationship status and testosterone in North American heterosexual and non-heterosexual men and women: Cross-sectional and longitudinal data. *Psychoneuroendocrinology, 31,* 715–723. (10)

van Avesaat, M., Troost, F. J., Ripken, D., Peters, J., Hendriks, H. F. J., & Masclee, A. A. M. (2015). Intraduodenal infusion of a combination of tastants decreases food intake in humans. *American Journal of Clinical Nutrition, 102,* 729–735. (9)

Van Cantfort, T. E., Gardner, B. T., & Gardner, R. A. (1989). Developmental trends in replies to Wh-questions by children and chimpanzees. In R. A. Gardner, B. T. Gardner, & T. E. Van Cantfort (Eds.), *Teaching sign language to chimpanzees* (pp. 198–239). Albany: State University of New York Press. (13)

van den Bos, W., Rodriguez, C. A., Schweitzer, J. B., & McClure, S. M. (2014). Connectivity strength of dissociable striatal tracts predicts individual differences in temporal discounting. *Journal of Neuroscience, 34,* 10298–10310. (4)

van den Heuvel, M. P., Mandl, R. C. W., Stam, C. J., Kahn, R. S., & Pol, H. E. H. (2010). Aberrant frontal and temporal complex network structure in schizophrenia: A graph theoretical analysis. *Journal of Neuroscience, 30,* 15915–15926. (14)

van den Pol, A. N. (1999). Hypothalamic hypocretin (orexin): Robust innervation of the spinal cord. *Journal of Neuroscience, 19,* 3171–3182. (9)

Van den Stock, J., De Winter, F.-L., de Gelder, B., Rangarajan, J. R., Cypers, G., Maes, F., . . . Vandenbulcke, M. (2015). Impaired recognition of body expressions in the behavioral variant of frontotemporal dementia. *Neuropsychologia, 75,* 496–504. (13)

Van den Stock, J., De Winter, F.-L., de Gelder, B., Rangarajan, J. R., Cypers, G., Maes, F., . . . Vandenbulcke, M. (2015). Impaired recognition of body expressions in the behavioral variant of frontotemporal dementia. *Neuropsychologia, 75,* 496–504. (13)

van der Klaauw, A. A., & Farooqi, I. S. (2015). The hunger genes: Pathways to obesity. *Cell, 161,* 119–132. (9)

van der Kloet, D., Merckelbach, H., Giesbrecht, T., & Lynn, S. J. (2012). Fragmented sleep, fragmented mind: The role of sleep in dissociative symptoms. *Perspectives on Psychological Science, 7,* 159–175. (8)

van de Rest, O., Wang, Y., Barnes, L. L., Tangney, C., Bennett, D. A., & Morris, M. C. (2016). *APOE* ε4 and the associations of seafood and long-chain omega-3 fatty acids with cognitive decline. *Neurology, 86,* 2063–2070. (9)

VanderLaan, D. P., Forrester, D. L., Petterson, L. J., & Vasey, P. L. (2013). The prevalence of Fa'afafine relatives among Samoan gynephilic men and fa'afafine. *Archives of Sexual Behavior, 42,* 353–359. (10)

van der Vinne, V., Zerbini, G., Siersema, A., Pieper, A., Merrow, M., Hut, R. A., . . . Kantermann, T. (2015). Timing of examinations affects school performance differently in early and late chronotypes. *Journal of Biological Rhythms, 30,* 53–60. (8)

van der Zwan, Y. G., Janssen, E. H. C. C., Callens, N., Wolffenbuttel, K. P., Cohen-Kettenis, P. T., van den Berg, M., . . . Beerendonk, C. (2013). Severity of virilization is associated with cosmetic appearance and sexual function in women with congenital adrenal hyperplasia: A cross-sectional study. *Journal of Sexual Medicine, 10,* 866–875. (10)

van Erp, T. G. M., Hibar, D. P., Rasmussen, J. M., Glahn, D. C., Pearlson, G. D., Andreassen, O. A., . . . Turner, J. A. (2016). Subcortical brain volume abnormalities in 2028 individuals with schizophrenia and 2540 healthy controls via the ENIGMA consortium. *Molecular Psychiatry, 21,* 547–553. (14)

van Haren, N. E. M., Schnack, H. G., Koevoets, M. G. J. C., Cahn, W., Pol, H. E. H., & Kahn, R. S. (2016). Trajectories of subcortical volume change in schizophrenia: A 5-year follow-up. *Schizophrenia Research, 173,* 140–145. (14)

van Honk, J., & Schutter, D. J. L. G. (2007). Testosterone reduces conscious detection of signals serving social correction. *Psychological Science, 18,* 663–667. (10)

van Honk, J., Schutter, D. J., Bos, P. A., Kruijt, A. W., Lentjes, E. G., & Baron-Cohen, S. (2011). Testosterone administration impairs cognitive empathy in women depending on second-to-fourth digit ratio. *Proceedings of the National Academy of Sciences (U.S.A.), 108,* 3448–3452. (10)

van Ijzendoorn, M. H., & Bakermans-Kranenburg, M. J. (2012). A sniff of trust: Meta-analysis of the effects of intranasal oxytocin administration on face recognition, trust to in-group, and trust to out-group. *Psychoneuroendocrinology, 37,* 438–443. (13)

van Leeuwen, M., Peper, J. S., van den Berg, S. M., Brouwer, R. M., Pol, H. E. H., Kahn, R. S., & Boomsma, D. I. (2009). A genetic analysis of brain volumes and IQ in children. *Intelligence, 37,* 181–191. (12)

van Meer, M. P. A., van der Marel, K., Wang, K., Otte, W. M., el Bouazati, S., Roeling, T. A. P., . . . Dijkhuizen, R. M. (2010). Recovery of sensorimotor function after experimental stroke correlates with restoration of resting-state interhemispheric functional activity. *Journal of Neuroscience, 30,* 3964–3972. (4)

van Praag, H., Kempermann, G., & Gage, F. H. (1999). Running increases cell proliferation and neurogenesis in the adult mouse dentate gyrus. *Nature Neuroscience, 2,* 266–270. (4)

van Praag, H., Schinder, A. F., Christie, B. R., Toni, N., Palmer, T. D., & Gage, F. H. (2002). Functional neurogenesis in the adult hippocampus. *Nature, 415,* 1030–1034. (4)

van Rooij, S. J. H., Kennis, M., Sjouwerman, R., van den Heuvel, M. P., Kahn, R. S., & Geuze, E. (2015). Smaller hippocampal volume as a vulnerability factor for the persistence of post-traumatic stress disorder. *Psychological Medicine, 45,* 2737–2746. (11)

Van Wanrooij, M. M., & Van Opstal, A. J. (2004). Contribution of head shadow and pinna cues to chronic monaural sound localization. *Journal of Neuroscience, 24,* 4163–4171. (6)

Van Wanrooij, M. M., & Van Opstal, A. J. (2005). Relearning sound localization with a new ear. *Journal of Neuroscience, 25,* 5413–5424. (6)

Van Zoeren, J. G., & Stricker, E. M. (1977). Effects of preoptic, lateral hypothalamic, or dopamine-depleting lesions on behavioral thermoregulation in rats exposed to the cold. *Journal of Comparative and Physiological Psychology, 91,* 989–999. (9)

van Zuijen, T. L., Plakas, A., Maassen, B. A. M., Maurits, N. M., & van der Leij, A. (2013). Infant ERPs separate children at risk of dyslexia who become good readers from those who become poor readers. *Developmental Science, 16,* 554–563. (13)

Vargas-Irwin, C. E., Shakhnarovich, G., Yadollahpour, P., Mislow, J. M. K., Black, M. J., & Donoghue, J. P. (2010). Decoding complete reach and grasp actions from local primary motor cortex populations. *Journal of Neuroscience, 30,* 9659–9669. (7)

Vasey, P. L., & VanderLaan, D. P. (2010). An adaptive cognitive dissociation between willingness to help kin and nonkin in Samoan *Fa'afafine. Psychological Science, 21,* 292–297. (10)

Vawter, M. P., Evans, S., Choudary, P., Tomita, H., Meador-Woodruff, J., Molnar, M., . . . Bunney, W. E. (2004). Gender-specific gene expression in post-mortem human brain. Localization to sex chromosomes. *Neuropsychopharmacology, 29,* 373–384. (10)

Velanova, K., Wheeler, M. E., & Luna, B. (2009). The maturation of task set-related activation supports late developmental improvements in inhibitory control. *Journal of Neuroscience, 29,* 12558–12567. (7)

Verhage, M., Maia, A. S., Plomp, J. J., Brussard, A. B., Heeroma, J. H., Vermeer, H., . . . Sudhof, T. C. (2000). Synaptic assembly of the brain in the absence of neurotransmitter secretion. *Science, 287,* 864–869. (4)

Veroude, K., Zhang-James, Y., Fernandez-Castillo, N., Bakker, M. J., Cormand, B., & Faraone, S. V. (2016). Genetics of aggressive behavior: An overview. *American Journal of Medical Genetics B, 171,* 3–43. (11)

Verrey, F., & Beron, J. (1996). Activation and supply of channels and pumps by aldosterone. *News in Physiological Sciences, 11,* 126–133. (9)

Vieland, V. J., Walters, K. A., Lehner, T., Azaro, M., Tobin, K., Huang, Y., & Brzustowicz, L. M. (2014). Revisiting schizophrenia linkage data in the NIMH repository: Reanalysis of regularized data across multiple studies. *American Journal of Psychiatry, 171,* 350–359. (14)

Villeda, S. A., Luo, J., Mosher, K. I., Zou, B., Britshgi, M., Bieri, G., . . . Rando, T. A. (2011). The ageing systemic milieu negatively regulates neurogenesis and cognitive function. *Nature, 477,* 90–94. (4)

Villeda, S. A., Plambeck, K. E., Middeldorp, J., Castellano, J. M., Mosher, K. I., Luo, J., . . . Wyss-Coray, T. (2014). Young blood reverses age-related impairments in cognitive function and synaptic plasticity in mice. *Nature Medicine, 20,* 659–663. (4)

Viñals, X., Moreno, E., Lanfumey, L., Cordomí, A., Pastor, A., de la Torre, R., . . . Robledo, P. (2015). Cognitive impairment induced by delta9-tetrahydrocannabinol occurs through heteromers between cannabinoid CB_1 and serotonin 5-HT_{2A} receptors. *PLoS Biology, 13,* e1002194. (6)

Virkkunen, M., DeJong, J., Bartko, J., Goodwin, F. K., & Linnoila, M. (1989). Relationship of psychobiological variables to recidivism in violent offenders and impulsive fire setters. *Archives of General Psychiatry, 46,* 600–603. (11)

Virkkunen, M., Eggert, M., Rawlings, R., & Linnoila, M. (1996). A prospective follow-up study of alcoholic violent offenders and fire setters. *Archives of General Psychiatry, 53,* 523–529. (11)

Virkkunen, M., Nuutila, A., Goodwin, F. K., & Linnoila, M. (1987). Cerebrospinal fluid monoamine metabolite levels in male arsonists. *Archives of General Psychiatry, 44,* 241–247. (11)

Visser, E. K., Beersma, G. M., & Daan, S. (1999). Melatonin suppression by light in humans is maximal when the nasal part of the retina is illuminated. *Journal of Biological Rhythms, 14,* 116–121. (8)

Viswanathan, A., & Freeman, R. D. (2007). Neurometabolic coupling in cerebral cortex reflects synaptic more than spiking activity. *Nature Neuroscience, 10,* 1308–1312. (3)

Vita, A., De Peri, L., Deste, G., & Sacchetti, E. (2012). Progressive loss of cortical gray matter in schizophrenia: A meta-analysis and meta-regression of longitudinal MRI studies. *Translational Psychiatry, 2,* Article e190. (14)

Viviani, D., Charlet, A., van den Burg, E., Robinet, C., Hurni, N., Abatis, M., . . . Stoop, R. (2011). Oxytocin selectively gates fear responses through distinct outputs from the central amygdala. *Science, 333,* 104–107. (11)

Vocci, F. J., Acri, J., & Elkashef, A. (2005). Medication development for addictive disorders: The state of the science. *American Journal of Psychiatry, 162,* 1432–1440. (14)

Volkow, N. D., Koob, G. F., & McLellan, A. T. (2016). Neurobiologic advances from the brain disease model of addiction. *New England Journal of Medicine, 374,* 363–371. (14)

Volkow, N. D., Wang, G.-J., Telang, F., Fowler, J. S., Logan, J., Childress, A.-R., . . . Wong, C. (2006). Cocaine cues and dopamine in dorsal striatum: Mechanism of craving in cocaine addiction. *Journal of Neuroscience, 26,* 6583–6588. (14)

Volman, I., Verlagen, L., den Ouden, H. E. M., Fernández, G., Rijpkema, M., Franke, B., Toni, I., & Roelofs, K. (2013). Reduced serotonin transporter availability decreases prefrontal control of the amygdala. *Journal of Neuroscience, 33,* 8974–8979. (11)

von Gall, C., Garabette, M. L., Kell, C. A., Frenzel, S., Dehghani, F., Schumm-Draeger, P. M., . . . Stehle, J. H. (2002). Rhythmic gene expression in pituitary depends on heterologous sensitization by the neurohormone melatonin. *Nature Neuroscience, 5,* 234–238. (8)

von Melchner, L., Pallas, S. L., & Sur, M. (2000). Visual behaviour mediated by retinal projections directed to the visual pathway. *Nature, 404,* 871–876. (4)

Voss, U., Holzmann, R., Hobson, A., Paulus, W., Koppehele-Gossel, J., Klimke, A., & Nitsche, M. A. (2014). Induction of self-awareness in dreams through frontal low current stimulation of gamma activity. *Nature Neuroscience, 17,* 810–812. (8)

Vrba, E. S. (1998). Multiphasic growth models and the evolution of prolonged growth exemplified by human brain evolution. *Journal of Theoretical Biology, 190,* 227–239. (4)

Vuga, M., Fox, N. A., Cohn, J. F., George, C. J., Levenstein, R. M., & Kovacs, M. (2006). Long-term stability of frontal electroencephalographic asymmetry in adults with a history of depression and controls. *International Journal of Psychophysiology, 59,* 107–115. (14)

Vuilleumier, P. (2005). Cognitive science: Staring fear in the face. *Nature, 433,* 22–23. (11)

Vuoksimaa, E., Panizzon, M. S., Chen, C. H., Fiecas, M., Eyler, L. T., Fennema-Notestine, C., . . . Kremen, W. S. (2015). The genetic association between neocortical volume and general cognitive ability is driven by global surface area rather than thickness. *Cerebral Cortex, 225,* 2127–2137. (12)

Vyadyslav, V. V., & Harris, K. D. (2013). Sleep and the single neuron: The role of global slow oscillations in individual cell rest. *Nature Reviews Neuroscience, 14,* 443–451. (8)

Vyazovskiy, V. V., Cirelli, C., Pfister-Genskow, M., Faraguna, U., & Tononi, G. (2008). Molecular and electrophysiological evidence for net synaptic potentiation in wake and depression in sleep. *Nature Neuroscience, 11,* 200–208. (8)

Wager, T. D., & Atlas, L. Y. (2013). How is pain influenced by cognition? Neuroimaging weighs in. *Perspectives on Psychological Science, 8,* 91–97. (3)

Wager, T. D., & Atlas, L. Y. (2015). The neuroscience of placebo effects: Connecting context, learning and health. *Nature Reviews Neuroscience, 16,* 403–418. (6)

Wager, T. D., Scott, D. J., & Zubieta, J.-K. (2007). Placebo effects on human μ-opioid activity during pain. *Proceedings of the National Academy of Sciences, USA, 104,* 11056–11061. (6)

Wagner, A. D., Schacter, D. L., Rotte, M., Koutstaal, W., Maril, A., Dale, A. M., . . . Buckner, R. L. (1998). Building memories: Remembering and forgetting of verbal experiences as predicted by brain activity. *Science, 281,* 1188–1191. (3)

Wagner, D. D., Boswell, R. G., Kelley, W. M., & Heatherton, T. F. (2012). Inducing negative affect increases the reward value of appetizing foods in dieters. *Journal of Cognitive Neuroscience, 24,* 1625–1633. (9)

Wagner, E. L., & Gleeson, T. T. (1997). Postexercise thermoregulatory behavior and recovery from exercise in desert iguanas. *Physiology & Behavior, 61,* 175–180. (9)

Wagner, U., Gais, S., Haider, H., Verleger, R., & Born, J. (2004). Sleep inspires insight. *Nature, 427,* 352–355. (8)

Wahl, A. S., Omlor, W., Rubio, J. C., Chen, J. L., Zheng, H., Schröter, A., . . . Schwab, M. E. (2014). Asynchronous therapy restores motor control by rewiring of the rat corticospinal tract after stroke. *Science, 344,* 1250–1255. (4)

Waisbren, S. R., Brown, M. J., de Sonneville, L. M. J., & Levy, H. L. (1994). Review of neuropsychological functioning in treated phenylketonuria: An information-processing approach. *Acta Paediatrica, 83*(Suppl. 407), 98–103. (4)

Waldherr, M., & Neumann, I. D. (2007). Centrally released oxytocin mediates mating-induced anxiolysis in male rats. *Proceedings of the National Academy of Sciences, USA, 104,* 16681–16684. (10)

Waldo, M. L. (2015). The frontotemporal dementias. *Psychiatric Clinics of North America, 38,* 193–209. (13)

Waldvogel, J. A. (1990). The bird's eye view. *American Scientist, 78,* 342–353. (5)

Walker, E. F., Savoie, T., & Davis, D. (1994). Neuromotor precursors of schizophrenia. *Schizophrenia Bulletin, 20,* 441–451. (14)

Wallen, K. (2005). Hormonal influences on sexually differentiated behavior in nonhuman primates. *Frontiers in Neuroendocrinology, 26,* 7–26. (10)

Wallis, J. D. (2012). Cross-species studies of orbitofrontal cortex and value-based decision-making. *Nature Neuroscience, 15,* 13–19. (3)

Wallman, J., & Pettigrew, J. D. (1985). Conjugate and disjunctive saccades in two avian species with contrasting oculomotor strategies. *Journal of Neuroscience, 5,* 1418–1428. (5)

Walsh, T., McClellan, J. M., McCarthy, S. E., Addington, A. M., Pierce, S. B., & Cooper, G. M. (2008). Rare structural variants disrupt multiple genes in neurodevelopmental pathways in schizophrenia. *Science, 320,* 539–543. (14)

Walum, H., Westberg, L., Henningsson, S., Neiderhiser, J. M., Reiss, D., Ige, W., . . . Lichtenstein, P. (2008). Genetic variation in the vasopressin receptor 1a gene (*AVPR1A*) associates with pair-bonding behavior in humans. *Proceedings of the National Academy of Sciences (U.S.A.), 105,* 14153–14156. (10)

Wan, N., & Lin, G. (2016). Parkinson's disease and pesticides exposure: New findings from a comprehensive study in Nebraska, USA. *Journal of Rural Health, 32,* 303–313. (7)

Wan, X., Takano, D., Asamizuya, T., Suzuki, C., Ueno, K., Cheng, K., . . . Tanaka, K. (2012). Developing intuition: Neural correlates of cognitive-skill learning in caudate nucleus. *Journal of Neuroscience, 32,* 17492–17501. (12)

Wang, A., Costello, S., Cockburn, M., Zhang, X., Bronstein, J., & Ritz, B. (2011). Parkinson's disease risk from ambient exposure to pesticides. *European Journal of Epidemiology, 26,* 547–555. (7)

Wang, A. Y., Miura, K., & Uchida, N. (2013). The dorsomedial striatum encodes net expected return, critical for energizing performance vigor. *Nature Neuroscience, 16,* 639–647. (7)

Wang, C.-H., Tsai, C. L., Tu, K.-C., Muggleton, N. G., Juan, C.-H., & Liang, W. K. (2015). Modulation of brain oscillations during fundamental visuo-spatial processing: A comparison between female collegiate badminton players and sedentary controls. *Psychology of Sport and Expertise, 16,* 121–129. (5)

Wang, D. O., Kim, S. M., Zhao, Y., Hwang, H., Miura, S. K., Sossin, W. S., & Martin, K. C. (2009). Synapse- and stimulus-specific local translation during long-term neuronal plasticity. *Science, 324,* 1536–1540. (12)

Wang, H., Goehring, A., Wang, K. H., Penmatsa, A., Ressler, R., & Gouaux, E. (2013). Structural basis for action by diverse antidepressants on biogenic amine transporters. *Nature, 503,* 141–145. (14)

Wang, J., Qin, W., Liu, F., Liu, B., Zhou, Y., Jiang, T., & Yu, C. (2016). Sex-specific mediation effect of the right fusiform face area volume on the association between variants in repeat length of *AVPR1A* RS3 and altruistic behavior in healthy adults. *Human Brain Mapping, 37,* 2700–2709. (10)

Wang, Q., Schoenlein, R. W., Peteanu, L. A., Mathies, R. A., & Shank, C. V. (1994). Vibrationally coherent photochemistry in the femtosecond primary event of vision. *Science, 266,* 422–424. (5)

Wang, S., Tudusciuc, O., Mamelak, A. N., Ross, I. B., Adolphs, R., & Rutishauer, U. (2014). Neurons in the human amygdala selective for perceived emotion. *Proceedings of the National Academy of Sciences (U.S.A.), 111,* E3100–E3119. (11)

Wang, T.-M., Holzhausen, L. C., & Kramer, R. H. (2014). Imaging an optogenetic pH sensor reveals that protons mediate lateral inhibition in the retina. *Nature Neuroscience, 17,* 262–268. (2)

Wang, T., Okano, Y., Eisensmith, R., Huang, S. Z., Zeng, Y. T., Lo, W. H. Y., & Woo, S. L. C. (1989). Molecular genetics of phenylketonuria in Orientals: Linkage disequilibrium between a termination mutation and haplotype 4 of the phenylalanine hydroxylase gene. *American Journal of Human Genetics, 45,* 675–680. (4)

Warach, S. (1995). Mapping brain pathophysiology and higher cortical function with magnetic resonance imaging. *The Neuroscientist, 1,* 221–235. (3)

Ward, B. W., Dahlhamer, J. M., Galinsky, A. M., & Joestl, S. S. (2014). Sexual orientation and health among US adults: National Health Interview Survey, 2013. *National Health Statistics Reports, 15,* 1–10. (10)

Ward, I. L., Bennett, A. L., Ward, O. B., Hendricks, S. E., & French, J. A. (1999). Androgen threshold to activate copulation differs in male rats prenatally exposed to alcohol, stress, or both factors. *Hormones and Behavior, 36,* 129–140. (10)

Ward, I. L., Romeo, R. D., Denning, J. H., & Ward, O. B. (1999). Fetal alcohol exposure blocks full masculinization of the dorsolateral nucleus in rat spinal cord. *Physiology & Behavior, 66,* 571–575. (10)

Ward, I. L., Ward, B., Winn, R. J., & Bielawski, D. (1994). Male and female sexual behavior potential of male rats prenatally exposed to the influence of alcohol, stress, or both factors. *Behavioral Neuroscience, 108,* 1188–1195. (10)

Ward, I. L., & Ward, O. B. (1985). Sexual behavior differentiation: Effects of prenatal manipulations in rats. In N. Adler, D. Pfaff, & R. W. Goy (Eds.), *Handbook of behavioral neurobiology* (Vol. 7, pp. 77–98). New York: Plenum Press. (10)

Ward, O. B., Monaghan, E. P., & Ward, I. L. (1986). Naltrexone blocks the effects of prenatal stress on sexual behavior differentiation in male rats. *Pharmacology Biochemistry and Behavior, 25,* 573–576. (10)

Ward, O. B., Ward, I. L., Denning, J. H., French, J. A., & Hendricks, S. E. (2002). Postparturitional testosterone surge in male offspring of rats stressed and/or fed ethanol during late pregnancy. *Hormones and Behavior, 41,* 229–235. (10)

Warman, G. R., Pawley, M. D. M., Bolton, C., Cheeseman, J. F., Fernando, A. T., Arendt, J., & Wirz-Justice, A. (2011). Circadian-related sleep disorders and sleep medication use in the New Zealand blind population: An observational prevalence study. *PLoS One,* 322073. (8)

Warren, R. M. (1999). *Auditory perception.* Cambridge, England: Cambridge University Press. (6)

Watanabe, D., Savion-Lemieux, T., & Penhune, V. B. (2007). The effect of early musical training on adult motor performance: Evidence for a sensitive period in motor learning. *Experimental Brain Research, 176,* 332–340. (4)

Watanabe, M., & Munoz, D. P. (2010). Presetting basal ganglia for volitional actions. *Journal of Neuroscience, 30,* 10144–10157. (7)

Watkins, K. E., Shakespeare, T. J., O'Donoghue, M. C., Alexander, I., Ragge, N., Cowey, A., & Bridge, H. (2013). Early auditory processing in area V5/MT+ of the congenitally blind brain. *Journal of Neuroscience, 33,* 18242–18246. (4)

Watrous, A. J., Tandon, N., Conner, C. R., Pieters, T., & Ekstrom, A. D. (2013). Frequency-specific network connectivity increases underlie accurate spatiotemporal memory retrieval. *Nature Neuroscience, 16,* 349–356. (12)

Waxman, S. G., & Ritchie, J. M. (1985). Organization of ion channels in the myelinated nerve fiber. *Science, 228,* 1502–1507. (1)

Weber, F., Chung, S., Beier, K. T., Xu, M., Luo, L., & Dan, Y. (2015). Control of REM sleep by ventral medulla GABAergic neurons. *Nature, 526,* 435–438. (8)

Weber-Fox, C. M., & Neville, H. J. (1996). Maturational constraints on functional specializations for language processing: ERP and behavioral evidence in bilingual speakers. *Journal of Cognitive Neuroscience, 8,* 231–256. (13)

Weeland, J., Overbeek, G., de Castro, B. O., & Matthys, W. (2015). Underlying mechanisms of gene-environment interactions in externalizing behavior: A systematic review and search for theoretical mechanisms. *Clinical Child and Family Psychology Review, 18,* 413–442. (11)

Wegener, D., Freiwald, W. A., & Kreiter, A. K. (2004). The influence of sustained selective attention on stimulus selectivity in macaque visual area MT. *Journal of Neuroscience, 24,* 6106–6114. (13)

Wei, W., Nguyen, L. N., Kessels, H. W., Hagiwara, H., Sisodia, S., & Malinow, R. (2010). Amyloid beta from axons and dendrites reduces local spine number and plasticity. *Nature Neuroscience, 13,* 190–196. (12)

Wei, Y., Krishnan, G. P., & Bazhenov, M. (2016). Synaptic mechanisms of memory consolidation during sleep slow oscillations. *Journal of Neuroscience, 36,* 4231–4247. (8)

Weidensaul, S. (1999). *Living on the wind.* New York: North Point Press. (9)

Weinberger, D. R. (1996). On the plausibility of "the neurodevelopmental hypothesis" of schizophrenia. *Neuropsychopharmacology, 14,* 1S–11S. (14)

Weindl, A. (1973). Neuroendocrine aspects of circumventricular organs. In W. F. Ganong & L. Martini (Eds.), *Frontiers in neuroendocrinology 1973* (pp. 3–32). New York: Oxford University Press. (9)

Weiskrantz, L., Warrington, E. K., Sanders, M. D., & Marshall, J. (1974). Visual capacity in the hemianopic field following a restricted occipital ablation. *Brain, 97,* 709–728. (5)

Weiss, A. H., Granot, R. Y., & Ahissar, M. (2014). The enigma of dyslexic musicians. *Neuropsychologia, 54,* 28–40. (13)

Weiss, A. P., Ellis, C. B., Roffman, J. L., Stufflebeam, S., Hamalainen, M. S., Duff, M., . . . Schacter, D. L. (2009). Aberrant frontoparietal function during recognition memory in schizophrenia: A multimodal neuroimaging investigation. *Journal of Neuroscience, 29,* 11347–11359. (14)

Weiss, P. (1924). Die funktion transplantierter amphibienextremitäten. Aufstellung einer resonanztheorie der motorischen nerventätigkeit auf grund abstimmter endorgane [The function of transplanted amphibian limbs. Presentation of a resonance theory of motor nerve action upon tuned end organs]. *Archiv für Mikroskopische Anatomie und Entwicklungsmechanik, 102,* 635–672. (4)

Weiss, P. H., & Fink, G. R. (2009). Grapheme-colour synaesthetes show increased grey matter volumes of parietal and fusiform cortex. *Brain, 132,* 65–70. (6)

Welchman, A. E., Stanley, J., Schomers, M. R., Miall, C., & Bülthoff, H. H. (2010). The quick and the dead: When reaction beats intention. *Proceedings of the Royal Society, B, 277,* 1667–1674. (7)

Weller, L., Weller, A., Koresh-Kamin, H., & Ben-Shoshan, R. (1999). Menstrual synchrony in a sample of working women. *Psychoneuroendocrinology, 24,* 449–459. (6)

Weller, L., Weller, A., & Roizman, S. (1999). Human menstrual synchrony in families and among close friends: Examining the importance of mutual exposure. *Journal of Comparative Psychology, 113,* 261–268. (6)

Wenker, S. D., Leal, M. C., Farías, M. I., Zeng, X., & Pitossi, F. J. (2016). Cell therapy for Parkinson's disease: Functional role of the host immune response on survival and differentiation of dopaminergic neuroblasts. *Brain Research, 1638, Part A,* 15–29. (7)

Wenzler, S., Levine, S., van Dick, R., Oertel-Knöckel, V., & Aviezer, H. (2016). Beyond pleasure and pain: Facial expression ambiguity in adults and children during intense situations. *Emotion, 16,* 807–814. (11)

Wessinger, C. M., VanMeter, J., Tian, B., Van Lare, J., Pekar, J., & Rauschecker, J. P. (2001). Hierarchical organization of the human auditory cortex revealed by functional magnetic resonance imaging. *Journal of Cognitive Neuroscience, 13,* 1–7. (6)

Weston, L., Hodgekins, J., & Langdon, P. E. (2016). Effectiveness of cognitive behavioural therapy with people who have autistic spectrum disorders: A systematic review and meta-analysis. *Clinical Psychology Review, 49,* 41–54. (14)

Whalen, P. J., Kagan, J., Cook, R. G., Davis, F. C., Kim, H., Polis, S., . . . Johnstone, T. (2004). Human amygdala responsivity to masked fearful eye whites. *Science, 306,* 2061. (11)

Wheeler, M. A., Smith, C. J., Ottolini, M., Barker, B. S., Purohit, A. M., Grippo, R. M., . . . Güler, A. D. (2016). Genetically targeted magnetic control of the nervous system. *Nature Neuroscience, 19,* 756–761. (3)

Whitesell, J. D., Sorensen, K. A., Jarvie, B. C., Hentges, S. T., & Schoppa, N. E. (2013). Interglomerular lateral inhibition targeted on external tufted cells in the olfactory bulb. *Journal of Neuroscience, 33,* 1552–1563. (5)

Whitwell, R. L., Milner, A. D., & Goodale, M. A. (2014). The two visual systems hypothesis: New challenges and insights from visual form agnostic patient DF. *Frontiers in Neurology, 5,* article 255. (5)

Wiesel, T. N. (1982). Postnatal development of the visual cortex and the influence of environment. *Nature, 299,* 583–591. (5)

Wiesel, T. N., & Hubel, D. H. (1963). Single-cell responses in striate cortex of kittens deprived of vision in one eye. *Journal of Neurophysiology, 26,* 1003–1017. (5)

Wilczek, F. (2015). A weighty mass difference. *Nature, 520,* 303–304. (0)

Wilhelm, B. G., Mandad, S., Truckenbrodt, S., Kröhnert, K., Schäfer, C., Rammner, B., . . . Rizzoli, S. O. (2014). Composition of isolated synaptic boutons reveals the amounts of vesicle trafficking proteins. *Science, 344,* 1023–1028. (2)

Willems, R. M., Hagoort, P., & Casasanto, D. (2010). Body-specific representations of action verbs: Neural evidence from right- and left-handers. *Psychological Science, 21,* 67–74. (13)

Willerman, L., Schultz, R., Rutledge, J. N., & Bigler, E. D. (1991). In vivo brain size and intelligence. *Intelligence, 15,* 223–228. (12)

Williams, C. L. (1986). A reevaluation of the concept of separable periods of organizational and activational actions of estrogens in development of brain and behavior. *Annals of the New York Academy of Sciences, 474,* 282–292. (10)

Williams, C. T., Barnes, B. M., Richter, M., & Buck, C. L. (2012). Hibernation and circadian rhythms of body temperature in free-living Arctic ground squirrels. *Physiological and Biochemical Zoology, 85,* 397–404. (8)

Williams, E. F., Pizarro, D., Ariely, D., & Weinberg, J. D. (2016). The Valjean effect: Visceral states and cheating. *Emotion, 16,* 897–902. (9)

Williams, G., Cai, X. J., Elliott, J. C., & Harrold, J. A. (2004). Anabolic neuropeptides. *Physiology & Behavior, 81,* 211–222. (9)

Williams, M. T., Davis, H. N., McCrea, A. E., Long, S. J., & Hennessy, M. B. (1999). Changes in the hormonal concentrations of pregnant rats and their fetuses following multiple exposures to a stressor during the third trimester. *Neurotoxicology and Teratology, 21,* 403–414. (10)

Williams, R. W., & Herrup, K. (1988). The control of neuron number. *Annual Review of Neuroscience, 11,* 423–453. (1, 7)

Willingham, D. B., Koroshetz, W. J., & Peterson, E. W. (1996). Motor skills have diverse neural bases: Spared and impaired skill acquisition in Huntington's disease. *Neuropsychology, 10,* 315–321. (7)

Wilson, B. A., Baddeley, A. D., & Kapur, N. (1995). Dense amnesia in a professional musician following herpes simplex virus encephalitis. *Journal of Clinical and Experimental Neuropsychology, 17,* 668–681. (12)

Wilson, J. D., George, F. W., & Griffin, J. E. (1981). The hormonal control of sexual development. *Science, 211,* 1278–1284. (10)

Wilson-Mendenhall, C. D., Barrett, L. F., & Barsalou, L. W. (2013). Neural evidence that human emotions share core affective properties. *Psychological Science, 24,* 947–956. (11)

Wimmer, R. D., Schmitt, L. I., Davidson, T. J., Nakajima, M., Deisseroth, K., & Halassa, M. M. (2015). Thalamic control of sensory selection in divided attention. *Nature, 526,* 705–707. (13)

Winder, B., Lievesley, R., Kaul, A., Elliott, H. J., Thorne, K., & Hocken, K. (2014). Preliminary evaluation of the use of pharmacological treatment with convicted sexual offenders experiencing high levels of sexual preoccupation, hypersexuality and/or sexual compulsivity. *Journal of Forensic Psychiatry & Psychology, 25,* 176–194. (10)

Windle, M., Kogan, S. M., Lee, S., Chen, Y. F., Lei, K. M., Brody, G. H., . . . Yu, T. Y. (2016). Neighborhood X serotonin transporter linked polymorphic region (5_HTTLPR) interactions for substance abuse from ages 10 to 24 years using a harmonized data set of African American children. *Development and Psychopathology, 28,* 415–431. (14)

Winer, G. A., Cottrell, J. E., Gregg, V., Fournier, J. S., & Bica. L. A. (2002). Fundamentally misunderstanding visual perception: Adults' belief in visual emissions. *American Psychologist, 57,* 417–424. (5)

Winfree, A. T. (1983). Impact of a circadian clock on the timing of human sleep. *American Journal of Physiology, 245,* R497–R504. (8)

Winocur, G., & Hasher, L. (1999). Aging and time-of-day effects on cognition in rats. *Behavioral Neuroscience, 113,* 991–997. (8)

Winocur, G., & Hasher, L. (2004). Age and time-of-day effects on learning and memory in a non-matching-to-sample test. *Neurobiology of Aging, 25,* 1107–1115. (8)

Winocur, G., Moscovitch, M., & Sekeres, M. (2007). Memory consolidation or transformation: Context manipulation and hippocampal representations of memory. *Nature Neuroscience, 10,* 555–557. (12)

Wirdefeldt, K., Gatz, M., Pawitan, Y., & Pedersen, N. L. (2005). Risk and protective factors for Parkinson's disease: A study in Swedish twins. *Annals of Neurology, 57,* 27–33. (7)

Wise, R. A. (1996). Addictive drugs and brain stimulation reward. *Annual Review of Neuroscience, 19,* 319–340. (14)

Wissman, A. M., & Brenowitz, E. A. (2009). The role of neurotrophins in the seasonal-like growth of the avian song control system. *Journal of Neuroscience, 29,* 6461–6471. (4)

Witelson, S. F., Beresh, H., & Kigar, D. L. (2006). Intelligence and brain size in 100 postmortem brains: Sex, lateralization and age factors. *Brain, 129,* 386–398. (12)

Witelson, S. F., & Pallie, W. (1973). Left hemisphere specialization for language in the newborn: Neuroanatomical evidence of asymmetry. *Brain, 96,* 641–646. (13)

Witthoft, N., & Winawer, J. (2013). Learning, memory, and synesthesia. *Psychological Science, 24,* 258–263. (6)

Wokke, M. E., Vandenbroucke, A. R. E., Scholte, H. S., & Lamme, V. A. F. (2013). Confuse your illusion: Feedback to early visual cortex contributes to perceptual completion. *Psychological Science, 24*, 63–71. (5)

Wohleb, E. S., Franklin, T., Iwata, M., & Duman, R. S. (2016). Integrating neuro-immune systems in the neurobiology of depression. *Nature Reviews Neuroscience, 17*, 497–511. (14)

Wohlgemuth, M. J., & Moss, C. F. (2016). Midbrain auditory selectivity to natural sounds. *Proceedings of the National Academy of Sciences (U.S.A.), 113*, 2508–2513. (6)

Wolf, M. E. (2016). Synaptic mechanisms underlying persistent cocaine craving. *Nature Reviews Neuroscience, 17*, 351–365. (14)

Wolf, S. (1995). Dogmas that have hindered understanding. *Integrative Physiological and Behavioral Science, 30*, 3–4. (11)

Wolff, V., Amspach, J.-P., Lauer, V., Rouyer, O., Bataillard, M., Marescaux, C., & Geny, B. (2013). Cannabis-related stroke: Myth or reality? *Stroke, 44*, 558–563. (4)

Wolkin, A., Rusinek, H., Vaid, G., Arena, L., Lafargue, T., Sanfilipo, M., . . . Rotrosen, J. (1998). Structural magnetic resonance image averaging in schizophrenia. *American Journal of Psychiatry, 155*, 1064–1073. (14)

Wolman, D. (2012). A tale of two halves. *Nature, 483*, 260–263. (13)

Wolpert, L. (1991). *The triumph of the embryo.* Oxford, England: Oxford University Press. (4)

Womelsdorf, T., Schoffelen, J.-M., Oostenveld, R., Singer, W., Desimone, R., Engel, A. K., & Fries, P.. (2007). Modulation of neuronal interactions through neuronal synchronization. *Science, 316*, 1609–1612. (13)

Wong, M., Gnanakumaran, V., & Goldreich, D. (2011). Tactile spatial acuity enhancement in blindness: Evidence for experience-dependent mechanisms. *Journal of Neuroscience, 31*, 7028–7037. (4)

Wong, P. C. M., Skoe, E., Russo, N. M., Dees, T., & Kraus, N. (2007). Musical experience shapes human brainstem encoding of linguistic pitch perception. *Nature Neuroscience, 10*, 420–422. (4)

Wong, L. E., Gibson, M. E., Arnold, H. M., Pepinsky, B., & Frank, E. (2015). Artemin promotes functional long-distance axonal regeneration to the brainstem after dorsal root crush. *Proceedings of the National Academy of Sciences (U.S.A.), 112*, 6170–6175. (4)

Wong, W. I., Pasterski, V., Hindmarsh, P. C., Geffner, M. E., & Hines, M. (2013). Are there parental socialization effects on the sex-typed behavior of individuals with congenital adrenal hyperplasia? *Archives of Sexual Behavior, 42*, 381–391. (10)

Wong, Y. K., & Wong, A. C. N. (2014). Absolute pitch memory: Its prevalence among musicians and dependence o the testing context. *Psychonomic Bulletin & Review, 21*, 534–542. (6)

Wooding, S., Kim, U., Bamshad, M J., Larsen, J., Jorde, L. B., & Drayna, D. (2004). Natural selection and molecular evolution in *PTC*, a bitter-taste receptor gene. *American Journal of Human Genetics, 74*, 637–646. (4)

Woodson, J. C., & Balleine, B. W. (2002). An assessment of factors contributing to instrumental performance for sexual reward in the rat. *Quarterly Journal of Experimental Psychology, 55B*, 75–88. (10)

Woodward, N. D. (2016). The course of neuro-psychological impairment and brain structure abnormalities in psychotic disorders. *Neuroscience Research, 102*, 39–46. (14)

Woodworth, R. S. (1934). *Psychology* (3rd ed.). New York: Holt. (1)

Wooley, A. W., Chabris, C. F., Pentland, A., Hashmi, N., & Malone, T. W. (2010). Evidence for a collective intelligence factor in the performance of human groups. *Science, 330*, 686–688. (11)

Woolf, N. J. (1991). Cholinergic systems in mammalian brain and spinal cord. *Progress in Neurobiology, 37*, 475–524. (3)

Woolf, N. J. (1996). Global and serial neurons form a hierarchically arranged interface proposed to underlie memory and cognition. *Neuroscience, 74*, 625–651. (8)

Workman, J. L., Barha, C. K., & Galea, L. A. M. (2012). Endocrine substrates of cognitive and affective changes during pregnancy and postpartum. *Behavioral Neuroscience, 126*, 54–72. (10)

Wright, I. C., Rabe-Hesketh, S., Woodruff, P. W. R., David, A. S., Murray, R. M., & Bullmore, E. T. (2000). Meta-analysis of regional brain volumes in schizophrenia. *American Journal of Psychiatry, 157*, 16–25. (14)

Wright, N. D., Bahrami, B., Johnson, E., DiMalta, G., Rees, G., Frith, C. D., & Dolan, R. J. (2012). Testosterone disrupts human collaboraton by increasing egocentric choices. *Proceedings of the Royal Society B, 279*, 2275–2280. (11)

Wu, L.-Q., & Dickman, J. D. (2012). Neural correlates of a magnetic sense. *Science, 336*, 1054–1057. (6)

Wulfeck, B., & Bates, E. (1991). Differential sensitivity to errors of agreement and word order in Broca's aphasia. *Journal of Cognitive Neuroscience, 3*, 258–272. (13)

Wurtman, J. J. (1985). Neurotransmitter control of carbohydrate consumption. *Annals of the New York Academy of Sciences, 443*, 145–151. (2)

Wyart, C., Webster, W. W., Chen, J. H., Wilson, S. R., McClary, A., Khan, R. M., & Sobel, N. (2007). Smelling a single component of male sweat alters levels of cortisol in women. *Journal of Neuroscience, 27*, 1261–1265. (6)

Wyatt, H. R. (2013). Update on treatment strategies for obesity. *Journal of Clinical Endocrinology and Metabolism, 98*, 1299–1306. (9)

Wylie, S. A., Claassen, D. O., Huizenga, H. M., Schewel, K. D., Ridderinkhof, K. R., Bashore, T. R., & van den Wildenberg, W. P. M. (2012). Dopamine agonists and the suppression of impulsive motor actions in Parkinson disease. *Journal of Cognitive Neuroscience, 24*, 1709–1724. (7)

Wynne, C. D. L. (2004). The perils of anthropomorphism. *Nature, 428*, 606. (0)

Wynne, L. C., Tienari, P., Nieminen, P., Sorri, A., Lahti, I., Moring, J., . . . Miettunen, J. (2006). Genotype-environment interaction in the schizophrenia spectrum: Genetic liability and global family ratings in the Finnish adoption study. *Family Process, 45*, 419–434. (14)

Xia, Z., Hoeft, F., Zhang, L., & Shu, H. (2016). Neuroanatomical anomalies of dyslexia: Disambiguating the effects of disorder, performance, and maturation. *Neuropsychologia, 81*, 68–78. (13)

Xie, J., & Padoa-Schioppa, C. (2016). Neuronal remapping and circuit persistence in economic decisions. *Nature Neuroscience, 19*, 855–861. (13)

Xu, H.-T., Pan, F., Yang, G., & Gan, W.-B. (2007). Choice of cranial window type for *in vivo* imaging affects dendritic spine turnover in the cortex. *Nature Neuroscience, 10*, 549–551. (4)

Xu, M., Chung, S., Zhang, S., Zhong, P., Ma, C., Chang, W.-C., . . . Dan, Y. (2015). Basal forebrain circuit for sleep-wake control. *Nature Neuroscience, 18*, 1641–1647. (8)

Xu, Y., Padiath, Q. S., Shapiro, R. E., Jones, C. R., Wu, S. C., Saigoh, N., . . . Fu, Y. H. (2005). Functional consequences of a *CKI delta* mutation causing familial advanced sleep phase syndrome. *Nature, 434*, 640–644. (8)

Yamaguchi, S., Isejima, H., Matsuo, T., Okura, R., Yagita, K., Kobayashi, M., . . . Okamura, H. (2003). Synchronization of cellular clocks in the suprachiasmatic nucleus. *Science, 302*, 1408–1412. (8)

Yamamoto, T. (1984). Taste responses of cortical neurons. *Progress in Neurobiology, 23*, 273–315. (6)

Yanagisawa, K., Bartoshuk, L. M., Catalanotto, F. A., Karrer, T. A., & Kveton, J. F. (1998). Anesthesia of the chorda tympani nerve and taste phantoms. *Physiology & Behavior, 63*, 329–335. (6)

Yang, G., Lai, C. S. W., Cichon, J., Ma, L., Li, W., & Gan, W.-B. (2014). Sleep promotes branch-specific formation of dendritic spines after learning. *Science, 344*, 1173–1178. (8)

Yang, G., Pan, F., & Gan, W.-B. (2009). Stably maintained dendritic spines are associated with lifelong memories. *Nature, 462*, 920–924. (4)

Yang, G., Wang, Y. Y., Sun, J., Zhang, K., & Liu, J. P. (2016). Ginkgo biloba for mild cognitive impairment and Alzheimer's disease: A systematic review and meta-analysis of randomized controlled trials. *Current Topics in Medicinal Chemistry, 16*, 520–528. (12)

Yano, H., Baranov, S. V., Baranova, O. V., Kim, J., Pan, Y., Yablonska, S., . . . Friedlander, R. M. (2014). Inhibition of mitochondrial protein import by mutant huntingtin. *Nature Neuroscience, 17*, 822–831. (7)

Yehuda, R. (2002). Post-traumatic stress disorder. *New England Journal of Medicine, 346,* 108–114. (11)

Yeo, G. S. H., & Heisler, L. K. (2012). Unraveling the brain regulation of appetite: Lessons from genetics. *Nature Neuroscience, 15,* 1343–1349. (9)

Yeomans, J. S., & Frankland, P. W. (1996). The acoustic startle reflex: Neurons and connections. *Brain Research Reviews, 21,* 301–314. (11)

Yetish, G., Kaplan, H., Gurven, M., Wood, B., Pontzer, H., Manger, P. R., . . . Siegel, J. M. (2015). Natural sleep and its seasonal variations in three pre-industrial societies. *Current Biology, 25,* 2862–2868. (8)

Yin, H. H., & Knowlton, B. J. (2006). The role of the basal ganglia in habit formation. *Nature Reviews Neuroscience, 7,* 464–476. (7)

Yolken, R. H., Dickerson, F. B., & Torrey, E. F. (2009). Toxoplasma and schizophrenia. *Parasite Immunology, 31,* 706–715. (14)

Yoo, S.-S., Hu, P. T., Gujar, N., Jolesz, F. A., & Walker, M. P. (2007). A deficit in the ability to form new human memories without sleep. *Nature Neuroscience, 10,* 385–392. (8)

Yoon, K. L., Hong, S. W., Joormann, J., & Kang, P. (2009). Perception of facial expressions of emotion during binocular rivalry. *Emotion, 9,* 172–182. (13)

Yoon, S.-H., & Park, S. (2011). A mechanical analysis of woodpecker drumming and its application to shock-absorbing systems. *Bioinspiration and Biomimetics, 6:* 016003. (4)

Yoshida, J., & Mori, K. (2007). Odorant category profile selectivity of olfactory cortex neurons. *Journal of Neuroscience, 27,* 9105–9114. (6)

Yoshida, K., Li, X., Cano, G., Lazarus, M., & Saper, C. B. (2009). Parallel preoptic pathways for thermoregulation. *Journal of Neuroscience, 29,* 11954–11964. (9)

Yousem, D. M., Maldjian, J. A., Siddiqi, F., Hummel, T., Alsop, D. C., Geckle, R. J., . . . Doty, R. L. (1999). Gender effects on odor-stimulated functional magnetic resonance imaging. *Brain Research, 818,* 480–487. (6)

Yttri, E. A., & Dudman, J. T. (2016). Opponent and bidirectional control of movement velocity in the basal ganglia. *Nature, 533,* 402–406. (7)

Yu, T. W., & Bargmann, C. I. (2001). Dynamic regulation of axon guidance. *Nature Neuroscience Supplement, 4,* 1169–1176. (4)

Yuval-Greenberg, S., & Heeger, D. J. (2013). Continuous flash suppression modulates cortical activity in early visual cortex. *Journal of Neuroscience, 33,* 9635–9643. (13)

Zadra, A., Desautels, A., Petit, D., & Montplaisir, J. (2013). Somnambulism: Clinical aspects and pathophysiological hypotheses. *Lancet Neurology, 12,* 285–294. (8)

Zadra, A., & Pilon, M. (2008). Polysomnographic diagnosis of sleepwalking: Effects of sleep deprivation. *Annals of Neurology, 63,* 513–519. (8)

Zakharenko, S. S., Zablow, L., & Siegelbaum, S. A. (2001). Visualization of changes in presynaptic function during long-term synaptic plasticity. *Nature Neuroscience, 4,* 711–717. (12)

Zanos, P., Moaddel, R., Morris, P. J., Georgiou, P., Fischell, J., Elmer, G. I., . . . Gould, T. D. (2016). NMDAR inhibition-independent antidepressant actions of ketamine metabolites. *Nature, 533,* 481–486. (14)

Zant, J. C., Kim, T., Prokai, L., Szarka, S., McNally, J., McKenna, J. T., . . . Basheer, R. (2016). Cholinergic neurons in the basal forebrain promote wakefulness by actions on neighboring non-cholinergic neurons: An opto-dialysis study. *Journal of Neuroscience, 36,* 2057–2067. (8)

Zatorre, R. J., Fields, R. D., & Johansen-Berg, H. (2012). Plasticity in gray and white: Neuroimaging changes in brain structure during learning. *Nature Neuroscience, 4,* 528–536. (4)

Zeki, S. (1980). The representation of colours in the cerebral cortex. *Nature, 284,* 412–418. (5)

Zeki, S. (1983). Colour coding in the cerebral cortex: The responses of wavelength-selective and colour-coded cells in monkey visual cortex to changes in wavelength composition. *Neuroscience, 9,* 767–781. (5)

Zeki, S., & Shipp, S. (1988). The functional logic of cortical connections. *Nature, 335,* 311–317. (5)

Zentner, M., & Mitura, K. (2012). Stepping out of the caveman's shadow: Nations' gender gap predicts degree of sex differentiation in mate preferences. *Psychological Science, 23,* 1176–1185. (10)

Zerwas, S., Lund, B. C., Von Holle, A., Thornton, L. M., Berrettini, W. H., Brandt, H., . . . Bulik, C. M. (2013). Factors associated with recovery from anorexia nervosa. *Journal of Psychiatric Research, 47,* 972–979. (9)

Zhang, G., Pizarro, I. V., Swain, G. P., Kang, S. H., & Selzer, M. E. (2014). Neurogenesis in the lamprey central nervous system following spinal cord transection. *Journal of Comparative Neurology, 522,* 1316–1332. (4)

Zhang, J., Ackman, J. B., Xu, H.-P., & Crair, M. C. (2012). Visual map development depends on the temporal pattern of binocular activity in mice. *Nature Neuroscience, 15,* 298–307. (5)

Zhang, J., Liu, J., & Xu, Y. (2015). Neural decoding reveals impaired face configural processing in the right fusiform face area of individuals with developmental prosopagnosia. *Journal of Neuroscience, 35,* 1539–1548. (5)

Zhang, L., Hirano, A., Hsu, P.-K., Jones, C. R., Sakai, N., Okuro, M., . . . Fu, Y.-H. (2016). A *PERIOD3* variant causes a circadian phenotype and is associated with a seasonal mood trait. *Proceedings of the National Academy of Sciences (U.S.A.),* (8)

Zhang, X., & Firestein, S. (2002). The olfactory receptor gene superfamily of the mouse. *Nature Neuroscience, 5,* 124–133. (6)

Zhang, Y., Cudmore, R. H., Lin, D. T., Linden, D. J., & Huganir, R. L. (2015). Visualization of NMDA receptor-dependent AMPA receptor synaptic plasticity *in vivo. Nature Neuroscience, 18,* 402–407. (12)

Zhang, Y., Proenca, R., Maffei, M., Barone, M., Leopold, L., & Friedman, J. M. (1994). Positional cloning of the mouse obese gene and its human homologue. *Nature, 372,* 425–432. (9)

Zhan, Y., Paolicelli, R. C., Sforazzini, F., Weinhard, L., Bolasco, G., Pagani, F., . . . Gross, C. T. (2014). Deficient neuron-microglia signaling results in impaired functional brain connectivity and social behavior. *Nature Neuroscience, 17,* 400–406. (1)

Zhao, Y., Terry, D., Shi, L., Weinstein, H., Blanchard, S. C., & Javitch, J. A. (2010). Single-molecule dynamics of gating in a neurotransmitter transporter homologue. *Nature, 465,* 188–193. (2)

Zheng, B., Larkin, D. W., Albrecht, U., Sun, Z. S., Sage, M., Eichele, G., . . . Bradley, A. (1999). The *mPer2* gene encodes a functional component of the mammalian circadian clock. *Nature, 400,* 169–173. (8)

Zhou, D., Lebel, C., Lepage, C., Rasmussen, C., Evans, A., Wyper, K., . . . Beaulieu, C. (2011). Developmental cortical thinning in fetal alcohol spectrum disorders. *NeuroImage, 58,* 16–25. (4)

Zhou, F., Zhu, X. W., Castellani, R. J., Stimmelmayr, R., Perry, G., Smith, M. A., & Drew, K. L. (2001). Hibernation, a model of neuroprotection. *American Journal of Pathology, 158,* 2145–2151. (8)

Zhu, Q., Zhang, J., Luo, Y. L. L., Dilks, D. D., & Liu, J. (2011). Resting-state neural activity across face-selective cortical regions is behaviorally relevant. *Journal of Neuroscience, 31,* 10323–10330. (5)

Zhu, Y., Fenik, P., Zhan, G. X., Mazza, E., Kelz, M., Aston-Jones, G., & Veasey, S. C. (2007). Selective loss of catecholaminergic wake-active neurons in a murine sleep apnea model. *Journal of Neuroscience, 27,* 10060–10071. (8)

Ziegler, J. C., & Goswami, U. (2005). Reading acquisition, developmental dyslexia, and skilled reading across languages: A psycholinguistic grain size theory. *Psychological Bulletin, 131,* 3–29. (13)

Zihl, J., & Heywood, C. A. (2015). The contribution of LM to the neuroscience of movement vision. *Frontiers in Integrative Neuroscience, 9,* article 6. (5)

Zihl, J., von Cramon, D., & Mai, N. (1983). Selective disturbance of movement vision after bilateral brain damage. *Brain, 106,* 313–340. (5)

Zimmerman, A., Bai, L., & Ginty, D. D. (2014). The gentle touch receptors of mammalian skin. *Science, 346,* 950–954. (6)

Zimmerman, C. A., Lin, Y.-C., Leib, D. E., Guo, L., Huey, E. L., Daly, G. E., . . . Knight, Z. A. (2016). Thirst neurons anticipate the homeostatic consequences of eating and drinking. *Nature, 537,* 680–684. (9)

Zipursky, R. B., Reilly, T. J., & Murray, R. M. (2013). The myth of schizophrenia as a progressive brain disease. *Schizophrenia Bulletin, 39,* 1363–1372. (14)

Zipser, B. D., Johanson, C. E., Gonzalez, L., Berzin, T. M., Tavares, R., Hulette, C. M., . . . Stopa, E. G. (2007). Microvascular injury and blood–brain barrier leakage in Alzheimer's disease. *Neurobiology of Aging, 28,* 977–986. (1)

Zola, S. M., Squire, L. R., Teng, E., Stefanacci, L., Buffalo, E. A., & Clark, R. E. (2000). Impaired recognition memory in monkeys after damage limited to the hippocampal region. *Journal of Neuroscience, 20,* 451–463. (12)

Zorzi, M., Priftis, K., & Umiltà, C. (2002). Neglect disrupts the mental number line. *Nature, 417,* 138. (13)

Zucker, K. J., Bradley, S. J., Oliver, G., Blake, J., Fleming, S., & Hood, J. (1996). Psychosexual development of women with congenital adrenal hyperplasia. *Hormones and Behavior, 30,* 300–318. (10)

Zuckerman, L, Rehavi, M., Nachman, R., & Weiner, I. (2003). Immune activation during pregnancy in rats leads to a post-pubertal emergence of disrupted latent inhibition, dopaminergic hyperfunction, and altered limbic morphology in the offspring: A novel neurodevelopmental model of schizophrenia. *Neuropsychopharmacology, 28,* 1778–1789. (14)

Zurif, E. B. (1980). Language mechanisms: A neuropsychological perspective. *American Scientist, 68,* 305–311. (13)

Name Index

Aarts, H., 364
Abate, P., 461
Abbott, N. J., 24
Abbott, S. B. G., 299
AbdelMalik, P., 484
Abe, A. S., 290
Abi-Dargham, A., 487
Abouy, P., 195
Abrahamsson, N., 434
Abrams, W., 139
Ackman, J. B., 170
Acri, J., 465
Acuna-Goycolea, C., 310
Adamantidis, A., 283
Adamec, R. E., 362
Adamo, M., 180
Adams, D. B., 330
Adams, H. L., 494
Adams, R. B., Jr., 368, 455
Adcock, R. A., 389
Addis, D. R., 397
Adeeb, N., 493
Adler, M., 472
Adler, N. T., 330
Admon, R., 368
Adolphs, R., 354, 359, 369, 370, *371*, 429
Adrien, J., 274
Agarwal, A. F., 321
Agarwal, N., 207
Aghajanian, G. K., 471
Aglioti, S., 141, 448
Agnew, L. L., 470
Agrati, D., 324
Agster, K. L., 398
Aguirre, G. K., 166
Aharon, I., 463
Ahissar, M., 437
Ahlskog, J. E., 312
Ahmed, E. I., 324
Ahmed, I. I., 325
Ahn, W., 459
Airaksinen, M. S., 123
Airan, R. D., 472
Airavaara, M., 251
Ajina, S., 166
Akers, K. G., 392
Al-Karawi, D., 475
Al-Rashid, R. A., 312
Alagiakrishnan, K., 390
Alain, C., 128
Alais, D., 443
Alanko, K., 342, 343
Alberini, C. M., 392
Alberts, J. R., 334
Albouy, G., 283, 402
Albrecht, D. G., 170
Albright, T. D., 181
Albuquerque, D., 314
Alcuter, S., 118
Aleman, A., 481
Alerstam, T., 281
Alexander, G. M., 327
Alexander, J. T., 310
Allaire, J. C., 392
Allan, D., 353
Allebrandt, K. V., 262

Allen, G. I., 221
Allen, H., 447
Allen, H. L., 105
Allen, J. S., 319, 417
Alleva, E., 123, 125
Allison, T., 282
Almazen, M., 433
Almeida, J., 127
Almli, C. R., 312
Almonte, J. L., 379
Alsop, D., 195
Altena, E., 275, 476
Alvarez-Buylla, A. A., 171
Alzmon, G., 132
Aman, J. E., 130
Amano, K., 181
Amanzio, M., 207
Amateau, S. K., 325
Ambady, N., 368
American Psychiatric Association, 480, 492
Amering, M., 371
Ames, M. A., 344
Amiry-Moghaddam, M., 24
Amlaner, C. J., 281
Amting, J. M., 370
An, Y., 392
Anaclet, C., 271, 273
Anand, P., 207
Anastasiya, A., 262
Andersen, J. L., 228
Andersen, R. A., 235
Andersen, T. S., 88
Anderson, C., 343
Anderson, D. J., 191, 310
Anderson, E., 444
Anderson, F., 362
Anderson, M. A., 139
Anderson, M. E., 241
Anderson, S., 196
Anderson, S. F., 469
Andrade, D. V., 290
Andreasen, N. C., 485
Andres, K. H., 200
Andrés-Pueyo, A., 363
Andrew, D., 208
Andrews, S. C., 237
Andrews, T. J., 153
Andrillon, T., 273
Angelucci, A., 124
Ansiau, D., 261
Antenor-Dorsey, J. A., 250
Anthony, T. E., 310
Aoki, C., 19, 493
Aplin, L. C., 260
Apostaolakis, E. M., 328
Applebaum, S., 220
Appleman, E. R., 283
Araneda, R. C., 219
Arango, V., 364
Araque, A., 22
Araripe, L. O., 323
Archer, J., 363
Archer, S. N., 265
Arcurio, L. R., 180
Arduino, C., 207
Arendt, D., 265

Arendt, J., 261
Ariely, D., 311
Armstrong, J. B., 303
Arnold, A. P., 323, 324, 326
Arnold, H. M., 139
Arnsten, A. F. T., 377
Arseneau, L. M., 291
Arun, S. P., 178, 179
Arver, S., 417
Arvidson, K., 211
Asai, M., 310
Åsberg, M., 364
Ascher, E. A., 456
Ascoli, G., 21, 406
Aserinsky, E., 269–270
Asher, B., 359
Ashida, H., 181
Ashley, R., 127
Ashmore, L. J., 265
Asmundson, G. J. G., 365
Assal, G., 429
Aston-Jones, G., 265, 310
Atherton, N. M., 474
Athos, E. A., 195
Atlas, L. Y., 96, 207
Attardo, A., 411
Attwell, D., 136
Atzei, A., 141
Aubin, H.-J., 465
Audero, E., 364
Avena, N. M., 316
Aviezer, H., 357
Avinun, R., 332
Axel, R., 119, 217
Axmacher, N., 443

Babich, F. R., 406
Babikian, T., 136
Babinet, C., 124
Babor, T. F., 461
Bachevalier, J., 367, 398
Backlund, E.-O., 251
Bäckman, J., 281
Baddeley, A. D., 384, 389
Baer, J. S., 461
Bagemihl, B., 342
Baghdoyan, H. A., 274
Bai, L., 200
Bailey, C. H., 408
Bailey, J. A., 128
Bailey, J. M., 342, 343, 344, 348
Bailey, K. G. D., 436
Baird, A. A., 368
Bajo-Grañeras, R., 22
Baker, B. N., 191
Baker, C. I., 129
Baker, G. B., 284
Baker, L., 109
Baker, S. W., 341
Bakermans-Kranenburg, M. J., 455
Bakken, T. E., 153, 418
Bakker, J., 325
Baldessarini, R. J., 471, 472
Bale, T. L., 107
Ball, W. A., 273
Ballard, P. A., 250

Maquet, P., 236, 274
Marcar, V. L., 182
Marcel, A. J., 447
March, S. M., 461
Marcinowska, A., 472
Marcus, D. K., 342
Marek, R., 368
Maret, S., 283
Marin, M. M., 195
Mariño, G., 199
Mark, A. L., 308
Mark, G. P., 316
Markou, A., 464
Markowitsch, H. J., 390
Markowitz, J. C., 473
Markulev, C., 474
Marlatt, M. W., 125
Marlin, B. J., 454
Marois, R., 221
Marquié, J.-C., 261
Marrett, S., 182
Marris, E., 12
Marsden, C. D., 487
Marsh, J. K., 459
Marshall, J., 166
Marshall, J. C., 448
Marshall, J. F., 142
Marsicano, G., 58
Marsman, A., 488
Martens, M. A., 433
Martin, A., 114
Martin, C. E., 346
Martin, G., 153
Martin, N. G., 109
Martin, P. R., 155
Martin, R., 22
Martin, R. C., 436
Martin, S. D., 473
Martindale, C., 154
Martinez, V., 259
Martínez-Horta, S., 249, 252
Martínez-Orgado, J., 137
Martinez-Vargas, M. C., 328
Martinowich, K., 471
Maruff, P., 280
Marvin, E., 195
Masal, E., 260
Mascaro, J. S., 333
Masland, R. H., 149
Maslen, H., 412
Mason, M. F., 96
Mason, P., 205
Mason, R. T., 290
Massimini, M., 273, 283, 457
Masterton, R. B., 191
Mataga, N., 219
Mathews, G. A., 340
Mathias, C. J., 354
Mathies, R. A., 153
Matrisciano, F., 472
Matson, J. L., 494
Matsubara, S., 488
Matsumoto, Y., 280
Matsunami, H., 214
Mattavelli, G., 367
Mattes, R. D., 213
Matthys, W., 363
Mattingley, J. B., 448
Matuszewich, L., 328, 330, 463
Maurer, D., 171, 173
Maurice, D., 284
Maurits, N. M., 437
Maxwell, J. S., 357
May, P. R. A., 136
Maya Vetencourt, J. F., 472

Mayberg, H. S., 476
Mayberry, R. I., 434
Maydeu-Olivares, A., 363
Mayer, A. D., 333
Mazoyer, B., 425
Mazur, A., 328
Mazza, E., 283
Mazziotta, J. C., 94
McAllister, A. K., 484
McBride, C. S., 187
McBride, J. L., 253
McBurney, D. H., 213
McCall, C., 424, 454
McCarley, R. W., 284
McCarthy, M., 325, *326*
McCarthy, M. M., 325, 326
McClarty, B., 372
McCleskey, E. W., 207
McClintock, M. K., 220
McClure, S. M., 131
McConnell, J. V., 406
McConnell, S. K., 124
McCormick, C. M., 342
McCoy, A. N., 168
McCrea, A. E., 344
McCullough, M., 455
McDermott, R., 363
McDonald, J. J., 443
McDonald, M. J., 321
McDonald, M. M., 359
McDonough, I. M., 132
McElroy, A. E., 211
McEwen, B., 376
McEwen, B. S., 292, 376, 381
McEwen, G. N., Jr., 295
McGaugh, J. L., 389
McGinty, D., 285
McGivern, R. F., 325
McGorry, P. D., 474
McGrath, J., 484
McGrath, J. J., 493
McGrillen, K., 214, 424
McGue, M., 417, 460, 461
McGuffin, P., 469
McGuire, S., 109
McGuire, S. A., 417
McHugh, P. R., 306
McIntyre, M., 328
McIntyre, R. S., 314
McKeever, W. F., 424
McKemy, D. D., 201
McKenzie, A., 130
McKenzie, I. A., 118
McKinnon, W., 379
McKnight, S. L., 265
McLellan, W. A., 294, 295, 464
McLeod, K., 469
McMenamin, B. W., 357
McMillan, K. A., 365
McNaughton, B. L., 93, 283, 399
McNay, E., 24
McNeil, R., 153
McNeill, D., 433
McQuilkin, M., 139
McStephen, M., 280
Meddis, R., 275
Mednick, S. A., 283, 484
Mednick, S. C., 269
Meduna, L., 473
Mehta, P. M., 365
Meier, M. H., 484
Meier, P. J., 23
Meijer, R. I., 24
Meiselman, H. L., 212
Meister, M., 122, 220

Meister, M. L. R., 453
Melby-Lervåg, M., 126
Melcher, J. R., 192
Melis, A. P., 418
Melloni, L., 443
Melone, M., 488
Meltzer, H. Y., 488
Meltzoff, A. N., 237
Melzack, R., 205, 208
Menaker, M., 263, 264
Menard, C., 469
Menchetti, M., 473
Mendel, G., 104
Mendelsohn, M., 119
Mendes, M. B., 359
Méndez-Bértolo, C., 368
Mendieta-Zéron, H., 309
Mendle, J., 324, 468
Menon, D. K., 136
Menon, V., 485
Mera, R. S., 392
Merad, M., 469
Merckelbach, H., 280
Mergen, H., 314
Mergen, M., 314
Merikangas, K. P., 476
Mérillat, S., 129
Merkley, T., 136
Merrow, M., 260, 262
Mertens, J., 476
Mervis, C. B., 433
Merzenich, M. M., 84, 140, 192
Mesgarani, N., 192, 196
Meshi, D., 119
Metcalf, S. A., 484
Metzinger, T., 88
Mevorach, C., 447
Meyer, B., 207
Meyer, J. R., 130
Meyer, K., 87, 191
Meyer-Bahlburg, H. F. L., 340, 341
Meyerhof, W., 214
Meyerhoff, J. M., 362
Meyer-Lindenberg, A., 433, 481, 484
Mezzanotte, W. S., 276
Miall, C., 244
Michalek, J., 328
Micheva, K. D., 56
Mickel, S. F., 390
Mierson, S., 213
Mihara, T., 454
Mika, A., 377
Milich, R., 304
Millan, M. J., 470
Miller, A., 363
Miller, A. C., 428
Miller, B. L., 456
Miller, C. A., 410
Miller, E. K., 447
Miller, G., 11, 331
Miller, G. A., 441
Miller, G. E., 379
Miller, I. N., 249
Miller, J., 245, 484
Miller, J. C., 474
Miller, J. F., 400, 453
Miller, L. A., 214, 424
Miller, R. J., 118
Miller, S. L., 220
Mills, R., 325
Milner, A. D., 177, 178, 235
Milner, B., 395
Milner, P., 462
Min, J., 314
Minard, A., 280

Subject Index/Glossary